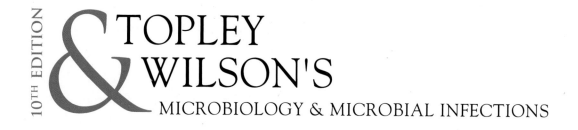

10TH EDITION

TOPLEY & WILSON'S

MICROBIOLOGY & MICROBIAL INFECTIONS

CUMULATIVE INDEX

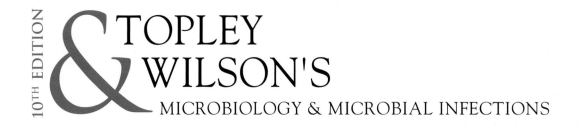

TOPLEY & WILSON'S
MICROBIOLOGY & MICROBIAL INFECTIONS

10ᵀᴴ EDITION

Topley & Wilson's Microbiology and Microbial Infections has grown from one to eight volumes since first published in 1929, reflecting the ever-increasing breadth and depth of knowledge in each of the areas covered. This tenth edition continues the tradition of providing the most comprehensive reference to microorganisms and the resulting infectious diseases currently available. It forms a unique resource, with each volume including examples of the best writing and research in the fields of virology, bacteriology, medical mycology, parasitology, and immunology from around the globe.

www.topleyandwilson.com

VIROLOGY Volumes 1 and 2

Edited by Brian W.J. Mahy and Volker ter Meulen
Volume 1 ISBN 0 340 88561 0; Volume 2 ISBN 0 340 88562 9; 2 volume set ISBN 0 340 88563 7

BACTERIOLOGY Volumes 1 and 2

Edited by S. Peter Borriello, Patrick R Murray, and Guido Funke
Volume 1 ISBN 0 340 88564 5; Volume 2 ISBN 0 340 88565 3; 2 volume set ISBN 0 340 88566 1

MEDICAL MYCOLOGY

Edited by William G. Merz and Roderick J. Hay
ISBN 0 340 88567 X

PARASITOLOGY

Edited by F.E.G. Cox, Derek Wakelin, Stephen H. Gillespie, and Dickson D. Despommier
ISBN 0 340 88568 8

IMMUNOLOGY

Edited by Stephan H.E. Kaufmann and Michael W. Steward
ISBN 0 340 88569 6

Cumulative index

ISBN 0 340 88570 X

8 volume set plus CD-ROM

ISBN 0 340 80912 4

CD-ROM only

ISBN 0 340 88560 2

For a full list of contents, please see the *Complete table of contents* on page vii

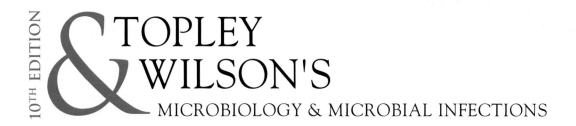

10TH EDITION

TOPLEY & WILSON'S

MICROBIOLOGY & MICROBIAL INFECTIONS

CUMULATIVE INDEX

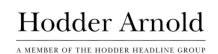

Hodder Arnold

A MEMBER OF THE HODDER HEADLINE GROUP

ASM
PRESS

First published in Great Britain in 1929
Second edition 1936; Third edition 1946
Fourth edition 1955; Fifth edition 1964
Sixth edition 1975; Seventh edition 1983 and 1984
Eight edition 1990; Ninth edition 1998
This tenth edition published in 2005 by
Hodder Arnold, an imprint of Hodder Education and a member of the Hodder Headline Group,
338 Euston Road, London NW1 3BH

http://www.hoddereducation.com   www.topleyandwilson.com

Distributed in the United States of America by ASM Press, the book publishing division of the American Society for
Microbiology, 1752 N Street, N.W. Washington, D.C. 20036, USA

Hodder Headline's policy is to use papers that are natural, renewable and recyclable products and made from wood
grown in sustainable forests. The logging and manufacturing processes are expected to conform to the
environmental regulations of the country of origin.

Whilst the advice and information in this book are believed to be true and accurate at the date of going to press,
neither the author[s] nor the publisher can accept any legal responsibility or liability for any errors or omissions that
may be made. In particular (but without limiting the generality of the preceding disclaimer) every effort has been
made to check drug dosages; however it is still possible that errors have been missed. Furthermore, dosage
schedules are constantly being revised and new side-effects recognized. For these reasons the reader is strongly
urged to consult the drug companies' printed instructions before administering any of the drugs recommended in
this book.

British Library Cataloguing in Publication Data
A catalogue record for this book is available from the British Library

Library of Congress Cataloging-in-Publication Data
A catalog record for this book is available from the Library of Congress

Index only	ISBN-10 0 340 88570 X	ISBN-13 978 0 340 88570 3
Complete set and CD-ROM	ISBN-10 0 340 80912 4	ISBN-13 978 0 340 80912 9
Indian edition	ISBN-10 0 340 88559 9	ISBN-13 978 0 340 88559 8

1 2 3 4 5 6 7 8 9 10

Commissioning Editor: Serena Bureau / Joanna Koster
Development Editor: Layla Vandenberg
Project Editor: Zelah Pengilley
Production Controller: Deborah Smith
Index: Merrall-Ross International Ltd.
Cover Designer: Sarah Rees

Cover image: Herpes simplex virus, TEM. Dr. Linda Stannard, UCT / Science Photo Library; Helicobacter pylori
bacteria. A.B. Dowsett / Science Photo Library; Candida albicans fungus, SEM. Stem Jems / Science Photo Library;
Toxocara roundworm. Jackie Lewin, EM Unit, Royal Free Hospital / Science Photo Library; Coloured SEM of
macrophage engulfing protozoan / Science Photo Library

Typeset in 9/11 Times New Roman by Lucid Digital, Salisbury, UK
Printed and bound in Italy

What do you think about this book? Or any other Hodder Arnold title? Please send your comments to
www.hoddereducation.com

Table of Contents

Complete table of contents for *Topley & Wilson's Microbiology and Microbial Infections*

VIROLOGY, VOLUMES 1 AND 2

PART I	GENERAL CHARACTERISTICS OF VIRUSES	1
1	**A short history of research on viruses** Leslie Collier	3
2	**The origin and evolution of viruses** Esteban Domingo and John J. Holland	11
3	**The nature and classification of viruses** Marc H.V. Van Regenmortel	24
4	**The classification of vertebrate viruses** Craig R. Pringle	38
5	**The morphology and structure of viruses** Rob W.H. Ruigrok, Guy Schoehn, and James F. Conway	57
6	**Propagation and identification of viruses** Dean D. Erdman	86
7	**The replication of viruses** David J. Rowlands	105
8	**Negative-strand RNA virus replication** Richard M. Elliott	127
9	**Positive-strand RNA virus replication in vertebrate hosts** Jo Ellen Brunner and Bert L. Semler	135
10	**DNA virus replication** Sandra K. Weller	147
11	**Genetics of vertebrate viruses** Craig R. Pringle	174
12	**Virus–host cell interactions** L. Andrew Ball	202
13	**Pathogenesis of viral infections** Neal Nathanson and Kenneth L. Tyler	236
14	**The immune response to viral infections** Anthony A. Nash and Bernadette M. Dutia	270
15	**The role of cytokines in viral infections** Paula M. Pitha and Myriam S. Künzi	292
16	**Viral evasion of the host immune response** Antonio Alcami	311
17	**Viral oncogenicity** James C. Neil and John A. Wyke	330
18	**The epidemiology of viral infections** Arnold S. Monto	353
19	**The order *Mononegavirales*** Andrew J. Easton and Craig R. Pringle	378
20	**The order *Nidovirales*** Eric J. Snijder, Stuart G. Siddell, and Alexander E. Gorbalenya	390
PART II	SPECIFIC VIRUSES AND VIRAL INFECTION	405
21	**Parvoviruses** Peter Tattersall and Susan F. Cotmore	407
22	**Adenoviruses** Willie Russell	439
23	**Papillomaviruses** Margaret Stanley and Mark Pett	448
24	**Polyomaviruses** Jessica Otte, Mahmut Safak, and Kamel Khalili	473
25	**Herpesviruses: general properties** Andrew J. Davison and J. Barklie Clements	488
26	**Alphaherpesviruses: herpes simplex and varicella-zoster** Anthony C. Minson	506
27	**Betaherpesviruses: cytomegalovirus, human herpesviruses 6 and 7** William J. Britt	520
28	**Human herpesvirus 8** Bernhard Fleckenstein and Frank Neipel	541
29	**Gammaherpesviruses: Epstein–Barr virus** M. Anthony Epstein and Dorothy H. Crawford	559
30	**Poxviruses** Geoffrey L. Smith	578
31	**Poxvirus replication** Richard C. Condit and Richard W. Moyer	594
32	**Orthomyxoviruses: influenza** Nancy J. Cox, Gabriele Neumann, Ruben O. Donis, and Yoshihiro Kawaoka	634
33	**General properties of the paramyxoviruses** Paul A. Rota, Bettina Bankamp, and William J. Bellini	699
34	**Morbilliviruses: measles virus** Sibylle Schneider-Schaulies and William J. Bellini	712

35   **Rubulavirus: mumps virus**   Wendy A. Knowles and Li Jin   744
36   **Respiroviruses: parainfluenza virus**   Richard W. Peluso and Anne Moscona   763
37   **Pneumovirus and Metapneumovirus: respiratory syncytial virus and
     human metapneumovirus**   Ralph A. Tripp   783
38   **Paramyxoviruses of animals**   Paul A. Rota and Thomas Barrett   807
39   **Coronaviruses, toroviruses, and arteriviruses**   Stuart G. Siddell,
     John Ziebuhr, and Eric J. Snijder   823
40   **Picornaviruses**   Philip Minor   857
41   **Human enteric RNA viruses: astroviruses**   Michael J. Carter and Margaret M. Willcocks   888
42   **Human enteric RNA viruses: Noroviruses and Sapoviruses**   Ian N. Clarke and
     Paul R. Lambden   911
43   **Reoviruses, orbiviruses, and coltiviruses**   Terence S. Dermody and Ulrich Desselberger   932
44   **Rotaviruses**   Ulrich Desselberger, Jim Gray, and Mary K. Estes   946
45   **Rubella**   Jennifer M. Best, Samantha Cooray, and Jangu E. Banatvala   959
46   **Flaviviruses**   John T. Roehrig and Duane J. Gubler   993
47   **Togaviruses**   Scott C. Weaver and Ilya V. Frolov   1010
48   **Bunyaviridae**   Alan D.T. Barrett and Robert E. Shope   1025
49   **Arenaviruses**   Maria S. Salvato and Juan D. Rodas   1059
50   **Filoviruses**   Heinz Feldmann and Hans-Dieter Klenk   1085
51   **Rhabdoviruses: rabies**   Noël Tordo, Pierre-Emmanuel Ceccaldi,
     Yves Gaudin, and Alex I. Wandeler   1102
52   **Borna disease virus**   Thomas Briese, Mady Hornig, and W. Ian Lipkin   1137
53   **Hepatitis A and E**   Betty Robertson   1160
54   **Hepatitis C virus**   Peter Simmonds and David Mutimer   1189
55   **Hepatitis B**   Wolfram H. Gerlich and Michael Kann   1226
56   **Hepatitis delta virus**   John M. Taylor   1269
57   **TT virus and other anelloviruses**   Mauro Bendinelli and Fabrizio Maggi   1276
58   **Retroviruses and associated diseases in humans**   Charlene S. Dezzutti, Walid Heneine,
     Roumiana S. Boneva, and Thomas M. Folks   1284
59   **Foamy viruses**   Axel Rethwilm   1304
60   **Human immunodeficiency virus**   Ulrich Schubert and Myra McClure   1322
61   **Prions of humans and animals**   Adriano Aguzzi   1346

PART III   SYNDROMES CAUSED BY A RANGE OF VIRUSES   1401
62   **Infections of the central nervous system**   Jürgen Schneider-Schaulies,
     Sibylle Schneider-Schaulies, and Volker ter Meulen   1403
63   **Viral infections of the fetus and neonate, other than rubella**   Gisela Enders   1443
64   **Virus infections in immunocompromised patients**   Anthony Simmons   1498

PART IV   PRINCIPLES OF DIAGNOSIS AND CONTROL   1513
65   **Safety in the virology laboratory**   Graham Lloyd and Michael P. Kiley   1515
66   **The laboratory diagnosis of viral infections**   Steven Specter and Mauro Bendinelli   1532
67   **Immunoprophylaxis of viral diseases**   Stephen C. Hadler and Jane F. Seward   1551
68   **Viral vectors for gene therapy**   R. Michael Linden and Kenneth I. Berns   1590
69   **Antiviral chemotherapy**   Hugh J. Field and Richard J. Whitley   1605
70   **The emergence and re-emergence of viral diseases**   Brian W.J. Mahy and
     Frederick A. Murphy   1646

BACTERIOLOGY, VOLUMES 1 AND 2

PART I   GENERAL BASIC CHARACTERISTICS   1
1   **The bacteria: historical introduction**   Bohumil S. Drasar   3
2   **Taxonomy and nomenclature of bacteria**   John T. Magee   15
3   **Bacterial growth and metabolism**   James P. Shapleigh   37
4   **Bacterial genetics**   Matthew B. Avison and Peter M. Bennett   80

| 5 | **Bacteriocins and bacteriophages**   Martin Day | **136** |
| 6 | **Molecular basis of bacterial adaptation to a pathogenic lifestyle**   Kim R. Hardie, Tom Baldwin, and Paul Williams | **146** |

PART II   GENERAL ECOSYSTEMS   **183**

7	**Airborne bacteria** Linda D. Stetzenbach	**185**
8	**Bacteriology of soils and plants** Guy R. Knudsen	**195**
9	**Bacteriology of water** Edwin E. Geldreich	**211**
10	**Bacteriology of milk and milk products** Frederick J. Bolton	**229**
11	**Bacteriology of foods, excluding dairy products** Diane Roberts	**263**
12	**Human microbiota** Patrick R. Murray	**293**

PART III   GENERAL EPIDEMIOLOGY, TRANSMISSION, AND THERAPY   **307**

13	**Epidemiology of infectious diseases** Stephen R. Palmer and Meirion R. Evans	**309**
14	**Theory of infectious disease transmission and control** Angus Nicoll, Nigel J. Gay, and Norman T. Begg	**335**
15	**Emergence and resurgence of bacterial infectious diseases** Ruth L. Berkelman and Keith P. Klugman	**359**
16	**Healthcare-associated infections** Mark H. Wilcox and R.C. Spencer	**368**
17	**Microbial susceptibility and resistance to chemical and physical agents** A. Denver Russell	**421**
18	**Antibacterial therapy** Ian M. Gould	**466**

PART IV   ORGAN AND SYSTEM INFECTIONS   **507**

19	**Bloodstream infection and endocarditis** Harald Seifert and Hilmar Wisplinghoff	**509**
20	**Bacterial meningitis** Keith A.V. Cartwright	**555**
21	**Other CNS bacterial infections** Fiona E. Donald	**581**
22	**Bacterial infections of the eye** Susan E. Sharp and Michael R. Driks	**598**
23	**Bacterial infections of the upper respiratory tract** Richard B. Thomson Jr	**606**
24	**Bacterial infections of the lower respiratory tract** Robert C. Read	**622**
25	**Bacterial infections of the genital tract** Catherine Ison	**657**
26	**Bacterial infections of the urinary tract** Sören G. Gatermann	**672**
27	**Bacterial infections of bones and joints** Anthony R. Berendt	**684**

PART V   LABORATORY ASPECTS   **709**

28	**Conventional laboratory diagnosis of infection** Joseph D.C. Yao	**711**
29	**Molecular laboratory diagnosis of infection** Robin Patel	**721**
30	**Bacterial immunoserology** Roger Freeman	**738**
31	**Biological safety for the clinical laboratory** Michael Noble	**760**

PART VI   ORGANISMS AND THEIR BIOLOGY   **769**

32	*Staphylococcus* Sharon J. Peacock	**771**
33	*Streptococcus* and *Lactobacillus* Mogens Kilian	**833**
34	*Enterococcus* Lúcia M. Teixeira and Richard R. Facklam	**882**
35	**Gram-positive anaerobic cocci** Michael W.D. Wren	**903**
36	*Bacillus anthracis, Bacillus cereus,* **and other aerobic endospore-forming bacteria** Niall A. Logan	**922**
37	**Listeria** Jim McLauchlin	**953**
38	*Erysipelothrix* Walter F. Schlech	**970**
39	**Corynebacteria and rare coryneforms** Guido Funke	**977**
40	*Tropheryma* Matthias Maiwald	**998**
41	*Actinomyces* **and related genera** Guido Funke	**1005**
42	*Bifidobacterium, Eubacterium,* **and** *Propionibacterium* William G. Wade and Julie F. Downes	**1023**
43	*Clostridium botulinum* **and** *Clostridium tetani* Eric A. Johnson	**1035**
44	*Clostridium perfringens, Clostridium difficile,* **and other** *Clostridium species* S. Peter Borriello and Klaus Aktories	**1089**

45	***Nocardia*** **and other aerobic actinomycetes** Patricia S. Conville and Frank G. Witebsky	**1137**
46	***Mycobacterium tuberculosis*** **complex,** ***Mycobacterium leprae,*** **and other slow-growing mycobacteria** Gaby E. Pfyffer and Véronique Vincent	**1181**
47	**Rapidly growing mycobacteria** Frank G. Witebsky and Patricia S. Conville	**1236**
48	***Neisseria*** Timothy A. Mietzner and Stephen A. Morse	**1270**
49	***Acinetobacter*** **and** ***Moraxella*** William Riley	**1301**
50	***Veillonella*** **and other anaerobic gram-negative cocci** Jonathan S. Brazier	**1312**
51	**The Enterobacteriaceae: general characteristics** J.J. Farmer III, M.K. Farmer, and Barry Holmes	**1317**
52	***Escherichia*** Tom Cheasty and Henry R. Smith	**1360**
53	***Shigella*** Phillippe J. Sansonetti	**1386**
54	***Salmonella*** E. John Threlfall	**1398**
55	***Proteus, Morganella,*** **and** ***Providencia*** Bernard W. Senior	**1435**
56	***Yersinia*** Audrey Wanger	**1458**
57	***Citrobacter, Klebsiella, Enterobacter, Serratia,*** **and other Enterobacteriaceae** Patrick R. Murray, Barry Holmes, and Hazel M. Auken	**1474**
58	***Vibrio*** Judith A. Johnson	**1507**
59	***Aeromonas*** Barbara J. Chang and J. Michael Janda	**1524**
60	***Campylobacter*** **and** ***Arcobacter*** Olivier Vandenberg, Martin B. Skirrow, and Jean-Paul Butzler	**1541**
61	***Helicobacter*** Robert J. Owen	**1563**
62	***Pseudomonas*** Norberto J. Palleroni	**1591**
63	***Burkholderia*** **spp. and related genera** Tyrone L. Pitt and David Dance	**1607**
64	***Pasteurella, Mannheimia, Actinobacillus, Eikenella, Kingella, Capnocytophaga,*** **and other miscellaneous gram-negative rods** William M. Janda and Reinier Mutters	**1649**
65	***Haemophilus*** Mary P.E. Slack	**1692**
66	***Brucella*** Patrick R. Murray and Michael J. Corbel	**1719**
67	***Francisella*** Francis E. Nano and Karen L. Elkins	**1752**
68	***Legionella*** Timothy G. Harrison	**1761**
69	***Bordetella*** Roger Parton	**1786**
70	***Borrelia*** Danièle Postic	**1818**
71	***Treponema*** Victoria Pope and Bret M. Steiner	**1838**
72	***Leptospira*** Ben Adler and Solly Faine	**1865**
73	***Bartonella*** **and** ***Afipia*** Anna Sander	**1885**
74	***Spirillum minus*** **and** ***Streptobacillus moniliformis*** Scott A. Martin	**1908**
75	***Bacteroides, Prevotella,*** **and** ***Porphyromonas*** Haroun N. Shah, Saheer E. Gharbia, and Ingar Olsen	**1913**
76	***Fusobacterium*** **and** ***Leptotrichia*** Tor Hofstad and Ingar Olsen	**1945**
77	***Mycoplasma*** Shmuel Razin	**1957**
78	***Chlamydia*** Per-Anders Mårdh	**2006**
79	***Rickettsia*** **and** ***Orienta*** Didier Raoult and J. Stephen Dumler	**2026**
80	***Ehrlichia*** **and** ***Anaplasma*** J. Stephen Dumler and Didier Raoult	**2048**
81	***Coxiella burnetii*** Nigel F. Lightfoot and Graham Lloyd	**2072**

MEDICAL MYCOLOGY

PART I	**BACKGROUND AND BASIC INFORMATION**	**1**
1	**Historical introduction: evolution of knowledge of the fungi and mycoses from Hippocrates to the twenty-first century** Edouard Drouhet	**3**
2	**Kingdom Fungi: fungal phylogeny and systematics** Thomas G. Mitchell	**43**
3	**Fungal structure and morphology** Paul F. Lehmann	**69**
4	**Laboratory diagnosis** Glenn D. Roberts and Norman L. Goodman	**82**
5	**Mycoserology and molecular diagnosis** Ruth Matthews and James P. Burnie	**97**
6	**Histopathological diagnosis of mycotic diseases** Henrik Elvang Jensen and Francis W. Chandler	**121**

PART II   THERAPEUTIC AGENTS AND VACCINES   145
7   **Antifungal agents and antifungal susceptibility testing**
          Sanjay G. Revankar, John R. Graybill, and Thomas F. Patterson   147
8   **Principles of antifungal therapy**   Peter G. Pappas   164
9   **Resistance to antifungal agents**   Sevtap Arikan and John H. Rex   168
10   **Management of superficial infections**   Jeff Weeks and Boni Elewski   182

PART III SUPERFICIAL AND OCULAR FUNGAL INFECTIONS   193
11   **White piedra, black piedra, and tinea nigra**   G. Sybren de Hoog and Eveline Guého   195
12   **Superficial diseases caused by *Malassezia* species**   Vicente Crespo Erchiga and
          Eveline Guého   202
13   **The dermatophytes**   Arvind A. Padhye and Richard C. Summerbell   220
14   **Dermatomycotic molds**   Colin K. Campbell and Elizabeth M. Johnson   244
15   **Superficial candidiasis**   Paul L. Fidel Jr and Karen L. Wozniak   255
16   **Oculomycosis**   Philip A. Thomas and P. Geraldine   273

PART IV   SUBCUTANEOUS MYCOSES   345
17   **Subcutaneous zygomycosis**   David H. Ellis   347
18   **Chromoblastomycosis**   Philippe Esterre   356
19   **Sporotrichosis**   Roberto Arenas   367
20   **Eumycetomas**   Roderick J. Hay   385
21   **Protothecosis**   R. Scott Pore   396
22   **Pythiosis**   Leonel Mendoza   412
23   **Lobomycosis**   Sinésio Talhari and Roger Pradinaud   430
24   **Rhinosporidiosis**   Sarath N. Arseculeratne and Leonel Mendoza   436

PART V   SYSTEMIC MYCOSES DUE TO DIMORPHIC FUNGI   477
25   **Blastomycosis**   Arthur F. Di Salvo and Bruce S. Klein   479
26   **Coccidioidomycosis**   Demosthenes Pappagianis   502
27   **Histoplasmosis**   Ram P. Tewari, L. Joseph Wheat, and L. Ajello   519
28   **Paracoccidioidomycosis**   Gil Benard and Marcello Franco   541
29   **Penicilliosis**   Maria Anna Viviani and Nongnuch Vanittanakom   560

PART VI   SYSTEMIC MYCOSES CAUSED BY OPPORTUNISTIC FUNGI   577
30   **Candidiasis**   Esther Segal and Daniel Elad   579
31   **Serious infections caused by uncommon yeasts**   Janine R. Maenza and William G. Merz   624
32   **Cryptococcosis**   John R. Perfect and Gary M. Cox   637
33   **Systemic zygomycosis**   David H. Ellis   659
34   **Aspergillosis**   Malcolm D. Richardson   687
35   **Deep phaeohyphomycosis**   Chester R. Cooper, Jr   739
36   **Deep hyalohyphomycosis**   Caroline B. Moore and David W. Denning   749
37   ***Pneumocystis* pneumonia**   Melanie T. Cushion   763

PART VII UNUSUAL DISEASE PRESENTATIONS BY FUNGI   807
38   **Adiaspiromycosis and other infections caused by *Emmonsia* species**   Lynne Sigler   809

PARASITOLOGY

PART I   GENERAL PARASITOLOGY   1
1   **History of human parasitology**   F.E.G. Cox   3
2   **World-wide importance of parasites**   Gabriel A. Schmunis and
          Francisco J. López-Antuñano   24
3   **Epidemiology of parasitic infections**   Roy M. Anderson   50
4   **Immunology and immunopathology of human parasitic infections**
          F.E.G. Cox and Derek Wakelin   67

5   Control of parasites, parasitic infections, and parasitic diseases
     David H. Molyneux   103
6   Diagnosis of parasitic infections   Stephen H. Gillespie   148

PART II   PROTOZOA   157
7   Cellular organization of parasitic protozoa   Heinz Mehlhorn   159
8   Classification and introduction to the parasitic protozoa   F.E.G. Cox   186
9   Amebiasis: *Entamoeba histolytica* infections   Adolfo Martínez-Palomo and
     Martha Espinosa-Cantellano   200
10   Other intestinal amebae   John P. Ackers   218
11   Opportunistic amebae   David T. John   226
12   Giardiasis   Lynne S. Garcia   241
13   *Trichomonas* infections   Donald E. Burgess   255
14   *Dientamoeba fragilis* and other intestinal flagellates   Jaroslav Kulda and
     Eva Nohýnková   266
15   *Balantidium coli*   Viqar Zaman and F.E.G. Cox   275
16   Old World leishmaniasis   Paul A. Bates and R.W. Ashford   283
17   New World leishmaniasis   Ralph Lainson and Jeffrey J. Shaw   313
18   African trypanosomiasis   Samuel J. Black and John Richard Seed   350
19   New World trypanosomiasis   Michael A. Miles   376
20   Intestinal coccidia: cryptosporidiosis, isosporiasis, cyclosporiasis   Vincent McDonald and
     M. Paul Kelly   399
21   Toxoplasmosis   J.P. Dubey   422
22   *Sarcocystis*   J.P. Dubey   443
23   Babesiosis of humans   Sam R. Telford III and Andrew Spielman   451
24   Malaria   Marcel Hommel and Herbert M. Gilles   464
25   Microsporidiosis   Alan Curry   529
26   *Blastocystis hominis*   Jeffrey J. Windsor   556

PART III   HELMINTHS   571
27   Nature and classification of parasitic helminths   David I. Gibson   573
28   Schistosomes: general   Somei Kojima and Andrew S. MacDonald   600
29   Schistosomes: African   Somei Kojima and Andrew S. MacDonald   610
30   Schistosomes: Asian   Somei Kojima   626
31   Lung and liver flukes   Melissa R. Haswell-Elkins   640
32   Intestinal tapeworms   Jørn Andreassen   658
33   Larval cestodes   Ana Flisser and Philip S. Craig   677
34   Gastrointestinal nematodes – *Ascaris*, hookworm, *Trichuris*, and *Enterobius*
     Celia V. Holland   713
35   *Stronglyloides* and *Capillaria*   Michael Cappello and Peter J. Hotez   737
36   *Toxocara*   Elena Pinelli, Laetitia M. Kortbeek, and Joke W.B. van der Giessen 750
37   *Trichinella*   Dickson D. Despommier   757
38   Lymphatic filariasis   Subash Babu and Thomas B. Nutman   769
39   Onchocerciasis   Janette E. Bradley, James A.G. Whitworth, and Maria-Gloria Basáñez 781
40   *Angiostrongylus* (*Parastrongylus*) and less common nematodes   Kentaro Yoshimura 802
41   Dracunculiasis   Ralph Muller   830

IMMUNOLOGY

PART I   INTRODUCTION   1
1   Introduction   Brigitte A. Askonas   3
2   History   Anne Marie Moulin   5

PART II   INNATE IMMUNITY AND INFLAMMATION   19
3   Phagocytes part 1: Macrophages   Gordon D. Brown and Siamon Gordon   21
4   Phagocytes part 2: Neutrophils   Antonio Ferrante   35

5	**Basophils and eosinophils** Edward E.S. Mitre and Thomas B. Nutman	**55**
6	**Natural killer cells** Klas Kärre and Jens Zerrahn	**79**
7	**Pattern recognition** Nicolas W.J. Schröder and Ralf R. Schumann	**109**
8	**Apoptosis** Antoine Galmiche and Arturo Zychlinsky	**131**
9	**Complement** B. Paul Morgan	**141**
10	**Antimicrobial peptides: defensins and cathelicidins** Robert I. Lehrer and Tomas Ganz	**165**
11	**Lipid mediators: leukotrienes, prostanoids and other lipids** Charles W. Parker	**181**
12	**The acute phase response** John G. Raynes	**193**

PART III   SOLUBLE MEDIATORS   **215**

13	**Chemokines** Marco Baggiolini and Pius Loetscher	**217**
14	**Type I interferons and receptors** Sidney Pestka	**237**
15	**Cytokines** Sergio Romagnani	**273**

PART IV   ACQUIRED IMMUNITY   **301**

16	**Antibodies and B lymphocytes** William Cushley and Gillian Borland	**303**
17	**The B-cell antigen receptor** Anthony L. DeFranco	**339**
18	**Monoclonal antibody therapy** Andrew J.T. George	**353**
19	**Processing and presentation of antigen by the class II histocompatibility system** Emil R. Unanue	**375**
20	**CD4$^+$ T lymphocytes** Allan M. Mowat and Paul Garside	**389**
21	**MHC class I antigen processing system** Jonathan W. Yewdell	**403**
22	**The role of CD8 T cells in the control of infectious disease and malignancies** Shiou-Chih Hsu (Stephen)	**419**
23	**Unconventional T cells** Adrian Hayday and Carrie Steele	**435**
24	**T-cell receptors** Marc Bonneville	**449**
25	**Lymphocyte-mediated cytotoxicity** Eckhard R. Podack	**471**
26	**Immunological memory** Shane Crotty and Rafi Ahmed	**487**
27	**Lymphocyte homing** Michel Aurrand-Lions and Beat A. Imhof	**503**
28	**The mucosal immune response** Kohtaro Fujihashi, Prosper N. Boyaka and Jerry R. McGhee	**519**
29	**Superantigens** Bernhard Fleischer	**555**
30	**Immunogenetics** Marie-Anne Shaw	**571**

PART V   INFECTION AND IMMUNITY   **615**

31	**Viral interference with the host immune response** Antonio Alcami, Ann B. Hill and Ulrich H. Koszinowski	**617**
32	**Evasion of immune responses by bacteria** Kingston H.G. Mills and Aoife P. Boyd	**645**
33	**Parasite evasion** Werner Solbach and Richard Lucius	**675**

PART VI   IMMUNOPATHOLOGY AND IMMUNODEFICIENCY   **693**

34	**Shock/sepsis** Daniela N. Männel	**695**
35	**DTH-associated pathology** Stefan Ehlers and Christoph Hölscher	**705**
36	**Airway hypersensitivity** Elizabeth R. Jarman and Jonathan R. Lamb	**731**
37	**Autoimmunity** Helena Crowley and Brigitte T. Huber	**747**
38	**The immunocompromised host** Alain Fischer	**765**
39	**Acquired immunodeficiencies** Ralf Ignatius and Thomas Schneider	**787**

PART VII   VACCINES   **817**

40	**New approaches to vaccine delivery** Charalambos D. Partidos	**819**
41	**New vaccine technologies** James P. Nataro and Myron M. Levine	**837**
42	**Peptide vaccines** Claude P. Muller and Mike M. Putz	**853**
43	**Live vaccine carriers** Gordon Dougan, Richard J. Aspinall, Frances Bowe and Liljana Petrovska	**895**
44	**Naked DNA vaccines** Linda S. Klavinskis	**909**
45	**Adjuvants and subunit vaccines** Giuseppe Del Giudice and Rino Rappuoli	**925**
46	**Mathematical models of vaccination** Graham F. Medley and D. James Nokes	**947**

Contributors

John P. Ackers MA DPHIL MSC
Professor of Postgraduate Education in Public Health
Department of Infectious and Tropical Diseases
London School of Hygiene and Tropical Medicine
London, UK

Ben Adler BSC BA PHD MASM
Director, ARC Centre for Microbial Genomics
Department of Microbiology
Monash University
Victoria, Australia

Adriano Aguzzi MD PHD hcFRCP FRCPATH
Institute of Neuropathology
University Hospital of Zürich
Zürich, Switzerland

Rafi Ahmed
Emory Vaccine Center; and
Department of Microbiology and Immunology
Emory University School of Medicine
Atlanta, GA, USA

L. Ajello† PHD
Formerly Adjunct Professor
Department of Ophthalmology
Emory University Eye Center
Atlanta, GA, USA

Klaus Aktories MD PHD
Director, Institute of Experimental and
Clinical Pharmacology and Toxicology
University of Freiburg
Freiburg, Germany

Antonio Alcami PHD
Department of Medicine
University of Cambridge
Addenbrooke's Hospital Cambridge, UK; and
Senior Research Assistant
Centro Nacional de Biotecnologia (CSIC)
Campus Universidad Autonoma
Madrid, Spain

Roy M. Anderson
Department of Infectious Disease Epidemiology
Imperial College School of Medicine
London, UK

Jørn Andreassen
Department of Population Biology
Biological Institute, University of Copenhagen
Copenhagen, Denmark

Roberto Arenas MD
Professor of Dermatology and
Medical Mycology
Hospital General 'Dr. Manuel Gea González'
University of Mexico
México D.F.

Sevtap Arikan MD
Professor of Microbiology
Head of Mycology Laboratory
Hacettepe University Faculty of Medicine
Department of Microbiology and Clinical Microbiology
Ankara Turkey

Sarath N. Arseculeratne MBBS (CEY) DIP BACT
(MANCH) DPHIL (OXON)
Department of Microbiology, Faculty of Medicine
University of Peradeniya
Peradeniya Sri Lanka

R.W. Ashford BSC PHD DSC
Liverpool School of Tropical Medicine
Liverpool, UK

Brigitte A. Askonas
Department of Biological Sciences
Imperial College London
London, UK

Richard J. Aspinall
Reader in Immunology
Division of Investigative Science and Medicine
Imperial College London
London, UK

Hazel M. Aucken MA PhD
Formerly Clinical Microbiologist
Specialist and Reference Microbiology Division
Health Protection Agency, Centre for Infections
London, UK

Michel Aurrand-Lions PhD
Senior Scientist
Department of Pathology and Immunology
Centre Medical Universitaire
Geneva, Switzerland

Matthew B. Avison BSc PhD
Lecturer in Microbiology
Department of Pathology and Microbiology
University of Bristol
Bristol, UK

Subash Babu MBBS PhD
Helminth Immunology Section
Laboratory of Parasitic Diseases
National Institutes of Health
Bethesda, MD, USA

Marco Baggiolini MD
Professor
University of Lugano (USI)
Lugano, Switzerland

Tom Baldwin
Institute of Infection, Immunity and Inflammation
Queen's Medical Centre
Nottingham, UK

L. Andrew Ball DPhil
Professor of Microbiology
University of Alabama at Birmingham
Birmingham, AL, USA

Jangu E. Banatvala CBE MA MD FRCP FRCPath
FMedSci
Emeritus Professor of Clinical Virology
Guy's, King's and St Thomas' Medical
and Dental School
London, UK

Bettina Bankamp PhD
Measles, Mumps, Rubella and Herpes Team
Respiratory and Enteric Viruses Branch
Division of Viral and Rickettsial Diseases
National Center for Infectious Diseases
Centers for Disease Control and Prevention
Atlanta, GA, USA

Alan D.T. Barrett PhD
Department of Pathology
University of Texas Medical Branch
Galveston, TX, USA

Thomas Barrett PhD
Institue for Animal Health
Pirbright Laboratory
Pirbright, UK

Maria-Gloria Basáñez MSc PhD FRES
Senior Lecturer and MSc Course Organiser
Department of Infectious Disease Epidemiology
Imperial College School of Medicine
London, UK

Paul A. Bates BA PhD
Senior Lecturer in Medical Parasitology
Liverpool School of Tropical Medicine
Liverpool, UK

Norman T. Begg
Director of Vaccines
GlaxoSmithKline
Welwyn Garden City, UK

William J. Bellini PhD
Chief, Measles, Mumps, Rubella and
Herpesviruses Team
Respiratory and Enteric Viruses Branch
Division of Viral and Rickettsial Diseases
National Center for Infectious Diseases
Centers for Disease Control and Prevention
Atlanta, GA, USA

Gil Benard
Medical Researcher, Laboratory of Dermatology and
Immunodeficiencies
Medical School of the University of São Paulo
São Paulo, Brazil

Mauro Bendinelli MD PhD
Professor of Microbiology; and
Director of Virology and Retrovirus Center
Department of Experimental Pathology
Virology Section, University of Pisa
Pisa, Italy

Peter M. Bennett BSc PhD
Professor of Bacterial Genetics
Department of Pathology and Microbiology
School of Medical Sciences
University of Bristol
Bristol, UK

Anthony R. Berendt BM BCH FRCP
Consultant Physician-in-Charge, Bone Infection Unit
Nuffield Orthopaedic Centre
Headington, Oxford, UK

Ruth L. Berkelman MD
Department of Epidemiology
Rollins School of Public Health
Emory University
Atlanta, GA, USA

Kenneth I. Berns MD PHD
Director, UF Genetics Institute; and
Professor, Molecular Genetics and Microbiology
College of Medicine
University of Florida
Gainesville, FL, USA

Jennifer M. Best PHD FRCPATH
Reader in Virology
Department of Infectious Diseases
King's College London
London, UK

Samuel J. Black BSC PHD
Head of Department
Department of Veterinary & Animal Sciences
University of Massachusetts
Amherst, MA, USA

Frederick A. Bolton
Director, Health Protection Agency Laboratory
Manchester Royal Infirmary
Manchester, UK

Roumiana S. Boneva MD PHD
Medical Epidemiologist
National Center for Infectious Diseases
Centers for Disease Control and Prevention
Atlanta, GA, USA

Marc Bonneville
Research Director, CNRS
INSERM U601
Institute of Biology
Nantes, France

Gillian Borland PHD
Division of Biochemistry & Molecular Biology
Institute of Biomedical & Life Sciences
University of Glasgow, UK

S. Peter Borriello PHD FRCPATH FFPH
Director, Specialist and Reference
Microbiology Division; and Interim Director
Health Protection Agency, Centre for Infections
London, UK

Frances Bowe
Centre for Molecular Microbiology and Infection
Department of Biological Sciences
Imperial College London
London, UK

Prosper N. Boyaka
Department of Microbiology
The University of Alabama at Birmingham
Birmingham, AL, USA

Aoife P. Boyd BA(Mod) PHD
Lecturer, Department of Microbiology
National University of Ireland
Galway, Ireland

Janette E. Bradley BSC PHD
School of Biology, University of Nottingham
Nottingham, UK

Jonathan S. Brazier MSC CBIOL MIBIOL PHD SRCS
Anaerobe Reference Laboratory
NPHS Microbiology Cardiff
University Hospital of Wales
Cardiff, UK

Thomas Briese PHD
Jerome L. and Dawn Greene
Infectious Disease Laboratory
Mailman School of Public Health
Columbia University
New York, NY, USA

William J. Britt MD
Department of Pediatrics
University of Alabama at Birmingham
Birmingham, AL, USA

Gordon D. Brown PHD
Institute of Infectious Disease and Molecular Medicine
Faculty of Health Sciences, CLS
University of Cape Town
Cape Town, South Africa

Jo Ellen Brunner PHD
Instructional Support Group
School of Biological Sciences
University of California
Irvine, CA, USA

Donald E. Burgess PHD
Collection Scientist, Protistology
American Type Culture Collection
Manassas, VA, USA

James P. Burnie DSc MD PhD FRCPath MRCP MSc
Professor of Medical Microbiology
University of Manchester; and
Chief Executive Officer, NeuTec Pharma plc
Manchester, UK

Jean-Paul Butzler MD PhD
Professor of Clinical Microbiology and Epidemiology
Department of Human Ecology, Faculty of Medicine
Vrije Universiteit Brussels
Brussels, Belgium

Colin K. Campbell BSc MSc PhD
Mycology Reference Laboratory and National
Collection of Pathogenic Fungi
Health Protection Agency
Specialist and Reference Microbiology
Division, HPA South West Laboratory
Bristol, UK

Michael Cappello MD
Associate Professor
Departments of Pediatrics and
Epidemiology and Public Health
Yale School of Medicine
New Haven, CT, USA

Michael J. Carter BA PhD
School of Biomedical and Molecular Sciences
University of Surrey
Guildford, UK

Keith A.V. Cartwright MA BM FRCPath FFPH
Head of Intervention Policy and Research and
Development Local and Regional Services
Health Protection Agency South West
Stonehouse, UK

Pierre-Emmanuel Ceccaldi PhD
Senior Scientist
Unit 'Epidémiologie et Physiopathologie
des Virus Oncogènes'
Institut Pasteur
Paris, France

Francis W. Chandler DVM PhD
Professor Emeritus
Department of Pathology
Medical College of Georgia
Augusta, GA, USA

Barbara J. Chang BSc PhD FASM
Associate Professor
Microbiology, School of Biomedical and
Chemical Sciences
The University of Western Australia
Nedlands, Western Australia

Tom Cheasty BSc
Head, ESYV Reference Unit
Laboratory of Enteric Pathogens
Specialist and Reference Microbiology Division
Health Protection Agency, Centre for Infections
London, UK

Ian N. Clarke BSc PhD
Professor of Virology
Division of Infection, Inflammation and Repair
School of Medicine
University of Southampton
Southampton, UK

J. Barklie Clements FRSE FMedSci
Professor of Virology
Division of Virology
Institute of Biological and Life Sciences
University of Glasgow
Glasgow, UK

Leslie Collier MD DSc FRCP FRCPath
Professor Emeritus of Virology
The London Hospital and Medical College, London;
Formerly Director, Vaccines and Sera Laboratories
The Lister Institute of Preventive Medicine
Elstree, Hertfordshire, UK

Richard C. Condit PhD
Department of Molecular Genetics and Microbiology
University of Florida College of Medicine
Gainesville, FL, USA

Patricia S. Conville MS MT(ASCP)
Medical Technologist, Microbiology Service
Department of Laboratory Medicine
National Institutes of Health Clinical Center
Bethesda, MD, USA

James F. Conway BSc PhD
Group Leader
Laboratoire de Microscopie Electronique Structurale
Institut de Biologie Structurale
Grenoble, France

Chester R. Cooper, Jr PhD
Associate Professor
Department of Biological Sciences
Youngstown State University
Youngstown, OH, USA

Samantha Cooray MBiochem PhD
Department of Virology
Wright Fleming Institute
Imperial College Faculty of Medicine
London, UK

Michael J. Corbel PHD DSC(Med) FIBiol FRCPATH
Head, Division of Bacteriology
National Institute of Biological Standards and Control
Potters Bar, Hertfordshire, UK

Susan F. Cotmore PHD
Senior Research Scientist
Department of Laboratory Medicine
Yale University School of Medicine
New Haven, CT, USA

F.E.G. Cox PHD DSC
Senior Visiting Research Fellow
Department of Infectious and Tropical Diseases
London School of Hygiene and Tropical Medicine
London, UK

Gary M. Cox MD
Associate Professor of Medicine
Duke University Medical Center
Durham, NC, USA

Nancy J. Cox PHD
Chief, Influenza Branch
Division of Viral and Rickettsial Diseases
Centers for Disease Control and Prevention
Atlanta, GA, USA

Philip S. Craig
Biosciences Research Institute
School of Environment and Life Sciences
University of Salford
Salford, UK

Dorothy H. Crawford MBBS PHD MD FRCP
DSC FRSE
Professor of Medical Microbiology
School of Biomedical & Clinical Laboratory Sciences
University of Edinburgh
Edinburgh, UK

Vicente Crespo Erchiga MD PHD
Head, Department of Dermatology
Hospital Reginal Universitario Carlos Haya
Málaga, Spain

Shane Crotty PHD
Assistant Member
Division of Vaccine Discovery
La Jolla Institute for Allergy & Immunology (LIAI)
San Diego, CA, USA

Helena Crowley
Department of Pathology
Tufts University School of Medicine
Boston, MA, USA

Alan Curry BSC PHD
Head of Unit, Electron Microscopy Unit
Manchester Royal Infirmary
Manchester, UK

Melanie T. Cushion
Professor, Department of Internal Medicine
University of Cincinnati College of Medicine and the
Cincinnati Veterans Affairs Medical Center
Cincinnati, OH, USA

William Cushley PHD
Division of Biochemistry & Molecular Biology
Institute of Biomedical & Life Sciences
University of Glasgow, UK

David A. Dance MB CHB MSC FRCPATH
Regional Microbiologist
Health Protection Agency (South West)
Plymouth, UK

Andrew J. Davison MA PHD
MRC Virology Unit
Institute of Virology
University of Glasgow
Glasgow, UK

Martin Day BSC PHD
Reader in Microbial Genetics
School of Biosciences
Cardiff University
Cardiff, UK

Anthony L. DeFranco
Department of Microbiology and Immunology
University of California
San Francisco, CA, USA

G. Sybren de Hoog PHD
Senior researcher
Centralbureau voor Schimmelcultures
Utrecht, The Netherlands; and
Professor, Institue for Biodiversity and
Ecosystem Dynamics, University of Amsterdam
Amsterdam, The Netherlands

Giuseppe Del Giudice MD
IRIS Research Center, Chiron SrI
Siena, Italy

David W. Denning FRCP FRCPATH
University of Manchester and
Wythenshawe Hospital
Manchester, UK

Terence S. Dermody MD
Professor of Pediatrics and Microbiology
and Immunology
Elizabeth B. Lamb Center for Pediatric Research
Vanderbilt University School of Medicine
Nashville, TN, USA

Dickson D. Despommier
Professor of Public Health and Microbiology
Department of Environmental Health Sciences
Mailman School of Public Health, Columbia University
New York, NY, USA

Ulrich Desselberger MD FRCPATH FRCP
Clinical Microbiology and Public Health Laboratory
Addenbrooke's Hospital
Cambridge, UK (until July 2002)

Charlene S. Dezzutti PHD
HIV and Retrovirology Branch
Division of AIDS, STD, and TB Laboratory Research
National Center for HIV, STD, and TB Prevention
Centers for Disease Control and Prevention
Atlanta, GA, USA

Arthur F. Di Salvo MD
Former South Carolina State Public
Health Laboratory Director
Reno, NV, USA

Esteban Domingo PHD
Professor CSIC
Centro de Biología Molecular "Severo Ochoa"
CSIC-UAM, Universidad Autónoma de Madrid
Cantoblanco, Madrid, Spain

Fiona E. Donald BMEDSCI BMBS FRCPATH
Consultant Medical Microbiologist
Department of Microbiology
University Hospital
Queen's Medical Centre
Nottingham, UK

Ruben O. Donis DVM PHD
Chief, Molecular Genetics Section
Influenza Branch
Division of Viral and Rickettsial Diseases
National Centers for Infectious Diseases
Centers for Disease Control and Prevention
Atlanta, GA, USA

Gordon Dougan
Professor and Director
Centre for Molecular Microbiology and Infection
Department of Biological Sciences
Imperial College London
London, UK

Julie F. Downes BSC
Research Assistant
Department of Microbiology
King's College London
London, UK

Bohumil S. Drasar PHD DSC FRCPATH CBIOL FBIOL
DFC DHE DIPHIC (Hon)
Emeritus Professor of Bacteriology
London School of Hygiene & Tropical Medicine
University of London
London, UK

Michael R. Driks MD
Baptist-Luthern Medical Center
Kansas City, MO, USA

Edouard Drouhet† MD
Formerly Professor of Mycology
Pasteur Institute, Mycology Unit
Paris, France

J.P. Dubey BVSC&AH MVSC PHD
Senior Scientist
United States Department of Agriculture
Beltsville Agricultural Research Centre
MD, USA

J. Stephen Dumler MD
Division of Medical Microbiology
Department of Pathology
The Johns Hopkins University School of Medicine
Baltimore, MD, USA

Bernadette M. Dutia BSC PHD
Senior Research Fellow
Laboratory for Clinical and Molecular Virology
Division of Veterinary Biomedical Sciences
University of Edinburgh
Edinburgh, UK

Andrew J. Easton BSC PHD
Professor of Virology
Department of Biological Sciences
University of Warwick
Coventry, UK

Stefan Ehlers MD
Professor, Division of Molecular Infection Biology
Research Center Borstel
Borstel, Germany

Daniel Elad DVM PHD
Head, Division of Bacteriological and Mycological
Laboratories
Kimron Veterinary Institute
Bet Dagan, Israel

Boni Elewski MD
Professor of Dermatology
Department of Dermatology
University of Alabama at Birmingham
Birmingham, AL, USA

Karen L. Elkins PhD
Senior Investigator, Laboratory of Mycobacteria
Division of Bacterial, Parasitic and Allergenic Products
CBER/US FDA
Bethesda, MD, USA

Richard M. Elliott BSc DPhil FRSE
Professor of Molecular Virology
Division of Virology
Institute of Biomedical and Life Sciences
University of Glasgow
Glasgow, UK

David H. Ellis BSc (Hons) MSc PhD FASM
FRCPA (Hon)
Associate Professor, Mycology Unit
Women's and Children's Hospital
North Adelaide, Australia

Gisela Enders MD
Professor of Virology
Head of the Institute of Virology
Infectiology and Epidemiology; and
Chief, Laboratory Prof. G. Enders and Partners
Stuttgart, Germany

M. Anthony Epstein MA MD DSc PhD FRS
Nuffield Department of Clinical Medicine
University of Oxford, John Radcliffe Hospital
Oxford, UK

Dean D. Erdman Dr PH
Team Leader
Respiratory Virus Diagnostics Section
Division of Viral and Rickettsial Diseases
National Center for Infectious Diseases
Centers for Disease Control and Prevention
Atlanta, GA, USA

Martha Espinosa-Cantellano MD DSc
Center for Research and Advanced Studies
Mexico City, Mexico

Philippe Esterre DVM PhD MSc
Head of Plasmodium Chemoresistance
Reference Center (CNRCP)
Institut Pasteur de Guyane
French Guiana, South America

Mary K. Estes PhD
Professor, Department of Molecular Virology
and Microbiology
Baylor College of Medicine
Houston, TX, USA

Meirion R. Evans BA MB BCh FRCP FFPH
Senior Lecturer
Department of Epidemiology, Statistics and
Public Health
College of Medicine, Cardiff Univeristy
Cardiff, UK

Richard R. Facklam PhD
Distinguished Consultant
Division of Bacterial and Mycotic Diseases
Centers for Disease Control and Prevention
Atlanta, GA, USA

Solly Faine
MediSci Consulting, Armadale; and Emeritus Professor
Department of Microbiology, Monash University
Melbourne, Australia

John J. Farmer III PhD
Scientist Director
United States Public Health Service (Retired)
Foodborne and Diarrheal Diseases Branch
Division of Bacterial and Mycotic Diseases
Center for Infectious Diseases
Centers for Disease Control and Prevention
Atlanta, GA, USA

Mary Katherine Farmer MD
Palmetto Health Richland
University of South Carolina School of Medicine
Columbia, SC, USA

Heinz Feldmann MD
Chief, Special Pathogens Program
National Microbiology Laboratory
Public Health Agency of Canada; and
Associate Professor
Department of Medical Microbiology
University of Manitoba
Winnipeg, MB, Canada

Antonio Ferrante FRCPath PhD
Director of Department of Immunopathology
Women's and Children's Hospital
South Australia; and
Professor, Department of Paediatrics
University of Adelaide; and
Professor of Immunopharmacology
School of Pharmacy and Medical Sciences
University of South Australia
Adelaide, Australia

Paul L. Fidel Jr PHD
Carl Baldridge Research Professor
Department of Microbiology, Immunology, and
Parasitology
Louisiana State University Health
Sciences Center
New Orleans, LA, USA

Hugh J. Field SCD FRCPATH
Reader in Comparative Virology
Centre for Veterinary Science
University of Cambridge
Cambridge, UK

Alain Fischer
Inserm U429
Necker University Hospital
Paris, France

Bernhard Fleckenstein MD
Professor and Chairman
Institute for Clinical and Molecular Virology
University of Erlangen-Nürnberg
Erlangen, Germany

Bernhard Fleischer
Bernhard Nocht Institute for Tropical Medicine
and Institute for Immunology
University Hospital Eppendorf
Hamburg, Germany

Ana Flisser
Directora de Investigacion
Hospital General 'Dr Manuel Gea Gonzalez'; and
SSA Investigadora Departamento de Microbiologia
y Parasitologia
Facultad de Medicina, UNAM
Mexico DF, Mexico

Thomas M. Folks PHD
HIV and Retrovirology Branch
Division of AIDS, STD, and
TB Laboratory Research
National Center for HIV, STD, and TB Prevention
Centers for Disease Control and Prevention
Atlanta, GA, USA

Marcello Franco MD PHD
Chairman, Department of Pathology
Federal University of São Paulo
Paulista School of Medicine
São Paulo, Brazil

Roger Freeman†
Formerly Director, Public Health Laboratory
General Hospital
Newcastle Upon Tyne, UK

Ilya V. Frolov PHD
Department of Microbiology and Immunology
University of Texas Medical Branch
Galveston, TX, USA

Kohtaro Fujihashi
Department of Pediatric Dentistry
Immnunobiology Vaccine Center
School of Dentistry
University of Alabama at Birmingham
Birmingham, AL, USA

Guido Funke MD
Director, Department of Medical Microbiology
and Hygiene; and
CEO, Gärtner and Colleagues Laboratories
Ravensburg, Germany

Antoine Galmiche MD PHD
Department of Cellular Microbiology
Max Planck Institute fur Ifektions Biologie
Berlin, Germany

Tomas Ganz PHD MD
Departments of Medicine and Pathology
David Geffen School of Medicine at UCLA
Los Angeles, CA, USA

Lynne S. Garcia MS MT FAAM
Director, LSG and Associates
Santa Monica, CA, USA

Paul Garside PHD
Professor of Immunobiology
Division of Immunology, Infection and Inflammation
University of Glasgow, Western Infirmary
Glasgow, UK

Sören G. Gatermann
Head, Department of Medical Microbiology
Ruhr-Universität Bochum
Bochum, Germany

Yves Gaudin PHD
Director
Laboratoire de Virologie Moléculaire et Structurale
UMR-CNRS 2472; UMR-INRA 1157 CNRS
Gif-sur-Yvette, Cedex, France

Nigel J. Gay
Modelling and Economics Unit
Communicable Diseases Surveillance Centre (CDSC)
Health Protection Agency, Centre for Infections
London, UK

Edwin E. Geldreich BS MS
Consulting Microbiologist, Retired Senior Microbiologist
US Environmental Protection Agency
Cincinnati, OH, USA

Andrew J.T. George MA PHD FRCPATH
Professor of Molecular Immunology
Department of Immunology
Division of Medicine
Imperial College London
Hammersmith Hospital
London, UK

P. Geraldine MSC MPHIL PHD
Department of Animal Science
Bharathidasan University
Tiruchirapalli, India

Wolfram H. Gerlich PHD
Professor and Director
Institute of Medical Virology
Justus Liebig University Giessen
Giessen, Germany

Saheer E. Gharbia BSC MSC PHD
Head, Genomics, Proteomics and
Bioinformatics Unit
Specialist and Reference Microbiology Division (SRMD)
Health Protection Agency, Centre for Infections
London, UK

David I. Gibson BSC PHD DSC
Head of Division, Parasitic Worms Division
Department of Zoology
The Natural History Museum
London, UK

Herbert M. Gilles MD DSC FRCP FFPH DTM&H
Professor Emeritus
Liverpool School of Tropical Medicine
University of Liverpool
Liverpool, UK

Stephen H. Gillespie MD FRCP(EDIN) FRCPATH
Professor of Medical Microbiology; and
Regional Microbiologist
Centre for Medical Microbiology
Royal Free and University College Medical School
London, UK

Norman L. Goodman
Professor Emeritus
Department of Pathology
College of Medicine, University of Kentucky
Lexington, KY, USA

Alexander E. Gorbalenya PHD DSCI
Associate Professor
Department of Medical Microbiology
Leiden University Medical Center
Leiden, The Netherlands

Siamon Gordon MB CHB FAMS PHD
Glaxo Wellcome Professor of Cellular Pathology
Sir William Dunn School of Pathology
University of Oxford
Oxford, UK

Ian M. Gould BSC PHD MBCHB FRCPE FRCPATH
Consultant Microbiologist
Department of Medical Microbiology
Aberdeen Royal Infirmary Aberdeen, UK; and
Honorary Full Professor of Microbiology
Epidemiology and Public Health
University of Trnava, Slovakia

Jim Gray FIBMS PHD FRCPATH
Head, Enteric Virus Unit
Virus Reference Department
Health Protection Agency, Centre for Infections
London, UK

John R. Graybill
Professor of Medicine
Division of Infectious Diseases
University of Texas Health Science Center
San Antonio, TX, USA

Duane J. Gubler SCD
Director of Asia-Pacific Institute for Tropical Medicine
and Infectious Diseases; and
Chair, Department of Medicine and
Medical Microbiology
John A. Burns School of Medicine
Honolulu, HI, USA

Eveline Guého PHD
Researcher INSERM
Formerly Pasteur Institute, Mycology Unit
Paris, France

Stephen C. Hadler MD
Senior Advisor for Strengthening Childhood
Immunization, Global Immunization Division
National Immunization Program
Centers for Disease Control and Prevention
Atlanta, GA, USA

Kim R. Hardie PGCAP PHD BSC(Hons)
Institute of Infection, Immunity and Inflammation
Centre for Biomolecular Sciences
Nottingham University
Nottingham, UK

Timothy G. Harrison BSc PhD
Deputy Director
Respiratory and Systemic Infection Laboratory
Specialist and Reference Microbiology Division
Health Protection Agency, Centre for Infections
London, UK

Melissa R. Haswell-Elkins PhD
Senior Lecturer, Indigenous Health and
Indigenous Stream Co-ordinator
Australian Integrated Mental Health Initiative
North Queensland Health Equalities Promotion Unit
School of Population Health
University of Queensland, Cairns
Queensland, Australia

Roderick J. Hay DM FRCP FRCPATH
Dean, Faculty of Medicine and Health Sciences
Queens University Belfast,
Belfast

Adrian Hayday BA MA PhD
Head of Division of Immunology, Infection
and Inflammatory Diseases
Kay Glendinning Professor, and Chair
The Peter Gorer Department of Immunobiology
Guy's, King's, and St Thomas' Medical School
King's College London
London, UK

Walid Heneine PhD
HIV and Retrovirology Branch,
Division of AIDS, STD, and TB Laboratory Research
National Center for HIV, STD, and TB Prevention
Centers for Disease Control and Prevention
Atlanta, GA, USA

Ann B. Hill MB BS FRACP PhD
Associate Professor
Department of Molecular Microbiology
and Immunology
Oregon Health and Science University
Portland, OR, USA

Tor Hofstad MD PhD
Emeritus Professor of Microbiology
Department of Microbiology and Immunology
The Gade Institute
University of Bergen
Bergen, Norway

Celia V. Holland PhD
Associate Professor and Head of Department
Department of Zoology, Trinity College
Dublin, Ireland

John J. Holland PhD
Emeritus Professor
Division of Biology and Institute of
Molecular Genetics, University of California
San Diego, La Jolla, CA, USA

Barry Holmes MSc PhD DSC FIBIOL
Head, National Collection of Type Cultures
Health Protection Agency, Centre for Infections
London, UK

Christoph Hölscher PhD
Junior Professor, Junior Research Group
Molecular Infection Biology, Research Center Borstel
Borstel, Germany

Marcel Hommel MD PhD
Professor of Tropical Medicine
Liverpool School of Tropical Medicine
Liverpool, UK

Mady Hornig MA MD
Director of Translational Research
Jerome L. and Dawn Greene Infectious Disease
Laboratory; and
Associate Professor of Epidemiology
Mailman School of Public Health
Columbia University
New York, NY, USA

Peter J. Hotez MD PhD
Professor and Chair
Department of Microbiology and
Tropical Medicine
The George Washington University
Washington, DC, USA

Shiou-Chih Hsu (Stephen) PhD
Postdoctoral Research Scientist
Institute of Animal Health
Compton, Berkshire, UK

Brigitte T. Huber PhD
Department of Pathology
Tufts University School of Medicine
Boston, MA, USA

Ralf Ignatius
Department of Medical Microbiology and Infection
Immunology, Charité University Medicine Berlin
Berlin, Germany

Beat A. Imhof PhD
Professor and Chairman
Department of Pathology and Immunology
Centre Medical Universitaire
Geneva, Switzerland

Catherine Ison PHD FRCPATH
Director
Sexually Transmitted Bacteria Reference
Laboratory
Specialist and Reference Microbiology Division
Health Protection Agency, Centre for Infections
London, UK

J. Michael Janda PHD
Chief, Microbial Diseases Laboratory
California Department of Health Services
Richmond, CA, USA

William M. Janda PHD
Department of Pathology
Division of Clinical Pathology
University of Illinois Medical Center at Chicago
Chicago, IL, USA

Elizabeth R. Jarman PHD
Wellcome Trust Research Laboratories
Malawi-Liverpool School of Tropical Medicine
Blantyre, Malawi

Henrik Elvang Jensen DVM DR VET SCI PHD
Diplomate, European College of Veterinary
Pathologists
The Royal Veterinary and Agricultural University
Copenhagen, Denmark

Li Jin MD PHD MRCPATH
Clinical Scientist, Enteric Virus Reference
Department, Health Protection Agency
Centre for Infections, London, UK

David T. John MSPH PHD
Professor of Microbiology/Parasitology; and
Associate Dean for Basic Sciences
and Graduate Studies
Oklahoma State University, Center for Health Studies
Tulsa, OK, USA

Elizabeth M. Johnson BSC PHD
Director, Mycology Reference Laboratory and
National Collection of Pathogenic Fungi
Health Protection Agency, Specialist and Reference
Microbiology Division, HPA, South West Laboratory
Bristol, UK

Eric A. Johnson SCD
Professor of Food Microbiology and Toxicology
Food Research Institute, University of Wisconsin
Madison, WI, USA

Judith A. Johnson PHD
Chief, Clinical Microbiology and Molecular Diagnostics
Veterans Affairs Maryland Health Care System; and

Associate Professor of Pathology
University of Maryland School of Medicine
Baltimore, MD, USA

Michael Kann MD
Professor of Virology
Justus Liebig University Giessen
Giessen, Germany

Klas Kärre
Microbiology and Tumorbiology Center (MTC)
Karolinska Institute
Stockholm, Sweden

Stefan H.E. Kaufmann PHD
Director, Department of Immunology
Max-Planck-Institute for Infection Biology
Berlin, Germany

Yoshihiro Kawaoka DVM PHD
Professor and Director
International Research Center for Infectious Diseases;
and Division of Virology
Department of Microbiology and Immunology
Institute of Medical Science
University of Tokyo, Tokyo, Japan; and
Professor, Department of Pathobiological Sciences
School of Veterinary Medicine
University of Wisconsin-Madison
Madison, WI, USA

M. Paul Kelly
Senior Lecturer (Wellcome Fellow)
Barts and the London School of Medicine
and Dentistry
Adult and Paediatric Gastroenterology
Digestive Disease Research Centre
London, UK

Kamel Khalili PHD
Professor and Director
Center for Neurovirology and Cancer Biology
Temple University
Philadelphia, PA USA

Michael P. Kiley PHD †
Formerly USDA, Agricultural Research Service
Animal Production, Product Value
Beltsville, MD, USA

Mogens Kilian DDS PHD
Professor of Bacteriology
Department of Medical Microbiology
and Immunology
University of Aarhus
Aarhus, Denmark

Linda S. Klavinskis BSC PHD
Senior Lecturer
Peter Gorer Department of Immunobiology
Guys, Kings' and St. Thomas' School of Medicine
Guys Hospital, London, UK

Bruce S. Klein
Professor of Pediatrics
Internal Medicine and Medical Microbiology and
Immunology
University of Wisconsin Medical School
Madison, WI, USA

Hans-Dieter Klenk MD
Institute of Virology Medical School
Philipps-University
Marburg, Germany

Keith P. Klugman MB BCH PHD
Professor of Global Health
The Rollins School of Public Health; and
Professor of Medicine
Division of Infectious Diseases, School of Medicine
Emory University
Atlanta, GA, USA

Wendy A. Knowles BSC PHD MIBIOL
Clinical Scientist, Enteric, Respiratory and
Neurological Virus Laboratory
Specialist and Reference Microbiology Division
Health Protection Agency, Centre for Infections
London, UK

Guy R. Knudsen BS MS PHD
Soil and Land Resources Division
University of Idaho
Moscow, ID, USA

Somei Kojima MD PHD
Professor Emeritus
The University of Tokyo, Tokyo, Japan; and
Deputy Director, Center for Medical Science
International University of Health and Welfare
Otawara, Tochigi Prefecture, Japan

Laetitia M. Kortbeek MD
Medical Microbiologist
Diagnostic Laboratory for Infectious Diseases
and Perinatal Screening (LIS)
National Institute of Public Health
and the Environment, Bilthoven
The Netherlands

Ulrich H. Koszinowski
Chair of Virology
Max von Pettenkofer-Institut
München, Germany

Jaroslav Kulda RNDR PHD
Professor of Parasitology
Department of Parasitology, Faculty of Science
Charles University in Prague
Prague, Czech Republic

Myriam S. Künzi PHD
Postdoctoral Fellow, John Hopkins Oncology Center
Baltimore, MD, USA

Ralph Lainson OBE FRS AFTWAS BSC PHD DSC
Department of Parasitology
Instituto Evandro Chagas
Belém, Pará, Brazil

Jonathan R. Lamb DSC FRCPATH FMEDSCI FRSE
GlaxoSmithKline Immunology Group
Translational Medicine and Technology
Clinical Pharmacology and Discovery Medicine
Greenford, UK

Paul R. Lambden BSC PHD
Senior Research Fellow, Molecular Microbiology
University Medical School
Southampton General Hospital
Southampton, UK

Paul F. Lehmann PHD
Professor, Department of Medical Microbiology and
Immunology
Medical College of Ohio
Toledo, OH, USA

Robert I. Lehrer MD
Department of Medicine
UCLA School of Medicine
Los Angeles, CA, USA

Myron M. Levine MD DTPH
Professor and Director
Center for Vaccine Development
University of Maryland School of Medicine
Baltimore, MD, USA

Nigel F. Lightfoot MBBS MRCPATH MSC
Director of Emergency Response
Centre for Emergency Preparedness and Response
Health Protection Agency, Porton Down
Salisbury, UK

R. Michael Linden PHD
Associate Professor
Department of Gene and Cell Medicine, and
Department of Microbiology
Mount Sinai School of Medicine
New York, NY, USA

W. Ian Lipkin MD
Jerome L. and Dawn Greene Infectious
Disease Laboratory
Mailman School of Public Health
Columbia University
New York, NY, USA

Graham Lloyd BSc MSc PhD FIBMS
Head, Special Pathogens Reference Unit
Novel and Dangerous Pathogens
Centre for Emergency Preparedness and Response
Health Protection Agency, Porton Dawn
Salisbury, UK

Pius Loetscher PD PhD
Novartis Institutes of Biomedical Research
Novartis Pharma AG
Basel, Switzerland

Niall A. Logan
Senior Lecturer and
University Biological Safety Adviser
Department of Biological and Biomedical Sciences
Glasgow Caledonian University
Glasgow, UK

Francisco J. López-Antuñano
Instituto Nacional de Salud Publica
Colonia Santa Maria Ahuacatitlan
Morelos, Mexico

Richard Lucius
Full Professor, Department of Molecular Parasitology
Institute of Biology
Humboldt-University Berlin
Berlin, Germany

Andrew S. MacDonald BSc PhD
MRC Research Fellow
Institute of Immunology and Infection Research
University of Edinburgh
Edinburgh, UK

Janine R. Maenza MD
Clinical Assistant Professor of Medicine
Division of Allergy and Infectious Diseases
Department of Medicine, University of Washington
Seattle, WA, USA

John T. Magee PhD
Scientific Officer, Cardiff Public Health Laboratory
Cardiff, UK

Fabrizio Maggi MD PhD
Assistant, Clinical Virology
Department of Experimental Pathology
Virology Section, University of Pisa
Pisa, Italy

Brian W.J. Mahy MA PhD ScD DSc
Senior Scientific Research Advisor
National Center for Infectious Diseases
Centers for Disease Control and Prevention
Atlanta, GA, USA

Matthias Maiwald MD PhD FRCPA D(ABMM)
Associate Professor and Consultant Microbiologist
Department of Microbiology and Infectious Diseases
Flinders University and Medical Centre
Bedford Park, Australia; and
Department of Microbiology and Immunology
Stanford University School of Medicine
Stanford, California, USA

Daniela N. Männel
Department of Immunology
University of Regensburg
Germany

Per-Anders Mårdh PhD MD
Department of Obstetrics and Gynecology
Lund University
Lund, Sweden

Scott A. Martin BS MS PhD
Professor, Department of Animal and Dairy Science
University of Georgia
Athens, GA, USA

Adolfo Martínez-Palomo MD DSc
Emeritus Professor
Center for Research and Advanced Studies
Mexico City, Mexico

Ruth Matthews MSc MD PhD FRCPATH
Professor of Infectious Diseases
University of Manchester; and
Research & Development Director, NeuTec Pharma plc
Manchester, UK

Myra McClure PhD DSc FRCPATH
Professor of Retrovirolgy and
Honorary Consultant in GU Medicine
Head of Section of Infectious Diseases
Jefferiss Research Trust Laboratories
Wright-Fleming Institute, Faculty of Medicine
Imperial College London
London, UK

Vincent McDonald PhD
Reader in Gastroenterology
Centre for Gastroenterology
Institute of Cell and Molecular Science
Barts and the London School of Medicine and Dentistry
Queen Mary College, University of London
London, UK

Jerry R. McGhee
Department of Microbiology
The University of Alabama at Birmingham
Birmingham, AL, USA

Jim McLauchlin PHD
Food Safety Microbiology Laboratory
Specialist and Reference Microbiology Division
Health Protection Agency Center for Infections
London, UK

Graham F. Medley BSC PHD
Professor of Infectious Disease Epidemiology
Department of Biological Sciences
University of Warwick
Coventry, UK

Heinz Mehlhorn
Department of Parasitology
University of Duesseldorf
Duesseldorf, Germany

Leonel Mendoza MSC PHD
Associate Professor, Medical Technology Program
Microbiology and Molecular Genetics
Michigan State University
East Lansing, MI, USA

William G. Merz PHD
Professor of Pathology,
Dermatology, Epidemiology, and Molecular
Microbiology and Immunology
The Johns Hopkins University
Baltimore, MD, USA

Timothy A. Mietzner PHD
Department of Molecular Genetics and Biochemistry
University of Pittsburgh School of Medicine
Pittsburgh, PA, USA

Michael A. Miles MSC PHD DSC FRCPATH
Professor of Medical Protozoology
Department of Infectious and Tropical Diseases
London School of Hygiene and Tropical Medicine
London, UK

Kingston H.G. Mills BA(Mod) PHD
Professor of Experimental Immunology
Department of Biochemistry
Trinity College Dublin
Ireland

Philip Minor BA PHD
National Institute for Biological Standards and
Control (NIBSC), Division of Virology
South Mimms, Potters Bar
Herts, UK

Anthony C. Minson BSC PHD
Professor of Virology, Virology Division
Department of Pathology, University of Cambridge
Cambridge, UK

Thomas G. Mitchell PHD
Associate Professor
Department of Molecular Genetics and Microbiology
Duke University Medical Center
Durham, NC, USA

Edward E.S. Mitre MD
Clinical Associate
Laboratory of Parasitic Diseases
National Institute of Allergy and Infectious Diseases
National Institutes of Health
Bethesda, MD, USA

David H. Molyneux MA PHD DSC
Director, Lymphatic Filariasis Support Centre
Liverpool School of Tropical Medicine
Liverpool, UK

Arnold S. Monto MD
Professor of Epidemiology, Director
The University of Michigan Bioterrorism
Preparedness Initiative
University of Michigan School of Public Health
Ann Arbor, MI, USA

Caroline B. Moore MSC PHD SRCS CBIOL
Senior Clinical Scientist
Regional Mycology Centre
Department of Microbiology, Hope Hospital
Salford, UK

B. Paul Morgan FRCPATH MRCP PHD
Department of Medical Biochemistry and
Immunology
University of Wales College of Medicine
Cardiff, UK

Stephen A. Morse MSPH PHD
Associate Director for Science
Bioterrorism and Preparedness and Response Program
National Center for Infectious Diseases
Centers for Disease Control and Prevention
Atlanta, GA, USA

Anne Moscona MD
Professor, Pediatrics and Microbiology/Immunology
Vice Chair of Pediatrics for Research
Weill Medical College
Cornell University
New York, NY, USA

Anne Marie Moulin MD PhD
Directeur de Recherche
Centre National de la Recherche Scientifique, CEDEJ
Le Caire, Egypte

Allan M. Mowat BSc(Hons) MBChB PhD FRCPath
Division of Immunology, Infection and Inflammation
University of Glasgow, Western Infirmary
Glasgow, UK

Richard W. Moyer PhD
Senior Associate Dean for Research
Development; and
Professor, Department of Molecular Genetics
and Microbiology
University of Florida College of Medicine
Gainesville, FL, USA

Claude P. Muller
Professor of Immunology
University of Trier, Trier, Germany; and
Institute of Immunology, LNS; and
Director, WHO Collaborating Center for Measles and
European Reference Laboratory for Measles
and Rubella
Luxembourg, Grand-Duchy of Luxembourg

Ralph Muller BSc PhD DSc FIBiol
Honorary Senior Lecturer
Department of Infectious and Tropical Diseases
London School of Hygiene and Tropical Medicine
London, UK

Frederick A. Murphy DVM PhD
School of Veterinary Medicine
University of California Davis
Davis, CA, USA

Patrick R. Murray PhD
Chief, Microbiology Service
Department of Laboratory Medicine
National Institutes of Health Clinical Center
Bethesda, MD, USA

David Mutimer MBBS MD FRACP FRCP
Reader in Hepatology, University of Birmingham; and
Consultant Hepatologist, Liver and Hepatobiliary Unit
Queen Elizabeth Hospital
Birmingham, UK

Reinier Mutters PhD
Professor, Institute of Medical Microbiology
and Hospital Hygiene
Philipps University
Marburg, Germany

Francis E. Nano PhD
Professor, Department of Biochemistry
and Microbiology
University of Victoria
Victoria, BC, Canada

Anthony A. Nash PhD FRSE
Laboratory for Clinical and Molecular Virology
Centre for Infectious Diseases
University of Edinburgh
Edinburgh, UK

James P. Nataro MD PhD
Professor of Pediatrics and Medicine
Center for Vaccine Development; and
Associate Chair for Research
Department of Pediatrics
University of Maryland School of Medicine
Baltimore, MD, USA

Neal Nathanson MD
Associate Dean, Global Health Programs
University of Pennsylvania School of Medicine
Philadelphia, PA, USA

James C. Neil BSc PhD FRSE
Professor of Virology and Molecular Oncology
Institute of Comparative Medicine
University of Glasgow Veterinary School
Glasgow, UK

Frank Neipel MD
Institute for Clinical and Molecular Virology
University of Erlangen-Nürnberg
Erlangen, Germany

Gabriele Neumann PhD
Department of Pathobiological Sciences
School of Veterinary Medicine
University of Wisconsin-Madison
Madison, WI, USA

Angus Nicoll CBE
Director, Communicable Disease Surveillance
Centre (CDSC)
Health Protection Agency Centre for Infections
London, UK

Michael Noble MD FRCPC
Associate Professor
Department of Pathology and
Laboratory Medicine
University of British Columbia; and
Medical Microbiology and Infection Control
Vancouver Hospital
Vancouver, BC, Canada

Eva Nohýnková RNDR PHD
Head, Department of Tropical Medicine
Faculty Hospital Bulovka, Charles University in Prague
Prague, Czech Republic

D. James Nokes BSC PHD
Senior Lecturer, Ecology and Epidemiology Group
Department of Biological Sciences
University of Warwick, Coventry, UK; and
Senior Research Officer
Centre for Geographic Medicine Research (Coast)
Kenya Medical Research Institute
Kilifi, Kenya

Thomas B. Nutman MD
Head, Helminth Immunology Section, and
Head, Clinical Parasitology Unit
Laboratory of Parasitic Diseases
National Institute of Allergy and Infectious Diseases
National Institutes of Health
Bethesda, MD, USA

Ingar Olsen DDS PHD
Professor, Department of Oral Biology; and
Dean of Research
Dental Faculty, University of Oslo
Oslo, Norway

Jessica Otte BS
Center for Neurovirology and Cancer Biology
Temple University
Philadelphia, PA, USA

Robert J. Owen PHD FRCPATH
Head, HPA Campylobacter and Heliobacter
Reference Unit
Specialist and Reference Microbiology Division
Health Protection Agency, Centre for Infections
London, UK

Arvind A. Padhye PHD
Guest Researcher, Mycotic Diseases Branch
Division of Bacterial and Mycotic Diseases
Centers for Disease Control and Prevention
Atlanta, GA, USA

Norberto J. Palleroni PHD
Research Professor
Department of Biochemistry and Microbiology
Cook College, Rutgers University
New Brunswick, NJ, USA

Stephen R. Palmer MA MB BCHIR FRCP FFPHM
Mansel Talbot Professor of Epidemiology
and Public Health
Department of Epidemiology
Statistics and Public Health
College of Medicine, Cardiff University
Cardiff, UK

Demosthenes Pappagianis MD PHD
Professor of Medical Microbiology and
Immunology, School of Medicine
University of California
Davis, CA, USA

Peter G. Pappas MD
Professor of Medicine
University of Alabama at Birmingham School of
Medicine
Birmingham, AL, USA

Charles W. Parker MD
Emeritus Professor of Medicine Microbiology/
Immunology
Washington University School of Medicine
St. Louis, MO, USA

Charalambos D. Partidos DVM MSc PHD
Senior Research Scientist
UPR 9021, CNRS
Immunologie et Chimie Thérapeutiques
Institut de Biologie Moléculaire et Cellulaire
Strasbourg, France

Roger Parton BSC PHD
Senior Lecturer
Division of Infection and Immunity
Institute of Biomedical and Life Sciences
University of Glasgow
Glasgow, UK

Robin Patel MD
Associate Professor of Medicine; and
Associate Professor of Microbiology
Division of Infectious Diseases,
Division of Clinical Microbiology
Mayo Clinic College of Medicine
Rochester, MN, USA

Thomas F. Patterson MD FACP
Professor of Medicine
Director, San Antonio Center for Medical Mycology
The University of Texas Health Science Center
at San Antonio
San Antonio, TX, USA

Sharon J. Peacock PHD FRCP FRCPATH
Wellcome Trust Career Development Fellow in
Clinical Tropical Medicine
Faculty of Tropical Medicine
Mahidol University
Bangkok, Thailand

Richard W. Peluso PHD
Vice President Process Sciences and
Manufacturing, Targeted Genetics
Seattle, WA, USA

John R. Perfect MD
Professor of Medicine
Duke University Medical Center
Durham, NC, USA

Sidney Pestka MD
Professor and Chairman
Department of Molecular Genetics
Microbiology and Immunology
University of Medicine and Dentistry
Robert Wood Johnson Medical School
Pistcataway NJ, USA; and Program Director
Cancer Institute of New Jersey
New Brunswick, NJ, USA; and
Chief Scientific Officer
PBL Biomedical Laborateries
Piscataway, NJ, USA

Liljana Petrovska DVM MSc PHD
Centre for Molecular Microbiology and Infection
Department of Biological Sciences
Imperial College London
London, UK

Mark Pett MA PHD
Postdoctoral Research Associate
MRC Cancer Cell Unit
Hutchinson MRC Research Centre
Cambridge, UK

Gaby E. Pfyffer PHD
Professor of Medical Microbiology
Head, Department of Medical Microbiology
Center for Laboratory Medicine; and
Member of the Board of Hospital Directors
Kantonsspital Luzern
Luzern, Switzerland

Elena Pinelli MSc PHD
Senior Scientist
Diagnostic Laboratory for Infections Diseases and
Perinatal Screening (LIS)
National Institute of Public Health
and the Environment (RIVM)
Bilthoven, The Netherlands

Paula M. Pitha MS PHD
Sidney Kimmel Comprehensive Cancer Centre
Johns Hopkins School of Medicine
Baltimore, MD, USA

Tyrone L. Pitt
Laboratory of Healthcare Acquired Infections
Specialist and Reference Microbiology Division
Health Protection Agency, Centre for Infections
London, UK

Eckhard R. Podack
Professor and Chairman
Department of Microbiology
and Immunology
University of Miami School of Medicine
Miami, FL, USA

Victoria Pope PHD
Team Leader, Syphilis Serology
Reference Laboratory
Laboratory Reference and Research Branch
Division of STD Prevention
National Center for HIV, STD, and
TB Prevention
Centers for Disease Control and Prevention
Atlanta, GA, USA

R. Scott Pore PHD
Professor of Microbiology, Immunology
and Cell Biology
West Virginia University School of Medicine
Morgantown, WV, USA

Danièle Postic MD
Laboratoire des Spirochètes, Institut Pasteur
Paris, France

Roger Pradinaud
Centre Hospitalier Andree Rosemon
Service de Dermatologie
Cayenne, Cedex, France

Craig R. Pringle BSC PHD
Emeritus Professor,
Biological Sciences Department
University of Warwick
Coventry, UK

Mike M. Putz MENG PHD
Department of Virology
Faculty of Medicine, Imperial College London
London, UK

Didier Raoult MD PHD
Unité des Rickettsies CNRS UMR 6020
Faculté de Médecine
Marseille, France

Rino Rappuoli PHD
IRIS Research Center, Chiron SrI
Siena, Italy

John G. Raynes BSC PHD
Senior Lecturer
London School of Hygiene and Tropical Medicine
London, UK

Shmuel Razin
The Jacob Epstein Professor of Bacteriology
Department of Membrane and
Ultrastructure Research
The Hebrew-University Hadassah Medical School
Jerusalem, Israel

Robert C. Read BMEDSCI MBCHB MD FRCP
Professor in Infectious Diseases
Division of Genomic Medicine
University of Sheffield and Royal Hallamshire Hospital
Sheffield, UK

Axel Rethwilm MD
Institut für Virologie und Immunbiologie
Universität Würzburg
Würzburg, Germany

Sanjay G. Revankar MD
Associate Professor of Medicine
Division of Infectious Diseases
Dallas VA Medical Center; and
Department of Medicine, UT Southwestern
Dallas, TX, USA

John H. Rex MD FACP
Vice President and Medical Director for Infection
Astra Zeneca Pharmaceuticals, Cheshire, UK; and
Adjunct Professor of Medicine,
University of Texas Medical School,
Houston, TX, USA

Malcolm D. Richardson BSC PHD FRCPATH FIBIOL
Associate Professor in Medical Mycology
Department of Bacteriology and Immunology
Haartman Institute, University of Helsinki
Helsinki, Finland

William Riley PHD D(ABMM)
Technical Director, Microbiology
Baptist Hospital of Miami
South Miami Hospital
Miami, FL, USA

Diane Roberts BSC PHD FIBIOL FIFST
Formerly Deputy Director of the PHLS
Food Safety Microbiology Laboratory

Glenn D. Roberts PHD
Consultant, Division of Clinical Microbiology
Department of Laboratery Medicine and Pathology
Mayo Clinic; and Professor of Microbiology and of
Laboratory Medicine, Mayo Clinic College of Medicine
Rochester, MN, USA

Betty Robertson PHD
Division of Viral Hepatitis
Centers for Disease Control and Prevention
Division of Viral Hepatitis
Atlanta, GA, USA

Juan D. Rodas DVM MSC PHD
Assistant Professor
Facultad de Ciencias Agrarias y
Laboratorio de Immunovirologia
Universidad de Antioquia
Medellin, Columbia

John T. Roehrig PHD
Chief, Arbovirus Diseases Branch
Division of Vector-Borne Infectious Diseases
National Center for Infectious Diseases
Centers for Disease Control
and Prevention Public Health Service
Fort Collins, CO, USA

Sergio Romagnani
Department of Internal Medicine
University of Florence, Italy

Paul A. Rota PHD
Measles, Mumps, Rubella and Herpesvirus Team
Respiratory and Enteric Viruses Branch
Division of Viral and Rickettsial Diseases
Centers for Disease Control and Prevention
Atlanta, GA, USA

David J. Rowlands PHD
School of Biochemistry and Microbiology
University of Leeds
Leeds, UK

Rob W.H. Ruigrok PHD
Laboratoire de Virologie Moléculaire et Structurale
FRE 2854 CNRS-Université Joseph Fourier
Grenoble, France

A. Denver Russell DSC PHD FRCPATH FRPHARMS†
Formerly Professor of Pharmaceutical Microbiology
Welsh School of Pharmacy, Cardiff University
Cardiff, UK

Willie Russell BSC PHD FRSE
Emeritus Research Professor
School of Biology
University of St Andrews
Fife, UK

Mahmut Safak PHD
Head, Laboratory of Molecular Virology
Center for Neurovirology and Cancer Biology
Temple University
Philadelphia, PA USA

Maria S. Salvato PHD
Professor, Institute of Human Virology
University of Maryland Biotechnology Institute
Baltimore, MD, USA

Anna Sander
Institut für Medizinische Mikrobiologie und Hygiene
Albert-Ludwigs Universität Freiburg
Freiburg, Germany

Phillippe J. Sansonetti MD
Professeur à l'Institut Pasteur
Unité de Pathogénie Microbienne Moléculaire
Unité INSERM 389, Institute Pasteur
Paris, France

Walter F. Schlech III MD FACP FRCPC
Head, Division of Infectious Diseases
Department of Medicine
Dalhousie University, QEII Health Sciences Center
Halifax, Nova Scotia, Canada

Gabriel A. Schmunis
Communicable Diseases Unit
Pan American Health Organization
Washington, DC, USA

Thomas Schneider
Gastroenterologie, Infektiologie, Rheumatologie
Charité, Campus Benjamin Franklin
Universitätsmedizin
Berlin, Germany

Jürgen Schneider-Schaulies PHD
Professor of Virology
Institute for Virology and Immunobiology
University of Würzburg, Würzburg, Germany

Sibylle Schneider-Schaulies PHD
Professor of Virology
Institute for Virology and Immunobiology
University of Würzburg
Würzburg, Germany

Guy Schoehn PHD
Laboratoire de Virologie Moléculaire et Structurale
FRE 2854 CNRS-Université Joseph Fourier
Grenoble, France

Nicolas W.J. Schröder MD
Institute for Microbiology and Hygiene
'Charité' University Medical Center
Medical Faculty of The Humboldt-University
Berlin, Germany

Ulrich Schubert PHD
Institute for Clinical and Molecular Virology
University of Erlangen-Nürnberg
Erlangen, Germany

Ralf R. Schumann MD PHD
Professor of Medicine and Microbiolobgy
Institute for Microbiology and Hygiene
'Charité' University Medical Center
Medical Faculty of The Humboldt-University
Berlin, Germany

John Richard Seed PHD
Professor, Department of Epidemiology
School of Public Health
University of North Carolina
Chapel Hill, NC, USA

Esther Segal PHD
Professor of Microbiology and Mycology,
Head, Department of Human Microbiology
Sackler School of Medicine, Tel-Aviv University
Tel Aviv, Israel

Harald Seifert MD
Professor of Medical Microbiology and Hygiene
Institute for Medical Microbiology
Immunology and Hygiene
University of Cologne
Cologne, Germany

Bert L. Semler PHD
Professor and Chair
Department of Microbiology and Molecular Genetics
University of California
Irvine, CA, USA

Bernard W. Senior BSC PHD FRCPATH
Senior Lecturer, Infection and Immunity Group
Department of Molecular and Cellular Pathology
University of Dundee Medical School
Ninewells Hospital
Dundee, UK

Jane F. Seward MBBS MPH
Chief, Viral Vaccine Preventable Diseases Branch
Epidemiology and Surveillance Division
National Immunization Program
Centers for Disease Control and Prevention
Atlanta, GA, USA

Haroun N. Shah BSC PHD FRCPATH
Head, Molecular Identification Services
Specialist and Reference Microbiology Division
Health Protection Agency, Centre for Infections
London, UK

James P. Shapleigh PHD
Department of Microbiology
Cornell University
Ithaca, NY, USA

Susan E. Sharp PHD
Assistant Professor, Department of Pathology
Oregon Health and Sciences University; and
Director of Microbiology, Kaiser Permanente-NW
Airport Regional Laboratory
Portland, OR, USA

Jeffrey J. Shaw OBE DSC PHD DAP&E
Parasitology Department
Biomedical Sciences Institute
São Paulo University, São Paulo, Brazil

Marie-Anne Shaw BSC PHD
Senior Lecturer in Human Genetics
School of Biology
University of Leeds
Leeds, UK

Robert E. Shope† MD
Formerly John S. Dunn Distinguished
Chair in Biodefense, Department of Pathology
University of Texas Medical Branch
Galveston, TX, USA

Stuart G. Siddell BSC PHD
Professor of Virology
Department of Pathology and Microbiology
University of Bristol
Bristol, UK

Lynne Sigler MSC
Professor and Curator,
University of Alberta Microfungus Collection &
Herbarium, Devonian Botanic Garden,
Edmonton, AB, Canada

Peter Simmonds BM PHD MRCPATH
Centre for Infectious Diseases
University of Edinburgh
Edinburgh, UK

Anthony Simmons MA MB BCHIR PHD
Professor, Pediatrics, Pathology, Microbiology
and Immunology, 2.330 Children's Hospital
University of Texas Medical Branch at Galveston
Galveston, TX, USA

Martin B. Skirrow MB PHD FRCPATH
Honorary Emeritus Consultant Microbiologist
Health Protection Agency Laboratory

Gloucestershire Royal Hospital
Gloucester, UK

Mary P.E. Slack MA MB BCHIR FRCPATH
Head, Haemophilus Reference Unit
Respiratory and Systemic Infection Laboratory
Specialist and Reference Microbiology Division
Health Protection Agency, London; and Head
WHO Collaborating Centre for Haemophilus influenzae

Geoffrey L. Smith PHD FRS
Professor of Virology; and
Wellcome Trust Research Fellow
Department of Virology
Faculty of Medicine
Imperial College London
London, UK

Henry R. Smith MA PHD
Director, Laboratory of Enteric Pathogens
Health Protection Agency, Centre for Infections
London, UK

Eric J. Snijder PHD
Associate Professor
Department of Medical Microbiology
Leiden University Medical Center
Leiden, The Netherlands

Werner Solbach MD
Professor and Chair
Institute for Medical Microbiology and Hygiene
University Luebeck
Luebeck, Germany

Steven Specter PHD
Professor, Medical Microbiology and Immunology and
Associate Dean for Admissions and Student Affairs
University of South Florida College of Medicine
Tampa, FL, USA

Robert C. Spencer MBBS MSC FRCPATH FRCP(G)
HONDIPHIC
Laboratory Director
Health Protection Agency
South West Regional Laboratory
Bristol Royal Infirmary
Bristol, UK

Andrew Spielman BS SCD MA(Hon)
Department of Immunology and Infectious Diseases
Harvard School of Public Health
Boston, MA, USA

Margaret Stanley PHD
Professor of Epithelial Biology
Department of Pathology
University of Cambridge, UK

Carrie Steele BA MSC PHD
The Peter Gorer Department of Immunology
Guy's, King's, and St Thomas' Medical School
King's College London
London, UK

Bret M. Steiner PHD
Laboratory Reference and Research Branch
Division of STD Prevention
National Center for HIV, STD, and TB Prevention
Centers for Disease Control and Prevention
Atlanta, GA, USA

Linda D. Stetzenbach PHD
Director, Microbiology Division
Harry Reid Center for Environmental Studies
University of Nevada, Las Vegas
Las Vegas, NV, USA

Michael W. Steward BSC PHD BSC
Emeritus Professor of Immunology
London School of Hygiene and Tropical Medicine
London, UK

Richard C. Summerbell
Centraalbureau voor Schimmelcultures
Utrecht, The Netherlands

Sinésio Talhari PHD
Chief, Department of Tropical Dermatology
Institute of Tropical Medicine
School of Medicine
University of Amazonas
Manaus, Brazil

Peter Tattersall PHD
Professor, Departments of Laboratory
Medicine and Genetics
Yale University School of Medicine
New Haven, CT, USA

John M. Taylor PHD
Senior Member
Fox Chase Cancer Center
Philadelphia, PA, USA

Lúcia M. Teixeira PHD
Associate Professor
Department of Medical Microbiology
Institute of Microbiology

Federal University of Rio de Janeiro
Rio de Janeiro, RJ, Brazil

Sam R. Telford III SCD
Associate Professor of Infectious Diseases
Tufts University School of Veterinary Medicine
North Grafton, MA, USA; and
Visiting Scientist in Immunology and
Infectious Diseases
Harvard School of Public Health
Boston, MA, USA

Volker ter Meulen MD
Professor Emeritus of Clinical Virology
and Immunology
Former Chairman of the Institute for Virology
and Immunbiology, University of Würzburg
Würzburg, Germany

Ram P. Tewari DVM MPH PHD
Professor of Microbiology
Department of Cell Biology and Neurosciences
Rutgers University
Piscataway, NJ, USA

Philip A. Thomas MD PHD MAMS FIMSA
Professor and Head of Ocular Microbiology
Institute of Ophthalmology, Joseph Eye Hospital
Tiruchirapalli, Tamilnadu, India

Richard B. Thomson PHD
Professor of Pathology
Northwestern University Feinberg
School of Medicine; and Director of Microbiology
Evanston Northwestern Healthcare
Evanston, IL, USA

E. John Threlfall PHD
Deputy Director, Laboratory of Enteric Pathogens
Specialist and Reference Microbiology Division
Health Protection Agency, Centre for Infections
London, UK

Noël Tordo PHD
Chief of Laboratory; and
Head, Unit 'Stratégies Antivirales'
Virology Department, Institut Pasteur
Paris, France

Ralph A. Tripp PHD
Professor and GRA Chair, University of Georgia,
College of Veterinary Medicine
Department of Infectious Diseases
Athens, GA, USA

Kenneth L. Tyler MD
Reuler-Lewin Family Professor of Neurology and
Professor of Medicine
Microbiology and Immunology
University of Colorado Health Sciences
Center and Chief, Neurology Service
Denver Veterans Affairs Medical Center
Denver, CO, USA

Emil R. Unanue MD
Professor and Chair
Department of Pathology and Immunology
Washington University School of Medicine
St Louis, MO, USA

Olivier Vandenberg MD
Department of Microbiology
Saint-Pierre University Hospital
Brussels, Belgium

Joke W.B. van der Giessen DVM PhD
Senior Scientist, Parasitic Zoonoses
Microbiological Laboratory for Health Protection
National Institute of Public Health and the
Environment (RIVM)
Bilthoven, The Netherlands

Nongnuch Vanittanakom Dr rer nat
Professor of Medical Microbiology
Department of Microbiology
Faculty of Medicine, Chiang Mai University
Chiang Mai, Thailand

Marc H.V. Van Regenmortel PhD
Emeritus Research Director, CNRS
Biotechnology School of the University of Strasbourg
Illkirch, France

Véronique Vincent PhD
Institute Pasteur
Reference Library for Mycobacteria
Paris, France

Maria Anna Viviani MD
Associate Professor of Hygiene
Laboratory of Medical Mycology
Institute of Hygiene and Preventive Medicine
School of Medicine, Universita degli Studi di Milano
Milano, Italy

William G. Wade BSc MSc DipBM PhD
Professor of Oral Microbiology and
Clinical Consultant Scientist
Department of Microbiology,
King's College London
London, UK

Derek Wakelin PhD DSc FRCPath
Professor Emeritus, University of Nottingham
Nottingham, UK

Alex I. Wandeler PhD
Canadian Food Inspection Agency
Ontario Laboratory Fallowfield
Nepean, Ontario,
Canada

Audrey Wanger PhD
Associate Professor
Department of Pathology
University of Texas-Houston,
Medical School
Houston, TX, USA

Scott C. Weaver PhD
Director for Tropical and Emerging
Infectious Diseases
UTMB Center for Biodefense and
Emerging Infectious Disease; and
Professor, Departments of Pathology
Microbiology & Immunology
University of Texas Medical Branch
Galveston, TX, USA

Jeff Weeks MD
University of Alabama at Birmingham
Department of Dermatology
Birmingham, AL, USA

Sandra K. Weller PhD
Professor and Chair
Molecular, Microbial and Structural Biology
University of Connecticut Health Center
Farmington, CT, USA

L. Joseph Wheat MD
President and Director
MiraVista Diagnostics &
MiraBella Technologies
Indianapolis, IN, USA

Richard J. Whitley MD
Professor of Pediatrics, Microbiology
Medicine and Neurosurgery
University of Alabama at Birmingham
Children's Hospital
Birmingham, AL, USA

James A.G. Whitworth MD FRCP MFPH DTM&H
Head of International Activities
Wellcome Trust
London, UK

Mark H. Wilcox BMEDSCI BM BS MD MRCPATH
Professor/Consultant
Professor of Medical Microbiology
Leeds General Infirmary and University of Leeds
Old Medical School
Leeds, UK

Margaret M. Willcocks BSC PHD
School of Biomedical and Molecular Sciences
University of Surrey
Guildford, UK

Paul Williams BPHARM PHD
Professor of Molecular Microbiology; and
Director, Institute of Infection, Immunity
and Inflammation, Centre for Biomolecular Sciences
University of Nottingham,
Nottingham UK

Jeffrey J. Windsor MSC CSCI FIBMS
Senior Biomedical Scientist
National Public Health Service for Wales
Microbiology Aberystwyth, Bronglais Hospital
Aberystwyth, Ceredigion, Wales, UK

Hilmar Wisplinghoff MD
Institute of Medical Microbiology
Immunology and Hygiene
University of Cologne
Cologne, Germany

Frank G. Witebsky MD
Assistant Chief, Microbiology Service
Department of Laboratory Medicine
National Institutes of Health Clinical Center
Bethesda, MD, USA

Karen L. Wozniak MS PHD
Department of Medicine
Section of Infectious Diseases
Boston University Medical Center
Boston, MA, USA

Michael W.D. Wren CSCI FIBMS CBIOL MIBIOL
FRIPH
Clinical Microbiologist
UCL Hospitals
London, UK

John A. Wyke MA, VETMB, PHD, MRCVS, FRSE
Senior Research Fellow
Institute of Comparative Medicine
University of Glasgow Veterinary School
Glasgow, UK

Joseph D.C. Yao MD
Division of Clinical Microbiology
Mayo Clinic
Rochester, MN, USA

Jonathan W. Yewdell
Laboratory of Viral Diseases
National Institute of Allergy and
Infectious Diseases
Bethesda, MD, USA

Kentaro Yoshimura DVM PHD
Professor Emeritus
Akita University School of Medicine
Akita, Japan

Viqar Zaman DSC FRCPATH
Honorary Visiting Professor
Department of Pathology & Microbiology
The Aga Khan University
Karachi, Pakistan

Jens Zerrahn PHD
Max-Planck-Institute for Infection Biology
Department of Immunology
Berlin, Germany

John Ziebuhr MD
Associate Professor, Institute of Virology
and Immunology, University of Würzburg
Würzburg, Germany

Arturo Zychlinsky
Max Planck Institut fur Infektions Biologie
Department of Cellular Microbiology
Berlin, Germany

Abbreviations

aa	amino acid	**ADC**	acquired immunodeficiency syndrome dementia complex
AA	arachidonic acid		
AAE	acquired angioedema	**ADCC**	antibody-dependent cell-mediated cytotoxicity; or antibody-dependent cellular cytotoxicity
AAFP	American Academy of Family Physicians		
AAP	American Academy of Pediatrics	**ADCI**	antibody-dependent cellular inhibition
AAV	adeno-associated virus	**ADCL**	anergic diffuse cutaneous leishmaniasis
Ab	antibody	**ADE**	antibody-dependent enhancement
Ab/HRP	antibody coupled to horseradish peroxidase	**ADH**	alcohol dehydrogenase; or arginine dihydrolase
		AdoMet	S-adenosylmethionine
AB	alcian blue; or asteroid bodies	**ADP**	adenosine diphosphate
ABC	ATP-binding cassette; or avidin–biotin enzyme complex	**Ad pol**	adenovirus polymerase
		ADRP	adenosine diphosphate-ribose1′-phosphatase
ABCD	amphotericin B colloidal dispersion	**AE**	alveolar echinococcosis; or attaching and effacing (lesions)
ABG	arterial blood gas		
ABLC	amphotericin B lipid complex	**AEC**	airway epithelial cell
ABLV	Australian bat lyssavirus	**AF-1**	accessory factor-1
ABMT	autologous bone marrow transplantation	**AFB**	acid-fast bacilli
ABPA	allergic bronchopulmonary aspergillosis	**AFLP**	amplified fragment length polymorphism
ABR	annual biting rate	**AFP**	α-fetoprotein
ABSV	Absettarov virus	**AFS**	allergic fungal sinusitis
AC	accessory chain; or adenylate cyclase	**Ag**	antigen
ACA	acrodermatitis chronica atrophicans	**Ag2**	antigen 2
ACE	accessory cholera enterotoxin	**AGE**	agarose gel electrophoresis
ACE2	angiotensin-converting enzyme 2	**AGG**	agglutinogen
ACES	N-2-acetamido-2-amino-ethanesulfonic acid	**AGMK**	African green monkey kidney
AC-Hly	adenylyl cyclase hemolysin toxin	**AGP**	acid glycoprotein
ACIP	Advisory Committee on Immunization Practices (USA)	**AGUS**	atypical glandular cells of undetermined significance
ACMHV-2	avian carcinoma virus Mill Hill virus 2	**AHC**	acute hemorrhagic conjunctivitis
ACMSF	Advisory Committee on the Microbiological Safety of Food	**AHL**	acylhomoserine lactone
		AHR	airway hyperresponsiveness
ACOG	American College of Obstetricians and Gynecologists	**AHSV**	African horse sickness virus
		AICD	activation-induced cell death; or antigen induced cell death
ACP	acyl carrier protein		
ACT	adenylate cyclase toxin	**AID**	activation-induced cytokine deaminase
α₁-ACT	α₁-antichymotrypsin	**AIDS**	acquired immune deficiency syndrome
ACTG	acquired immunodeficiency syndrome clinical trial group	**AIM**	dichlorodiphenyltrichloroethane
		AIP	autoinducing peptide
ACTH	adrenocorticotropic hormone	**ALA**	δ-aminolevulinic acid
ACV	aciclovir; or acyclovir	**ALAT**	alanine aminotransferase
ACV-MP	acyclovir monophosphate	**ALDH**	aldehyde dehydrogenase
ACV-TP	acyclovir triphosphate	**ALFV**	Alfuy virus
AD	atopic dermatitis; or autodisable	**ALP**	alkaline phosphatase; or alkaline protease
Ad35	adenovirus type 35	**ALPS**	autoimmune lymphoproliferative syndrome
ADA	adenosine deaminase deficiency	**ALS**	antilymphocyte serum

Als1p   agglutin-like sequence-1
ALT   alanine amino transferase
ALV   avian leukosis virus
ALV-E   avian leukosis virus subgoup E
AM   'aseptic' meningitis
AMA   apical membrane antigen
AMB   amphotericin B
AMDV   Aleutian mink disease virus
AMP   adenosine monophosphate
AMP-RT   amplified reverse transcriptase
αMSH   α-melanocyte-stimulating hormone
AMV   avian myeloblastosis virus
ANCA   antineutrophil cytoplasmic antibody
AND   anaphylactic degranulation
ANP   acyclic nucleoside phosphonate
ANT   adenine nucleotide translocator
anti-GST   anti-glutathione *S*-transferase
ANV   avian nephritis virus
AP   antiproliferative activity
APAAP   alkaline phosphatase-antialkaline phosphatase
Apaf-1   apoptosis protease-activating factor-1
APC   amino acid-polyamine choline; or antigen-presenting cell
APD   average pore diameter
APECED   autoimmune polyendocrinopathy–candidiasis–ectodermal dystrophy
APEX   arrayed primer extension
APOBEC3G   apolipoprotein B mRNA editing enzyme
APOC   African Programme for Onchocerciasis Control
APOIV   Apoi virus
APP   acute phase proteins; or amyloid precursor protein
AP-PCR   arbitrary primer PCR
APR   acute phase response
APRF   acute phase response factor
APS   adenyl sulfate
APS-1   autoimmune polyendocrine syndrome type 1
APV   avian pneumovirus
Ara-A   adenine arabinoside
Ara-C   1-β-D-arabinofuranosylcytosine
Ara-MP   adenine arabinoside-monophosphate
Ara-TP   adenine arabinoside-triphosphate
ARD   antimicrobial removal device
ARDRA   amplified 16S ribosomal DNA restriction analysis
ARDS   acute respiratory distress syndrome; or adult respiratory distress syndrome
ARIMA   autoregressive integrated moving average
AROAV   Aroa virus
ART   antiretroviral therapy
ARV   Adelaide river virus
As₂O₃   arsenic trioxide
ASAT   aspartate aminotransferase
ASC   antibody-secreting cell
ASCUS   atypical squamous cells of undetermined significance
ASFV   African swine fever virus

ASHP   accelerated and stabilized hydrogen peroxide
ASM   airway smooth muscle mass
ASP   acylation stimulating protein; or amnesic shellfish poisoning
AST   alkaline phosphatase
ASWS   alkali-soluble water-soluble
AT   adenine–thymine; or ataxia telangiectasia
A+T   adenine and thymine
ATCC   American Type Culture Collection
ATF   ambient temperature fimbriae
α-TIF   α-*trans*-inducing factor
ATL   acute T-cell leukemia; or adult T-cell leukemia/lymphoma
ATP   adenosine 5′ triphosphate; or annual transmission potential
ATPase   adenosine triphosphatase
ATP/GTP   adenosine 5′-triphosphate/guanosine 5′-triphosphate
ATR   anthrax toxin receptor
ATS   American Thoracic Society
AUIC   area under the curve inhibitory concentration
AV   antiviral activity; or arterio-venous; or atrioventricular
AVL   American visceral leishmaniasis
AVP   arginine vasopressin
AZT   azidothymidine; or 3′-azido-3′-deoxythymidine
AZT-DP   azidothymidine diphosphate
AZT-TP   azidothymidine triphosphate

B19   human parvovirus B19
BA   bacillary angiomatosis; or Bayesian analysis
BAD1   blastomyces adhesin 1
BaEV   baboon endogenous virus
BAGV   Bagaza virus
BAL   bronchoalveolar lavage
BALF   bronchoalveolar lavage fluid
BALT   bronchus-associated lymphoepithelial tissue
BANV   Banzi virus
BAP   bacillary angiomatosis peliosis
BAstV   bovine astrovirus
BB   biobreeding; or mid-borderline (leprosy)
BBB   blood–brain barrier
BBV   Bukalasa bat virus
BC   blood culture
BCA-1   B-cell-attracting chemokine
BCC   basal cell carcinoma
BCDMH   bromo-chloro-dimethyldantoin
BCESM   *B. cepacia* epidemic strain marker
BCG   bacille Calmette-Guérin
BCoV   bovine coronavirus
BCP   bromocresol purple; or bromocresol-purple agar lactose
BcR   B-cell antigen receptor complex
BCR   B-cell receptor
BCRF   B-cell regulatory factor
BCV   Batu Cave virus
BCYE   buffered charcoal yeast extract

BD	borna disease
BDCL	borderline disseminated cutaneous leishmaniasis
bDNA	branched DNA; or branched-chain DNA
BDPV	Barbarie duck parvovirus
BDV	Border disease virus; or borna disease virus
BE	bile–esculin
BEFV	bovine ephemeral fever virus
BFDV	beak and feather disease virus
BFP	biological false-positives; or bundle-forming pilus
BfPAI	*B. fragilis* pathogenicity island
BFPyV	budgerigar fledgling polyomavirus
BFT	*B. fragilis* toxin
BFU-E	burst-forming units erythroid
BFV	Barmah Forest virus; or bovine foamy virus
BG	Bordet–Gengou
BGH	bovine growth hormone
Bgp1	biliary glycoprotein 1
BGS	buffered glycerol saline
BH	Bcl-2 homology; or black-hooded
BHC	benzene hexachloride
BHI	brain–heart infusion
BHIA	brain–heart infusion agar
BHK	baby hamster kidney
bHLH	basic-loop-helix
BI	biological indicators; or bacterial index
BIG	botulism immune globulin
BIR	baculoviral IAP repeat
BIV	bovine immunodeficiency virus
BKPyV	BK polyomavirus
BKV	BK virus
BKVN	BKV-associated nephropathy
BL	Burkitt's lymphoma
BLIS	bacteriocin-like inhibitory substance
BLNAR	β-lactamase-negative, ampicillin resistant
BLP	bacterial lipoprotein
BLS	bare lymphocyte syndrome
BLV	bovine leukemia virus
BMI	body mass index
BMT	bone marrow transplant
BOD	biochemical oxygen demand
BOUV	Bouloui virus
bp	base pair
BPF	Brazilian purpuric fever
BPI	bactericidal/permeability-increasing protein
BPL	β-propiolactone
BPSU	British Paediatric Surveillance Unit
BPV	bovine parvovirus; or bovine papillomavirus
BPV-1	bovine papillomavirus type 1
BPyV	bovine polyomavirus
BrkA	*Bordetella* resistance to killing protein A
BR-PCR	broad-range polymerase chain reaction
BSA	bovine serum albumin
BSAC	British Society for Antimicrobial Chemotherapy
BSAP	early B cell factor
BSC	biological safety cabinet
BSE	bovine spongiform encephalopathy
BSI	bloodstream infection

BSL	biosafety level
BSQV	Bussuquara virus
BSS	balanced salt solution
BT	borderline tuberculoid (leprosy)
Bti	*Bacillus thuringiensis israeliensis* H–14 serotype toxin
Btk	Bruton's tyrosine kinase
BToV	bovine torovirus
BTV 10	bluetongue virus type 10
5-BU	5-bromouracil
BV	bacterial vaginosis
BVaraU	bromovinylarabinosyl-uracil
BVDU	bromovinyl deoxyuridine
BVDU-DP	bromovinyl deoxyuridine-diphosphate
BVDU-MP	bromovinyl deoxyuridine-monophosphate
BVDV	bovine viral diarrhea virus
BVU	bromovinylarabinosyl-uracil
C	complement; or cytosine
C3NeF	C3 nephritic factor
C4NeF	C4 nephritic factor
CA	capsid
CAA	circulating anodic antigen; or cold agglutinin antibody
CAB-2	C activation blocker-2
CABG	coronary artery bypass graft
CAdV	canine adenovirus
CAEP	ceramide aminoethyl phosphonate
CAH	chronic active hepatitis
CAM	cell adhesion molecule; or chorioallantoic membrane
CAMHB-LHB	cation-adjusted Mueller-Hinton broth with 2–5 percent lysed house blood
cAMP	cyclic adenosine 5′-monophosphate
CAMP	Christie–Atkins–Munch-Petersen (test)
CAP	catabolite gene activator protein
CAPD	continuous ambulatory peritoneal dialysis
CAR	Cobas Amplicor, Roche; or coxsackie adenovirus receptor
CARD	caspase-recruitment domain
CARE	candidal DNA repetitive element
CART	combined antiretroviral therapy
CAT	chloramphenicol acetyl transferase; or computer-assisted tomography; or computerized axial tomography
CATT	card agglutination test for trypanosomiasis
CAV	chicken anemia virus
Cbp	Csk-binding protein
CbpA	choline binding protein A
CCA	chimpanzee coryza agent; or circulating cathodic antigen
ccc	covalently closed circular
cccDNA	covalently closed circular DNA
CCDC	consultant for communicable disease control
CCE	cornified cell envelope
CCHFV	Crimean–Congo hemorrhagic fever virus
CCoV	canine enteric coronavirus

CCP	critical control point
CcpA	catabolite control protein
CCPA	chronic cavitary pulmonary aspergillosis
CCPP	contagious caprine pleuropneumonia
ccu	color-changing unit
CCV	channel catfish virus
CD	circular dichroism
CDAD	*Clostridium difficile*-associated disease
CDC	Centers for Disease Control and Prevention (USA)
CDD	community directed distributors
CDI	conformation-dependent immunoassay
CDKI	cyclin-dependent kinase inhibitor
cDNA	complementary DNA
CDP	cytidine 5′-diphosphate
CDR	*Communicable Disease Report*; or complementarity determining region
CDSC	Communicable Disease Surveillance Center
CDT	cytolethal distending toxin
CDTI	community-directed treatment with ivermectin
CDV	canine distemper virus
CE	cystic echinococcosis
CEA	carcinoembryonic antigen
CEC	cation-exchange capacity
CEE	central European encephalitis
CETP	cholesterol ester-transfer protein
CEV	cell-associated enveloped virus
CF	complement-fixation; or cystic fibrosis
CFA	cellular fatty acid; or colonization factor antigen; or complete Freund's adjuvant; or culture filtrate antigen
CFPA	chronic fibrosing pulmonary aspergillosis
CFT	complement-fixation text
CFTR	cystic fibrosis transmembrane conductance regulator
cfu	colony-forming unit
CFU-E	colony-forming units erythroid
CGD	chronic granulomatous disease
CGI	complicated gonococcal infection
cGMP	cyclic guanosine monophosphate
CGRP	calcitonin gene-related peptide
CHEF	contour-clamped homogeneous electrical field (electrophoresis)
CHH	cartilage hair hypoplasia
CHIKV	Chikungunya virus
CHO	Chinese hamster ovary
CHS	Chédiak–Higashi syndrome
CI	complementation index
CIC	circulating immune complex
CID	cytomegalic inclusion disease
CIE	countercurrent immunoelectrophoresis
CIEBOV	Côte d'Ivoire ebola virus
CIITA	class II transactivator
CIN	cefsulodin-Irgasan-novobiocin; or cervical intra-epithelial neoplasia
CIV	Carey island virus
CJD	Creutzfeldt–Jakob disease
CK II	casein kinase II
CL	cutaneous leishmaniasis
CLA	cutaneous lymphocyte-associated antigen
CLC	Charcot–Leyden crystal
CLIP	class II-associated invariant chain peptide
CLO	*campylobacter*-like organism
CLP	common lymphoid progenitor cells; or core-like particle
3CLp	3C-like protease; or 3C-like proteinase
CLR	collagen-like region
CM	cerebral malaria
cma	chromosome-mobilizing ability
CMA	corn meal agar
CMBCS	continuously monitoring blood culture system
CMC	carboxymethylcellulose; or chronic mucocutaneous candidiasis; or critical micelle concentration
CMFL	community microfilarial load
CMGS	cooked meat medium containing glucose and starch
CMI	cell mediated immunity
CMIS	common mucosal immune system
CML	chronic myelogenous leukemia
CMP	common myeloid progenitor cells; or cytidine monophosphate
CMR	chloroform–methanol residue
CMRNG	chromosomally-mediated resistant *Neisseria gonorrhoeae*
CMV	cytomegalovirus
CNA	colistin sulfate and nalidixic acid; or colistin–nalidixic acid
CNF1	cytotoxic necrotizing factor 1
CnMV	canine minute virus
CNPA	chronic necrotizing pulmonary aspergillosis
CNS	central nervous system
CNTF	ciliary neurotropic factor
CO$_2$	carbon dioxide
COI	cytochrome C oxidase I
COL	chronic obstructive lung
Con A	concanavalin A
CoNS	coagulase-negative staphylococci
COP	circum oval precipitin
COP-1	coat protein 1
COPD	chronic obstructive pulmonary disease
COPV	canine oral papillomavirus
COWP	cryptosporidial oocyst wall protein
COX-2	cyclooxygenase 2
cp	cytopathic
CP	capsular polysaccharide
CPCV	Cacipacore virus
CPD	cyclic phosphodiesterase
CPE	cytopathic effect
CpG	cytidine phosphate-guanosine dinucleotide
CPH	chronic persistent hepatitis
CPMV	cowpea mosaic virus
CPS	carbohydrate phosphotransferase system
CPSF	cleavage and polyadenylation specificity factor

CPT	cycling probe technology		**CVA**	cefoperazone–vancomycin–amphotericin
CPV	canine parvovirus		**CVB3**	coxsackie virus B3
CPXV	cowpox virus		**CVC**	central venous catheter
CQR	Chloroquine-resistant		**cVDPV**	circulating vaccine-derived poliovirus
CQS	chloroquine-sensitive		**CVF**	cobra venom factor
CR	complement receptor		**CVID**	common variable immunodeficiency
CR2	complement receptor 2		**CVS**	challenge virus standard; or chorionic villi
CR3	complement receptor 3			sampling; or congenital varicella syndrome
CRA	chlorine-releasing agent		**CWD**	chronic wasting disease
CRAMP	cathelin-related antimicrobial peptide		**CypA**	cyclophilin A
CRBSI	catheter-related bloodstream infection			
CRD	Cross-reacting determinant		**D**	aspartate
CRE	*cis*-acting replication element		**2D**	two-dimensional
CREB	cyclic AMP-responsive element-binding protein		**2-DIE**	two-dimensional immunoelectrophoresis
CRF	circulating recombinant form; or coagulase-		**3D**	three-dimensional
	reacting factor; or corticotropin-releasing factor		**D4T**	2′,3′-didehydro-2′-deoxythymidine; or
CRM	chromosome region maintenance; or cross-			didehydrodeoxyuridine
	reacting material		**D4T-DP**	D4T diphosphate
CrmA	cytokine response modifier A		**D4T-TP**	D4T triphosphate
CRMOX	Congo red magnesium oxalate		**DA**	dopamine
CRP	C-reactive protein; or cAMP receptor protein;		**dAb**	domain antibody
	or confluent and reticulate papillomatosis of		**DAEC**	diffusely adhering *Escherichia coli*
	Gougerot–Carteaud		**DAF**	decay accelerating factor
CRPV	cottontail rabbit papillomavirus		**DAG**	diacylglygerol
CRS	chronic rhinosinusitis; or congenital rubella		**DALY**	disability-adjusted life years
	syndrome		**DANA**	2,3-didehydro-2-deoxy-N-acetylneuraminic
CRV	Cowbone Ridge virus			acid
cryo-EM	cryo-electron microscopy		**DAP**	diaminopimelic acid
CS	coli surface		**DAPI**	4′, 6′-diamino-2-phenylindole hydrochloride
CS-1	corticostatin-1		**DARC**	Duffy antigen receptor for chemokines
CsA	cyclosporin A		**DAT**	direct agglutination test
CSA	*Coccidioides*-specific antigen		**DBM**	diazobenzyloxymethyl
CSD	Cambridge Structural Database (UK)		**DBNPA**	2,2-dibromo-3-nitropropionamide
CSE	conserved sequence element		**DBP**	DNA-binding protein
CSF	cerebrospinal fluid; or colony stimulating factor;		**DBS**	dried blood spots
	or competence and sporulation factor		**DBV**	Dakar bat virus
CSFV	classical swine fever virus		**DC**	dendritic cell; or disseminated candidiasis
CSL	circumsporozoite-like antigen		**DCL**	Diffuse (more correctly 'disseminated')
CSO	civil society organizations			cutaneous leishmaniasis
CSP	circum sporozoite protein; or competence stimu-		**DC-SIGN**	cell-specific ICAM-grabbing nonintegrin
	lating peptide		**DD**	death domain; or double diffusion
CSR	class switch recombination		**DDA-TP**	dideoxyadenosine 5′ triphosphate
CSS	chlorhexidine silver sulfadiazine		**DDC**	dideoxycytidine
CT	cholera enterotoxin; or cholera antitoxin; or		**DDI**	2′,3′-dideoxyinosine
	cholera toxin; or computed tomography; or		**DDI-MP**	2′,3′-dideoxyinosine monophosphate
	covert toxocariasis		**ddNTP**	dideoxynucleotide triphosphate
CTA	cystine trypticase agar		**DDT**	dichlorodiphenyltrichloroethane
CTACK	cutaneous T-cell attracting chemokine		**DEAC**	di-ethyl aluminum chloride
CTAPIII	connective tissue-activating peptide III		**DED**	death effector domain
CT-B	cholera toxin B		**DEET**	diethylmethylbenzamide; or
CTBA	cystine-tellurite blood agar			diethyltoluamide
CTE	constitutive RNA transport element		**DEFRA**	Department of the Environment, Food and
CTFV	Colorado tick fever virus			Rural Affairs (UK)
CTL	cytotoxic T-lymphocyte		**DENV**	dengue virus
CTP	cytidine triphosphate		**DETC**	dendritic epidermal T cells
Cu/Zn SOD	copper and zinc-containing superoxide dismutase		**DFA**	direct fluorescent or immunofluorescent-
CV	cowpox virus			antibody

DFA-TP direct fluorescent antibody test for *Treponema pallidum*

DFMO α-difluoromethylornithine

DGI disseminated gonococcal infection

DGlcDAG diglucosyl diacylglycerol

DHBV duck hepatitis B virus

DHF dengue hemorrhagic fever

DHF/DDS dengue hemorrhagic fever/dengue shock syndrome

DHFR dihydrofolate reductase

DHPS dihydropteroate synthase

DI defective interfering

DIC disseminated intravascular coagulation

DISC death-inducing signal complex

DMSO dimethyl sulfoxide

DMV dolphin morbillivirus; or double membrane vesicle

DN dominant negative; or double negative

DNA deoxyribonucleic acid

DNA-PK DNA-dependent protein kinase

DNApol DNA polymerase

DNCB dinitrochlorobenzene

DNP 2,4-dinitrophenol

DNT dermonecrotic toxin

DoH Department of Health (UK)

DOTS diseases other than syphilis; or directly observed therapy, short-course

DPA dipicolinic acid

DPG diphosphatidylglycerol

DR direct repeat

DRADA double-stranded RNA adenosine deaminase activity

DRAG dinitrogenase reductase-activating glycohydrolase

DRAT dinitrogenase reductase ADP-ribosyltransferase

DRD2 dopamine receptor D2

DRiP defective ribosomal products

DRM detergent-resistant membrane

DS double sandwich; or double-stain

DSB double-strand break

dsDNA double-stranded DNA

DSO double-strand origin

DSP deep-seated phaeohyphomycosis; or diarrhetic shellfish poison

dsRNA double-stranded RNA

DSS dengue shock syndrome

DT definitive phage type; or diphtheria toxin or toxid; or dye test

DTaP diphtheria and tetanus toxoids and acellular pertussis vaccine

DTH delayed-type hypersensitivity

DTM dermatophyte test medium

DTP diphtheria/tetanus/pertussis

dUMP deoxyuridine 5′-monophosphatase

DY drowsy

E glutamate

EA early antigen

EAE erythema arthriticum epidemicum; or experimental allergic encephalomyelitis; or experimental autoimmune encephalomyelitis

EAF EPEC adherence factor

EAggEC enteroaggregative *Escherichia coli*

EANMAT East African Network for Monitoring Antimalarial Treatment

EAST enteroaggregative heat-stable enterotoxin

EAV equine arteritis virus; or endogenous avian virus

EB elementary body; or ethidium bromide

EBA erythrocyte binding antigen

EBER Epstein–Barr virus-encoded small RNA

EBF terminal deoxynucleotidyl transferase

EBHSV European brown hare syndrome virus

EBLV European bat lyssavirus

EBNA Epstein–Barr virus nuclear antigen

EBOV Ebola virus

EBSS Earle's balanced salt solution

EBV Epstein–Barr virus

EC *Escherichia coli*

EC50 effective concentration

ECG eletrocardiograph or eletrocardiogram

ECM extracellular material; or extracellular matrix; or extracellular matrix component

ECP eosinophil cationic protein; or extracellular product

ECSIT evolutionarily conserved signaling intermediate in Toll pathways

ECTV ectromelia virus

ED Entner–Doudoroff

EDB electron-dense bodies

EDF eosinophil differentiating factor

EDN eosinophil derived neurotoxin

EDTA ethylene diamine tetraacetic acid

EEEV eastern equine encephalomyelitis virus

EEV extracellular enveloped virus

EF edema factor

EF-1α elongation factor 1 alpha

EF-2 elongation factor 2

EF-3 elongation factor 3

EFV equine foamy virus

EGF epidermal growth factor

EGIA evoked gamma interferon assay

EGTA ethyleneglycol-bis(b-aminoethylether)-N,N,N′,N′-tetraacetic acid

Eh redox potential

EHDV epizootic hemorrhagic disease virus

EHEC enterohemorrhagic *Escherichia coli*

EHV Edge hill virus

EHV-2 equine herpesvirus 2

EI erythema infectiosum

EIA enzyme immunoassay

EIAV equine infectious anemia virus

EIC extracellular induction component

EIEC entero-invasive *Escherichia coli*

eIF-2α eukaryotic translation initiation factor 2α

eIF-3 eukaryotic translation initiation factor 3

EIPV	enhanced potency inactivated poliovirus vaccine
ELAM	endothelial leukocyte adhesion molecule 1
ELC	Epstein–Barr virus-induced receptor ligand chemokine
ELISA	enzyme-linked immunosorbent assay
ELVIS	enzyme-linked virus-inducible system
EM	electron microscope; or erythema migrans
EMB	eosin methylene blue
EMCV	encephalomyocarditis virus
EMP	Embden–Meyerhof–Parnas; or erythrocyte membrane protein
EN	endemic normal
ENL	erythema nodosum leprosum
ENT	ear, nose, and throat
EntFM	enterotoxin FM
EntK	enterotoxin K
EntT	enterotoxin T
ENTV	Entebbe bat virus
EOP	efficiency of plating
EORTC	European Organization for Research in the Treatment of Cancer
EP	early palindrome
EPEC	enteropathogenic *Escherichia coli*
epg	eggs per gram
EPI	expanded program of immunization
EPM	equine protozoal encephalomyelitis
EPO	erythropoietin; or eosinophil peroxidase
EpoR	erythropoietin receptor
EPP	exposure prone procedure
EPS	exopolysaccharide; or extracellular polysaccharide
ER	endoplasmic reticulum
ERAD	endoplasmic reticulum-associated degradation
ERCP	endoscopic retrograde cholangio-pancreatography
ERG	electroretinograms
ERGIC	endoplasmic reticulum–Golgi intermediate compartment
ERIC	enterobacterial repetitive intergenic consensus
ERIC-PCR	enterobacterial repetitive intergenic consensus polymerase chain reaction
ERK	extracellular regulated kinase; or extracellular signal-regulated kinase
ES	embryonic stem; or excretory/secretory
ESAG	expression site associated genes
ESAT6	early secretory antigen type 6
ESBL	extended spectrum beta-lactamase
ESC	extracellular sensing component
ESM	extended-spectrum macrolide
Esp	enterococcal surface protein
ESR	erythrocyte sedimentation rate
EST	expressed sequence tag
ESV	encystation-specific vesicles
ET	electrophoretic type; or epidermolytic toxin
ETA	exfoliatin A
ETB	exfoliatin B
ETBF	enterotoxigenic *B. fragilis*

ETEC	enterotoxigenic *Escherichia coli*
ETO	ethylene oxide
EToV	equine torovirus
EU	European Union
EV	ectromelia virus; or epidermodysplasia verruci-formis
EWGLI	European Working Group for *Legionella* Infections
F	fusion; or phenylalanine
FA	fluorescent antibody
FACS	fluorescence activated cell sorter
FAD	flavin adenine dinucleotide
FADD	Fas-associated death domain
FAE	follicle-associated epithelium
FAFLP	fluorescence-based amplified fragment length polymorphism
FAK	focal adhesion kinase
FAME	fatty acid methyl ester
FasL	Fas ligand
FAstV	feline astrovirus
FAT	fluorescent antibody test
FBP	ferripyochelin-binding protein; or ferrous sulfate–sodium metabisulfite–sodium pyruvate; or fructose-1,6-biphosphate
5-FC	5-fluorocytosine
FcαRI	Fcα receptor
FcγR	Fcγ receptor
FCoV	feline coronavirus
FcR	Fc receptor
FCV	famciclovir; or feline calicivirus
FDA	Food and Drug Administration (USA)
FDC	follicular dendritic cell
FeLV	feline leukemia virus
FFI	fatal familial insomnia
ffu	focus-forming unit
FFV	feline foamy virus
FGF	fibroblast growth factor
FHA	filamentous hemagglutinin
FHL	familial hemophagocytic lymphohistiocytosis
fHL-1	fH-like-1
FIGE	field-inversion gel electrophoresis
FILCO	Filariasis Control Movement
FIPV	feline infectious peritonitis virus
FI-RSV	formalin-inactivated respiratory syncytial virus
FISH	fluorescent in situ hybridization
FITC	fluorescein isothiocyanate
FIV	feline immunodeficiency virus
FLIP	FLICE-inhibitory protein
FLK2	fetal liver kinase 2
FMDV	foot-and-mouth disease virus
FML	fucose—mannose ligand
fMLP	formyl-methionine-leucine-phenylalanine
FMN	flavin adenine mononucleotide
FNA	fine-needle aspiration
FP	flavoprotein
FPLV	feline panleukopenia virus

FPV	feline panleukopenia virus; or fowlpox virus
FRET	fluorescence resonance energy transfer
FrMLV	friend murine leukemia virus
FSA	Food Standards Agency (UK)
FSE	feline spongiform encephalopathy
FTA	fluorescent treponemal antibody
FTA-ABS	fluorescent treponemal antibody-absorption
FTIR	fourier-transformed infrared
5-FU	5-fluorouracil
5-FUTP	5-fluorouracil triphosphate
FUO	fever of unknown origin
FV	foamy virus
FYSA	formalized yolk-sac antigen
G6PD	glucose-6-phosphate dehydrogenase
G6PDH	glucose-6-phosphate dehydrogenase (reduced)
Gab1	Grb-2-associated binding protein 1
GABA	γ-amino butyric acid
GAD	glutamic acid decarboxylase
GAE	granulomatous amebic encephalitis
GAG	glycosaminoglycan
GalC	galactosylceramide
GALT	gut-associated lymphoepithelial tissues
GAP	GTPase-activating proteins
GAPDH	glyceraldehyde-3-phosphate-dehydrogenase
GAV	gill-associated virus
GAVI	Global Alliance for Vaccines and Immunization
gB	glycoprotein B
GBP	glycophorin-binding protein
GBS	group B streptococci; or Guillain–Barré syndrome
GBV-A	GB virus A
GBV-B	GB virus B
GBV-C	GB virus C
GC	germinal center
G+C	guanine and cytosine
3GC	third generation cephalosporin
GCAT	glycerophospholipid cholesterol acetyltransferase
GCFT	gonococcal complement fixation test
GC-MS	gas chromatography-mass spectrometry
GCP-2	granulocyte chemoattractant protein 2
G-CSF	granulocyte colony stimulating factor
GCV	ganciclovir
GCV-MP	ganciclovir monophosphate
GCV-TP	ganciclovir triphosphate
GDD	glycine–aspartic acid–aspartic acid
GDI	guanine nucleotide dissociation inhibitor
GEF	guanine nucleotide exchange factor
GERD	gastroesophageal disease; or gastroesophageal reflux disease
GETV	Getah virus
GF	Gridley's fungus
GFP	green fluorescent protein
gG	glycoprotein G
GGTP	γ-glutamyl transpeptidase
GGYV	Gadget's gully virus
GH	growth hormone
GI	gastrointestinal
GIS	geographic information system
GIT	gastrointestinal tract
GLC	gas–liquid chromatography
GLP	glycolipoprotein
GM	granulocyte-macrophage; or growth medium
GM-CSF	granulocyte/macrophage or monocyte colony stimulation factor
GmDNV	*Galleria mellonella* densovirus
GMS	Gomori's methenamine silver nitrate
GnRH	gonadotropin-releasing hormone
Gp	glycoprotein
GPA	glucose peptone agar
GPAC	gram-positive anaerobic cocci
GPCR	G-protein-coupled receptor
GPELF	Global Program to Eliminate Filariasis
GPI	glycosyl-phosphatidyl-inositol; or glucose-6-phosphate isomerase
GPV	Goose parvovirus
GR	glutathione reductase; or glycine–arginine-rich
GRE	glucocorticoid-responsive element
GREP	Global Rinderpest Eradication Programme
gRNA	guide RNA
GRO	growth-related oncogene
GROα/β	growth-related gene product α/β
GSH	glutathione
GSHV	ground squirrel hepatitis virus
GSP	general secretory pathway
GSS	Gerstmann–Sträussler–Scheinker
GSSG	glutathione reductase substrate glutathione disulphide
GST	glutathione *S*-transferase
GTP	guanosine $5'$-triphosphate
GTPase	guanosine triphosphatase
4-GuDANA	4-guanidino-Neu5Ac2en
GUM	genitourinary medicine
GUS	glucuronidase
GVHD	graft-versus-host disease
H	hemagglutinin; or histidine
H$_2$	hydrogen
HA	hemagglutination; or hemagglutinin
HAA	human T-cell leukemia virus-associated arthropathy
HAART	highly active antiretroviral therapy
HAD	human immunodeficiency virus-associated dementia
HAE	hereditary angioedema
HAI	hemagglutination inhibition; or hospital-acquired infection
HAM	human T-cell leukemia virus-associated myelopathy
HAMA	human anti-mouse (or rat) antibody
HAM/TSP	human T-cell leukemia virus-1-associated myelopathy/tropical spastic paraparesis
HANV	Hanzalova virus

HaPyV	hamster polyomavirus
HAstV	human astrovirus
HAV	hepatitis A virus
Hb	hemoglobin
HBcAg	hepatitis B virus core antigen
HBD	human β-defensin
HBD-1	human β-defensin-1
HBeAg	hepatitis B e antigen
HBIG	hepatitis B immunoglobulin
Hbl	hemolysin BL
HbS	hemoglobin S
HBsAg	hepatitis B surface antigen
HBSP	hepatitis B spliced protein
HBSS	Hank's balanced salt solution
HBV	hepatitis B virus
HCC	hepatocellular carcinoma
HCFC	hydrochlorofluorocarbon
hCG	human chorionic gonadotropin
HCMV	human cytomegalovirus
HCoV	human coronavirus OC43, 229E, or NL63
HCV	hepatitis C virus; or hog cholera virus
HD	helper dependent; or Hodgkin's disease; or human intestinal defensin
HDCS	human diploid cell strain
HDL	high-density lipoprotein
HDV	hepatitis delta virus
HE	hektoen enteric; or hematoxylin–eosin; or hemagglutinin–esterase
H&E	hematoxylin and eosin
HECoV	human enteric coronavirus
HEF	hemagglutinin–esterase fusion
HEK	human embryonic kidney
HEL	hen egg white lysozyme
HEPA	high efficiency particulate air
HERV	human endogenous retrovirus
HES	hematoxylin–eosin–saffron
5-HETE	5-Hydroxyeicosatetraenoic acid
HEV	hepatitis E virus; or high endothelial venule
HF	host factor; or hydrops fetalis
HFMD	hand-foot-and-mouth disease
Hfr	high frequency recombination
HFRS	hemorrhagic fever with renal syndrome
HFT	high-frequency transduction
HFV	human foamy virus
HG	hybridization group
HGE	human granulocytic ehrlichiosis
HGF	hemopoietic growth factor
HGH	human grown hormone
HGSIL	high-grade squamous intraepithelial lesion
HGV	hepatitis G virus
Hh	hemopoietic histocompatibility
HHBV	heron hepatitis B virus
HHT	12-hydroxy-5, 8, 10-heptadecatraenoic acid
HHV-1	human herpesvirus 1
HHV-6	human herpesvirus 6
HHV-7	human herpesvirus 7

HHV-8	human herpesvirus 8
HI	hemagglutination inhibition
Hib	*Haemophilus influenzae* type b
HIES	hyper-IgE syndrome
HIgM	hyper-IgM syndrome
HiPIP	high-potential iron protein
HIR	humoral immune response
HIV	human immunodeficiency virus
HIV-1	human immunodeficiency virus type 1
HIV-2	human immunodeficiency virus type 2
HIVA	HIV-1 clade A
HL	hemolysis; or human lung
HLA	human leukocyte antigen
HLE	heat-labile enterotoxin
hLPO	human lactoperoxidase
HLR	high-level resistance
HlyA	α-haemolysin
HM	hexose monophosphate
HME	human monocytic (or monocytotropic) ehrlichiosis
HMGB1	high mobility group 1 protein
HMO	health maintenance organization
HMP	hexose monophosphate pathway
hMPV	human metapneumovirus
HN	hemagglutinin-neuraminidase
HNE	hemagglutinin noose epitope
HNF	hepatonuclear factor
HNIG	human normal immunoglobulin
HNP	human neutrophil peptide
hnRNP	heterogeneous nuclear ribonucleoprotein
Hoc	highly antigenic outer capsid
HPA	Health Protection Agency (UK)
5-HPETE	5-hydroperoxide eicosatetraenoate
HPI	high-pathogenicity island
HPIV-3	human parainfluenza virus type 3
HPLC	high-performance or high-pressure liquid chromatography
HPMPC	hydroxyphonosphonylmethoxycytosine
HPRT	hypoxanthine–guanine phosphoribosyl transferase
HPS	hemophagocytic syndrome
HPV	human papilloma virus
HR	heptad repeat
HRF	histamine-releasing factor
HR-HPV	high-risk human papillomavirus
HRIG	human anti-rabies immunoglobulin
HRP	horseradish peroxidase
HRR	haplotype relative risk
HRSV	human respiratory syncytial virus
HRT	human rectal tumor
HRV	human rhinovirus
HS	heparan sulfate
Hsc	heat-shock cognate
HSC	hematopoietic or hemopoietic stem cell
HSE	heat-stable enterotoxin
HSK	herpes simplex virus-induced keratitis; or herpetic stromal keratitis

HSP	heat shock protein		**iCJD**	iatrogenic Creutzfeldt–Jakob disease
HSP90	heat shock protein 90		**ICLN**	infection control link nurse
HSPG	heparan sulfate protein glycoconjugates; or heparan sulfate proteoglycans		**ICN**	infection control nurse
hSPO	human salivary peroxidase		**ICNV**	International Committee on Nomenclature of Viruses
HSSA	heat-stable somatic antigen		**iCOS**	inducible co-stimulatory molecule
HST	heat-stable toxin		**ICS**	immunochromatographic strip
HSV	herpes simplex virus; or herpesvirus saimiri		**ICSB**	International Committee for Systematic Bacteriology
HSV-1	herpes simplex virus type 1		**ICSP**	International Committee on Systematics of Prokaryotes
HSV-2	herpes simplex virus type 2			
HT	hemorrhagic toxin		**ICT**	infection control team
5HT	serotonin		**ICTV**	International Committee on Taxonomy of Viruses
HTE	hamster trachea epithelial			
HTH	helix–turn–helix		**ICTVdB**	International Committee on Taxonomy of Viruses database
HTIG	human tetanus immunoglobulin			
HTLV	human T-cell leukemia virus; or human T-cell lymphotropic virus		**ICU**	intensive care unit
			Id	idiotypic
HTLV-1	human T-cell leukemia or lymphocyte virus-1		**ID**	immunodiffusion; or infective dermatitis
HTLV-2	human T-cell leukemia virus-2		**iDC**	immature dendritic cell
HTM	*Haemophilus* test medium		**IDCF**	immunodiffusion complement fixation
HToV	human torovirus		**IDDM**	insulin-dependent diabetes mellitus
HTST	high temperature, short time		**IDSA**	Infectious Diseases Society of America
Hu	human		**idt**	indeterminate (leprosy)
HU	human T-cell leukemia virus-associated uveitis		**IDTP**	immunodiffusion tube precipitin
huIgG	unspecific pooled human immunoglobulin		**IDU**	idoxuridine; or injecting drug user
HuR	human RNA-binding protein		**IDU-TP**	idoxuridine triphosphate
HUS	hemolytic-uremic syndrome		**IE**	immediate–early
HUVS	hypocomplementemic urticarial vasculitis		**IEBC**	International Entomopathogenic *Bacillus* Centre
HV4	hypervariable region 4		**IEC**	intestinal epithelial cell
HVAC	heating, ventilation, and air-conditioning		**IEF**	isoelectric focusing
HVEM	herpesvirus entry mediator		**IEL**	intraepithelial lymphocyte
HVR	hypervariable region		**IEM**	immunoelectron microscopy
HVR1	hypervariable region 1		**IEOP**	immunoelectro-osmophoresis
HVS	herpesvirus saimiri		**IEV**	intracellular enveloped virus
HWP-1	hyphal wall protein-1		**IF**	immunofluorescence; or inactivation factor; or intermediate filament
HY	hyper			
HYPRV	Hypr virus		**IFA**	immunofluorescence assay; or indirect fluorescent antibody assay; or incomplete Freund's adjuvant
I	isoleucine			
IAA	infection-associated antigen		**IFAT**	immunofluorescent antibody test; or indirect immunofluorescent antibody test
IAP	inhibitor of apoptosis protein			
IATA	International Air Transport Association		**IFN**	interferon
IATS	International Antigenic Typing Scheme		**IFN-α**	interferon-alpha
IAVI	International AIDS Vaccine Initiative		**IFN-β**	interferon-beta
IBD	identical by descent; or inflammatory bowel disease		**IFN-γ**	interferon-gamma
			IFNGR1	interferon γ receptor β_1 subunit
IBS	identical by state; or irritable bowel syndrome		**IFT**	immunofluorescence testing
IBV	infectious bronchitis virus		**Ig**	immunoglobulin
i.c.	intracerebral		**IgA**	immunoglobulin A
ICA	islet cell antibody		**IGF-1**	insulin-like growth factor 1
ICAM	intracellular adhesion molecule		**IgG**	immunoglobulin G
ICAM-1	intercellular adhesion molecule 1		**IgM**	immunoglobulin M
ICAO	International Civil Aviation Organization		**IGS**	intergenic spacer
ICC	Infection Control Committee		**IHA**	indirect hemagglutination assay
ICD	infection control doctor		**IHAT**	indirect hemagglutination test
ICE	integrative conjugative element; or interleukin-1β-converting enzyme		**IHC**	immunohistochemical

IHSS	idiopathic hypertophic subaortic stenosis
IID	infectious intestinal disease
IJSB	*International Journal of Systematic Bacteriology*
IJSEM	*International Journal of Systematic and Evolutionary Microbiology*
IL	interleukin
IL-1	interleukin-1
IL-1β	interleukin-1β
IL-1R	interleukin-1 receptor
IL-1Ra	IL-1 receptor antagonist
IL-2	interleukin-2
IL-3	interleukin-3
IL-4	interleukin-4
IL-6	interleukin-6
IL-10	interleukin-10
IL-12	interleukin-12
ILF	isolated lymphocyte follicle
ILHV	Ilhéus virus
IM	infectious mononucleosis
IMA	inhibitory mold agar
IMDM	Iscove's modified Dulbecco's medium
IMP	inflammation modulatory protein; or inosine-5′-phosphate
IMS	immunomagnetic separation
IMV	intracellular mature virus
IN	integrase
indels	insertions or deletions
iNOS	inducible nitric oxide synthetase/synthase
Int	integrase
Int1p	integrin-like protein-1
IOM	Institute of Medicine (USA)
IP	inflammatory protein; or internal promoter; or intraperitoneally
IP$_3$	inositol triphosphate
IP10	interferon-inducible protein 10
IPA	immunoperoxidase assay
IPO	immunoperoxidase
IPT	Intermittent presumptive treatment
IPTG	isopropyl-β-D-galactopyranoside
IPV	inactivated poliovirus vaccine
IR	inverted repeat; or intercept ratio
IRES	internal ribosomal entry site
IRF	interferon regulatory factor
IRF-1	interferon-regulatory factor-1
IRF-3	interferon regulatory factor-3
IRF-7	interferon regulatory factor-7
IRMA	immunoradiometric assay
IS	insertion sequence
ISAGA	immunosorbent agglutination assay
ISAV	infectious salmon anemia virus
ISCAR	immunostimulatory carrier
ISCOM	immunostimulating complex
ISDR	interferon-sensitivity determining region
ISF	immunosuppressive fraction
ISG	interferon-stimulated gene; or invariable surface glycoprotein
ISHAM	International Society for Human and Animal Mycology
ISRE	interferon-specific response element
ISS	immunostimulatory sequence
ISVP	infectious subvirion particle
I-TAC	interferon-inducible T-cell α-chemoattractant
ITAM	immunoreceptor tyrosine based activation motif
ITFDE	International Task Force for Disease Eradication
ITIM	immunoreceptor tyrosine-based inhibitory motif
ITN	insecticide-treated nets
ITR	inverted terminal repeat
ITS	internal transcribed spacer
ITS1	internal transcribed spacer 1
ITS2	internal transcribed spacer 2
ITV	Israel turkey meningo-encephalitis virus
IU	international unit
IUDR	iodoxyuridine
IUMS	International Union of Microbiological Societies
IUTLD	International Union Against Tuberculosis and Lung Disease
IV	immature virion; or intravenous
IVDU	intravenous drug user
IVET	in vivo expression technology
IVF	in vitro fertilization
IVIG	intravenous immunoglobulin
IVN	nucleoid-containing IV
JAK	Janus kinase
Jaks	Janus-family kinase
JAM1	junctional adhesion molecule 1
JCPyV	JC polyoma virus
JCV	Jamestown Canyon virus
JEV	Japanese encephalitis virus
JI	jet injector
JLP	juvenile laryngeal papillomatosis
JMVM	*Journal of Medical and Veterinary Mycology*
JNK	c-Jun NH$_2$-terminal kinase
JSRV	jaagsiekte sheep retrovirus
JUGV	Jugra virus
JUTV	Jutiapa virus
JV	Jena virus
K	lysine
KADV	Kadam virus
KAP	knowledge, attitudes, and practice
kb	kilobase
kDNA	kinetoplast DNA
KDO	keto-deoxy-octulonate; or 2-keto-3-deoxy-D-manno-oct-2-ulosonic acid; or 2-keto-3-deoxyoctonic acid
KDPG	2-keto-3-deoxy-6-phosphogluconate
KE	*Klebsiella/Enterobacter*
KEDV	Kedougou virus
KFDV	Kyasanur Forest disease virus

KIA	Kligler's iron agar	**LGL**	large granular lymphocyte
KIR	killer cell immunoglobulin-like receptor; or killer inhibitory receptor	**LGSIL**	low-grade squamous intraepithelial lesion
		LGTV	Langat virus
KIVI	kit for in vitro isolation	**LGV**	lymphogranuloma venereum
KL	kit ligand	**LH**	light-harvesting
KLH	keyhole limpet hemocyanin	**LHB**	percent lysed horse blood
KO	knock-out	**LHR**	late phase response
KOH	potassium hydroxide	**LHRH**	luteinizing hormone-releasing hormone
KOKV	Kokobera virus	**LIF**	leukemia inhibitory factor
KOUV	Koutango virus	**LIP**	lymphoid interstitial pneumonitis
KRV	Kilham rat virus	**LIR-1**	leukocyte immunoglobulin-like receptor 1
KS	Kaposi's sarcoma	**LIV**	Louping ill virus
KSHV	Kaposi's sarcoma herpesvirus	**LJP**	localized juvenile periodontitis
KSIV	Karshi virus	**lktA**	leukotoxin A
KTR	killer toxin receptor	**LL**	borderline lepromatous (leprosy)
KUMV	Kumlinge virus	**LLAP**	*Legionella*-like amebal pathogen
KUNV	Kunjin virus	**LLO**	cytolysin listeriolysin O; or listeriolysin O
		LMI	leukocyte migration inhibition
L	large; or late; or leucine	**LMP**	last menstrual period; or latent membrane protein; or low-molecular-weight protein
LA	latex agglutination		
LAB	linker for activation of B cells	**LMP1**	latent membrane protein 1
LAD	leukocyte adhesion deficiency	**LNYV**	lettuce necrotic yellows virus
LAF	laminar air flow	**L-OasA**	lipidated outer surface protein A
LAH	left anterior hemiblock	**LOD**	logarithm of odds
LAIV	live-attenuated influenza vaccine	**LOS**	lipo-oligosaccharide
LAK	L-associated kinase; or lymphokine-activated killer	**LP**	lamina propria; or leader protein; or lipopoly-saccharide; or lactoperoxidase
LAM	lipoarabinomannan	**LPD**	lymphoproliferative disease
L-AMB	liposomal amphotericin B	**LPG**	lipophosphoglycan
LAMPf	*Mycoplasma fermentans* lipoprotein		
LAP	latency-associated protein; or leukemia-associated protein	**LPL**	lamina propria lymphocyte
		LPMV	La-Piedad Michoacan-Mexico virus
LASIK	laser-in-situ keratomileusis	**LPR**	lipoprotein receptor-related; or lymphoprolifera-tive responses
LAT	latency-associated transcript; or latex particle agglutination; or linker for activation of T cells		
		LPS	lipopolysaccharide
LB	laminated (multilamellar) body; or Lyme borre-liosis	**LPV**	lymphotropic papovavirus
		LR	leishmaniasis recidivans
LBP	lipopolysaccharide-binding protein	**LRC**	leukocyte receptor cluster
LBSN	List of Bacterial names with Standing in Nomenclature	**LR-HPV**	low-risk human papillomavirus
		LRN	Laboratory Response Network
LC	Langerhans' cell	**LRR**	leucin-rich repeat
LCL	localized forms of cutaneous leishmaniasis; or lymphoblastoid cell line	**LRSV**	lychnis ringspot virus
		LRT	lower respiratory tract
LCMV	lymphocytic choriomeningitis virus	**LS-A**	liver-stage antigen
LCR	ligase chain reaction	**LSA-1**	liver stage-specific antigen 1
LD	Legionnaires' disease	**LSA-3**	liver stage-specific antigen 3
LD50	median lethal dose	**LSC**	lymphoid stem cell
LDC	lysine decarboxylase	**LSU**	large subunit
LDH	lactate/lactic dehydrogenase	**LT**	lethal toxin; or lymphotoxin; or leukotriene; or heat-labile enterotoxin
LDL	low density lipoprotein		
LDLR	low density lipoprotein-related; or low-density lipoprotein receptor	**LT-α**	lymphotoxin α
		LTA	lipoteichoic acid
LDV	lactate dehydrogenase-elevating virus	**LT-B**	heat-labile enterotoxin B subunit
LEM	leukocyte-endogenous mediator	**LTB₄**	leukotriene B$_4$
LF	lethal factor	**LTBI**	latent TB infection
LFA-1	lymphocyte function-associated antigen 1	**LT-βR**	LT-β receptor
LFA-1α	leukocyte function antigen-1α	**LT-βR-IgFcγ**	LT-βR-immunoglobulin fusion protein

LTC$_4$	leukotriene C$_4$
LTD$_3$	leukotriene D$_3$
LTNP	long-term non-progressing
LTR	long terminal repeat
LTSF	low-temperature steam with formaldehyde
LVS	live vaccine strain
M	matrix; or methionine; or microfold
MA	matrix; or membrane antigen
mAb	monoclonal antibody
MAC	*Mycobacterium avium* complex; or membrane attack complex; or multiple antigen construct
MACPF	membrane attack complex/perforin
MadCAM-1	mucosal addressin-cell adhesion molecule-1
MADT	morphological alteration and disintegration test
MAF	macrophage activating factor
MAGUK	phospholipase
MAIDS	murine AIDS model
MALDI-TOF-MS	matrix-assisted laser desorption/ionization time of flight mars spectrometry
MALP	mycoplasmal lipopeptide
MALT	mucosa-associated lymphoepithelial or lymphoid tissue
MAM	*M. arthritidis* mitogen
Map	mitochondrial associated protein
MAP	mitogen-activated protein; or multiple antigenic peptide
MAPK	mitogen-activated protein kinase
MAR	monoclonal antibody-resistant
MARV	Marburg virus
MAS	*M. arthritidis* superantigen
MASP	mannose-binding protein-associated serine protease
MAT	microscopic or modified agglutination test
MATE	multidrug and toxic compound extrusion
MAYV	Mayaro virus
Mb	megabase
MBC	minimal bactericidal concentration
MBL	mannan- or mannose-binding lectin
MBM	meat and bone-meal
MBP	major basic protein; or mannan-binding protein; or myelin basic protein
MBR	monthly biting rate
MCA	middle cerebral artery
McAbs	monoclonal antibodies
MCD	multifocal Castleman disease
M cells	membranous epithelial cell
MCGF	mast cell growth factor
MCL	mucocutaneous lesion
MCLO	*Mycobacterium chelonae*-like organism
MCMV	murine cytomegalovirus
MCP	membrane co-factor protein; or monocyte chemoattractant protein; or methyl-accepting chemotaxis protein
MCP-1	monocyte chemoattractant protein-1
MCP-2	monocyte chemoattractant protein-2
MCP-3	monocytic chemoattractant protein-3

MCS	multiple cloning site
M-CSF	macrophage colony-stimulating factor
mCT	mutant cholera toxin
MCV	molluscum contagiosum virus
***m*-dap**	*meso*-diaminopimelic acid
MDBK	Madin–Darby bovine kidney
mDC	myeloid dendritic cell
MDC	monocyte-derived chemokine
MDCK	Madin–Darby canine kidney
MDH	malate dehydrogenase
MDP	muramyl dipeptide
MDPV	muscovy duck parvovirus
MDR	multidrug resistance
MDT	multidrug therapy
ME	myalgic encephalomyelitis
2ME	2-mercaptoethanol
MEAV	Meaban virus
MEC	minimal effective concentration
medRNA	mini-exon derived RNA
MEE	multienzyme electrophoresis; or multilocus enzyme electrophoresis
MEK	MAPK/ERK kinase
MEM	minimal Eagle medium; or minimal essential medium
MenA	*Neisseria meningitidis* group A
MenB	*Neisseria meningitidis* group B
MenC	*Neisseria meningitidis* group C
MenW135	*Neisseria meningitidis* group W135
MenY	*Neisseria meningitidis* group Y
methyl-CoM	methyl-coenzyme M
MeV	measles virus
MEV	Meaban virus
MF	*Malassezia* folliculitis; or membrane-filter; or mitogenic factor
MFC	minimum fungicidal concentration
MFP	membrane-fusion protein
MFS	major facilitator superfamily
MGF	myxoma growth factor
MGlcDAG	monoglucosyl diacylglycerol
MGP	methyl-α-D-glucopyranoside
MHA-TP	microhemagglutination assay for antibodies to *Treponema pallidum*
MHC	major histocompatibility complex
MHC I	major histocompatibility complex class I
MHC II	major histocompatibility complex class II
MHRA	Medicines and Healthcare Products Regulatory Agency (UK)
MHV	murine hepatitis virus; or mouse hepatitis virus
MHV-68	murine gammaherpesvirus 68
MHVR	mouse hepatitis virus receptor
MI	morphological index; or myocardial infarction
MIBE	measles inclusion body encephalitis
MIC	minimal inhibitory concentration
MIDV	Middelburg virus
MIF	macrophage inhibition factor; or migration inhibitory factor; or microimmunofluorescence
mIg	membrane immunoglobulin

Mig	monokine induced by interferon γ
MIM	Multilateral Initiative on Malaria
Mip	macrophage infectivity potentiator
MIP	macrophage inflammatory protein
MIP-1α	macrophage infectivity potentiator or inflammatory protein 1α
MIP-2	macrophage inflammatory protein-2
MIP-α/β	macrophage inflammatory protein 1-α/β
MIRU	mycobacterial interspersed repetitive unit
MK	monkey kidney
ML	maximum likelihood
MLC	minimum lethal concentration
MLEE	multilocus enzyme electrophoresis
MLN	mesenteric lymph node
MLO	*Mycoplasma*-like organism
MLRT	multilocus restriction typing
Mls	minor lymphocyte-stimulating antigen
MLST	multilocus sequence typing
mLT	mutant labile toxin
MLV	murine leukemia virus
MM	maintenance medium
MMLV	Montana myotis leukoencephalitis virus
MMO	methane monooxygenase
MMP	matrix metalloprotease or metalloproteinase
MMR	macrophage mannose receptor; or measles, mumps, and rubella
MMTV	mouse mammary tumor virus
MMV	Medicines for Malaria Venture; or mice minute virus
Mo	mouse
MOCV	molluscum contagiosum virus
MODV	Modoc virus
MOF	multiple organ failure
MOG	myelin oligodendrocyte glycoprotein
MOH	Ministry of Health
MOI	multiplicity of infection
MOM	mitochondrial outer membrane
MoMLV	Moloney murine leukemia virus
MOMP	major outer-membrane protein
MOPS	3-[*N*-morpholino]-propanesulfonic acid
MOTT	mycobacteria other than tubercle
MP	maximum parsimony
Mφ	macrophage
MPD	maximum pore diameter
MPGN	membranoproliferative glomerulonephritis
MPL	monophosphoryl lipid A
MPL-TDM	monophosphoryl lipid A/trehalose dicorynomycolate
MPMV	Mason–Pfizer monkey virus
MPN	most probable number
MPO	myeloperoxidase
MPS	mononuclear phagocytic system
MPT	mitochondria-permeability transition
MPTR	major polymorphic tandem repeat
MPV	murine pneumonia virus
MPyV	murine polyomavirus
MR	mannose-resistant; or methyl red; or minocycline-rifampin; or multiresistant; or magnetic resonance
MRA	microbiological risk assessment
MR/K	mannose-resistant *Klebsiella*-like
MR/P	mannose-resistant *Proteus*-like
MREHA	mannose-resistant and eluting hemagglutinin
MRI	magnetic resonance imaging
mRNA	messenger RNA
MRSA	methicillin resistant *Staphylococcus aureus*
MRSE	methicillin-resistant *Staphylococcus epidermidis*
MRSP	mapped restriction site polymorphism
MS	macrolide, lincosamide, and streptogramin; or mannose-sensitive; or multiple sclerosis
MSCRAMM	microbial surface components recognizing adhesive matrix molecule
MSF	Médecins Sans Frontières
MSHA	mannose-sensitive hemagglutinin
MSM	men who have sex with men
MSP	merozoite surface protein
MSP-1	major merozoite surface protein-1
MSR	MSG-related proteins
MSSA	methicillin-sensitive *Staphylococcus aureus*
MST	mean survival time
MT	methyltransferase
mtDNA	mitochondrial DNA
MTOC	microtubule organizing center
MTP	monthly transmission potential
MTT	3-4,5-dimethyl-2-thiazolyl-2,5-diphenyl-2*H*-tetrazolium bromide
MULT-1	mouse ULBP-like transcript-a
MuLV	murine leukemia virus
MuV	mumps virus
MV	measles virus; or myxoma virus
MVA	modified vaccinia virus Ankara
MVB	multivesicular body
MVEV	Murray valley encephalitis virus
MVM	minute virus of mice
MW	molecular weight
MYXV	myxoma virus
N	asparagine; or nucleocapsid; or nucleoprotein
N$_0$	initial number
NA	neuraminidase
NAA	nucleic acid amplification
NAAT	nucleic acid amplification test
nAChR	nicotinic acetylcholine receptor
NACI	National Advisory Committee on Immunization (Canada)
NACM	*Naegleria* ameba cytopathogenic material
NAD	nicotinamide adenine dinucleotide
NADP+	nicotinamide adenine dinucleotide phosphate
NADPH	nicotinamide adenine dinucleotide phosphate (reduced)
NAF	non agglutinating fimbriae
NAG	*N*-acetylglucosamine; or nonagglutinable
NAH	naphthalene

NALC-NaOH	*N*-acetyl-L-cysteine-sodium hydroxide		**NMSC**	nonmelanoma skin cancer
NALT	nasopharyngeal-associated lymphoepithelial tissue		**NNA**	neomycin nalidixic acid
			NNIS	National Nosocomial Infection Surveillance (USA)
NANB	non-A, non-B		**NNN**	Novy, MacNeal, Nicolle
NANBH	non-A, non-B hepatitis		**NNRTI**	nonnucleoside reverse transcriptase inhibitor
NANP	asparagine−alanine−asparagine−proline		**NNS**	nonsegmented negative-strand
NAO	nucleus-associated organelle		**NO**	nitric oxide
NAP	*p*-nitro-α-acetylamino-*β*-propiophenone		**NOD**	non-obese diabetic; or nucleotide-binding oligomerization domain
NAP-2	neutrophil-activating protein 2			
NaPTA	sodium phosphotungstate		**noncp**	noncytopathic
NAS	nuclear addressing signal		**2NOS-2**	nitric oxide synthase
NASBA	nucleic acid sequence based amplification		**NP**	nucleocapsid-associated protein; or nucleoprotein
NAT	nucleic acid amplification technique			
NBS	nigmegen breakage syndrome		**NPC**	nasopharyngeal carcinoma; or nuclear pore complex
NBT	nitroblue tetrazolium			
NBTE	nonbacterial thrombotic endocarditis		**n-PCR**	nested polymerase chain reaction
NC	nucleocapsid		**NPHS-ARL**	National Public Health Service Anaerobe Reference Laboratory for England and Wales
NCAM	neuronal cell adhesion molecule			
NCBI	National Center for Biotechnology Information		**NPL**	nonparametric linkage
			NPS	nasopharyngeal secretion
NCCLS	National Committee for Clinical Laboratory Standards (USA)		**Nramp-1**	natural resistance-associated macrophage protein-1
NCHI	noncapsulate *Hemophilus influenzae*		**NRE**	negative regulatory element
NCL	neotropical cutaneous leishmaniasis		**NRTI**	nucleoside reverse transcriptase inhibitor
NCR	noncoding region		**nRT-PCR**	nested reverse transcription-polymerase chain reaction
NCV	noncholera vibrios			
NDUV	Ndumu virus		**nS**	nanosiemen
NDV	Newcastle disease virus		**NS**	nonstructural
NE	neutralizing epitope; or norepinephrine		**NSAID**	nonsteroidal antiinflammatory drug
NEGV	Negishi virus		**NSP**	neurotoxic shellfish poison; or nonstructural protein
NEP	nuclear export protein			
NES	nuclear export signal		**NspA**	neisserial surface protein A
NF	nuclear factor		**nt**	nucleotide
NF1	nuclear factor I		**NT**	virus-neutralizing
NF-κB	nuclear factor kappa B		**NTAL**	non-T cell activation linker
NFAT	nuclear factor activated T cell		**NTAV**	Ntaya virus
NFT	neurofibrillary tangles		**NTM**	nontuberculous mycobacteria
NGDO	nongovernmental development organization		**NTNH**	nontoxic nonhemagglutinating protein
NGF	nerve growth factor		**NTR**	non-translated region; or noncoding region; or non-translated RNA
NGO	nongovernmental organization			
NGU	non-gonoccocal urethritis		**NtRTI**	nucleotide reverse transcriptase inhibitor
Nhe	non-hemolytic enterotoxin		**NUD**	nonulcer dyspepsia
NHEJ	nonhomologous end joining		**NV**	Nipah virus; or nonvirion; or Norwalk virus
NHP	nonhuman primate			
NHS	National Health Service (UK)		**nvCJD**	new variant Creutzfeldt–Jakob disease
NIBSC	National Institute of Biological Standards and Control (UK)		**NVCP**	Norwalk virus capsid protein
			NVDP	asparagine−valine−aspartate−proline
NID	national immunization days		**NVFA**	non-volatile fatty acid
NIH	National Institutes of Health (USA)		**NVS**	nutritionally variant streptococci
NIV	Nipah virus		**NZB**	New Zealand black
NJ	neighbor-joining		**NZW**	New Zealand white
NJLV	Naranjal virus			
NK	natural killer		**OA**	oleic acid–albumin
NLS	nuclear localization sequence or signal		**OAE**	otoacoustic emission
NLV	Norwalk-like viruses		**OAS**	2′,5′-oligoadenylate synthetase
NMR	nuclear magnetic resonance		**2′-OAS**	2′,5′-oligoadenylate system
			OAstV	ovine astrovirus

OAT	ornithine aminotransferase
OC	Outbreak Committee
OCP	Onchocerciasis Control Programme
OD	optical denisty
ODC	ornithine carbamoyltransferase or decarboxylase
ODN	oligodeoxynucleotide
ODRS	oxygen-derived reactive species
OE	outer envelope
OEPA	Onchocerciasis Elimination Program for the Americas
OF	opacity factor; or oxidation–fermentation
OHFV	Omsk hemorrhagic fever virus
OHPAT	outpatient and home parenteral antibiotic therapy
OI	opportunistic infection
OIE	World Organization for Animal Health
OL	ornithine amine lipid
OLM	ocular lava migrans
OLT	orthotopic liver transplantation
OM	outer membrane
OMP	outer membrane protein
OMV	outer membrane vesicle
ONCHOSIM	onchocerciasis simulation model
ONNV	O'nyong-nyong virus
ONPG	orthonitrophenol-β-D-galactopyranoside
ONS	Office for National Statistics (UK)
OOA	oxoline–esculin agar
OPAT	outpatient parenteral antibiotic therapy or treatment
OPC	oropharyngeal candidiasis
OPCS	Office of Population Censuses and Surveys (UK)
OPN	osteopontin
OPV	oral poliovirus vaccine
orf	open reading frame
ORI	origin of replication
oriT	origin of transfer
oriV	origin of vegetative replication
ORS	oral rehydration solution
Osp	outer surface protein
OspA	outer surface protein A
OVA	ovalbumin
P	phosphoprotein; or pneumonia; or proline
PA	phosphatidic acid; or platelet-aggregating; or protective antigen
pABA	*para*-aminobenzoic acid
PABP	poly(A) binding protein
PABPII	poly(A) binding protein II
PAD	phage antibody display
PAE	post antibiotic effect
PAF	platelet-activating factor
PAGE	polyacrylamide gel electrophoresis
PAHO	Pan American Health Organization
PAI	pathogenicity island
PAI-1	plasminogen activator inhibitor type I
PAIR	percutaneous aspiration–injection–re-aspiration

PAL	peptidoglycan-associated lipoprotein
PAM	primary amebic meningoencephalitis
PAMP	pathogen-associated microbial or molecular patterns
Pap	papanicolaou; or pyelonephritis-associated pili
PAP	peroxidase–antiperoxidase
PARP	poly-ADP-ribose-polymerase
PAS	periodic acid–Schiff
PAstV	porcine astrovirus
PBL	peripheral blood leukocyte or lymphocyte
PBMC	peripheral blood mononuclear cell
PBP	penicillin-binding protein
PBS	phosphate-buffered saline; or primer binding site
PC	phosphorylcholine
P3C	tripalmitoyl-*S*-glyceryl-cysteinylserylserine
PCBP	poly(rC) binding protein
PCBP1	poly(rC) binding protein 1
PCBP2	poly(rC) binding protein 2
PCD	propamidine isothionate; or programmed cell death
PcG	polycomb group
PCMS	*p*-chloromercuriphenylsulfonic acid
PCNA	proliferating cell nuclear antigen
PCoV	puffinosis coronavirus
PCP	*Pneumocystis* pneumonia
PCR	polymerase chain reaction
PCR-EIA	polymerese chain reaction-enzyme immunoassay
PCR-REA	polymerase chain reaction-restriction enzyme amplification
PCR-SSCP	polymerase chain reaction single-strand conformation polymorphism
PCT	procalcitonin
PCV	porcine circovirus; or penciclovir
PCV-MP	penciclovir-monophosphate
PCV-TP	penciclovir-triphosphate
PD	prenatal diagnosis
PDA	potato dextrose agar
PDB	protein database
pDC	plasmacytoid dendritic cell
PDGF	platelet derived growth factor
PDH	pyruvate dehydrogenase complex
PDR	Physicians' Desk Reference (USA)
PDV	phocine distemper virus
PE	phosphatidylethanolamine; or Pro-Glu
PECAM-1	platelet endothelial cell adhesion molecule-1
PEDV	porcine epidemic diarrhea virus
PEG	polyethylene glycol
PEI	polyethyleneimine
PEL	primary effusion lymphoma
PEMS	poult enteritis mortality syndrome
PEP	phosphoenolpyruvate; or post-exposure prophylaxis
PET	positron emission tomography; or pyrogenic exotoxin
PFA	phosphonoformic acid
PfEMP1	P. falciparum erythrocyte membrane protein 1

PFGE	pulsed field gel electrophoresis
Pfk	phosphofructokinase
pfu	plaque forming unit
PFV	prototype foamy virus
PG	prostaglandin
6-PGD	6-phosphate gluconate dehydrogenase
PGD$_2$	prostaglandin D$_2$
PGE$_2$	prostaglandin E$_2$
PGL-I	phenolic glycolipid I
PGM	phosphoglucomutase
PGN	peptidoglycan
PGPR	plant growth-promoting rhizobacteria
PGRS	polymorphic GC-rich repetitive sequence
PGU	post-gonococcal urethritis
PHA	phytohemagglutinin
PHB	poly-β-hydroxybutyrate
PHC	primary hepatocellular carcinoma
PHCoV	pheasant coronavirus
PHEV	porcine haemagglutinating encephalomyelitis virus
PHI	primary HIV-1 infection
PHLS	Public Health Laboratory Service, now HPA (UK)
PHMB	polyhexamethylene biguanide
pI	isoelectric point
PI	gonococcal protein; or propamidine isethionate; or protein I; or phosphatidyl inositol; or protease inhibitor
P&I	pneumonia and influenza
PI3K	phosphatidylinositol 3-kinase
PI-9	protease inhibitor 9
PIA	polysaccharide intercellular adhesin
PIC	polymorphism information content; or preintegration complex
PICC	peripherally inserted central catheter
PID	pelvic inflammatory disease
PIE	postinfectious encephalitis
PIF	parvoviral initiation factor
pIgA	polymeric IgA
pIgR	polymeric immunoglobulin receptor
PIM	prototheca isolation medium
PIP$_2$	phosphatidylinositol biphosphate
PIP$_3$	phosphatidylinositol 3,4,5-triphosphate
PIV2	parainfluenza virus 2
PKC	protein kinase C
PKCε	protein kinase Cε
PKDL	post kala-azar dermal leishmaniasis
PKH	paroxysmal cold hemoglobinuria
PKR	protein kinase dsRNA
PLA$_2$	phospholipase A$_2$
PLC-β-1	phosphatidylinositol 4,5,-bisphosphate
PLCγ1	phospholipase Cγ1
PLCγ2	phospholipase Cγ2
pLDH	parasite lactate dehydrogenase
PLET	polymyxin-lysozyme EDTA-thallous acetate
PLG	poly(lactide-co-glycolide)
PLP	proteolipid protein
PLpro	papainlike cysteine proteinase
PLSP	polymeric lamellar substrate particle
PLTP	phospholipid-transfer protein
PMA	phorbol myristate acetate
PMC	pseudomembraneous colitis
PMD	piecemeal degranulation
PMEA	9-(2-phosphonylmethoxyethyl) adenine
pmf	proton motive force
PMF	*Proteus mirabilis* fimbriae
PMKC	primary cynomolgus or rhesus monkey kidney cell
PML	polymorphonuclear leukocyte; or progressive multifocal leukoencephalopathy
PMLP	promyelocyte leukemia protein
PMMA	polymethylmethacrylate
PMN	polymorphonuclear cell; or polymorphonuclear neutrophil; or polymorphonucleated neutrophilic granulocyte
PMNL	polymorphonuclear leukocyte
PMPA	R-9-(2-phosphonylmethoxypropyl) adenine
PMS	pyrolysis mass spectrometry
PMTV	potato mop-top virus
PMV	porpoise morbillivirus
PNG	Papua New Guinea; or polymorphonuclear granulocyte
PNH	paroxysmal nocturnal hemoglobinuria
PNP	Purine nucleoside phosphorylase
PNSG	poly-N-succinyl beta-1-6 glucosamine
pO$_2$	partial pressure of oxygen
PoEV	porcine endogenous retrovirus
POGS	Parinaud's oculoglandular syndrome
poly(A)	polyadenylate
POP	persistent organic pollutants
POPG	palmitoyloleoylphosphatidylglycerol
POTV	Potiskum virus
POWV	Powassan virus
PP	Peyer's patch
PPARα	peroxisome proliferator receptor α
PPBV	Phnom Penh bat virus
PPD	purified protein derivative of tuberculin
PPDK	pyruvate phosphate dikinase
PPE	Pro-Pro-Glu
PPi	inorganic pyrophosphate
PPI	proton pump inhibitor
PPi-PFK	inorganic pyrophosphate-dependent phosphofructokinase
PPIase	peptidyl-prolyl isomerase
PPNG	penicillinase-producing *Neisseria gonorrhoeae*
PPP	public–private partnerships
PPRV	peste des petits ruminants virus
PPS	postpolio syndrome
PPV	porcine parvovirus
PQS	pseudomonas quinolone signal
PR	peptide-receptive; or protease
PRA	polymerase chain reaction/restriction enzyme analysis; or proline-rich antigen
PRAS	pre-reduced, anaerobically sterilized (media)

PRCoV	porcine respiratory coronavirus	**Q**	glutamine
PRE	post-transcriptional regulatory element	**QAC**	quarternary ammonium compound
PRN	pertactin; or plaque reduction neutralization	**QBC**	quantitative buffy coat
PRNT	plaque reduction neutralization test	**QPCR**	quantitative polymerase chain reaction
pro-IL-1β	proinflammatory cytokine IL-1β	**QRDR**	quinolone resistance determining region
PROM	premature rupture of the membrane	**QRNG**	quinolone-resistant *Neisseria gonorrhoeae*
PROS	pathogen-related oral spirochetes		
PrP	prion protein	**R**	arginine; or direct repeat
PRP	penicillin resistant pneumonia; or polyribose-phosphate; or polyribosyl ribitol phosphate	**RA**	rheumatoid arthritis
		RABV	rabies virus
PRR	pattern recognition receptor	**r-Ad**	recombinant adenovirus
PRRSV	porcine reproductive and respiratory syndrome virus	**RAE**	retinoic acid early inducible
		RAG	recombinant-activating gene
PR-RT/RN	protease-reverse transcriptase/RNase H	**RaLPS**	detoxified lipopolysaccharide
PsaA	pilus adhesin	**RANTES**	regulated upon activation of normal T cell expressed and secreted
PSG	peripheral sensory ganglia; or promastigote secretory gel		
		RAPD	random amplified polymorphic DNA
PSLV	poa semilatent virus	**RAPD-PCR**	random amplified polymorphic DNA polymerase chain reaction
PSP	paralytic shellfish poison; or promastigote surface protease		
		RAPLOA	rapid assessment of prevalence of eye worm
PspA	pneumococcal surface protein	**RAST**	radioallergoabsorbent test
PSV	peak systolic velocity	**RB**	reticulate body
PT	pertussis toxin; or phage type	**RBBB**	right bundle branch block
PTA	phosphotungstate	**RBC**	red blood cell
PTB	polypyrimidine tract binding	**rBCG**	recombinant BCG
PTd	pertussis toxoid	**RBL-1**	rat basophilic leukemia cell
Ptd Ins (3,4,5) P3	phosphatidylinositol 3,4,5-trisphosphate	**RBM**	Roll Back Malaria
		RBS	ranitidine bismuth citrate; or ribosome binding sequence; or rep binding site
PtdSer	phosphatidylserine		
PTHrP	parathyroid hormone-related protein	**RBV**	Rio Bravo virus; or ribavirin
PTK	protein tyrosine kinase	**rc**	relaxed circular
Ptl	pertussis toxin liberation	**RC**	repeat cluster; or rolling circle
PTLD	post-transplant lymphoproliferative disease	**RCA**	regulators of C activation
		RCCS	random cloned chromosomal sequence
PTM	peritrophic matrix	**RCI**	reaction center I
PToV	porcine torovirus	**RCII**	reaction center II
pTP	precursor of the terminal protein	**RD**	rhabdomyosarcoma cells
PTS	phosphoenolpyruvate phosphotransferase; or phosphoenolpyruvate-dependent phosphotransferase system; or phosphotransferase transport system	**r-det**	resistance determinant
		rDNA	ribosomal DNA
		RdRp	RNA-dependent RNA polymerase
		RE	restriction enzyme
PT/SAP	Pro–Thr/Ser–Ala–Pro	**REA**	restriction endonuclease or enzyme analysis
PTX3	long pentraxin		
PUO	pyrexia of unknown origin	**REAC**	restriction endonuclease digestion of chromosomal DNA
PV	papillomavirus; or polyomavirus; or parasitophorous vacuole; or pityriasis versicolor		
		REAP	restriction endonuclease digestion of plasmid DNA
PVA	polyvinyl alcohol		
PVC	polvinylchloride	**REBOV**	Reston ebola virus
PVE	prosthetic valve endocarditis	**REMO**	rapid epidemiological mapping of onchocerciasis
PVL	Panton–Valentine leukocidin		
PVM	parasitophorous vacuole membrane; or pneumonia virus of mice	**REP**	repetitive element sequence; or repetitive extragenic palindromic
PVR	poliovirus receptor	**rep-PCR**	repetitive DNA PCR; or repetitive extragenic palindromic element typing; or repetitive-element polymerase chain reaction
PYD	pyrin domain		
PYG	peptone yeast glucose; or peptone–yeast extract–glucose		
		rER	rough endoplasmic reticulum
PYR	pyrrolidonyl-β-naphthylamide	**RESA**	ring-infected erythrocyte surface antigen
PYV	polyomavirus		

RF	recombination frequency; or replicative form; or retroperitoneal fibromatosis; or rheumatoid factor
RF-C	replication factor C
RFLP	restriction fragment length polymorphism
RFMS	rapid field assessment process
RFV	Royal Farm virus
RGD	Arg-Gly-Asp; or arginine-glycine-asparagine
RGM	rapidly growing mycobacteria
RH	relative humidity
RHDV	rabbit hemorrhagic disease virus
RHR	rolling hairpin replication
RI	replicative intermediate
RIA	radioimmunoassay
RID	receptor internalization and degradation
RIL	rabbit ileal loop
Ris	regulator of intracellular stress
RIT	rabbit infectivity testing
RITARD	removable intestinal tie adult rabbit diarrhea
RIVET	recombinase-based IVET
RK	rabbit kidney; or receptor kinase
RKV	rabbit kidney vacuolating virus
RML	Rocky Mountain Laboratory
RMP	reduction-modifiable protein
RMVM	*Review of Medical and Veterinary Mycology*
RNA	ribonucleic acid
RNAi	RNA inhibition; or RNA interference
RNAP	RNA polymerase
RND	resistance/nodulation/cell-division family
RNI	reactive nitrogen intermediate
RNP	ribonucleocapsid particle; or ribonucleoprotein
ROCV	Rocio virus
RODAC	replicate organism detection and counting
ROI	reactive oxygen intermediate
ROS	reactive oxygen species
RPA	replication protein A
RPC	replication protein C
RPCFT	Reiter protein complement fixation test
RPLA	reverse passive latex agglutination
RPR	rapid plasma reagin
rpsU	ribosomal protein subunit
RPV	rinderpest virus; or rabbitpox virus
RPXV	rabbitpox virus
RR	ribonucleotide reductase
RRE	rev responsive element
RREID	rapid rabies enzyme immunodiagnosis
rRNA	ribosomal RNA
RRP	recurrent respiratory papillomatosis
RRV	rhesus monkey rhadinovirus; or Ross river virus
rSJPM	recombinant *S. japonicum* paramyosin
RSP	recombinant subviral particle
RSS	recombination signal sequence; or recurrent nontyphoidal salmonella septicemia
RSSE	Russian spring–summer encephalitis
RSV	respiratory syncytial virus
RT	reverse transcriptase
RTA	replication and transcription activator
RTC	reverse transcription complex
RtCoV	rat coronavirus
RTD	rhesus theta (θ) defensin; or routine test dilution
RTF	reduced transport fluid; or resistance transfer factor
RT-PCR	reverse transcriptase polymerase chain reaction
RTX	repeat-in-toxin
RUBV	rubella virus
RuMP	ribulose monophosphate
RV	rabies virus
RVV	rhesus–human reassortant rotavirus
RVVC	recurrent VVC
S	serine
SA	sialic acid; or splice acceptor
SA12	simian agent 12
SAA	serum amyloid A
SABV	Saboya virus
SAC	Staphylococcus aureus Cowan strain I
SAF	scrapie-associated fibril; or sodium-acetate acetic-acid formalin
SAFLP	single-enzyme amplified fragment length polymorphism fingerprinting
SAg	superantigen
SAG	surface antigen
SAGE	serial analysis of gene expression
SaHV-1	herpes saimiri
SAI	sexually acquired infection
SAK	staphylokinase
SAL	sterility assurance level
SALT	skin-associated lymphoid tissue
SAM	*S*-adenosyl-L-methionine
SAM:SMT	*S*-adenosyl-Lmethionine:sterol C-24 methyl-transferase
SAP	secretory aspartyl protease; or SLAM-associated protein; or serum amyloid P
SAPA	shared acute phase antigen
SAR	secondary attack rate; or structure–activity relationship
SARA	sexually acquired reactive arthritis
SARS	severe acute respiratory syndrome
SARS-CoV	severe acute respiratory syndrome coronavirus
SASP	small acid-soluble protein
SAT	standard tube-agglutination test
SBA	sheep blood agar
sBCYE	selective buffered charcoal yeast extract agar
SBE	subacute bacterial endocarditis
SBHI	Sabouraud's brain–heart infusion
SBT	serum bactericidal titer
SC	secretory component; or stratum corneum
SCBV-IM	sugarcane bacilliform virus-Ireng Maleng
SCC	squamous cell carcinoma
SCF	Save the Children Fund; or stem cell factor
SCID	severe combined immunodeficiency disease
SCIDS	severe combined immunodeficiency disease syndrome

SCIEH	Scottish Centre for Infection and Environmental Health	**SIL**	squamous intraepithelial lesion
sCJD	sporadic Creutzfeldt–Jakob disease	**SIN**	self-inactivating
SCN	severe congenital neutropenia	**SINV**	Sindbis virus
SCR	short consensus repeat	**SIR**	susceptible, infectious, resistant
sCR1	soluble form of the C receptor CR1	**SIRPα**	signal regulatory protein alpha
SCV	small colony variant	**SIRS**	systemic inflammatory response syndrome
SD	seborrheic dermatitis; or smooth domed; or Shine–Dalgarno; or splice donor	**SIV**	simian immunodeficiency virus
SDA	Sabouraud's dextrose agar; or strand displacement amplification	**s.l.**	*sensu lato*
		SL	stem-loop
SDAV	sialodacryoadenitis virus	**SLAM**	signaling lymphocyte activation molecule
SDD	selective decontamination of the digestive tract; or serine–aspartic acid–aspartic acid	**SLC**	secondary lymphoid tissue chemokine
		SLE	systemic lupus erythematosus
SDF-1	stromal cell-derived factor 1	**SLEV**	St. Louis encephalitis virus
SDF-1α	stromal cell-derived factor 1α	**SLN**	solitary lymph node
SDH	succinate dehydrogenase	**SLPI**	secretory leukocyte protease inhibitor
SDS	sodium dodecyl sulfate	**SLT**	Shiga-like toxin
SDS-PAGE	sodium dodecyl sulfate polyacrylamide gel electrophoresis	**SLV**	Sapporo-like virus
		SMAC	sorbitol MacConkey; or supramolecular activation cluster
SE	staphylococcal enterotoxin	**SmD**	streptomycin dependent
SEA	soluble egg antigen; or staphylococcal enterotoxin A	**SMD**	smooth domed (colony morphology)
		SMEZ	streptococcal mitogenic exotoxin Z
SEB	staphylococcal enterotoxin B	**SMG**	*Streptococcus milleri* group
SEBOV	Sudan ebola virus	**SMRF**	small multidrug resistance family
SEC	serpin enzyme complex	**SMT**	smooth transparent (colony morphology)
SED	subepithelial dome	**SN**	serum neutralization
SELP	simian virus 40 early leader protein	**SNHL**	sensorineural hearing loss
SEM	scanning electron microscope or microscopy	**SNP**	single nucleotide polymorphism
SEPV	Sepik virus	**snRNAs**	small nuclear RNA
sER	smooth endoplasmic reticulum	**SNS**	segmented negative-stranded
SERA	serine rich antigen	**Soc**	small outer capsid
SERP	serine-rich protein	**SOCS**	suppressors of cytokine synthesis
serpin	serine protease inhibitor	**SOD**	superoxide dismutase
SF	splicing factor; or steel factor	**SOFA**	sequential organ failure assessment
SFA	sanglifehrin A	**SOKV**	Sokoluk virus
SFFV	spleen focus-forming virus	**SOM**	soil organic matter
SFG	spotted fever group	**SP**	structural protein; or surfactant protein
SFGF	Shope fibroma growth factor	**SP-A**	surfactant protein A
SFV	Semliki Forest virus; or simian foamy virus	**SPC**	standard plate count
		SP-D	surfactant protein D
sg	subgenomic	**SPDP**	*N*-succinimidyl-3-(2-pyridyldithio) propionate
SGA	Sabouraud's glucose (dextrose) agar	**SPDV**	salmon pancreas disease virus
SH	small hydrophobic	**SPE**	streptococcal pyrogenic exotoxin
SHa	Syrian hamster	**SPEB**	streptococcal erythrogenic toxin B
SHa/Mo	Syrian hamster/mouse	**SPECT**	single photon emission computed tomography
SHFV	simian haemorrhagic fever virus	**SPG**	sucrose phosphate glutamate
SHIV	simian–human immunodeficiency virus	**SPI**	*Salmonella* pathogenicity island
SHM	somatic hypermutation	**SPIEM**	solid-phase immunoelectron microscopy
SHP-1	-SH2-domain-containing tyrosine phosphatase	**SPOV**	Spondweni virus; or sporophorous vesicle
SI	stimulation indices	**SPS**	sodium polyanethol sulfonate
SIB	single-step immunoblot	**SPV**	San Perlita virus
SICA	schizont-infected cell agglutination antigen	**SRA**	serum resistance associated
sICAM	soluble intercellular adhesion molecule	**SRBC**	sheep erythrocyte
SIDS	sudden infant death syndrome	**SRE**	serum response element; or small repetitive element
sIgA	secretory IgA		
SIGN	specific intracellular adhesion molecule-3 grabbing nonintegrin	**SREHP**	serine-rich *E. histolytica* protein
		SREV	Saumarez Reef virus

SRF	serum-response factor		**TA**	transaldolase
SRH	single radial hemolysis		**TAA**	tumor-associated antigen
SRL	*Shigella* resistance locus		**TABM**	T-cell-derived antigen-binding molecule
SRP	signal recognition particle		**TABV**	Tamana bat virus
SRS	slow-reacting substance		**TAN**	total adenine nucleotide
SRSV	small round structured virus		**TAO**	thyroid-associated ophthalmopathy
SRV	Saumarez Reef virus; or simian type D virus; or small round virus		**TAP**	transporter associated with antigen presentation or processing
SS	Stainer–Scholte		**TAstV**	turkey astrovirus
SSA	streptococcal superantigen		**TAT**	twin arginine translocation
SSAT	spermidine/spermine-N^1-acetyltransferase		**Tb**	Tbilisi
SSB	single-strand break		**TB**	tuberculosis
SSCP	single-strand conformational polymorphism		**TBA**	traditional birth attendants
ssDNA	single-stranded DNA		**TBE**	tick-borne encephalitis
SSI	surgical site infection		**TBEV**	tick-borne encephalitis virus
SSp	streptomycin/spectinomycin		**TBF**	thick blood film
SSP	serotype-specific plasmid		**TBP**	TATA-binding protein
SSPE	subacute sclerosing panencephalitis		**TbpB**	transferrin-binding protein B
ssRNA	single-stranded RNA		**TBSA**	tuberculostearic acid
SSSS	staphylococcal scalded skin syndrome		**TBW**	tracheobronchial washing
SST	sodium silicotungstate		**3TC**	2′-deoxy-3′-thiacytidine
SSU	small subunit		**Tc**	cytotoxic T cell
SSUrRNA	small subunit ribosomal RNA		**TCA**	tricarboxylic acid; or trichloracetic acid
ST	Shiga toxin		**TCBS**	thiosulfate-citrate-bile salts-sucrose
STAT	signal transducer and activator of transcription		**TCC**	terminal C complex
STAT6	signal transducer and activator of transcription 6		**TCF**	tracheal colonization factor
STD	sexually transmitted disease		**TCGF**	T-cell growth factor
STE	surface tubule element		**TCI**	transcutaneous immunization
STEC	Shiga toxin producing *E. coli*		**TCNA**	*T. cruzi* neuraminidase
STI	sexually transmitted infection		**TCoV**	turkey coronavirus
STIKO	German Vaccinee Commission		**TCP**	toxin coregulated pilus
STLV	simian T-lymphotropic virus		**TCR**	T cell receptor
STM	signature tagged mutagenesis		**TCR⁺**	T cell receptor positive
STMV	stump-tailed macaque virus		**TCRβ**	T cell receptor β
sTNFR2	TNF receptor 2		**TCSTS**	two-component signal transduction system
STORCH	syphilis, toxoplasma, other diseases, rubella, cytomegalovirus, herpes simplex virus		**TCT**	tracheal cytotoxin
			TDA	thymus-dependent area
STRV	Stratford virus		**TDE**	transmissible degenerative encephalopathy
SU	surface		**TDHT**	5-thyminyl-5,6-dihydrothymine
suPAR	soluble urokinase plasminogen activator receptor		**TDM**	trehalose dimycolate
SV	subvirion		**TDP**	thermal death point
SV-5	simian virus 5		**TdT**	X-linked agammaglobulinemia; or terminal deoxynucleotidyl transferase
SV40	simian vacuolating virus 40; or simian virus 40		**TDT**	thermal death time; or transmission disequilibrium test
svCAM	soluble vascular cell adhesion molecule			
SVDV	swine vesicular disease virus		**TE**	toxoplasmic encephalitis
SVP	subviral particle		**TEA**	T-early α
SVV	Sal Vieja virus		**TEC**	thymic medullary epithelial cell
SWAP	sector-wide approaches to financing; or soluble worm antigen preparation		**TECK**	thymus-expressed chemokine
			TEE	transesophageal echocardiography
			TEM	transmission electron microscopy
T	thymine		**TF**	tissue factor; or transferrin; or transcription factor
T3	triiodothyronine			
T3D	type 3 Dearing (virus)		**TfR**	transferrin receptor
T4	thyroxine		**TFSS**	type IV secretion system
T$_{CM}$	central memory T cell		**TFT**	trifluridine; or trifluorothymidine
T$_{EM}$	effector memory T cell		**Tg**	transgenic
T$_{FH}$	follicular B-helper T			

TG	typhus group		**TPE**	tropical pulmonary eosinophilia
TGEV	transmissible gastroenteritis virus		**TPHA**	*Treponema pallidum* haemagglutination assay
TGF	transforming growth factor		**TPI**	*Treponema pallidum* immobilization; or triose
TGF-β	transforming growth factor beta			phosphate isomerase
TGF-β1	transforming growth factor-β1; or tumor growth		**TPO**	thrombopoietin
	factor β1		**TPP**	thiamine pyrophosphate
TGN	trans Golgi network		**TPPII**	tripeptidyl peptidase
Th	T helper [cell]		**TPPA**	*Treponema pallidum* particle assay; or *Treponema pallidum* particle agglutination
TH	tyrosine hydroxylase			
Th1	T helper 1		**TPx-1**	thioredoxin peroxidase-1
Th2	T helper 2		**Tr**	T-regulatory
ThCE	T-helper cell epitope		**TR**	terminal repeat; or trypanothione reductase
Ti	tumor-inducing		**Tr1**	T-regulatory 1
TI	B-cell stimulatory/activatory protein		**TRAF**	tumor necrosis factor receptor activating factor
TIBO	thiobenzimidazolone		**TRAF-6**	tumor necrosis factor receptor-associated factor 6
TIMP	tissue inhibitors of metalloprotease		**TRAIL**	tumor necrosis factor-related, apoptosis-inducing
Tir	translocated intimin receptor			ligand
TIR	terminal inverted sequence region; or Toll/inter-leukin-1 receptor		**TRAP**	thrombospondin related adhesion protein
			TRBP	tat region binding protein
T2J	type 2 Jones (virus)		**TRE-1**	tax response element 1
TK	thymidine kinase; or transketolase		**TREC**	T-cell receptor excition circle
TL	thymus leukemia		**Treg**	T-regulatory
T1L	type 1 Lang (virus)		**TR-FIA**	time-resolved fluoroimmunoassay
TLC	thin-layer chromatography		**TRH**	thyrotropin-releasing hormone
TLMV	TTV-like minivirus		**TRIS**	tris(hydroxymethyl)amino-methane
TLR	Toll-like receptor		**TRITC**	tetra-methylrhodamine isothiocyanate
TLR 2	Toll-like receptor 2			isomer R
TLR 4	Toll-like receptor 4		**TRLA**	treatment-resistant Lyme arthritis
TLR 9	Toll-like receptor 9		**tRNA**	transfer RNA
TLTF	trypanosome-derived lymphocyte triggering		**TRNG**	tetracycline-resistant *Neisseria gonorrhoeae*
	factor		**TROCV**	Trocara virus
Tm	DNA pseudo-melting point		**TRS**	terminal resolution sequence; or transcription-regulating sequence
TM	transmembrane			
TMA	transcription-mediated amplification		**TRUST**	toluidine red unheated serum test
TMAF	trypanosomal macrophage activating factor		**ts**	temperature-sensitive
TMEV	Theiler's murine encephalomyelitis virus		**TS**	thymidylate synthase
TMN	tubular membranous network		**T[S]$_2$**	trypanothione disulfide
TMUV	Tembusu virus		**TSB**	tryptic or trypticase soy-broth
TMV	tobacco mosaic virus		**TSE**	transmissible spongiform encephalopathy
TNF	tumor necrosis factor		**TSG**	tumor suppressor gene
TNF-α	tumor necrosis factor-alpha		**TSH**	thyroid-stimulating hormone
TNF-β	tumor necrosis factor-beta		**T[SH]$_2$**	dihydrotrypanothione
TNFR	tumor necrosis factor receptor		**TSI**	triple sugar iron (agar)
TOC	total organic carbon		**TSP**	tropical spastic paraparesis
TOL	toluene		**TSP/HAM**	tropical spastic paraparesis/human T-cell
TOP	termination of pregnancy			leukemia virus-I associated myelopathy
topo	topoisomerase		**TSS**	toxic shock syndrome
topo I	topoisomerase I		**TSST-1**	toxic shock syndrome toxin-1
TORCH	toxoplasma gondii, other diseases, rubellavirus, cytomegalovirus, herpes simplex virus		**TST**	tuberculin skin test
			TT	tetanus toxoid; or tuberculoid
TORCHES-CLAP	toxoplasma gondii, other diseases, rubellavirus, cytomegalovirus, herpes simplex virus, entero-virus, syphilis, chickenpox virus, Lyme disease, AIDs, parvovirus B19		**TTE**	transthoracic echocardiography
			TTGA	taurocholate tellurite gelatin agar
			TTMV	torque-teno-minivirus
			TTP	thrombotic thrombocytopenic purpura; or thymidine triphosphate
TP	terminal protein; or tube precipitin			
TPA	tetradecanoylphorbol acetate		**TTSS**	type III secretion system
TPD	transdermal powder delivery		**TTV**	torque-teno-virus

TUT	terminal uridylate transferase
TxA₂	thromboxane A$_2$
TxB₂	thromboxane B$_2$
TYUV	Tyuleniy virus
UBT	urea breath test
UCA	uroepithelial cell adhesin
UCLA	University of California, Los Angeles
UCS	upstream conserved sequence
UEV	ubiquitin E2 variant
UGI	uncomplicated gonococcal infection
UGSV	Uganda S virus
UHT	ultra-heat-treated
ULBP	UL16 binding protein
UMP	uridine 5′-monophosphate
UNG	uracil-*N*-glycosylase
UNICEF	United Nations International Children's Emergency Fund
uPAR	urokinase-type plasminogen activator receptor
UPEC	uropathogenic *E. coli*
UPGMA	unweighted pair-group method with arithmetic mean
UPRTase	uracil phosphoribosyltransferase
UPS	ubiquitin proteasome system
UPU	Universal Postal Union
URR	upstream regulatory region
URT	upper respiratory tract
US	ultrasonography
USDA	United States Department of Agriculture
USF-1	upstream stimulatory factor-1
USR	unheated serum reagin
USUV	Usutu virus
UTI	urinary tract infection
UTR	untranslated region
UV	ultraviolet
V	valine
VA	virus-associated
VACV	vaccinia virus; or valaciclovir
VAERS	vaccine adverse events reporting system
VAP	ventilator-associated pneumonia; or virus attachment protein
VAPP	vaccine-associated paralytic poliomyelitis
VAT	variable antigen type
VBNC	viable but nonculturable
VCAM	vascular cell adhesion molecule
VCAM-1	vascular cell adhesion molecule 1
vCJD	variant Creutzfeldt–Jakob disease
vCKBP	viral chemokine binding protein
vCKR	viral chemokine receptor
VCP	viral complement control protein
VCRC	Vector Control Research Centre
VD	venereal disease
VDRL	Venereal Disease Research Laboratory
VE	vaccine efficacy
VEEV	Venezuelan equine encephalitis virus

VEGF	vascular endothelial growth factor
VETF	viral early transcription factor
vFLIP	viral FLICE inhibitory protein
VGF	vaccinia growth factor
VHDL	very high density lipoprotein
vhs	viral host protein shut off
VHSV	viral hemorrhagic septicemia virus
VHW	village health worker
Vif	virus infectivity factor
vIFN-γR	viral IFN-γ receptor
VIG	vaccinia immunoglobulin
vIL-6	IL-6 homolog
vIL-10	IL-10 homolog
vIL-17	IL-17 homolog
vIL-18BP	viral interleukin-18 binding protein
vIL-1βR	viral interleukin-1β receptor
VIM	Verona imipenemase
VIPR	vasoactive intestinal peptide receptor
VITF	viral intermediate transcription factor
VL	viral load; or visceral leishmaniasis
VLA-4	very late activated antigen-4
VLBW	very low birth weight
VLDL	very-low-density lipoprotein
VLM	visceral larva migrans
VLP	virus-like particle
VLTF	viral late transcription factor
VMK	vervet monkey kidney
VN	virus neutralization
VNA	virus-neutralizing antibody
VNTR	variable number tandem repeat
VP	ventriculoperitoneal; or Voges–Proskauer
VPI	vibrio pathogenicity island
Vpr	viral protein R
Vpu	viral protein U
VRE	vancomycin resistant enterococci
VRSA	vancomycin-resistant *Staphylococcus aureus*
vSag	viral superantigen
vSEMA	semaphorin homologue
VSG	variable surface glycoprotein
VSIV	vesicular stomatitis Indiana virus
VSP	variable small protein; or variant-specific surface protein
VSV	vesicular stomatitis virus
VT	verotoxin
VTEC	Vero cytotoxin-producing *Escherichia coli*
VTF	viral termination factor
VTM	viral transport medium
vTNFR	viral TNF receptor
VV	vaccinia virus
VVC	vulvovaginal candidiasis
VZIG	varicella-zoster immune globulin
VZV	varicella zoster virus
W	Tryptophan
WABO	Whipple's-associated bacterial organism
WAS	Wiskott–Aldrich syndrome

WASP	Wiscott–Aldrich syndrome protein	**X-SCID**	X-linked severe combined immunodeficiency
Wb	Weybridge	**XTT**	2,3-bis-2-methoxy-4-nitro-5-sulphophenyl-5-
WB	western blot		[phenylaminocarbonyl]-2*H*-tetrazo-lium hydroxide
WBC	white blood cell count; or white blood cell		
WCE	Wolff–Chaikoff effect	**Y**	tyrosine
WCP	whole-cell protein	**YAC**	yeast artificial chromosome
WEEV	western equine encephalomyelitis virus	**YAOV**	Yaounde virus
WESSV	Wesselsbron virus	**YFV**	yellow fever virus
WG	week of gestation	**YHV**	yellow head virus
WHO	World Health Organization	**YLDV**	yaba-like disease virus
WHV	woodchuck hepatitis virus	**YMTV**	yaba monkey tumor virus
WMD	weapons of mass destruction	**YOKV**	yokose virus
WNV	West Nile virus	**YPM**	*Y. pseudotuberculosis* mitogen
WR	Wassermann reaction		
		ZAP	ζ-associated protein
XLA	X-linked agammaglobulinemia	**ZDV**	zidovudine
XLAAD	X-linked autoimmunity-allergic disregulation syndrome	**ZEBOV**	Zaire ebola virus
		ZF	zinc-finger
XLD	xylose-lysine-deoxycholate	**ZIG**	zoster immunoglobulin
XLP	X-linked lymphoproliferative	**ZIKV**	Zika virus
XLPS	X-linked lymphoproliferative syndrome	**ZOT**	zonula occludens toxin

Index

Notes

Each page reference is preceded by a code in bold showing the volume that the entry can be found in:
V1: Virology volume 1
V2: Virology volume 2
B1: Bacteriology volume 1
B2: Bacteriology volume 2
M: Medical mycology
P: Parasitology
I: Immunology

References to whole chapters are indicated in bold. (Fig.) and (Tab.) refer to figures and tables respectively. *vs.* indicates a comparison or differential diagnosis.

To save space in the index, the following abbreviations have been used

APCs - antigen-presenting cells
BCE - B-cell epitope
BCR - B-cell receptor
CNS - central nervous system
CTL - cytotoxic T cell (lymphocyte)
EBV - Epstein–Barr virus
EIA - enzyme immunoassay
ELISA - enzyme-linked immunosorbent assay
G-CSF - granulocyte colony stimulating factor
GM-CSF - granulocyte-macrophage colony stimulating factor
HAART - highly active antiretroviral therapy
HCMV - Human cytomegalovirus
HHV - human herpesvirus
HIV - human immunodeficiency virus
HLA - human leukocyte antigen
HPV - human papillomavirus
HSV - herpes simplex virus
HTLV - Human T-cell leukemia (lymphotrophic) virus
ICAM - intracellular adhesion molecule

IFN - interferon
Ig - immunoglobulin
IL - interleukin
LCMV - Lymphocytic choriomeningitis virus
LPS - lipopolysaccharide
LT - *Escherichia coli* heat labile enterotoxin
M-CSF - macrophage colony stimulating factor
MHC - major histocompatibility complex
NK cells - natural killer cells
PCP - *Pneumocystis* pneumonia
PCR - polymerase chain reaction
SCF - stem cell factor
SLE - systemic lupus erythematosus
SV40 - Simian virus 40
TCE- T-cell epitope
TCR - T-cell receptor
Th1 - T helper cells type 1
Th2 - T helper cells type 2
VZV - varicella-zoster virus

A18R gene, **V1**.611

A20 protein, poxvirus replication, **V1**.169 (Tab.)

A50 protein, poxvirus replication, **V1**.169 (Tab.)

AA amyloidosis, **I**.209

A antigen, *Brucella melitensis* LPS, **B2**.1725, **B2**.1726 (Fig.)

Aardvarks, histoplasmosis, **M**.521–2

Abacavir, **V2**.1620–1
adverse reactions, **V2**.1621
HIV infection, **V2**.1334
point mutations resistance, **V2**.1337 (Fig.)
resistance to, **V2**.1621
structure, **V2**.1620 (Fig.)

Abattoir workers, erysipeloid, **B2**.971

Abdominal actinomycosis, **M**.140 (Fig.)

Abdominal pain
giardiasis, **P**.242
opisthorchiasis, **P**.649

Abelcet, **M**.612
aspergillosis therapy, **M**.721–2

Abiotrophia, **B2**.833–5, **B2**.862–3
infection, endocarditis, **B1**.528–9, **B1**.537
metabolism, **B2**.838
normal microbiota, **B1**.296 (Tab.)
see also individual species

Abiotrophia adjacens, **B2**.862

Abiotrophia balaenopterae, **B2**.862

Abiotrophia defectiva, **B2**.862
infection, endocarditis, **B1**.529, **B1**.533

Abiotrophia para-adiacens, **B2**.862

Abortion
in animals, **B2**.1549
Arcobacter, **B2**.1557
bacterial vaginosis association, **B1**.668
Campylobacter infection, **B2**.1549
Chlamydia psittaci infection, **B2**.2015
Clostridium perfringens infection, **B2**.1111
filovirus infection, **V2**.1094
HCMV infection, **V2**.1447

HSV-2 infection, **V2**.1463
Parvovirus B19 virus infection, **V2**.1468
rubella, **V2**.977
VZV infection, **V2**.1454

Abscess(es)
gram-positive anaerobic cocci, **B2**.910–11
mycetoma, **M**.385
oral cavity, **B1**.618–19
peritonsillar, **B1**.629
specimens, **M**.84
subcutaneous, histoplasmosis, **M**.565 (Fig.)
upper respiratory tract, **B1**.608–9

Absettarov virus (ABSV), **V2**.998 (Tab.)

Absidia, **M**.9, **M**.20, **M**.660, **M**.660 (Tab.)

Absidia corymbifera, **M**.659–62, **M**.674
histopathology, **M**.128 (Tab.), **M**.136 (Fig.)
identification, **M**.661–2, **M**.662 (Fig.), **M**.676 (Fig.)
infection, **M**.661, **M**.674
experimental, **M**.677
keratitis, **M**.301–2

Absidia corymbifera,
  infection (*Continued*)
    meningitis, **M**.661
    nosocomial, **M**.536 (Fig.)
    oculomycoses, **M**.281 (Tab.), **M**.287
    otitis externa, **M**.247–8
    rhino-orbital-cerebral zygomycosis, **M**.290
    scleritis, **M**.316
Acalculous cholecystitis, **P**.539
Acanthamoeba, **P**.187, **P**.226
  antibacterial susceptibility/resistance, **B1**.434
  cell differentiation, **P**.229
  classification, **P**.197, **P**.226
  culture, **P**.235
  cysts, **P**.227–8, **P**.228 (Fig.)
  encystment, **P**.229–30
  genetics, **P**.231
  immune response, **P**.87, **P**.232
  infection
    clinical features, **P**.231–2
    CNS, **P**.226, **P**.229
    diagnosis, **P**.235
    epidemiology/control, **P**.235–6
    keratitis *see Acanthamoeba* keratitis
    route, **P**.231
  infection, vaccination, **P**.237
  life-cycle, **P**.229, **P**.229 (Fig.)
  reproduction, **P**.227, **P**.231
  structure, **P**.227–8, **P**.228 (Fig.)
  see also individual species
Acanthamoeba castellanii, **P**.229–30
  antibacterial susceptibility/resistance, **B1**.445
Acanthamoeba culbertsoni, **P**.235, **P**.237
  treatment of infection, **P**.237
Acanthamoeba hatchetti, **P**.238
Acanthamoeba keratitis, **P**.226, **P**.229
  chemotherapy, **P**.237
  clinical features, **P**.231–2
  diagnosis, **P**.235
  epidemiology/control, **P**.236
  HSV keratitis *vs.,* **P**.235
  pathology, **P**.234
  prevention, **P**.238
Acanthamoeba palestinensis, **P**.235, **P**.237
Acanthamoeba polyphaga, **P**.238
Acanthamoeba rhysodes, **P**.235, **P**.237
Acanthella, **P**.596
Acanthocephala, **P**.596–8
  classification, **P**.597
    Archiacanthocephala, **P**.597
    Palaeacanthocephala, **P**.597–8
  structure/characteristics, **P**.596, **P**.596 (Fig.)
Acanthocephalans, **P**.573
Acanthocephalus, **P**.598
Acanthopodia, **P**.227
Acanthor, **P**.596
Acanthosis, onchocerciasis, **P**.794
Acaricides, babesiosis control, **P**.460
Accelerated and stabilized hydrogen peroxide,
    hard surface cleaning agent, **B1**.429
'Accessory proteins'
  arteriviruses, **V1**.835–6
  coronaviruses, **V1**.395, **V1**.835–6
  Equine arteritis virus, **V1**.835–6

Equine torovirus (EToV: Berne virus),
    V1.835–6
  Murine hepatitis virus, **V1**.835–6
  Porcine epidemic diarrhea virus, **V1**.835–6
  Severe acute respiratory syndrome
    coronavirus, **V1**.835–6
AccuProbe *Enterococcus* probe, **B2**.887
ACE gene
  meningococcal meningitis association, **I**.594
  periodontitis association, **I**.595
Acellular pertussis vaccine, recombinant DNA
    techniques, **I**.937–8
Acetabula, tapeworms, **P**.659
Acetate
  production, *Bifidobacterium,* **B2**.1024
  utilization, **B1**.52
    as carbon and energy source, **B1**.53–4
    Enterobacteriaceae identification,
      B2.1319 (Tab.)
Acetoacetyl-CoA, **B1**.42, **B1**.56
Acetobacter, carbohydrate catabolism, **B1**.60
Acetylcholinesterase, intestinal nematode
    secretion, **I**.686
Acetyl-CoA, **B1**.42, **B1**.55–6
Acetyl-CoA acetyltransferase, **B1**.56
Acetylethyleneimine, inactivated vaccines,
    V2.1553
N-Acetylglucosamine, **B1**.42–3
  Borrelia culture, **B2**.1827
N-Acetyl-β-glucosaminidase, **B2**.1924 (Tab.)
N-Acetylmuramic acid, **B1**.42–3
Acholeplasma
  characteristics, **B2**.1958 (Tab.)
  classification, **B2**.1967, **B2**.1969
  genetics, **B2**.1967–8
    genome structure, **B2**.1973–4
  metabolism and biochemical properties,
    B2.1969, **B2**.1994
Acholeplasma laidlawii, **B1**.296 (Tab.)
  cell culture contamination, **B2**.1964–5
  cellular morphology, **B2**.1959 (Fig.)
  colonial morphology, **B2**.1958 (Fig.)
  genetic analysis, transposition, **B2**.1981
  membrane lipids, **B2**.1971
Achorion, **M**.220
Achorion schoenleinii, **M**.220
Achromobacter, **B2**.1787
Achromobacter xylosoxidans, nosocomial
    infection, **B1**.401 (Tab.)
Aciclovir (ACV), **V2**.1611–12
  development, **V2**.1605
  discovery, **V1**.9
  herpes encephalitis, **V1**.507, **V2**.1421
  historical aspects, **V1**.9 (Tab.)
  HSV infection, **V1**.511–12, **V2**.1501
    immunodeficient patients (non-HIV),
      V2.1506
    latent infection, **V2**.1638
    neonatal infection, **V2**.1467
    in pregnancy, **V2**.1466–7
  infection use, **V2**.1612
  mechanism of action, **V1**.217–18, **V1**.511–12,
    V2.1611–12, **V2**.1612 (Fig.)
  pharmacokinetics/pharmacodynamics,
    V1.511–12

resistance, **V2**.1634
  immunocompromised, **V2**.1635
resistance, HSV, **V1**.512, **V2**.1501
structure, **V1**.511–12, **V2**.1611 (Fig.),
    V2.1613 (Fig.)
VZV infection, **V1**.516–17, **V2**.1507
  in HIV infection, **V2**.1502, **V2**.1505
  immunodeficient patients (non-HIV),
    V2.1506
  neonate, **V2**.1461
  in pregnancy, **V2**.1458, **V2**.1460
Acidaminococcus, **B2**.1312
  biochemical detection, **B2**.1312, **B2**.1314–15
  differential characteristics, **B2**.1313 (Tab.)
  historical perspective, **B2**.1312
  possible infection, **B2**.1314
Acidaminococcus fermentans, **B1**.296 (Tab.)
  culture, **B2**.1314
  habitats, **B2**.1313
Acid environments, *Brucella,* **B2**.1728–9
Acid-fast bacteria, **B2**.1190
  historical aspects, **B1**.6
Acid-fast stains/staining, **B1**.713 (Tab.),
    B1.714, **B2**.1190
  modified, **B2**.1139–40
  reagents, **B2**.1140
Acid-heat treatment, **B1**.454
Acid phosphatase, Q fever pathogenesis,
    B2.2077
Acids
  antibacterial, **B1**.422, **B1**.423 (Tab.)
  sugar metabolism, **B1**.23, **B1**.23 (Fig.)
Acidulants, **B1**.422
Acinetobacter, **B2**.1302–5
  airborne, **B1**.189
  antibacterial susceptibility/resistance, **B1**.442
    β-lactam antibiotic resistance, **B1**.472–3
    genetic resistance, **B2**.1304–5
  antibacterial susceptibility testing, **B2**.1304
  cell wall/outer membrane structure,
    B2.1303–4
    LPS, **B2**.1303–4
  characteristics, **B2**.1302, **B2**.1303 (Tab.)
  classification, **B2**.1271, **B2**.1301–2
    taxonomic delineation, **B2**.1301–2
  conjugation, **B1**.103
  epidemiology, **B2**.1303
  in foods
    fish, **B1**.279
    meat and meat products, **B1**.273
    milk, **B1**.233
    poultry, **B1**.277–8
  identification, **B2**.1302–3
  infection
    bacteremia, **B1**.521–2
    clinical significance, **B2**.1304
    endocarditis, **B1**.532
    keratitis, **B1**.601
    management/therapeutic options, **B2**.1304
    nosocomial, **B1**.401 (Tab.), **B2**.1302 (Tab.),
      B2.1303
    pneumonia, **B1**.640–1
    sinusitis, **B1**.615
  normal microbiota, **B1**.296 (Tab.), **B1**.301
  siderophores, **B2**.1304

Acinetobacter, (Continued)
  soil pathogens, **B1**.203
  typing, **B2**.1303
  virulence factors, **B2**.1303–4
  waterborne, **B1**.211, **B1**.221
  see also individual species
Acinetobacter baumannii
  bacteremia, **B1**.521–2
  nosocomial infection, **B1**.371, **B1**.401 (Tab.),
    B2.1302 (Tab.), **B2**.1303, **B2**.1304
Acinetobacter calcoaceticus, **B2**.1302 (Tab.)
  classification, **B2**.1301
  natural competence, **B1**.99
  nosocomial infection, **B1**.401 (Tab.)
Acinetobacter haemolyticus, nosocomial
    infection, **B2**.1302 (Tab.), **B2**.1303
Acinetobacter johnsonii, nosocomial infection,
    B2.1302 (Tab.), **B2**.1303
Acinetobacter lwoffi, nosocomial infection,
    B2.1302 (Tab.), **B2**.1303
Acinetobacter radioresistens, **B2**.1302 (Tab.)
Acne vulgaris, *Propionibacterium acnes,*
    B2.1032
Aconitase, **B1**.52
Acquired angioedema (AAE), **I**.154
Acquired immune response *see* Adaptive
    immune response
Acquired immunodeficiency syndrome (AIDS)
    see AIDS
Acremonium
  antifungal susceptibility, **M**.752 (Tab.)
  ecology, **M**.758
  histopathology, **M**.128 (Tab.)
  identification, **M**.390, **M**.392 (Tab.)
  infection, **M**.189, **M**.758
    dacryocystitis, **M**.298
    diagnosis, **M**.752
    endophthalmitis, **M**.317, **M**.326
    keratitis, **M**.303, **M**.328
    oculomycoses, **M**.275 (Tab.), **M**.283
    onychomycosis, **M**.246
    scleritis, **M**.316
    therapy, **M**.758
  morphology, **M**.757
Acremonium falciforme, **M**.89 (Tab.), **M**.390
Acremonium kiliense, **M**.89 (Tab.), **M**.390
  endophthalmitis, **M**.326
  keratitis, **M**.328
Acremonium recifei, **M**.89 (Tab.), **M**.390
Acremonium strictum, **M**.248, **M**.249 (Fig.)
  onychomycosis, **M**.246
Acridine dyes, **B1**.427–8, **B1**.438
  action, **B1**.438
  frame-shift mutations, **B1**.85
Acridine orange
  cerebrospinal fluid examination, **B1**.559
  quantitative buffy coat (QBC) technique,
    African trypanosomiasis diagnosis,
    P.366–7
Actin
  Candida gene, **M**.103, **M**.608
  cytoskeleton, **I**.37
  neutrophil function disorders, **I**.769
  polymerization, **I**.37
Actinobacillus, **B2**.1658–66
  animal associations, **B2**.1659, **B2**.1665–6

characteristics, **B2**.1653, **B2**.1659–61,
    B2.1659 (Tab.)
  habitats, **B2**.1649–50
  as normal microbiota, **B1**.296 (Tab.)
  taxonomy, **B2**.1658–61
  virulence factors, **B2**.1661–2
  see also individual species
Actinobacillus actinomycetemcomitans,
    B2.1549–50, **B2**.1661–3, **B2**.1693–4
  antibacterial susceptibility/resistance,
    B2.1664
  characteristics, **B2**.1660 (Tab.), **B2**.1661,
    B2.1664
  culture and identification, **B2**.1663–4
  habitats, **B2**.1649–50
  infection
    endocarditis, **B1**.532, **B2**.1663
    gingivitis, **B1**.614
    localized juvenile periodontitis, **B2**.1662,
      B2.1663
    periodontal, **B2**.1662–3
    treatment, **B2**.1664
  virulence factors, **B2**.1661–2
    cytolethal distending toxin, **B2**.1661
    fimbriae, **B2**.1661
    immunosuppressive fraction, **B2**.1662
    leukotoxin, **B2**.1661, **B2**.1662
Actinobacillus arthritidis
  characteristics, **B2**.1659 (Tab.)
  classification, **B2**.1658–9
  habitats, **B2**.1665–6
Actinobacillus capsulatus
  characteristics, **B2**.1660 (Tab.)
  classification, **B2**.1658–9
  habitats, **B2**.1659
Actinobacillus delphinicola
  characteristics, **B2**.1660 (Tab.)
  classification, **B2**.1658–9
  habitats, **B2**.1659
  infection in sea mammals, **B2**.1665–6
Actinobacillus equuli
  characteristics, **B2**.1659 (Tab.)
  classification, **B2**.1658–9
  habitats, **B2**.1659
  infection
    in animals, **B2**.1665–6
    in humans, **B2**.1666
  subspecies *haemolyticus,* **B2**.1658–9
Actinobacillus hominis, **B2**.1665
  characteristics, **B2**.1659 (Tab.)
  classification, **B2**.1658–9
Actinobacillus indolicus
  characteristics, **B2**.1660 (Tab.), **B2**.1661
  classification, **B2**.1658–9
  habitats, **B2**.1659, **B2**.1665–6
Actinobacillus lignieresii
  characteristics, **B2**.1659 (Tab.)
  classification, **B2**.1658–9
  habitats, **B2**.1659, **B2**.1665–6
  infection
    in animals, **B2**.1665–6
    in humans, **B2**.1666
Actinobacillus minor
  characteristics, **B2**.1660 (Tab.), **B2**.1661
  classification, **B2**.1658–9

habitats, **B2**.1659, **B2**.1665–6
Actinobacillus muris
  characteristics, **B2**.1660 (Tab.)
  classification, **B2**.1658–9
  habitats, **B2**.1659
Actinobacillus pleuropneumoniae, **B1**.151,
    B2.1662, **B2**.1694
  animal infection, **B2**.1662
  characteristics, **B2**.1659 (Tab.)
  classification, **B2**.1658–9
  habitats, **B2**.1659
Actinobacillus porcinus
  characteristics, **B2**.1660 (Tab.), **B2**.1661
  classification, **B2**.1658–9
  habitats, **B2**.1659, **B2**.1665–6
Actinobacillus rossii
  characteristics, **B2**.1660 (Tab.)
  classification, **B2**.1658–9
  habitats, **B2**.1659
Actinobacillus salpingitidis, reclassification,
    B2.1658–9
Actinobacillus scotiae
  characteristics, **B2**.1660 (Tab.)
  classification, **B2**.1658–9
  habitats, **B2**.1659
  infection in sea mammals, **B2**.1665–6
Actinobacillus seminis
  characteristics, **B2**.1660 (Tab.)
  classification, **B2**.1658–9
  habitats, **B2**.1659
Actinobacillus succinogenes
  characteristics, **B2**.1660 (Tab.)
  classification, **B2**.1658–9
  habitats, **B2**.1659, **B2**.1665–6
Actinobacillus suis
  characteristics, **B2**.1659 (Tab.)
  classification, **B2**.1658–9
  habitats, **B2**.1659
  infection
    animals, **B2**.1665–6
    humans, **B2**.1666
Actinobacillus ureae, **B2**.1665
  characteristics, **B2**.1659 (Tab.), **B2**.1665
  classification, **B2**.1650, **B2**.1658–9, **B2**.1665
  infection in humans, **B2**.1665
Actinobacteria, **B2**.1024
  classification, **B2**.998
Actinobaculum schaalii, **B2**.1007 (Tab.),
    B2.1016 (Tab.)
Actinobaculum suis
  antibacterial susceptibility/resistance,
    B2.1011
  biochemical properties, **B2**.1009
  cell wall composition, **B2**.1005,
    B2.1010 (Tab.)
  characteristics, **B2**.1016 (Tab.)
  classification, **B2**.1005
  culture, **B2**.1008
  habitats, **B2**.1007 (Tab.)
  metabolism, **B2**.1009
  pathogenicity, **B2**.1007 (Tab.), **B2**.1018
Actinobaculum urinale, **B2**.1007 (Tab.)
Actinomadura, **B2**.1137–8, **B2**.1150
  antibacterial susceptibility/resistance,
    B2.1145, **B2**.1150

Actinomadura, (Continued)
  characteristics, **B2**.1150
  classification, **B2**.1137–8
  diaminopimelic acid and sugars, **B2**.1145
  infection, **B2**.1150, **B2**.1159–60
  microscopic morphology, **B2**.1143
Actinomadura latina, **B2**.1150
Actinomadura madurae, **M**.128 (Tab.),
    B2.1150, **B2**.1159–60
Actinomadura pelletieri, **M**.128 (Tab.),
    M.140 (Fig.), **B2**.1150
Actinomyces, **B2**.1005
  antibacterial susceptibility/resistance,
    B2.1011
    metronidazole, **B1**.495
  antigens, **B2**.1005, **B2**.1009–11, **B2**.1011 (Fig.)
  biochemical properties, **B2**.1008–9
  cell wall composition, **B2**.1005, **B2**.1009,
    B2.1009–11, **B2**.1010 (Tab.)
  characteristics, **B2**.1014 (Tab.)
  classification, **B2**.1005–6, **B2**.1011–12
  definition, **B2**.1005
  habitats, **B2**.1006
  identification, **B2**.1012–17
    biochemical tests, **B2**.1013
    commercial tests, **B2**.1013–17
    culture, **B2**.1007–8
    phenotypic tests, **B2**.1013
    protein electrophoresis, **B2**.1013
    serodiagnosis, **B2**.1017
  infection
    genital tract, **B1**.669
    intracranial abscess, **B1**.585
    mastitis, **B1**.230
    oral cavity abscess, **B1**.618
  isolation, **B2**.1012–13, **B2**.1012–17
    selective media, **B2**.1013
  metabolism, **B2**.1008–9
  morphology, **B2**.1006–7
    cellular morphology, **B2**.1006,
      B2.1008 (Fig.)
    colonial morphology, **B2**.1006–7,
      B2.1008 (Fig.)
  in normal microbiota, **B1**.296 (Tab.), **B1**.303,
    B2.1017–18
    oropharynx, **B1**.301, **B1**.609, **B1**.614
    vagina, **B1**.303
  pathogenicity, **B2**.1018
  stains, **M**.123 (Tab.), **M**.124–5
  typing, **B2**.1017
    genetic typing, **B2**.1017
    serological cross-reactions in,
      B2.1010 (Tab.)
  see also individual species
Actinomyces bernardiae, cell wall composition,
    B2.1009
Actinomyces bovis
  cellular morphology, **B2**.1006
  cell wall composition, **B2**.1005, **B2**.1009,
    B2.1010 (Tab.)
  characteristics, **B2**.1014 (Tab.)
  classification, **B2**.1005–6
  culture, **B2**.1008
  habitats, **B2**.1007 (Tab.)
  pathogenicity, **B2**.1007 (Tab.), **B2**.1018
  serological cross-reactions, **B2**.1010 (Tab.)

Actinomyces bowdenii, **B2**.1007 (Tab.),
    B2.1016 (Tab.)
Actinomyces canis, **B2**.1007 (Tab.),
    B2.1016 (Tab.)
Actinomyces cardiffensis, **B2**.1007 (Tab.),
    B2.1016 (Tab.)
Actinomyces catuli, **B2**.1007 (Tab.),
    B2.1016 (Tab.)
Actinomyces coleocanis, **B2**.1007 (Tab.),
    B2.1016 (Tab.)
Actinomyces denticolens
  antigens, **B2**.1009–11
  cell wall composition, **B2**.1010 (Tab.)
  characteristics, **B2**.1014 (Tab.)
  classification, **B2**.1012
  habitats, **B2**.1007 (Tab.)
  pathogenicity, **B2**.1007 (Tab.)
  serotyping, **B2**.1017
Actinomyces europaeus, **B2**.1007 (Tab.)
Actinomyces funkei, **B2**.1007 (Tab.),
    B2.1016 (Tab.)
Actinomyces georgiae
  cell wall composition, **B2**.1010 (Tab.)
  characteristics, **B2**.1014 (Tab.)
  classification, **B2**.1012
  habitats, **B2**.1007 (Tab.)
  pathogenicity, **B2**.1007 (Tab.)
Actinomyces gerencseriae
  antigens, **B2**.1009–11
  cell wall composition, **B2**.1009,
    B2.1010 (Tab.)
  characteristics, **B2**.1014 (Tab.)
  classification, **B2**.1012
  culture, **B2**.1007–8
    colonial morphology, **B2**.1006–7
  genetic typing, **B2**.1017
  habitats, **B2**.1007 (Tab.)
  pathogenicity, **B2**.1007 (Tab.), **B2**.1018
  serological cross-reactions, **B2**.1010 (Tab.)
Actinomyces graevenitzii, **B2**.1016 (Tab.)
  colonial morphology, **B2**.1006–7
  habitats, **B2**.1007 (Tab.)
  pathogenicity, **B2**.1007 (Tab.)
Actinomyces hongkongensis, **B2**.1007 (Tab.),
    B2.1016 (Tab.)
Actinomyces hordeovulneris
  antibacterial susceptibility/resistance,
    B2.1011
  cell wall composition, **B2**.1010 (Tab.)
  characteristics, **B2**.1014 (Tab.)
  classification, **B2**.1012
  culture, **B2**.1007–8
  habitats, **B2**.1007 (Tab.)
  pathogenicity, **B2**.1007 (Tab.), **B2**.1018
  serotyping, **B2**.1017
    cross-reactions, **B2**.1010 (Tab.)
Actinomyces howellii
  antigens, **B2**.1009–11
  cell wall composition, **B2**.1010 (Tab.)
  characteristics, **B2**.1014 (Tab.)
  classification, **B2**.1012
  habitats, **B2**.1007 (Tab.)
  pathogenicity, **B2**.1007 (Tab.)
  serotyping, **B2**.1017
Actinomyces humiferus, **B2**.1012

Actinomyces hyovaginalis
  cell wall composition, **B2**.1009,
    B2.1010 (Tab.)
  characteristics, **B2**.1014 (Tab.)
  colonial morphology, **B2**.1006–7
  habitats, **B2**.1007 (Tab.)
  pathogenicity, **B2**.1007 (Tab.), **B2**.1018
Actinomyces israelii, **B2**.1014 (Tab.)
  antigens, **B2**.1009–11, **B2**.1011 (Fig.)
  biochemical properties, **B2**.1008–9
  cellular morphology, **B2**.1006, **B2**.1008 (Fig.)
  cell wall composition, **B2**.1009,
    B2.1010 (Tab.)
  classification, **B2**.1006, **B2**.1012
  culture, **B2**.1007–8
    colonial morphology, **B2**.1006–7,
      B2.1008 (Fig.)
  genetic typing, **B2**.1017
  habitats, **B2**.1006, **B2**.1007 (Tab.)
  histopathology, **M**.128 (Tab.), **M**.140 (Fig.)
    stains, **M**.122
  identification, **B2**.1017
    serological cross-reactions, **B2**.1010 (Tab.)
  infection, endophthalmitis, **B1**.603
  isolation, **B2**.1013
  metabolism, **B2**.1008–9
  pathogenicity, **B2**.1007 (Tab.), **B2**.1018
Actinomyces marimammalium, **B2**.1007 (Tab.),
    B2.1016 (Tab.)
Actinomyces meyeri, **M**.128 (Tab.)
  antibacterial susceptibility/resistance,
    B2.1011
  biochemical properties, **B2**.1009
  cell wall composition, **B2**.1010 (Tab.)
  characteristics, **B2**.1014 (Tab.)
  classification, **B2**.1012
  culture, **B2**.1007–8
  genetic typing, **B2**.1017
  habitats, **B2**.1007 (Tab.)
  metabolism, **B2**.1009
  pathogenicity, **B2**.1007 (Tab.)
Actinomyces naeslundii, **M**.128 (Tab.),
    B2.1014 (Tab.)
  antigens, **B2**.1009–11, **B2**.1011 (Fig.)
  biochemical properties, **B2**.1008–9
  cellular morphology, **B2**.1006, **B2**.1008 (Fig.)
  cell wall composition, **B2**.1009,
    B2.1010 (Tab.)
  classification, **B2**.1012
  culture, **B2**.1007–8
    colonial morphology, **B2**.1006–7,
      B2.1008 (Fig.)
  habitats, **B2**.1007 (Tab.)
  identification, **B2**.1017
    genetic typing, **B2**.1017
  isolation, **B2**.1013
  metabolism, **B2**.1008–9
  as normal microbiota, **B2**.1017–18
  pathogenicity, **B2**.1007 (Tab.), **B2**.1018
  serotyping, **B2**.1017
    cross-reactions, **B2**.1010 (Tab.)
Actinomyces nasicola, **B2**.1007 (Tab.),
    B2.1016 (Tab.)
Actinomyces neuii
  antibacterial susceptibility/resistance,
    B2.1011

Actinomyces neuii (*Continued*)
  cell wall composition, **B2**.1010 (Tab.)
  characteristics, **B2**.1014 (Tab.)
  colonial morphology, **B2**.1006–7
  habitats, **B2**.1007 (Tab.)
  pathogenicity, **B2**.1007 (Tab.)
Actinomyces odontolyticus, **M**.128 (Tab.)
  antigens, **B2**.1009–11
  cellular morphology, **B2**.1006
  cell wall composition, **B2**.1009,
    B2.1010 (Tab.)
  characteristics, **B2**.1014 (Tab.)
  classification, **B2**.1012
  colonial morphology, **B2**.1006–7
  culture, **B2**.1007–8
  genetic typing, **B2**.1017
  habitats, **B2**.1007 (Tab.)
  isolation, **B2**.1013
  pathogenicity, **B2**.1007 (Tab.), **B2**.1018
  serological cross-reactions, **B2**.1010 (Tab.)
Actinomyces oricola, **B2**.1007 (Tab.),
    B2.1016 (Tab.)
Actinomyces pyogenes
  cell wall composition, **B2**.1009
  reclassification, **B2**.1005
Actinomyces radicidentis
  characteristics, **B2**.1016 (Tab.)
  habitats, **B2**.1007 (Tab.)
  pathogenicity, **B2**.1007 (Tab.)
Actinomyces radingae
  cell wall composition, **B2**.1009,
    B2.1010 (Tab.)
  characteristics, **B2**.1014 (Tab.)
  habitats, **B2**.1007 (Tab.)
  pathogenicity, **B2**.1007 (Tab.), **B2**.1018
Actinomyces slackii
  antigens, **B2**.1009–11
  cell wall composition, **B2**.1010 (Tab.)
  characteristics, **B2**.1014 (Tab.)
  classification, **B2**.1012
  habitats, **B2**.1007 (Tab.)
  pathogenicity, **B2**.1007 (Tab.)
  serotyping, **B2**.1017
Actinomyces suimastitidis, **B2**.1007 (Tab.),
    B2.1016 (Tab.)
Actinomyces turicensis
  cell wall composition, **B2**.1010 (Tab.)
  characteristics, **B2**.1014 (Tab.)
  habitats, **B2**.1006, **B2**.1007 (Tab.)
  pathogenicity, **B2**.1007 (Tab.), **B2**.1018
Actinomyces urinale, **B2**.1016 (Tab.)
Actinomyces urogenitalis, **B2**.1007 (Tab.),
    B2.1016 (Tab.)
Actinomyces vaccimaxillae, **B2**.1007 (Tab.),
    B2.1016 (Tab.)
Actinomyces viscosus, **M**.128 (Tab.)
  antigens, **B2**.1009–11, **B2**.1011 (Fig.)
  biochemical properties, **B2**.1008–9
  cell wall composition, **B2**.1009,
    B2.1010 (Tab.)
  characteristics, **B2**.1014 (Tab.)
  classification, **B2**.1012
  culture, **B2**.1007–8
  habitats, **B2**.1007 (Tab.)
  identification, **B2**.1017
    genetic typing, **B2**.1017

  serological cross-reactions, **B2**.1010 (Tab.)
  isolation, **B2**.1013
  metabolism, **B2**.1008–9
  morphology, **B2**.1006
    colonies, **B2**.1006–7
  normal oral flora, **B1**.609
  pathogenicity, **B2**.1018
Actinomycetales, **B2**.1181
  see also individual species
Actinomycetes
  aerial hyphae, **B2**.1143
  airborne dispersal, **B1**.189
  antibacterial susceptibility/resistance,
    B2.1138, **B2**.1145
  biochemical testing, **B2**.1141–5
    acetamide hydrolysis, **B2**.1143
    arylsulfatase, **B2**.1143
    carbohydrates, **B2**.1143–4
    gelatin hydrolysis, **B2**.1144
    lysozyme, **B2**.1144
    Middlebrook opacification, **B2**.1144
    substrate decomposition, **B2**.1144
  cell wall and cell membrane composition,
    B2.1145–6
  classification, **B2**.1137–9
    strain typing, **B2**.1148–9
    taxonomic relationships, **B2**.1139
    see also individual genus/species
  conidia, **B2**.1143
  diaminopimelic acid, **B2**.1145
  histopathology, **M**.128 (Tab.)
    stains, **M**.123 (Tab.), **M**.124–5
  identification
    microscopic morphology, **B2**.1141–3
    molecular, **B2**.1146–8
    other systems and methods, **B2**.1144–5
    phenotypic, **B2**.1141–3
    serologic testing, **B2**.1149–50
  isolation and cultivation, **B2**.1138–41
  lipids, **B2**.1145–6
  menaquinones, **B2**.1145
  pathogenicity, **B2**.1149
  serology, **M**.391–2
  spores, **M**.5 (Fig.)
  staining properties, **B2**.1139–40
  temperature studies, **B2**.1144
  thermophilic, **B2**.1170
  waterborne, **B1**.220
Actinomycetoma, **M**.27, **M**.385, **M**.386–7
  clinical features, **M**.388
  geographical distribution, **M**.387–8
  histopathology, **M**.128 (Tab.)
  infection *see* Actinomycoses
Actinomycetoma
  etiologic agents, **B2**.1159–60
  treatment, **B2**.1159–60
Actinomycin, **P**.179
Actinomycoses
  abdominal, **M**.140 (Fig.)
  diagnosis, **M**.389
  histopathology, **M**.140 (Fig.)
  human, **B2**.1018
  mycetoma, **M**.140 (Fig.)
  therapy, **M**.389
  thoracic, **M**.140 (Fig.)

Activated protein C, septic shock therapy,
    I.702–3
Activation factors, **P**.70–2
Activation-induced cell death (AICD)
  CD4+ T cells in HIV infection, **I**.792
  IL-16, **I**.289
  peripheral tolerance, **I**.750
Acute adult T-cell leukemia, **V2**.1289–90
Acute atrophic candidiasis, **M**.598
Acute bronchiolitis, **V1**.776–7
  clinical manifestations, **V1**.776–7
  etiology, **V1**.776
  pathogenesis, **V1**.776
    host immune response, **V1**.776
  risk factors, **V1**.777
  treatment, **V1**.777
Acute cytokine release syndromes,
    interferon-γ, **I**.288
Acute dermatotolymphangitis, lymphatic
    filariasis, **P**.773
Acute epidemic hemorrhagic conjunctivitis
    (AHC), **V2**.872
  Coxsackie virus, **V2**.872
  Enterovirus 70 infection, **V2**.872
Acute gastritis, *Helicobacter pylori* infection,
    B2.1578, **B2**.1579
Acute infection (viral)
  duration, **V1**.258
  immune clearance, **V1**.258
Acute inflammatory reactions, opisthorchiasis,
    P.651
Acute lymphocytic leukemia (ALL),
    I.788 (Tab.)
Acute mastoiditis, pathogenesis, **B1**.617
Acute motor axonal neuropathy (AMAN),
    B2.1551
Acute myeloid leukemia (AML)
  immunodeficiency, **I**.788 (Tab.)
  TCE peptide vaccines, **I**.865 (Tab.)
Acute phase proteins (APPs), **I**.193, **I**.198–206,
    B1.739
  clinical use, **I**.206
  deficiencies, **I**.209
  evolutionary conservation, **I**.198–9
  inhibitory factors, **I**.197
  innate immune response, **I**.199–202
  microbial delivery, **I**.201 (Fig.), **I**.202 (Fig.)
  negative type, **I**.205
  procoagulant/fibrinolytic proteins, **I**.203–4
  production
    IL-1, **I**.284–5
    IL-6, **I**.285
    IL-11, **I**.279
  protease inhibitors, **I**.200–2
  regulatory molecules, **I**.204
  timing of production, **I**.198
  transport proteins, **I**.202–3
  see also individual types; specific types
Acute phase response, **I**.194 (Tab.), **B1**.739–40,
    I.193–214
  behavioral changes, **I**.209
  control, **I**.209
  C-reactive protein, **B1**.739
  definition, **I**.193
  disadvantage, **B1**.739

Acute phase response (*Continued*)
  disorders, **I.**209–10
    see also specific diseases/infection
  Escherichia coli infection, **B1.**740
  fever, **I.**209
  hemopoietic responses, **I.**198, **I.**206–7
    lymphocytes, **I.**206
    monocytes, **I.**207
    platelets, **I.**207
    polymorphonuclear cells, **I.**206–7
    red cells, **I.**207
  hormonal changes, **I.**208–9
    arginine vasopressin, **I.**208
    catecholamines, **I.**208
    corticotropin-releasing factor, **I.**208
    glucagon, **I.**208
    glucocorticoids, **I.**198 (Fig.), **I.**208
    growth hormone, **I.**208
    insulin-like growth factor 1, **I.**208
    leptin, **I.**208–9
    procalcitonin, **I.**208
    prolactin, **I.**208
    thyroxine, **I.**208
    triiodothyronine, **I.**208
  induction, **I.**194–8
    injury, **I.**194
    LPS, **I.**196–7
    nutrient deficiency, **I.**197
    proinflammatory cytokines, **I.**195–7
    signal transduction, **I.**196 (Fig.)
    systemic inflammation, **I.**194–5
    timing, **I.**194–5, **I.**195 (Fig.)
    TLRs, **I.**194
  interpretation, **B1.**739–40
    organ failure effects, **B1.**739–40
    species-specific effects, **B1.**740
  liver protective responses, **I.**205–6
  local hyperemia, **B1.**739
  measurement, **B1.**740
    neutrophil responses, **B1.**740
    nitroblue tetrazolium reduction, **B1.**740
    procalcitonin levels, **B1.**740
  metabolic changes, **I.**207–8
    lipid metabolism, **I.**207
    micronutrients, **I.**207–8
    protein metabolism, **I.**207
  neutrophils, **B1.**739
  signs/symptoms, **I.**193
    anorexia, **I.**198
    fever, **I.**197–8, **I.**198 (Fig.)
    somnolence, **I.**198, **I.**209
  Staphylococcus aureus infection, **B1.**740
  see also Acute phase proteins (APPs);
    Immune response; Proinflammatory
    cytokines
Acute pseudomembranous candidiasis, **M.**598
Acute pulmonary histoplasmosis capsulati *see*
    Histoplasmosis
Acute pulmonary invasive aspergillosis,
    M.698–9, **M.**699 (Fig.), **M.**705–6,
    M.719–26
Acute respiratory distress syndrome (ARDS),
    B1.633–4
Acute schistosomiasis, **I.**718–19
Acute sinusitis, **B1.**615

Acute suppurative otitis media, **B1.**617
Acute suppurative parotitis, melioidosis,
    B2.1628, **B2.**1628 (Fig.)
N-Acylated-D-perosamine, *Brucella* LPS,
    B2.1725
Acylation, influenza hemagglutinin, **V1.**652
Acylation stimulating protein (ASP), **I.**147
Acyl carrier protein (ACP), **B1.**61
N-Acylhomoserine lactones, **B1.**170–1,
    B1.171 (Fig.)
Acylureidopenicillins, *Proteus*, **B2.**1443–4
Adamson's fringe, **M.**238
Adanson, M, **B1.**11
Adaptive immune response, **B1.**177, **I.**403–4
  bacterial infection, **I.**646–7, **I.**646 (Fig.)
  Balantidium coli infection, **P.**279–80
  candidiasis *see specific infection*
  complement *see* Complement
  defects, **I.**575
  immune evasion, **V1.**311–12
    viral infection, **I.**630–9
  immunodeficiency diseases/disorders,
    I.773–82
  innate immunity *vs.*, **I.**377 (Tab.)
  parasitic infection
    malaria, **P.**486
    schistosomiasis, **P.**605
    trichomoniasis, **P.**258–9
  prion diseases, **V2.**1384–6
  time scales, **V1.**271 (Fig.)
  viral infection, **I.**618
    HSV infection, **V1.**284–5
    Human respiratory syncytial virus
      infection, **V1.**794–6
    immune interference, **I.**630–9
    influenza, **V1.**663
  see also specific mechanisms
ADAR1, microbial recognition, **I.**24 (Tab.)
Adcaris lumbricoides, **I.**682–3
Addison's disease, **M.**550
Additions, **B1.**87
Adefovir
  hepatitis B therapy, **V2.**1261, **V2.**1629
  HIV infection, **V2.**1334–6
  resistance, **V2.**1637
  structure, **V2.**1617 (Fig.)
Adelaide River virus (ARV)
  classification, **V1.**385–6
  genome structure, **V2.**1112 (Fig.)
Adenine arabinoside *see* Vidarabine
Adeno-associated viruses (AAV), **V1.**440,
    V1.441 (Fig.)
  discovery, **V1.**409–10
  DNA strand polarization, **V1.**42
  epidemiology, **V1.**427–8
    non-human primates, **V1.**427–8
  gene repertoire, **V1.**408
  gene therapy vectors, **V1.**428–9,
    V2.1595 (Tab.), **V2.**1598–602
    animal models, **V2.**1600–1
    clinical trials, **V2.**1601–2
    diseases, **V1.**428, **V2.**1600–1
    immune response, **V2.**1600–1
    Rep gene deletion, **V2.**1599–600
    'self-complementary' vectors, **V1.**428–9
    S phase cell targeting, **V1.**428

    stable vertical transmission, **V1.**428
    tissue specificity limitation, **V1.**429
    transgene size limitation, **V1.**429
    vector production, **V2.**1600
  genome, **V2.**1598
    sequencing, **V1.**409–10
  heparan sulfate binding, **V1.**416–17
  historical aspects, **V1.**427
  infection *see* Adeno-associated viruses
    (AAV), infection
  life cycle, **V2.**1598–9
    cell entry, **V1.**416–17
    platelet derived growth factor binding,
      V1.416–17
  replication, **V1.**148 (Tab.), **V1.**159–60,
    V1.408, **V1.**418–20, **V2.**1599
    cellular proteins, **V1.**159
    helper virus requirement, **V1.**160
    initiation, **V1.**159
    inverted terminal repeat (ITR) structures,
      V1.159–60, **V2.**1599
    leading-strand replication, **V1.**159
    origin of replication, **V1.**159
    proteins, **V1.**159
    Rep40 protein, **V1.**159, **V2.**1599
    Rep52 protein, **V1.**159, **V2.**1599
    Rep68 protein, **V1.**159, **V1.**418–19,
      V2.1599
    Rep78 protein, **V1.**159, **V1.**418–19,
      V2.1599
    site specific integration, **V2.**1599
    'terminal resolution,' **V1.**419
    viral proteins, **V1.**149 (Tab.)
  structural proteins, **V2.**1599
  structure/morphology, **V2.**1598
  see also Dependovirus
Adeno-associated viruses (AAV), infection
  adenovirus coinfection, **V2.**1598–9
  gene integration, **V1.**423–4
  herpesvirus coinfection, **V2.**1598–9
  infection routes, **V1.**428
  nuclear targeting, **V1.**424
Adeno-associated virus 2 (AAV-2)
  capsids, **V1.**420–1
  gene transcription, **V1.**414 (Fig.)
  genome structure, **V1.**414 (Fig.)
  morphology/structure, **V1.**412, **V1.**413 (Fig.)
  type species, **V1.**409–10
Adeno-associated virus-5 (AAV-5)
  gene transcription, **V1.**414 (Fig.)
  genome structure, **V1.**414 (Fig.)
Adenocarcinomas
  BCE peptide vaccines, **I.**855 (Tab.)
  TCE peptide vaccines, **I.**865 (Tab.)
Adenolymphangitis, lymphatic filariasis, **P.**773
Adenophorea, **P.**588–9
  features, **P.**588
  Trichinelloidea, **P.**588–9
Adenosine-deaminase ADAR1, interferon
    actions, **V1.**295
Adenosine deaminase deficiency (ADA), **I.**774
Adenovir *see* Penciclovir
Adenoviridae
  characteristics, **V1.**177 (Tab.)
  classification, **V1.**27 (Tab.), **V1.**43 (Tab.),
    V1.45, **V2.**1594–5

Adenoviridae (*Continued*)
  see also Adenoviruses; *Atadenovirus;*
    Aviadenovirus; Mastadenovirus;
    Siadenovirus; *specific viruses*
Adenoviruses, **V1.439–47**
  adeno-associated virus replication, **V1**.160
  alternate splicing, **V1**.180
  antigens, **V1**.443
    serotype-specific, **V1**.443
  classification, **V1**.439, **V1**.443
    subgroups by disease, **V1**.444 (Tab.)T
  directed mutagenesis, **V1**.183–4
  discovery/historical aspects, **V1**.439,
    V2.1594–5
  enteric, **V1**.444
  fecal-oral transmission, **V1**.445
  fecal shedding, **V1**.444
  gene expression, **V1**.115 (Fig.)
  gene therapy vectors, **V2**.1594–7,
    V2.1595 (Tab.)
    examples, **V2**.1597
    helper-dependent vectors, **V2**.1597
    vector design, **V2**.1595–6
  as gene vector, cystic fibrosis gene therapy,
    B1.651
  genome, **V1**.160–1, **V1**.439–41, **V2**.1595
    inverted terminal repeats (ITRs), **V1**.441
    sequencing, **V1**.442
  genome replication, **V1**.123, **V1**.123 (Fig.),
    V1.160–2, **V1**.163 (Fig.), **V1**.218,
    V1.441–2
    cellular proteins, **V1**.160, **V1**.161–2
    DNA-binding protein (DBP), **V1**.160,
      V1.161, **V1**.162
    DNA polymerase, **V1**.147–8, **V1**.149 (Tab.),
      V1.160, **V1**.162
    elongation, **V1**.162
    helicase lack, **V1**.149
    initiation, **V1**.162
    nuclear factor I (NF1), **V1**.160, **V1**.161–2
    nuclear factor 2 (NF2), **V1**.160
    Oct-1 protein, **V1**.160–2
    origin of replication, **V1**.160, **V1**.161
    priming mechanisms, **V1**.162
    pTP, **V1**.149 (Tab.), **V1**.161, **V1**.162
    replication compartments/centers,
      V1.170–1
    strand displacement synthesis, **V1**.162
    terminal protein, **V1**.160
    viral proteins, **V1**.160–161
  host cell interactions
    double-strand break repair mechanisms,
      V1.169–70
    host protein synthesis, **V1**.121, **V1**.203,
      V1.224
    S-phase entry, **V1**.217
  immune evasion, **V1**.298 (Tab.), **V2**.1596–7
    antigen presentation, **V1**.229–30
    apoptosis interference, **V1**.323, **V1**.324–5,
      I.627, **V2**.1595
    cytokines, **V1**.298 (Tab.), **V1**.316, **I**.623,
      V2.1596–7
    death-receptor inhibitors, **I**.626
    IFN interference, **V1**.230, **V1**.315, **I**.619,
      V2.1596–7
    MHC interference, **V1**.287, **V1**.321,
      V1.322, **I**.634, **I**.637

peptide-loading complex, **I**.633–4
infection *see* Adenovirus infection
isolation/propagation and identification,
  V1.95, **V1**.96 (Tab.), **V1**.446
  cytospinning, **V2**.1540–1
  genotypes, **V1**.443
  mixed cell culture, **V1**.88
  monoclonal antibodies, **V1**.443
  serotypes, **V1**.439
  tissue/organ culture, **V1**.446
morphology/structure, **V1**.68 (Fig.),
  V1.439–40, **V1**.440 (Fig.), **V1**.442 (Fig.)
  capsid morphology and structure, **V2**.1595
  pentons and hexons, **V1**.439–40, **V1**.443
polypeptides, **V1**.439–40, **V1**.442–3,
  V1.443 (Tab.)
  'early' proteins, **V1**.441, **V1**.445
  'late' proteins, **V1**.442
  non-structural, **V1**.442
  see also specific proteins
properties, **V1**.439–43
protease, **V1**.442
protein synthesis/translation, **V1**.442
  splicing mechanisms, **V1**.114–15
  temporal control, **V1**.118
receptors, **V1**.212
recombination, herpesviruses, **V1**.187
replication, **V1**.440
  cell entry mechanisms, **V1**.106–7,
    V1.107 (Fig.), **V1**.108–9, **V1**.213,
    V1.215–16, **V1**.241 (Tab.), **V1**.441
  genome *see above*
  maturation of virion, **V1**.442–3
  mRNA synthesis, **V1**.110, **V1**.441
  stability and resistance, **V1**.439–40
  terminal protein (TP), **V1**.439–40
    precursor (pTP), **V1**.441–2
  transcription, **V1**.441
    alternate start sites, **V1**.180
  transcription factors, **V1**.441, **V1**.442
  as vaccine vectors, **I**.897–8, **I**.897 (Tab.),
    I.899, **I**.902, **I**.903
    attenuated vaccine vectors, **I**.830–1
    skin application, **I**.823
  see also Adenoviridae
Adenovirus infection, **V1**.160, **V1**.443–6
  abortive, **V1**.443–4
  adeno-associated virus coinfection,
    V2.1598–9
  in AIDS/HIV infection, **V2**.1499 (Tab.),
    V2.1504
  animal infection, **V1**.444–5
  cell entry, **V1**.241 (Tab.)
  children, **V1**.445
  clinical features, **V1**.443–5
    cytopathic effects, **V1**.94 (Fig.)
    epidemic keratoconjunctivitis (shipyard
      eye), **V1**.444, **V1**.444 (Tab.)T
    gastrointestinal disease, **V1**.444
    respiratory disease, **V1**.443–4
  control, **V1**.446
  diagnosis, **V1**.446
    cytopathology, **V2**.1534 (Tab.)
  epidemiology, **V1**.368, **V1**.445
  immune response, **V1**.445–6, **V2**.1596
    cell-mediated, **V1**.445–6

defensin actions, **I**.168
'early' proteins role, **V1**.445
humoral, **V1**.445
IFN-α effects, **V1**.295
IFNs, **I**.260 (Tab.)
IL-1, **V1**.296–7
immunocompromised patients, **V1**.444
immunodeficient patients (non-HIV),
  V2.1508–9
oncogenesis, **V1**.337–8, **V1**.338 (Tab.),
  V2.1594–5
tumors associated, **V1**.332 (Tab.)
pathogenesis/pathology, **V1**.445, **V2**.1596–7
subgroups of adenoviruses, **V1**.444 (Tab.)
SV40 co-infection, **V2**.1596
therapy
  antiviral chemotherapy, **V2**.1631
  imiquimod, **V2**.1631
vaccination, **V1**.446
Adenovirus polymerase (Ad pol), **V1**.160
Adenovirus type 2
  genome structure, **V1**.441
  polypeptides, **V1**.443 (Tab.)
Adenovirus type 5, **V1**.445
Adenovirus type 8 infection, **V1**.444
  keratoconjunctivitis due to, **B1**.386
Adenovirus type 11 infection, **V1**.444
Adenovirus type 35 infection, **V1**.445
Adenovirus type 40, **V1**.446
Adenovirus type 41, **V1**.446
Adenylate cyclase toxin (ACT), *Bordetella,*
  B2.1789, **B2**.1789 (Tab.), **B2**.1796–7
Adenylyl cyclase hemolysin toxin (AC-Hly),
  I.654–5
ADEPT (Antibody Directed Enzyme Pro-drug
  Therapy), **I**.360
  advantages, **I**.360
  amplification step, **I**.360
  drawbacks, **I**.360
  pharmacokinetics, **I**.360
adhE gene, *E. coli* K-12, **B1**.55
Adherence
  eukaryotic receptors, **B1**.147
  host-and species-specific tropisms, **B1**.147–8
  Mycoplasma, **B2**.1986
  nonspecific, **B1**.147
  pathogenicity mechanism, **B1**.147
  specific, **B1**.147
Adhesins, **B1**.147–9
  Aeromonas, **B2**.1536
  Bordetella, **B1**.627, **B2**.1799
  Enterococcus, **B2**.897
  Helicobacter, **B2**.1577–8
  Pseudomonas aeruginosa, **B1**.627
  Streptococcus pneumoniae, **B1**.627
  tissue specificity, **B1**.147–8
  see also specific types
Adhesion molecules
  basophils, **I**.58, **I**.59 (Tab.)
  CNS expression, **V2**.1409
  Entamoeba histolytica, **P**.205
  eosinophils, **I**.59 (Tab.), **I**.60
  expression, TLR stimulus, **I**.697
  induction, lymphotoxin, **I**.286–7
  lymphocyte migration, **I**.505

Adhesion molecules (*Continued*)
  SCF effects, **I**.275
  TCR–superantigen binding, **I**.560
  vascular cell adhesion molecule 1, **I**.275
Adhesion ring
  CTL killing mechanisms, **I**.474, **I**.474 (Fig.)
  lymphocyte-mediated cytotoxicity,
    I.474 (Fig.), **I**.477–8
Adiaspiromycosis, **M**.809
  AIDS, **M**.809, **M**.813, **M**.814–15, **M**.821
  causative agents, **M**.809
    see also Emmonsia; individual species
  clinical presentation, **M**.813–15
  diagnosis, **M**.125, **M**.127, **M**.809, **M**.814,
    M.817–21, **M**.818
    cytochemistry, **M**.816
    direct examination, **M**.817
    histopathology, **M**.815
    immune response, **M**.816–17
    radiology, **M**.814, **M**.814 (Fig.)
  differential diagnosis, **M**.821
  epidemiology, **M**.812–13
  histopathology, **M**.128 (Tab.), **M**.135 (Fig.)
  history, **M**.26–7, **M**.811–12
  therapy, **M**.821
    amphotericin B, **M**.821
    flucytosine, **M**.821
    ketoconazole, **M**.821
    thiabendazole, **M**.821
  unconfirmed reports, **M**.815
Adiaspores, *Emmonsia,* **M**.809–11,
    M.815 (Fig.), **M**.816, **M**.817 (Fig.)
Adipocytes, IL-11 effects, **I**.279
Adjuvants, **I**.926–32, **I**.928 (Tab.), **V2**.1555–7
  attenuated tetanus toxin, **I**.925
  definition, **I**.925
  delivery routes, **I**.926–7
  DNA vaccines, **I**.918–19, **I**.918 (Tab.)
  history, **I**.925
  IL-2, **I**.878–9
  IL-12, **I**.879
  immunostimulating particles
    structure, **I**.930
    vaccine models, **I**.930–1
    see also Immunostimulating particles
      (ISCOMs)
  inactivated diphtheria toxin, **I**.925
  inactivated (killed) vaccines, **V2**.1552–3
  intranasal vaccination, **I**.830, **I**.831–2
  mechanism of action, **I**.896, **I**.926–7
    APC activation, **I**.926
    depot effects, **I**.926
    MHC class II expression, **I**.926
    Th1/Th2 cell polarization, **I**.926
    TLRs, **I**.926
  mutated bacterial toxins, **I**.931–2
    development, **I**.931–2
    intranasal administration, **I**.932
    oral administration, **I**.932
    vaccine models, **I**.932
  necessity in attenuated vaccines, **I**.896
  new types, **I**.927–32
    see also individual types
  purified vaccine components, **I**.925
  TCE peptide vaccines, **I**.878–9

transcutaneous immunization, **I**.837–8
  virosomes, **I**.929
  see also individual types
Adolescents
  hepatitis A, **V2**.1173
  vaccination programs, **V2**.1559
Adonitol fermentation, Enterobacteriaceae
  identification, **B2**.1319 (Tab.)
ADP-ribose 1'-phosphatase, coronaviruses,
  V1.832–3
ADRBR gene, **I**.580
Adrenal glands
  histoplasmosis capsulati, **M**.523–4,
    M.524 (Fig.)
  Pneumocystis carinii infection, **M**.785
Adrenaline injection, gas gangrene after,
  B2.1111, **B2**.1113
Adrenocorticotrophic hormone (ACTH),
  I.169
Adressins, intracellular bacteria, **I**.649
Adult respiratory distress syndrome (ARDS),
  I.699–700
  blastomycosis, **M**.489
  C5 blocking antibody therapy, **I**.158
  soluble complement receptor 1 therapy,
    I.158
Adults
  Human respiratory syncytial virus infection,
    V1.791, **V1**.797–8
  influenza, **V1**.660–1
  Paragonimus heterotremus, **P**.641 (Fig.)
Adult T-cell leukemia/lymphoma (ATL),
    I.801–2, **V2**.1289–90, **V2**.1429
  diagnosis, **V2**.1289–90
  IFN-α therapy, **V2**.1291–2
  subtypes, **V2**.1289–90
Advanced medical care, emerging infection,
  V2.1660
Adventitious agents, inactivated (killed)
  vaccines, **V2**.1556
Aedes vector
  California encephalitis, **V2**.1048–9
  Chikungunya virus, **V2**.1021
  dengue fever, **V1**.372
  Dengue virus, **V2**.1000
  Eastern equine encephalitis virus, **V2**.1019
  La Crosse virus, **V2**.1048–9
  Murray Valley encephalitis, **V2**.1003
  Ross River virus, **V2**.1022
  Semliki Forest virus, **V2**.1023–4
  Sindbis virus, **V2**.1023
  Western equine encephalitis virus, **V2**.1020
  yellow fever, **V1**.372, **V2**.999
Aequorea victoria, green fluorescent protein,
  B1.207
Aeration tanks, airborne bacteria,
  B1.186 (Tab.)
Aerial disinfection, **B1**.430, **B1**.435 (Tab.)
Aerobacter, nitrification, **B1**.200
Aerobactin, **B1**.151
Aerobic blood cultures, **B1**.513–14
Aerobic endospore formers
  Bacillus see Bacillus
  habitats, **B2**.924
  non-*Bacillus* derived, **B2**.922–3
Aerobic pathways, larval cestodes, **P**.681

Aerobic respiration, **B1**.63–5
Aerococcus, as normal microbiota,
  B1.296 (Tab.)
Aerococcus viridans, as normal microbiota,
  B1.296 (Tab.)
  skin colonization, **B1**.304
Aerodigestive tract, HPV infection,
  V1.463 (Tab.), **V1**.464, **V1**.465 (Fig.),
  V1.465 (Tab.)
Aeromonadaceae, **B2**.1532
Aeromonas, **B2**.1524–40
  antibacterial susceptibility/resistance,
    B2.1532–4
    acquired, **B2**.1534
    ampicillin, **B2**.1532–4
    β-lactam antibiotics, **B1**.472–3, **B2**.1534
    cephalosporin, **B2**.1532–4
    plasmids, **B2**.1530
  bacteriophages, **B2**.1535
  characteristics, **B2**.1330 (Tab.), **B2**.1512–13,
    B2.1513 (Tab.)
  classification, **B2**.1507, **B2**.1524,
    B2.1525 (Tab.), **B2**.1530–1
    controversies, **B2**.1531
    molecular methods, **B2**.1531
    phylogenetics, **B2**.1530
  culture, **B2**.1529
    mesophilic strains, **B2**.1529
    pigment formation, **B2**.1529
    psychrophillic strains, **B2**.1529
  genetics, **B2**.1529–30
    ahsA gene, **B2**.1525
    plasmids, **B2**.1529–30
    vapA gene, **B2**.1525
  habitats, **B2**.1524–5
    foods, **B2**.1524–5
    freshwater, **B2**.1524–5
  identification, **B2**.1532, **B2**.1533 (Tab.)
    commercial assays, **B2**.1532
    conventional assays, **B2**.1532
    dihydrolase reactions, **B2**.1532
    Møarboxylase test, **B2**.1532
    molecular methods, **B2**.1532
    PCR, **B2**.1532
    screening reactions, **B2**.1532
    selective media, **B2**.1532
    Voges–Proskauer test, **B2**.1532
  infection
    endophthalmitis, **B1**.603
    nosocomial, **B1**.401 (Tab.)
  isolation, **B2**.1531–2
    blood samples, **B2**.1531
    cerebrospinal fluid, **B2**.1531
    gastrointestinal samples, **B2**.1531–2
  metabolism, **B2**.1529
  morphology, **B2**.1525–9
    bundle-forming pili (Bfp), **B2**.1528
    capsules, **B2**.1527
    flagella, **B2**.1527–8
    flagellin, **B2**.1527–8
    LPS, **B2**.1527, **B2**.1535
    pili, **B2**.1528
    porins, **B2**.1528–9
    S-layers, **B2**.1525, **B2**.1526 (Fig.)
  in normal microbiota, **B1**.296 (Tab.)

Aeromonas, (Continued)
pathogenicity, **B2**.1535–6
adhesins, **B2**.1536
β-hemolysin, **B2**.1535–6
cytotonic enterotoxins, **B2**.1536
enterotoxin, **B2**.1535–6
gasteroenteritis, **B2**.1535–6
secreted enzymes, **B2**.1536
typing, **B2**.1534–5
biotyping, **B2**.1534
conventional methods, **B2**.1534
molecular methods, **B2**.1535
serotyping, **B2**.1535
vegetables, **B1**.282
waterborne, **B1**.220, **B1**.221, **B1**.223
see also individual species
Aeromonas allosaccharophilia,
B2.1525 (Tab.)
Aeromonas bestarium, **B2**.1525 (Tab.)
culture, **B2**.1529
identification, **B2**.1533 (Tab.)
Aeromonas caviae, **B2**.1525 (Tab.)
antibacterial susceptibility/resistance,
B2.1532–4
β-lactams, **B2**.1534
classification, **B2**.1530, **B2**.1531
habitats, **B2**.1524–5
identification, **B2**.1533 (Tab.)
PCR assays, **B2**.1532
metabolism, **B2**.1529
morphology
flagella, **B2**.1527–8
LPS, **B2**.1527
pathogenicity, **B2**.1524, **B2**.1536
adhesins, **B2**.1536
β-hemolysin, **B2**.1535–6
secreted enzymes, **B2**.1536
Aeromonas culiciola, **B2**.1525 (Tab.)
classification, **B2**.1531
Aeromonas encheleia, **B2**.1525 (Tab.)
Aeromonas eucrenophila, **B2**.1525 (Tab.)
culture, **B2**.1529
identification, **B2**.1533 (Tab.)
Aeromonas hydrophila, **B2**.1525 (Tab.)
antibacterial susceptibility/resistance,
B2.1532–4
β-lactams, **B2**.1534
classification, **B2**.1530, **B2**.1531
genetics, **B2**.1529
plasmids, **B2**.1529–30
habitats, **B2**.1524–5
identification, **B2**.1533 (Tab.)
PCR assays, **B2**.1532
metabolism, **B2**.1529
morphology
capsules, **B2**.1527
flagella, **B2**.1527–8
LPS, **B2**.1527
pili, **B2**.1528
porins, **B2**.1528–9
S-layers, **B2**.1525, **B2**.1526 (Fig.)
nosocomial infection, **B1**.376
pathogenicity, **B2**.1524, **B2**.1536
adhesins, **B2**.1536
β-hemolysin, **B2**.1535–6

cytotonic enterotoxins, **B2**.1536
secreted enzymes, **B2**.1536
pili, **B2**.1511
viable but nonculturable state, **B2**.1529
Aeromonas jandei, **B2**.1525 (Tab.)
antibacterial susceptibility/resistance,
B2.1532–4
β-lactams, **B2**.1534
identification, **B2**.1533 (Tab.)
PCR assays, **B2**.1532
pathogenicity, **B2**.1536
secreted enzymes, **B2**.1536
Aeromonas media, **B2**.1525 (Tab.)
culture, **B2**.1529
identification, **B2**.1533 (Tab.)
Aeromonas molluscorum, **B2**.1525 (Tab.),
B2.1531
Aeromonas popoffi, **B2**.1524–5, **B2**.1525 (Tab.)
Aeromonas salmonicida, **B2**.1525 (Tab.)
antibacterial susceptibility/resistance,
acquired, **B2**.1534
classification, **B2**.1531
culture, **B2**.1529
genetics, **B2**.1529–30
identification, **B2**.1532, **B2**.1533 (Tab.)
morphology
capsules, **B2**.1527
flagella, **B2**.1528
LPS, **B2**.1527
pili, **B2**.1528
porins, **B2**.1528–9
S-layers, **B1**.155, **B2**.1525
viable but nonculturable state, **B2**.1529
virulence plasmids, **B2**.1529–30
Aeromonas salmonischuberticida,
B2.1525 (Tab.)
Aeromonas schubertii
classification, **B2**.1531
identification, **B2**.1532, **B2**.1533 (Tab.)
PCR assays, **B2**.1532
morphology, S-layers, **B2**.1525
pathogenicity, **B2**.1536
adhesins, **B2**.1536
Aeromonas simiae, **B2**.1525 (Tab.)
classification, **B2**.1531
Aeromonas sobria, **B2**.1525 (Tab.)
classification, **B2**.1530, **B2**.1531
pathogenicity, **B2**.1536
Aeromonas trota, **B2**.1525 (Tab.)
antibacterial susceptibility/resistance,
B2.1532–4
identification, **B2**.1532, **B2**.1533 (Tab.)
PCR assays, **B2**.1532
LPS, **B2**.1527
pathogenicity, β-hemolysin, **B2**.1535–6
Aeromonas veronii, **B2**.1525 (Tab.)
antibacterial susceptibility/resistance,
B2.1532–4
classification, **B2**.1531
habitats, **B2**.1524–5
identification, **B2**.1533 (Tab.)
metabolism, **B2**.1529
morphology
flagella, **B2**.1527–8
pili, **B2**.1528

porins, **B2**.1528–9
S-layers, **B2**.1525, **B2**.1526 (Fig.)
pathogenicity, **B2**.1524
adhesins, **B2**.1536
β-hemolysin, **B2**.1535–6
secreted enzymes, **B2**.1536
Aerosol transmission
bacteria *see* Airborne bacteria; Bioaerosols
viruses, **V1**.354, **V1**.355, **V2**.1403–4
filovirus, **V2**.1093–4
influenza, **V1**.667
norovirus infection, **V2**.919
Venezuelan equine encephalitis virus,
V2.1018
Aeruginocins, **B1**.136–7
pyocins, **B1**.138
Aeruginosin A/B, **B2**.1596–7
'Afferent' activation, CD8 T cells, **I**.404
Affinity maturation, memory B cells, **I**.491
Afipia, **B2**.1900–3, **B2**.1901 (Tab.)
antibacterial susceptibility/resistance,
B2.1903
biochemistry, **B2**.1903
cell walls, **B2**.1903
characteristics, **B2**.1902 (Tab.)
culture, **B2**.1901–3
epidemiology, **B2**.1900–1
infection, **B2**.1900
clinical significance, **B2**.1901–3
morphology, **B2**.1901 (Fig.)
reservoirs, **B2**.1900–1
staining, **B2**.1903
see also individual species
Afipia birgiae, **B2**.1901 (Tab.), **B2**.1902 (Tab.)
Afipia broomeae, **B2**.1901 (Tab.),
B2.1902 (Tab.)
Afipia clevelandensis, **B2**.1901 (Tab.),
B2.1902 (Tab.)
Afipia felis, **B2**.1901 (Tab.), **B2**.1902 (Tab.)
Afipia massiliensis, **B2**.1901 (Tab.),
B2.1902 (Tab.)
Aflatoxins
cheeses, **B1**.252
nuts, **B1**.287
AFLP® Microbial Fingerprinting, **B1**.736
Africa
food-borne botulism, **B2**.1069
'meningitis belt', **B1**.562, **B1**.562 (Fig.)
microsporidiosis, **P**.538
parasitic disease importance, **P**.27 (Fig.)
African histoplasmosis *see* Histoplasmosis
African horse sickness virus (AHSV), **V2**.942
emerging infection, **V2**.1651 (Tab.)
African Initiative on Malaria (AIM), **P**.518
African Programme for Onchocerciasis
Control (APOC), **P**.110, **P**.121, **P**.788
African swine fever virus (ASFV), **V1**.44
emerging infection, **V2**.1651 (Tab.)
immune evasion
apoptosis mitochondrial pathways,
V1.324–5
caspase inhibition, **V1**.324, **I**.627
cytokine expression/activation, **V1**.316,
I.623
inflammation inhibition, **V1**.286

African tick-bite fever, clinical manifestations, **B2**.2039 (Tab.)

African trypanosomiasis *see* Trypanosomiasis, African

Agammaglobulinemia, **I**.779–80
autosomal recessive, **I**.780
bronchiectasis, **I**.780
respiratory tract infection, **B1**.626, **I**.780
viral CNS infection, **V2**.1411–12
X-linked, **I**.779

Agar dilution susceptibility testing, **B1**.717
antifungal testing, **M**.158

Age
emerging viral infection, **V2**.1655
enterovirus infection, **V2**.870
hepatitis B, **V2**.1255
hepatitis C disease progression, **V2**.1204
Newcastle disease virus infection, **V1**.815
rhinovirus infection, **V2**.873
susceptibility to infection, **V1**.263–4
transmission effects, **V1**.356–7
vaccination models *see* Vaccination, mathematical models
vaccination program effects, **B1**.345
vaccine response, **V2**.1557–8
see also Adolescents; Children; Elderly patients; Neonatal infection

Age at infection, vaccination models, **I**.949, **I**.960

Age gateways, vaccination models, **I**.962

Agenerase *see* Amprenavir

Age-related prevalence
Clonorchis, **P**.648
gastrointestinal nematodes, **P**.722–3, **P**.722 (Fig.)
Opisthorchis, **P**.648
Trichuris trichiuria, **P**.722–3, **P**.722 (Fig.)

Agglutination tests, **B1**.718, **B1**.748–9
antibodies detected, **B1**.749
brucellosis diagnosis, **B1**.744–5
chromophores, **B1**.748–9
H antigens, **B1**.748
O antigens, **B1**.748
passive, **B1**.748

Agglutin-like sequence-1 (Als1p), **M**.259

Agricultural development projects
epidemics, **P**.117
malaria epidemiology, **P**.34, **P**.512–13

Agriculture/agricultural workers infection
airborne bacteria, **B1**.186 (Tab.)
bacteria exposure, **B1**.185–7, **B1**.186 (Tab.)
emerging viral infection, **V2**.1660–1
endotoxin exposure, **B1**.186 (Tab.), **B1**.189
erysipeloid, **B2**.971
mycetoma, **M**.388
paracoccidioidomycosis, **M**.544, **M**.545
prototheccosis, **M**.397, **M**.399
sporotrichosis, **M**.367–8

Agrobacterium
glucose catabolism, **B1**.60
phytopathogenicity, **B1**.202

Agrobacterium tumefaciens
biocontrol, **B2**.1994
nucleic acid composition, **B2**.1729 (Tab.)
phytopathogenicity, **B1**.202

plant genetic modification, **B1**.202
virulence factors, **B1**.115

ahsA gene, **B2**.1525

AICD *see* Activation-induced cell death (AICD)

Aichi virus, classification, **V1**.50–2

AID gene mutations, hyper-IgM syndromes, **I**.781

AIDS, **M**.12, **I**.791
antifungal resistance, **M**.168
behavioural control, **B1**.354
bodily spillages, cleaning, **B1**.424
cause of death, **I**.791
epidemiology, modeling approaches, **B1**.337–8
fluconazole *see* Fluconazole
historical aspects/re-evaluation, **I**.6–9
IL-15 therapy, **I**.282–3
ketoconazole absorption, **M**.611
measles vaccination, **V1**.736
molecular epidemiology, **V1**.198
progressive multifocal leucoencephalopathy (PML), **V1**.478, **V2**.1416–18
superantigens, **I**.564
surveillance, **B1**.318–19
TNF-α, **I**.286
see also HIV infection

AIDS, concomitant infection
adiaspiromycosis, **M**.809, **M**.813–15, **M**.818, **M**.821
alveolar echinococcosis, **P**.691
aspergillosis, **M**.12, **M**.700, **M**.705–6
sino-orbital, **M**.294–5
babesiosis, **P**.458
bacillary angiomatosis, **B2**.1894
bartonellosis
bacillary angiomatosis, **B2**.1894
endocarditis, **B2**.1894
Blastocystis hominis infection, **P**.563
blastomycosis, **M**.490, **M**.492, **M**.497
Bordetella, **B2**.1811
bronchiectasis, **B1**.645
bronchitis, **B1**.645
candidiasis, **M**.11–12, **M**.328, **M**.580, **M**.591, **M**.593, **M**.597
C. dubliniensis infection, **M**.580, **M**.585
CNS, **M**.600
as defining illness, **M**.256
ketoconazole, **M**.611
oral, **M**.189, **M**.256, **M**.262–3, **M**.598, **M**.599
therapy, **M**.189, **M**.610
Chagas' disease, **I**.678
coccidioidomycosis, **M**.113, **M**.508–10, **M**.516
cryptococcosis, **M**.11–12, **M**.18, **M**.109, **M**.324–5, **M**.328, **M**.644
cutaneous, **M**.647–8
genitourinary, **M**.648
HAART, **M**.644, **M**.651–3
intraocular infection, **M**.324–5
meningoencephalitis, **M**.645–6, **M**.646 (Tab.), **M**.647 (Tab.), **M**.649, **M**.651
prognosis, **M**.653
pulmonary, **M**.647, **M**.650

cryptosporidiosis, **P**.45, **P**.76, **B1**.403, **P**.404–5, **I**.677
clinical aspects, **P**.404–5
prevalence, **P**.409–10
cysticercosis, **P**.691
Dientamoeba fragilis infection, **P**.267–8
EBV, **V1**.336–8, **V1**.345
echinococcosis, **P**.691
emergence/resurgence, **B1**.362
Encephalitozoon cuniculi infection, **M**.69, **P**.539, **P**.541
Endolimax nana infection, **P**.223
Enterocytozoon bieneusi infection, **P**.538
folliculitis, **M**.15
giardiasis, **P**.76, **P**.247, **P**.251
HCMV infection, **V1**.52–2, **V2**.1498, **V2**.1499 (Tab.), **V2**.1502–3
cell-mediated immune response, **V1**.524–5
in children, **V2**.1505
HAART effects, **V2**.1502
natural history, **V1**.523
progression effects, **V2**.1499–500
herpesvirus infection, EBV-associated lymphomas, **V1**.571
HHV-6 infection, **V1**.528–9, **V2**.1499 (Tab.), **V2**.1503
contribution to pathology, **V1**.531
HHV-7 infection, **V1**.528–9, **V2**.1503
contribution to pathology, **V1**.531
HHV-8 infection, **V1**.551, **V2**.1499 (Tab.), **V2**.1503
prevention/treatment, **V2**.1503
histoplasmosis, **M**.11–2, **M**.23, **M**.112, **M**.530–1, **M**.535–7
ocular, **M**.288, **M**.325, **M**.329
HPV infection, **V1**.338, **V2**.1499 (Tab.), **V2**.1503–4
hyalohyphomycosis, **M**.751
intracranial abscesses, **B1**.583, **B1**.584 (Tab.), **B1**.586
isosporiasis, **P**.97, **P**.412–14
Kingella kingae, **B2**.1670
leishmaniasis, **P**.298–9, **P**.301, **P**.339, **P**.341
lung infection, **B1**.645
see also individual types
malaria interactions, **P**.494–5
Malassezia sympodialis infection, **M**.627
microsporidiosis, **I**.8–9, **P**.45, **P**.189, **P**.529, **P**.536, **P**.539, **P**.541, **P**.543
diagnosis, **P**.545
disease indicator, **P**.538
fecal tumor necrosis factor-α, **P**.539
mycoplasma, **B2**.1964–5
Nocardia asteroides, **B2**.1157
non-tuberculous mycobacteria, **B2**.1205–6, **B2**.1206 (Tab.)
M. avium complex, **B2**.1205–6, **B2**.1208–9
disseminated, **B2**.1208, **B2**.1208 (Fig.), **B2**.1209
entry and infection route, **B2**.1208–9
epidemiology, **B2**.1208
immune response, **B2**.1209
risk factors, **B2**.1209
treatment, **B2**.1209
M. celatum, **B2**.1214

AIDS
non-tuberculous mycobacteria (*Continued*)
M. genavense, **B2**.1209–10
M. haemophilum, **B2**.1210
M. kansasii, **B2**.1211
nosocomial infection, **B1**.382–3
oculomycoses, **M**.328–9
paracoccidioidomycosis, **M**.550, **M**.553–4
Pasteurella multocida, **B2**.1654–5
PCP, **M**.764, **M**.783–4, **M**.789, **M**.791
clinical presentation, **M**.784
diagnosis, **M**.786 (Fig.), **M**.787
histopathology, **M**.785–6
immune response, **M**.792, **M**.793–4,
M.794–6
TMP-SMX therapy, **M**.764, **M**.784, **M**.789,
M.790
penicilliosis marneffei, **M**.12, **M**.21, **M**.27,
M.560, **M**.562–3 (Tab.), **M**.566,
M.567 (Fig.), **M**.569, **M**.570–1
diagnosis, **M**.569–70
therapy, **M**.571
phaeohyphomycosis, **M**.740, **M**.743
Pneumocystis carinii, ocular infection,
M.327, **M**.329
pneumonia, **B1**.645
protothecosis, **M**.399
protozoal infection with, **P**.74–5
Pseudomonas aeruginosa, **B2**.1593
rapidly growing mycobacteria, **B2**.1249,
B2.1250, **B2**.1255, **B2**.1256
rhinoscleroma, **B1**.616–17
Rhodococcus equi, **B2**.1167–8
Saccharomyces cerevisiae infection, **M**.628
Salmonella, **B2**.1424–5
schistosomiasis, **P**.97
sclerosing cholangitis, **P**.405
seborrheic dermatitis, **M**.212
sinusitis, **B1**.645
Sporobolomyces salmonicolor, **M**.628
sporotrichosis, **M**.28, **M**.368, **M**.371, **M**.375,
M.380
ocular, **M**.325–6
Stenotrophomonas maltophilia, **B2**.1636
stomatitis, **B1**.614
Streptococcus pneumoniae, **B1**.630–1
syphilis with, **B1**.662–3, **B2**.1843, **B2**.1856–7
systemic zygomycosis, **M**.661, **M**.674–5
tetanus, **B2**.1065
toxoplasmosis, **P**.85–6, **P**.432, **I**.676
trichomoniasis with, **P**.261
Trichosporon cutaneum (*T. beigelii*)
infection, **M**.629
tuberculosis, **I**.592–3, **B2**.1199, **B2**.1201–2
testing, **B2**.1185
AIDS-dementia complex (ADC), **V2**.1426–8
autoimmunity in, **V2**.1428
cytokines, **V1**.304, **V2**.1428
pathogenesis, **V2**.1428
pathology, **V2**.1427 (Fig.), **V2**.1428
symptoms, **V2**.1427–8
AIDS-related lymphoma, **I**.795–6
Ainsworth, G C, **M**.32
Aiolös, B cell development, **I**.324–5
Air, bacteria in *see* Airborne bacteria

Airborne bacteria, **B1**.310, **B1**.185–94
adverse human health effects, **B1**.188–9
types of causative agent, **B1**.188–9
infection spread, **B1**.329
laboratory precautions, *Mycobacterium
tuberculosis*, **B2**.1189
LPS *see* Lipopolysaccharide (LPS)
monitoring, **B1**.189–91
settling factors, **B1**.187
survival factors, **B1**.187
water sources, **B1**.185–7
see also Bioaerosols; *individual species*
Air conditioning systems, **B1**.186 (Tab.),
B1.189
Legionnaires' disease transmission, **B1**.634–5
Air control measures, aspergillosis prevention,
M.730
Air-cooling towers, Legionnaires' disease,
B1.376
AIRE gene, **I**.779
Air pollution, respiratory tract infection,
B1.626
'Airport malaria,' **P**.29, **P**.511, **P**.514–15
Air sampling, bacteria monitoring, **B1**.189–91
Air sterilization
filtration, **B1**.453
UV radiation, **B1**.452
Air travel
emerging bacterial infection, **B1**.360
parasitic disease spread, **P**.29
Airway hypersensitivity/hyperactivity,
I.731–45
airway remodeling, **I**.732
extracellular matrix deposition, **I**.731–2
APCs, **I**.736–7
complement, **I**.738
early acute phase response, **I**.732
eosinophils, **I**.731–2, **I**.735–6
animal models, **I**.735–6
inflammatory mediators, **I**.735
passive transfer experiments, **I**.736
recruitment, **I**.735
γδ T cells, **I**.737–8
IgE-mediated pathology, **I**.732–3
IL-4, **I**.732–3, **I**.735
IL-10, **I**.737, **I**.739–40
IL-12, **I**.740–1
animal models, **I**.740–1
Th1/Th2 balance, **I**.740
IL-13, **I**.732–3, **I**.733–4, **I**.734–5
chemokine expression, **I**.736
immunoregulatory networks, **I**.738–41
see also Hygiene hypothesis
late phase response, **I**.732
mast cells, **I**.731–2, **I**.735
mechanisms, **I**.731–2
Th2 cell pathology, **I**.731–5, **I**.734
chemokine receptors, **I**.734
chemokines, **I**.734
deficient mouse models, **I**.733
FcεRII (CD23) upregulation, **I**.733–4
IgE production, **I**.733–4
RAG-1 deficient mice, **I**.734
vascular adhesion molecule, **I**.733–4
see also individual interleukins

see also Asthma
Airway remodeling
airway hypersensitivity *see* Airway
hypersensitivity/hyperreactivity
chronic asthma, **I**.732
Airways *see* Respiratory tract
Ajello, L, **M**.32
Ajellomyces, **M**.77, **M**.811–12, **M**.819–20
ascocarps, **M**.819, **M**.820 (Fig.)
ascospores, **M**.813, **M**.819–20, **M**.821 (Fig.)
Ajellomyces capsulatus, **M**.23, **M**.77, **M**.819–20
Ajellomyces crescens, **M**.819–20, **M**.820 (Fig.),
M.821 (Fig.)
Ajellomyces dermatitidis, **M**.24, **M**.77, **M**.486,
M.521, **M**.819–20
Akabane virus infection, **V2**.1043
Akadon
arenaviruses associated, **V2**.1060 (Tab.),
V2.1061
Leishmania braziliensis, **P**.326
Akt protein kinase, BCR signaling, **I**.345
Alamar blue, **M**.157
Alanine aminotransferase (ALT)
acute hepatitis B, **V2**.1246, **V2**.1251
chronic hepatitis B, **V2**.1248
hepatitis A, **V2**.1171
Alaska, food-borne botulism, **B2**.1066–7
Albendazole
alveolar echinococcosis treatment, **P**.696–7,
P.699
Capillaria philippiensis control, **P**.747
cystic echinococcosis treatment, **P**.698–9
cysticercosis treatment, **P**.697–8
Enterobius vermicularis infection, **P**.732
Gnathostoma spinigerum control, **P**.822
lymphatic filariasis treatment, **P**.777
microsporidiosis, **P**.548–50
Oesophagostomum control, **P**.812
schistosomiasis control, **P**.125
Ternidens deminutus control, **P**.811
toxocariasis therapy, **P**.755
Alcaligenaceae, **B2**.1787
Alcaligenes, **B2**.1787
in milk, **B1**.233
waterborne, **B1**.211, **B1**.221
Alcaligenes denitrificans, **B1**.442
Alcaligenes faecalis, **B2**.1787
as airborne bacteria, **B1**.189
Alcaligenes xylosoxidans, keratitis, **B1**.601
Alcelaphine herpesvirus 1, **V1**.542 (Tab.)
genome sequences, **V1**.494 (Tab.)
infection, **V1**.279 (Tab.)
Alcian blue stain, **M**.124
Alcohol(s), **B1**.423 (Tab.), **B1**.427
handwash preparations, **B1**.766–7
resistance to, **B1**.442
see also Ethanol
Alcohol dehydrogenase (ADH), **B1**.55
CoA-linked, **B1**.55
Entamoeba histolytica, **P**.204
Alcohol fermentation, **B1**.54
acetyl-CoA formation, **B1**.56
Alcoholism
Erysipelothrix rhusiopathiae infection,
B2.971

Alcoholism (*Continued*)
  immunodeficiency, **I**.788 (Tab.)
  paracoccidioidomycosis, **M**.545
Aldehyde dehydrogenase (ALDH), *Entamoeba histolytica*, **P**.204
Aldehydes, **B1**.423 (Tab.), **B1**.426–7
  viruses, effects on, **B1**.439–40
Aldolase, **B1**.51, **B1**.58, **B1**.59
Aldopentoses, **B1**.59
Alemtuzumab, licensing, **I**.355 (Tab.)
Alenquer virus infection, **V2**.1047
Aleppo button, **P**.313
Aleurioconidia, **M**.79 (Fig.)
  Emmonsia, **M**.811–12, **M**.818, **M**.819 (Fig.)
Aleutian mink disease virus (AMDV), **V1**.412
  capsids, **V1**.413
  infection
    chronic infection, **V1**.426
    fetal/neonatal hosts, **V1**.425–6
    immunopathology, **V1**.279 (Tab.)
    infectious immune complexes, **V1**.262
    passive viremia, **V1**.241
  pathogenic potential, **V1**.422
Alexidine, **B1**.426
  action, **B1**.437 (Tab.), **B1**.438
Algorithms, fungal classification, **M**.48
Alkaline nuclease, HSV-1 replication, **V1**.165 (Tab.)
Alkalis, **B1**.422–4, **B1**.423 (Tab.)
Alkhurma virus, **V2**.1648 (Tab.)
Alkylamines, γδ T cell binding, **I**.439, **I**.440 (Fig.)
Alkylating agents, **B1**.423 (Tab.)
  action, **B1**.437 (Tab.), **B1**.438
  as mutagen, **B1**.84–5
  as mutagens, **V1**.183
  see also specific types
Allelic exclusion, TCR gene assembly, **I**.456–7
Allergic bronchopulmonary aspergillosis (ABPA), **M**.105, **M**.693
  cystic fibrosis and, **M**.693–4, **M**.712
  diagnosis, **M**.693, **M**.710 (Fig.), **M**.712
  history, **M**.18–9
  immune response, **M**.707, **M**.708
    cellular response, **M**.709
    humoral response, **M**.708
  prognosis, **M**.717–18
  therapy, **M**.718
Allergic contact dermatitis, **I**.826
Allergies
  airborne bacteria, **B1**.188
  aspergillosis *see* Aspergillosis
  Aspergillus fumigatus, **M**.692–3
  asthma *see* Asthma
  basophils, **I**.57
  CCR3, **I**.227
  cystic echinococcosis, **P**.688
  inflammation, IL-9, **I**.283 (Fig.)
  passive immunization, **V2**.1568
  rhinosinusitis, **M**.296
  sinusitis *see* Sinusitis, allergic fungal
  toxocariasis, **P**.754
  see also Atopy
Allescheria, **M**.19

Allexivirus, **V1**.27 (Tab.)
Allied Vaccine Group, **V2**.1583
Alloiococcus otitis, **B1**.296 (Tab.)
Allolactose, **B1**.70–1
Allopurinol
  Chagas disease, **P**.380, **P**.393
  Old World leishmaniasis, **P**.307
Alloreactivity, TCR–MHC–peptide interactions, **I**.463
Allotropic specificity
  parvoviruses, **V1**.422
  porcine parvovirus, **V1**.422
Allspice, **B1**.287
Allylamines, **M**.169 (Tab.), **M**.183 (Tab.), **M**.184, **M**.233
  dermatophytoses therapy, **M**.184
  mechanism of action, **M**.70, **M**.184
  resistance, **M**.175
α3 domain, MHC class I, **I**.405
α₁-acid glycoprotein (AGP), **I**.205
  acute phase response, **I**.195 (Fig.)
  drug binding, **I**.205
α heavy chain, IgA structure, **I**.307
α-linked glycolipids, αβ T cell recognition, **I**.441–2, **I**.443 (Fig.)
α₁-antichymotrypsin, **I**.202
  acute phase response, **I**.195 (Fig.)
α₁-antitrypsin, **I**.201–2
A-structures, Hepatitis B virus, **V1**.65
αβ T-cells, **V1**.274
  CD1a/b/c-reactive cells, **I**.442–3
    glycolipid antigens, **I**.442–3 (Fig.)
  CD1d-reactive cells, **I**.441–2
    α-linked glycolipid recognition, **I**.441–2, **I**.443 (Fig.)
    CD161 expression, **I**.441
    cytokine secretion, **I**.442
    Th1/Th2 balance effects, **I**.442
  intraepithelial lymphocytes, **I**.441, **I**.529
    IL-16 expression, **I**.441
    nonclassic MHC recognition, **I**.441
    'stress antigen' recognition, **I**.441
    TLRs expression, **I**.441
  MR1-reactive cells, **I**.443, **I**.444 (Fig.)
  TCR *see* T-cell receptor (TCR)
  tonsils, **I**.533
  unconventional peptide-reactive, **I**.445
    N-formylated peptides, **I**.445
  vulvovaginal candidiasis, **M**.265
  see also T cell(s)
α/δ locus, TCR, **I**.450 (Fig.), **I**.451
Alpha fetoprotein (AFP), hepatitis B diagnosis, **V2**.1249
Alphaherpesvirinae
  characteristics, **V1**.177 (Tab.)
  classification, **V1**.43 (Tab.), **V1**.488–9
  evolution, **V1**.175–6
  host range, **V1**.489
  see also Alphaherpesviruses
Alphaherpesviruses, **V1.506–19**
  genome sequences, **V1**.494 (Tab.)
  immune evasion, **V1**.320

infection
  CNS infection, **V2**.1418, **V2**.1418–22
  latency, **V1**.206
  see also Alphaherpesvirinae
α₂-Macroglobulin, **I**.202
  defensin binding, **I**.168
  LDL receptor-related protein, **I**.202
  lectin pathway regulation, **I**.149–51
  microbial delivery, **I**.202 (Fig.)
Alpha-methyl-D-glucoside fermentation, Enterobacteriaceae identification, **B2**.1319 (Tab.)
Alphanodavirus, **V1**.53
α₁-protease inhibitor, **I**.201–2
Alpharetrovirus
  classification, **V1**.46, **V2**.1286 (Tab.)
  tumors associated, **V1**.331 (Tab.)
Alphaviridae
  neural spread, **V1**.244 (Tab.)
  see also specific viruses
Alphavirus
  classification, **V1**.53, **V2**.1010
  see also Alphaviruses
Alphaviruses
  6K protein, **V2**.1014
  capsid (C) protein, **V2**.1014
  cell receptors, **V1**.213, **V2**.1015
  classification, **V2**.1010–12
    phylogenetic tree, **V2**.1012 (Fig.)
  E1 glycoprotein, **V2**.1012, **V2**.1014–15
    neutralizing antibodies, **V2**.1015
  E2 glycoprotein, **V2**.1012, **V2**.1014–15
    heparan sulfate binding, **V2**.1015
  E3 protein, **V2**.1014
  genome replication, **V1**.141 (Fig.)
  genome structure, **V2**.1012–14, **V2**.1013 (Fig.)
    conserved sequence element (CSE), **V2**.1014
    conserved sequences, **V2**.1014
  geographical distribution, **V2**.1017–18
  immune evasion, **V2**.1015–16
  infection *see* Alphavirus infection
  members, **V2**.1011 (Tab.)
  nsP1 protein, **V2**.1012–14
  nsP2 protein, **V2**.1012–14
  protein synthesis, **V1**.141 (Fig.)
  replication, **V2**.1012–14, **V2**.1013 (Fig.)
    cellular entry, **V1**.108–9
    nonstructural protein regulation, **V2**.1012–14
    particle assembly/release, **V1**.144
  structural proteins, **V2**.1014–15
    see also individual proteins
  virion structure, **V2**.1012
  see also Alphavirus
Alphavirus infection, **V2**.1010, **V2**.1018
  control, **V2**.1018–19
    equine vaccines, **V2**.1019
    transmission interruption, **V2**.1018
    vector control, **V2**.1018–19
  diagnosis, **V2**.1018
    serology, **V2**.1547
  encephalitis, **V1**.244 (Tab.)
  host cell interactions, **V2**.1015–16
    cell receptors, **V2**.1015

Alphavirus infection
host cell interactions (*Continued*)
metabolism, **V2**.1015
transcription downregulation, **V2**.1015–16
host range, **V2**.1015, **V2**.1016–17
immune response, **V2**.1018
humoral immunity, **V2**.1018
neural spread, **V1**.244 (Tab.)
pathogenesis, **V2**.1018
CNS infection, **V2**.1018
insect host, **V2**.1018
skeletal muscle replication, **V2**.1018
transmission cycles, **V2**.1016–18,
V2.1016 (Fig.), **V2**.1017 (Fig.)
arthropods, **V2**.1010
mosquitoes, **V2**.1018
reservoir hosts, **V2**.1017
'Altered self-model,' TCR, **I**.449–50
Alternaria
in cereals, **B1**.284
in fruit, **B1**.282, **B1**.283
infection *see Alternaria* infection
Alternaria alternaria, **M**.248–9
onychomycosis, **M**.246
Alternaria citri, **B1**.282
Alternaria infection
allergic fungal sinusitis, **M**.696
CNS, **M**.743
oculomycoses, **M**.278 (Tab.), **M**.283–4
contact lens contamination, **M**.331
dacryocanaliculitis, **M**.298
endophthalmitis, **M**.323
voriconazole therapy, **M**.153
Alternate reading frames, respirovirus
transcription, **V1**.771
Alternate splicing
adenoviruses, **V1**.180
genomes, **V1**.180
Minute virus of mice (MVM), **V1**.157–8
Alternate start sites, **V1**.180
Alternate termination sites, **V1**.180
Alternative complement pathway *see*
Complement
Alternative initiation sites, **V1**.116–17
Alternative open reading frames, **V1**.116–17,
V1.224
Alterococcus agarolyticus, **B2**.1330 (Tab.)
Alteromonas
fish, **B1**.279
poultry, **B1**.277–8
Aluminum hydroxide adjuvant, **I**.928 (Tab.),
V2.1552–3
Aluminum phosphate adjuvant, **I**.928 (Tab.)
Aluminum salt adjuvants, **I**.925, **I**.926
monophosphoryl lipid combination, **I**.929–30
Th2 cell response, **I**.926
Alveolar macrophages, **V1**.793–4
Alysiella, classification, **B2**.1271
Alzheimer's disease
BCE peptide vaccines, **I**.855 (Tab.), **I**.875–6
design, **I**.875–6
complement pathology, **I**.155 (Tab.), **I**.156
macrophages, **I**.31
pathogenesis, **I**.875
prion diseases *vs.*, **V2**.1367

AMAC-1 (CCL18), **I**.218 (Tab.)
Amantidine, **V2**.1625–6
Borna disease virus infection, **V2**.1153
historical aspects, **V1**.9 (Tab.)
influenza, **V1**.679–80, **V2**.1625–6
mechanism of action, **V1**.657, **V1**.679,
V2.1626
resistance, **V1**.679–80
influenza A virus, **V2**.1636
structure, **V2**.1626 (Fig.)
toxicity, **V2**.1637–8
Amapari virus, **V2**.1060 (Tab.)
Amastigotes, **P**.285–6
Leishmania see Leishmania
Ambisense coding, **V1**.181, **V1**.181 (Fig.)
arenaviruses, **V1**.181
bunyaviruses, **V1**.181
circoviruses, **V1**.181
phleboviruses, **V1**.181, **V1**.181 (Fig.),
V2.1033–5
Punta Toro virus, **V1**.181, **V1**.181 (Fig.)
tospoviruses, **V2**.1035
AmBisome, **M**.612
aspergillosis therapy, **M**.720–1, **M**.725
neonates, **M**.726
Amblyomma africanum, **B2**.2040
Amblyomma americanum, **B1**.362, **B2**.2050–1
Amblyomma cajennense, **B2**.2038
Amblyomma hebraeum, **B2**.2040
Amdinocillin, *Enterobacter*, **B2**.1484–5
Amdovirus, **V1**.412
infection *see Amdovirus* infection
members, **V1**.411 (Tab.)
Amdovirus infection, **V1**.425–7
epidemiology, **V1**.425
pathogenesis, **V1**.425–6
fetal/neonatal hosts, **V1**.425–6
immunocompromised hosts, **V1**.426
mature hosts, **V1**.426
Amebae
classification, **P**.197, **P**.201, **P**.226
anomalies/changes, **P**.200–1
facultative, **P**.187–8
historical aspects, **P**.13, **P**.200
Legionella, **B2**.1767
lobopodia/filopodia, **P**.178 (Fig.), **P**.179,
P.201–2
motility, **P**.170 (Fig.), **P**.227
parasitic, **P**.187
Amebae, intestinal, **P.218–25**
biochemistry/molecular biology, **P**.219
classification, **P**.201, **P**.218, **P**.219 (Fig.)
epidemiology, **P**.219–20
hematophagous, **P**.210
immune response, **P**.75, **P**.218–19
multiple infection, **P**.218–19
life cycles, **P**.219–20
cyst output, **P**.219–20
nonpathogenic, **P**.200–1
see also individual species
Amebae, opportunistic, **P.226–40**
biochemistry, **P**.229–31
cell differentiation, **P**.229–30
classification, **P**.226

infection
chemotherapy, **P**.236–7
clinical features, **P**.231–2
diagnosis, **P**.234–5
epidemiology/control, **P**.235–6
immunology, **P**.87, **P**.232
pathology, **P**.232–4
vaccination, **P**.237
see also Amebiasis
integrated control, **P**.237
life-cycles, **P**.228–9
molecular biology/genetics, **P**.229–31
structure, **P**.227–9
'Ameba-like' division, **P**.181, **P**.183 (Fig.)
Amebapore, **P**.205–6
Amebiasis, **P**.187, **P**.200, **P**.206
carriers, **P**.212–13
chemotherapy, **P**.213–14
drugs of choice, **P**.213
resistance, **P**.213
see also individual drugs
clinical features, **P**.207–8, **P**.220–4
complications, **P**.210–11
control, **P**.37, **P**.39, **P**.130, **P**.214–15
see also individual methods
cutaneous, **P**.208
diagnosis, **P**.211–12, **P**.220
brain biopsies, **P**.153
cysts in healthy people, **P**.211
fecal examination, **P**.220
fecal samples, **P**.150
immunoassays, **P**.154
indirect hemagglutination assay, **P**.154
indirect immunofluorescence assay, **P**.154
isoenzyme patterns, **P**.200–1, **P**.211
molecular biology, **P**.220
returning travelers, **P**.149
serological, **P**.211–12
epidemiology, **P**.37, **P**.46 (Tab.), **P**.211–12
incidence, **P**.212, **P**.213
serological surveys, **P**.212, **P**.213
extraintestinal, **P**.207–8
cellular immunity in, **P**.210
historical aspects, **P**.13, **P**.200–1
immunology, **P**.208–10
antibody prevalence, **P**.212
cellular response, **P**.209–10
humoral response, **P**.208–9
incubation period, **P**.207
intestinal, **P**.207
amoeboma, **P**.207
appendicitis, **P**.207
diagnosis, **P**.211
dysentery, **P**.207
fulminating colitis, **P**.207
ulcerations in, **P**.206 (Fig.), **P**.207, **P**.210,
P.210 (Fig.)
'invasive', **P**.200–1, **P**.206
incidence, **P**.213
'luminal', **P**.206
epidemiology, **P**.213
mortality, **P**.37
pathology, **P**.210–11
public health importance, **P**.105 (Tab.)
travellers/immigrants, **P**.29

Amebiasis (*Continued*)
  surgery, **P**.213
  susceptibility, **P**.212–13
  transmission, **P**.207, **P**.214
    prevention, **P**.214
      see also Above, control
  vaccines/vaccination, **P**.75, **P**.214
    development status, **I**.933 (Tab.)
    recombinant peptides, **P**.214
    Vibrio cholerae vectors, **I**.844
Amebic colitis, fulminating, **P**.207
Amebic dysentery, **P**.207
  Balantidium coli infection *vs.*, **P**.279
  historical aspects, **P**.13
  incidence, **P**.212
Amebicides, **P**.213
Amebic liver abscess, **P**.208, **P**.208 (Fig.)
  chemotherapy, **P**.213
  clinical features, **P**.208
  diagnosis, **P**.211
  experimental studies, **P**.210
  incidence, **P**.213
  pathology, **P**.208 (Fig.)
  recurrence, **P**.213
Amebida, **I**.675–6
Ameboflagellates, classification, **P**.197
Ameboid forms, *Blastocystis hominis*, **P**.557–9,
  P.559 (Fig.), **P**.560 (Fig.)
American Academy of Pediatrics, measles
  vaccination recommendations, **V1**.735–6
American Thoracic Society (ATS), pneumonia
  treatment guidelines, **B1**.638,
  B1.639 (Tab.)
American Type Culture Collection, **V1**.86
American visceral leishmaniasis (AVL) *see*
  Leishmaniasis, New World
Amidinopenicillins, spectrum of activity,
  B1.475
Amikacin, **B1**.482, **B1**.499 (Tab.)
  Brucella, **B2**.1742
  Cedecea, **B2**.1491
  Enterobacter, **B2**.1484–5
  Listeria, **B2**.957–8
  Nocardia, **B2**.1145, **B2**.1165–6
  Serratia, **B2**.1488–9
  structure, **B1**.483 (Fig.)
Amino acids
  Enterobacteriaceae culture, **B2**.1345
  synthesis, **B1**.60
    Trypanosoma brucei, **P**.360
  utilization
    Fusobacterium, **B2**.1945, **B2**.1948
    Neisseria, **B2**.1274–5
α-Aminoadipic acid, **M**.44
P-Amino-benzaldehyde, 3-thiosemicarbazone,
  V1.9
p-Aminobenzoic acid, **B1**.490 (Fig.)
Aminobisphosphonates, γδ T cell binding,
  I.440 (Fig.)
Aminoglycosides, **B1**.482
  mode of action, **B1**.482
  modifying enzymes, **B1**.484 (Tab.)
  pharmacodynamics, **B1**.469–70
  pharmacology, **B1**.482

  resistance, **B1**.482
    Enterococcus, **B2**.891–2, **B2**.892 (Tab.),
      B2.893
    Staphylococcus, **B2**.794 (Tab.), **B2**.804
  spectrum of activity, **B1**.482
    Actinobacillus actinomycetemcomitans,
      B2.1664
    Actinomyces, **B2**.1011
    Campylobacter, **B2**.1548
    Capnocytophaga, **B2**.1677
    Cardiobacterium hominis, **B2**.1672–3
    Citrobacter, **B2**.1476
    Clostridium, **B2**.1064–5
    gonorrhea treatment, **B1**.662
    Lactobacillus, **B2**.866
    Listeria, **B2**.957–8
    Pasteurella multocida, **B2**.1655
    Proteus, **B2**.1443–4
    Streptococcus, **B2**.861
    Vibrio, **B2**.1514
    see also specific types
  structure, **B1**.482, **B1**.483 (Fig.)
  toxicity/adverse effects, **B1**.482
Aminopeptidases, antigen processing, **I**.412
4-Aminoquinaldinium derivatives, **B1**.428
Aminosidine, Old World leishmaniasis, **P**.307
Ammonia, **B2**.1446
Ammonification, **B1**.65, **B1**.66
Ammonium chloride, viral cell entry, **V1**.213
Ammonium salts
  Bifidobacterium bifidum, **B2**.1027
  soil bacteria fixation, **B1**.200
Amnesic shellfish poisoning (ASP), **B1**.280
Amniocentesis, **V2**.1445, **V2**.1445 (Tab.)
  fetal HCMV infection, **V2**.1451
  VZV infection, **V2**.1457
Amocarzine, onchocerciasis, **P**.790
Amodiaquine, malaria therapy, **P**.506
Amoeboma, **P**.207
Amoebostomes, **P**.227
Amorofine, **M**.233, **M**.234
  onychomycosis/dermatomycosis therapy,
    M.252
Amoxicillin
  history, **B1**.473
  spectrum of activity, **B1**.499 (Tab.)
    Actinobacillus actinomycetemcomitans,
      B2.1664
    Bacillus anthracis, **B2**.938
    Borrelia, **B2**.1831 (Tab.)
    Chlamydia trachomatis, **B2**.2021
    Eikenella corrodens, **B2**.1668
    Haemophilus, **B2**.1702 (Tab.)
    Helicobacter pylori, **B2**.1574–5
    Listeria, **B2**.957–8
    otitis media treatment, **B1**.617–18
    Pasteurella multocida, **B2**.1655
    in syphilis, **B2**.1858
  structure, **B1**.474 (Fig.)
Amoxicillin-clavulanate
  Actinobacillus actinomycetemcomitans,
    B2.1664
  Klebsiella, **B2**.1480
  Nocardia, **B2**.1145, **B2**.1165–6
  Pasteurella multocida, **B2**.1655

Amphistosomes, **P**.583–4
Amphocil, **M**.612
  aspergillosis therapy, **M**.721
Amphotericin B, **M**.148–9, **M**.182,
  M.183 (Tab.), **P**.237
  adverse effects, **I**.49
  aspergillosis therapy, **M**.719–20
    empirical therapy, **M**.724–5
    empirical treatment, **M**.724–5
    itraconazole *vs.*, **M**.728
    low-dose, **M**.727
    lung transplants, **M**.703, **M**.704
    neonates, **M**.725–6
  azole antifungal agents combination, **M**.153
  colloidal dispersion (ABCD),
    M.721
  deoxycholate, **M**.148–9
  flucytosine combination, **M**.149–50, **M**.612,
    M.651–2
  historical aspects, **M**.147–8
  intravitreal injection, **M**.319
  kidney effects, **M**.612
  lipid complexes *see* Amphotericin B lipid
    complex (ABLC)
  mechanism of action, **M**.70, **M**.148–9, **M**.172,
    M.172 (Tab.)
  mucocutaneous/mucosal leishmaniasis,
    P.341–2
  Old World leishmaniasis, **P**.307
  primary amebic meningoencephalitis,
    P.236–7
  prophylaxis, **M**.726–9
  recent modifications, **M**.147–8
  resistance, **M**.149, **M**.171, **M**.171 (Tab.)
    Candida, **M**.1702–3, **M**.611
    commonly reported fungi, **M**.171 (Tab.),
      M.172
    Condidiobolus, **M**.352
    Fusarium solani, **M**.172
    molecular aspects, **M**.173
    primary and secondary, **M**.172
    Scedosporium, **M**.172, **M**.757
    significant incidence, **M**.171 (Tab.)
    Trichosporon, **M**.172
  side-effects, **M**.511, **M**.611–12
  susceptibility testing, **M**.170–2
  therapy
    Acremonium infection, **M**.758
    adiaspiromycosis, **M**.821
    blastomycosis, **M**.497
    Blastoschizomyces capitatus infection,
      M.626
    blepharitis, **M**.297
    candidiasis, **M**.610 (Fig.), **M**.611, **M**.613
    coccidioidomycosis, **M**.511
    conjunctivitis, **M**.299
    cryptococcosis, **M**.651–2
    dacryocanaliculitis, **M**.298
    endophthalmitis, **M**.319–24, **M**.326–7
    Fusarium, **M**.755
    Hansenula anomala, **M**.626
    histoplasmosis, **M**.529–30, **M**.530 (Tab.),
      M.531, **M**.531 (Tab.)
    keratitis, **M**.307–8, **M**.312
    Malassezia infection, **M**.627
    mycetoma, **M**.393

Amphotericin B
  therapy (*Continued*)
    Paecilomyces infection, **M**.758
    paracoccidioidomycosis, **M**.551
    penicilliosis marneffei, **M**.571
    protothecosis, **M**.402
    pythiosis, **M**.425–6
    rhino-orbital-cerebral zygomycosis, **M**.293
    rhino-orbital infection, **M**.294
    Rhodotorula infection, **M**.627–8
    Saccharomyces cerevisiae infection, **M**.628
    Scopulariopsis infection, **M**.758–9
    sino-orbital aspergillosis, **M**.295
    Sporobolomyces infection, **M**.628
    sporotrichosis, **M**.380
    systemic zygomycosis, **M**.677–8
    Trichosporon infection, **M**.629–30
    white piedra, **M**.197
    zygomycosis, **M**.352
  toxicity, **M**.148–9
  visceral leishmaniasis, **P**.341
Amphotericin B colloidal dispersion (ABCD),
    aspergillosis therapy, **M**.721
Amphotericin B lipid complex (ABLC),
    M.149, **M**.149 (Tab.), **M**.171–2, **M**.612,
    M.613, **M**.721–2
  aspergillosis therapy, **M**.721–2
    empirical therapy, **M**.725
    prophylaxis, **M**.727
  diseases treated, **M**.149
  empirical therapy, **M**.149
  rhino-orbital-cerebral zygomycosis, **M**.293
Amphoteric surfactants, **B1**.423 (Tab.),
    B1.425
Ampicillin
  pharmacology, **B1**.475
    blood–brain barrier, **B1**.475–6
  resistance
    Aeromonas resistance, **B2**.1532–4
    Burkholderia pseudomallei, **B2**.1620
    Enterococcus, **B2**.892, **B2**.892 (Tab.)
    Salmonella Typhi, **B2**.1416
  spectrum of activity, **B1**.473
    Cardiobacterium hominis, **B2**.1672–3
    Citrobacter, **B2**.1476
    Eikenella corrodens, **B2**.1668
    Enterobacter, **B2**.1484–5
    Escherichia, **B2**.1369–70
    Haemophilus, **B2**.1702–4, **B2**.1702 (Tab.),
      B2.1703 (Tab.)
    intracranial abscess, **B1**.588
    Klebsiella, **B2**.1480
    Leclercia, **B2**.1495
    Leminorella, **B2**.1496
    Listeria, **B2**.957–8
    Pasteurella multocida, **B2**.1655
    Proteus, **B2**.1441–3
    Serratia, **B2**.1488–9
    in syphilis, **B2**.1858
    typhoid fever, **B2**.1416
  structure, **B1**.474 (Fig.)
Amplicons, HSV, **V2**.1598
Amplicor®, **B1**.722
  applications, **B1**.723 (Tab.)
Amplicor Monitor®, **B1**.723 (Tab.)

Amplified® MTD, **B1**.723 (Tab.)
Amplified fragment length polymorphisms
    (AFLPs)
  fungi, **M**.47
  Helicobacter, **B2**.1570
  Legionella, **B2**.1776, **B2**.1776 (Fig.)
  Malassezia, **M**.215–16
  Mycoplasma, **B2**.1995
  soil bacteria, **B1**.206
  Vibrio, **B2**.1516
Amprenavir, **V2**.1624
  resistance, **V2**.1624
    HIV, **V2**.1337 (Fig.)
  structure, **V2**.1625 (Fig.)
Amputations, gas gangrene after, **B2**.1112–13
AmrAB-OprA multidrug efflux system,
    B2.1620
Amur virus (AMRV), **V2**.1666 (Tab.)
Amycolata, **B2**.1150
Amycolata autotrophica, **B2**.1150
Amycolatopsis, **B2**.1150
  microscopic morphology, **B2**.1143
Amycolatopsis orientalis, **B2**.1150
iso-Amylamine, systemic $\gamma\delta$ T cell binding,
    I.440 (Fig.)
Amyloid-β 42 residue peptide (Aβ_{42}), vaccine
    design, **I**.875–6
Amyloid plaques, **V2**.1365
  see also Prion protein (PrP)
Amylopectin, storage elements, **P**.179
Anaerobes, aerotolerant, *Giardia*, **P**.243
Anaerobic bacteria
  catalase-negative gram-positive cocci,
    B2.883 (Tab.)
  denitrification, **B1**.200
  Enterococcus, **B2**.882, **B2**.883 (Tab.)
  infection
    aspiration pneumonia, **B1**.643 (Tab.)
    bacteremia, **B1**.516 (Fig.)
  as normal microbiota, **B1**.303
    colonization of oropharynx/tonsils,
      B1.294–5, **B1**.301
    on skin, **B1**.304
  soil aeration, **B1**.196–7
  see also individual species
Anaerobic blood cultures, **B1**.513–14
Anaerobic conditions, *Balantidium coli*,
    P.278–9
Anaerobic glycolysis, *Plasmodium*, **P**.476
Anaerobic pathways, larval cestodes, **P**.681
Anaerobic respiration, **B1**.65–7
  electron donors, **B1**.65–7
  nitrate reduction, **B1**.66
  sulfate reduction, **B1**.66
  terminal electron acceptors, **B1**.65, **B1**.67
Anaerobiosis, *Entamoeba histolytica*, **P**.204
Anaerococcus, **B2**.912–13
  biochemical characteristics, **B2**.908 (Tab.)
  classification, **B2**.904, **B2**.905 (Tab.)
  identification, **B2**.906–7, **B2**.908 (Tab.)
  as normal microbiota, **B1**.296 (Tab.)
  taxonomy, **B2**.913
Anaerococcus hydrogenalis, **B2**.908 (Tab.),
    B2.912
Anaerococcus lactolyticus, **B2**.912
  biochemical characteristics, **B2**.908 (Tab.)

classification, **B2**.904–5
Anaerococcus octavius, **B2**.912
  biochemical characteristics, **B2**.908 (Tab.)
  classification, **B2**.905
Anaerococcus prevotii, **B2**.913
  biochemical characteristics, **B2**.908 (Tab.)
  classification, **B2**.904–5
  clinical importance, **B2**.910
  as normal microbiota, **B2**.907–10
Anaerococcus tetradius, **B2**.913
  biochemical characteristics, **B2**.908 (Tab.)
Anaerococcus vaginalis, **B2**.913
  biochemical characteristics, **B2**.908 (Tab.)
  classification, **B2**.904–5
  normal microbiota, **B2**.910
Anaeroglobulus germinatus, **B2**.1312
Anaeroplasma, **B2**.1958 (Tab.)
  classification, **B2**.1967
  culture, **B2**.1963
Anaerorhabdus furcosus, **B1**.296 (Tab.)
Anajatuba virus, **V2**.1666 (Tab.)
Anal intercourse, viral infection, **V1**.237
Anal swabs, *Taenia saginata saginata* diagnosis,
    P.667
Anamorph(s), **M**.77, **M**.78 (Fig.), **M**.79 (Fig.),
    M.221 (Tab.)
  classification, **M**.45
  dermatophytes, **M**.45–6, **M**.221 (Tab.)
  history, **M**.10–1
Anaphylatoxin inactivator (carboxypeptidase
    N), **I**.147
Anaphylaxis, vaccines, **V2**.1564
Anaplasma
  antibacterial susceptibility/resistance,
    B2.2065–6
  antigens, **B2**.2055–7
    diversity, **B2**.2053–5
  classification, **B2**.2026, **B2**.2048–9, **B2**.2053
  culture, **B2**.2052
  genome, **B2**.2053–5
    gene cloning, **B2**.2053–5
  habitats, **B2**.2049 (Tab.), **B2**.2050–1
  identification and typing methods, **B2**.2057
  identification, staining procedures, **B2**.2051–2
  infection, **B2**.2049 (Tab.), **B2**.2059–61
    tick transmission, **B2**.2066–7
  isolation, **B2**.2052
  metabolism, **B2**.2053
  microenvironment, **B2**.2051
  morphology, **B2**.2051
  replication, **B2**.2052
Anaplasma bovis, **B2**.2049 (Tab.)
Anaplasma centrale
  antigens
    genes, **B2**.2053–5
    MSP5, **B2**.2056
  identification and typing methods, **B2**.2057
  nomenclature, **B2**.2049–50
Anaplasma marginale
  antigens, **B2**.2056–7
    diversity, **B2**.2055
    major surface proteins, **B2**.2053–6
    MSP5, **B2**.2056
  classification, **B2**.2027 (Fig.)
  genome, **B2**.2053

Anaplasma marginale (*Continued*)
  habitats, hosts and diseases, **B2**.2049 (Tab.)
  identification and typing methods, **B2**.2057
  nomenclature, **B2**.2049–50
Anaplasma ovis, **B2**.2053–5
Anaplasma phagocytophilum (*Ehrlichia phagocytophilia*)
  antibiotic sensitivity, **B2**.2065–6
  antigens, **B2**.2056–7
    diversity, **B2**.2055
    genes, **B2**.2055
    major surface protein-2, **B2**.2053–6
    morphology, **B2**.2052 (Fig.)
  Borrelia burgdorferi co-transmission, **B2**.2060, **B2**.2063–4, **B2**.2066
  classification, **B2**.2027 (Fig.), **B2**.2050–1
  habitats, hosts and diseases, **B2**.2049 (Tab.), **B2**.2050–1
  identification and typing methods, **B2**.2057
  infection *see below*
Anaplasma phagocytophilum (*Ehrlichia phagocytophilia*), infection (human anaplasmosis), **B2**.2058 (Tab.), **B2**.2059–61
  cells infected, **B2**.2059–60
  clinical presentation, **B2**.2060
  diagnosis, **B2**.2059–60, **B2**.2063–5
    culture-based assays, **B2**.2065
    molecular diagnostic assays, **B2**.2064–5
    serological assays, **B2**.2063–4
    specimen collection, **B2**.2063–5
  emerging bacterial infection, **B1**.362
  epidemiology and natural history, **B2**.2062–3
    reforested areas, **B1**.362
  histopathologic changes, **B2**.2060–1
  prevention, **B2**.2066
  severity, **B2**.2060
  tick testing as predictor of disease, **B2**.2053–5
  transmission, pathogenesis, and clinical manifestations, **B2**.2057–61, **B2**.2058 (Tab.)
  treatment, **B2**.2066
Anaplasma platys, **B2**.2049 (Tab.)
Anaplasmataceae
  antigens, **B2**.2055–7
    immune reactions toward, **B2**.2056–7
    Surface_Ag_2 proteins, **B2**.2053–6
  cell wall composition, **B2**.2051, **B2**.2055–7
  classification, **B2**.2048–9, **B2**.2053
    phylogenetic relationship, **B2**.2053, **B2**.2054 (Fig.)
  genome, **B2**.2053–5
  historical perspectives, **B2**.2049–50
  identification and typing methods, **B2**.2057
    serological tests, **B2**.2057
    staining procedures, **B2**.2051–2
  microenvironment and morphology, **B2**.2051
Anaplasmosis (human) *see Anaplasma phagocytophilum* (*Ehrlichia phagocytophilia*), infection (human anaplasmosis)
Anatomical barriers, host resistance, **B1**.175–6
Ancylistaceae, **M**.347, **M**.348 (Tab.), **M**.349

Ancylostoma, **P**.589, **I**.682–3
  classification, **P**.715
  life cycle, **P**.589
  structure, **P**.587 (Fig.), **P**.589
  zoonotic infection, **P**.715 (Tab.)
  see also individual species
Ancylostoma brasiliense, **P**.715 (Tab.)
Ancylostoma caninum, **P**.715 (Tab.)
  biology/feeding, **P**.719
Ancylostoma ceylanicum, **P**.715 (Tab.)
Ancylostoma duodenale, **P**.713
  biology/feeding, **P**.714 (Tab.), **P**.718, **P**.719
  epidemiology/population biology, **P**.722
    global distribution/abundance, **P**.722
    prevalence, **P**.713–14
  historical aspects, **P**.8–9
  infection, **P**.719, **P**.720–1
    cross-placenta, **P**.720–1
    vaccines, **I**.933 (Tab.)
  life cycle, **P**.718 (Tab.), **P**.720 (Fig.)
  life expectancy, **P**.60 (Tab.)
  morphology, **P**.717
    buccal capsules, **P**.717 (Fig.)
    eggs, **P**.720
    Necator americanus vs., **P**.717
  as opportunistic species, **P**.720–1
  see also Hookworm infection
Ancylostoma japonicum, **P**.715 (Tab.)
Ancylostoma malayanum, **P**.715 (Tab.)
Ancylostomatidae, **P**.589
  features, **P**.589
Ancylostomatoidea, **P**.589
  features, **P**.589
Ancylostoma tubaeforme, **P**.715 (Tab.)
Andes virus, **V2**.1666 (Tab.)
Anellovirus
  characteristics, **V1**.177 (Tab.)
  classification, **V1**.27 (Tab.), **V1**.42, **V2**.1277, **V2**.1278 (Tab.)
Anelloviruses, **V2**.**1276–83**
Anemia
  aplastic, chloramphenicol, **B1**.484–5
  babesiosis, **P**.454
  falciparum malaria, **P**.481
  hemolytic, *Mycoplasma pneumoniae* infection, **B1**.634
  iron-deficiency *see* Iron-deficiency anemia
  malaria, **P**.498–9, **P**.501 (Tab.)
    in children, **P**.482–3
    mechanisms, **P**.495
  pernicious, *Diphyllobothrium latum* infection, **P**.672, **P**.673
Anergic diffuse cutaneous leishmaniasis (ADCL) *see* Leishmaniasis, New World
Anergy *see* Clonal anergy
Anesthesia, leprosy, **B2**.1204, **B2**.1205
Aneurinibacillus, **B2**.922–3
Aneurinibacillus aneurinilyticus, **B2**.922–3
Aneurysms, in Chagas disease, **P**.386, **P**.386 (Fig.)
Angiostrongylidae, **P**.592
Angiostrongylus, **P**.592
  infection, eosinophils, **I**.57
  see also Parastrongylus; individual species

Angiostrongylus cantonensis, **P**.802–8
  classification/morphology, **P**.802, **P**.803 (Fig.)
    females, **P**.802
    males, **P**.802
  control, **P**.807–8
    prevention, **P**.808
  geographical distribution, **P**.804
  infection *see below*
  life cycle, **P**.803–4
    intermediate hosts, **P**.803
    paratenic hosts, **P**.803
    transmission/epidemiology, **P**.804
Angiostrongylus cantonensis infection
  clinical manifestations, **P**.804–5
    animal model, **P**.805, **P**.806 (Fig.)
    eosinophilic meningocephalitis, **P**.803
    eosinophilic myelomeningoencephalitis, **P**.804–5
    eosinophilic radiculomyelocephalitis, **P**.804–5
    ocular angiostrongyliasis, **P**.805
    self-limiting, **P**.804
    symptom frequency, **P**.805 (Tab.)
  diagnosis, **P**.806–7, **P**.807 (Tab.)
    cerebrospinal fluid eosinophilia, **P**.807
    eosinophilia, **P**.806
    magnetic resonance imaging, **P**.806
    serology, **P**.806–7
  pathogenesis/pathology, **P**.805–6
    eosinophil infiltrates, **P**.805, **P**.806 (Fig.)
    leukocyte infiltrates, **P**.805–6
Angiostrongylus costaricensis, **P**.808–10
  control, **P**.810
    prevention, **P**.810
  infection *see below*
  life cycle, **P**.808–9
    intermediate host, **P**.808–9
    migratory pathway, **P**.809
    natural host, **P**.808–9
  morphology, **P**.808, **P**.808 (Fig.)
  transmission/epidemiology, **P**.809
Angiostrongylus costaricensis infection
  clinical manifestations, **P**.809
    symptom frequency, **P**.809 (Tab.)
  diagnosis, **P**.810
  pathogenesis/pathology, **P**.810
    granulomas, **P**.810
Angiostrongylus mackerrase, **P**.802
Angiostrongylus malaysiensis, **P**.802
Angiotensin-converting enzyme 2 (ACE2), **V1**.838
Angiotensin-converting enzyme gene *see ACE* gene
Angiotensinogen, **I**.204
Angular cheilitis, **M**.598
  candidiasis, **M**.598
Anidulafungin, **M**.154
  characteristics, **M**.155 (Tab.)
Anilides, **B1**.428
Animal(s)
  listeriosis in, **B2**.953–4
    experimental models, **B2**.962–3
  Lyme borreliosis, **B2**.1822–3
  melioidosis, **B2**.1628–9
  normal gut flora, **B2**.1934

Animal(s) (*Continued*)
  parasitic disease control, **P**.115–16
  pathogens, **B1**.202–4
  as reservoir hosts *see* Reservoir hosts
  as source of bacterial infection, **B1**.329
    wastes, **B1**.212, **B1**.223–4
  toxoplasmosis, **P**.436, **P**.439–40
  vaccination, **P**.439–40
Animal domestication
  gastrointestinal nematodes, **P**.713–14
  Leishmania braziliensis, **P**.326–7
Animal facilities, airborne bacteria,
  B1.186 (Tab.), **B1**.189
Animal infection
  Chlamydia psittaci infection, **B2**.2014
  coronaviruses, **V1**.392
  rabies *see* Rabies
  Salmonella Typhi infection, **B2**.1425
Animal models
  adeno-associated virus gene vectors,
    V2.1600–1
  antiviral chemotherapy, **V2**.1609–10,
    V2.1609 (Tab.)
  autoimmune disease *see* Autoimmune
    diseases/disorders; *specific diseases/
    infection*
  Avian pneumovirus, **V1**.790
  Blastocystis hominis, **P**.564
  Burkholderia thailandensis infection,
    B2.1625–6
  cryptosporidiosis, **P**.405–7
  ebolaviruses, **V2**.1095
  filovirus infection, **V2**.1095
  gastrointestinal candidiasis, **M**.262
  genetic susceptibility to viral infection,
    I.588–9
  hepatitis B, **V2**.1233
  Human metapneumovirus, **V1**.790
  Human respiratory syncytial virus, **V1**.790
  leishmaniasis, **I**.596
  linkage, **I**.572–3
  Marburg virus, **V2**.1095
  measles pathogenesis, **V1**.725
  Metapneumovirus, **V1**.790
  microsporidiosis, **P**.540
  NK cell ablation, **I**.82, **I**.85
  oropharyngeal candidiasis, **M**.263
  PCP, **M**.793, **M**.795–6
  Pneumovirus, **V1**.790
  Pseudomonas aeruginosa infection, **I**.593–4
  rhinosporidiosis, **M**.456–7, **M**.472
  schistosomiasis, **P**.605–6
  tuberculosis granulomas, **I**.714–15,
    I.715 (Fig.), **I**.716 (Fig.)
  virucidal activity, **B1**.435–6
  vulvovaginal candidiasis, **M**.264, **M**.265–6
Anisakidae, **P**.590–1
Anisakis, **P**.590, **P**.813–18
  classification/morphology, **P**.813–14,
    P.814 (Fig.), **P**.815 (Fig.), **P**.817 (Fig.)
  control, **P**.818
  infection *see Anisakis* infection
  life cycle, **P**.590–1, **P**.814, **P**.815 (Fig.)
  transmission/epidemiology, **P**.814
  see also Pseudoterranova decipens

Anisakis infection
  clinical manifestations, **P**.815–16,
    P.816 (Tab.)
    gastric infection, **P**.816
    granulomas, **P**.816–17
    hypersensitivity reaction, **P**.815–16
    intestinal infection, **P**.816
  diagnosis, **P**.817–18
    endoscopy, **P**.817
    immunodiagnosis, **P**.817–18
    radiology, **P**.817
    ultrasound, **P**.817
  pathology, **P**.816–17
  public health importance, **P**.44–5
*Anixiopsis stercoraria (Aphanoascus
    fulvescens),* **M**.247
Ankylosing spondylitis, *HLA-B27* association,
  I.577, **I**.594–5, **I**.752, **I**.752 (Tab.)
Annual transmission potential (ATP),
  onchocerciasis, **P**.785–6
Anogenital cancers, HPV infection,
  V1.463 (Tab.), **V1**.465–7
Anopheles, **P**.470
  DDT resistance, **P**.126
  feeding habits, **P**.469, **P**.470
  indoor feeding (endophagy), **P**.470
  infection by *Plasmodium,* **P**.470
  lymphatic filariasis transmission, **P**.9
  O'nyong-nyong virus transmission, **V2**.1022
  outdoor feeding (exophagy), **P**.470
  Plasmodium development, **P**.469–70
  vectorial competence, **P**.470
Anoplocephalidae, **P**.577
Anorectal infection, gonorrhea, **B1**.658
Anorexia, acute phase response, **I**.198
Anterior nares, *Staphylococcus,* **B2**.777–9
Anthelmintic drugs
  Enterobius vermicularis control, **P**.732
  gastrointestinal nematode control, **P**.730
  liver fluke control, **P**.653–4
  lung fluke control, **P**.653–4
Anthrax, **B1**.203, **B2**.930–8
  in animals, **B2**.930
    forms and symptoms, **B2**.930
    herbivores, **B2**.930
    specimens for diagnosis, **B2**.933–4
  bioterrorism, **B1**.364
  diagnosis, **B2**.934–7
    specimens for, **B2**.932–3, **B2**.947
  etiology, **B2**.930
  in humans, **B2**.930–1
    clinical features, **B2**.932
    cutaneous, **B2**.931–2
    gastrointestinal, **B2**.931–2
    inhalation, **B2**.931–2
    meningitis, **B2**.931
    milk-borne transmission, **B1**.242
    non-industrial, **B2**.930–1
    oropharyngeal, **B2**.931– 2
    prophylaxis, **B2**.937–8
    specimens for diagnosis, **B2**.932–4
    treatment, **B2**.937–8
    vaccination, **B2**.938
  organism entry, **B1**.203
  pneumonia, **B1**.637

TNF-α suppression, **I**.652
  vaccines, **I**.933 (Tab.)
Anthraxin (trade mark) skin test, **B2**.937
Anthropophilic dermatophytes, **M**.45–6,
  M.223–5, **M**.227–8, **M**.227 (Tab.)
Anti-amebic antibodies, **P**.209
Anti-antigen 5 antibodies
  alveolar echinococcosis, **P**.689
  cystic echinococcosis, **P**.689
  neurocysticercosis, **P**.689
Anti-antigen B antibodies, cystic
  echinococcosis, **P**.689–90
Anti-antigen B (paramyosin) antibodies,
  cysticercosis, **P**.689–90
Antibacterial agents/therapy, **B1**.421–45,
  B1.466–505
  activity
    evaluation, **B1**.435–6, **B1**.435 (Tab.)
    factors affecting, **B1**.430–3
  classification by mode of action, **B1**.470,
    B1.470 (Tab.)
    cell membrane agents, **B1**.470 (Tab.),
      B1.496–7
    cell wall synthesis, **B1**.470–81,
      B1.470 (Tab.)
    nucleic acid synthesis inhibitors,
      B1.470 (Tab.), **B1**.490–6
    protein synthesis inhibitors, **B1**.470 (Tab.),
      B1.481–90
  combinations, **B1**.470
  concentration, **B1**.430–1, **B1**.431 (Fig.),
    B1.431 (Tab.)
  control of, **B1**.468–9
    education, **B1**.468
    formulary, **B1**.468
    guidelines, **B1**.468
    laboratory testing, **B1**.468–9
    primary *vs.* secondary care, **B1**.468–9
    use restriction, **B1**.468
    WHO essential drugs, **B1**.467,
      B1.467 (Tab.)
  ecological issues, **B1**.466–7
    environmental pollution, **B1**.466
    resistance generation, **B1**.466–7
  food, **B1**.267
  future prospects, **B1**.466
  laboratory control, **B1**.497–500
    antibiotic assays, **B1**.500
    see also Antibacterial susceptibility testing
  mechanisms of action, **B1**.436–40,
    B1.437 (Tab.)
  natural antibacterial systems, **B1**.430
  pharmacodynamics, **B1**.469–70
    dose variation, **B1**.469–70
    dosing interval, **B1**.469–70
  physical agents, **B1**.454
  principles, **B1**.469
    clinical assessments, **B1**.469
  resistance *see below*
  terminology, **B1**.421
  in treatment, **B1**.422–30
    upper respiratory tract infection, **B1**.608
    *see also specific diseases/infection; specific
      types*
  see also Antibiotic(s); *specific antibacterial
    agents*

Antibacterial defense mechanisms, *Ascaris lumbricoides,* **P**.719
Antibacterial susceptibility/resistance, **B1**.440–5, **B1**.441 (Tab.)
  bacterial evolution, **B1**.33
  control of, **B1**.468
  generation in community, **B1**.467
  generation in hospitals, **B1**.466–7, **B1**.467–8
  resistance gene conjugation, **B1**.103–4
  use *vs.,* **B1**.467–8
  see also individual species
Antibacterial susceptibility testing, **B1**.497–500, **B1**.716–18
  antibiotic titrations, **B1**.497–8
    E-test, **B1**.498
    indications for, **B1**.500
    MIC titrations, **B1**.498
  breakpoint method, **B1**.498
  clinical relevance, **B1**.500
  disk diffusion, **B1**.498
  DNA probes, **B1**.498–500
  Enterobacteriaceae, **B2**.1352–4
  semi-automated methods, **B1**.498
Antibiotic(s)
  aerosolized, **B1**.650–1
  historical perspective, **B1**.371–2
  opportunistic infection, **M**.12
  organisms
    Campylobacter, **B2**.1548
    Cedecea, **B2**.1491
    Citrobacter, **B2**.1476
    Edwardsiella, **B2**.1491–2
    Enterobacter, **B2**.1484–5
    Escherichia, **B2**.1369–70
    Ewingella, **B2**.1493
    Haemophilus, **B2**.1702–4, **B2**.1710
    keratitis, **B1**.602
    Klebsiella, **B2**.1480
    Kluyvera, **B2**.1494
    Lactobacillus, **B2**.866
    Leclercia, **B2**.1495
    Legionella, **B2**.1776–7
    Leminorella, **B2**.1496
    Listeria, **B2**.957–8
    Moellerella, **B2**.1496
    Mycobacterium, **B2**.1217–19
    Nocardia, **B2**.1165–6
    Rahnella, **B2**.1497
    Serratia, **B2**.1488–9
    Staphylococcus, **B2**.793–805, **B2**.794 (Tab.)
    Streptococcus, **B2**.861–2
    Tatumella, **B2**.1497
    Yokenella, **B2**.1498
  prophylaxis
    Clostridium difficile infection, **B2**.1122–3
    endocarditis, **B1**.539
    meningococcal meningitis, **B1**.567
    pneumococcal meningitis, **B1**.572
    in surgery, **B1**.387–8
  resistance
    bacterial evolution, **B1**.30, **B1**.31
    drug efflux, **B1**.440
    nosocomial infection, **B1**.371
    plasmid genes, **B1**.110–11
    repeat exposure, **B1**.441

transposons, **B1**.111
synthesis, plasmids, **B1**.113–14
in therapy
  conjunctivitis, **B1**.600
  in cystic fibrosis, **B1**.650–1
  endocarditis, **B1**.533
  endophthalmitis, **B1**.604
  in intracranial abscess, **B1**.587–9, **B1**.589 (Tab.)
  joint prostheses, **B1**.392
  pneumococcal meningitis, **B1**.571
Antibiotic prophylaxis, neutrophil disorders, **I**.50
Antibodies, **P**.69–70, **V1**.276–8, **I.303–38**
  analysis, **V2**.1545–7
    avidity measurement, **V2**.1547
    isotype determination, **V2**.1546–7
    paired sample titration, **V2**.1545–6
    specimens, **V2**.1533 (Tab.), **V2**.1547
    viral epitope mapping, **V2**.1546
    virus neutralization assays, **V2**.1545
    see also specific assays
  assays
    histoplasmosis, **M**.111–12
    penicilliosis marneffei, **M**.570
  bacterial infection, **I**.647
    candidiasis, **M**.607
    degradation/modification, **I**.662
  classical complement pathway activation, **I**.142–3
  detection, **P**.153–4
    enterovirus infection, **V2**.877
    rubella, **V2**.978–81
  discovery, **B1**.7
  functions, **B1**.743
    basophil activation, **I**.354, **I**.357
  helminth infection
    blocking, **I**.685–6
    class switching, **I**.686
    destruction, **I**.685–6
  immune evasion, **V1**.287, **V1**.313 (Fig.)
    bacterial evasion, **B1**.177
    blocking, **B2**.1282
  infected cell destruction, **V1**.278
    ADCC *see* Antibody-dependent cellular cytotoxicity (ADCC)
    complement-mediated lysis, **V1**.278
    in vivo, **V1**.278
  isotypes
    gastrointestinal nematode infection, **P**.725
    see also individual isotypes
  kinetics, **I**.492, **I**.492 (Fig.)
  levels during infection *see* Humoral immune response
  neutralization mechanisms, **V1**.277
    penetration inhibition, **V1**.277
    virus–receptor blockade, **V1**.277
    see also Neutralizing antibodies
  in parasitic infection, **P**.68
    lymphatic filariasis, **P**.776
    malaria immunology/immunity, **P**.488–9
    trichomoniasis, **P**.258
  protein A-binding, **I**.661–2
  protein G-binding, **I**.661–2
  structure *see* Immunoglobulin structure

vaccines, **V2**.1556
viral infection, **I**.638
  HCMV infection, **V1**.524, **V1**.525
  HTLV-1-associated myelopathy/tropical spastic paraparesis, **V2**.1429–30
  Human respiratory syncytial virus, **V1**.794–5
  immune interference, **I**.638
  virion release inhibition, **V1**.278
  see also Humoral immune response; Immunoglobulin(s); *specific antibodies; specific immunoglobulins*
Antibody-binding proteins, bacterial immune interference, **I**.661–2
Antibody-binding sites, influenza hemagglutinin, **V1**.664
Antibody-dependent cellular cytotoxicity (ADCC), **P**.70, **V1**.278, **I**.354, **I**.357
  CD4 cells, **I**.791
  helminth infection, **P**.88, **P**.90, **I**.683
    filarial nematode infection, **P**.91
    Schistosoma, **I**.683
    schistosomiasis, **P**.94, **P**.617–18, **P**.617 (Fig.), **P**.631–2
  histoplasmosis capsulati, **M**.525–6, **M**.529
  in HIV infection, **I**.791
  macrophages, **V1**.273
  malaria immunity, **P**.490
  NK cells, **I**.627, **I**.796
    in cancer, **I**.101
  structure–function relationship, **I**.311–12
Antibody-dependent cellular inhibition (ADCI), malaria immunity, **P**.489
Antibody-dependent enhancement (ADE), **V2**.1413
Antibody Directed Enzyme Pro-drug Therapy *see* ADEPT (Antibody Directed Enzyme Pro-drug Therapy)
Antibody fragments *see* Monoclonal antibodies, therapy
Antibody-induced antigenic modulation, **V2**.1413
Antibody-mediated absorption, **V1**.211
Antibody-mediated neutralization, *Mononegavirales* order, **V1**.381
Anti-CD40 antibodies, tumor therapy, **I**.358
α1-Antichymotrypsin, IL-6 effects, **I**.285
Anticoagulants, *Ancylostoma,* **P**.719
Anticonvulsive drugs, subacute sclerosing panencephalitis treatment, **V1**.734
Anti-cysticercus antibodies, **P**.689
Anti-disease immunity, malaria, **P**.486, **P**.492–3
Anti-DNA antibody induction, DNA vaccines, **I**.920
AntiDNase B assays, *Streptococcus pyogenes* detection, **B1**.750–1
Anti-epileptic drugs, neurocysticercosis treatment, **P**.696
Antifolates
  mechanism of action, **P**.509
  resistance
    Plasmodium, **P**.479–80
    point mutations, **P**.480
Antifungal agents, **M**.182–5, **M.147–63**
  clinical trial design for, **M**.165–7
  current use, **M**.148–55
  empiric therapy, **M**.165

Antifungal agents (*Continued*)
  fungicidals and fungistatics, **M**.156
  future drugs, **M**.155
    new targets, **M**.155
  historical aspects, **M**.147–8
  mechanisms of action, **M**.148, **M**.148 (Tab.)
  principles of therapy, **M**.164
  prophylactic and preemptive therapy,
    M.164–5
  resistance, **M**.155–6, **M**.168
    AIDS, **M**.168
    allylamines, **M**.175
    azoles, **M**.170, **M**.173, **M**.173 (Tab.)
    correlations with clinical resistance, **M**.171
    definitions of, **M**.168–9
    detection, **M**.169–71
    echinocandins, **M**.176
    flucytosine, **M**.176
    griseofulvin, **M**.177
    mechanisms of, **M**.171–7
    origin of, **M**.169
    polyenes, **M**.170–1
    primary and secondary, **M**.169
    see also individual species
  specific therapy, **M**.165
  for superficial fungal infection, **M**.182
  susceptibility, **M**.752 (Tab.)
  susceptibility testing *see* Susceptibility
    testing, antifungal agents
  topical, **M**.182–5
  see also individual agents; individual species;
    specific diseases/infection
Antigen(s)
  Aspergillus fumigatus, **M**.694, **M**.712
  BCR binding, **I**.342, **I**.348
  candidiasis, **M**.590–1, **M**.607
  complexity in parasites, **I**.680
  cryptococcosis, **M**.641, **M**.649
  detection, **P**.154, **B1**.718
    clonorchiasis, **P**.653
    histoplasmosis, **M**.112
    malaria diagnosis, **P**.504
    opisthorchiasis, **P**.653
    penicilliosis marneffei diagnosis, **M**.571
  'dummy antigens' as controls, **V1**.91
  extraction procedures, **V1**.91–2
  historical aspects, **B1**.12
  infection diagnosis, **V2**.1535
    HTLV, **V2**.1294
  intranasal vaccination, **I**.830
  malaria, **P**.486–8, **P**.487 (Tab.)
    diversity, **P**.491–2
  microfold (M) cell uptake, **I**.530
  monoclonal antibody therapy, **I**.362
  mucosal vaccination, **I**.827
  persistence, seroepidemiology, **B1**.743
  preparation, **V1**.90–1
  presentation, **P**.68
  processing, **P**.68
  specificity of antibodies for, **B1**.12
  TCR recognition, **I**.461–3
  in urine, **B1**.673
  variation
    bacterial immune interference *see* Immune
      evasion, bacteria

  protozoa, **I**.680–1
  see also individual species
Antigen B (paramyosin), *Taenia solium,*
  P.682–3
Antigen-dependent immunological memory,
  I.496, **I**.497 (Tab.)
Antigenic change, transmission dynamics, **P**.62
Antigenic drift, **B1**.324
  influenza, **V1**.367, **V1**.668–9
  see also Influenza viruses
Antigenic modulation, **V2**.1413
Antigenic shift, **B1**.324
  influenza, **V1**.367, **V1**.669–71
  see also Influenza virus A
Antigenic variation
  discovery, **P**.15
  enterovirus infection, **V2**.876–7
  Giardia, **P**.245, **P**.246
  HIV-1, **V1**.262
  influenza hemagglutinin, **V1**.653,
    V1.670 (Fig.)
  malaria, **P**.492
  noroviruses *see* Noroviruses
  Plasmodium, **P**.82, **P**.492
  smoldering infection, **V1**.262
  Trypanosoma brucei, **P**.80, **P**.169
  variable surface glycoprotein, **P**.353–5, **P**.362
Antigen-independent immunological memory,
  I.496–8, **I**.497 (Tab.)
Antigen presentation, **I**.29, **I**.381–3
  bacterial immune interference *see* Immune
    evasion, bacteria
  basophils, **I**.66
  CD1, **I**.29
  to CD4 T cells *see* CD4+ T-cell(s)
  definition, **I**.375
  dendritic cells, **I**.29, **I**.903
  eosinophils, **I**.67
  historical aspects/re-evaluation, **I**.12
  immune evasion *see* Immune evasion
  Langerhans' cells, **I**.821
  macrophages, **I**.29–30
  malaria immunity, **P**.489–90
  MHC I *see* Major histocompatibility
    complex (MHC) class I
  MHC II *see* Major histocompatibility
    complex (MHC) class II
  MHC class I, **V1**.275
  MHC class II, **V1**.274–5
  MHC restriction, **I**.375, **I**.379, **I**.379 (Tab.),
    I.426, **I**.427 (Fig.)
  mucosal immune response, **I**.524
    common mucosal immune system, **I**.534–5
  orthopoxviruses, **V1**.619
  pattern recognition, **I**.123
  peripheral lymphoid organs, **I**.378–9
  poxvirus immune evasion, **V1**.229–30,
    V1.619, **V1**.622–3
  second signal, **I**.29
  TCRs, **I**.555
  thymus, **I**.378–9
  vaccines, **V2**.1556
  see also Antigen processing
Antigen-presenting cells (APCs), **P**.68, **I**.112,
  I.376–8, **I**.555
  activation, adjuvant effects, **I**.926

  airway hypersensitivity, **I**.736–7
  asthma, **I**.736–7
  CD8 T cell activation, **I**.404, **I**.426–7
  hematopoiesis, **I**.112, **I**.113 (Fig.)
  IFN-γ effects, **I**.288
  IL-27, **I**.284
  immunological synapse, **I**.465
  measles-induced immunosuppression,
    V1.727–9, **V1**.728 (Tab.)
  mucosal immune response, **I**.538
  pattern recognition, **I**.112 (Fig.)
  Peyer's patches, **I**.532
  schistosomiasis, **P**.617
  superantigens, **B1**.157
  T cell interactions, **I**.383–4
    'two-signal' hypothesis, **I**.383
  Th1/Th2 differentiation, **I**.399
  transcutaneous immunization, **I**.837
  transfection, DNA vaccines, **I**.914,
    I.915 (Fig.), **I**.916
  tuberculosis, **B2**.1202
Antigen processing, **P**.68, **I**.377, **I**.377 (Fig.),
  I.382, **I**.382 (Tab.)
  chaperones, **I**.415
  common mucosal immune system, **I**.534–5
  defective ribosomal products, **I**.410
  definition, **I**.409
  entry into cell, **I**.382
  exogenous peptides, **I**.414–15
    cell membrane crossing, **I**.414
    endoplasmic reticulum-associated
      degradation, **I**.414
    endosomal compartments, **I**.414–5
  exogenous proteins, **I**.414–15
  immune evasion *see* Immune evasion
  orthopoxviruses, **V1**.619
  poxvirus immune evasion, **V1**.229–30,
    V1.619, **V1**.622–3
  proteasomes, **I**.412
  secretory proteases, **I**.414
  TAP-independent, **I**.413–14
  trimming enzymes, **I**.412–13
    aminopeptidases, **I**.412
  vaccines, **V2**.1556
  viral immune interference, **I**.633, **I**.633 (Fig.),
    I.635 (Fig.)
  see also Antigen presentation; Major
    histocompatibility complex (MHC) class
    I; Major histocompatibility complex
    (MHC) class II; Ubiquitin–proteasome
    pathway
Anti-HBc test, **V2**.1246, **V2**.1251–4
Anti-HBs antibodies, **V2**.1254
Anti-heat shock protein antibodies, *Chlamydia*
  infection, **B2**.2009
Anti-herpes drugs, **V1**.511–12
Anti-idiotypic antibodies
  autoimmune disease therapy, **I**.864
  vaccines, **V2**.1553
Anti-idiotypic vaccination, candidiasis, **M**.267
Anti-inflammatory cytokines, **I**.274 (Tab.),
  I.292–7
Anti-interleukin 6 antibodies, **V1**.554
Anti-La antibodies, SLE, **I**.758
Antimalarial drugs *see* Malaria

Antimicrobial peptides, **I.165–79**
  cathelicidins *see* Cathelicidins
  defensins *see* Defensins
  definition, **I**.165
  in neutrophils, **I**.165
Antimicrobial susceptibility, *Basidiobolus ranarrum*, **M**.352
Antimonials, pentavalent, **P**.306, **P**.341
Antimony, resistance to, **B1**.114
Antinaeglerial agents, **P**.236–7
Antioxidant secretion, *Ascaris* immune evasion, **I**.686
Antiparasite drug resistance *see* Drug resistance
Antiphagocytic activity, *Aspergillus fumigatus*, **M**.707
Antiphospholysin test, staphylococci detection, **B1**.750
Antiport, **B1**.49
Antiproliferative activity, interferon-α, **I**.245, **I**.245 (Tab.)
Anti-RNP antibodies, SLE, **I**.758
Anti-Ro antibodies, SLE, **I**.758
Antisepsis, definition, **B1**.421
Antiseptics
  Burkholderia cepacia complex survival, **B2**.1610
  historical aspects, **B1**.6
  mode of action, **B1**.497
  total-body treatment, **B1**.387
Anti-Sm antibodies, SLE, **I**.758
Antistrepsolysin O titer (ASOT), **B1**.750–1
Anti-swarming agents, *Proteus* culture, **B2**.1438–9
Anti-TAC monoclonal antibody, IL-2 blocking, **I**.280
Antithrombin III, **I**.204
  septic shock therapy, **I**.701–2
α₁-Antitrypsin
  in airway secretion, **B1**.623
  deficiency, **B1**.623
Antituberculous drugs
  in drug-resistant TB, **B2**.1199–200
  see also Tuberculosis
Anti-tyvelose reactions, *Trichinella*, **P**.764
Antiviral chemotherapy, **V2.1605–45**
  clinical trials, **V2**.1610
  combination, **V2**.1639
  controlled trials, **V1**.365
  discovery/assessment, **V2**.1606–10
    animal models, **V2**.1609–10, **V2**.1609 (Tab.)
    molecular targets, **V2**.1606, **V2**.1607–10
    rational drug design, **V2**.1606–7
    serendipitous, **V2**.1606
    structure–activity relationships, **V2**.1609
    tissue culture, **V2**.1608–9
    virus enzyme screens, **V2**.1608
  effective concentration (EC₅₀), **V2**.1608–9
  historical aspects, **V1**.8–9, **V1**.9 (Tab.)
    year(s) of introduction, **V1**.9 (Tab.)
  IFN-α, **I**.245, **I**.245 (Tab.), **I**.260 (Tab.)
  immune system, **V2**.1606
  infection
    congenital HCMV infection, **V2**.1453
    HCMV infection, **V1**.526–7
    hepatitis B treatment, **V2**.1260–1

hepatitis C control, **V2**.1215–16
HIV infection, **V2**.1473
HTLV-associated myelopathy(HAM)/ tropical spastic paraparesis (TSP), **V2**.1290
influenza, **V1**.679–80
latent infection, **V2**.1638–9
poxvirus therapy, **V1**.590
Kaposi's sarcoma therapy, **V1**.553
mechanism of action, **V2**.1607 (Fig.), **V2**.1610–31
  herpesvirus inhibitors, **V2**.1611–19
new strategies, **V1**.19–20
  error catastrophe, **V1**.19–20
prophylactic, tumor virus infection, **V1**.349
selective index, **V2**.1610
selective toxicity, **V2**.1605
  animal models, **V2**.1610
specific diagnosis, **V2**.1605–6
therapeutic index, **V2**.1610
toxicity, **V2**.1637–8
  toxic concentration, **V2**.1608–9
type I INFs, **I**.260 (Tab.)
Antiviral chemotherapy resistance, **V2**.1632–7
  acquired, **V2**.1634 (Tab.)
  biochemical *vs.* clinical, **V2**.1633
  definition, **V2**.1632, **V2**.1632 (Fig.)
  detection of, **V2**.1633 (Tab.)
  error-prone RNA polymerases, **V2**.1632–3
  genetic analysis, **V1**.194
  HIV-1 *see* HIV-1
  in laboratory, **V2**.1634 (Tab.)
  modeling, **V2**.1633
  mutations, **V2**.1633
  study of, **V2**.1634 (Tab.)
  viral evolution, **V2**.1632
  virus fitness, **V2**.1633–4
  see also specific antivirals
Antiviral susceptibility testing, **V2**.1543–4
  genotypic assays, **V2**.1543
  HIV, **V2**.1543
  HSV, **V2**.1543
  PCR, **V2**.1543
  phenotypic assays, **V2**.1543
Aonchotheca, **P**.589
Aortic stenosis, *Chlamydia pneumoniae* infection, **B2**.2016
aP-1 transcription factor, **V1**.335–6
Aphanoascus fulvescens, **M**.247, **M**.249
  culture, **M**.245
  onychomycosis, **M**.247
Aphthovirus, **V1**.50–2
  see also Aphthoviruses
Aphthoviruses
  cell entry, receptors, **V2**.867 (Tab.)
  characteristics, **V2**.861 (Tab.)
  classification, **V2**.858, **V2**.859 (Fig.)
  genome structure, **V2**.865
  properties, **V2**.1162 (Tab.)
  protein processing, **V1**.140
  protein synthesis, **V1**.115–16
  see also Aphthovirus
Apical complexes
  Cryptosporidium parvum, **P**.402
  Plasmodium, **P**.466

Apical complex organelles, *Cryptosporidium parvum*, **P**.402
Apicomplexa, **P**.422, **P**.443, **I**.675–6
Apicoplast, *Plasmodium*, **P**.479
API system, *Enterococcus* identification, **B2**.889–90
Aplastic anemia, chloramphenicol, **B1**.484–5
Apoi virus, **V2**.998 (Tab.)
Apolipoprotein B mRNA editing enzyme (APOBEC3G)
  antiretroviral activity, **V2**.1325–6
  Vif (virus infectivity factor) phosphoprotein interaction, **V2**.1325–6, **V2**.1328
Apolipoproteins, trypanosomes, effect on, **P**.352–3
Apophysomyces, **M**.20, **M**.660 (Tab.), **M**.662
Apophysomyces elegans, **M**.21, **M**.662, **M**.675
  identification, **M**.662–3, **M**.662 (Fig.), **M**.676–7
  infection
    necrotizing fasciitis, **M**.21, **M**.21 (Fig.)
    oculomycoses, **M**.281 (Tab.), **M**.287
    rhino-orbital-cerebral zygomycosis, **M**.290, **M**.291
Apoptosis, **V1**.334, **I**.617, **I**.623–7, **I.131–9**
  bacterial immune interference *see* Immune evasion, bacteria
  bacterial-induced, **I**.136–8
    bacterial toxins, **I**.136–7
    Pseudomonas aeruginosa, **I**.138
    Salmonella, **I**.137–8
    Salmonella typhimurium, **I**.138
    Shigella, **I**.137–8
    Yersinia, **I**.138
  basophils, **I**.57
  caspase activation
    death-inducing signal complex, **I**.623–4
    death receptors, **I**.623–4
    mitochondria, **I**.624
    see also Caspase(s)
  CD4+ T cells in HIV infection, **I**.791–2
  cellular regulation, **I**.624–6
    caspase activity, **I**.624
    mitochondrial apoptosis, **I**.624, **I**.626
  CNS, **V2**.1408
  complement *see* Complement
  debris removal, **I**.136
    complement, **I**.354
    phosphatidylserine, **I**.131, **I**.136
    Rac GTPase, **I**.136
    Rho, **I**.136
  definition, **V1**.229, **I**.623
  eosinophils *see* Eosinophil(s)
  Fas ligand, **I**.477
  historical aspects/re-evaluation, **I**.13–4
  IL-1β, **V1**.621
  immune evasion *see* Immune evasion
  induction, **I**.131–2, **V1**.658, **V1**.662
    bacterial infection *see above*
    CTLs, **I**.422–3
    death receptors, **I**.131
    extrinsic *vs.* intrinsic pathways, **I**.131–2, **I**.132 (Fig.)
    LTα, **I**.286–7
    organelle disruption, **I**.131
    transcriptional control changes, **I**.131

Apoptosis (*Continued*)
  lymphocyte-mediated cytotoxicity, **I**.471–2
  macrophages, **I**.27
  mechanisms/regulation, **I**.135–6, **I**.135 (Fig.)
    caspase-acyivated DNase, **I**.136
    cytoskeleton, **I**.136
    decoy proteins, **I**.135
    FLICE-inhibitory proteins, **I**.135
    Golgi apparatus, **I**.136
    granzyme M, **I**.476
    inhibitors of apoptosis, **I**.135
    NF-κB, **I**.135
    plectin, **I**.136
    ubiquitinylation, **I**.135
  mitochondria, **I**.132–3, **I**.624
    Bcl-2 proteins, **I**.132
    cytochrome *c,* **I**.132
    endonuclease G, **I**.132
    HtrA2/Omni, **I**.132
    mitochondria-permeability transition, **I**.133
    pro-caspases, **I**.132
    Smac/Diablo, **I**.132
  morphological alterations, **I**.131, **I**.135 (Fig.)
  MX protein, **V1**.662
  Mycoplasma hyorhinis inducing, **B2**.1985
  neutrophils *see* Neutrophil(s)
  nuclear DNA cleavage, **I**.131
  p53 induction role, **V1**.334
  peripheral tolerance, **I**.750
  prevention, **V1**.773–4
    Chlamydia pneumoniae infection, **B2**.2009
  pro-apoptosis molecules, **I**.133, **I**.133 (Fig.)
    BH1–3 subfamily, **I**.133
    BH3 subfamily, **I**.133
    mitochondria-permeability transition, **I**.133
  prosurvival molecules, **I**.132–3
    Bcl-2, **I**.132–3, **I**.133 (Fig.)
  reovirus σ1 protein, **V2**.936–7
  signal blocking, **V2**.1595
  transforming growth factor-β, **I**.297
  Ureaplasma urealyticum inducing, **B2**.1985
  viral infection
    adenovirus immune evasion, **V2**.1595
    enterovirus, **V2**.869
    flavivirus, **V2**.997
    HTLV-1-associated myelopathy/tropical
      spastic paraparesis (HAM/TSP), **V2**.1430
    immune interference *see* Immune evasion,
      viruses
    influenza viruses, **V1**.658, **V1**.662
    nonproductive infection, **V1**.205
    papillomavirus E6 protein, **V1**.459–60
    poxviruses *see* Poxviruses
    rabies, **V2**.1123
    reovirus infection, **V2**.936–7
    respiroviruses, **V1**.773–4
    Rubella virus, **V2**.965
    see also Cell–virus interactions
Apoptosis protease-activating factor-1
  (Apaf-1), **I**.135
Apoptosomes
  assembly, **I**.135
  caspase-9 activation, **I**.134, **I**.135
Appendicitis
  amebic, **P**.207

Balantidium coli infection, **P**.279
Enterobius vermicularis infection, **P**.731
Appendix, as inductive site, **I**.530
Apples, black rot, **B1**.282
Approved Lists of Bacterial Names, **B1**.18
Aptamers, **B1**.755
AqpZ, facilitated diffusion, **B1**.48–9
Aquabirnavirus, **V1**.48
Aquareovirus, **V1**.47–8, **V2**.932
Aquarium employees, lobomycosis, **M**.430,
  M.431
Aquatic mammals, morbillivirus infection,
  V1.812–15
Arabinitol, *Candida,* **M**.101, **M**.608
1-β-D-Arabinofuranosylcytosine (ARA-C),
  Borna disease virus infection, **V2**.1153
Arabinose
  fermentation, **B1**.57
  operon, *Escherichia coli,* **B1**.71–2
L-Arabinose fermentation, Enterobacteriaceae
  identification, **B2**.1319 (Tab.)
D-Arabitol fermentation, Enterobacteriaceae
  identification, **B2**.1319 (Tab.)
Arachidonic acid
  eosinophils, **I**.57, **I**.66
  metabolism pathways, **I**.181–4
  metabolites, **I**.181–9
  production
    cyclooxygenases, **I**.181–4
    lipoxygenases, **I**.181–4
    neutrophils, **I**.46
    phospholipase A$_2$, **I**.181–4
  structure, **I**.181
Arachnia propionica, histopathology,
  M.128 (Tab.)
Arachnoiditis, meningeal, **P**.686–7
Araraquara virus, **V2**.1666 (Tab.)
Ara system, plasmid cloning vectors, **B1**.122–3
Aravan virus (ARAV), **V2**.1104
Arboviruses
  epidemiology, **V1**.372–3
  infection *see* Arbovirus infection
  isolation/propagation and identification,
    V1.95, **V1**.96 (Tab.)
  transmission, **V1**.249
Arbovirus infection
  infection process, **V1**.237–9
  laboratory-acquired, **V2**.1516
Arcanobacterium, **B2**.994
  cell wall composition, **B2**.1010 (Tab.)
  classification, **B2**.978 (Tab.), **B2**.1005
  habitats, **B2**.978
  as normal microbiota, **B1**.296 (Tab.)
Arcanobacterium bernardiae, **B2**.994
  disease associations, **B2**.981 (Tab.)
  habitats, **B2**.978
Arcanobacterium haemolyticum, **B2**.994
  biochemical characteristics, **B2**.993 (Tab.)
  disease associations, **B2**.981 (Tab.)
  habitats, **B2**.978
  pharyngitis, **B1**.611–12
Arcanobacterium pyogenes, **B2**.994
  biochemical characteristics, **B2**.993 (Tab.)
  disease associations, **B2**.981 (Tab.)
  habitats, **B2**.978

Archaebacteria, **B1**.11
  cell walls, **B1**.44
  chaperones, **B1**.47
  metabolism, **B1**.68–70
    methanogenesis, **B1**.68–9
    see also Methanogens
    nonmethanogenic, **B1**.69–70
  nonmethanogenic metabolism, **B1**.69–70
  phylogeny, **B1**.30–1
Archezoa
  classification, **P**.195–6, **P**.196, **P**.218
  flagellated, **P**.196–7
Archiacanthocephala
  classification, **P**.597
    Moniliformida, **P**.597
    Oligacanthorhynchida, **P**.597
  features, **P**.597
Archiascomycetes, **M**.55 (Tab.), **M**.62 (Fig.)
Arcitumomab, licensing, **I**.355 (Tab.)
Arcobacter
  antibacterial susceptibility/resistance,
    B2.1556–7
  antigens, structure, **B2**.1555
  cell wall composition, **B2**.1555
  classification, **B2**.1553–4
  culture, **B2**.1555–6
  definition, **B2**.1553
  habitats, **B2**.1554–5
  historical perspective, **B2**.1553–4
  isolation/identification, **B2**.1555–6
    food and environmental specimens,
      B2.1555–6
  morphology, **B2**.1554–5, **B2**.1554 (Fig.)
  pathogenicity, **B2**.1557
    bovine mastitis, **B2**.1557
    diarrheal disease, **B2**.1557
    reproductive disease, **B2**.1557
  physical/chemical agent susceptibility/
    resistance, **B2**.1555
  species, **B2**.1543 (Tab.), **B2**.1557–8
  typing methods, **B2**.1556
Arcobacter butzleri (Campylobacter butzleri),
  B2.1543 (Tab.), **B2**.1557–8
  antibacterial susceptibility/resistance,
    B2.1556–7
  classification, **B2**.1554
  habitats, **B2**.1554
  isolation/identification, **B2**.1556
    culture, **B2**.1555
    typing methods, **B2**.1556
  morphology, **B2**.1554 (Fig.)
  pathogenicity, **B2**.1557
  physical/chemical agent
    susceptibility/resistance, **B2**.1555
Arcobacter cryaerophilus, **B2**.1543 (Tab.),
  B2.1557–8
  antibacterial susceptibility/resistance,
    B2.1556
  classification, **B2**.1553–4
  culture, **B2**.1555
  habitats, **B2**.1554
  isolation/identification, **B2**.1556
  pathogenicity, **B2**.1557
Arcobacter nitrofigilis, **B2**.1557–8
  classification, **B2**.1553–4
  culture, **B2**.1555

Arcobacter nitrofigilis, (Continued)
  habitats, **B2**.1554
Arcobacter skirrowii, **B2**.1543 (Tab.),
    B2.1557–8
  antibacterial susceptibility/resistance,
    B2.1556
  classification, **B2**.1554
  culture, **B2**.1555
  pathogenicity, **B2**.1557
Arenaviridae
  characteristics, **V1**.129 (Tab.), **V1**.177 (Tab.)
  classification, **V1**.27 (Tab.), **V1**.49 (Tab.),
    V1.50, **V2**.1060–1
  see also Arenaviruses; *specific viruses*
Arenavirus
  characteristics, **V1**.129 (Tab.)
  see also Arenaviruses
Arenaviruses, **V2**.**1059–84**
  aerosol stability, **V2**.1071
  antibodies, **V2**.1069
    detection, **V2**.1076
    monoclonal, **V2**.1069
  antigens, **V2**.1068–9
  classification
    cross-reactivities between viruses, **V2**.1069
    New World group, **V2**.1060–1,
      V2.1060 (Tab.)
    Old World group, **V2**.1060 (Tab.)
    phylogenetic tree, **V2**.1061 (Fig.)
    serological techniques, **V2**.1069
  defective interfering (DI) particles, **V2**.1062
  epidemiology
    animal reservoirs, **V2**.1060 (Tab.), **V2**.1061
    geographical distribution, **V2**.1060 (Tab.),
      V2.1061, **V2**.1062 (Fig.)
    host range, **V2**.1064–5
    reservoir hosts, **V2**.1060 (Tab.), **V2**.1061
  genome, **V2**.1062–4
    ambisense coding, **V1**.181, **V2**.1064,
      V2.1064 (Fig.), **V2**.1065
    bisegmented genome, **V2**.1060–2
    non-coding regions, **V2**.1066
    panhandles, **V2**.1064
    secondary structures, **V2**.1064
    segmentation, **V1**.180–1
  glycoproteins (GP), **V2**.1064 (Fig.),
    V2.1067–8
    envelope, **V2**.1061–2
    transcription and synthesis, **V2**.1065–6
  historical aspects, **V2**.1059
  infection *see* Arenavirus infection
  isolation/propagation and identification,
    V1.95, **V1**.96 (Tab.), **V2**.1075–6
    nucleic acid detection, **V2**.1075–6
    tissue specimens, **V2**.1076 (Tab.)
  life cycle, **V2**.1065 (Fig.)
  L RNA segment, **V2**.1062, **V2**.1064 (Fig.)
    RNA synthesis, **V2**.1066, **V2**.1068
  monoclonal antibodies, **V2**.1069
  morphology and structure, **V2**.1061–2,
    V2.1063 (Fig.)
  nucleocapsid proteins (NP/N), **V2**.1064 (Fig.),
    V2.1067
    RNA synthesis, **V2**.1066
    transcription and synthesis, **V2**.1065–6

  polypeptides
    non-structural, **V2**.1068
    structural, **V2**.1067–8
  prototype, **V2**.1059
  purification, **V2**.1061–2
  reassortant viruses, **V2**.1064
  replication, **V2**.1064–7
    gene expression, **V2**.1065–6
    host cell nucleus role, **V2**.1066
    host cell ribosomes/enzymes role,
      V2.1066–7
    infection process, **V1**.241 (Tab.)
    mRNA transcription, **V2**.1065–6
    RNA synthesis, **V1**.131–2
    tropism and virus entry, **V2**.1064–5
    virus-host interactions during, **V2**.1066–7
  RNA polymerase (L), **V2**.1067
  spikes, GP-1 and GP-2 in, **V2**.1067–8
  S RNA segment, **V2**.1062, **V2**.1064 (Fig.)
  zinc-binding protein, **V2**.1068
  Z protein, **V2**.1064 (Fig.), **V2**.1067, **V2**.1068
    antibodies, **V2**.1069
    promyelocyte leukemia protein binding,
      V2.1068
    transcription and synthesis, **V2**.1065–6
  see also Arenaviridae
Arenavirus infection, **V2**.1069–78
  carriers, **V2**.1070–1
  clinical features, **V2**.1069–70
    animals, **V2**.1069–70
    humans, **V2**.1070
  diagnosis, **V2**.1075–6
  differential diagnosis, **V2**.1075–6
  emerging infection, **V2**.1060
  epidemiology, **V2**.1070–1
  immune response, **V2**.1072–5
    IFN activity, **I**.260 (Tab.)
  immunopathology, **V2**.1073–5
    CNS pathology, **V2**.1073–4
    effectors in, **V2**.1073
  immunosuppression in, **V2**.1074–5
    cell-mediated, **V2**.1074
    humoral, **V2**.1075
  pathogenesis, **V2**.1071–2
    animals, **V2**.1071
    humans, **V2**.1071–2
  persistent, **V2**.1066, **V2**.1071
  prophylaxis, **V2**.1076–7
  transmission, **V1**.371–2, **V1**.371 (Tab.),
    V2.1070–1
  treatment, **V2**.1077–8
    antiviral agents, **V2**.1078
    immunotherapy, **V2**.1077–8
    vaccine, **V2**.1076–7
Argentine hemorrhagic fever, **V2**.1070
Arginase, **V1**.272–3
  granuloma formation, **I**.708
  schistosomiasis, **I**.722
Arginine dihydrolase
  Enterobacteriaceae identification,
    B2.1319 (Tab.)
  pathway, **B2**.1598
Arginine, *Pseudomonas* growth, **B2**.1598
Arginine vasopressin, acute phase response,
    I.208

Argyll-Robertson, Douglas, **P**.10
Arizona hinshawii see Salmonella
Armadillo(s)
  leprosy, **B2**.1182, **B2**.1204
  Paracoccidioides brasiliensis, **M**.544
  sporotrichosis, **M**.370–1
  Trypanosoma cruzi host, **P**.391
AroC gene, **I**.842
AroD gene, **I**.842
Aromatic diamidines, Old World
    leishmaniasis, **P**.306–7
Arrayed primer extension, aspergillosis
    diagnosis, **M**.718
Arsenic trioxide, HTLV type 1 (HTLV-1)
    infection, **V2**.1292
Arsenophonus, characteristic, **B2**.1330 (Tab.)
Arsenophonus nasonae, **B2**.1337
Artemether, schistosomiasis, **P**.607, **P**.635–6
Arterial blood gases, PCP diagnosis, **M**.788
Arteriosclerosis
  Chlamydia pneumoniae infection,
    B2.2016–17
  endocarditis in, **B1**.525–6
Arteriviridae, **V1**.26, **V1**.378
  characteristics, **V1**.177 (Tab.)
  classification, **V1**.27 (Tab.), **V1**.51 (Tab.),
    V1.53, **V1**.390, **V1**.824, **V1**.825
  genome size, **V1**.395
  type species, **V1**.825
  see also Arteriviruses; *specific viruses*
Arterivirus
  classification, **V1**.53, **V1**.392
  morphology, **V1**.391 (Fig.)
Arteriviruses
  accessory proteins, **V1**.835–6
  classification, **V1**.824, **V1**.824 (Tab.)
    characteristics, **V1**.823
  envelope (E) protein, **V1**.827, **V1**.836 (Tab.),
    V1.837, **V1**.840
  genome, **V1**.825
    common leader sequence, **V1**.395
    expression strategies, **V1**.829 (Fig.)
    non-translated region, **V1**.825–7
    open reading frames, **V1**.827
    overlaps, **V1**.827–8
    packaging, **V1**.827
    pseudoknot, **V1**.827–8
    regulatory elements, **V1**.825–6
    structure, **V1**.828 (Fig.)
    transcription-regulating sequence,
      V1.826–7
  glycoproteins, **V1**.827
    see also specific types
  GP₂ glycoprotein, **V1**.836 (Tab.), **V1**.839–40
  GP₃ glycoprotein, **V1**.836 (Tab.), **V1**.839–40
  GP₄ glycoprotein, **V1**.836 (Tab.), **V1**.839–40
    antibodies, **V1**.840
  GP₅ glycoprotein, **V1**.836 (Tab.), **V1**.839–40
    neutralizing antibodies, **V1**.840
  helicases, **V1**.834
  infection *see* Arterivirus infection
  major surface glycoprotein (MSG), **V1**.827
    cell entry, **V1**.838
  membrane (M) protein, **V1**.827,
    V1.836 (Tab.), **V1**.837
    antibodies, **V1**.840

Arteriviruses (*Continued*)
  morphology/structure, **V1**.395, **V1**.825,
    V1.826 (Fig.)
  nonstructural proteins, **V1**.827–8, **V1**.832–6
  nucleocapsid (N) protein, **V1**.827, **V1**.836–7,
    V1.836 (Tab.)
    cell-mediated immunity, **V1**.840
  replicase (RNA polymerase), **V1**.398,
    V1.827–8, **V1**.832–5, **V1**.833 (Fig.)
    intracellular localization, **V1**.835
    nsp10, **V1**.834
    post-translational modification, **V1**.832,
      V1.834
    proteinase domain, **V1**.832
    ribosomal frameshifting, **V1**.832
    RNA-dependent RNA polymerase
      activity, **V1**.833–4
    sequence analysis, **V1**.832
  replication, **V1**.828–9
    RNA synthesis, **V1**.396
  reverse genetics, **V1**.830–1
  size, **V1**.825
  structural proteins, **V1**.836 (Tab.)
    see also specific types
  subgenomic RNA, **V1**.828–30
    'discontinuous minus strand synthesis,'
      V1.401
  transcription, **V1**.829–30
  translation, **V1**.831–2
  see also Arteriviridae; Coronaviruses;
    Toroviruses
Arterivirus infection, **V1**.392, **V1**.823,
  V1.841–8, **V1**.841 (Tab.), **V1**.846–8
  IFN activity, **I**.260 (Tab.)
  immune response, **V1**.840–1
    cell-mediated, **V1**.840
    humoral, **V1**.840
Arthralgia
  chikungunya, **V2**.1021–2
  rubella, **V2**.969–70
    vaccination, **V2**.984
Arthritis
  Chlamydia trachomatis infection, **B2**.2013
  mumps, **V1**.750
  prostaglandin E$_2$, **I**.188
  septic, **B1**.244–5
Arthrobacter, **B2**.991
  biochemical characteristics, **B2**.993 (Tab.)
    glucose catabolism, **B1**.60
    nitrification, **B1**.200
  chemotaxonomic characteristics,
    B2.978 (Tab.)
  disease associations, **B2**.981 (Tab.)
Arthrobacter cumminsii, **B2**.991
  habitats, **B2**.978
Arthroconidia, **M**.78–9, **M**.79 (Fig.), **M**.251–2
  Coccidioides immitis, **M**.503, **M**.503 (Fig.),
    M.504, **M**.504 (Fig.), **M**.506–7, **M**.509
Arthroderma, **M**.77, **M**.221 (Tab.)
Arthroderma otae, mating types, **M**.223
Arthroderma simii, **M**.223, **M**.230–1
Arthrodermataceae, **M**.61
Arthrographis kalrae, oculomycoses,
  M.275 (Tab.), **M**.283
Arthropathy
  Parvovirus B19 virus infection, **V1**.430

rubella vaccine, **V2**.1566
Arthropods
  bacterial pathogens, **B1**.203–4
  pathogenicity of mycoplasmas in, **B2**.1965
Arthropod vectors, **V1**.237–9, **V2**.1403–4
  alphavirus transmission, **V2**.1010
  in emerging viral infection, **V2**.1658
  orbivirus infection, **V2**.942
  rhabdoviruses, **V2**.1102
  see also Vector(s); *individual species*
Arthus reaction, African trypanosomiasis,
  P.365
Artificial competence, **B1**.99, **B1**.100
  Bacillus subtilis, **B1**.99–100
  covalently closed circle DNA, **B1**.100
  electroporation, **B1**.100
  Escherichia coli, **B1**.99
  Haemophilus influenzae, **B1**.99–100
  Neisseria gonorrhoeae, **B1**.100
  plasmid DNA, **B1**.100
  Salmonella Typhimurium, **B1**.99
  Staphylococcus aureus, **B1**.99
  Streptococcus pneumoniae, **B1**.99–100
Artificial replication systems, **V2**.1093
AS04 *see* Monophosphoryl lipid (MPL)
  adjuvant
Asalimumab, licensing, **I**.355 (Tab.)
Asbestos filters, **B1**.453
Ascariasis
  basophils, **I**.68
  clinical manifestations, **P**.725–7
    acute complications, **P**.726–7, **P**.726 (Tab.)
    childhood malnutrition, **P**.727
    chronic ascariasis, **P**.727
    crypt hyperplasia, **P**.727
    growth retardation, **P**.727
    hypersensitivity, **P**.726
    morbidity, **P**.725, **P**.726 (Tab.)
    pulmonary ascariasis, **P**.726
    seasonal infection, **P**.726
    villous atrophy, **P**.727
  control, **P**.130
    community-based chemotherapy, **P**.64–5,
      P.64 (Fig.)
    school-age children, **P**.125
  diagnosis, **P**.730
  epidemiology, **P**.42, **P**.46 (Tab.)
    age-relation, **P**.42
    geographical distribution, **P**.42
  establishment, **P**.720
    transmission routes, **P**.720
  historical aspects, **P**.6
  host genetic factors, **P**.55
  immunogenetics, **I**.600
    HLA genes, **I**.600–1
  morbidity, **P**.42
  mortality, **P**.28 (Tab.), **P**.29 (Tab.), **P**.42
  prevalence *vs.* age, **P**.54 (Fig.)
  public health importance, **P**.42–3,
    P.105 (Tab.)
  treatment, ivermectin, **P**.789
Ascaridiidae, **P**.590
  features, **P**.590
Ascaridoidea, **P**.590–1
  Anisakidae, **P**.590–1

Ascaridiidae, **P**.590
Ascaris, **P**.590
  historical aspects, **P**.6
  immune evasion, antioxidant secretion, **I**.686
  infection *see* Ascariasis
  structure/life cycle, **P**.590
  zoonotic infection, **P**.715 (Tab.)
  see also individual species
Ascaris lumbricoides, **P**.713
  biology/feeding, **P**.714 (Tab.), **P**.718–19
    antibacterial defense mechanisms, **P**.719
  epidemiology/population biology, **P**.722
    age-related prevalence, **P**.722–3,
      P.722 (Fig.)
    global distribution/abundance, **P**.722
    infection predisposition, **P**.724–5
    intensity, **P**.723–4, **P**.723 (Fig.)
    number of worms per host, **P**.724,
      P.724 (Fig.)
    prevalence, **P**.713–14
  historical aspects, **P**.5, **P**.6
  immunity, **P**.729
  infection *see* Ascariasis
  life cycle, **P**.715, **P**.717, **P**.718 (Tab.),
    P.720 (Fig.)
    egg production, **P**.720
    tissue migration, **P**.718–19
  life expectancy, **P**.60 (Tab.)
  morphology, **P**.715, **P**.717
    cuticle, **P**.717
    eggs, **P**.715, **P**.716 (Fig.)
Ascaris suum, **P**.715 (Tab.)
Ascaroside, *Ascaris lumbricoides* eggs, **P**.715
Ascending cholestasis, liver fluke infection,
  P.649
Ascites, liver fluke infection, **P**.649
Ascocarps, *Ajellomyces*, **M**.819–20, **M**.820 (Fig.)
Ascoli test, **B2**.937
Ascomycetes, *Pneumocystis*, **M**.772–4, **M**.778,
  M.778 (Tab.), **M**.796
Ascomycetous yeast, **M**.631, **M**.631 (Tab.)
Ascomycota, **M**.44 (Fig.), **M**.49–51,
  M.50 (Tab.), **M**.52 (Fig.), **M**.53–63,
  M.55 (Tab.)
Ascospore(s)
  Ajellomyces, **M**.813, **M**.819–20, **M**.820 (Fig.),
    M.821 (Fig.)
  Aspergillus, **M**.688, **M**.691–2
  Aspergillus nidulans, **M**.691
  Histoplasma capsulatum var. *capsulatum*,
    M.520
Ascoviridae, **V1**.27 (Tab.), **V1**.43 (Tab.)
  see also specific viruses
Aseptic meningitis (viral)
  coxsackieviruses, **V2**.1423–4
  echoviruses, **V2**.863
  enteroviruses, **V2**.1423
  enterovirus infection, **V2**.870
  HSV, **V1**.507
  LCMV, **V2**.1070
  mumps, **V1**.750, **V2**.1430
  mumps vaccine, **V2**.1570
  Tacaribe virus, **V2**.1070
Aseptic packaging, **B1**.271

Asexual reproduction
  anamorphs, **M**.45, **M**.77, **M**.78 (Fig.), **M**.79 (Fig.), **M**.221, **M**.221 (Tab.)
  classification, **M**.45, **M**.51
  Cryptococcus neoformans, **M**.639
Asfarviridae
  characteristics, **V1**.177 (Tab.)
  classification, **V1**.27 (Tab.), **V1**.43 (Tab.), **V1**.44
  see also specific viruses
Asfivirus, **V1**.44
Ashbya gossypii, growth, **M**.71–2
Ashford, Richard, **P**.18
Asia, food-borne botulism, **B2**.1067–9
Asialo glycoprotein receptor, **V2**.1092
Aspartate, transport, **B1**.49
Aspergillin, **M**.93 (Tab.)
Aspergilloma, **M**.104–6, **M**.696, **M**.697 (Fig.)
  diagnosis, **M**.712
  hemopytsis, **M**.696
  histopathology, **M**.711 (Fig.)
  history, **M**.18–9
  immune response, **M**.709
    humoral response, **M**.708–9
  therapy, **M**.718–19
Aspergillosis, **M**.659, **M.687–738**
  aetiological agents, **M**.692
  AIDS *see* AIDS, concomitant infection
  allergic, **M**.694, **M**.695, **M**.696
    allergic bronchopulmonary *see* Allergic bronchopulmonary aspergillosis (ABPA)
    allergic fungal sinusitis, **M**.694, **M**.695, **M**.696
    Aspergillus fumigatus, **M**.693
    prednisone, **M**.718
    Pseudomonas aeruginosa, **M**.693–4
  causative agents, **M**.63, **M**.687–9, **M**.692
    see also individual species
  clinical presentation, **M**.692–706
    bone, **M**.700, **M**.719
    bronchopleural fistulae, **M**.704
    bronchopneumonia, **M**.698–9
    chronic granulomatous disease, **I**.48, **I**.770
    chronic rhinosinusitis, **M**.696
    CNS, **M**.137 (Fig.), **M**.697, **M**.700, **M**.705
    ears *see below*
    endophthalmitis, **M**.322, **M**.700, **M**.719
    esophagus, **M**.701
    external auditory canal, **M**.700–1
    gastrointestinal tract, **M**.701, **M**.705
    heart, **M**.700, **M**.705
    infective endocarditis, **M**.700, **M**.705, **M**.711, **M**.719
    liver, **M**.701
    meningitis, **M**.697
    myocarditis, **M**.141 (Fig.), **M**.700
    nose, **M**.694–5
    onychomycosis, **M**.246
    orbit, **M**.694, **M**.695, **M**.700
    osteomyelitis, **M**.700
    otomycoses *see below*
    paranasal sinuses *see* Paranasal sinuses, aspergillosis
    peritonitis, **M**.701–2
    pulmonary *see below*

  skin infection, **M**.701
  spleen, **M**.701
  tracheobronchitis, **M**.704
  ulceration, **M**.701
  cystic fibrosis, **M**.693–4, **M**.712
  diabetes mellitus, **M**.694–5
  diagnosis, **M**.125–7, **M**.709–18
    arrayed primer extension, **M**.718
    bronchoalveolar lavage *see* Bronchoalveolar lavage (BAL)
    calcofluor white, **M**.711, **M**.711 (Fig.)
    cerebrospinal fluid, **M**.697
    diagnostic criteria, **M**.710
    DNA-Chip technology, **M**.718
    EIAs, **M**.106–7
    ELISA *see* Enzyme-linked immunosorbent assay (ELISA)
    fungemia, **M**.699–700
    histopathology, **M**.128 (Tab.), **M**.137 (Fig.), **M**.141 (Fig.), **M**.710–11, **M**.710 (Fig.), **M**.711 (Fig.), **M**.717
    nucleic acid sequence based amplification, **M**.718
    reverse transcriptase PCR, **M**.718
    serology, **M**.92, **M**.93 (Tab.), **M**.104–9, **M**.712–15
    skin tests, **M**.711–12
  disseminated, **M**.137 (Fig.)
  epidemiology, **M**.11, **M**.12, **M**.706
    birds, **M**.18
    building works, **M**.692–3, **M**.729
    construction work, **M**.692, **M**.729
    construction workers, **M**.692, **M**.729
    contact lens contamination, **M**.330–1
    heart transplants, **M**.704–5
    kidney transplants, **M**.701
    liver transplants, **M**.701
    lung transplants *see below*
    orthotopic liver transplantation, **M**.701
    renal transplants, **M**.701–2
    transplantation recipients, **M**.107–8, **M**.701–5
  eye infection *see below*
  fungemia, **B1**.523
  history, **M**.18–9, **M**.19 (Fig.)
  immune response, **M**.705, **M**.706–9
    colony-stimulating factors, **M**.709, **M**.724
    defensins, **M**.708
    G-CSF, **M**.724
    GM-CSF, **M**.709, **M**.724
    granulocytopenia, **M**.698
    IFN-γ, **M**.708
    IL-25, **I**.292
    ILs, **M**.724
    monocyte chemotactic protein-1/CC chemokine ligand-2 (MCP-1/CCL2), **M**.707–8
    neutropenia, **M**.724–5
    NK cells, **M**.707–8
    phagocytes, **M**.707, **M**.724
    polymorphonuclear neutrophils, **M**.707
    regulation, **M**.709
    skin tests, **M**.711–12
    T cells, **M**.709

  immunosuppression of infections, **M**.19, **M**.694, **M**.698, **M**.699–700, **M**.705, **M**.709
    cyclosporin A, **M**.708
  invasive, **M**.104–6, **M**.697–8
    acute pulmonary, **M**.698–9, **M**.699 (Fig.), **M**.705–6, **M**.719–26
    AIDS, **M**.699–700, **M**.705
    bone marrow recipients, **M**.698
    bronchoalveolar lavage, **M**.698
    cell-mediated immune response, **M**.709
    cellular immune response, **M**.709
    CNS, **M**.697, **M**.700, **M**.705
    cutaneous, **M**.701, **M**.719
    endocarditis, **M**.700, **M**.705, **M**.711, **M**.719
    fungemia, **M**.699–700
    gastrointestinal, **M**.701, **M**.705
    hepatic, **M**.701, **M**.705
    history, **M**.19
    humoral immune response, **M**.709
    myocarditis, **M**.700, **M**.705
    neonates, **M**.705–6
    ocular, **M**.700, **M**.705
    osteomyelitis, **M**.700, **M**.719
    otomycosis, **M**.700–1
    splenic, **M**.701, **M**.705
    transplants, **M**.701–5
    see also individual transplants
  lung transplants, **M**.701, **M**.702–4, **M**.703
    amphotericin B therapy, **M**.703, **M**.704
    bronchopleural fistulae, **M**.704
    etiological agents, **M**.703
    incidence, **M**.702
    mortality, **M**.703
    radiology, **M**.704
    single lung, **M**.702, **M**.703–4
    therapy, **M**.703, **M**.704
    time of onset, **M**.702
    tracheobronchitis, **M**.704
    types of infections, **M**.702
  necrotizing, chronic, **M**.696, **M**.717, **M**.719
  neonates *see* Neonatal infection
  nosocomial, **B1**.403
  nosocomial infection, **M**.692, **M**.706, **M**.729
  oculomycoses, **M**.274, **M**.279, **M**.294–5, **M**.295–6, **M**.700, **M**.719
    dacryocystitis, **M**.298
    endophthalmitis, **M**.317, **M**.318, **M**.320, **M**.322
    keratitis, **M**.300, **M**.301, **M**.302, **M**.306, **M**.307–9, **M**.312, **M**.313 (Fig.), **M**.316
      post surgical, **M**.327
    scleritis, **M**.316, **M**.317
  otomycoses (ear infection), **M**.700–1
    econazole therapy, **M**.700–1
    invasive, **M**.700–1
    nystatin therapy, **M**.700–1
    otitis externa, **M**.247–8
  prevention, **M**.729–31
    air control measures, **M**.730
    laminar air flow, **M**.730
  prognosis, **M**.717–18
  prophylaxis, **M**.726–9
    itraconazole, **M**.727–9

Aspergillosis (*Continued*)
  pulmonary, **M**.137 (Fig.), **M**.141 (Fig.)
    acute invasive, **M**.698–9, **M**.699 (Fig.),
      M.719–26
  risk factors, **M**.706
  surfactant proteins, **M**.707
  therapy, **M**.718–26
    abelcet, **M**.721–2
    AmBisome *see* AmBisome
    amphocil, **M**.721
    amphotericin B *see* Amphotericin B
    amphotericin B *vs.* itraconazole, **M**.728
    caspofugin, **M**.724, **M**.726
    combination therapy, **M**.726
    corticosteroids, **M**.695, **M**.698, **M**.707
    cyclosporin A, **M**.708
    echinocandins, **M**.155
    empirical therapy, **M**.724–5
    fluconazole *vs.* itraconazole, **M**.728
    itraconazole, **M**.719, **M**.722–3
    itraconazole *vs.* fluconazole, **M**.728
    neonates, **M**.725–6
    patient selection criteria, **M**.710
    voriconazole, **M**.153, **M**.723–4
Aspergillus, **M**.687–738
  antigens, **M**.694, **M**.706, **M**.712, **M**.717
    detection, **M**.713–15, **M**.717
    β-1,3-D-glucan, **M**.716–17
  biochemistry
    elastase, **M**.688, **M**.692, **M**.706, **M**.707
    galactofuran, **M**.712, **M**.713
    galactomannan, **M**.712, **M**.713, **M**.714,
      M.717
    β-1,3-D-Glucan, **M**.716–17
    heat shock proteins, **M**.106, **M**.107, **M**.694
    metabolites, **M**.713
    oxalic acid, **M**.713
    phialides, **M**.687
    proteases, **M**.688, **M**.692, **M**.706
  cereal spoilage, **B1**.284
  classification, **M**.63, **M**.687–9
    groups, **M**.688
  ecology, **M**.692, **M**.706, **M**.729
  environmental source identification, **M**.95
  food contamination, **M**.729
  genetic analysis
    18S rRNA genes, **M**.688–9
    28S rRNA genes, **M**.688–9
    in situ DNA hybridization, **M**.94
    internal transcribed spacer regions,
      M.688–9
    mitochondrial DNA, **M**.715
    ribosomal DNA, **M**.108, **M**.715
    single-strand conformational
      polymorphisms, **M**.715
    species-specific probes, **M**.715
  growth rate, **M**.688, **M**.690
  herbs and spices spoilage, **B1**.287–8
  histopathology, **M**.89 (Tab.), **M**.127 (Tab.),
    M.128 (Tab.), **M**.141 (Fig.), **M**.710–11,
    M.711 (Fig.), **M**.717
  history, **M**.18–9
  identification, **M**.688–9, **M**.689 (Tab.)
    blood culture, **M**.711
    culture, **M**.91 (Tab.), **M**.688, **M**.689–90,
      M.711

GenBank, **M**.689
genus/strain, **M**.94
immunoblotting, **M**.712–13
inhibition EIA, **M**.714–15
Pastorex test, **M**.107–8, **M**.713
PCR *see* Polymerase chain reaction (PCR)
serology, **M**.712–15
specimen site selection, **M**.83 (Tab.)
infection *see* Aspergillosis
meat, **B1**.276
morphology, **M**.688, **M**.689–92, **M**.689 (Tab.)
  anamorphs, **M**.687
  colony characteristics, **M**.689–90,
    M.689 (Tab.)
  conidia, **M**.687, **M**.691
  conidial head, **M**.689–90, **M**.690–1,
    M.690 (Fig.), **M**.691 (Fig.)
  conidiophores, **M**.687, **M**.689–90, **M**.690–1
  hyphae, **M**.689–90, **M**.717
  mycelium, **M**.690
  phialides, **M**.687, **M**.689–91
  teleomorphs, **M**.687
pathogenicity, **M**.688, **M**.692–3
reproduction
  asexual, **M**.687, **M**.688
  sexual, **M**.688, **M**.691–2
resistance, **M**.169
  fluconazole, **M**.169
  flucytosine, **M**.176
Aspergillus candidus, **M**.249
  onychomycosis, **M**.246
Aspergillus clavatus, **M**.691 (Fig.)
Aspergillus ferreus, **M**.691 (Fig.)
Aspergillus flavus
  cereal spoilage, **B1**.284
  cheese spoilage, **B1**.252
  contact lens contamination, **M**.330–1
  infection, **M**.687
    histopathology, **M**.128 (Tab.)
    keratitis, **M**.302 (Fig.), **M**.312, **M**.313 (Fig.),
      M.327–8
    lung transplants, **M**.703
    retinitis, **M**.323
    serology, **M**.93 (Tab.), **M**.105
    see also Aspergillosis
  morphology, **M**.689 (Fig.)
Aspergillus fumigatus
  ecology, **M**.692, **M**.706
  genetic analysis
    antigens, **M**.694
    DNA hybridization, **M**.692
    mitochondrial DNA, **M**.715
    PCR, **M**.108, **M**.715–16
    ribosomal DNA, **M**.108, **M**.715
  histopathology, **M**.128 (Tab.), **M**.137 (Fig.),
    M.141 (Fig.), **M**.711 (Fig.)
  history, **M**.18–9, **M**.19 (Fig.)
  infection *see* Aspergillosis; *below*
  morphology, **M**.689 (Fig.), **M**.690 (Fig.)
  outside air, **M**.706, **M**.729
  phagocytes, **M**.707, **M**.724
  proteins
    cilo-inhibitory, **M**.707
    elastase, **M**.688, **M**.692, **M**.707
    galactofuran, **M**.712

galactomannan, **M**.107, **M**.712, **M**.714
gliotoxin, **M**.707, **M**.709
proteases, **M**.692, **M**.707
tritrpticin sensitivity, **I**.172
virulence factors, **M**.79
Aspergillus fumigatus infection, **M**.687, **M**.692
  allergic aspergillosis, **M**.693
  cattle abortion, **M**.692
  dacryocanaliculitis, **M**.298
  endophthalmitis, **M**.317, **M**.323, **M**.330 (Fig.)
  in HIV infection, **I**.795
  immune response, **M**.706–9
    allergic reaction, **M**.692–3
    antigens, **M**.712
    antiphagocytic activity, **M**.707
    cyclosporin A, **M**.708
    fibrinogen binding, **M**.706
    phospholipids, **M**.709
    skin tests, **M**.711–12
  keratitis, **M**.303, **M**.305, **M**.327–8
  lung transplants, **M**.703
  otomycosis, **M**.700–1
  route, **M**.692
  scleritis, **M**.317
  serology, **M**.93 (Tab.)
  virulence, **M**.688, **M**.692, **M**.707
  voriconazole therapy, **M**.153
  see also Aspergillosis
Aspergillus glaucus, **M**.249, **M**.690–1
  fruit, **B1**.283
  herbs and spices, **B1**.287
  onychomycosis, **M**.246
Aspergillus hollandicus, **M**.246
  onychomycosis, **M**.246
Aspergillus nidulans
  ascospores, **M**.691–2
  growth, **M**.71–2
    mycelium development, **M**.72–3
  histopathology, **M**.89 (Tab.), **M**.128 (Tab.),
    M.139 (Fig.)
  infection, **M**.687
    lung transplants, **M**.703
    mycetoma, **M**.392 (Tab.)
    see also Aspergillosis
  virulence factors, **M**.79–80
Aspergillus niger
  chitin-lacking mutants, **M**.71
  fruit, **B1**.283
  genetic analysis, **M**.71
  herbs and spices, **B1**.287
  histopathology, **M**.128 (Tab.), **M**.137 (Fig.)
  history, **M**.8–9
  infection, **M**.687, **M**.710 (Fig.)
    lung transplants, **M**.703
    otitis externa, **M**.247–8
    otomycosis, **M**.700–1
    serology, **M**.93 (Tab.), **M**.105
    see also Aspergillosis
  morphology, **M**.690 (Fig.)
  temperature, **M**.74
Aspergillus ornatus, **M**.691–2
Aspergillus oryzae, infection, **M**.687
  see also Aspergillosis
Aspergillus parasiticus
  cheese spoilage, **B1**.252

Aspergillus parasiticus (*Continued*)
  in wheat, **B1**.284
Aspergillus restrictus
  mitogillin, **M**.694
  onychomycosis, **M**.246
  see also Aspergillosis
Aspergillus sclerotiorum, onychomycosis,
    M.246
Aspergillus sydowi, **M**.729–30
  onychomycosis, **M**.246
  see also Aspergillosis
Aspergillus terreus, **M**.687
  amphotericin B resistance, **M**.172
  infection
    endophthalmitis, **M**.322
    lung transplants, **M**.703
    see also Aspergillosis
Aspergillus unguis, onychomycosis, **M**.246
Aspergillus ustus, **M**.687
Aspergillus versicolor, **M**.246, **M**.249,
    M.250 (Fig.), **M**.687
  lung transplants, **M**.703
Asp fI protein, **M**.672
Aspirin, Reye's syndrome, **B1**.323
Asplenia
  Connexin 43 gene mutation, **I**.771
  Streptococcus pneumoniae infection, **I**.771
  ZIC3 gene mutations, **I**.771
Aspoxicillin, *Pasteurella multocida,* **B2**.1655
Assiminea, fluke intermediate host, **P**.646
Astacus, Paragonimus intermediate host, **P**.646
Asteroid bodies, **M**.122
  Sporothrix schenckii, **M**.375, **M**.376 (Fig.),
    M.377
Asteroleplasma, **B2**.1958 (Tab.)
  classification, **B2**.1967
  culture, **B2**.1963
Asthma
  allergic, **I**.731, **I**.733
    IL-9, **I**.735
    Th1 immune correlations, **I**.738–9
  APCs, **I**.736–7
  Chlamydia pneumoniae infection, **B2**.2016
  chronic, **I**.731
    airway remodeling, **I**.732
  endotoxin exposure, **B1**.189
  genetic linkage, **I**.580, **I**.733
  hygiene hypothesis *see* Hygiene hypothesis
  IL-4 receptor, **I**.581–2
  IL-5, **I**.735, **I**.736
  IL-13 receptor, **I**.581–2
  immunogenetics, **I**.580
  prevalence, **I**.731
  prostaglandin E$_2$, **I**.188
  Sporobolomyces, **M**.628
  Th2 cell pathology, **I**.733–5
  see also Airway hypersensitivity/
    hyperreactivity
Asthmatic manifestations, toxocariasis, **P**.754
Astrakhan fever, **B2**.2030–1, **B2**.2031 (Tab.)
  clinical manifestations, **B2**.2039 (Tab.)
Astrocytes, in progressive multifocal
    leucoencephalopathy (PML), **V2**.1404/,
    V2.1417 (Fig.)
Astrocytomas, JC virus association, **V1**.479

Astrotactin, domains, **I**.476 (Fig.)
Astroviridae
  characteristics, **V1**.177 (Tab.)
  classification, **V1**.27 (Tab.), **V1**.51 (Tab.),
    V1.53
  see also Astroviruses; *specific viruses*
Astroviruses, **V2.888–910**
  animal strains, **V2**.903
  biophysical properties, **V2**.890
    resistance to physical agents, **V2**.890,
      V2.900
  capsid antigen
    conservation, **V2**.899
    detection of, **V2**.895
  classification, **V2**.889–90, **V2**.890 (Tab.)
    serology, **V2**.899
  evolution, **V2**.900
  genome, **V2**.894 (Tab.)
    cross-species transfer evidence, **V2**.900
    frameshift signal, **V2**.894 (Fig.)
    nuclear localization signal, **V2**.896
    nucleotide sequences, **V2**.899–900
    open reading frames, **V2**.892–3,
      V2.894 (Tab.)
    organization, **V2**.892–5, **V2**.893 (Fig.)
    recombination, **V2**.900
    sequencing, **V2**.892–3
  historical aspects, **V2**.889–90
  immunity to, **V2**.905
  importance, **V2**.888–9
  infection *see* Astrovirus infection
  infectivity, **V2**.897–8
  morphology/structure, **V1**.138, **V2**.888–9,
    V2.888 (Fig.), **V2**.890–2
    alkaline conditions, **V2**.891
    cryo-electron microscopy, **V2**.891–2,
      V2.892 (Fig.)
    electron microscopy, **V2**.890–1
    particle size, **V2**.891
    surface projections, **V2**.891
  nonstructural proteins, **V2**.892–3, **V2**.896
    processing, **V2**.896–7, **V2**.897 (Fig.)
    see also specific types
  picornaviruses *vs.,* **V2**.861
  prevalence, **V2**.901–3
    feces, **V2**.902
    nosocomial infection, **V2**.902–3
    seasonality, **V2**.902
    seroprevalence, **V2**.901–2
    serotype differences, **V2**.902
  protein coding/expression, **V2**.896–9
  replication, **V2**.893–5
    cell penetration, **V2**.893–4
    cell-surface receptors, **V2**.893–4
    nuclear involvement, **V2**.894–5
    subgenomic RNA, **V2**.895, **V2**.895 (Fig.)
  RNA-dependent RNA-polymerase,
    V2.892–3, **V2**.896
    conservation, **V2**.899
    synthesis, **V2**.897
  in seafood, **V2**.900–1
  sequence phylogeny, **V2**.899–900,
    V2.900 (Fig.)
  PCR, **V2**.899
  serine protease, **V2**.896

structural proteins, **V2**.896
  processing, **V2**.891, **V2**.897–9,
    V2.898 (Fig.)
  see also specific types
transmission, **V2**.900–1
  environmental, **V2**.901
  fecal–oral route, **V2**.900
  food borne, **V2**.900–1
  person-to-person, **V2**.900
  in water, **V2**.901
Astrovirus infection
  in AIDS/HIV infection, **V2**.1504
  at-risk groups, **V2**.904
  clinical manifestations, **V2**.903–5
    avian, **V2**.904–5
    gastroenteritis, **V2**.903
    incubation period, **V2**.903–4
    mammalian, **V2**.903–4
    non-humans, **V2**.904
  detection/diagnosis, **V2**.905–7
    cell culture, **V2**.889, **V2**.906
    EIAs, **V2**.906
    electron microscopy, **V2**.889, **V2**.905–6
    in feces, **V2**.889
    molecular methods, **V2**.889, **V2**.906–7
  IFN activity, **I**.260 (Tab.)
  immunodeficient patients (non-HIV),
    V2.1508–9
  outbreaks, **V2**.904
    avian, **V2**.904–5
  pathogenesis, **V2**.905
  volunteer studies, **V2**.904
Asymptomatic infection
  acute hepatitis C, **V2**.1202–3
  Balantidium coli, **P**.279
  Candida albicans, **M**.257–8
  Chlamydia screening, **B2**.2009–10, **B2**.2021
  cystic echinococcosis, **P**.688
  cysticercosis, **P**.700
  Dientamoeba fragilis infection, **P**.267–8
  giardiasis, **P**.251
  lymphatic filariasis, **P**.773
  observational studies, **V1**.364
Atadenovirus, **V1**.45
  see also Atadenoviruses
Atadenoviruses, **V1**.439
  see also Atadenovirus
Ataxia telangiectasia, **I**.776–7
  TCR recombination, **I**.454
Atazanavir, **V2**.1625
  HIV resistance, **V2**.1337 (Fig.)
  structure, **V2**.1624 (Fig.)
Atherosclerosis
  Chlamydia pneumoniae association, **B1**.365
  HCMV infection association, **V1**.521
  macrophages, **I**.31
Atmospheric pollution, denitrification process,
    B1.200
Atopic dermatitis
  causative agents, **M**.213
  clinical condition, **M**.213
  immunological aspects, **M**.213
  ketoconazole therapy, **M**.213
  superantigens, **I**.562

Atopobium, **B2**.904, **B2**.917
  classification, **B2**.905 (Tab.)
  identification, **B2**.906–7
Atopy
  genetic linkage, **I**.580
  immunogenetics, **I**.580
  see also Allergies
Atovaquone®, **M**.781, **M**.789, **M**.790–1, **M**.796
  babesiosis, **P**.459
  mechanism of action, **P**.478
  toxoplasmosis, **P**.437
Atovaquone®–proguanil (Malarone®),
    malaria therapy, **P**.506
ATPase, Old World *Leishmania,* **P**.295–6
ATP-binding cassette (ABC transporters),
    B1.48, **B1**.49
ATP-phosphoglyceric transphosphorylase,
    B1.51
ATP synthase, **B1**.64–5
Attachment proteins (viral), **V1**.207–9
  CNS, **V2**.1405–6, **V2**.1406 (Tab.)
  glycoprotein spikes, **V1**.208
  multiple copies, **V1**.206
  paramyxoviruses, **V1**.701–2, **V1**.706–7
  Pneumovirinae, **V1**.706, **V1**.707
  see also Cellular receptors; *specific viruses*
Attack rate
  definition, **B1**.310
  secondary
    definition, **B1**.310
    vaccine efficacy studies, **B1**.324–5
Attenuated parasite vaccine model,
    schistosomiasis, **P**.605–6
Attenuation
  biosynthetic operon regulation, **B1**.72
  viruses
    cell culture, **V1**.251
    cold-adapted, **V1**.251–2
    genetic analysis, **V1**.195
    by mutagenesis, **V1**.251–2, **V1**.254–5
    negative-strand RNA viruses, **V1**.195
    selection after, **V1**.252
    see also Vaccines, live
Audouin, V, **M**.6
Aura virus (AURAV), **V2**.1011 (Tab.)
Aureobasidium pullulans, **M**.199, **B1**.282
  oculomycoses, **M**.278 (Tab.), **M**.283–4
Australian bat lyssavirus (ABLV), **V2**.1104,
    V2.1120
  emerging infection, **V2**.1648 (Tab.)
Austrian's syndrome, **B1**.530
Autoantibodies
  C3 complement protein, **I**.153
  SLE, **I**.155
  therapeutic type I INFs, due to, **I**.261
  see also individual types
Autoantigens, systemic γδ T cells, **I**.441
Autochthonous infection, *Retortamonas
    intestinalis,* **P**.273
Autoclaving, **B1**.447, **B1**.447 (Fig.)
  microsporidians, **P**.550
Autofluorescence, *Legionella,* **B2**.1762 (Tab.)
Autoimmune diseases/disorders, **I**.**747–63**
  animal models, **I**.757–9
    disadvantages, **I**.757–8

NK cells, **I**.103
CD4 T cells, **I**.390
complement deficiency associations, **I**.771
definition, **I**.747–8
discovery, **I**.748
DNA vaccines, **I**.920
environmental factors, **I**.752–6
  twin studies, **I**.752
etiology, **I**.747 (Fig.)
genetics, **I**.751–2
  HLA-DR alleles, **I**.751
  MHC genes, **I**.751–2
  non-MHC genes, **I**.752
historical aspects/re-evaluation, **I**.12, **I**.13
immune dysregulation, **I**.756
immunization cause, **I**.759–60
lymphocyte-mediated cytotoxicity, **I**.472
neutrophil phagocytosis, **I**.40
NK cells *see* Natural killer (NK) cells
pathogen-induced, **I**.752–3, **I**.753–6,
    I.753 (Tab.)
  bystander activation, **I**.755–6
  epitope spreading, **I**.756
  molecular mimicry, **I**.753–4
  superantigen activation, **I**.754–5
perforin deficiency, **I**.480
prevalence, **I**.748, **I**.748 (Tab.)
pyrogenic exotoxins, **I**.562
signs/symptoms, **I**.747
superantigens, **I**.562
systemic *vs.* organ-specific, **I**.748
therapy, **I**.760
  anti-idiotope antibodies, **I**.864
  gene therapy, **I**.760
  immune system modification, **I**.760
  immunosuppression, **I**.760
tissue destruction mechanisms, **I**.757
see also Tolerance; *specific diseases/infection*
Autoimmune lymphoproliferative syndrome
    (ALPS), **I**.750, **I**.756
Autoimmune polyendocrine syndrome type 1
    (APS-1), **I**.752
Autoimmune polyendocrinopathy–candidiasis–
    ectodermal dystrophy (APECED), **I**.779
Autoimmune thyroid disease, **I**.757
Autoimmunity
  in Chagas disease, **P**.385–8, **P**.393–4
  HTLV-1-associated myelopathy/tropical
      spastic paraparesis (HAM/TSP),
      V2.1429–30
  malaria, **P**.501 (Tab.)
  in neuro-AIDS, **V2**.1428
  virus-induced in CNS, **V2**.1414–15
Autoinducer, **B1**.72, **B1**.169–70
Autoinduction, **B1**.72
Autoinfection
  Capillaria philippiensis, **P**.745
  Strongyloides, **P**.739
Autologous bone marrow transplantation,
    GM-CSF therapy, **I**.277
Autolysins, **B1**.40, **B1**.42–3
Autolysosomes, **P**.177
Autosomal recessive agammaglobulinemia,
    I.780
Autotransporter proteins, **B1**.174–5,
    B1.174 (Tab.)

Auxiliary regions, DNA virus replication,
    V1.148
Avacuolar forms, *Blastocystis hominis,* **P**.557,
    P.559–60, **P**.560 (Fig.)
Avastin, licensing, **I**.355 (Tab.)
Avastrovirus, **V1**.53
Average pore diameter, viruses, **V1**.5
Avery, O, **B1**.12, **B1**.13
Aviadenovirus, **V1**.45
  see also Aviadenoviruses
Aviadenoviruses, **V1**.439
  see also Aviadenovirus
Avian B cell lymphomas, oncogenesis, **V1**.340
Avian botulism, **B2**.1038–9, **B2**.1058,
    B2.1070–1, **B2**.1074
Avian carcinoma virus Mill Hill virus-2
    (ACMHV-2), **V1**.345–6
Avian infection, microsporidiosis, **P**.544
Avian infectious bronchitis virus (IBV),
    V1.843–4
Avian infectious bronchitis virus (IBV)
    infection, **V1**.843–4
  diagnosis, **V1**.844
  immune response, **V1**.843–4
  management, **V1**.844
  vaccination, **V1**.844
Avian influenza viruses, **V2**.1651 (Tab.)
Avian leukosis virus (ALV)
  oncogenesis mechanism, **V1**.338
  receptors, **V1**.246 (Fig.)
Avian leukosis virus subgroup E (ALV-E),
    V2.1297
Avian myeloblastosis virus (AMV), **V1**.345–6
Avian nephritis virus (ANV)
  classification, **V2**.890 (Tab.)
  genome, **V2**.894 (Tab.)
  infection, **V2**.904–5
  isolation, **V2**.889–90
Avian paramyxovirus 1 *see* Newcastle disease
    virus
Avian paramyxovirus 2, **V1**.744
Avian paramyxovirus 6
  phylogeny, **V1**.388
  small hydrophobic proteins, **V1**.708
Avian paramyxovirus 9, **V1**.744
Avian pneumovirus (APV), **V1**.784
  animal models, **V1**.790
  classification, **V1**.385
  fusion (F) protein, **V1**.787
  genome structure, **V1**.785 (Fig.), **V1**.789
  glycoprotein (G), **V1**.787–8
  infection, **V1**.784
  in vitro culture, **V1**.790
  large (L) protein, **V1**.788
  matrix (M) protein, **V1**.788–9
  morphology, **V1**.787, **V1**.788 (Fig.)
  nucleocapsid (N) protein, **V1**.788
  phosphoprotein (P), **V1**.788
  type species, **V1**.784
Avibirnavirus, **V1**.48
Avidin, food, **B1**.267, **B1**.268 (Tab.)
Avidity, antibody analysis, **V2**.1547
Avihepadnavirus, **V2**.1227
  classification, **V1**.46–7
Avipoxvirus, **V1**.589
  classification, **V1**.579 (Tab.), **V1**.582, **V1**.594

Avipoxvirus, (Continued)
  genome size, **V1**.583, **V1**.589
  phylogenetic comparisons, **V1**.583
  taxonomy, **V1**.595 (Tab.)
Avsunviroidae, **V1**.54 (Tab.)
Avulavirus
  characteristics, **V1**.129 (Tab.), **V1**.702 (Tab.)
  classification, **V1**.48–9, **V1**.382, **V1**.700 (Tab.),
    V1.808 (Fig.)
  genome, **V1**.387 (Tab.), **V1**.700, **V1**.701 (Fig.)
  phylogeny, **V1**.388
  see also Avulaviruses
Avulaviruses
  animal infection, **V1**.815–16
  attachment (HN) protein, **V1**.706–7
    conservation, **V1**.706–7
  P protein, **V1**.704
  see also Avulavirus
Axenic cultures, *Trypanosoma brucei,* **P**.358
Axenization, **P**.200–1
Axilla
  Staphylococcus, **B2**.777
  white piedra, **M**.196
Axonal loss, multiple sclerosis, **I**.757
Axonal transport
  Rabies virus, **V2**.1122
  retrograde, **V2**.1405, **V2**.1412
Axonemes, **P**.179–80
Axostyles, **P**.170–2
5-Azacytidine, mutagen, **V1**.183
Azathioprine
  African trypanosomiasis, **P**.371
  immunodeficiency, **I**.788 (Tab.)
Azidothymidine (AZT), **V2**.1619, **M**.709
  discovery, **V1**.9
  foamy virus therapy, **V2**.1315–16
  historical aspects, **V1**.9 (Tab.)
  HIV infection, **V2**.1334
    neonates, **V2**.1473–4
    point mutation resistance, **V2**.1337 (Fig.)
    in pregnancy, **V2**.1473
    resistance, **V2**.1636
  HTLV-associated myelopathy
    (HAM)/tropical spastic paraparesis
    (TSP), **V2**.1290
  resistance, **V2**.1636
  structure, **V2**.1335 (Fig.), **V2**.1620 (Fig.)
Azithromycin
  Actinobacillus actinomycetemcomitans,
    B2.1664
  babesiosis, **P**.459
  Bordetella infection, **B2**.1793–4
  Borrelia susceptibility/resistance,
    B2.1831 (Tab.)
  Chlamydia trachomatis infection therapy,
    B2.2018
  gonorrhea treatment, **B1**.661–2
  Haemophilus, **B2**.1702 (Tab.),
    B2.1703 (Tab.), **B2**.1710
  Mycobacterium, **B2**.1222–3
  Mycoplasma pneumoniae pneumonia, **B1**.634
  Pasteurella multocida, **B2**.1655
  pharmacology, **B1**.487
  primary amebic meningoencephalitis,
    P.236–7
  structure, **B1**.486 (Fig.)

  in syphilis, **B2**.1858
  toxoplasmosis, **P**.437
  trachoma therapy, **B2**.2021
  typhoid fever treatment, **B2**.1416
Azlocillin
  Listeria, **B2**.957–8
  structure, **B1**.474 (Fig.)
Azoles, **M**.150–3, **M**.169 (Tab.)
  adverse effects, **M**.151 (Tab.), **M**.152,
    M.183–4, **M**.511
  amphotericin B with, **M**.153
  drug interactions, **M**.151–2, **M**.152 (Tab.),
    M.183
  ergosterol with, **M**.173
  historical aspects, **M**.147
  mechanism of action, **M**.70, **M**.150, **M**.173,
    M.182–3
  pharmacokinetics, **M**.150, **M**.150 (Tab.)
  resistance, **M**.170, **M**.173, **M**.173 (Tab.)
    Candida, **M**.169, **M**.170, **M**.174, **M**.611,
      M.612
    Candida glabrata, **M**.170–1, **M**.174
    Candida krusei, **M**.169, **M**.173, **M**.174
    commonly reported fungi, **M**.171 (Tab.)
    mechanisms, **M**.173 (Tab.), **M**.174
    significant incidence, **M**.171 (Tab.)
  spectrum of activity, **M**.151 (Tab.)
  therapy
    black piedra, **M**.198
    blastomycosis, **M**.497
    candidiasis, **M**.12, **M**.182–3, **M**.257,
      M.609–10, **M**.612
    coccidioidomycosis, **M**.511
    cryptococcosis, **M**.651–2
    dermatophytoses, **M**.182–3, **M**.183 (Tab.)
    keratitis, **M**.308–9
    Malassezia infection, **M**.182–3
    paracoccidioidomycosis, **M**.551
    phaeohyphomycosis, **M**.745
    pityrosporal folliculitis, **M**.185–6
    prototheosis, **M**.402
    white piedra, **M**.197
    zygomycosis, **M**.352
    topical, **M**.182–3, **M**.183 (Tab.)
Azospirillum, nitrogen fixation, **B1**.201
Azotobacter, **B1**.9
  glucose catabolism, **B1**.60
  nitrogen fixation, **B1**.201
  radiation-resistance, **B1**.46
Azotobacter vinelandii
  natural competence, **B1**.99
  nitrogenases, **B1**.63
AZT *see* Azidothymidine (AZT)
Aztreonam, **B1**.480
  Enterobacter, **B2**.1484–5
  Haemophilus, **B2**.1702 (Tab.)
  Klebsiella, **B2**.1480
  Serratia, **B2**.1488–9
  structure, **B1**.479 (Fig.)
Azurophil granules
  cathelicidins, **I**.174
  neutrophils, **I**.165–6
Azygospores, **M**.659
  zygomycete, **M**.669

B1 cells, B cells, **I**.435
B1 protein, poxvirus replication, **V1**.168–9,
  V1.169 (Tab.)
B2 cells, B cells, **I**.435
B7–1 (CD80)
  antigen presentation, **I**.29, **I**.383–4
  CD4 T cells/APC interactions, **I**.392 (Fig.)
    dendritic cells, **I**.394
  CD28 interactions
    B cell activation, **I**.326–7
    T-cell activation, **I**.404
  DNA vaccine co-administration, **I**.919 (Tab.)
  expression, CpG adjuvant effects, **I**.931
  inhibition, IL-10 effects, **I**.292–3
  upregulation, CpG stimulation, **I**.911
B7–2 (CD86)
  antigen presentation, **I**.29, **I**.383–4
  CD4 T cells/APC interactions, **I**.392 (Fig.)
    dendritic cells, **I**.394
  CD28 interactions
    B cell activation, **I**.326–7
    T-cell activation, **I**.404
  DNA vaccine co-administration, **I**.919 (Tab.)
  expression, CpG adjuvant effects, **I**.931
  inhibition, IL-10 effects, **I**.292–3
  upregulation, CpG stimulation, **I**.911
B7-related ligand, CD4 T cells, **I**.395
  APC interactions, **I**.392 (Fig.)
b12 anti-HIV-gp120 monoclonal antibody,
  I.319–20
  antigen-binding site, **I**.319–20
  asymmetrical structure, **I**.319
  heavy chain constant domain interactions,
    I.319
  hinge region, **I**.319
  normal structure *vs.*, **I**.320
B19 virus *see* Parvovirus B19 virus
Babesia, **P**.189
  'accordion-like' gametocytes, **P**.451, **P**.453
  apical complex organelles, **P**.452
  biochemistry, **P**.453
  classification, **P**.198, **P**.451–2
  exoerythrocytic forms, **P**.451, **P**.453
  historical aspects, **P**.451
  infection *see* Babesiosis
  intraerythrocytic forms, **P**.451, **P**.452, **P**.453
  isoenzymes, **P**.453
  life cycle, **P**.452–3
  molecular biology/genetics, **P**.453
  pre-erythrocytic cycle absence, **P**.451, **P**.452
  replication, **P**.453
  ribosomal RNA genes, **P**.452
  species, **P**.452
  sporozoites, **P**.452
  structure, **P**.452–3
  Theileria relationship, **P**.451–2
  transmission, **P**.452–3
  vectors, **P**.458
    ticks, **P**.453, **P**.458–9
  virulence-associated gene *(Bm13)*, **P**.453
  see also individual species
Babesia bovis, **P**.189
  discovery, **P**.451
  immune response, **P**.85

Babesia canis
structure, **P**.171 (Fig.)
see also Babesiosis
Babesia divergens
epizootiology, **P**.458–9
infection *see* Babesiosis
molecular biology/genetics, **P**.453
vector, **P**.458–9
Babesia equi, **P**.451–2
life cycle, **P**.453
see also Babesiosis
Babesia gibsoni-like WA-1 parasite, **P**.454
infection
blood films, **P**.458 (Fig.)
clinical features, **P**.455
diagnosis, **P**.457
epidemiology, **P**.459
treatment, **P**.460
reservoir, **P**.459
vector, **P**.458, **P**.459
Babesia microti, **P**.189, **P**.451–2
biochemistry, **P**.453
hosts, **P**.458
infection *see* Babesiosis
life cycle, **P**.458
strains/genetics, **P**.453
Babesiosis, **P**.454–60
blood transfusions, **P**.27–9, **P**.459
carriers, **P**.456
chemotherapy, **P**.459–60
emergency, **P**.459–60
clinical features, **P**.454–5
Babesia divergens, **P**.454–5
Babesia gibsoni-like WA-1, **P**.455
Babesia microti, **P**.454
fulminant, **P**.454–5
initial symptoms, **P**.454
subclinical infection, **P**.454
control, **P**.458–9
diagnosis, **P**.456–7, **P**.457 (Fig.)
blood films, **P**.455, **P**.457 (Fig.), **P**.458 (Fig.)
PCR, **P**.457
serological, **P**.457
differential diagnosis, malaria, **P**.454
emergency treatment, **P**.459–60
epidemiology, **P**.458–9
epizootiology, **P**.458–9
geographical distribution, **P**.459
patterns, **P**.458
historical aspects, **P**.451
first infection, **P**.454
in HIV infection, **P**.458
treatment, **P**.459
immunology, **P**.69, **P**.85, **P**.455, **P**.455–6
antibody response, **P**.456
immunity, **P**.456
T cell response, **P**.456
integrated control, **P**.460
tick density reduction, **P**.460
tick repellents, **P**.460
mortality, **P**.454, **P**.459–60
pathology, **P**.456
public health significance, **P**.44, **P**.45, **P**.454
reinfection, **P**.455–6, **P**.456
severity/age relationship, **P**.454

splenectomy association, **P**.454–5
susceptibility, experimental, **P**.455–6
vaccination, **P**.460
Baboon endogenous virus (BaEV),
xenotransplantation, **V2**.1297
Bacampicillin, pharmacology, **B1**.475
BAC degradation, papillomavirus E6 protein,
V1.460 (Tab.)
Bacillaceae, cereals, **B1**.284–5
Bacillary angiomatosis (BA), **B2**.1894
as AIDS-defining illnesses, **B2**.1894
erythromycin treatment, **B2**.1899
histology, **B2**.1898
HIV infection, **B2**.1894
Bacille Calmette–Guérain *see* BCG vaccine
Bacillus
antibacterial susceptibility/resistance,
B2.946
antigens, **B2**.928–30
flagellar antigens, **B2**.929
small acid-soluble proteins, **B2**.927–8
somatic antigens, **B2**.928
characteristics, **B2**.922, **B2**.935 (Tab.)
classification/nomenclature
evolution of, **B2**.1335
species, **B2**.923
classification, taxonomy, **B2**.922–3
clinical testing use, **B2**.923
colonies, **B2**.924–5, **B2**.926 (Fig.),
B2.925 (Fig.)
commercial importance, **B2**.923–4
antibiotic production, **B2**.923
competence and sporulation factor, **B2**.927
definition, **B2**.922
endospores, **B2**.926–8
L-alanine germinant, **B2**.928, **B2**.931–2
antigens, **B2**.929–30
dormancy, **B2**.924
formation, **B2**.927–8
germination, **B2**.928, **B2**.931–2
morphologies, **B2**.943 (Fig.), **B2**.946
resistance, **B2**.924, **B2**.927–8
glutamate transporters, **B1**.49
habitats, **B2**.924
herbs and spices, **B1**.287
waterborne, **B1**.220, **B1**.221
identification, **B2**.928–30, **B2**.940–1,
B2.944–6
DNA hybridization, **B1**.25
specimens and isolation, **B2**.938–9
importance, **B2**.923–4
infection, **B2**.938–47
nosocomial infection, **B1**.401 (Tab.)
opportunistic pathogens, **B2**.938–47
life cycle, **B2**.924–6
morphology, **B2**.925
L-forms, **B2**.925–6
as normal microbiota, **B1**.296 (Tab.)
nuts, **B1**.287
pasteurization, **B1**.232–3
as soil bacteria, **B1**.199–200
sporulation, **B2**.927–8
cell division, **B2**.927
process, **B2**.927
triggers, **B2**.927

sterilization
heat, **B1**.446, **B1**.446 (Tab.), **B1**.454 (Tab.)
ionizing radiation, **B1**.450, **B1**.454 (Tab.)
typing, **B2**.928–30
vitamin production, **B2**.923
Bacillus amyloliquefaciens, **B2**.935 (Tab.)
Bacillus anthracis
antibacterial susceptibility/resistance,
B2.937–8
antibiotics, **B2**.937–8
antigens, **B2**.928, **B2**.929–30, **B2**.937
cell wall polysaccharide, **B2**.928
endospores, **B2**.929–30
toxin components, **B2**.937
bioterrorism/biological warfare, **B1**.189,
B1.203, **B1**.364–5, **B1**.768
capsules, **B2**.934–7, **B2**.934 (Fig.)
composition, **B1**.44
'ghosts,' **B2**.932–3
characteristics, **B2**.935 (Tab.)
endospores
anthrax transmission, **B2**.930–1
antigen detection, **B2**.929–30
germination, **B2**.931–2
infective doses, **B2**.930–1
mailed in the USA, **B1**.364–5
sample handling safety, **B2**.933
survival in environment, **B2**.930
unintentional release from Soviet
bioweapons facility, **B1**.364–5
genes, for toxins, **B2**.931–2
habitats, **B2**.924
humans, **B1**.203
identification and isolation, **B2**.933–4
Anthraxin (trade mark) skin test,
B2.937
antigens, **B2**.928, **B2**.929–30, **B2**.937
colonies, **B2**.926 (Fig.), **B2**.934–7, **B2**.948
culture, **B2**.934, **B2**.948
diagnosis kits, **B2**.945
EIA systems, **B2**.937
microscopy, **B2**.934 (Fig.), **B2**.947
monoclonal antibody tests, **B2**.937
morphology, **B2**.934 (Fig.)
real-time PCR assays, **B2**.937
specimens for, **B2**.932–3
staining, **B2**.934–7, **B2**.947
immune evasion, **B1**.154
infection *see* Anthrax
medical and veterinary significance, **B1**.203
livestock, **B1**.203
in milk, **B1**.242
pathogenicity, **B2**.930–8
pXO1 and pXO2 genes, **B2**.931–2
research importance, **B2**.923
sunlight, **B1**.452
toxin
edema factor, **B2**.931–2, **B2**.937, **B2**.938
genetics, **B2**.931–2
lethal factor, **B2**.931–2, **B2**.937, **B2**.938
mechanism of action, **B1**.156 (Tab.),
B2.931–2
protective antigen, **B2**.931–2, **B2**.937,
B2.938

Bacillus anthracis (*Continued*)
  virulence factors
    exopolysaccharides, **B1**.154
    spreading determinants, **B1**.153 (Tab.)
Bacillus brevis, **B1**.287
Bacillus cereus, **B2**.939
  antibacterial susceptibility/resistance,
    B2.942–3, **B2**.946
  characteristics, **B2**.935 (Tab.), **B2**.940–2
  endospore survival, **B2**.939
  in foods, **B2**.939
    hazard analysis, **B1**.288
    herbs and spices, **B1**.287, **B1**.288
    milk, **B1**.242, **B2**.923–4
    milk powder, **B1**.248
    rice, **B1**.285, **B2**.929
    spoilage, **B2**.923–4
    vegetables, **B1**.282
    wheat, **B1**.284–5
  habitats, **B2**.924
  health and clinical uses, **B2**.923
  identification, **B2**.944–5
    colonies, **B2**.926 (Fig.), **B2**.934, **B2**.940–1,
      B2.945–6
    culture, **B2**.940–1, **B2**.947
    endospore antigens, **B2**.930
    H antigens, **B2**.928, **B2**.929, **B2**.941
    microscopy, **B2**.943 (Fig.), **B2**.946
    morphology, **B2**.943 (Fig.), **B2**.946
    serotypes and biotypes, **B2**.929
    typing, **B2**.928, **B2**.929
  infection *see Bacillus cereus* infection
  sterilization
    heat, **B1**.446 (Tab.)
    ionizing radiation, **B1**.446 (Tab.)
  toxins, **B2**.939–40
    emetic toxin, **B2**.940
    enterotoxins, **B2**.939–42
Bacillus cereus infection
  endophthalmitis, **B1**.603, **B1**.604, **B2**.940
  food poisoning
    diarrheal-type, **B2**.939
    emetic-type, **B2**.939
    infective dose, **B2**.939
    investigations, **B2**.938–9
    specimens, **B2**.939
  gastroenteritis
    cream, **B1**.248
    rice, **B1**.285
  keratitis, **B1**.601
  mastitis, **B1**.230, **B2**.940
  milk-borne, **B1**.242
  neonates, **B2**.940
  treatment, **B2**.942–3
  wounds, **B2**.940, **B2**.942–3
Bacillus circulans
  characteristics, **B2**.935 (Tab.)
  colonies, **B2**.926 (Fig.), **B2**.945–6
  infection, **B2**.944
    treatment, **B2**.946–7
  microscopy, **B2**.943 (Fig.)
  morphology, **B2**.943 (Fig.)
Bacillus coagulans
  canning process, **B1**.271, **B1**.283
  characteristics, **B2**.935 (Tab.)

  food spoilage, **B2**.923–4
  infection, **B2**.944
Bacillus fusiformis, **B2**.1945
Bacillus halodurans, **B2**.923
Bacillus licheniformis, **B2**.935 (Tab.)
  antibacterial susceptibility/resistance, **B2**.946
  colonies, **B2**.945–6
  in food, **B2**.923–4
    herbs and spices, **B1**.287–8
    wheat, **B1**.285
  habitats, **B2**.924
  identification, **B2**.944–5
    microscopy, **B2**.943 (Fig.)
    morphology, **B2**.943 (Fig.)
  infection, **B2**.943–4
    treatment, **B2**.946
  L-forms, **B2**.925–6
Bacillus megaterium, **B2**.935 (Tab.)
  catabolite repression, **B1**.73–4
  colonies, **B2**.926 (Fig.)
  endospore germination, **B2**.928
  habitats, **B2**.924
  herbs and spices, **B1**.287
  identification, **B2**.944–5
    microscopy, **B2**.943 (Fig.), **B2**.946
    morphology, **B2**.943 (Fig.), **B2**.946
  megacins, **B1**.136–7, **B1**.139
  waterborne, **B1**.211–12
Bacillus mycoides, **B2**.935 (Tab.)
  fish infection, **B2**.944
  waterborne, **B1**.211–12
Bacillus necrophorus, **B2**.1945–6
Bacillus polymyxa, **B1**.287
Bacillus popilliae, **B1**.203–4
Bacillus pumilus
  characteristics, **B2**.935 (Tab.)
  colonies, **B2**.926 (Fig.)
  herbs and spices, **B1**.287
  infection, **B2**.944
    treatment, **B2**.946
  microscopy, **B2**.943 (Fig.), **B2**.946
  morphology, **B2**.943 (Fig.), **B2**.946
  sterilization
    heat, **B1**.446 (Tab.)
    ionizing radiation, **B1**.446 (Tab.), **B1**.450,
      B1.454 (Tab.)
Bacillus schlegelii, **B2**.924
Bacillus sphaericus, **B2**.935 (Tab.)
  colonies, **B2**.926 (Fig.)
  endospores, resistance, **B2**.924
  flagella serotyping, **B2**.929
  habitats, **B2**.924
  infection, **B2**.944
  microscopy, **B2**.943 (Fig.), **B2**.946
  morphology, **B2**.943 (Fig.), **B2**.946
  mosquitocidal strains, **B2**.929
*Bacillus stearothermophilus (Geobacillus
    stearothermophilus)*
  sterilization
    canning process, **B1**.271, **B1**.283
    heat, **B1**.446, **B1**.446 (Tab.), **B1**.454 (Tab.)
    ionizing radiation, **B1**.446 (Tab.)
  transport of solutes, **B1**.49
  *see also Geobacillus stearothermophilus
    (Bacillus stearothermophilus)*

Bacillus subterraneus, **B2**.924
Bacillus subtilis, **B2**.935 (Tab.)
  antibacterial agents, **B1**.438, **B1**.454 (Tab.)
    spores, **B1**.433, **B1**.439
  artificial competence, **B1**.99–100
  biochemistry
    catabolite repression, **B1**.50, **B1**.73–4
    ion gradient-linked transport, **B1**.49
    nitrate reduction, **B1**.66
    sigma (σ) factors, **B1**.75
    TCA cycle, **B1**.61
  biological control agents against plant
    pathogens, **B1**.202–3
  colonies, **B2**.926 (Fig.), **B2**.945–6
  endospores, **B2**.926–7
  in food
    herbs and spices, **B1**.287
    wheat, **B1**.284–5
  food spoilage, **B2**.923–4
  genetics, chromosomes, **B1**.81
  habitats, **B2**.924
  H-antigens, **B2**.929
  health and clinical uses, **B2**.923
  identification, **B2**.944–5
    microscopy, **B2**.943 (Fig.)
    morphology, **B2**.943 (Fig.)
  ilv-leu operon, **B1**.72
  infection, **B2**.944
    treatment, **B2**.946
  morphology, L-form, **B2**.925–6
  natural competence, **B1**.99
  quorum sensing, **B1**.72, **B1**.172
  risk categorization, **B1**.762
  signal transduction, **B1**.167–8
  sporulation, **B1**.75, **B2**.927
  starvation, **B1**.75
  sterilization
    ethylene oxide, **B1**.454 (Tab.)
    heat, **B1**.446 (Tab.), **B1**.454 (Tab.)
    ionizing radiation, **B1**.446 (Tab.)
  typing, **B2**.929
  waterborne, **B1**.211–12
Bacillus thuringiensis
  antibacterial susceptibility/resistance, **B2**.942
  biological control agent, **B1**.203–4, **B2**.923
    Bt pesticides, **B1**.203–4, **B2**.923, **B2**.940
    resistance, **B1**.203–4
  characteristics, **B2**.935 (Tab.)
  colonies, **B2**.926 (Fig.), **B2**.934
  σ-endotoxins, **B2**.923, **B2**.940
  habitats, **B2**.924
  identification
    endospore antigens, **B2**.930
    H antigens, **B2**.928, **B2**.929
    heat-stable somatic antigens, **B2**.928
    microscopy, **B2**.940–1, **B2**.943 (Fig.),
      B2.946
    morphology, **B2**.940–1, **B2**.943 (Fig.),
      B2.946
    serovars, **B2**.929
    typing, **B2**.928, **B2**.929
  infection, **B2**.940
  mosquito pathogenic strain, **B2**.929
  transgenic crop plants development, **B2**.923,
    B2.940

Bacillus tusciae, **B2**.924

Bacitracin, **B1**.481

   Streptococcus, **B2**.862

Bactenecin-5 (Bac5), **I**.173

Bactenecin-7 (Bac7), **I**.173

Bacteremia, **B1**.509

  acquisition and classification, **B1**.510–11

  antibiotic susceptibility/resistance, **B1**.524

  causative organisms, **B1**.516, **B1**.519, **B1**.522

    Acinetobacter baumannii, **B1**.521–2

    anaerobic bacteria, **B1**.523

    Bartonella, **B1**.524

    Brucella, **B1**.523

    Enterobacteriaceae, **B1**.520–1

    Enterococcus, **B1**.518, **B2**.896

    Erysipelothrix rhusiopathiae, **B2**.971

    Escherichia coli, **B1**.520

    fungi, **B1**.522–3

    gram-negative, **B1**.516 (Fig.), **B1**.520–2,

      B1.522, **B1**.523

    gram-positive, **B1**.516 (Fig.), **B1**.517–20

    human brucellosis, **B2**.1737

    Leptospira, **B1**.524

    Lyme borreliosis, **B2**.1828–9

    melioidosis, **B2**.1629

    Mycobacteria, **B1**.524

    Mycobacterium, **B1**.524

    Mycobacterium abscessus, **B2**.1247,

      B2.1249

    Mycobacterium aurum, **B2**.1251

    Mycobacterium neoaurum, **B2**.1259

    Mycobacterium smegmatis, **B2**.1261

    Neisseria, **B1**.522

    Pasteurella multocida, **B2**.1654–5

    Pseudomonas aeruginosa, **B1**.521

    special requirements, **B1**.523–4

    Staphylococci, coagulase-negative, **B1**.518

    Staphylococcus aureus, **B1**.517–18, **B1**.524

    Streptococcus pneumoniae, **B1**.519, **B1**.569,

      B1.570 (Fig.)

    see also specific infection

  classification, **B1**.510–11

  clinical presentation, **B1**.510

  community-acquired, **B1**.510–11

  continuous, **B1**.510

  definition, **B1**.510–11, **B1**.511 (Tab.)

  intermittent, **B1**.510, **B1**.511–12

  mortality, **B1**.392–3

  nosocomial, **B1**.392–3, **B1**.509

    after catheterization, **B1**.510, **B1**.512

    classification, **B1**.510–11

    false-positive culture impacts, **B1**.510

  perioperative, **B1**.388–9

  predisposing conditions, **B1**.512

  primary, **B1**.510

  secondary, **B1**.393, **B1**.509–10

  specimens, **B1**.512–14

    blood collection, **B1**.512

    contamination, **B1**.512

    disinfection, **B1**.512

    timing, **B1**.512

    transport, **B1**.512

    volume, **B1**.513

  technical issues, **B1**.511–12

  transient, **B1**.510, **B1**.527

  treatment, **B1**.524

  see also Blood cultures

Bacteria

  adaptation/changes causing

    emergence/resurgence of infection,

    B1.362–4

  in air *see* Airborne bacteria

  carbon:nitrogen ratios, **B1**.200

  cell counts, **B1**.38

    methods, **B1**.38

    total, **B1**.38

    viable, **B1**.38

  cell length, **B1**.40–1

  cell mass, **B1**.38

  chromosome replication, **B1**.46

  colonization, **B1**.294–5

  composition, **B1**.42

    capsules, **B1**.44

    carbohydrate and lipid, **B1**.42

    cellular polymers, **B1**.42

    cytoplasmic membrane, **B1**.44–5

    enzymes and pathways, **B1**.45–6

    flagella and pili, **B1**.44

    protein, **B1**.42

    RNA and DNA, **B1**.42

  infection *see* Infection(s)

  nutrition, **B1**.37–8

  response to stress, **B1**.74

  resting cells, **B1**.40

  starvation, **B1**.75

  structure, **B1**.42–6

  water content, **B1**.42

  weight, **B1**.42

  see also individual species

Bacterial vaginosis (BV), **B1**.665–8

  causative organisms, **B1**.665, **B2**.911

  'clue cells,' **B1**.665, **B1**.666

  diagnosis, **B1**.666

    four composite criteria (Amsel's criteria),

    B1.666

    gram stained vaginal smears, grading,

    B1.666, **B1**.667 (Fig.), **B1**.667 (Tab.)

  predisposing factors, **B1**.665

  sequelae, **B1**.668

  synonyms, **B1**.665

  treatment, **B1**.666–8

Bactericidal/permeability increasing protein

  (BPI), **I**.114–15, **I**.114 (Tab.)

  neutrophils, **I**.115

  as therapy target, **I**.124

Bacteriochlorophylls, chemotaxonomy, **B1**.24

Bacteriocins, **B1**.136–9

  assay, **B1**.137

  biosynthesis, **B1**.138–9

  characteristics, **B1**.136–7

  classification, **B1**.136–7

  definition, **B1**.136, **B2**.894–5

  host range, **B1**.139

  immunity to, **B1**.139

  importance of, **B1**.139

  modes of action, **B1**.137–8

    membrane potential destruction, **B1**.137–8

    nucleolysis, **B1**.138

    protein synthesis inhibition, **B1**.138

  nomenclature, **B1**.136–7

  release, **B1**.138

  resistance, **B1**.138–9

  tolerance, **B1**.138–9

  typing, **B1**.139

    Burkholderia cepacia, **B2**.1614

    Clostridium perfringens, **B2**.1093

    Enterococcus, **B2**.893–5

    Haemophilus, **B2**.1706

    Proteus, **B2**.1445

    Providencia, **B2**.1451

    Pseudomonas aeruginosa, **B1**.136–8

    Staphylococcus, **B2**.790

    Streptococcus, **B2**.850–2

    Yersinia, **B2**.1467–8

  uptake, **B1**.138–9

Bacteriological Code, **B1**.16–8

Bacteriological warfare, **I**.7

Bacteriology

  'pure', **B1**.9–10

  systematic, **B1**.10–4

Bacteriophage(s), **B1**.139–43

  analysis, **B1**.141–3

    assays, **B1**.141–2

    environmental role, **B1**.142–3

    plaque morphology, **B1**.142

    transduction, **B1**.142

  antibody display, **B1**.755

  as cloning vectors, **B1**.119–20, **B1**.120–1

  definition, **B1**.136

  discovery, **B1**.9

  double-stranded DNA, **B1**.141

  environmental role, **B1**.142–3

  historical aspects, **B1**.13

  identification, **B1**.143

  inhibition, plasmids, **B1**.115–16

  morphology, **B1**.140

  receptors

    O antigen, **B2**.1341

    pili, **B1**.102

  single-stranded DNA, **B1**.140–1

  single-stranded RNA, **B1**.140

  tox⁺, **B2**.984

  typing, **B1**.143

    Aeromonas, **B2**.1535

    Brucella, **B2**.1730–1, **B2**.1732 (Tab.)

    Burkholderia cepacia, **B2**.1614

    Burkholderia thailandensis, **B2**.1623

    Clostridium, **B2**.1093

    Enterobacteriaceae, **B2**.1344

    Enterococcus, **B2**.893–5, **B2**.895

    Escherichia, **B2**.1370

    Listeria, **B2**.956, **B2**.962

    Mycoplasma arthritidis, **B2**.1974, **B2**.1986

    Salmonella Agona, **B2**.1416–17

    Salmonella Paratyphi B, **B2**.1421

    Salmonella Typhi, **B2**.1408

    Staphylococcus, **B2**.792

    Streptococcus, **B2**.839

    Vibrio, **B2**.1511, **B2**.1512, **B2**.1518

  virucidal activity, **B1**.434–6, **B1**.440

Bacteriophage СТХΦ, **B2**.1511, **B2**.1512,

  B2.1518

  Vibrio cholerae, **B1**.149

Bacteriophage K139, **B2**.1512

Bacteriophage λ, **B1**.120–1, **B1**.141–142
  specialized transduction, **B1**.105–6,
    B1.105 (Fig.)
Bacteriophage M13, **B1**.120
Bacteriophage MAV1, **B2**.1974, **B2**.1986
Bacteriophage MS2 *(Leviviridae),* **B1**.140
Bacteriophage Mu, as transposable element,
  B1.91
Bacteriophage P1, **B1**.142–3
  generalized transduction, **B1**.104
Bacteriophage P22, **B1**.142
Bacteriophage ΦX174 *(Microviridae),*
    B1.140–1
  laboratory glove penetration studies, **B1**.765
Bacteriophage PRD1, **V1**.68 (Fig.)
Bacteriophage T4, **V1**.60 (Fig.)
Bacteriorhodopsin, **B1**.69–70
Bacteriuria
  asymptomatic significant, **B1**.679
  definition, **B1**.677
  of elderly, **B1**.394
  of pregnancy, **B1**.679
Bacteroidaceae, **B2**.1913–14, **B2**.1952
  normal microbiota, **B2**.1932–4
    in animals, **B2**.1934
    gastrointestinal tract, **B2**.1933
    oral cavity, **B2**.1932–3
    vaginal, **B2**.1933–4
Bacteroides, **B2**.1917–20
  antibacterial susceptibility/resistance,
    B2.1930–1, **B2**.1935–6
    mechanisms, **B2**.1935
  antigens, **B2**.1937
  cell wall composition, **B2**.1915
  classification, **B2**.1913–17
    criteria, **B2**.1914–15
    current status, **B2**.1929–30
    rRNA sequence analysis, **B2**.1915–17
  conjugation, **B1**.103
  fatty acids, **B2**.1915
  genus definition, **B2**.1918–20
  LPS, **B2**.1937
  menaquinones, **B2**.1915
  molecular analysis, **B2**.1931–2
  normal microbiota, **B1**.296 (Tab.), **B1**.301–3,
    B2.1932–4
    in animals, **B2**.1934
    bifidobacteria relationship, **B2**.1933
    gastrointestinal tract, **B2**.1933
    vagina, **B2**.1934
  normal nasopharyngeal flora, **B1**.609
  nosocomial bacteremia, **B1**.393
  pathogenicity, **B2**.1936–8
  phylogenetic tree, **B2**.1917 (Fig.)
  pigments, **B2**.1915, **B2**.1916 (Fig.)
  plasmids, **B2**.1931
  propionic acid fermentation, **B1**.56
  species
    current status, **B2**.1929–30
    G + C range, **B2**.1915
    type strains, **B2**.1918 (Tab.)
  sphingolipids, **B2**.1915
  transposons, **B1**.93–4, **B2**.1931
Bacteroides amylophilus, **B2**.1930
Bacteroides caccae, **B2**.1920

Bacteroides distasonis, **B2**.1920
  as normal microbiota, **B2**.1933
Bacteroides eggerthii, **B2**.1920
  as normal microbiota, **B2**.1933
Bacteroides fragilis, **B2**.1918
  antibacterial susceptibility/resistance,
    B1.499 (Tab.)
  capsular antigen, **B2**.1918
  cell wall, **B2**.1918
  classification, **B2**.1913–17
  fecal flora, **B2**.1918
  infection
    bacteremia, **B1**.523
    endocarditis, **B1**.533
    intracranial abscess, **B1**.583–5
  pathogenicity, **B2**.1936–8
    abscess formation, **B2**.1938
    exotoxins, **B2**.1937
    LPS, **B2**.1937
Bacteroides furcosus, **B2**.1930
Bacteroides gracilis, **B2**.1929
Bacteroides hypermegas, **B2**.1930
Bacteroides melaninogenicus, **B2**.1913–15
Bacteroides merdae, **B2**.1920
Bacteroides microfusus, **B2**.1930
Bacteroides multiacidus, **B2**.1930
Bacteroides nodosus, **B2**.1930
Bacteroides ochraceus, **B2**.1915, **B2**.1930
Bacteroides ovatus, **B2**.1920
Bacteroides pneumosintes, **B2**.1929–30
Bacteroides praeacutus, **B2**.1929
  intracranial abscess, **B1**.584–5
Bacteroides putredinis, **B2**.1930
Bacteroides splanchnicus, **B2**.1920
Bacteroides stercoris, **B2**.1920
Bacteroides succinogenes, **B2**.1930
Bacteroides termitidis, **B2**.1930
Bacteroides thetaiotaomicron, **B2**.1920
  bacteremia, **B1**.523
  normal microbiota, **B2**.1933
Bacteroides uniformis, **B2**.1920
Bacteroides ureolyticus, **B2**.1552–3
  classification, **B2**.1929
Bacteroides variabilis, **B2**.1920
Bacteroides vulgatus, **B2**.1920
  as normal microbiota, **B2**.1933
Baculoviridae, **V1**.27 (Tab.), **V1**.43 (Tab.)
  hepatitis E virus ORF2 as antigen for HEV
    assays, **V2**.1179–80
  see also specific viruses
Baculovirus
  immune evasion
    caspase inhibitors, **I**.627
    inhibitors of apoptosis, **I**.135, **I**.624, **I**.627
  production systems, virus-like particles,
    I.840
  see also Baculoviridae
Bad protein, **I**.133
  structure, **I**.133 (Fig.)
'Baggage malaria,' **P**.511, **P**.514–15
Bailing, airborne bacteria, **B1**.186 (Tab.)
Bak protein, **I**.133
Balamuthia
  classification, **P**.190–1
  diagnosis, **P**.235

  immune response, **P**.87, **P**.232
  infection
    chemotherapy, **P**.237
    clinical features, **P**.231
    route, **P**.231
  pathogenesis, **P**.233–4
Balamuthia mandrillaris, **P**.187, **P**.226
  classification, **P**.226
  epidemiology/control, **P**.236
  life-cycle, **P**.229
  structure, **P**.228, **P**.228 (Fig.)
Balantidium, classification, **P**.197
Balantidium coli, **P**.189, **P.275–82**
  biochemistry, **P**.278–9
    anaerobic conditions, **P**.278–9
    hyaluronidase, **P**.278–9
  classification, **P**.275
  historical aspects, **P**.275
  infection *see Balantidium coli* infection
  life cycle, **P**.277–8
    binary fission, **P**.277, **P**.279 (Fig.)
    excystation, **P**.277
    sexual union (syngamy), **P**.277–8,
      P.279 (Fig.)
    transmission, **P**.278
  locomotion, **P**.276
  nutrition, **P**.276
  structure, **P**.275–7
    cilia, **P**.276, **P**.277 (Fig.)
    contractile vacuoles, **P**.276, **P**.277 (Fig.)
    cyclopharynx, **P**.275–6
    cyst, **P**.277, **P**.278 (Fig.), **P**.279 (Fig.)
    cystosome, **P**.275–6
    cytopyge, **P**.277 (Fig.)
    macronucleus, **P**.276–7, **P**.277 (Fig.),
      P.278 (Fig.)
    micronucleus, **P**.276–7, **P**.278 (Fig.)
    peristome, **P**.275–6, **P**.276 (Fig.)
    trophozoite, **P**.275–6, **P**.276 (Fig.),
      P.277 (Fig.), **P**.278 (Fig.)
Balantidium coli infection
  amebic dysentery *vs.,* **P**.279
  appendicitis *vs.,* **P**.279
  chemotherapy, **P**.281
  clinical aspects, **P**.279–80
    acute disease, **P**.279
    asymptomatic carrier, **P**.279
    chronic disease, **P**.279
  diagnosis, **P**.280
    biopsy, **P**.280
    fecal examination, **P**.280
  epidemiology, **P**.280–1
    animal reservoirs, **P**.275, **P**.280–1
    distribution, **P**.280–1
    human outbreaks, **P**.281
  immunology, **P**.76, **P**.279–80
    acquired immunity, **P**.279–80
    HIV infection, **P**.279–80
  integrated control, **P**.281
  pathology, **P**.280, **P**.280 (Fig.)
    Campylobacter coli co-infection, **P**.280
  BALB/c mice, babesiosis, **P**.455–6
  Baltimore classification, **V1**.180
    negative-strand RNA viruses classification,
      V1.127, **V1**.128 (Fig.)

Baltimore classification (*Continued*)
  positive-strand RNA viruses, **V1**.135
  viral classification, **V1**.109, **V1**.109 (Fig.)
Bamboo rat, *Penicillium marneffei* in, **M**.26,
  M.560–1, **M**.561 (Figs.), **M**.561 (Tab.),
  M.562
*Bam*HI (restriction enzyme), EBV genome
  characterization, **V1**.560, **V1**.560 (Fig.)
Bangui virus infection, **V2**.1047
Banzi virus (BANV), **V2**.998 (Tab.)
Barbarie duck parvovirus (BDPV), **V1**.410
Bare lymphocyte syndrome (BLS)
  immunogenetics, **I**.575
    MHC class II, **I**.575
  NK cells, **I**.103
  pathology, **I**.575
Bare skin immunization *see* Vaccination, bare
  skin
Barmah Forest virus, **V2**.1011 (Tab.), **V2**.1023
Barnaviridae, **V1**.27 (Tab.), **V1**.51 (Tab.)
  see also specific viruses
Barrier nursing, **B1**.328–9
  hepatitis B control, **V2**.1257
Bartenders, candidiasis, **M**.597
Bartonella, **B2**.1885–900
  antibacterial susceptibility/resistance,
    B2.1898–9
  classification, **B2**.1886–7, **B2**.1886 (Tab.),
    B2.2026
    biochemistry, **B2**.1895, **B2**.1896 (Tab.)
    electron microscopy, **B2**.1887
    microscopy, **B2**.1887
    PCR, **B2**.1895–7
  culture, **B2**.1895
    samples, **B2**.1895
    solid media, **B2**.1895
  historical perspective, **B2**.1885–6
  infection *see* Bartonellosis
  morphology, flagella, **B2**.1887
  pathogenicity, **B2**.1899
  reservoirs, **B2**.1887–8
    species association, **B2**.1887
  transmission, **B2**.1887–8
    ectoparasites, **B2**.1887
Bartonella alsatica
  characteristics, **B2**.1886 (Tab.)
  fimbriae, **B2**.1887
Bartonella bacilliformis
  antibacterial susceptibility/resistance,
    B2.1891
  biochemistry, **B2**.1889–90, **B2**.1896 (Tab.)
    deformin, **B2**.1891
  characteristics, **B2**.1886 (Tab.)
  classification, **B2**.1886, **B2**.2027 (Fig.)
  culture, **B2**.1889–90
  genotyping, **B2**.1890
  geographical distribution, **B2**.1888
  infection, **B2**.1888 (Tab.)
    see also Bartonellosis; Carrión's disease
  morphology, **B2**.1890
    flagella, **B2**.1887
  nucleic acid composition, **B2**.1729 (Tab.)
  pathogenicity, **B2**.1899
  transmission, **B2**.1887, **B2**.1888
Bartonella birtlesii, **B2**.1886 (Tab.)
Bartonella bovis, **B2**.1886 (Tab.)

Bartonella capreoli
  characteristics, **B2**.1886 (Tab.)
  flagella, **B2**.1887
Bartonella chomelii, **B2**.1886 (Tab.)
Bartonella clarridgeiae, **B2**.1886 (Tab.)
  biochemistry, **B2**.1896 (Tab.)
  infection, **B2**.1888 (Tab.), **B2**.1899–900
    see also Bartonellosis
  morphology, **B2**.1887 (Fig.)
  flagella, **B2**.1887
Bartonella doshiae, **B2**.1886 (Tab.)
  classification, **B2**.1886
Bartonella elizabethae, **B2**.1886 (Tab.)
  biochemistry, **B2**.1896 (Tab.)
  infection, **B2**.1888 (Tab.), **B2**.1899
    see also Bartonellosis
  isolation, **B1**.524
Bartonella grahamii, **B2**.1886 (Tab.)
  classification, **B2**.1886
  infection, **B2**.1888 (Tab.), **B2**.1900
    see also Bartonellosis
Bartonella henselae, **B2**.1886 (Tab.)
  biochemistry, **B2**.1896 (Tab.)
  classification, **B2**.2027 (Fig.)
  culture, **B2**.1895
    solid media, **B2**.1895
  geographical distribution, **B2**.1897
  infection, **B2**.1888 (Tab.)
    bacillary angiomatosis, **B2**.1894
    conjunctivitis, **B1**.598–9
    endocarditis, **B1**.536, **B2**.1894
    immunoassays, **B2**.1897
    peliosis hepatitis, **B2**.1894
    see also Bartonellosis; Cat-scratch disease
  isolation/identification
    culture media, **B1**.524
    PCR, **B2**.1897
  morphology, **B2**.1887 (Fig.)
    pili, **B2**.1887
  pathogenicity, **B2**.1899
  transmission, **B2**.1887
Bartonella koehlerae, **B2**.1886 (Tab.)
Bartonella peromysci, **B2**.1886 (Tab.)
Bartonella quintana, **B2**.1886 (Tab.)
  biochemistry, **B2**.1896 (Tab.)
  classification, **B2**.2026, **B2**.2027 (Fig.)
  culture
    growth media/conditions, **B1**.524
    solid media, **B2**.1895
  immunoassays, **B2**.1897
  infection, **B2**.1888 (Tab.)
    bacillary angiomatosis, **B2**.1894
    endocarditis, **B2**.1894
    peliosis hepatitis, **B2**.1894
    see also Bartonellosis; Trench fever
  nucleic acid composition, **B2**.1729 (Tab.)
  pathogenicity, **B2**.1899
  pili, **B2**.1887
  transmission, **B2**.1887
Bartonella schoenbuchii, **B2**.1886 (Tab.)
  flagella, **B2**.1887
Bartonella talpae, **B2**.1886 (Tab.)
  classification, **B2**.2027 (Fig.)
Bartonella taylorii, **B2**.1886 (Tab.)
  classification, **B2**.1886

Bartonella tribocorum, **B2**.1886 (Tab.)
  fimbriae, **B2**.1887
  pathogenicity, **B2**.1899
Bartonella vinsonii
  subspecies *arupensis*, **B2**.1886 (Tab.),
    B2.1888 (Tab.), **B2**.1900
  subspecies *berkhoffii*, **B2**.1886 (Tab.),
    B2.1888 (Tab.), **B2**.1900
  subspecies *vinsonii*, **B2**.1886 (Tab.)
Bartonella washoensis
  characteristics, **B2**.1886 (Tab.)
  infection, **B2**.1888 (Tab.), **B2**.1900
Bartonellosis, **B2**.1888 (Tab.), **B2**.1899–900
  in AIDS *see* AIDS, concomitant infection
  animals, **B2**.1887–8
  bacteremia, **B1**.524
  endocarditis, **B1**.533, **B1**.534, **B1**.537
  identification, **B1**.524
    see also Cat-scratch disease; Trench fever
Basal body *see* Kinetosome (basal body)
Basal cell carcinoma (BCC), HPV association,
  V1.464
Base analogues
  incorporation, point mutations, **B1**.84–5
  mutagens, **V1**.183
Base pair substitutions
  point mutations *see* Point mutations
  suppression, **B1**.86–7
Basic fuschin dye, *Brucella* species
  differentiation, **B2**.1735
Basic reproduction number (R_0)
  bacterial infection, **B1**.337–8, **B1**.340,
    B1.340 (Tab.)
    estimation, **B1**.341
  parasitic infection *see* Epidemiology of
    infection, parasitic infection
  see also Infection(s), mathematical models
Basidiobolaceae, **M**.348 (Tab.)
Basidiobolus, **M**.347–8, **M**.348 (Tab.)
  classification, **M**.53
  identification
    culture, **M**.352
    hematoxylin and eosin stain, **M**.351–2,
      M.351 (Fig.)
  infection, **M**.350
    diagnosis, **M**.351–2
    histopathology, **M**.351–2
    immune response, **M**.350–2
    microscopy, **M**.351–2
    Splendore–Hoeppli phenomenon,
      M.351–2, **M**.351 (Fig.)
Basidiobolus haptosporus, **M**.347–8
Basidiobolus meristosporus, **M**.347–8
Basidiobolus ranarum, **M**.347–8,
  M.348 (Fig.)
  antimicrobial susceptibility, **M**.352
  classification, **M**.53, **M**.347–8
  histopathology, **M**.128 (Tab.)
  morphology, **M**.348–9, **M**.348 (Fig.)
  subcutaneous infection, **M**.348, **M**.350–1,
    M.351 (Fig.)
  therapy, **M**.352
Basidiobolus ranarum, **M**.351 (Fig.)
Basidiomycetous yeast, **M**.631, **M**.632 (Tab.)
  see also individual species

Basidiomycota, **M**.44 (Fig.), **M**.49–51,
 M.50 (Tab.), **M**.52 (Fig.), **M**.63,
 M.65 (Tab.), **M**.197
 see also individual species
Basidiospores, *Cryptococcus neoformans*,
 M.639, **M**.640 (Fig.), **M**.644–5
Basiliximab, **I**.333
Basogranulin, basophils, **I**.64
Basophilia, **I**.67
 infectious diseases, **I**.68 (Tab.)
Basophils, **I**.55
 activation, **I**.62–3
 antibody binding, **I**.354, **I**.357
 IgE-mediated, **I**.62
 markers, **I**.63
 non-IgE-mediated, **I**.62
 basic biology, **I**.55–8
 cell trafficking, **I**.58–61
 adhesion, **I**.58, **I**.59 (Tab.)
 chemotaxis, **I**.58, **I**.60
 see also individual chemokines
 chemokines, **I**.59 (Tab.)
 cytokine production, **I**.59 (Tab.), **I**.66
 eotaxin effects, **I**.66
 IL-4, **I**.66, **I**.280
 IL-13, **I**.66
 leukotriene B$_4$ production, **I**.185
 platelet-activating factor, **I**.191
 Th1/Th2 differentiation, **I**.399
 degranulation, **I**.62–3
 anaphylactic *vs.* piecemeal, **I**.63
 IL-1, **I**.63
 potentiators, **I**.63
 effector molecules, **I**.63–4, **I**.63 (Tab.)
 basogranulin, **I**.64
 histamine, **I**.62, **I**.63–4
 LTC$_4$, **I**.64
 MIP-1α, **I**.64
 functions, **I**.61–6, **I**.66–7
 in allergic reactions, **I**.57
 antigen presentation, **I**.66
 apoptosis, **I**.57
 Ig class switching, **I**.66
 growth/differentiation, **I**.55–7
 GM-CSF, **I**.57
 IL-3, **I**.55–7, **I**.66
 IL-5, **I**.55, **I**.57, **I**.278
 IL-6, **I**.57
 nerve growth factor, **I**.57
 TGF-β, **I**.57
 TNF-α, **I**.57
 helminth infection, **I**.55, **I**.57, **I**.67–8
 Ascaris, **I**.68
 Fasciola, **I**.68
 Nippostrongylus brasiliensis, **I**.68
 Onchocerca, **I**.68
 Schistosoma, **I**.68
 Strongyloides, **I**.68
 Toxocara, **I**.68
 Trichinella spiralis, **I**.68
 Trochostrongylus colubriformis, **I**.68
 Wuchereria, **I**.68
 in infectious disease, **I**.67–71, **I**.68 (Tab.)
 helminth infection *see above*
 viral infection *see below*

integrins, **I**.59 (Tab.)
 morphology, **I**.55, **I**.56 (Fig.)
 natural history, **I**.57
 receptors
 C3a receptor, **I**.146
 CC chemokines, **I**.223–4
 chemokine, **I**.220
 FcεRI, **I**.62, **I**.316
 FcγRIIb, **I**.62
 selectins, **I**.59 (Tab.)
 vascular cell adhesion molecule 1 binding,
 I.58
 viral infection, **I**.70–1
 HIV, **I**.55, **I**.70–1
 respiratory viruses, **I**.71
 rhinovirus 16, **I**.71
Bassi, A, **M**.6
Bats
 histoplasmosis, **M**.520–21, **M**.535–6
 rabies, **V2**.1120
Bavay, Arthur, **P**.9
Bax protein, **I**.133
 structure, **I**.133 (Fig.)
BAY-57-1293, **V2**.1617–18
 structure, **V2**.1618 (Fig.)
Bayesian analysis (BA), **M**.48–9
Bayou virus, **V2**.1666 (Tab.)
 emerging infection, **V2**.1646–7
 recognition, **V2**.1653 (Tab.)
Bay-sore, **P**.323
Bazin, E, **M**.6
Bc$_1$ complex, **B1**.64
BCA-1 *see* B-cell-attracting chemokine
 (BCA-1:CXCL13)
B cell(s), **I.303–38**
 activation, **I**.326–7
 antigen effects, **I**.326
 B7–1 (CD80)–CD28 interactions,
 I.326–7
 B7–2 (CD86)–CD28 interactions,
 I.326–7
 CD4 T cell interactions, **I**.326
 CD5 effects, **I**.348
 CD22 effects, **I**.348
 CD40–CD40L interactions, **I**.326–7,
 I.348–9
 CD72 effects, **I**.348
 FcγRIIB effects, **I**.347
 follicular dendritic cell interactions,
 I.326–7
 germinal centers, **I**.401
 GM-CSF production, **I**.277
 IL-4, **I**.348–9
 IL-5, **I**.348–9
 intercellular adhesion molecule 1, **I**.326
 leukocyte function-associated antigen-1,
 I.326
 mucosal vaccination, **I**.827
 PIR-B effects, **I**.348
 activation markers, **V1**.565
 as APCs, **I**.376, **I**.378
 antigen uptake, **I**.382
 CD4 T cells, **I**.394
 B1 cells, **I**.435
 B2 cells, **I**.435

complement receptors, **I**.147
 complement receptor 1, **I**.151
 complement receptor 2 (CR2:CD21), **I**.148
 cytokines produced
 GM-CSF, **I**.277
 IL-10, **I**.292
 lymphotoxin, **I**.286
 development *see below*
 diseases/infection *see specific diseases/
 infection*
 DNA vaccine priming, **I**.914
 genetic diversity, **I**.8
 homing
 BLC (CXCL13), **I**.226
 CCR7, **I**.226
 chemokines, **I**.226
 CXCR4, **I**.226
 EBV-induced receptor ligand chemokine,
 I.226
 SLC, **I**.226
 IL-9 effects, **I**.282
 IL-10 effects, **I**.293–4
 IL-13 effects, **I**.294–7
 IL-21 effects, **I**.283–4
 in infection
 acute viral infection clearance, **V1**.258
 bacterial infection, **I**.646
 depletion in African trypanosomiasis,
 P.80–1
 EBV infection, **V1**.248–9, **V1**.565, **V1**.570
 HIV infection *see* HIV infection
 HTLV-1-associated myelopathy/tropical
 spastic paraparesis (HAM/TSP),
 V2.1429–30
 hyperendemic malaria, **V1**.570
 kinetics, **I**.492 (Fig.)
 parasitic infection, **P**.69
 prion diseases, **V2**.1376–7, **V2**.1379
 viruses replicating in, **V1**.243 (Tab.)
 measles-induced immunosuppression,
 V1.728 (Tab.)
 naive
 CXCR5 expression, **I**.400
 memory B cells *vs.*, **I**.491 (Tab.)
 Peyer's patches, **I**.532
 receptors
 complement receptors *see above*
 CXCR5, **I**.225–6
 Fcα/μR, **I**.317–18
 see also B-cell receptor (BCR)
 respiratory tract, **B1**.608
 secondary lymphoid tissue, **I**.512
 T cells *vs.*, **I**.490 (Tab.)
 tolerance development, **I**.323
 tonsils, **I**.533
B-cell adapter for PI 3-kinase (BCAP), **I**.345
B-cell-attracting chemokine (BCA-1:CXCL13),
 I.218 (Tab.)
 B cell homing, **I**.226
 Helicobacter pylori infection, **I**.230
B cell development, **I**.322, **I**.322 (Fig.)
 antigen-dependent, **I**.326
 antigen-independent, **I**.322–3
 Igh allelic exclusion, **I**.324
 Igh gene rearrangement, **I**.323
 Igl gene rearrangement, **I**.323, **I**.324

B cell development
  antigen-independent (*Continued*)
    IL-7, **I**.323
    lymphoid stem cells, **I**.323
    negative selection, **I**.323, **I**.324
    pre-BcR formation, **I**.323–4
    RAG degradation, **I**.324
    selection, **I**.323–4
  BCR effects, **I**.340–1, **I**.340 (Fig.)
    see also B-cell receptor
  class switching, **I**.491
  Ig surface expression, **I**.323
  IL-4 effects, **I**.280
  IL-7 effects, **I**.281, **I**.341
  M-CSF effects, **I**.277
  positive selection, **I**.491
  prostaglandin E_2 effects, **I**.188
  transcriptional control, **I**.324–6
    Aiolös, **I**.324–5
    E2A gene, **I**.325
    E12 protein, **I**.325
    E47 protein, **I**.325
    EBF (early B-cell factor), **I**.325
    Ikaros, **I**.324
    PAX5/BSAP, **I**.326
    PU.1, **I**.324
  see also Immunoglobulin(s), synthesis
B-cell epitopes (BCEs), **I**.853
  peptide vaccines *see* Peptide vaccines
  Rubella virus, **V2**.967
B-cell lymphomas, avian, **V1**.340
B-cell receptor (BCR), **I.339–52**
  antigen uptake, **I**.348
    Igα/Igβ, **I**.348
  B cell development/activation, **I**.348–9
    Fas-induced death protection, **I**.348–9
    T helper cells, **I**.348–9
    tolerance, **I**.348
    VJ recombination, **I**.348
  diversity, **I**.748–9
  high-order structure, **I**.341–2
    antigen binding effects, **I**.342
    clustering hypothesis, **I**.342
    tonic signaling, **I**.342
  Ig structure, **I**.311
  membrane form
    secreted form *vs.,* **I**.339
    synthesis, **I**.339
  pre-BCR, **I**.323–4, **I**.340–1
    functions, **I**.341
    Igα, **I**.340–1
    Igβ, **I**.340–1
    Ig heavy chain, **I**.332, **I**.340–1
    λ5, **I**.340–1
    mutations, **I**.341
    signaling, **I**.341
    structure, **I**.340–1, **I**.340 (Fig.)
    surrogate light chains, **I**.340–1
    Vpre-B, **I**.340–1
  secreted form
    membrane form *vs.,* **I**.339
    synthesis, **I**.339
  signaling, **I**.342–8
    BLNK (SLP-65), **I**.343–5
    co-receptors, **I**.347–8

downstream transcription factor activation,
      I.346–7
    lipid raft associations, **I**.342
    PI 3-kinase activation, **I**.345
    protein tyrosine kinase activation, **I**.342–3
    Ras, **I**.346
    sequences, **I**.341
    signal complex formation, **I**.343–5
    Vav, **I**.345–6
  structure, **I**.339–42, **I**.340 (Fig.)
    high-order *see above*
    Igα (CD79a), **I**.339
    Igβ (CD79b), **I**.339
    Ig domains, **I**.339
    immunoreceptor tyrosine-based activation
      motifs, **I**.341
B-cell stimulating/activatory protein (BSAP),
      I.326
BCG vaccine, **B2**.1219
  controversy, **B2**.1219
  laboratory workers, **B1**.767
  leprosy prevention, **B2**.1219, **B2**.1221
  as vector *see* Vaccines, live
Bcl-2 protein
  apoptosis prevention, **I**.132–3, **I**.133 (Fig.),
      I.624, **I**.626
    mechanism of action, **I**.133
  CD8 T cell activation, **I**.428
  IL-10 effects, **I**.293–4
  mitochondria apoptosis, **I**.132
  structure, **I**.133 (Fig.)
Bcl-10 protein
  BCR signaling, **I**.346–7
  structure, **I**.346–7
Bcl-X_L protein
  apoptosis prevention, **I**.132–3
  structure, **I**.133 (Fig.)
BcrA multidrug resistance pump,
      B2.1610–11
BDProbe Tec®, **B1**.723 (Tab.)
Beansprouts, *Salmonella* Enteritidis
      bacteriophage type 4b from, **B1**.322
Beauveria bassiana, **M**.6, **M**.220
Beauveria bassiana infection
  keratitis, **M**.328
  oculomycoses, **M**.275 (Tab.)
Beauveria, histopathology, **M**.128 (Tab.)
Bebaru virus (BEBV), **V2**.1011 (Tab.)
Bedpans, nosocomial infection, **B1**.379–80
Beef, intestinal *Sarcocystis* infection, **P**.448
Beet farming, waterborne bacteria, **B1**.212,
      B1.219
Beetles, bacterial pathogens, **B1**.203–4
Behavioral factors
  cross-sectional surveys, **P**.56–7
  emerging bacterial infection, **B1**.360–1
  sexually transmitted diseases, **B1**.354
Behavioral Risk Factor Surveillance System,
      vaccine uptake, **B1**.326
von Behring, E A, **B1**.7
Beijerinckii, **B1**.201
Beijerinck, M W, **V1**.3, **B1**.201
  viral filterability, **V1**.24
Bejel *see* Syphilis, endemic (Bejel)
Belgian red, *Giardia* detection, **P**.250–1
Benethamine penicillin, **B1**.473

Benign anogenital lesions, HPV associations,
      V1.463 (Tab.)
Benign tertian malaria *see* Malaria, vivax/ovale
      (benign tertian)
1,2-Benisothiazol-3-one (BIT), **B1**.427
Benomyl resistance gene, *Candida albicans,*
      M.608
Benyvirus, **V1**.27 (Tab.)
Benzathine penicillin, **B1**.473
Benzene, bioremediation, **B1**.201
Benzimadoles, hepatitis C therapy, **V2**.1216
Benzimidazole, Chagas disease, **P**.392–3
Benzodiazepines, in tetanus, **B2**.1066
Benzoic acid, **B1**.422
  pH, **B1**.432
Benzothiadiazines, hepatitis C therapy,
      V2.1216
Benzyl alcohol, **B1**.427
Benzylpenicillin (penicillin G), **B1**.473
  in gas gangrene, **B2**.1116
  meningococcal disease, **B1**.566
  pharmacology, **B1**.475
    blood–brain barrier, **B1**.475–6
  in pneumococcal meningitis, **B1**.571
  spectrum of activity, **B1**.499 (Tab.)
    Actinobacillus actinomycetemcomitans,
      B2.1664
    Actinomyces, **B2**.1011
    Bacillus anthracis, **B2**.937–8
    Borrelia, **B2**.1831 (Tab.)
    Gram-positive anaerobic cocci, **B2**.911
    Klebsiella, **B2**.1480
    Streptococcus, **B2**.861–2
    Tropheryma whippelii, **B2**.1002
  structure, **B1**.474 (Fig.)
*Bergey's Manual of Systematic Bacteriology
      (Bergey's Manual),* **B1**.15, **B1**.16–8,
      B1.20, **B1**.26
    Fusobacterium, **B2**.1945–6
    nomenclature changes, **B1**.32
Bermejo virus, **V2**.1666 (Tab.)
Berne virus *see* Equine torovirus (EToV:
      Berne virus)
Berrimah virus, **V1**.385–6
Bertiella, **P**.577, **P**.673
Beta-adrenergic agonists, acute bronchiolitis
      therapy, **V1**.777
β_2-microglobulin, MHC class I, **I**.405, **I**.408–9,
      I.428–9
β locus, TCR, **I**.450–1, **I**.450 (Fig.)
β pleated sheets, Ig structure, **I**.305
Betaherpesvirinae
  characteristics, **V1**.177 (Tab.)
  classification, **V1**.43 (Tab.), **V1**.488–9
  evolution, **V1**.175–6, **V1**.520
  see also Betaherpesviruses
Betaherpesviruses, **V1.520–40**
  conserved proteins, **V1**.520
  gene expression, regulation, **V1**.499
  genome, **V1**.494 (Tab.), **V1**.520
  immune evasion, **V1**.502–3
  infection
    cell restriction, **V1**.520
    host range, **V1**.489
    human infection, **V1**.520
    immune response, **V1**.285

Betaherpesviruses (*Continued*)
  see also *Betaherpesvirinae; specific viruses*
Betanodavirus, **V1**.53
Betaretrovirus, **V1**.46, **V2**.1286 (Tab.)
  see also Betaretroviruses
Betaretroviruses
  insertional mutagenesis, **V1**.340
  tumors associated, **V1**.331 (Tab.)
  see also *Betaretrovirus*
Bet protein, foamy viruses *see* Foamy viruses
Bevacizumab, licensing, **I**.355 (Tab.)
Bexxar, licensing, **I**.355 (Tab.)
BH1–3 subfamily, **I**.133
BH3 subfamily, **I**.133
Bhanja virus infection, **V2**.1047
BHK-21 cells, arenaviruses in, **V2**.1063 (Fig.),
  V2.1064–5
Bias
  in case–control studies, **B1**.316
  in cohort studies, **B1**.315
  loss to follow-up, **B1**.315
  misclassification, **B1**.315
  rumination, **B1**.316
Biased hypermutation
  measles inclusion body encephalitis (MIBE),
    V1.193
  Measles virus, **V1**.193
  negative-strand RNA viruses, **V1**.193
  RNA virus evolution, **V1**.17
  subacute sclerosing panencephalitis (SSPE),
    V1.193
  variability, **V1**.193
Bicarbonate requirement, *Neisseria,*
  B2.1274–5
Bicozamycin, **B2**.906
Bid (BH3 domain binding B-cell lymphoma)
  protein, **I**.133
  granzyme M cleavage, **I**.476
  structure, **I**.133 (Fig.)
Bifidobacterium, **B2**.1011–12, **B2**.1023–7
  antibacterial susceptibility/resistance,
    B2.1024–5
  cell wall, **B2**.1024
  cell walls, **B2**.1024
  classification, **B2**.1025, **B2**.1025 (Tab.),
    B2.1026 (Tab.)
    isoenzyme patterns, **B2**.1026
    oligonucleotide probes, **B2**.1025–6
    polyacrylamide gel electrophoresis,
      B2.1025–6
  culture, **B2**.1024
    fermentation tests, **B2**.1025–6
    nonselective media, **B2**.1025
  genus definition, **B2**.1023
  habitats, **B2**.1024
  heterolactic acid fermentation pathway,
    B1.58
  historical perspective, **B2**.1024
  isolation, **B2**.1025–6
  metabolism, **B2**.1024
    acetic acid production, **B2**.1024
  morphology, **B2**.1024
  as normal microbiota, **B1**.296 (Tab.),
    B1.302–3, **B2**.1026
    Bacteroides relationship, **B2**.1933
  pathogenicity, **B2**.1026

ultrastructure, **B2**.1024
virulence factors, **B2**.1026
Bifidobacterium adolescentis, **B2**.1025 (Tab.)
  classification, **B2**.1025
    oligonucleotide probes, **B2**.1025–6
  fermentation tests, **B2**.1025–6
  in normal microbiota, **B2**.1026
Bifidobacterium angulatum, **B2**.1025 (Tab.)
  classification, **B2**.1025
  morphology, **B2**.1024
Bifidobacterium animalis, **B2**.1025 (Tab.)
Bifidobacterium asteroides, **B2**.1025 (Tab.)
  morphology, **B2**.1024
Bifidobacterium bifidum, **B2**.1023,
  B2.1025 (Tab.), **B2**.1026–7
  ammonium salt utilization, **B2**.1027
  antigens, **B2**.1027
  carbohydrate fermentation, **B2**.1027
  classification, **B2**.1025
    oligonucleotide probes, **B2**.1025–6
  morphology, **B2**.1024, **B2**.1026
Bifidobacterium boum, **B2**.1025 (Tab.)
Bifidobacterium breve, **B2**.1025 (Tab.)
  in normal microbiota, **B2**.1026
  oligonucleotide probe classification,
    B2.1025–6
Bifidobacterium catenulatum, **B2**.1025 (Tab.)
  classification, **B2**.1025
Bifidobacterium choerium, **B2**.1025 (Tab.)
Bifidobacterium coryneforme, **B2**.1025 (Tab.)
Bifidobacterium cuniculi, **B2**.1025 (Tab.)
Bifidobacterium dentium, **B2**.1025 (Tab.)
  classification, **B2**.1025
  fermentation tests, **B2**.1025–6
  in normal microbiota, **B2**.1026
  pathogenicity, **B2**.1026
Bifidobacterium gallicum, **B2**.1025 (Tab.)
Bifidobacterium gallinarum, **B2**.1025 (Tab.)
Bifidobacterium indicum, **B2**.1025 (Tab.)
Bifidobacterium infantis, **B2**.1025
Bifidobacterium longum, **B2**.1025 (Tab.)
  classification, **B2**.1025
    oligonucleotide probes, **B2**.1025–6
  fermentation tests, **B2**.1025–6
  in normal microbiota, **B2**.1026
Bifidobacterium magnum, **B2**.1025 (Tab.)
Bifidobacterium merycicum, **B2**.1025 (Tab.)
Bifidobacterium minimum, **B2**.1025 (Tab.)
Bifidobacterium pseudocatenulatum,
  B2.1025 (Tab.)
  classification, **B2**.1025
  in normal microbiota, **B2**.1026
Bifidobacterium pseudolongum, **B2**.1025 (Tab.)
Bifidobacterium pullorum, **B2**.1025 (Tab.)
Bifidobacterium ruminantium, **B2**.1025 (Tab.)
Bifidobacterium saeculare, **B2**.1025 (Tab.)
Bifidobacterium scardovii, **B2**.1025 (Tab.)
Bifidobacterium subtile, **B2**.1025 (Tab.)
Bifidobacterium suis, **B2**.1025
Bifidobacterium thermacidophilum,
  B2.1025 (Tab.)
Bifidobacterium thermophilum, **B2**.1025 (Tab.)
Bifonazole, **M**.235
Biguanides, **B1**.423 (Tab.), **B1**.426
Bik protein, structure, **I**.133 (Fig.)

Bile duct cancer
  clonorchiasis, **P**.641, **P**.648–9, **P**.651
  opisthorchiasis, **P**.641, **P**.648–50
Bile salts, Enterobacteriaceae culture, **B2**.1345
Bile shunts
  alveolar echinococcosis treatment, **P**.696
  cystic echinococcosis treatment, **P**.696
Bilharz, T., **P**.11
Biliary disease, cryptosporidiosis, **P**.405
Bill and Melinda Gates Foundation, **P**.103–6
Bilophila wadsworthia, **B1**.296 (Tab.)
Bimp2 (CARD14), **I**.347
Bim protein, **I**.133
  structure, **I**.133 (Fig.)
Binary fission
  Balantidium coli, **P**.277, **P**.279 (Fig.)
  Blastocystis hominis, **P**.560–1
  homothetogenic, **P**.181, **P**.183 (Fig.)
  microsporidians, **P**.531–2, **P**.532–4
  Trachipleistophora, **P**.534
  protozoa, **P**.181, **P**.183 (Fig.)
Binomial nomenclature, viral classification,
  V1.35–6
Binucleate forms, *Dientamoeba fragilis,* **P**.267
Bioaerosols, **B1**.185–8
  definition, **B1**.185
  generation activities, **B1**.185, **B1**.186 (Tab.)
  particulate size, **B1**.185–7
  rafting cells, **B1**.185–7
  see also Airborne bacteria
Biochemical tests, **B1**.22 (Tab.), **B1**.23–4,
  B1.23 (Fig.), **B1**.32–3
  bi-state results, **B1**.23
  Enterobacteriaceae, **B2**.1319 (Tab.),
    B2.1330 (Tab.), **B2**.1348
  thresholding, **B1**.24
  viral definition, **V1**.25
Biocides, **B1**.421–2
Biodegradation, *Burkholderia,* **B2**.1612–13
Biofilms, **B1**.149–50, **B1**.432–3
  bacteriophage density, **B1**.140
  Candida albicans see Candida albicans
  curli, **B1**.148–9
  extracellular polysaccharide production,
    B1.149–50, **B1**.150 (Fig.)
  formation, **B1**.149, **B1**.150 (Fig.)
  pathogenicity effects, **B1**.149–50
  plant root surface, **B1**.199, **B1**.205–7
  resistance, **B1**.443
  vegetables, **B1**.282
  Vibrio, **B2**.1508–9
  water, **B1**.220
Bioinformatics, fungal classification, **M**.49
Biological indicators (BIs), sterilization
  validation and monitoring, **B1**.454–5,
  B1.454 (Tab.)
Biological safety cabinets (BSC), **B1**.764–5,
  B1.765 (Tab.)
Biological safety officer, **V2**.1520–3
Biological transmission, **V1**.355
Biological warfare, **V2**.1018
  Bacillus anthracis, **B1**.203
  see also Bioterrorism
BIO-PCR, soil bacteria analysis, **B1**.206–7
Biopsy, **P**.153, **P**.153 (Tab.)
  Balantidium coli infection, **P**.280

Biopsy (*Continued*)
  brain, **P**.153, **P**.153 (Tab.)
  fetal viral infection diagnosis, **V2**.1445 (Tab.)
  giardiasis diagnosis, **P**.150
  Leishmania donovani diagnosis, **P**.153
  muscle, **P**.153, **P**.153 (Tab.)
  PCP, **M**.787
  skin, **P**.153, **P**.153 (Tab.)
  toxocariasis diagnosis, **P**.754–5
Bioremediation, **B1**.212, **B2**.1166–7
  definition, **B1**.202
  in situ, **B1**.202
  soil bacteria, **B1**.199, **B1**.201–2
Biosafety *see* Laboratory safety
Biosafety level 1 *see* Laboratories
Biosafety level 2 *see* Laboratories
Biosafety level 3 *see* Laboratories
Biosafety level 4 *see* Laboratories
Bioterrorism, **B1**.189, **B1**.364–5, **B1**.767–8
  airborne bacteria, **B1**.189
  Burkholderia mallei, **B2**.1634–5
  Burkholderia pseudomallei, **B2**.1634–5
  emerging infection, **V2**.1660
  Francisella tularensis, **B2**.1752
  poxviruses, **V1**.581, **V1**.589–90
  smallpox, **V1**.589–90
  specimen preparation, **B1**.724–5
  see also Biological warfare; *individual species*
Biotyping *see individual species*
Bipolaris
  histopathology, **M**.89 (Tab.)
  infection
    allergic fungal sinusitis, **M**.675
    CNS, **M**.743
    keratitis, **M**.301–2
    oculomycoses, **M**.278 (Tab.), **M**.283–4,
      M.294, **M**.295
    voriconazole therapy, **M**.153
  pigment production, **M**.742
Bipolaris hawaiiensis, **M**.294, **M**.295, **M**.329
Bipolaris spicifera
  histopathology, **M**.128 (Tab.)
  oculomycoses, **M**.295
  pigment production, **M**.742
Bird pathogens, rhabdoviruses, **V2**.1105
Birds
  aspergillosis, **M**.18
  botulism, **B2**.1038–9, **B2**.1058, **B2**.1070–1,
    B2.1074
  Campylobacter transmission, **B1**.239
  candidiasis, **M**.586, **M**.601–2
  Chlamydia psittaci infection, **B2**.2014
  cryptococcosis, **M**.643
  histoplasmosis, **M**.520, **M**.535–6
  infection, *Pasteurella*, **B2**.1654
  rhinosporidiosis, **M**.447, **M**.457, **M**.470,
    M.472
Birnaviridae
  characteristics, **V1**.177 (Tab.)
  classification, **V1**.27 (Tab.), **V1**.47 (Tab.),
    V1.48
  genome segmentation, **V1**.180–1
  see also specific viruses
Birnaviruses *see Birnaviridae*

BIR serine/threonine protein kinase,
    poxviruses, **V1**.605
Bispecific antibodies *see* Monoclonal
    antibodies, therapy
Bisphenols, **B1**.422, **B1**.423 (Tab.)
Bites
  cat
    Pasteurella dagmatis infection, **B2**.1657
    Pasteurella multocida infection, **B2**.1654–5
    Pasteurella pneumotropica infection,
      B2.1655–6
  dogs
    Capnocytophaga canimorsus infection,
      B2.1674–5
    Pasteurella canis infection, **B2**.1656
    Pasteurella dagmatis infection, **B2**.1657
    Pasteurella multocida infection, **B2**.1654–5
    Pasteurella pneumotropica infection,
      B2.1655–6
  horses
    Actinobacillus infection, **B2**.1666
    Pasteurella caballi infection, **B2**.1657
Bithynia, fluke intermediate host, **P**.646
Biverticillium, **M**.565
BKV-associated nephropathy (BKVN), **V1**.481
BK virus (BKV), **V1**.480–2
  genome structure, **V1**.480–1
BK virus (BKV) infection
  cancer association, **V1**.481–2
    animal models, **V1**.481
    humans, **V1**.481–2
  diagnosis, cytopathology, **V2**.1534 (Tab.)
  epidemiology, **V1**.480–1
  hemorrhagic cystitis, **V1**.481
  hemorrhagic nephritis, **V1**.481
  in HIV infection, **V2**.1499 (Tab.)
  immunodeficient patients (non-HIV),
    V2.1509–10
  immunohistochemistry, **V1**.480 (Fig.)
  infection routes, **V1**.480–1
  lytic infection process, **V1**.480–1
  NF-1 effects, **V1**.480–1
  NFκB, **V1**.480–1
  in pregnancy, **V1**.480–1
  reactivation, **V1**.480–1
  species infected, **V1**.473
Black Creek Canal virus, **V2**.1666 (Tab.)
  budding/transport, **V2**.1040
Black fluids, **B1**.422
  water hardness, **B1**.432
Black-hooded (BH) rats, Borna disease virus
    infection, **V2**.1145
Blackleg, cattle and sheep, **B1**.203
Black piedra, **M**.77, **M**.197–8
  causative agents, **M**.195, **M**.198
  see also individual species
  clinical presentation, **M**.197–8, **M**.198 (Fig.)
  history, **M**.11
  therapy, **M**.186, **M**.198
Bladder
  bacteriuria, **B1**.388–9
  catheterization, **B1**.388
    alternatives, **B1**.389
  colonization
    indwelling catheters, **B1**.388
    nosocomial, **B1**.388

  prevention, **B1**.388
  dysfunction, urinary infection, **B1**.672
  nosocomial infection, **B1**.388
  stones, **B2**.1446
Bladder cancer, TCE peptide vaccines,
    I.865 (Tab.)
Blanching, vegetables, **B1**.281–2
Blankophor whitening agent, **M**.123 (Tab.),
    M.125
Blast cells, GM-CSF production, **I**.277
Blastic conidiogenesis, **M**.77, **M**.78 (Fig.)
Blastocladiales, **M**.51, **M**.53
Blastocondidium, *Paracoccidioides brasiliensis*,
    M.542
Blastocrithidia triatomae, **P**.388–9
Blastocystis, classification, **P**.190–1, **P**.198
Blastocystis hominis, **P**.556–70
  biochemistry, **P**.561–3
    carbohydrates, **P**.561
    cardiolipin, **P**.561
    hydrogenosomes, **P**.561
    isoenzyme analysis, **P**.561
    lipids, **P**.561
  classification, **P**.556–7
    taxonomy, **P**.556
  epidemiology, **P**.566
    animal reservoirs, **P**.557
    developed countries, **P**.566
    developing countries, **P**.566
    ubiquity, **P**.557
  genetics, **P**.561–3
    diversity, **P**.562
    karyotyping, **P**.562
  historical aspects, **P**.556
  infection *see below*
  life cycle, **P**.560–1, **P**.562 (Fig.)
    binary fission, **P**.560–1
    endodyogeny, **P**.560–1
    plasmotomy, **P**.560–1
    schizogony, **P**.560–1
  molecular biology, **P**.561–3
    elongation factor gene, **P**.562–3
    small subunit rRNA genes, **P**.562
    strain differences, **P**.563
  structure, **P**.557–60
    ameboid form, **P**.557, **P**.558–9, **P**.559 (Fig.),
      P.560 (Fig.)
    avacuolar form, **P**.557, **P**.559–60,
      P.560 (Fig.)
    cyst form, **P**.557, **P**.559, **P**.559 (Fig.),
      P.560–1
    granular form, **P**.557, **P**.558, **P**.558 (Fig.)
    hydrogenosomes, **P**.557
    in vivo (trophozoite form), **P**.559–60
    multivacuolar form, **P**.557, **P**.560,
      P.560 (Fig.), **P**.561 (Fig.)
    vacuolar form, **P**.557, **P**.557 (Fig.),
      P.558 (Fig.)
Blastocystis hominis infection
  chemotherapy, **P**.566–7
    furazolidone, **P**.566–7
    iodoquinol, **P**.566–7
    mebendazole, **P**.566–7
    metronidazole, **P**.566–7
    nitazoxanide, **P**.567
    traditional Chinese medication, **P**.567

Blastocystis hominis infection
 chemotherapy (*Continued*)
  trimethoprim–sulfamethaxazole, **P**.567
 clinical aspects, **P**.563
  in AIDS, **P**.563
  immunosuppressed patients, **P**.563
  irritable bowel syndrome, **P**.563–4
  signs/symptoms, **P**.563
  travelers diarrhea, **P**.563
 diagnosis, **P**.565–6
  culture, **P**.565–6
  fluorescent staining, **P**.566
  stained preparations, **P**.565, **P**.565 (Fig.)
  unstained preparations, **P**.565
 differential diagnosis, **P**.565
 immunology, **P**.563–4
  serological detection, **P**.563–4
 pathogenicity, **P**.564–5
  animal models, **P**.564
  in vitro, **P**.564
 pathology, **P**.564–5
Blastomyces
 infection *see* Blastomycosis
 PCR, **M**.94
Blastomyces dermatitidis, **M**.479, **M**.480, **M**.485,
  M.487 (Fig.), **M**.488, **M**.492–3, **M**.495–6
 biochemistry, **M**.487–8
 classification, **M**.486–7
 colonies, **M**.819 (Fig.)
 culture, **M**.485, **M**.495
 ecology, **M**.480–3
 Emmonsia, **M**.810 (Tab.), **M**.811–12, **M**.817,
  M.818–20, **M**.819 (Fig.), **M**.821
 epidemiology, **M**.480, **M**.483–5
 genetics
  DNA probe, **M**.496
  manipulation, **M**.493
 geographical distribution, **M**.482,
  M.482 (Fig.), **M**.483 (Fig.), **M**.486–7
 growth, **M**.73
 histopathology, **M**.125, **M**.126 (Tab.),
  M.128 (Tab.), **M**.132 (Fig.)
  stains, **M**.122, **M**.124, **M**.125
 history, **M**.24, **M**.479–80
 identification, **M**.485, **M**.492, **M**.495–7
  exoantigen test, **M**.495–6
  hematoxylin and eosin stain, **M**.491
  histopathology, **M**.89 (Tab.), **M**.491,
   M.492 (Fig.)
  Histoplasma capsulatum var. *capsulatum*
   vs., **M**.531, **M**.532, **M**.534
  immunofluorescence, **M**.491, **M**.492, **M**.496
  microscopy, **M**.485–6, **M**.486 (Fig.),
   M.487 (Fig.), **M**.495
  nucleic acid probes, **M**.91
  serology, **M**.92
 meiotic stage, **M**.486, **M**.811–12, **M**.819–20
 morphology, **M**.126 (Tab.), **M**.485,
  M.485 (Fig.), **M**.486 (Fig.), **M**.487 (Fig.),
  M.491–2, **M**.492 (Fig.)
  dimorphism, **M**.25 (Fig.), **M**.480, **M**.485,
   M.487 (Fig.), **M**.488, **M**.492–3, **M**.495–6
  size variation, **M**.492, **M**.492 (Fig.)
 nomenclature, **M**.485
 PCR, **M**.491
 serology, **M**.93 (Tab.), **M**.112–13, **M**.496

 specimens, **M**.83 (Tab.), **M**.495
 teleomorph, **M**.486, **M**.811–12, **M**.819–20
 transmission, **M**.483, **M**.484
 vaccines, **M**.494–5, **I**.933 (Tab.)
Blastomycetes, classification, **M**.49, **M**.51
Blastomycosis, **M**.479, **M**.479–501
 adult respiratory distress syndrome, **M**.489
 AIDS, **M**.490, **M**.492, **M**.497
 animal infection, **M**.480–1, **M**.483–4
  dogs, **M**.480–1, **M**.483–4, **M**.488
 bone, **M**.489–90
  osteomyelitis, **M**.489–90
 causative agents *see Blastomyces dermatitidis*
 clinical presentation, **M**.488–95
  cutaneous, **M**.488, **M**.489 (Fig.), **M**.492
  miliary, **M**.489
  opportunistic, **M**.490
  pulmonary, **M**.489, **M**.490–2, **M**.497
  reactivation, **M**.490
  subclinical, **M**.490
  systemic, **M**.489
 CNS infection, **M**.489–90
 diagnosis, **M**.125–7, **M**.492, **M**.495–7
  EIAs, **M**.112–13
  histopathology, **M**.128 (Tab.), **M**.132 (Fig.),
   M.491, **M**.492 (Fig.)
  immunofluorescence, **M**.491, **M**.492, **M**.496
 epidemiology, **M**.480, **M**.483–5
 genitourinary tract infection, **M**.489
 geographical distribution, **M**.482,
  M.482 (Fig.), **M**.483 (Fig.), **M**.486–7
 history, **M**.24, **M**.479–80
 host-pathogen interactions, **M**.492–3
 immune response, **M**.494, **M**.496–7
 miliary, **M**.489
 oculomycoses, **M**.275 (Tab.), **M**.287–8,
  M.295, **M**.324
  blepharitis, **M**.297
  endophthalmitis, **M**.317, **M**.324
  keratitis, **M**.305
 pathology, **M**.491
 pneumonia, **M**.489
 prostate gland, **M**.489, **M**.495
 pulmonary, **M**.489, **M**.490–2, **M**.497
 serology, **M**.92, **M**.93 (Tab.), **M**.112–13,
  M.496
 skin infection, **M**.488, **M**.489 (Fig.), **M**.492
  testing, **M**.484
 specimens, **M**.83 (Tab.), **M**.495
 therapy, **M**.497
  amphotericin B, **M**.497
  azoles, **M**.497
  polyenes, **M**.497
 transmission, **M**.483, **M**.484
 urinary tract infection, **M**.489, **M**.495
 veterinarians, **M**.484, **M**.488
Blastoschizomyces
 characteristics, **M**.631, **M**.632 (Tab.)
 infection, **M**.625 (Tab.)
Blastoschizomyces capitatus
 characteristics, **M**.631
 infection, **M**.624–5
  clinical presentation, **M**.625
  diagnosis, **M**.626
  fungemia, **M**.625

  infective endocarditis, **M**.625
  meningitis, **M**.625–6
  myocarditis, **M**.625
  therapy, **M**.626
Blau syndrome, **I**.115, **I**.125
BL cells (Burkitt lymphoma cells), **V1**.566
Bleeding
 Bolivian and Argentine hemorrhagic fevers,
  V2.1070
 Lassa fever, **V2**.1070
Bleomycin, Kaposi's sarcoma therapy, **V1**.553
Blepharitis, **M**.296–8
 causative agents, **M**.296
  Blastomyces dermatitidis, **M**.297
  Candida, **M**.257, **M**.601
  Cryptococcus neoformans, **M**.296, **M**.297
  dermatophytoses, **M**.297
  dimorphic fungi, **M**.287–8
  Malassezia, **M**.296–7
  Microsporum, **M**.297
  Paracoccidioides brasiliensis, **M**.297
  Trichosporon, **M**.297
 dermatophytic, **M**.297
 diagnosis, **M**.297
 therapy, **M**.297
  amphotericin B, **M**.297
  fluconazole, **M**.297
  ketoconazole, **M**.297
  nystatin, **M**.297
  terbinafine, **M**.297
Blights, plant disease source, **B1**.202
Blind loop syndrome, **B1**.293–4
Blindness
 protothecosis, **M**.400
 trachoma, **B2**.2013–14
Blk tyrosine kinase, BCR signaling, **I**.342
BLNK (SLP-65)
 autosomal recessive agammaglobulinemia,
  I.780
 BCR signaling, **I**.343–5
Blood
 contamination, nosocomial infection, **B1**.384
 hepatitis A transmission, **V2**.1172–3
 hepatitis B transmission, **V1**.369, **V2**.1255–6
 hepatitis C transmission, **V2**.1203, **V2**.1208
 microscopy, bacterial meningitis, **B1**.559
 normal microbiota, **B1**.305
 virus shedding, **V1**.249
Bloodborne infection, **V1**.369–70
 see also specific disease/infection
Blood-borne transmission, definition,
  I.951 (Tab.)
Blood–brain barrier (BBB), **V1**.261,
  V2.1404–5, **V2**.1410–11
 ampicillin, **B1**.475–6
 bacterial meningitis development, **B1**.556–7
 cefotaxime, **B1**.478
 ceftriaxone, **B1**.478
 cephalosporins, **B1**.478
 disruption by bacteria, **B1**.557
 inflammatory cell crossing, **V2**.1409
 penicillins, **B1**.475–6
Blood cells, viruses replicating in,
  V1.243 (Tab.)

Blood concentration, African trypanosomiasis diagnosis, **P.**366–7
Blood cultures
 bacteria, **B1.**716
  aerobic/anaerobic bottles, **B1.**513
  children, **B1.**513
  contamination, **B1.**512–13
  false-positive, **B1.**510, **B1.**512
  growth detection, **B1.**514
  incubation, **B1.**514
  indications, **B1.**511–12
   bacterial meningitis, **B1.**559
   mycobacterial, **B1.**524
  media, **B1.**514
  neonates, **B1.**512–13
  numbers used, **B1.**513–14
  removal of antibacterial agents, **B1.**514
  results interpretation, **B1.**516
  sample processing, **B1.**514–16, **B1.**515 (Tab.)
   automated, **B1.**515–16
   manual, **B1.**515
   quantitative, **B1.**516
  skin preparation, **B1.**512
  transport, **B1.**514
  volume of blood, **B1.**513
 mycology, **M.**85, **M.**86–7
  Aspergillus, **M.**711
  Candida, **M.**606
  Cryptococcus neoformans, **M.**86–7, **M.**649–50
  Penicillium marneffei, **M.**569, **M.**570 (Fig.)
  specimen collection, **M.**83 (Tab.), **M.**84
 parasites, *Leishmania donovani* diagnosis, **P.**152–3
Blood films
 HTLV transmission, **V2.**1290 (Fig.)
 leishmaniasis, **P.**301
 malaria diagnosis, **P.**152, **P.**501 (Fig.)
 Trypanosoma cruzi, **P.**388
Blood group P antigen, Parvovirus B19 virus binding, **V1.**432
Bloodland Lake virus, **V2.**1666 (Tab.)
Blood meals, *Simulium*, **P.**785
Blood products
 emerging bacterial infection, **B1.**362
 HCMV infection, **V2.**1507
 hepatitis A, **V2.**1172–3
 hepatitis B, **V1.**369, **V2.**1257–8
 hepatitis C, **V2.**1203, **V2.**1208
 see also Blood transfusions
Blood samples, *Aeromonas* isolation, **B2.**1531
Blood stage targets, malaria vaccination, **P.**515–16
Blood-tissue barrier, viral penetration, **V1.**242–3
Blood transfusions, **P.**27–9
 babesiosis, **P.**27–9, **P.**459–60
 bacterial infection transmitted by, **B1.**362, **B1.**380–1
 Chagas disease transmission, **P.**27–9, **P.**379, **P.**392, **P.**395–6
 donor screening, hepatitis C, **V2.**1208–9, **V2.**1213, **V2.**1216
 hepatitis B transmission, **B1.**380–1
 hepatitis C transmission, **B1.**380–1

HIV transmission, **B1.**380–1
 malaria PCR diagnosis, **P.**506
 neutrophil disorders, **I.**50
 toxoplasmosis after, **P.**437
 Trypanosoma cruzi transmission, **P.**27–9, **P.**379, **P.**392, **P.**395–6
 viral infection transmission, **V1.**239
 West Nile virus transmission, **V2.**1002
 see also Blood products
Blood vessel contraction, leukotrienes, **I.**185
Bloody diarrhea
 amebic dysentery, **P.**207
 food-borne disease outbreak
  meat, **B1.**273–4
  see also Escherichia coli
Bloom syndrome, **I.**777
'Blue baby' syndrome, nitrate levels excess, **B1.**200
Bluetongue virus
 core-like particles (CLPs), **V2.**941 (Fig.)
 emerging infection, **V2.**1651 (Tab.)
 infection
  clinical manifestations, **V2.**942
  epidemiology, **V2.**942
  pathogenesis, **V2.**942
 proteins, orbivirus proteins *vs.*, **V2.**941 (Tab.)
 vaccines, **V2.**942
 virus-like particles (VLPs), **V2.**941 (Fig.)
B lymphocytes *see* B cell(s)
B lymphoma, BCE peptide vaccines, **I.**855 (Tab.)
B lymphoproliferative disease, latent EBV gene expression, **V1.**566 (Tab.)
BM2 protein, Influenza virus B, **V1.**657–8
Bmf protein, **I.**133
 structure, **I.**133 (Fig.)
Bocavirus, **V1.**412
 genome structure, **V1.**412
 infection *see below*
 members, **V1.**411 (Tab.)
Bocavirus infection, **V1.**425–7
 epidemiology, **V1.**425
 pathogenesis, **V1.**425–6
  fetal/neonatal hosts, **V1.**425–6
  immunocompromised hosts, **V1.**426
  mature hosts, **V1.**426
Body fluids
 normal microbiota, **B1.**305
 physical flushing of bacteria, **B1.**176
Body fluid transmission, HCMV, **V1.**522
Body tissues, normal microbiota, **B1.**305
Bolbosoma, **P.**598
 structure, **P.**596 (Fig.)
Bolivian hemorrhagic fever, **V2.**1070
Bolomys lasiurus, *Leishmania braziliensis*, **P.**326
Bombay phenotype, leukocyte adhesion deficiency type II, **I.**769
Bone
 adiaspiromycosis, **M.**818
 aspergillosis, **M.**700, **M.**719
 blastomycosis, **M.**489–90
 mycetoma, **M.**389
 penicilliosis marneffei, **M.**567
 pythiosis, **M.**418–19, **M.**419 (Fig.)

rhinosporidiosis, **M.**461, **M.**462, **M.**462 (Fig.)
 specimens, **M.**83 (Tab.)
Bone cement, **B1.**392
Bone defects, congenitally acquired rubella, **V2.**975
Bone/joint infection
 antibacterial treatment, **B1.**698–700
  duration, **B1.**700–1
  intravenous, **B1.**698–9
  systemic: oral, **B1.**699
  topical, **B1.**699–700, **B1.**700 (Fig.)
 challenges, **B1.**684
 children, **B1.**690
  Kingella kingae, **B2.**1669–70
 clinical features, **B1.**684, **B1.**691–2
 diagnosis, **B1.**692–6
  culture, **B1.**695–6
  histology, **B1.**696
  imaging, **B1.**693
  isotope scanning, **B1.**694
  laboratory, **B1.**692–3
  MRI, **B1.**694–5
  PCR, **B1.**696
  radiology, **B1.**693–4, **B1.**693 (Fig.)
  ultrasound, **B1.**694
 epidemiology, **B1.**684–5
 future directions, **B1.**703
 Gram-positive anaerobic cocci infection, **B2.**910
 human brucellosis, **B2.**1738
 inflammatory responses, **B1.**689–90
  bone responses, **B1.**689
  cell and molecular basis of joint destruction, **B1.**690
  molecular basis of bone resorption, **B1.**689
 microbiology, **B1.**690–1
 neonates, **B1.**690
 pathogenesis, **B1.**685–90
  access of organisms, **B1.**686–8
  biofilm formation, **B1.**685–6, **B1.**688–9
  mechanisms of persistence, **B1.**688–9
  quorum sensing, **B1.**688
  post-operative hematomas, **B1.**691
 prevention, **B1.**691
 prognosis, **B1.**701
 surgical treatment, **B1.**697–8
  dead space management and reconstruction, **B1.**697–8
  debridement and excision, **B1.**697
  soft tissue cover, **B1.**691, **B1.**697
 treatment, **B1.**696–701
  adjunctive, **B1.**701
  antibacterial *see above*
  surgical *see above*
 vaccine candidates, **B1.**691
 see also Osteomyelitis; *specific infection*
Bone marrow
 Pneumocystis carinii infection, **M.**785
 specimens, **M.**83 (Tab.), **M.**86 (Tab.)
Bone marrow failure, in HIV infection, **I.**792
Bone marrow sequestration, *Plasmodium*, **P.**472
Bone marrow transplantation (BMT), **I.**50
 aspergillosis, **M.**698
  amphotericin B therapy, **M.**727

Bone marrow transplantation (BMT)
(*Continued*)
  CMV intravenous Ig prophylaxis, **V2**.1566–7
  EBV infection, **V2**.1507
  HSV infection, **V2**.1506
  intracranial abscess, **B1**.582
  Nocardia infection after, **B2**.1155–6, **B2**.1163
  polyomavirus infection, **V2**.1509
  VZV infection, **V2**.1506
Bonferroni correction method, **I**.574
'Bootstrapping,' phylogenetic analysis of fungi,
  M.48, **M**.52 (Fig.)
Border disease, *Pestivirus* infection, **V2**.1005
Border disease virus (BDV), **V2**.993
Borderline disseminated cutaneous
  leishmaniasis, **P**.338–9
Bordetella, **B2**.**1786–817**
  adhesion, **B2**.1799, **B2**.1806–7
  antibacterial susceptibility/resistance,
    B2.1793–4
    antibiotic resistance plasmids, **B2**.1794
  bacteriophage, **B2**.1805
  biochemistry, **B2**.1793
  BrkA, **B2**.1801
  classification, **B2**.1787–8
    evolutionary considerations, **B2**.1787–8
    genus level, **B2**.1787
    phylogeny, **B2**.1787–8
    species, **B2**.1786
    species designations, **B2**.1787
    whole-genome sequences, **B2**.1786–7,
      B2.1793, **B2**.1805
  culture, **B2**.1789–90
    variation during growth, **B2**.1790
  definition, **B2**.1786
  filamentous hemagglutinin, **B2**.1789
  fimbriae, **B2**.1789, **B2**.1799
  genome organization, **B2**.1805
  growth requirements, **B2**.1790–1, **B2**.1793
    iron, **B2**.1793
    media, **B2**.1790–1
  habitats and pathogenicity, **B2**.1806–11
  host specificity, **B2**.1806–7, **B2**.1806 (Tab.)
  isolation/identification, **B2**.1791–2
    differential characteristics, **B2**.1788 (Tab.)
    nasopharyngeal swabs/aspirates, **B2**.1791
    serological tests, **B2**.1792
    transport medium, **B2**.1791
    typing methods, **B2**.1792–3
  LPS, **B2**.1789 (Tab.), **B2**.1796
  metabolism, **B2**.1793
  morphology and ultrastructure, **B2**.1789,
    B2.1790 (Fig.)
  motility, **B2**.1789
  R factors, **B2**.1794
  transposon mutagenesis, **B2**.1794–5
  virulence factors, **B2**.1789 (Tab.),
    B2.1790 (Fig.), **B2**.1794–801
    adenylate cyclase toxin, **B1**.156 (Tab.),
      B2.1789, **B2**.1796–7
    BrkA, **B2**.1801
    dermonecrotic toxin, **B2**.1795–6
    endotoxin, **B2**.1796
    filamentous hemagglutinin, **B2**.1789,
      B2.1792, **B2**.1799–800
    fimbriae, **B2**.1799

  pertactin, **B2**.1789, **B2**.1800–1
  pertussis toxin *see* Pertussis toxin (PT)
  regulation *see below*
  tracheal colonization factor, **B2**.1801
  tracheal cytotoxin, **B2**.1795
  Type III secretion system, **B2**.1789 (Tab.),
    B2.1801
  virulence regulation, **B2**.1801–5
    bvg locus, **B2**.1802, **B2**.1803 (Fig.), **B2**.1806
    phase variation, **B2**.1804 (Fig.)
    phase variation and phenotypic
      modulation, **B2**.1802
    regulator of intracellular stress (ris),
      B2.1804–6
    serotype variation, **B2**.1801–2
    significance, **B2**.1802–5, **B2**.1803 (Fig.)
    virulence-activated genes *(vag)*, **B2**.1802,
      B2.1803 (Fig.)
    virulence-repressed genes *(vrg)*, **B2**.1802,
      B2.1803 (Fig.)
Bordetella avium, **B2**.1786–7, **B2**.1810–11
  antibacterial susceptibility/resistance,
    B2.1794
  bacteriophages, **B2**.1805
  classification, **B2**.1787
  growth requirements, **B2**.1790–1
  habitats and pathogenicity, **B2**.1806–7
  infection, **B2**.1810–11
  isolation/identification, **B2**.1791–2
    culture characteristics, **B2**.1790
    differential characteristics, **B2**.1788 (Tab.)
  osteotoxin, **B2**.1810–11
  pathogenicity, **B2**.1789 (Tab.)
  phylogeny, **B2**.1788
  virulence factors, **B2**.1789 (Tab.)
    dermonecrotic toxin, **B2**.1795, **B2**.1810–11
    endotoxin, **B2**.1796
    filamentous hemagglutinin, **B2**.1799–800
  virulence regulation
    bvg locus, **B2**.1802–3
    phenotypic modulation, **B2**.1802
Bordetella avium-like group, **B2**.1786
Bordetella bronchiseptica, **B2**.1786–7, **B2**.1810
  antibacterial susceptibility/resistance,
    B2.1794
  bacteriophages, **B2**.1805
  biochemical activities and metabolism,
    B2.1793
    urease activity, **B2**.1793
  classification, **B2**.1787
    phylogeny, **B2**.1788
    species designation, **B2**.1787
  differential characteristics, **B2**.1788 (Tab.)
  genetics
    genome organization, **B2**.1805
    nucleic acid composition, **B2**.1729 (Tab.)
  growth requirements, **B2**.1790–1
  habitats and pathogenicity, **B2**.1810
  infection, **B1**.647, **B2**.1810
    animal, **B2**.1810
    atrophic rhinitis in swine, **B2**.1795, **B2**.1810
    human, **B2**.1810
  isolation/identification, **B2**.1791–2
  motility, **B2**.1789
  pathogenicity, **B2**.1789 (Tab.)
  signal transduction, **B1**.168

  virulence factors, **B2**.1789 (Tab.)
    adenylate cyclase toxin, **B2**.1796–7
    BrkA, **B2**.1801
    dermonecrotic toxin, **B2**.1795
    endotoxin, **B2**.1796
    filamentous hemagglutinin, **B2**.1799,
      B2.1800
    fimbriae, **B2**.1799
    pertactin, **B2**.1800–1
    tracheal cytotoxin, **B2**.1810
    Type III secretion system, **B2**.1801
  virulence regulation
    bvg locus, **B2**.1802–5
    phenotypic modulation, **B2**.1802
    regulator of intracellular stress, **B2**.1804–5
    significance, **B2**.1802–5
    virulence-repressed genes, **B2**.1802
Bordetella bronchiseptica, lysosomal killing
  resistance, **I**.651
Bordetella hinzii, **B2**.1786–7, **B2**.1811
  classification, **B2**.1787
  differential characteristics, **B2**.1788 (Tab.)
  endotoxin, **B2**.1796
  habitats and pathogenicity, **B2**.1806
  isolation/identification, **B2**.1791–2
Bordetella holmesii, **B2**.1786, **B2**.1787, **B2**.1811
  classification, **B2**.1787
  culture characteristics, **B2**.1790
  differential characteristics, **B2**.1788 (Tab.)
  endotoxin, **B2**.1796
  habitats and pathogenicity, **B2**.1806
  isolation/identification, **B2**.1791–2
    isolation from blood, **B2**.1786
Bordetella parapertussis, **B2**.1786–7, **B2**.1810
  antibacterial susceptibility/resistance,
    B2.1794
  bacteriophage, **B2**.1805
  biochemical activities and metabolism,
    B2.1793
  Bordetella pertussis vs., **B2**.1810
  classification, **B2**.1787
    phylogeny, **B2**.1788
  culture characteristics, **B2**.1790
  differential characteristics, **B2**.1788 (Tab.)
  genome organization, **B2**.1805
  growth requirements, **B2**.1790–1
  habitats and pathogenicity, **B2**.1810
  infection, **B1**.647
  isolation/identification, **B2**.1791–2
    EIAs, **B1**.752
    species designation, **B2**.1787
  lambs, **B2**.1810
  pathogenicity, **B2**.1789 (Tab.)
  virulence factors, **B2**.1789 (Tab.)
    adenylate cyclase toxin, **B2**.1796–7
    BrkA, **B2**.1801
    dermonecrotic toxin, **B2**.1795
    endotoxin, **B2**.1796
    filamentous hemagglutinin, **B2**.1799
    fimbriae, **B2**.1799
    pertactin, **B2**.1800
    Type III secretion system, **B2**.1801
  virulence regulation
    bvg locus, **B2**.1802
    phenotypic modulation, **B2**.1802

Bordetella pertussis, **B1**.645, **B2**.1786, **B2**.1807–10
adhesins, **B1**.627
agglutinogens, **B2**.1792
antigens
  antigenic shifts, **B2**.1809–10
  modulation, **B2**.1802
  serotype antigens, **B2**.1801–2
biochemical activities and metabolism, **B2**.1793
C (cyanic) and X (xanthic) mode, **B2**.1802
classification, **B2**.1787
  phylogeny, **B2**.1788
  species designation, **B2**.1787
culture, **B1**.646, **B2**.1790–1
differential characteristics, **B2**.1788 (Tab.)
genome organization, **B2**.1805
growth requirements, **B2**.1790–1
habitats, **B2**.1807–10
immune evasion
  chemotaxis inhibition, **I**.648
  dendritic cell effects, **I**.656, **I**.667–8
  IL-12 suppression, **I**.652
  outer membrane protein variation, **I**.661
  pore-forming toxins, **I**.655
  regulatory T cells, **I**.666
  Th1/Th2 balance, **I**.666
  TNF-α suppression, **I**.652
infection *see* Pertussis
isolation/identification, **B1**.646, **B2**.1791
  PCR analysis, **B2**.1792
  typing methods, **B2**.1792–3
pathogenicity, **B2**.1789 (Tab.), **B2**.1807–10
slime layer, **B2**.1789
vaccine *see* Pertussis
as vaccine vector, **I**.897 (Tab.)
virulence factors, **B1**.627, **B1**.646, **B2**.1789 (Tab.)
  adenylate cyclase toxin, **B2**.1796–7
  BrkA, **B2**.1801
  dermonecrotic toxin, **B2**.1795
  endotoxin, **B2**.1796
  filamentous hemagglutinin, **B2**.1789, **B2**.1799–800
  fimbriae, **B2**.1789, **B2**.1799
  pertactin, **B2**.1800–1
  pertussis toxin *see* Pertussis toxin (PT)
  spreading determinants, **B1**.153 (Tab.)
  tracheal colonization factor, **B2**.1801
  tracheal cytotoxin, **B2**.1795
  Type III secretion system, **B2**.1801
virulence regulation
  phase variation, **B2**.1802, **B2**.1804, **B2**.1804 (Fig.)
  serotype variation, **B2**.1801–2
  significance, **B2**.1802–4
Bordetella petrii, **B2**.1786, **B2**.1787
classification, **B2**.1787
culture characteristics, **B2**.1790
differential characteristics, **B2**.1788 (Tab.)
habitats and pathogenicity, **B2**.1806
Bordetella trematum, **B2**.1786, **B2**.1787, **B2**.1811
classification, **B2**.1787
culture characteristics, **B2**.1790

differential characteristics, **B2**.1788 (Tab.)
endotoxin, **B2**.1796
habitats and pathogenicity, **B2**.1806
motility, **B2**.1789
Bore hole water, **B1**.214–15
Boric acid, urine specimen transport, **B1**.677
Borna disease virus (BDV), **V2**.1433, **V2.1137–59**
characteristics, **V1**.129 (Tab.)
gene expression regulation, **V2**.1137
genome, **V2**.1137–8
  map and transcripts, **V2**.1138 (Fig.)
  open reading frames, **V2**.1137–8
  size, **V2**.1137–8
  subgenomic RNA, **V2**.1139
glycoprotein (G), **V2**.1137–8, **V2**.1142
  cell entry, **V2**.1142
  functional motifs, **V2**.1141 (Fig.)
  posttranslational modifications, **V2**.1142
  splicing, **V2**.1139–40
historical aspects, **V2**.1142–3
infection *see* Borna disease virus (BDV) infection
matrix (M) protein, **V2**.1137–8, **V2**.1141–2
  functional motifs, **V2**.1141 (Fig.)
  neutralizing antibodies, **V2**.1141–2
  splicing, **V2**.1139–40
molecular biology, **V2**.1137–42
nucleoprotein (N), **V2**.1137–8, **V2**.1140
  functional motifs, **V2**.1141 (Fig.)
  isoforms, **V2**.1140
  soluble (s) antigen, **V2**.1140
phosphoprotein (P), **V2**.1137–8, **V2**.1140–1
  functional motifs, **V2**.1141 (Fig.)
  phosphorylation pattern, **V2**.1141
  soluble (s) antigen, **V2**.1140
proteins, **V2**.1140–2
  functional motifs, **V2**.1141 (Fig.)
  see also specific proteins
replication, **V2**.1138–9
  mRNA splicing, **V2**.1139–40
RNA-dependent RNA polymerase (large (L) protein), **V2**.1137–8, **V2**.1142
  functional motifs, **V2**.1141 (Fig.)
  splicing, **V2**.1139–40
type species, **V1**.382, **V2**.1137
X-protein, **V2**.1137–8, **V2**.1140
  functional motifs, **V2**.1141 (Fig.)
  ribonucleoprotein interaction, **V2**.1140
Borna disease virus (BDV) infection, **V2**.1142–53
antiviral compounds, **V2**.1153
CNS infection, **V2**.1149–50, **V2**.1410, **V2**.1433
epidemiology, **V2**.1142–3
  geographical distribution, **V2**.1142–3
  reservoirs, **V2**.1143
  transmission, **V2**.1143
experimental models, **V2**.1143–8
  adult rat model, **V2**.1145–7
  behavioral features, **V2**.1146
  clinical features, **V2**.1146
  dopamine circuits, **V2**.1146–7
  mouse, **V2**.1148
  neonatal rat model, **V2**.1147–8

  nonhuman primates, **V2**.1148
  tree shrews *(Tupaia),* **V2**.1148
human infection, **V2**.1150–3
  associated diseases/infection, **V2**.1150, **V2**.1151 (Tab.)
  immune complexes, **V2**.1150
  molecular detection, **V2**.1150–3, **V2**.1152 (Tab.)
  RT-PCR, **V2**.1150–3
  serology, **V2**.1150, **V2**.1151 (Tab.)
immune response, **V2**.1149–50
  CNS infiltrates, **V2**.1149
  cytokines, **V2**.1149–50
  experimental models, **V2**.1146
  inflammation, **V2**.1148
  mechanism of damage, **V2**.1148
  neutralizing antibodies, **V2**.1141–2
  Th1/Th2 ratio, **V2**.1149–50
natural infection, **V2**.1143
  infection course, **V2**.1143
  persistence, **V2**.1143
  species infected, **V2**.1144 (Tab.)
vaccines, **V2**.1153
Bornaviridae, **V1**.26
characteristics, **V1**.129 (Tab.), **V1**.177 (Tab.), **V1**.382
classification, **V1**.27 (Tab.), **V1**.49 (Tab.), **V1**.127–8
  characteristics, **V1**.380 (Tab.)
phylogeny, **V1**.388
type species *see* Borna disease virus (BDV)
see also Bornaviruses; *specific viruses*
Bornavirus
classification, **V1**.127–8
genome structure, **V1**.387 (Tab.)
replication, nucleus, **V1**.182
Bornaviruses
genome structure, **V1**.387 (Tab.)
host range, **V1**.381–2
IFN activity, **I**.260 (Tab.)
morphology/structure, **V1**.128–30
see also Bornaviridae
Bornholm disease (pleurodynia), **V2**.871
Borrelia, **B2.1818–37**
antibacterial susceptibility/resistance, **B2**.1830–2, **B2**.1831 (Tab.)
  cephalosporins, **B2**.1830
  clarithromycin, **B2**.1830
  macrolides, **B2**.1830
  species differences, **B2**.1830–2
  tetracyclines, **B2**.1830
culture, **B2**.1827–8
  growth temperature, **B2**.1828
  selective media, **B2**.1828
genetics, **B2**.1823–5
  gene families, **B2**.1823–4
  genome sequences, **B2**.1823, **B2**.1824 (Fig.)
  major outer surface proteins, **B2**.1824–5
  open reading frames, **B2**.1825
  plasmids, **B2**.1823–5
  pseudogenes, **B2**.1823–4
  virulence factors, **B2**.1825
history, **B2**.1818–19
host–vector relationships, **B2**.1825–7
  antigenic variants, **B2**.1826, **B2**.1827

Borrelia,
  host–vector relationships (*Continued*)
    DNA microarray studies, **B2**.1826
    gene conversion, **B2**.1826
    physiological adaptations, **B2**.1825
    transmission to host, **B2**.1825–6
    vector acquisition, **B2**.1825
  immune evasion, **B2**.1822–3, **B2**.1827
  infection *see* Lyme borreliosis; Relapsing
    fever *(Borrelia)*
  isolation/identification, **B2**.1828–32
    EIAs, **B1**.753
  metabolism, **B2**.1827–8
    carbohydrates, **B2**.1827–8
    lipids, **B2**.1827–8
    proteins, **B2**.1827–8
  morphology, **B2**.1819, **B2**.1819 (Fig.)
    darkfield microscopy, **B2**.1819
  pathogenicity, **B2**.1825–7
    plasmid loss, **B2**.1825
    surface protein expression, **B2**.1826
    tissue invasion, **B2**.1826
  species characteristics, **B2**.1820 (Tab.)
  taxonomy, **B2**.1819–22
    genetic diversity, **B2**.1821
    nonpathogenic species, **B2**.1819–21
    PCR-methods, **B2**.1821
Borrelia afzelii
  animal reservoirs, **B2**.1822–3
  antibacterial susceptibility/resistance,
    B2.1830–2
  characteristics, **B2**.1820 (Tab.)
  genome sequences, **B2**.1824 (Fig.)
  geographical distribution, **B2**.1819
Borrelia andersonii, **B2**.1820 (Tab.)
  geographical distribution, **B2**.1819
Borrelia anserina, **B2**.1820 (Tab.)
  relapsing fever, **B2**.1822
Borrelia bissettii, **B2**.1820 (Tab.)
  chromosomes, **B1**.81
  geographical distribution, **B2**.1819–21
Borrelia burgdorferi
  Anaplasma phagocytophilum co-
    transmission, **B2**.2060, **B2**.2063–4,
    B2.2066
  antibacterial susceptibility/resistance,
    B2.1830–2
  characteristics, **B2**.1820 (Tab.)
  genome sequence, **B2**.1823, **B2**.1824 (Fig.)
  geographical distribution, **B2**.1819
  immune evasion
    IL-10 induction, **I**.653
    immunosuppression, **I**.665
    outer membrane protein variation, **I**.661
    Th1/Th2 balance, **I**.666
  infection *see* Lyme borreliosis
  taxonomy, **B2**.1819–21
    genetic diversity, **B2**.1821
    PCR-methods, **B2**.1821
  vaccine *see* Lyme borreliosis
Borrelia caucasica, **B2**.1820 (Tab.)
Borrelia coriaceae, **B2**.1820 (Tab.)
  animal infection, **B2**.1823
  relapsing fever, **B2**.1822

Borrelia crocidurae, **B2**.1820 (Tab.)
  immune evasion, **B2**.1827
  relapsing fever, **B2**.1822, **B2**.1827
  transmission, **B2**.1823
Borrelia diplodilli, **B2**.1820 (Tab.)
Borrelia duttonii, **B2**.1820 (Tab.)
  human reservoirs, **B2**.1823
  relapsing fever, **B2**.1822, **B2**.1827
  transmission, **B2**.1823
Borrelia garinii, **B2**.1820 (Tab.)
  animal reservoirs, **B2**.1822–3
  antibacterial susceptibility/resistance,
    B2.1830–2
  genome sequences, **B2**.1824 (Fig.)
  geographical distribution, **B2**.1819
Borrelia hermsii, **B2**.1820 (Tab.)
  antigenic variation, **B2**.1827
  relapsing fever, **B2**.1822
Borrelia hispanica, **B2**.1820 (Tab.)
Borrelia japonica, **B2**.1820 (Tab.)
  geographical distribution, **B2**.1819
Borrelia latyschewii, **B2**.1820 (Tab.)
Borrelia lonestari, **B2**.1820 (Tab.), **B2**.1821–2
  relapsing fever, **B2**.1822
Borrelia lusitaniae, **B2**.1820 (Tab.)
  geographical distribution, **B2**.1819
Borrelia mazzottii, **B2**.1820 (Tab.)
Borrelia merionesi, **B2**.1820 (Tab.)
Borrelia microti, **B2**.1820 (Tab.)
Borrelia miyamotoi, **B2**.1820 (Tab.), **B2**.1821
  relapsing fever, **B2**.1822
Borrelia parkeri, **B2**.1820 (Tab.)
  relapsing fever, **B2**.1822
Borrelia persica, **B2**.1820 (Tab.)
Borrelia recurrentis, **B2**.1820 (Tab.)
  epidemic relapsing fever, **B2**.1823
  human reservoirs, **B2**.1823
  relapsing fever, **B2**.1822, **B2**.1827
  transmission, **B2**.1823
Borrelia sinica, **B2**.1820 (Tab.)
  geographical distribution, **B2**.1819
Borrelia tanukii, **B2**.1820 (Tab.)
  geographical distribution, **B2**.1819
Borrelia theileri, **B2**.1820 (Tab.)
  animal infection, **B2**.1823
  relapsing fever, **B2**.1822
Borrelia turdi, **B2**.1820 (Tab.)
  antigenic variation, **B2**.1827
  geographical distribution, **B2**.1819
Borrelia turicatae, **B2**.1820 (Tab.)
  relapsing fever, **B2**.1822
Borrelia valaisiana, **B2**.1820 (Tab.)
  animal reservoirs, **B2**.1822–3
  geographical distribution, **B2**.1819
Borrelia venezuelensis, **B2**.1820 (Tab.)
Borrelia vincentii, stomatitis, **B1**.614
Borreliosis *see* Lyme borreliosis
'Bosch-yaws,' **P**.329
Botanical Nomenclature, fungi, **M**.51
'Bot cook ,' **B2**.1044
Bothria, tapeworms, **P**.659
Botryomyces caespitosus, **M**.357
Botrytis
  fruit, **B1**.282–3
  in vegetables, **B1**.281

Botrytis cinerea, **B1**.281
Botrytis parasiticus, **B1**.281
Bottled water, **B1**.215–7 (Tab.), **B1**.224–5
Botulinum antitoxin, **B2**.1049, **B2**.1062–3
Botulinum toxin, **B2**.1060–2
  animal resistance, **B2**.1073–4
  bioterrorism, **B1**.364
  canning process, **B1**.265–6, **B1**.270–1, **B1**.275,
    B1.283
  clostridial species producing, **B2**.1039 (Tab.),
    B2.1042–3, **B2**.1046, **B2**.1059–60
  culture, **B2**.1047, **B2**.1049, **B2**.1062
  detection, **B2**.1062–3
    bioassay in animals, **B2**.1049,
      B2.1062–3
    culturing of organisms for recovery,
      B2.1049
    immunological, **B2**.1063
    intravenous time-to-death method,
      B2.1063
    quantitative, **B2**.1063
  domains, **B2**.1061–2
  flaccid paralysis due to, **B2**.1061–2, **B2**.1071,
    B2.1072 (Fig.)
  genes, **B2**.1038–40
  homology to *C. tetani* toxin, **B2**.1061
  isolation, **B2**.1040
  lethal dose, **B2**.1036, **B2**.1060–1, **B2**.1072
  mechanism of action, **B1**.156 (Tab.),
    B2.1040, **B2**.1061–2
  medicinal use, **B2**.1040, **B2**.1076
  membrane translocation, **B2**.1061–2
  molecular weight, **B2**.1061
  production control, **B2**.1062
  protein complex, **B2**.1040
  safety precautions for laboratory workers,
    B2.1076
  serotypes, **B2**.1039–40, **B2**.1039 (Tab.),
    B2.1043, **B2**.1061, **B2**.1071
    food-borne botulism and risk, **B2**.1066,
      B2.1069
    infant botulism and risk, **B2**.1069–70
    intestinal infection and risk, **B2**.1070
  structure, **B2**.1040, **B2**.1061
  toxin complexes, **B2**.1062
  see also Clostridium botulinum
Botulism, **B2**.1066–76
  animal, **B2**.1038–9, **B2**.1041 (Tab.), **B2**.1058,
    B2.1061, **B2**.1073–4
    cattle, **B2**.1074
    horses, **B2**.1074
    mink and fox farming, **B2**.1074
    outbreaks, **B2**.1070–1
  bioterrorism, **B1**.364
  clinical aspects, **B2**.1036, **B2**.1071–4
  diagnosis, **B2**.1075–6
  epidemiology, **B2**.1041 (Tab.), **B2**.1066–71
  food-borne, **B2**.1071–2
    Africa, **B2**.1069
    Alaska, **B2**.1066–7
    Asia, **B2**.1067–9
    Canada, **B2**.1067
    China, **B2**.1067
    clinical features, **B2**.1071–2
    Clostridium botulinum strains, **B2**.1042–3,
      B2.1055–6, **B2**.1059–60

Botulism
food-borne (*Continued*)
convalescence and recovery, **B2**.1071–2
costs, **B2**.1067
Europe, **B2**.1069
geographical distribution, **B2**.1066–9
Japan, **B2**.1067–9
outbreaks, **B2**.1068 (Tab.)
risk with spore type, **B2**.1066, **B2**.1069
UK, **B2**.1069
USA, **B2**.1066–7
yogurt, **B1**.249
historical perspective, **B2**.1037–40
immunization, **B2**.1075–6
infant, **B2**.1047, **B2**.1069–70, **B2**.1072–3
C. botulinum strains, **B2**.1042–3,
B2.1055–7, **B2**.1059–60, **B2**.1070
clinical features, **B2**.1072–3,
B2.1072 (Fig.)
geographical distribution, **B2**.1069–70
incidence, **B2**.1070
misdiagnosis, **B2**.1072
intestinal infection, **B2**.1070
recovery, **B2**.1073
treatment, **B2**.1075–6
wound, **B2**.1072 (Fig.), **B2**.1073, **B2**.1112–3
'Bouba,' **P**.327
Bovine astrovirus (BAstV)
classification, **V2**.890 (Tab.)
infection, pathogenesis, **V2**.905
replication, **V2**.894–5
Bovine brucellosis *see* Brucellosis, bovine
Bovine coronavirus (BCoV), **V1**.392
genome
non-translated region, **V1**.827
packaging, **V1**.827
hemagglutinin-esterase (HE), **V1**.838–9
infection, **V1**.241 (Tab.), **V1**.841 (Tab.)
Bovine diarrhea virus (BDV), **V2**.993
Bovine ephemeral fever virus (BEFV)
classification, **V1**.385–6
genome structure, **V2**.1112 (Fig.)
type species, **V2**.1104
Bovine foamy virus (BFV), **V2**.1304–5
Bovine herpesvirus 1, **V1**.494 (Tab.)
Bovine herpesvirus 2, **V1**.492
Bovine herpesvirus 4, **V1**.494 (Tab.),
V1.542 (Tab.)
Bovine immunodeficiency virus (BIV),
V2.1592–3
Bovine leukemia virus (BLV)
oncogenic mechanisms, **V1**.342 (Tab.)
receptors, **V1**.246 (Fig.)
transformation by, **V1**.336
Bovine mastitis, prototothecosis, **M**.399–400,
M.407
Bovine mycotic abortion
Aspergillus fumigatus, **M**.692
Candida, **M**.602
Bovine papillomavirus(es)
oncogenesis, **V1**.338 (Tab.)
oncogenic, **V1**.342 (Tab.)
Bovine papillomavirus type 1 (BPV-1),
V1.449–50
genome organization, **V1**.451 (Fig.)
latent infection, **V1**.453

Bovine papular stomatitis virus, **V1**.583–5
Bovine parainfluenza virus 3, **V1**.763
classification, **V1**.382–3
hemagglutinin-neuraminidase, **V1**.766
V protein, **V1**.763–4
Bovine parvovirus (BPV), **V1**.412
infection, **V1**.426
Bovine polyomavirus (BPyV), **V1**.473
Bovine respiratory syncytial virus
classification, **V1**.385
NS1/2 proteins, **V1**.708
transcription, **V1**.702–3
Bovine rhinovirus type 1, **V2**.873
Bovine rhinovirus type 3, **V2**.873
Bovine serum albumin, as carrier protein,
I.862–3
Bovine spongiform encephalopathy (BSE),
V2.1347, **V2**.1362–3
chronic wasting disease (CWD) of deer and
elk *vs.*, **V2**.1363
emerging infection, **V2**.1651 (Tab.)
experimental transmission, **V2**.1362–3
historical aspects, **V1**.7
incidence, **V2**.1363 (Fig.)
kuru *vs.*, **V2**.1363
oral transmission, **V2**.1363
pathogenesis, **V2**.1373–4
transmission, **V2**.1348
UK epidemic (1986), **V2**.1348, **V2**.1362
variant Creutzfeldt–Jakob disease *vs.*,
V2.1369–70
Bovine torovirus (BToV)
hemagglutinin-esterase (HE), **V1**.838–9
infection, **V1**.841 (Tab.), **V1**.845–6
seroepidemiology, **V1**.845–6
tissue culture, **V1**.846
Bovine viral diarrhea, *Pestivirus* infection,
V2.1004–5
Bovine viral diarrhea virus (BVDV)
classification, **V1**.53–4
host transcript recombination, **V1**.190
Bowel cancer, γδ T cells, **I**.438
Bowel decontamination, selective, **B1**.390
Bowens disease, HPV associations,
V1.463 (Tab.)
Boyden chamber, neutrophils, **I**.51
Brachiola
classification, **P**.190–1, **P**.198, **P**.535
historical aspects, **P**.535–6
structure/life cycle, **P**.535
see also Microsporidians; Microsporidiosis
Brachiola algerae
in vitro culture, **P**.548
multilayered interlaced network, **P**.529–31
Bradyzoites
Sarcocystis, **P**.443–5
Toxoplasma gondii, **P**.425–6, **P**.425 (Fig.),
P.426 (Fig.)
T-263 bradyzoites, **P**.439
Brain
abscesses *see* Intracranial abscess (brain
abscess)
autoimmunity, **V2**.1414–15
chemokine expression, **V2**.1409–10
cytokine expression, **V2**.1409–10
immunologically privileged site, **V1**.261

lymphocyte trafficking, **V2**.1410–11,
V2.1411 (Fig.)
MHC expression, **V2**.1410
see also Central nervous system (CNS)
Brain atrophy, in syphilis, **B2**.1843
Brain biopsy, **P**.153, **P**.153 (Tab.)
Echinococcus multilocularis infection, **P**.153
Entamoeba histolytica infection, **P**.153
Taenia solium diagnosis, **P**.153
Brain damage, prion diseases, **V2**.1372–3
Brainstem herniation, **B1**.557–8
BRAK (CXCL14), **I**.218 (Tab.)
Branched DNA assay, **B1**.731, **B1**.733 (Fig.)
Branched DNA probes, **V2**.1537
viral load measurement, **V2**.1214
Branhamella, **B2**.1271
Brazil
New World leishmaniasis incidence,
P.313–14
rubella vaccination policy, **B1**.351
Brazilian Purpuric Fever (BPF), **B2**.1693
emerging bacterial infection, **B1**.362–3
Breakpoint method, antibacterial susceptibility
testing, **B1**.498
Breast cancer
BCE peptide vaccines, **I**.855 (Tab.)
TCE peptide vaccines, **I**.865 (Tab.)
Breastfeeding
giardiasis protection, **P**.250
HCMV infection, **V2**.1450, **V2**.1452
hepatitis B transmission, **V2**.1474–6
hepatitis C transmission, **V2**.1478,
V2.1479–81
HIV transmission, **V2**.1471, **V2**.1473–4
Mycobacterium leprae transmission, **B2**.1204
virus shedding, **V1**.249
VZV infection, **V2**.1461
Breathing, **B1**.607–8
Brenneria, **B2**.1330 (Tab.)
Brevibacillus
identification, **B2**.945
infection, **B2**.944
taxonomy, **B2**.922–3
Brevibacillus agri, **B2**.935 (Tab.)
infection, **B2**.944
Brevibacillus brevis, **B2**.935 (Tab.)
colonies, **B2**.926 (Fig.)
infection, **B2**.944
microscopy, **B2**.943 (Fig.)
morphology, **B2**.943 (Fig.)
taxonomy, **B2**.922–3
Brevibacillus laterosporus, **B2**.935 (Tab.)
colonies, **B2**.926 (Fig.)
infection, **B2**.944
microscopy, **B2**.943 (Fig.), **B2**.946
morphology, **B2**.943 (Fig.), **B2**.946
taxonomy, **B2**.922–3
Brevibacterium, **B2**.991
biochemical characteristics, **B2**.993 (Tab.)
chemotaxonomic characteristics,
B2.978 (Tab.)
disease associations, **B2**.981 (Tab.)
nuts, **B1**.287
Brevibacterium casei, **B1**.296 (Tab.), **B1**.304

Brevibacterium epidermidis, **B1**.296 (Tab.), **B1**.304
Brevibacterium linens, **B1**.252
Brevundimonas diminuta, **B2**.1637–8
   waterborne, **B1**.224–5
Brevundimonas vesicularis, **B2**.1637–8
Bricklayers, paracoccidioidomycosis, **M**.545
Brill–Zinsser disease (recrudescent typhus), **B2**.2041
Brisgaard's taxa, **B2**.1658–9
British Paediatric Association Surveillance Unit, **B1**.318–19
British Thoracic Society, pneumonia treatment guidelines, **B1**.638, **B1**.639 (Tab.)
Brivudin, **V2**.1614
   HSV-2 infection, **V2**.1614
   structure, **V2**.1611 (Fig.)
   VZV infection in pregnancy, **V2**.1460
BrkA, *Bordetella,* **B2**.1789 (Tab.), **B2**.1801
Broad host range vectors, **B1**.121
Brochothrix, **B2**.958
Brochothrix campestris, **B2**.958
Brochothrix thermosphacta, **B2**.958
   meat and meat products, **B1**.273, **B1**.275
   poultry, **B1**.277–8
Brodies abscess, **B1**.693, **B1**.740, **B1**.747
Brodimorprim, **B1**.491
Bromocresol purple (BCP)-casein-yeast extract agar, **M**.236–7
5-Bromodeoxyuridine, mutagen, **V1**.183
5-Bromouracil (5-BU), **B1**.83
Bromovinylarabinosyl-uracil *see* Sorivudine
Bromovinylarauridine, structure, **V2**.1611 (Fig.)
Bromovinyldeoxyuridine *see* Brivudin
Bromoviridae
   classification, **V1**.27 (Tab.), **V1**.51 (Tab.)
   see also specific viruses
Bronchial asthma, IL-9, **I**.283 (Fig.)
Bronchial brushings, **M**.84
Bronchiectasis, **B1**.649
   causative organisms, **B1**.649
   diagnosis, **B1**.649, **B1**.649 (Fig.)
   in HIV infection, **B1**.645
   management, **B1**.649
Bronchiectasis, agammaglobulinemia, **I**.780
Bronchi, normal microbiota, **B1**.302
Bronchitis
   acute, **B1**.647
   chronic, **B1**.647–9
      bacterial infection/exacerbation, **B1**.648
      Chlamydia pneumoniae infection, **B2**.2015–16
      definition, **B1**.647–8
      in HIV infection, **B1**.645
      Nocardia cyriacigeorgica infection, **B2**.1160–1
      pathogenesis, **B1**.648
      therapy, **B1**.648–9
   rhinovirus infection association, **V2**.873
Bronchoalveolar lavage (BAL)
   aspergillosis, **M**.711–12, **M**.715
      ELISA, **M**.715
      invasive, **M**.698
      PCR, **M**.715
   HSV infection, **V2**.1506
   mycology, **M**.84

PCP, **M**.784, **M**.787, **M**.792, **M**.794
Bronchodilators, acute bronchiolitis therapy, **V1**.777
Broncholithiasis, histoplasmosis capsulati, **M**.524–5
Bronchopleural fistulae, aspergillosis, **M**.704
Bronchopneumonia
   acute aspergillosis, **M**.698–9
   cattle, **B2**.1653–4
   pigs, **B2**.1810
   virus infection, **V2**.942
Bronchus-associated lymphoid tissue (BALT), **I**.529–30
Bronopol, **B1**.427
   action of, **B1**.437 (Tab.), **B1**.438
Broth dilution susceptibility testing, **B1**.717
Brovavir *see* Sorivudine
Broviac catheters, infection, **B1**.391
Brown and Brenn stain, **M**.124–5
Brown-Hopps stain, **M**.123 (Tab.)
Brownlee, J, **B1**.336–7
Bruce D., **P**.15
Brucella, **B2**.**1719–51**
   acid environments, **B2**.1728–9
   antibacterial susceptibility/resistance, **B2**.1742
      antibiotics, **B1**.433
      tetracycline resistance, **B2**.1730
      trimethoprim resistance, **B2**.1730
   antigens, **B2**.1725–9
      intracellular antigens, **B2**.1728
      in vivo antigens, **B2**.1728–9
      LPS, **B2**.1724–6, **B2**.1726 (Fig.)
      outer membrane proteins, **B2**.1724, **B2**.1728
      polysaccharides, **B2**.1726–8
   cellular composition, **B2**.1723–5
      lipids, **B2**.1724–5
      lipoproteins, **B2**.1724
      lysozyme resistance, **B2**.1723–4
      outer membrane proteins, **B2**.1724
      polysaccharide B, **B2**.1724, **B2**.1728
      porins, **B2**.1724, **B2**.1728
   characteristics, **B2**.1720–1
   classification, **B2**.1721
      restriction enzyme analysis, **B2**.1729–30
   culture, **B2**.1733–5
      biohazard aspects, **B2**.1733–4
      carbon dioxide, **B2**.1735
      dyes, **B2**.1735
      isoerythritol, **B2**.1734
      morphology, **B2**.1734, **B2**.1734 (Fig.)
      nutritional requirements, **B2**.1734
      pH, **B2**.1735
      selective media, **B2**.1734–5, **B2**.1739
      species differentiation, **B2**.1735
      temperature, **B2**.1735
   defensin resistance, **I**.168
   epidemiology, **B2**.1721–2
      sources, **B2**.1721–2
      transmission, **B2**.1721–2
   genetics, **B2**.1729–31
      bacteriophages, **B2**.1730–1, **B2**.1732 (Tab.)
      DNA–DNA hybridization studies, **B2**.1729
      genetic exchange, **B2**.1730

   genome composition, **B2**.1729–30
   genome map, **B2**.1729
   molecular cloning, **B2**.1730
   nucleic acid composition, **B2**.1729 (Tab.)
   plasmids, **B2**.1730
   restriction enzyme analysis, **B2**.1729–30
   RNA analysis, **B2**.1730
habitats, **B2**.1721–2
historical perspective, **B2**.1719–20
identification, serology, **B1**.757
immune evasion, **B2**.1736, **B2**.1737
infection
   in cattle *see* Brucellosis, bovine
   in humans *see* Brucellosis, human
metabolism/biochemistry, **B2**.1720–1, **B2**.1731
   as aerobes, **B2**.1731
   hydrogen sulfide production, **B2**.1731
   iron-restriction, **B2**.1728
   nitrate reductase, **B2**.1731
   oxidative activity, **B2**.1731, **B2**.1733 (Tab.)
   superoxide dismutase, **B2**.1731
   urease, **B2**.1731
   Voges–Proskauer test, **B2**.1731
morphology, **B2**.1719, **B2**.1723, **B2**.1724 (Fig.)
   differential diagnosis, **B2**.1723
   stains/staining, **B2**.1723
nonlysosomal organelles, **I**.650–1
physical/chemical agent susceptibility/resistance, **B2**.1733
   disinfectants, **B2**.1733
   heat, **B2**.1733
reference strains, **B2**.1744 (Tab.)
species, **B2**.1743–5
   see also individual species
virulence/pathogenicity, **B2**.1735–43
   host preferences, **B2**.1735–6
   HtrA stress-induced protein, **B2**.1736
   intracellular growth, **B2**.1736
   LPS, **B2**.1736
   rodents, **B2**.1736
   superoxide dismutase, **B2**.1736
   survival within macrophages, **B2**.1736
Brucella abortus, **B2**.1727 (Tab.)
   cellular composition
      in vivo antigens, **B2**.1728
      outer-membrane proteins, **B2**.1724
      porins, **B2**.1724
   complement surface masking, **I**.662–3
   culture
      carbon dioxide, **B2**.1735
      dyes, **B2**.1735
      isoerythritol, **B2**.1734
      samples, **B2**.1735
   epidemiology, **B2**.1721
      in cheese, **B1**.253
      in cream, **B1**.248
      eradication by country, **B2**.1719–20
      geographical distribution, **B2**.1721
   genetics
      bacteriophages, **B2**.1730–1, **B2**.1732 (Tab.)
      nucleic acid composition, **B2**.1729 (Tab.)
   glucose metabolism, **B1**.57
   hosts, **B2**.1719–20

Brucella abortus, (Continued)
  infection
    camels, **B2**.1722
    in cattle *see* Brucellosis, bovine
    in humans *see* Brucellosis, human
    intracellular growth, **B2**.1736
    mastitis, **B1**.230
    pathogenesis, **B2**.1719
  LPS, **B2**.1725
    B. melitensis vs., **B2**.1725
  metabolism/biochemistry
    oxidative metabolism, **B2**.1733 (Tab.)
    respiratory system, **B2**.1731
  morphology, **B2**.1720, **B2**.1723,
    B2.1723 (Fig.), **B2**.1724 (Fig.)
  nonlysosomal organelles, **I**.650
  reference strains, **B2**.1744 (Tab.)
  virulence/pathogenicity, **B2**.1720
    host preferences, **B2**.1735–6
Brucella canis
  characteristics, **B2**.1727 (Tab.), **B2**.1744–5
  epidemiology, **B2**.1720
    geographical distribution, **B2**.1722
  genetics
    bacteriophages, **B2**.1730–1, **B2**.1732 (Tab.)
    nucleic acid composition, **B2**.1729 (Tab.)
  infection, **B2**.1722
  morphology, **B2**.1720
  oxidative metabolism, **B2**.1733 (Tab.)
  reference strains, **B2**.1744 (Tab.)
  virulence/pathogenicity, **B2**.1720
    host preferences, **B2**.1735–6
Brucella maris, **B2**.1727 (Tab.)
Brucella melitensis
  characteristics, **B2**.1727 (Tab.), **B2**.1743
  in cheese, **B1**.253
  classification, **B2**.2027 (Fig.)
    reference strains, **B2**.1744 (Tab.)
  culture, **B2**.1734
    dyes, **B2**.1735
    isoerythritol, **B2**.1734
    samples, **B2**.1735
  epidemiology, geographical distribution,
    B2.1721
  genetics
    bacteriophages, **B2**.1730–1, **B2**.1732 (Tab.)
    nucleic acid composition, **B2**.1729 (Tab.)
  infection
    camels, **B2**.1722
    in cattle *see* Brucellosis, bovine
    dairy products, **B2**.1722
    goats, **B2**.1722
    hosts, **B2**.1719
    in humans *see* Brucellosis, human
    intracellular growth, **B2**.1736
    sheep, **B2**.1722
  LPS, **B2**.1725
    A antigen, **B2**.1725, **B2**.1726 (Fig.)
    B. abortus vs., **B2**.1725
    M antigen, **B2**.1725, **B2**.1726 (Fig.)
  in milk, **B1**.231
  morphology, **B2**.1720–3
  outer-membrane proteins, **B2**.1724
  oxidative metabolism, **B2**.1733 (Tab.)

    physical/chemical agent
      susceptibility/resistance, **B2**.1733
    virulence/pathogenicity, **B2**.1720
      host preferences, **B2**.1735–6
Brucella neotomae
  characteristics, **B2**.1727 (Tab.), **B2**.1744
  culture, dyes, **B2**.1735
  epidemiology, **B2**.1720
  genetics
    bacteriophages, **B2**.1730–1, **B2**.1732 (Tab.)
    nucleic acid composition, **B2**.1729 (Tab.)
  host preferences, **B2**.1735–6
  oxidative metabolism, **B2**.1733 (Tab.)
  reference strains, **B2**.1744 (Tab.)
Brucella ovis, **B2**.1727 (Tab.), **B2**.1744–5
  culture
    carbon dioxide, **B2**.1735
    selective media, **B2**.1735
  epidemiology, **B2**.1720
  genetics
    bacteriophages, **B2**.1730–1, **B2**.1732 (Tab.)
    nucleic acid composition, **B2**.1729 (Tab.)
  host preferences, **B2**.1735–6
  metabolism/biochemistry
    nitrogen metabolism, **B2**.1731
    oxidative metabolism, **B2**.1733 (Tab.)
  in milk, **B1**.231
  morphology, **B2**.1720
  reference strains, **B2**.1744 (Tab.)
Brucella suis, **B2**.1727 (Tab.), **B2**.1743–4
  culture, **B2**.1734
    dyes, **B2**.1735
    isoerythritol, **B2**.1734
  genetics
    bacteriophages, **B2**.1730–1, **B2**.1732 (Tab.)
    nucleic acid composition, **B2**.1729 (Tab.)
  geographical distribution, **B2**.1720, **B2**.1722
  immune evasion, TNF-α suppression, **I**.652
  infection
    cattle, **B2**.1722
      see also Brucellosis, bovine
    intracellular growth, **B2**.1736
    pigs, **B2**.1722
  metabolism/biochemistry
    nitrogen metabolism, **B2**.1731
    oxidative metabolism, **B2**.1733 (Tab.)
  morphology, **B2**.1720, **B2**.1723
  physical/chemical agent
    susceptibility/resistance, **B2**.1733
  reference strains, **B2**.1744 (Tab.)
  virulence/pathogenicity, **B2**.1720
    host preferences, **B2**.1735–6
Brucellosis, bovine, **B1**.229
  causative organisms, **B2**.1722
    *see also Brucella abortus; Brucella
      melitensis*
  epidemiology, **B2**.1721, **B2**.1722
    eradication by country, **B2**.1719–20
    geographical distribution, **B2**.1722
  intracellular growth, **B2**.1736
  mastitis, **B1**.230
  pathogenesis, **B2**.1719
Brucellosis, human
  chronic, **B2**.1738

  clinical manifestations, **B1**.744, **B2**.1737–8
    acute phase, **B2**.1737–8
    bacteremia, **B1**.523
    bone and joint infection, **B1**.690–1,
      B2.1738
    CNS effects, **B2**.1738
    endocarditis, **B1**.532, **B1**.536, **B2**.1738
    epididymoorchitis, **B2**.1738
    febrile phase, **B2**.1738
    fever, **B2**.1737–8
    focal hepatitis, **B2**.1738
    granulomatous response, **B1**.741
    hyperpyrexia, **B2**.1737–8
    splenomegaly, **B2**.1738
    thrombophlebitis, **B2**.1738
  diagnosis, **B1**.744–5, **B2**.1738–41
    agglutination tests, **B1**.744–5
    cell-mediated immunity tests, **B1**.745,
      B2.1741
    complement-fixation assays, **B1**.745
    culture, **B1**.744–5, **B2**.1739
    differential diagnosis, **B2**.1741
    exposure history, **B2**.1738–9
    PCR, **B2**.1739
    serology, **B1**.744–5, **B2**.1739–41
  epidemiology
    cheese, **B1**.253
    dairy products, **B2**.1722
    geographical distribution, **B2**.1721
    laboratory-acquired, **B1**.760, **B1**.765,
      B2.1721, **B2**.1733–4
    milk, **B1**.231, **B1**.253
    occupational transmission, **B2**.1721–2
    as zoonosis, **B2**.1721
  immune evasion, **B2**.1736–7
  immune response, **B2**.1737
    cell-mediated responses, **B2**.1737
    humoral responses, **B1**.744–5, **B2**.1737
    IFN-γ, **B2**.1737
    macrophages, **B2**.1737
  incubation period, **B2**.1737–8
  pathogenesis, **B2**.1736–7
    bacteremia, **B2**.1737
    granulomatous reaction, **B2**.1737
    infective process, **B2**.1736–7
    intracellular habitats, **B2**.1737
    LPS, **B2**.1737
  prophylaxis, **B2**.1741–2
    contact avoidance, **B2**.1741–2
    vaccine development, **B2**.1742
  risk categorization, **B1**.762
  treatment, **B2**.1742–3
    chronic, **B2**.1743
    co-trimoxazole, **B2**.1743
    doxycycline, **B2**.1742–3
    rifampicin, **B2**.1742–3
    tetracycline, **B2**.1743
  vaccine development, **B2**.1742
Brugia, **P**.591
  immune evasion
    cystatin, **I**.687
    cytokine destruction, **I**.686
    migration inhibitory factor homologue,
      I.687
    T cell inhibition, **I**.683

Brugia,
immune evasion (*Continued*)
transforming growth factor-β homologue,
I.687
infection *see* Lymphatic filariasis
life cycle
intermediate hosts, **P.**771
vectors, **P.**772
structure/life cycle, **P.**591
see also individual species
Brugia malayi, **I.**683, **P.**769
characteristics, **P.**771 (Tab.)
epidemiology, **P.**39, **P.**769
genomics, **P.**772
historical aspects, **P.**9, **P.**769–71
infection *see* Lymphatic filariasis
life cycle, **P.**758 (Fig.), **P.**771–2
morphology, **P.**769
Brugia timori, **P.**769
characteristics, **P.**771 (Tab.)
epidemiology, **P.**769
historical aspects, **P.**9, **P.**769–71
infection *see* Lymphatic filariasis
life cycle, **P.**758 (Fig.)
morphology, **P.**769
Brumpt, E, **M.**32–3
Bruton's disease *see* X-linked
agammaglobulinemia (Bruton's disease)
BSAC method, antibacterial susceptibility
testing, **B1.**498
BSL-4, henipavirus infection, **V1.**818
Btk tyrosine kinase
BCR signaling, **I.**344–5
gene mutations, **I.**780
structure, **I.**343 (Fig.)
'Buba,' **P.**327
'Bubo,' lymphogranuloma venereum, **B2.**2012
Buccal capsules, *Ancylostoma duodenale,*
P.717 (Fig.)
Buchnera aphidicola, **B2.**1330 (Tab.)
possible human infection, **B2.**1337
Buchnera, genome structure, **B2.**1973–4
Budding
Measles virus, **V1.**720–1
respiroviruses, **V1.**773
Budding yeasts, **M.**70 (Fig.), **M.**73
Budgerigar fledgling polyomavirus (BFPyV),
V1.473
'Bud scar,' **M.**73
Budvicia aquatica, **B2.**1319 (Tab.)
Buffaloes, leprosy, **B2.**1182
Buffered Charcoal Yeast Extract (BCYE)
agar, *Legionella* culture, **B2.**1768–9,
B2.1772
Building works, aspergillosis, **M.**692–3, **M.**729
Bulbar poliomyelitis, **V2.**870
Bulleidia, **B2.**1028
Bulleidia extructa, **B2.**1029 (Tab.)
Bundle-forming pili (Bfp), *Aeromonas,*
B2.1528
Bunyamwera virus
genome structure, **V2.**1031 (Tab.)
immune evasion, **V1.**199
immune evasion mechanisms, **V1.**199
NS_M protein, **V2.**1039
reverse genetics, **V1.**189–90

transcription, **V2.**1035–6
type species, **V2.**1025–6
Bunyaviridae, **V2.1025–58**
characteristics, **V1.**129 (Tab.), **V1.**177 (Tab.)
classification, **V1.**27 (Tab.), **V1.**49 (Tab.),
V1.50, **V1.**127–8, **V2.**1026
historical aspects, **V2.**1025
type species, **V2.**1025
see also Hantavirus; Nairovirus;
Orthobunyavirus; Phlebovirus;
Tospovirus; specific viruses
Bunyavirus
genome structure, **V2.**1033 (Fig.)
NS_M protein, **V2.**1038
see also Bunyaviruses
Bunyaviruses
antigens, **V2.**1041–2
G1 glycoprotein, **V2.**1026–8, **V2.**1030 (Fig.),
V2.1038
as antigen, **V2.**1041
cell attachment/entry, **V2.**1034
Golgi system retention, **V2.**1039–40
post-translational modification, **V2.**1038
G2 glycoprotein, **V2.**1026–8, **V2.**1030 (Fig.),
V2.1038
as antigen, **V2.**1041
cell attachment/entry, **V2.**1034
Golgi system retention, **V2.**1039–40
post-translational modification, **V2.**1038
genome, **V2.**1031–4
ambisense coding, **V1.**181
consensus sequences, **V2.**1031 (Tab.)
gene organization, **V2.**1033 (Fig.)
L (large) segment, **V2.**1028–31, **V2.**1039
M (medium) segment, **V2.**1028–31,
V2.1038–9
panhandle structures, **V2.**1032 (Fig.)
S (small) segment, **V2.**1028–31, **V2.**1038
subunit reassortment, **V1.**191
Golgi system transport, **V2.**1040
human pathogens, **V2.**1025, **V2.**1027 (Tab.)
isolation/propagation and identification,
V1.95, **V1.**96 (Tab.)
large (L) protein, **V2.**1030 (Fig.), **V2.**1031,
V2.1039
conserved sequences, **V2.**1039
morphology/structure, **V2.**1026–31,
V2.1030 (Fig.)
nonstructural proteins, **V2.**1031
see also specific types
NS_S protein, **V2.**1038
as IFN antagonist, **V2.**1038
nucleocapsid (N) protein, **V2.**1028–30,
V2.1030 (Fig.), **V2.**1038
as antigen, **V2.**1041
replication, **V2.**1034–41, **V2.**1036 (Fig.)
assembly/release, **V2.**1040–1
'cap-snatching,' **V1.**110, **V1.**131–2
cell attachment, **V2.**1034–5
cell entry, **V1.**213, **V2.**1034–5
genome replication, **V2.**1037–8
Golgi transport, **V2.**1039–40
protein synthesis/processing, **V2.**1038–9
transcription *see below*
reverse genetics, **V1.**133–4, **V1.**189
ribonucleocapsids, **V2.**1030–1, **V2.**1030 (Fig.)

RNA synthesis, **V1.**131–2
structural proteins, **V2.**1031
see also specific types
transcription, **V2.**1035–7, **V2.**1036 (Fig.)
capping, **V2.**1035
host cell functions, **V2.**1036–7
large (L) protein, **V2.**1035
termination, **V2.**1037
veterinary pathogens, **V2.**1042
virulence determinants, **V1.**255
large RNA segment and polymerase,
V1.255
middle RNA segment and glycoprotein
G1, **V1.**255
Bunyavirus infection, **V2.**1042–51
clinical manifestations, **V2.**1042–8
gastrointestinal symptoms, **V2.**1042
rash, **V2.**1042
diagnosis, **V2.**1050
serology, **V2.**1547
epidemiology, **V2.**1048–50
transmission, **V2.**1048
as zoonoses, **V2.**1048
immune response, **V2.**1041–2, **V2.**1050
cell-mediated, **V2.**1041
humoral, **V2.**1041
IFN activity, **I.**260 (Tab.)
INFs, **V2.**1041–2
infection process, **V1.**241 (Tab.)
pathogenesis, **V2.**1050
prevention/control, **V2.**1050–1
transmission, **V1.**371 (Tab.)
vaccines, **V2.**1050–1
Bunyavirus, infection *see* Bunyavirus infection
Burkholderia, **B2.1607–48**
in biodegradation/biocontrol, **B2.**1612–13
classification, **B2.**1607
defensin resistance, **I.**168
historical perspective, **B2.**1607
phytopathogenicity, **B1.**202
pseudomallei group, **B2.**1618
Burkholderia ambifara
classification, **B2.**1609
origins, **B2.**1608 (Tab.)
Burkholderia andropogonis, **B2.**1608 (Tab.)
Burkholderia anthina
classification, **B2.**1609
origins, **B2.**1608 (Tab.)
Burkholderia caledonica, **B2.**1608 (Tab.)
Burkholderia capacia complex, **B2.**1607
Burkholderia caribensis, **B2.**1608 (Tab.)
Burkholderia caryophylli, **B2.**1608 (Tab.)
Burkholderia cenocepacia
classification, **B2.**1609
genome sequence, **B2.**1610
origins, **B2.**1608 (Tab.)
Burkholderia cepacia
B. pseudomallei vs., **B2.**1618–19
chlorhexidine resistance, **B1.**442
classification, **B2.**1607–9
in cystic fibrosis, **B1.**650
infection
chronic granulomatous disease, **I.**770
nosocomial infection, **B1.**377,
B1.401 (Tab.), **B2.**1611

Burkholderia cepacia (*Continued*)
    origins, **B2**.1608 (Tab.)
    pathogenicity, metalloprotease, **B2**.1615
    waterborne, **B1**.630–1
Burkholderia cepacia complex, **B1**.296 (Tab.),
        B2.1607–17
    antibacterial susceptibility/resistance,
        B2.1610–11
        antiseptic survival, **B2**.1610
        BcrA multidrug resistance pump,
            B2.1610–11
        β-lactam resistance, **B2**.1610–11
        chloramphenicol, **B2**.1610
        trimethoprim–sulfamethoxazole, **B2**.1610
    cell surface structures, **B2**.1613–14
        cellular lipids, **B2**.1613
        exopolysaccharides, **B2**.1614
        flagella, **B2**.1614
        LPSs, **B2**.1613–14, **B2**.1617
        outer membrane proteins, **B2**.1613
        pili, **B2**.1614
    classification, **B2**.1608–9
        DNA–DNA hybridization, **B2**.1609
        recA gene, **B2**.1609
        restriction fragment length polymorphisms,
            B2.1609
        tRNA intergenic length polymorphism
            analysis, **B2**.1609
    culture, **B2**.1609–10
        selective media, **B2**.1609–10
    in cystic fibrosis, **B2**.1611–13
        cell entry/survival, **B2**.1616
        clinical outcomes, **B2**.1611
        environmental acquisition, **B2**.1612–13
        genomovars, **B2**.1611–12
        infection control measures, **B2**.1611
        prevalence, **B2**.1611
        Pseudomonas aeruginosa co-infection,
            B2.1617
        transmissibility factors, **B2**.1612
        transmission, **B2**.1611
    genomics, **B2**.1610
        genomovars, **B2**.1609
        replicons, **B2**.1610
    isolation/identification, **B2**.1609–10
        automated biochemistry assays, **B2**.1610
        ELISA, **B2**.1613
        LPS serotyping, **B2**.1613–14
        morphology, **B2**.1609
    members, **B2**.1609
    pathogenicity, **B2**.1615–17
        cell entry/survival, **B2**.1615–16
        endotoxin, **B2**.1617
        hemolysin, **B2**.1615
        lipases, **B2**.1615
        metalloprotease, **B2**.1615
        quorum sensing, **B2**.1617
        siderophores, **B2**.1616–17
        virulence factors, **B2**.1615
    taxonomy, **B2**.1607–9
    typing, **B2**.1614–15
        bacteriocins, **B2**.1614
        bacteriophages, **B2**.1614
        DNA analysis, **B2**.1614–15
        multilocus enzyme electrophoresis,
            B2.1615

    multilocus restriction typing, **B2**.1615
    PCR, **B2**.1614–15
    plasmids, **B2**.1615
    ribotyping, **B2**.1614–15
Burkholderia cocovenenans, **B2**.1608 (Tab.)
Burkholderia dolosa
    intracellular infection, **B2**.1615–16
    origins, **B2**.1608 (Tab.)
Burkholderia fungorum, **B2**.1608 (Tab.)
Burkholderia gladioli, **B2**.1607, **B2**.1617
    differential diagnosis, **B2**.1617
    nosocomial infection, **B2**.1617
    origins, **B2**.1608 (Tab.)
Burkholderia glathei, **B2**.1608 (Tab.)
Burkholderia graminis, **B2**.1608 (Tab.)
Burkholderia hospita, **B2**.1608 (Tab.)
Burkholderia kururensis, **B2**.1608 (Tab.)
Burkholderia mallei, **B2**.1607, **B2**.1632–3
    antibacterial susceptibility/resistance,
        B2.1632
    antigenic structure, **B2**.1632–3
        LPS, **B2**.1632–3
    as bioterrorist agent, **B2**.1634–5
    culture, **B2**.1632, **B2**.1634
    genomics, **B2**.1632
        B. pseudomallei vs., **B2**.1632
        DNA–DNA hybridization, **B2**.1632
    infection *see* Glanders
    morphology, **B2**.1632
    origins, **B2**.1608 (Tab.)
    waterborne, **B1**.224–5
Burkholderia multivorans
    classification, **B2**.1609
    infection, in cystic fibrosis, **B2**.1611–12
    origins, **B2**.1608 (Tab.)
Burkholderia phenazium, **B2**.1608 (Tab.)
Burkholderia phymatum, **B2**.1608 (Tab.)
Burkholderia pickettii, nosocomial infection,
    B1.376–7
Burkholderia pseudomallei, **B2**.1607,
        B2.1618–20
    antibacterial susceptibility/resistance,
        B2.1620
        ampicillin resistance, **B2**.1620
        AmrAB-OprA multidrug efflux system,
            B2.1620
        clavulanate-sensitive β-lactamase, **B2**.1620
    as bioterrorist agent, **B2**.1634–5
    culture, **B2**.1618–19, **B2**.1618 (Fig.), **B2**.1630
    flagellin, **B2**.1614
    genomics, *B. mallei vs.,* **B2**.1632
    habitats, **B2**.1618
    historical aspects, **B2**.1618
    infection *see* Melioidosis
    isolation/identification, **B2**.1618–20
        B. cepacia vs., **B2**.1618–19
        B. thailandensis vs., **B2**.1622
        confirmation, **B2**.1619
        culture, **B2**.1618–19
        latex agglutination test, **B2**.1619
        non-culture methods, **B2**.1619–20
        oligonucleotide probes, **B2**.1619–20
        PCR, **B2**.1619–20
    morphology, **B2**.1618, **B2**.1618 (Fig.)
    nomenclature, **B2**.1618

    origins, **B2**.1608 (Tab.)
    pathogenicity, metalloprotease, **B2**.1615
    physical /chemical susceptibility/resistance,
        B2.1620
Burkholderia pyrrocinia
    classification, **B2**.1609
    origins, **B2**.1608 (Tab.)
Burkholderia sacchari, **B2**.1608 (Tab.)
Burkholderia stabilis
    classification, **B2**.1609
    origins, **B2**.1608 (Tab.)
Burkholderia tericola, **B2**.1608 (Tab.)
Burkholderia thailandensis, **B2**.1620–6
    antibacterial susceptibility/resistance
        ampicillin resistance, **B2**.1621
        tetracycline resistance, **B2**.1621
    capsule, **B2**.1622
    cell surface structures, **B2**.1621–3
        cellular lipids, **B2**.1621
        exopolysaccharides, **B2**.1622
        flagella, **B2**.1622–3
        LPSs, **B2**.1621–2
        outer membrane proteins, **B2**.1621
    classification, **B2**.1620–1
    clinical isolates, **B2**.1620–1
    genomics, **B2**.1621
        LPS genes, **B2**.1622
    historical aspects, **B2**.1620–1
    infection
        animal models, **B2**.1625–6
        diabetes mellitus, **B2**.1626
        intracellular, **B2**.1624–5
        multinucleated giant cells, **B2**.1625
        vaccine development, **B2**.1621, **B2**.1623
        see also Melioidosis
    isolation/identification
        B. pseudomallei vs., **B2**.1622
        ELISA, **B2**.1621
        PCR, **B2**.1620–1
    origins, **B2**.1608 (Tab.)
    pathogenicity, **B2**.1624–6
        cell entry/survival, **B2**.1624–5
        cytokine induction, **B2**.1625–6
        extracellular enzymes, **B2**.1624
        siderophores, **B2**.1624
        toxic products, **B2**.1624
    typing, **B2**.1623–4
        bacteriophages, **B2**.1623
        DNA analysis, **B2**.1623–4
        DNA probes, **B2**.1623
        multilocus sequence typing, **B2**.1623–4
        random amplifies polymorphic DNA
            analysis, **B2**.1623
        ribotyping, **B2**.1623
Burkholderia ubonensis
    classification, **B2**.1609
    origins, **B2**.1608 (Tab.)
Burkholderia vietnamiensis
    antibacterial susceptibility/resistance,
        B2.1610
    classification, **B2**.1609
    intracellular infection, **B2**.1615–16
    origins, **B2**.1608 (Tab.)
Burkitt lymphoma (BL), **V1**.559
    cells, **V1**.566

Burkitt lymphoma (BL) (*Continued*)
 chromosomal translocation, **V1**.570
 clinical features, **V1**.569–70
 diagnosis, **V1**.570
 EBV, **V1**.248 (Fig.), **V1**.336–8, **V1**.569
  latent gene expression, **V1**.566,
   V1.566 (Tab.)
 endemic ('African'), **V1**.569–70
 immune response, **V1**.570
 malaria, **P**.501 (Tab.)
 malaria association, **V1**.570
 pathogenesis, **V1**.570
 protozoal infection, **P**.97
 sporadic ('American'), **V1**.569
 TCR recombination, **I**.454
 treatment, **V1**.570
Burns, infection after, **B1**.385–6, **B1**.399
 Proteus mirabilis, **B2**.1447
'Bursatee,' **M**.412
Burulin, **B2**.1185
Buruli ulcer, emerging bacterial infection,
 B1.362
Buschke, A, **M**.16, **M**.17 (Fig.)
Buschke–Lowenstein tumors, HPV association,
 V1.463 (Tab.), **V1**.465
Busse, O, **M**.16, **M**.17 (Fig.), **M**.18 (Fig.)
Bussuqara virus (BSQV), **V2**.998 (Tab.)
Butaconazole, candidiasis therapy, **M**.257
Butanediol, formation, **B1**.55
Butanol, fermentation, **B1**.55–6
Butcher, Eugene, **I**.505
Butchers, erysipeloid, **B2**.971
Butenafine, **M**.183 (Tab.), **M**.184
 dermatophytoses therapy, **M**.184
 mechanism of action, **M**.184
 tinea manuum, **M**.186–7
 tinea pedis, **M**.186–7
Butter, **B1**.250
Buttiauxella
 antibacterial susceptibility/resistance,
  B2.1352 (Tab.)
 DNA–DNA analysis, **B2**.1338
Buttiauxella agrestis, **B2**.1319 (Tab.)
Buttiauxella brennerae, **B2**.1319 (Tab.)
Buttiauxella ferragutiae, **B2**.1319 (Tab.)
Buttiauxella izardii, **B2**.1319 (Tab.)
Buttiauxella noackiae, **B2**.1319 (Tab.)
Buttiauxella warmboldiae, **B2**.1319 (Tab.)
iso-Butylamine, γδ T cell binding, **I**.440 (Fig.)
Butyrate fermentation, **B1**.55–6
Butyrivibrio fibrisolvens, **B1**.296 (Tab.)
Butyryl-CoA, **B1**.56
B-virus, emerging infection, **V2**.1648 (Tab.)
Bwamba virus infection, **V2**.1047
BXH-2 virus, myeloid leukemia, **V1**.339–40
Byssochlamys, fruit, **B1**.283
Bystander activation, autoimmune disease,
 I.755–6

C1 complement protein, **I**.143 (Tab.)
 antibody binding, **I**.142
 C1q, **I**.142–3
  classical pathway activation, **I**.145 (Fig.)
  deficiencies, **I**.149
  deficiency, **I**.752

 IgG interaction, **I**.312
 IgM interaction, **I**.312
 microbial recognition, **I**.24 (Tab.)
 MLV binding, **V1**.273
 SLE, **I**.149, **I**.155
 C1r, **I**.142–3
  classical pathway activation, **I**.145 (Fig.)
 C1s, **I**.142–3
  C4 cleavage, **I**.143
  classical pathway activation, **I**.145 (Fig.)
 classical pathway activation, **I**.142–3,
  I.145 (Fig.)
 cleavage, **I**.142
 deficiencies, **I**.151
 Ig binding, **I**.142–3
 immune complex clearance, **I**.155
 inhibition by *Taenia solium*, **P**.682–3
 regulation, **I**.149–51
  deficiency, **I**.153–4
 structure, **I**.142–3
C1-inhibitor, **I**.149–51, **I**.150 (Tab.)
 deficiency, **I**.153–4
 mechanism of action, **I**.149
C1q complement protein *see* C1 complement
 protein
C1r *see* C1 complement protein
C1s *see* C1 complement protein
C2 complement protein, **I**.143 (Tab.), **I**.144
 C4b binding, **I**.144
 classical pathway activation, **I**.144,
  I.145 (Fig.)
 cleavage, **I**.144
  lectin pathway activation, **I**.146
 deficiencies, **I**.151
  immunogenetics, **I**.579–80
 lectin pathway activation, **I**.145 (Fig.)
C2 domain, **I**.476 (Fig.)
C2 gene, **I**.579–80
C3a receptor (C3aR), **I**.147
C3b complement protein *see* C3 complement
 protein
C3 complement protein, **I**.143 (Tab.), **V2**.1384
 acute phase response, **I**.200
 alternative pathway activation, **I**.144–5
 C3a, **I**.144, **I**.146–7
  airway hypersensitivity, **I**.738
  basophil chemotaxis, **I**.60
  basophil degranulation, **I**.62–3
  eosinophil chemotaxis, **I**.60, **I**.61
  pathological effects, **I**.154
  receptor (C3aR), **I**.147
  viral infection, **V1**.273
 C3b, **I**.144, **I**.146
  alternative pathway activation, **I**.145,
   I.145 (Fig.)
  opsonization, **I**.39, **I**.146–7
  receptor binding, **I**.146–7
 classical pathway activation, **I**.144,
  I.145 (Fig.)
 cleavage, **I**.144
 deficiency, **I**.153, **I**.770–1
  acquired, **I**.153
  autoantibodies, **I**.153
  infection, **I**.770–1
  inherited, **I**.153

 lectin pathway activation, **I**.145 (Fig.)
 microbial recognition, **I**.24 (Tab.)
 regulation, **I**.151
 septic shock, **I**.698
C3 nephritic factors, **I**.153
C4a complement protein *see* C4 complement
 protein
C4A gene, **I**.579–80
C4b2a3b complex, **I**.144
C4b2a complex, **I**.144
C4b complement protein *see* C4 complement
 protein
C4B gene, **I**.579–80
C4-binding protein (C4BP), **I**.150 (Tab.), **I**.151
 deficiency, **I**.154
C4 complement protein, **I**.143–4, **I**.143 (Tab.),
 V2.1384
 C4a, **I**.143–4, **I**.147
  basophil histamine release, **I**.62
 C4b, **I**.143–4, **I**.146
  C2 binding, **I**.144
  opsonization, **I**.146–7
  receptor binding, **I**.146–7
 classical pathway activation, **I**.143–4,
  I.145 (Fig.)
 cleavage, **I**.143
 deficiencies, **I**.151
 immune complex clearance, **I**.155
 isotypes, **I**.143
 lectin pathway activation, **I**.145 (Fig.)
C5a receptor (C5aR:CD88), **I**.147
C5b complement protein, **I**.144
C5 complement protein, **I**.143 (Tab.), **I**.144
 airway hypersensitivity, **I**.738
 alternative pathway activation, **I**.145
 basophil histamine release, **I**.62
 blocking antibodies as therapy, **I**.158,
  I.158 (Tab.)
 C5a, **I**.144, **I**.146–7
  basophil chemotaxis, **I**.60
  basophil degranulation, **I**.63
  eosinophil chemotaxis, **I**.60–1
  inflammation, **I**.154
  intracellular signaling, **I**.222
  neutrophil apoptosis, **I**.149
  neutrophil recruitment, **I**.37
  pathological effects, **I**.154
  receptor (C5aR:CD88), **I**.147
  septic shock/organ damage, **I**.698–9
  viral infection, **V1**.273
 C5b, **I**.144
 classical pathway activation, **I**.144
 cleavage, **I**.144
 deficiency, **I**.153
 regulation, **I**.151
 septic shock, **I**.698
C6 complement protein, **I**.143 (Tab.), **I**.146
 deficiency, **I**.153
 regulation, **I**.151
 structure, **I**.476 (Fig.)
C7 complement protein, **I**.143 (Tab.), **I**.146
 deficiency, **I**.153
 regulation, **I**.151
 structure, **I**.476 (Fig.)
 see also Membrane attack complex (MAC)

C8 complement protein, **I**.143 (Tab.), **I**.146
  deficiency, **I**.153
  regulation, **I**.151
  structure, **I**.476 (Fig.)
  see also Membrane attack complex (MAC)
C9 complement protein, **I**.143 (Tab.), **I**.146
  deficiency, **I**.153
  regulation, **I**.151
  structure, **I**.476 (Fig.)
  see also Membrane attack complex (MAC)
Cabassou viru (CABV), **V2**.1011 (Tab.)
Cable pili, *Burkholderia*, **B2**.1614
Cache Valley virus infection, **V2**.1047
Cachexia, TNF-α, **I**.286
Cadidiasis, in HIV infection, **I**.795
Cadmium resistance, **B1**.114
  Staphylococcus, **B2**.794 (Tab.), **B2**.804–5
cagA gene, **B2**.1570
CagA pathogenicity island, **B2**.1577
CagA protein, **B1**.175
Calabazo virus, **V2**.1666 (Tab.)
Calcareous corpuscles, **P**.681–2
Calcifluor staining, microsporidiosis, **P**.546,
  P.547 (Fig.)
Calcium channels, defensin activation, **I**.170
Calcium hydroxide, **B1**.422–4
Calcium ions, *Plasmodium*, **P**.477
Calcium, perforin interaction, **I**.475, **I**.477 (Fig.)
Calcium phosphate, as adjuvant, **I**.928 (Tab.)
Calcofluor white, **M**.87, **M**.88 (Tab.),
  M.123 (Tab.), **M**.125, **M**.203, **M**.236
  aspergillosis, **M**.711, **M**.711 (Fig.)
  Coccidioides immitis, **M**.513
  Penicillium staining, **M**.245 (Fig.)
Calf lymph vaccine, smallpox eradication,
  V1.581
Caliciviridae
  characteristics, **V1**.139 (Tab.), **V1**.177 (Tab.)
  classification, **V1**.27 (Tab.), **V1**.51 (Tab.),
    V1.52, **V2**.1175, **V2**.1175 (Tab.)
  phylogenetic relationships, **V2**.917 (Fig.)
  see also Caliciviruses; *specific viruses*
Caliciviruses
  classic
    hepatitis E virus relationship, **V2**.1175,
      V2.1175 (Tab.)
    isolation/propagation and identification,
      V1.96 (Tab.)
    properties, **V2**.1175 (Tab.)
  genome organization, **V1**.135–6, **V1**.136 (Fig.)
  infection *see* Calicivirus infection
  morphology/structure, **V1**.138
  mRNA structure, **V1**.139, **V1**.140 (Tab.)
  picornaviruses *vs.,* **V2**.861
  see also Caliciviridae; Sapoviruses
Caliciviruses, mollusks, **B1**.280
Calicivirus infection
  IFN activity, **I**.260 (Tab.)
  immunodeficient patients (non-HIV),
    V2.1508–9
  vaccine, **I**.840
California encephalitis
  clinical manifestations, **V2**.1042–3
  epidemiology, **V2**.1048–9
  incubation period, **V2**.1043
  prevalence, **V2**.1042–3

  transmission, **V1**.372 (Tab.), **V2**.1043,
    V2.1048–9
Calmodulin, activation of adenylate cyclase
  toxin in *Bordetella*, **B2**.1797
Calnexin
  influenza hemagglutinin assembly, **V1**.650
  MHC class I assembly, **I**.408
Calodium, **P**.589
Calomys, arenaviruses association,
  V2.1060 (Tab.), **V2**.1061
Calpain, schistosomiasis vaccines, **P**.621,
  P.633 (Tab.), **P**.634–5
Calreticulin
  MHC class I assembly, **I**.408
  Rubella virus interaction, **V2**.964
Calvin cycle, **B1**.62
Calymmatobacterium granulomatis see
  Klebsiella granulomatis
Cambodia, schistosomiasis control programs,
  P.636–7
Camelpox virus
  classification, **V1**.583
  phylogenetics, **V1**.585
Camels
  antibodies, **I**.368–9
  Brucella infection, **B2**.1722
Campath, licensing, **I**.355 (Tab.)
Camphor degradation, plasmids, **B1**.114
Campylobacter
  antibacterial susceptibility/resistance, **B1**.433,
    B2.1548
    ciprofloxacin resistance, **B1**.363
    quinolone resistance, **B1**.493 (Tab.)
  antigens, **B2**.1546, **B2**.1555
    heat-stable LPS antigens, **B2**.1546
    surface antigens, **B2**.1546
  cell wall composition, **B2**.1546
  characteristics, **B2**.1543 (Tab.), **B2**.1547
  chemical/physical agent
    susceptibility/resistance, **B2**.1545–6
  classification, **B2**.1541–2, **B2**.1929
  conjugation, **B1**.103
  culture, **B2**.1543 (Tab.), **B2**.1544–5
  definition, **B2**.1541
  flagella, **B2**.1550–1
  in food
    meat and meat products, **B1**.273–5
    milk, **B1**.231–2, **B1**.235 (Tab.), **B1**.238–9
    vegetables, **B1**.282
  genetics, **B2**.1546
  habitats, **B1**.212, **B1**.218–19, **B2**.1542
  historical perspective, **B2**.1541–2
  infection, **B2**.1549–51
    animals, **B2**.1550
    cell association and invasion, **B2**.1550
    in day-care centers, **B1**.361
    enteritis, **B2**.1550
    periodontal disease, **B2**.1549–50
    reproductive disease, **B2**.1549
    systemic, **B2**.1549
    waterborne, **B1**.218–19
  isolation/identification, **B2**.1543 (Tab.),
    B2.1544–8
    biochemistry, **B2**.1547
    culture, **B2**.1547
    direct detection in feces, **B2**.1547

    food/environmental specimens, **B2**.1547
    serodiagnosis, **B2**.1547–8
  morphology, **B2**.1544
  motility, **B2**.1550–1
  normal microbiota, **B1**.296 (Tab.)
  pathogenicity, **B2**.1549–51
  physical/chemical agent
    susceptibility/resistance, **B2**.1545–6
  species, **B2**.1543 (Tab.), **B2**.1551–3
  toxins, **B2**.1551
  typing, **B2**.1548–9
    bacteriophage typing, **B2**.1549
    biotyping, **B2**.1548–9
    genotyping, **B2**.1549
    serotyping, **B2**.1548–9
  virulence factors, **B2**.1549–51
Campylobacter coli, **B2**.1543 (Tab.), **B2**.1547,
  B2.1553
  antibacterial susceptibility/resistance,
    B2.1548
  antigens, **B2**.1546
  classification, **B2**.1541–2
  culture, **B2**.1544–5
  flagella and motility, **B2**.1551
  genetics, **B2**.1546
  habitats, **B2**.1542
  infection
    Balantidium coli co-infection, **P**.280
    case-control study, **B1**.316
    cell association and invasion, **B2**.1550
    in poultry, **B1**.276–7
    isolation/identification, **B2**.1547
    typing methods, **B2**.1549
  pathogenicity, **B2**.1549–50
Campylobacter concisus, **B2**.1543 (Tab.),
  B2.1552–3
  culture, **B2**.1544, **B2**.1547
  habitats, **B2**.1542
  isolation/identification, **B2**.1547
  pathogenicity, **B2**.1549–50
Campylobacter cryaerophilia, **B2**.1553–4
  antibacterial susceptibility/resistance,
    B2.1556
  typing methods, **B2**.1556
Campylobacter curvus, **B2**.1543 (Tab.),
  B2.1552–3
  culture, **B2**.1544, **B2**.1547
  isolation/identification, **B2**.1547
  pathogenicity, **B2**.1549–50
Campylobacter fetus, **B2**.1543 (Tab.),
  B2.1551–2
  antibacterial susceptibility/resistance,
    B2.1548
  antigens, **B2**.1546
  classification, **B2**.1542
  culture, **B2**.1542 (Fig.), **B2**.1544–5
  genetics, **B2**.1546
  habitats, **B2**.1542
  infection, endocarditis, **B1**.532
  morphology, **B2**.1544
  outer membrane protein variation, **I**.661
  pathogenicity, **B2**.1549
Campylobacter (Bacteroides) gracilis,
  B2.1543 (Tab.), **B2**.1547, **B2**.1552–3
  habitats, **B2**.1542
  morphology, **B2**.1544

Campylobacter (Bacteroides) gracilis,
(Continued)
  pathogenicity, **B2**.1549–50
Campylobacter helveticus, **B2**.1543 (Tab.),
  B2.1553
Campylobacter hominis, **B2**.1543 (Tab.),
  B2.1552–3
Campylobacter hyoilei, **B2**.1543 (Tab.),
  B2.1553
  pathogenicity, **B2**.1550
Campylobacter hyointestinalis, **B2**.1543 (Tab.),
  B2.1551–2
  culture, **B2**.1544, **B2**.1547
  isolation/identification, **B2**.1547
  pathogenicity, **B2**.1550
Campylobacter jejuni, **B2**.1543 (Tab.), **B2**.1547,
  B2.1553
  antibacterial susceptibility/resistance,
    B2.1548
    quinolone resistance, **B1**.492–3
  antigens, **B2**.1546
  classification, **B2**.1541–2
  culture, **B2**.1544–6, **B2**.1544 (Fig.)
  flagella and motility, **B2**.1551
  in food
    milk, **B1**.230–1, **B1**.235 (Tab.), **B1**.238–9
    offal, **B1**.273
    poultry *see below*
  genetics, **B2**.1546
  habitats, **B2**.1542
  infection, **B2**.1549
    case-control study, **B1**.316
    cell association and invasion, **B2**.1550
    Guillain–Barré syndrome association,
      B1.365
    mastitis, **B1**.230, **B1**.239
    milk-borne, **B1**.238–9
  isolation/identification, **B2**.1547
    EIAs, **B1**.751–2
    serology and immunoassays, **B2**.1547–8
    typing methods, **B2**.1548–9
  LPS variation, **I**.661
  lysosomal killing resistance, **I**.651
  morphology, **B2**.1544
  pathogenicity, **B2**.1549–50
  in poultry
    chill drying, **B1**.277
    colonization, **B1**.276
    eggs, internal contamination, **B1**.276
    irradiation, **B1**.278
    oral inoculation and single chick
      contamination, **B1**.276
    slaughter operations, **B1**.277
    transportation and transmission, **B1**.277
  siderophores, **B2**.1551
  virulence factors, **B2**.1550–51
Campylobacter lamienae, **B2**.1543 (Tab.),
  B2.1551–2
Campylobacter lari, **B2**.1543 (Tab.), **B2**.1553
  antibacterial susceptibility/resistance,
    B2.1548
  antigens, **B2**.1546
  culture, **B2**.1544–5
  habitats, **B2**.1542
  morphology, **B2**.1544
  pathogenicity, **B2**.1550

typing methods, **B2**.1549
Campylobacter mucosalis, **B2**.1543 (Tab.),
  B2.1552–3
  culture, **B2**.1544, **B2**.1547
  isolation/identification, **B2**.1547
  pathogenicity, **B2**.1550
Campylobacter nitrofigilis, **B2**.1553–4
Campylobacter rectus, **B2**.1543 (Tab.),
  B2.1552–3
  antigens, **B2**.1546
  culture, **B2**.1544, **B2**.1547
  habitats, **B2**.1542
  isolation/identification, **B2**.1547
  pathogenicity, **B2**.1549–50
Campylobacter showae, **B2**.1543 (Tab.),
  B2.1552–3
  habitats, **B2**.1542
  morphology, **B2**.1544
  pathogenicity, **B2**.1549–50
Campylobacter sputorum, **B2**.1543 (Tab.),
  B2.1552–3
  culture, **B2**.1544, **B2**.1547
  habitats, **B2**.1542
  isolation/identification, **B2**.1547
  pathogenicity, **B2**.1549–50
Campylobacter upsaliensis, **B2**.1543 (Tab.),
  B2.1553
  pathogenicity, **B2**.1550
Canada, food-borne botulism, **B2**.1067
Canarypox virus, **V1**.614
  as vaccine vector, **I**.846, **I**.898, **I**.902
Canavan disease, gene therapy, **V2**.1601
Canavanine resistance, *Cryptococcus
  neoformans,* **M**.638, **M**.638 (Tab.)
Cancer(s)
  CD8 T cells, **I**.421
  clusters, **V1**.344
  concept, **V1**.334
  disorder of cellular control, **V1**.334
  historical aspects/re-evaluation, **I**.14
  immune evasion, **I**.483
  immune surveillance hypothesis, **I**.421
  incidence, **V1**.330–3
    of viral risk factors, **V1**.330–3, **V1**.331 (Fig.)
  initiation, **V1**.345–6
  JC virus *see* JC virus (JCV)
  multi-step development, **V1**.345–6
  NK cells *see* Natural killer (NK) cells
  perforin deficiency, **I**.480
  proto-oncogenes role, **V1**.340
  recessive mutations in, **V1**.334
  rejection
    dendritic epidermal γδ T cells, **I**.437
    granzymes, **I**.482 (Tab.)
    IFN-γ, **I**.478
    lymphocyte-mediated cytotoxicity, **I**.483
    perforin, **I**.482 (Tab.), **I**.483
  retroviruses, **V2**.1297–8
  SV40 *see* Simian virus 40 (SV40)
  therapy
    anti-CD40 antibodies, **I**.358
    bispecific antibodies, **I**.361
    IFN-α, **I**.258
    IL-2, **I**.280
    immunotherapy, **I**.421

  type I INFs, **I**.258
  TNF-α effects, **I**.286
  vaccines, **I**.421
    BCE peptides, **I**.855 (Tab.), **I**.876
    monophosphoryl lipid adjuvant, **I**.929–30
    TCE peptide vaccines, **I**.879
Cancer patients
  gastrointestinal candidiasis, **M**.256
  spinal epidural abscess, **B1**.592
Candida, **M**.579
  adherence, **M**.13–4, **M**.587
  biochemistry/physiology, **M**.583
    arabinitol, **M**.608
    carbohydrate metabolism, **M**.583, **M**.605
    coenzyme Q, **M**.580
    cytochrome P450 14α-demethylase, **M**.608
    enolase, **M**.100, **M**.591, **M**.607
    heat shock proteins, **M**.100, **M**.102–3,
      M.591, **M**.594, **M**.607
    mannan, **M**.587, **M**.590–1, **M**.607
    myeloperoxidase, **M**.590, **M**.593
    phospholipases, **M**.587–8
    proteases, **M**.100, **M**.103, **M**.583–4,
      M.587
    ubiquinones, **M**.580
  biofilm formation, **M**.588
  cell wall, **M**.590–1
  classification, **M**.46, **M**.54, **M**.61
  culture, **M**.581–2, **M**.603, **M**.606
    blood culture, **M**.606
    morphological media, **M**.604
  ecology, **M**.584–6
    environmental source identification, **M**.95
  fruit, **B1**.282–3
  genetics, **M**.583, **M**.605–6, **M**.608
    chitin synthase gene, **M**.608
    DNA probes, **M**.605–6, **M**.608
    karyotype analysis, **M**.583–4
    mitochondrial DNA, **M**.608
    PCR, **M**.101–2, **M**.584
    ribosomal DNA, **M**.103
    ribosomal RNA, **M**.580, **M**.608
    ribosome proteins (r-proteins), **M**.591
    SAP gene, **M**.103, **M**.584, **M**.587, **M**.605–6
  growth, **M**.73
    temperature, **M**.583
  history, **M**.13–4, **M**.14 (Fig.), **M**.579–80
  identification, **M**.602–8
    biochemical tests, **M**.605, **M**.605 (Fig.)
    blood culture, **M**.606
    culture *see Candida,* culture
    genus/strain, **M**.94
    histopathology, **M**.89 (Tab.), **M**.125,
      M.126 (Tab.), **M**.128 (Tab.), **M**.134 (Fig.),
      M.594–5
    in situ DNA hybridization, **M**.94
    microscopy, **M**.602, **M**.606
    Pastorex test, **M**.100, **M**.607
    PCR *see* Polymerase chain reaction (PCR)
    reverse passive latex agglutination,
      M.98–100
    serology, **M**.92, **M**.93 (Tab.), **M**.97–8,
      M.605
    specimens, **M**.602–3, **M**.606
  infection *see* Candidiasis

Candida, (Continued)
  morphology, **M**.126 (Tab.), **M**.581–4,
      M.588–9
    differentiation, **M**.604, **M**.606
    dimorphism, **M**.74, **M**.583
  nomenclature, **M**.580
  as normal microbiota, **B1**.302
  nosocomial infection *see* Candidiasis
  pathogenicity, **M**.586–90
  phenotypic switching, **M**.76, **M**.76 (Fig.),
      M.589
  resistance
    amphotericin B, **M**.611
    azoles, **M**.611–2
    fluconazole, **M**.169–70, **M**.174, **M**.585–6,
        M.611–2
    flucytosine, **M**.176, **M**.585
    polyenes, **M**.170–1, **M**.611
    susceptibility testing, **M**.169–70,
        M.170 (Tab.), **M**.608
  susceptibility testing, **M**.170, **M**.170 (Tab.),
      M.608, **M**.610 (Fig.)
  taxonomy, **M**.580–1
  tissue penetration, **M**.588
  ubiquinones, **M**.580
  virulence factors, **M**.586–7, **M**.598–9
Candida albicans
  adherence, **M**.4, **M**.587
  antibacterial susceptibility/resistance, **B1**.439,
      B1.444
  biochemistry
    heat shock proteins, **M**.101, **M**.102–3
    mannan, **M**.99
    phospholipases, **M**.588
    proteases, **M**.100, **M**.588
  biofilms, **M**.588
    morphology in, **M**.75–6
  classification, **M**.580–1
    Chlamydoconidia, **M**.74, **M**.604–5
  as commensal organism, **M**.257–8
    asymptomatic carriers, **M**.257–8
    colonization, **M**.258
    sites, **M**.257–8
  complement receptors, **M**.593
  culture, **M**.604, **M**.604 (Fig.)
    growth temperature, **M**.583
  ecology, **M**.584–5, **M**.589
  epidemiology, **M**.584–5
  fibrinogen binding, **M**.588
  genetics, **M**.580, **M**.583
    benomyl resistance gene, **M**.608
    gene sequencing, **M**.583
    karyotype analysis, **M**.583–4
    mitochondrial DNA, **M**.103
    morphology, **M**.74–5
    mutants, **M**.584, **M**.584 (Fig.), **M**.587
    PCR, **M**.101–2
    ribosomal DNA, **M**.103
    SAP gene, **M**.103
  histopathology, **M**.87 (Fig.), **M**.128 (Tab.),
      M.134 (Fig.), **M**.142 (Fig.)
  history, **M**.5, **M**.7 (Fig.), **M**.13–4, **M**.14 (Fig.),
      M.579–80
  identification, germ tube test, **M**.604–5
  infection *see* Candidiasis

  morphology, **M**.582, **M**.588–9
    biofilms, **M**.75–6
    chlamydoconidia, **M**.74, **M**.604–5
    dimorphism, **M**.74–6, **M**.75 (Fig.)
    genetic analysis, **M**.74–5
  as pathogen, **M**.255, **M**.258–9
    environmental factors, **M**.258–9
    hyphal form, **M**.258–9
    virulence factors, **M**.79–80, **M**.258–9
  phenotypic switching, **M**.76, **M**.76 (Fig.),
      M.589
  prevalence, **M**.584–5
  reference cultures, **B1**.29
  resistance
    amphotericin B, **M**.173
    azoles, **M**.169, **M**.170, **M**.174
    fluconazole, **M**.152, **M**.611, **M**.612
    flucytosine, **M**.176, **M**.585
  susceptibility testing, **M**.608–9, **M**.610 (Fig.)
  transmission, **M**.589
  vegetables, **B1**.281
  virulence factors, **M**.79–80, **M**.258–9
    agglutin-like sequence-1, **M**.259
Candida dubliniensis
  adherence, **M**.588
  classification, **M**.44–5, **M**.581
  discovery, **M**.580
  ecology, **M**.585
  epidemiology, **M**.585
  morphology, **M**.582
    chlamydoconidia, **M**.604–5
  nosocomial infection, **B1**.403
Candida fumigatus, genetic analysis, **M**.104
Candida glabrata
  adherence, **M**.588
  classification, **M**.580
  as commensal organism, **M**.257–8
  ecology, **M**.584–6
  epidemiology, **M**.584–6
  genetic analysis, **M**.583, **M**.584
    PCR, **M**.102, **M**.103
  histopathology, **M**.126 (Tab.), **M**.128 (Tab.),
      M.134 (Fig.), **M**.142 (Fig.)
  infection
    animal, **M**.601
    fungemia, **B1**.523
    gastrointestinal, **M**.599
    nosocomial, **B1**.403
    ocular, **M**.601
    oral, **M**.598
    proinflammatory cytokines, **M**.589–90
    vaginal, **M**.599
    see also Candidiasis
  mannan, **M**.99
  morphology, **M**.126 (Tab.), **M**.582
    dimorphism, **M**.75
  phenotypic switching, **M**.76
  phospholipases, **M**.588
  resistance
    azoles, **M**.170–1, **M**.174
    fluconazole, **M**.169, **M**.174, **M**.585–6
    flucytosine, **M**.176
  serology, **M**.99–101
  ubiquinones, **M**.580

Candida guilliermondii
  amphotericin B resistance, **M**.172
  classification, **M**.580–1
  ecology, **M**.584–5
  epidemiology, **M**.584–5
  histopathology, **M**.128 (Tab.)
  infection
    cutaneous, **M**.595
    keratitis, **M**.328
    nosocomial, **M**.585
    onychomycosis, **M**.597
    oral, **M**.598
    see also Candidiasis
  mannan, **M**.99
  morphology, **M**.582
  serology, **M**.99
  ubiquinones, **M**.580
Candida kefyr
  classification, **M**.580–1
  cutaneous infection, **M**.595
    see also Candidiasis
  ecology, **M**.584–6
  epidemiology, **M**.584–6
  morphology, **M**.582
  ubiquinones, **M**.580
Candida krusei
  classification, **M**.580–1
  as commensal organism, **M**.257–8
  culture, **M**.604, **M**.604 (Fig.)
  ecology, **M**.584–6
  epidemiology, **M**.584–6
  genetic analysis, **M**.585
    PCR, **M**.102–4
  histopathology, **M**.128 (Tab.)
  infection
    animal, **M**.602
    cutaneous, **M**.595
    ocular, **M**.601
    serology, **M**.99–101
    ubiquinones, **M**.580
    see also Candidiasis
  mannan, **M**.99
  morphology, **M**.582
    teleomorph, **M**.582
  nosocomial infection, **B1**.403
  phospholipases, **M**.588
  resistance, **M**.169
    amphotericin B, **M**.172
    azoles, **M**.169, **M**.173–4
    fluconazole, **M**.586
  see also Candidiasis
Candida lusitaniae, **M**.583
  amphotericin B resistance, **M**.172, **M**.611
  classification, **M**.580–1
  ecology, **M**.584–6
  epidemiology, **M**.584–6
  morphology, **M**.583
  serology, **M**.99
  teleomorph, **M**.583
  ubiquinones, **M**.580
Candida parapsilosis
  biochemistry
    heat shock proteins, **M**.101, **M**.102–3
    mannan, **M**.99
    phospholipases, **M**.588

Candida parapsilosis
biochemistry (*Continued*)
proteases, **M**.588
classification, **M**.580, **M**.581
ecology, **M**.584–6
epidemiology, **M**.584–6
genetic analysis, **M**.584
PCR, **M**.102–4
ribosomal DNA, **M**.103–4
guano, **M**.586
histopathology, **M**.128 (Tab.)
infection
animal, **M**.602
cutaneous infection, **M**.595
endocarditis, **M**.600
endophthalmitis, **M**.330
fungemia, **B1**.523
keratitis, **M**.328, **M**.331
nosocomial, **B1**.403, **M**.586
ocular, **M**.586, **M**.601
oculomycoses, **M**.280 (Tab.), **M**.286–7, **M**.327
onychomycosis, **M**.597
oral, **M**.598
serology, **M**.99, **M**.101
see also Candidiasis
morphology, **M**.583
phenotypic switching, **M**.76
Candida pseudotropicalis, **M**.128 (Tab.)
Candida (Torulopsis) stellata, fruit, **B1**.282
Candidate gene testing, **I**.572
Candida tropicalis
adherence, **M**.588
amphotericin B resistance, **M**.611
classification, **M**.580–1
as commensal organism, **M**.257–8
culture, **M**.604, **M**.604 (Fig.)
ecology, **M**.584–6
epidemiology, **M**.584–6
genetic analysis, **M**.584
PCR, **M**.102, **M**.103–4
ribosomal DNA, **M**.103–4
histopathology, **M**.128 (Tab.)
infection
animal, **M**.602
cutaneous infection, **M**.595
endocarditis, **M**.600
fungemia, **B1**.523, **M**.586
gastrointestinal, **M**.599
nosocomial, **B1**.403
oral, **M**.598
serology, **M**.99
ubiquinones, **M**.580
vaginal, **M**.599
see also Candidiasis
mannan, **M**.99
morphology, **M**.583
phenotypic switching, **M**.76
phospholipases, **M**.588
proteases, **M**.588
Candidatus, classification, **B2**.1964, **B2**.1967–8
Candidatus Helicobacter bovis, **B2**.1582–3
Candidatus Helicobacter suis, **B2**.1582–3
Candida viswanatii, **M**.580

Candidiasis, **M**.601, **B1**.679, **M.579–623**
animal infection, **M**.601, **M**.601–2
birds, **M**.586, **M**.601–2
bovine abortion, **M**.602
cell-mediated immune response, **M**.261, **M**.261 (Tab.), **M**.590, **M**.592–3, **M**.597
CTL, **M**.261
delayed-type hypersensitivity, **M**.261
T helper cells, type 1 (Th1), **M**.261
clinical presentation, **M**.595–601
angular cheilitis, **M**.598
cerebrospinal fluid, **M**.600
CNS infection *see below*
endocarditis, **M**.98, **M**.595, **M**.600
gallbladders, **M**.600
granulomas, **M**.597
hepatic, **M**.595, **M**.596 (Fig.), **M**.599–600
hepatosplenic, **M**.599–600
interdigital, **M**.189
liver, **M**.595, **M**.596 (Fig.), **M**.599–600
lung, **M**.600
mastitis, **M**.602
mucocutaneous *see* Candidiasis, cutaneous/mucocutaneous
oculomycoses *see below*
onychomycosis, **M**.189, **M**.597, **M**.602, **M**.609–11
otitis externa, **M**.247–8
pancreas, **M**.600
peritonitis, **M**.600
pulmonary, **M**.134 (Fig.)
renal, **M**.134 (Fig.), **M**.595, **M**.600
respiratory tract, **M**.600
skin infection *see* Candidiasis, cutaneous/mucocutaneous
spleen, **M**.595, **M**.599–600
urinary tract infection *see* Genitourinary tract infection
vaginal *see* Vulvovaginal candidiasis (VVC)
CNS infection, **M**.600
AIDS, **M**.600
meningitis, **M**.600, **M**.612
colony-stimulating factors, **M**.259–60, **M**.593, **M**.613
G-CSF, **M**.613
GM-CSF, **M**.593
concomitant zygomycosis, **M**.142 (Fig.)
cutaneous/mucocutaneous, **M**.189, **M**.255, **M**.584, **M**.595, **M**.602, **M**.609
acute infection, **M**.256
causative agents, **M**.595
chronic, **M**.13, **M**.255, **M**.256, **M**.597, **M**.610–11, **I**.779
clinical symptoms, **M**.256
diagnosis, **M**.258 (Tab.)
epidemiology, **M**.256
immune response, **M**.261–2, **M**.267 (Tab.)
skin testing, **M**.592
symptoms, **M**.258 (Tab.)
therapy, **M**.189, **M**.258 (Tab.)
cytokines, **M**.259–60, **M**.589–90
IFN-γ, **M**.593
ILs, **M**.592–3

diagnosis, **M**.97, **M**.125–7, **M**.602–8
biochemical tests, **M**.605, **M**.605 (Fig.)
DNA fingerprinting, **M**.257
EIAs, **M**.99, **M**.103–4
genus/strain, **M**.94
histopathology, **M**.89 (Tab.), **M**.125, **M**.126 (Tab.), **M**.128 (Tab.), **M**.134 (Fig.), **M**.142 (Fig.), **M**.594–5,
immunodiagnostic tests, **M**.591, **M**.606
in situ DNA hybridization, **M**.94
microscopy, **M**.602–3, **M**.606
Pastorex test, **M**.100, **M**.607
PCR *see* Polymerase chain reaction (PCR)
serology, **M**.92–3 (Tab.), **M**.97–104, **M**.605
serology/serological diagnosis *see below*
specimens, **M**.83 (Tab.), **M**.602–3, **M**.606
epidemiology, **M**.11–4, **M**.584–6
in AIDS *see* AIDS, concomitant infection
bartenders, **M**.597
children, **M**.596, **M**.609
dishwashers, **M**.597
fruit cannery workers, **M**.597
heroin addicts, **M**.12–3
prevalence, **M**.584
epithelial cells, **M**.260
fungemia, **B1**.522–4
antibacterial susceptibility/resistance, **B1**.524
history, **M**.5, **M**.7 (Fig.), **M**.13–4, **M**.14 (Fig.), **M**.579–80
humoral immunity, **M**.260–1, **M**.267 (Tab.)
IgA, **M**.260–1
immune response, **M**.590–4, **M**.597
acquired immunity, **M**.255–6
antibodies, **M**.607
antigens, **M**.590–1, **M**.607
CTL, **M**.261
cytokines *see above*
delayed-type hypersensitivity, **M**.261
dendritic cells, **M**.260
fungemia, **M**.13, **M**.586
humoral immunity *see above*
immunity, **M**.592, **M**.597
immunodiagnostic tests, **M**.97, **M**.591, **M**.606
immunosuppressive effect, **M**.589
innate resistance *see below*
leukoplakia, **M**.598
neutrophils, **I**.40, **I**.44
T cells, **M**.590, **M**.592–3, **M**.597
immunogenetics, **I**.595–6
immunosuppression, **M**.13, **M**.580, **M**.585, **M**.589
immunotherapy, **M**.267, **M**.597, **M**.611
anti-idiotypic vaccination, **M**.267
monoclonal antibodies, **M**.267
protease inhibitors, **M**.267
innate resistance, **M**.255–6, **M**.259–60, **M**.267 (Tab.)
cytokines, **M**.259–60
dendritic cells, **M**.260
epithelial cells, **M**.260

Candidiasis
  innate resistance (*Continued*)
    neutrophils, **M**.259
    NK cells, **M**.260
    phagocytosis, **M**.260
  nosocomial, **B1**.403, **M**.584–6, **M**.752
    epidemiological typing, **B1**.404–5
    spread by contact with staff, **B1**.378
    urine of catheterized patients, **B1**.679
  oculomycoses, **M**.280 (Tab.), **M**.286–7,
      M.586, **M**.601
    blepharitis, **M**.601
    Candida glabrata, **M**.601
    Candida parapsilosis, **M**.586, **M**.601
    chorioretinitis, **M**.320–1
    conjunctivitis, **M**.257, **M**.258 (Tab.), **M**.299,
      M.601
    contact lens contamination, **M**.331–2
    dacryocanaliculitis, **M**.298
    dacryocystitis, **M**.298, **M**.299
    endophthalmitis, **M**.317, **M**.318–19,
      M.320–1, **M**.329–30, **M**.586, **M**.601
    keratitis, **M**.257, **M**.258 (Tab.), **M**.300–3,
      M.305, **M**.307–9, **M**.312–15, **M**.328,
      M.601
    lacrimal canaliculitis, **M**.601
    oculomycoses, **M**.280 (Tab.)
    scleritis, **M**.317
    ulcerative blepharitis, **M**.296–7
  pathogenesis, **M**.589
  pathology, **M**.594–5
  prophylaxis, **M**.610–11, **M**.613, **M**.752
    fluconazole, **M**.586, **M**.610–11, **M**.613
  risk factors, **M**.594
  serology/serological diagnosis, **M**.92,
      M.93 (Tab.), **M**.97–104, **M**.605
  serotypes, **M**.581, **M**.585, **M**.590–1
  susceptibility, **M**.592
  therapy, **M**.580, **M**.609
    amphotericin B, **M**.610 (Fig.), **M**.611,
      M.613
    antibiotics, **M**.11–2
    azoles, **M**.12, **M**.257
    butaconazole, **M**.257
    caspofugin, **M**.613
    clotrimazole, **M**.609–10
    echinocandins, **M**.154–5
    fluconazole, **M**.257, **M**.610–11, **M**.610 (Fig.),
      M.612
    flucytosine, **M**.612
    immunotherapy *see above*
    itraconazole, **M**.611–13
    ketoconazole, **M**.609–10
    kidney, **M**.595, **M**.600
    miconazole, **M**.609–10
    nystatin, **M**.609, **M**.611
    susceptibility testing, **M**.608
    ubiquinones, **M**.580
    voriconazole, **M**.613
  transmission, **M**.589
  types of infection
    acute atrophic, **M**.598
    acute pseudomembranous, **M**.598
    chronic atrophic, **M**.598
    chronic hyperplastic, **M**.598
    cutaneous *see* Candidiasis, cutaneous/
      mucocutaneous
    deep-seated, **M**.13, **M**.595, **M**.597, **M**.599,
      M.606, **M**.611
    disseminated, **M**.134 (Fig.), **M**.601, **M**.612
    esophageal *see* Candidiasis, gastrointestinal
    gastrointestinal *see* Candidiasis,
      gastrointestinal
    genitourinary tract infection *see*
      Genitourinary tract infection;
      Vulvovaginal candidiasis (VVC)
    neonatal, **M**.13, **M**.14 (Fig.)
    oral *see* Oropharyngeal candidiasis (OPC)
    oropharyngeal (thrush) *see* Oropharyngeal
      candidiasis (OPC)
  vaccines, **M**.591, **M**.593–4, **M**.613, **I**.933 (Tab.)
Candidiasis, gastrointestinal, **M**.12–3,
    M.14 (Fig.), **M**.599
  as AIDS-defining illness, **M**.256
  animal infection, **M**.601
  animal models, **M**.262
  cancer patients, **M**.256
  causative agents, **M**.599
  colonization, **M**.584, **M**.589, **M**.594, **M**.599,
      M.613
  diagnosis, **M**.258 (Tab.)
  epidemiology, **M**.256
  esophageal, **M**.11, **M**.255, **M**.598, **M**.599,
      M.610–11
    animal infection, **M**.601
    host defenses, **M**.262
  immune response, **M**.262, **M**.267 (Tab.)
    animal models, **M**.262
    intraepithelial lymphocytes, **M**.262
    T helper cells, type 1 (Th1), **M**.262
  symptoms, **M**.258 (Tab.)
  therapy, **M**.258 (Tab.)
Candidiasis, superficial, **M**.13, **M.255–72**,
    M.594
  cutaneous *see* Candidiasis, cutaneous/
    mucocutaneous
  diagnosis, **M**.258 (Tab.)
  epidemiology, **M**.256–7
  gastrointestinal *see* Candidiasis,
    gastrointestinal
  general diagnosis, **M**.257
  mucocutaneous *see* Candidiasis, cutaneous/
    mucocutaneous
  ocular *see* Candidiasis, oculomycoses
  oropharyngeal *see* Oropharyngeal
    candidiasis (OPC)
  symptoms, **M**.258 (Tab.)
  therapy, **M**.182, **M**.183 (Tab.), **M**.189, **M**.257,
      M.258 (Tab.)
    azoles, **M**.182–3, **M**.257
    butaconazole, **M**.257
    fluconazole, **M**.189, **M**.257
    imidazoles, **M**.189
    itraconazole, **M**.189, **M**.257
    ketoconazole, **M**.257
    nystatin, **M**.257
    polyenes, **M**.182
    terbinafine, **M**.189
  vaginal *see* Vulvovaginal candidiasis (VVC)
Candidids, **M**.597
Candidin test, **M**.592
Candiduria, **M**.600

Candiru virus infection, **V2**.1047
Cand-Tech latex agglutination assay, **M**.98–9,
    M.607
Canine adenovirus (CAV), **V1**.444–5
Canine astrovirus (CAstV), **V2**.890 (Tab.)
Canine distemper virus, **V1**.712–13, **V1**.811–12
  cell attachment/penetration, **V1**.701–2
  classification, **V1**.382–3
  clinical manifestations, **V1**.811–12
  control, **V1**.812
    live vaccines, **V1**.812
    vaccines, **V1**.814–15, **I**.855 (Tab.)
  epizootiology, **V1**.812
  laboratory diagnosis, **V1**.812
  neurohoming, **V1**.811
  pathology, **V1**.811–12
  species affected, **V1**.811
    seals, **V1**.813–14
Canine enteric coronavirus (CCoV)
  infection, **V1**.841 (Tab.)
  membrane (M) protein, **V1**.837
Canine Minute virus (CnMV), **V1**.412
Canine oral papillomavirus (COPV)
  genome organization, **V1**.451 (Fig.)
  infection, **V1**.453
    temporal/spatial expression patterns,
      V1.453, **V1**.456 (Fig.)
  structure/morphology, **V1**.450 (Fig.)
Canine parvovirus (CPV)
  infection *see* Canine parvovirus (CPV)
    infection
  morphology/structure, **V1**.412, **V1**.413 (Fig.)
  vesicle trafficking, **V1**.417
Canine parvovirus (CPV) infection
  cell entry, **V1**.416–17
  emerging infection, **V2**.1651 (Tab.)
    mutation, **V2**.1653
    species-barrier crossing, **V2**.1657 (Tab.)
  endosomal bilayer penetration, **V1**.417–18
  neutralizing antibodies, **V1**.407–8
  nuclear targeting, **V1**.424
  pathogenesis, **V1**.426
  vaccines, **I**.855 (Tab.), **I**.871–2
  vesicle trafficking, **V1**.417
Canned products
  Clostridium botulinum spores destruction,
    B1.265–6, **B1**.270–1, **B1**.275, **B1**.283
  container integrity, **B1**.271, **B1**.283
  cured meats, **B1**.275
  fruit, **B1**.283
  meat and meat products, **B1**.275
  spoilage, **B1**.271, **B1**.283
  vegetables, **B1**.283
Caño Delgadito virus, **V2**.1666 (Tab.)
Canonical discriminant variates, **B1**.28
Cantaloupes, **B1**.283
Capillaria, **P**.589, **P**.743–7
  classification, **P**.743
  control, **P**.747
  general biology, **P**.743–4
  historical aspects, **P**.743
  infection
    clinical manifestations, **P**.746
    diagnosis, **P**.746
    immune response, **P**.746

Capillaria,
  infection (*Continued*)
    location in host, **P**.745
    pathogenesis/pathology, **P**.746
    transmission/epidemiology, **P**.745
  life cycle, **P**.744–5
  morphology/structure, **P**.743
  see also individual species
Capillaria aerophila
  classification, **P**.743
  control, **P**.747
  general biology, **P**.744
  historical aspects, **P**.743
  infection
    clinical manifestations, **P**.746
    diagnosis, **P**.746
    location in host, **P**.745
    pathogenesis/pathology, **P**.746
    transmission/epidemiology, **P**.745
  life cycle, **P**.745
  morphology/structure, **P**.743
Capillaria hepatica
  classification, **P**.743
  control, **P**.747
  general biology, **P**.744
  historical aspects, **P**.743
  infection
    clinical manifestations, **P**.746
    diagnosis, **P**.746
    location in host, **P**.745
    pathogenesis/pathology, **P**.746
    transmission/epidemiology, **P**.745
  life cycle, **P**.745
    eggs, **P**.744 (Fig.)
  morphology/structure, **P**.743
Capillaria philippiensis
  classification, **P**.743
  control, **P**.747
  general biology, **P**.743
  historical aspects, **P**.743
  infection
    clinical manifestations, **P**.746
    diagnosis, **P**.746
    location in host, **P**.745
    pathogenesis/pathology, **P**.746
    transmission/epidemiology, **P**.745
  life cycle, **P**.744–5
    autoinfection, **P**.745
    eggs, **P**.744 (Fig.)
    hyperinfection, **P**.745
  morphology/structure, **P**.743
  public health importance, **P**.44
Capillovirus, **V1**.27 (Tab.)
Capnocytophaga, **B2**.1930
  antibacterial susceptibility/resistance,
    B2.1677
  characteristics, **B2**.1675–7, **B2**.1676 (Tab.)
  culture, **B2**.1675–7
  habitats, **B2**.1649–50
  infection, **B2**.1674–5
    clinical significance, **B2**.1674–5
    gingivitis, **B1**.614
    nosocomial, **B1**.401 (Tab.)

isolation/identification, **B2**.1675–7
    differentiating characteristics,
      B2.1949 (Tab.)
  as normal microbiota, **B1**.296 (Tab.)
  species, **B2**.1930
  taxonomy, **B2**.1673–4
  virulence factors, **B2**.1674–5
Capnocytophaga canimorsus, **B2**.1675–7,
    B2.1676 (Tab.)
  antibacterial susceptibility/resistance,
    B2.1677
  classification, **B2**.1673–4
  culture, **B2**.1675–7
  identification, **B2**.1675–7
  infection in humans, **B2**.1674–5
Capnocytophaga cynodegmi, **B2**.1675–7,
    B2.1676 (Tab.)
  classification, **B2**.1673–4
  identification, **B2**.1675–7
Capnocytophaga gingivalis, **B2**.1676 (Tab.)
  classification, **B2**.1673
Capnocytophaga granulosa, **B2**.1676 (Tab.)
  classification, **B2**.1673
Capnocytophaga haemolytica, **B2**.1676 (Tab.)
  classification, **B2**.1673
Capnocytophaga ochracea, **B2**.1676 (Tab.)
  classification, **B2**.1673
Capnocytophaga sputigena, **B2**.1676 (Tab.)
  classification, **B2**.1673
Capping, **P**.180
  bunyavirus transcription, **V2**.1035
  gene expression, **V1**.112–13
Capping enzyme, poxviruses, **V1**.599 (Tab.)
Capravirine, **V2**.1623
  structure, **V2**.1622 (Fig.)
Capripoxvirus, **V1**.588
  classification, **V1**.579 (Tab.), **V1**.582, **V1**.594
  genome structure, **V1**.583
  phylogenetics, **V1**.583
  taxonomy, **V1**.595 (Tab.)
CA protein *see* HIV
Capsid(s), **V1**.6
  assembly
    foamy viruses, **V2**.1310
    isocahedral viruses, **V1**.65–7
    scaffolds, **V1**.65–7
  herpesviruses, **V1**.501
  HIV, **V1**.78–9, **V1**.78 (Fig.)
  HSV, **V2**.1597
  parvoviruses *see* Parvoviruses
  respiroviruses *see* Respiroviruses
  retroviruses, **V1**.78–9, **V1**.78 (Fig.)
  self-assembly, **V1**.65
Capsid (C) protein
  alphaviruses, **V2**.1014
  astroviruses *see* Astroviruses
  noroviruses *see* Noroviruses
  Rubella virus *see* Rubella virus (RV)
  sapoviruses, **V2**.923
Capsids, **B1**.140
'Cap-snatching'
  arenaviruses, **V1**.131–2
  bunyaviruses, **V1**.110, **V1**.131–2
  negative-strand RNA viruses, **V1**.131–2
  orthomyxoviruses, **V1**.110, **V1**.131–2

Capsules
  bacterial
    Aeromonas, **B2**.1527
    antigenic variation, **I**.660–1
    Burkholderia thailandensis, **B2**.1622
    composition, **B1**.44
    Enterobacter, **B2**.1343
    Enterobacteriaceae, **B2**.1339–40, **B2**.1343
    Escherichia coli, **B2**.1343
    Haemophilus, **B2**.1698
    Klebsiella, **B2**.1343
    polysaccharides, **I**.935
    Streptococcus pneumoniae, **B1**.608–9
  mycology, *Cryptococcus neoformans*,
    M.93 (Tab.), **M**.639 (Fig.), **M**.641–2
Carbacefem, structure, **B1**.471 (Fig.)
Carbacephems, **B1**.478–80
  structure, **B1**.479 (Fig.)
  see also specific types
Carbanilides, **B1**.428
Carbapenemases, *Bacteroides/Prevotella/*
    Porphyromonas, **B2**.1936
Carbapenems, **B1**.478–80
  resistance, **B1**.478–80
    verona imipenemase, **B1**.478–80
  resistance to, **B1**.478–80
  spectrum of activity
    Eikenella corrodens, **B2**.1668
    Klebsiella, **B2**.1480
    Proteus, **B2**.1443–4
    Vibrio, **B2**.1514
  structure, **B1**.471 (Fig.), **B1**.479 (Fig.)
  see also specific types
Carbenicillin
  history, **B1**.473
  pharmacology, **B1**.475
  spectrum of activity
    Citrobacter, **B2**.1476
    Enterobacter, **B2**.1484–5
    Escherichia, **B2**.1369–70
    Ewingella, **B2**.1493
    Kluyvera, **B2**.1494
    Leclercia, **B2**.1495
    Leminorella, **B2**.1496
  structure, **B1**.474 (Fig.)
Carbohydrate(s)
  bacterial, **B1**.42
  Bifidobacterium bifidum metabolism,
    B2.1027
  Blastocystis hominis, **P**.561
  Borrelia metabolism, **B2**.1827–8
  immune response, **I**.376, **I**.376 (Tab.)
  metabolism
    Plasmodium see Plasmodium
    tapeworms, **P**.662
  Pseudomonas metabolism, **B1**.59–60
  storage in vacuoles of protozoa, **P**.179
  subunit vaccines, **I**.424–5
Carbohydrate metabolism, *Candida*
    physiology, **M**.583, **M**.605
Carbon compounds
  five-carbon, metabolism, **B1**.57
  one-carbon incorporation into cellular
    material, **B1**.61–3
Carbon cycling, soil bacteria, **B1**.199–200

Carbon dioxide
  antibacterial properties, **B1**.430
  in atmosphere
    fruit, **B1**.283
    poultry, **B1**.277–8
    vegetables, **B1**.282
  Brucella culture, **B2**.1735
  fixation, **B1**.61–3
    Calvin cycle, **B1**.62
    other pathways, **B1**.62
    reductive TCA cycle, **B1**.62
  formation in glucose fermentations, **B1**.54,
    B1.58
  methane formation, **B1**.68
  Neisseria culture, **B2**.1274–5
Carbonic anhydrase production, *Neisseria,*
  B2.1270
Carbovir *see* Abacavir
Carboxypenicillins, *Proteus,* **B2**.1443–4
Carboxypeptidase N (anaphylatoxin
    inactivator), **I**.147
Carcinoembryonic antigen-related cell
    adhesion molecules, **V1**.246 (Fig.)
Carcinogens/carcinogenesis, **V1**.330
  clonorchiasis, **P**.651
  nitrosamines formation, **B1**.200
  opisthorchiasis, **P**.651
  poxviruses, **V1**.257
  see also Oncogenes; Oncogenesis
CARD10 (Mimp1), **I**.347
CARD11 (CARMA1), **I**.347
CARD14 (Bimp2), **I**.347
Card agglutination test for trypanosomes
    (CATT), **P**.129–30, **P**.367
Cardiac disease
  enterovirus infection, **V2**.871
  Whipple's disease, **B2**.999
Cardiac surgery
  bacterial infection after, **B1**.385
  fungal endophthalmitis after, **M**.318
Cardiac toxicity, diphtheria, **B2**.985
Cardiobacterium
  antibacterial susceptibility/resistance,
    B2.1672–3
  habitats, **B2**.1649–50
Cardiobacterium hominis, **B2**.1671–3
  antibacterial susceptibility/resistance,
    B2.1672–3
  characteristics, **B2**.1668 (Tab.), **B2**.1672
  classification, **B2**.1671
  culture, **B2**.1672
  identification, **B2**.1672
  infection, **B2**.1671–2
    clinical significance, **B2**.1671–2
    endocarditis, **B1**.532
  as normal microbiota, **B1**.296 (Tab.)
  taxonomy, **B2**.1671
Cardiolipin, *Blastocystis hominis,* **P**.561
Cardiovascular syphilis, **B2**.1855,
  B2.1855 (Tab.)
Cardioviruses
  cell entry, **V2**.867 (Tab.)
  characteristics, **V2**.861 (Tab.)
  classification, **V2**.858, **V2**.859 (Fig.)
  genome structure, **V2**.865
  morphology/structure, **V2**.862, **V2**.863

properties, **V2**.1162 (Tab.)
  size, **V2**.859
Carlavirus, **V1**.27 (Tab.)
CARMA1, **I**.347
Carotid artery stenosis, *Chlamydia
    pneumoniae* infection, **B2**.2016
Carrier proteins
  BCE peptide vaccines *see* Peptide vaccines,
    B-cell epitopes
  conjugate vaccines, **I**.935
  measles peptide vaccine, **I**.868–9
Carriers, **B1**.310, **B1**.338
  counseling, **V2**.1256
  hepatitis B *see* Hepatitis B
Carrión's disease, **B2**.1888–91
  clinical manifestations, **B2**.1888–9
    immunosuppression, **B2**.1888–9
  diagnosis, **B2**.1889–91
    culture, **B2**.1889–90
    histopathology, **B2**.1890–1
    PCR, **B2**.1890
    serology, **B2**.1890
  dormancy/latency, **B2**.1889
  geographical distribution, **B2**.1888
  historical perspective, **B2**.1885
  pathogenesis, **B2**.1891
  in pregnancy, **B2**.1889
  seroprevalence, **B2**.1889
  transmission, **B2**.1888
  treatment, **B2**.1891
    public health control measures, **B2**.1889
  see also Oroya fever; Verruga peruana
Cartilage hair hypoplasia (CHH), **I**.777
CART regime, protease inhibitors, **V2**.1336
Casamino acids-erythritol-albumin medium,
  M.236–7
Caseation, tuberculosis granulomas, **I**.713,
  I.715 (Fig.)
Case clusters, adverse reactions to vaccines,
  B1.325–6
Case–control studies
  bacterial infection, **B1**.315–16, **B1**.315 (Fig.)
    adverse reactions to vaccines, **B1**.325–6
    bias, **B1**.316
    disadvantages, **B1**.316
    outbreak investigation, **B1**.330
    statistical analysis, **B1**.316
    vaccine efficacy, **B1**.324–5
  immunogenetics, **I**.574
  viral infection, **V1**.361–3
    advantages/disadvantages, **V1**.362 (Tab.)
    cohort studies *vs.,* **V1**.361–2
    design, **V1**.362
    rubella epidemiology, **V1**.362–3
Case definition, in outbreak investigation,
  B1.327
Case-finding
  infection control, **B1**.347
  nosocomial infection surveillance, **B1**.405,
    B1.406 (Tab.)
Case identification, outbreaks, **B1**.327–8
Case management, cysticercosis control, **P**.119
Case series analyses, adverse reactions to
    vaccines, **B1**.325–6
Caspase(s), **I**.133–5
  bacterial immune interference, **I**.655

executioners, **I**.133–4
herpesvirus infection, **I**.776
inhibition, **I**.135, **V1**.324
  viral infection, **I**.625 (Fig.), **I**.627
initiators, **I**.133–4
protein–protein interactions, **I**.134–5
proteolytic cleavage, **I**.134
  granzyme M, **I**.476
structure, **I**.133, **I**.134 (Fig.)
subcellular compartmentalization, **I**.135
see also individual types
Caspase-1
  in macrophage apoptosis, **I**.137–8
  structure, **I**.134 (Fig.)
Caspase-2, **I**.134 (Fig.)
Caspase-3
  apoptosis initiation, **I**.134
  structure, **I**.134 (Fig.)
Caspase-5, **I**.134 (Fig.)
Caspase-8
  activation, **I**.134
  deficiency, **I**.776
  structure, **I**.134 (Fig.)
Caspase-9
  apoptosome activation, **I**.134–5
  structure, **I**.134 (Fig.)
Caspase-11, **I**.134 (Fig.)
Caspase-activated DNase (CAD)
  apoptosis, **I**.136
  granzyme M cleavage, **I**.476
Caspase activation and recruitment domain
    (CARD), **I**.134
  Bcl-10, **I**.346–7
  mitochondrial apoptosis, **I**.624
  as PPR, **I**.115
  signal transduction, **I**.115
  single nucleotide polymorphisms, **I**.125
Caspofungin, **M**.154
  characteristics, **M**.155 (Tab.)
  mechanism of action, **M**.70–1
  resistance, **M**.176
  therapy
    Acremonium infection, **M**.758
    aspergillosis, **M**.724, **M**.726
    candidiasis, **M**.613
    Paecilomyces infection, **M**.758
    Scopulariopsis infection, **M**.758–9
Castelo dos Sonhos virus, **V2**.1666 (Tab.)
Cat(s)
  Bartonella henselae reservoir, **B1**.536
  bites *see* Bites
  leprosy, **B2**.1182
  protothecosis, **M**.398, **M**.400
  rhinosporidiosis, **M**.456–7, **M**.464, **M**.466,
    M.472
  sporotrichosis, **M**.367–8, **M**.369 (Tab.),
    M.370
  toxoplasmosis
    prevention, **P**.439
    transmission, **P**.433, **P**.436
    vaccination, **P**.439
Catabolite control protein (CcpA), **B1**.73–4
Catabolite gene activator protein (CAP),
  B1.73

Catabolite repression, **B1**.72–3
  Escherichia coli and other enteric bacteria, **B1**.73
  mechanisms, **B1**.73
  role of phosphoenolpyruvate phosphotransferase system, **B1**.50, **B1**.73
Catabolite-responsive elements (CRE), **B1**.73–4
Catalase(s)
  conditions in soil, **B1**.196–7
  Helicobacter pathogenicity, **B2**.1576
  parasite immune avoidance mechanisms, **I**.686
  Porphyromonas identification, **B2**.1924 (Tab.)
  Prevotella identification, **B2**.1924 (Tab.)
Catalase-negative gram-positive cocci, **B2**.883 (Tab.)
Cataracts
  nosocomial infection, **B1**.386
  rubella, **V2**.973, **V2**.974 (Fig.)
  Spiroplasma, **B2**.1966
Cat bites *see* Bites
Catecholamines
  acute phase response, **I**.208
  degradation, *Cryptococcus neoformans*, **M**.642
Catfish *(Pangasius hypophthalmus)*, *Bacillus* infection, **B2**.944
Cathelicidins, **I**.172–5
  bactenecins, **I**.173
  genetics, **I**.174–5
  hCAP-18 *see* HCAP-18
  indolicidin, structure, **I**.172
  mechanism of action, **I**.172
  PR-39, **I**.173
    genes, **I**.174
  prophenins, **I**.173
  protegrins, **I**.172, **I**.174
    genes, **I**.174
  SMAP-29, **I**.173
  structure, **I**.172
    α-helical domains, **I**.173
    amino acid sequences, **I**.173 (Tab.)
    β-sheet domains, **I**.172
    proline-rich domains, **I**.172–3
    short antimicrobial domains, **I**.172
  synthesis/storage, **I**.173–4
    azurophilic granules, **I**.174
    neutrophil elastase, **I**.174
  tritrpticin *see* Tritrpticin
  see also individual types
Cathelin-related antimicrobial peptide (CRAMP), **I**.521
  expression, **I**.174
  genes, **I**.175
  structure, **I**.174
Cathepsin C deficiency, **I**.482–3
Cathepsin D, phagosome, **I**.25
Cathepsin G, neutrophil production, **I**.41
Cathepsin L inhibitor *see* Cathelicidins
Cathepsin L-like proteases, liver/lung flukes, **P**.652
Cathepsin S, **I**.382–3
Catheter(s)
  colonization, **B1**.391
    prevention, **B1**.391

infection associated, **B1**.388
  bacteremia, **B1**.510, **B1**.512–13
  elderly, **B1**.394
  Gordania sputi, **B2**.1152
  Gordania terrae, **B2**.1152–3
  Malassezia, **M**.626–7
  prevention, **B1**.388
  rapidly growing mycobacteria, **B2**.1250, **B2**.1253, **B2**.1255, **B2**.1261
  trichosporonosis, **M**.629
  Ustilago, **M**.630
  urinary, **B1**.674
    cultures, **B1**.679
    infection, **B1**.388
    sample collection, **B1**.677
    unacceptable specimens/deprecated procedures, **B1**.679
Cation exchange capacity (CEC), clay soils, **B1**.196
Cationic amino acid transporter, structure, **V1**.246 (Fig.)
Cationic liposomes, DNA vaccine encapsulation, **I**.913
Cat-scratch disease
  clinical manifestations, **B2**.1891–3, **B2**.1892 (Fig.), **B2**.1893 (Tab.)
    disseminated, **B2**.1892–3
    fever of unknown origin, **B2**.1892–3
    lymphadenitis, **B2**.1891
    neurology, **B2**.1892
    ocular, **B2**.1892
    regional lymphadenopathy, **B2**.1891–2
  diagnosis, **B2**.1894–8
    biochemistry, **B2**.1895
    culture, **B2**.1895
    histopathology, **B2**.1898
    PCR, **B2**.1895–7
  differential diagnosis, **B2**.1891
  epidemiology, **B2**.1891
  historical perspective, **B2**.1891
  serology, **B2**.1897–8
  treatment, **B2**.1898–9
Cattle
  abortion, **B2**.1549
    Aspergillus fumigatus, **M**.692
    Candida, **M**.602
  actinomycosis or 'lumpy jaw,' **B2**.1018
  botulism, **B2**.1074
  bronchopneumonia, **B2**.1653–4
  campylobacter mastitis, **B2**.1550
  Escherichia coli, O157:H7 reservoirs, **B1**.274
  Johne's disease, **B2**.1182
  listeriosis in, **B2**.963
  mastitis, **B1**.230, **B1**.239, **B1**.243–5, **M**.399–400, **M**.407
    Arcobacter, **B2**.1557
    Campylobacter, **B2**.1550
  pathogens
    Actinobacillus lignieresii, **B2**.1665–6
    Brucella, **B1**.229, **B1**.536
    Campylobacter, **B2**.1549
    Mannheimia haemolytica, **B2**.1654
    Mycobacterium bovis, **B2**.1200
    Mycobacterium paratuberculosis, **B2**.1182
    Pasteurella multocida, **B2**.1653–4

    pneumonic pasteurellosis/shipping fever, **B2**.1654
  prototheosis, **M**.399–400, **M**.407
  rhinosporidiosis, **M**.439, **M**.456–7, **M**.460, **M**.472
  septicemia, hemorrhagic, **B2**.1653–4
  tuberculosis, **B1**.229
  waterborne bacteria, **B1**.212, **B1**.218, **B1**.223–4
  wooden tongue disease, **B2**.1665–6
Cattle plague *see* Rinderpest
Caudovirales order, **V1**.26, **V1**.378
  classification, **V1**.42, **V1**.43 (Tab.), **V1**.390–2
Caulimoviridae
  classification, **V1**.27 (Tab.), **V1**.45–6, **V1**.46 (Tab.), **V1**.47
  see also Caulimoviruses; *specific viruses*
Caulimoviruses
  evolution, **V1**.13
  reverse transcription, **V1**.181–2
  see also Caulimoviridae
Caveolae, *Plasmodium*, **P**.473–5
Cavitary lesions, **M**.699
cblA, *Burkholderia* infection in cystic fibrosis, **B2**.1612
CC16 gene, IgE production, **I**.582
CC chemokine(s), **I**.217, **I**.218 (Tab.)
  basophil chemotaxis, **I**.58, **I**.60
  basophil histamine release, **I**.62
  eosinophil chemotaxis, **I**.61
  Human respiratory syncytial virus infection, **V1**.793–4
  macrophage production, **I**.28–9
  motif ligand, **I**.582
  receptors *see below*
  structure, **I**.217–19
  viral analogues, HHV-8, **V1**.550
CC chemokine receptors, **I**.220, **I**.510 (Tab.)
  CCR1, **I**.510 (Tab.)
    cell expression, **I**.223–4
    dendritic cells, **I**.224, **I**.393–4
    inflammatory disease, **I**.227
    ligands, **I**.224
    NK cells, **I**.224
    synthetic antagonists, **I**.231
    T cells, **I**.224
  CCR2
    CCR2b gene deletions, **I**.585
    cell expression, **I**.223–4
    deletion effects, **I**.228
    dendritic cells, **I**.224, **I**.393–4
    inflammatory disease, **I**.227
    ligands, **I**.224
    NK cells, **I**.224
    synthetic antagonists, **I**.231
    T cells, **I**.224
  CCR3 (eotaxin receptor), **I**.224–5, **I**.510 (Tab.)
    airway hypersensitivity, **I**.736
    allergic reactions, **I**.227
    cell expression, **I**.223–4, **I**.224–5
    chemokine antagonists, **I**.232
    CTLs, **I**.225
    dendritic cells, **I**.224
    eotaxin binding, **I**.60–1
    ligands, **I**.224

CC chemokine receptors
  CCR3 (eotaxin receptor) (*Continued*)
    NK cells, I.224
    synthetic antagonists, I.231
    T cells, I.224
    Th2 cells, I.224–5, I.400
  CCR4, I.510 (Tab.)
    CTLs, I.225
    memory T cells, I.227
    Th2 cells, I.225
  CCR5, I.510 (Tab.)
    CCR5 gene deletions, I.585
    cell expression, I.223–4
    CTLs, I.225
    dendritic cells, I.224, I.393–4
    HIV coreceptor, V1.106, I.227–8, V1.247, V1.253, I.585, V2.1323
    inactive variant expression, I.229
    inflammatory disease, I.227
    ligands, I.224
    memory lymphocytes, I.225
    memory T cells, I.225
    NK cells, I.224
    polymorphisms, HIV infection, V1.265, V1.265 (Tab.)
    structure, V1.246 (Fig.)
    synthetic antagonists, I.231
    T cells, I.224
    Th1 cells, I.225, I.400
  CCR6, I.510 (Tab.)
  CCR7, I.510 (Tab.)
    B cell homing, I.226
    CD4+CD45RO+ T cells, I.225–6
    deficient mice models, I.226
    dendritic cells, I.377–8, I.393–4
    lymphoid tissue homing, I.226
    memory lymphocytes, I.225
  CCR8, I.510 (Tab.)
    CTLs, I.225
    Th2 cells, I.225
  CCR9, I.510 (Tab.)
    memory T cells, I.227
    thymus expressed chemokine binding, I.227
  CCR10, I.510 (Tab.)
    cutaneous T-cell attracting chemokine (CTACK:CCL27), I.218 (Tab.), I.227
    memory T cells, I.227
  cell expression, I.220
  monocytes, I.223–4
  phagocytes, I.223–4
C chemokines, macrophage production, I.28–9
CCL1 (I-309), I.218 (Tab.)
CCL2 *see* Monocyte chemoattractant protein 1 (MCP-1: CCL2)
CCL3 *see* Macrophage inflammatory protein 1α (MIP-1α)
CCL3L1 (LD78β), I.218 (Tab.)
CCL4 *see* Macrophage inflammatory protein 1β (MIP-1β: CCL4)
CCL5 *see* RANTES (CCL5)
CCL7 *see* Monocyte chemoattractant protein 3 (MCP-3: CCL7)
CCL8 *see* Monocyte chemoattractant protein 2 (MCP-2: CCL8)

CCL11 (eotaxin-1), I.218 (Tab.)
CCL13 *see* Monocyte chemoattractant protein 4 (MCP-4: CCL13)
CCL14 (HCC-1), I.218 (Tab.)
CCL15 (HCC-2), I.218 (Tab.)
CCL16 (HCC-4), I.218 (Tab.)
CCL17 (TARC), I.218 (Tab.)
  CCR4 binding, I.227
CCL18 (DC-CK1), I.218 (Tab.)
CCL19 *see* Epstein–Barr virus-induced receptor ligand chemokine (ELC:CCL19)
CCL20, I.218 (Tab.)
  defensin competition, I.169
CCL21 *see* Secondary lymphoid tissue chemokine (SLC:CCL21)
CCL22 (MDC: STCP-1), I.218 (Tab.)
CCL23 (CKβ8), I.218 (Tab.)
CCL24 *see* Eotaxin-2 (CCL24)
CCL25 *see* Thymus expressed chemokine (TECK: CCL25)
CCL26 (eotaxin-3), I.61, I.218 (Tab.)
CCL27 *see* Cutaneous T-cell attracting chemokine (CTACK:CCL27)
CCL28 *see* MEC (CCL28)
CCR1 *see* CC chemokine receptors
CCR2 *see* CC chemokine receptors
CCR2b gene deletions, I.585
CCR3 *see* CC chemokine receptors
CCR4 *see* CC chemokine receptors
CCR5 *see* CC chemokine receptors
CCR5 gene deletions, I.585
CCR6, I.393–4, I.510 (Tab.)
CCR7 *see* CC chemokine receptors
CCR8 *see* CC chemokine receptors
CCR9 *see* CC chemokine receptors
CD1
  antigen presentation, I.29
  dendritic cell expression, I.442
  non-epidermal γδ T cells, I.438
CD1a/b/c-reactive T cells *see* αβ T-cells
CD1d-reactive T cells *see* αβ T-cells
CD2
  antigen presentation, I.384
  CD4 T cells, I.392 (Fig.), I.396
  NK cell development, I.85
  T cell development, I.455–6
  TCR–superantigen binding, I.560
CD3
  αβ TCRs interactions, I.460–1
  CD4 T cells, I.389, I.395
  deficiency, I.775
  HIV infection, I.793
  structure, I.395
  transduction complex, I.459 (Fig.), I.460
CD4
  BCR signaling, I.347
  CD4 T cells/APC interactions, I.392 (Fig.)
  degradation, Vpu protein, V2.1327–8
  downregulation, Nef protein, V2.1329
  HIV cellular receptor, V2.1323
  HIV entry into cells, I.389
  Nef expression downregulation, I.789
  structure, V1.211 (Fig.)
  T cell development, I.455–6

  TCR structure, I.460
  viral receptor, V1.209
CD4+CD45RO+ T cells
  chemokine receptors, I.225–6
  IL-9 production, I.281–2
CD4+ T-cell(s), V1.274–5, **I.389–402**
  accessory/co-stimulatory molecules, I.392 (Fig.), I.395–6, I.399
    4–1BBL, I.396
    B7–1 (CD80), I.392 (Fig.), I.394
    B7–2 (CD86), I.392 (Fig.), I.394
    B7-related ligand, I.392 (Fig.), I.395
    CD2, I.392 (Fig.), I.396
    CD3, I.389, I.395
    CD28, I.392 (Fig.), I.395, I.399
    CD40, I.392 (Fig.)
    CD40 ligand, I.396
    CD45, I.392 (Fig.)
    CD48, I.392 (Fig.)
    CD402, I.392 (Fig.)
    CTLA-4, I.399
    ICAM-1, I.392 (Fig.)
    ICAM-3, I.396
    ICOS, I.392 (Fig.), I.395, I.399
    leukocyte function antigen, I.392 (Fig.), I.396
    MHC class II, I.392 (Fig.)
    OX-40, I.392 (Fig.), I.396
    OX40-ligand, I.392 (Fig.)
    TCR, I.392 (Fig.), I.395
    TRANCE, I.396
  activation, I.392
  antigen presentation to, I.390, I.393–4
    B cells, I.394
    by dendritic cells, I.393
    epithelial cells, I.394
    macrophages, I.394
    MHC class II, I.389–90, I.392–3, I.426, I.877
    see also Major histocompatibility complex (MHC) class II
    MHC restriction, I.375, I.426, I.427 (Fig.)
    Th1/Th2 differentiation, I.399
  chemokine effects, I.224
  cytokines produced, I.395
    IL-5, I.57
  deficiency, V1.276
  dendritic cell interactions, I.393–4
    co-stimulatory molecules, I.394
    long-term persistence, I.392
    see also above antigen presentation
  development, I.390–2, I.391 (Fig.)
    negative selection, I.390, I.392
    positive selection, I.390, I.392
    thymus-dependent areas, I.393
  functions/role, I.389–90, I.390 (Fig.), I.404
    antibody-dependent cell-mediated cytotoxicity, I.791
    autoimmune diseases, I.390
    B-cell activation, I.326, I.400–1
    see also Germinal centers (GCs)
    CD8 T cell activation, I.426
    extracellular pathogens, I.390
    IgA synthesis, I.536

CD4+ T-cell(s)
functions/role (*Continued*)
memory B cell development, **I**.493
soluble antigen recognition, **I**.375
tolerance induction *see below*
granulomas, **I**.706–7
tuberculosis, **I**.713
IL-12 effect, **V1**.298
infection
cryptococcosis, **M**.645
histoplasmosis capsulati, **M**.527–8
Pneumocystis carinii infection, **M**.792,
M.793, **M**.796
subacute sclerosing panencephalitis,
V1.731
viruses *see below*
long-term persistence, **I**.392
lymphocytopenia, **I**.776, **I**.779
memory, chemokine receptors, **I**.225–6
MHC class II antigen presentation, **V1**.274–5
phenotypic markers, **I**.389
primary infection, kinetics, **I**.493–4,
I.494 (Fig.)
signaling, **I**.395
phosphatidyl-3-kinase, **I**.395
superantigens, **I**.394–5
TCE peptide vaccines, **I**.878
T helper cells type 1 *see* T-helper cells type 1
(Th1)
T helper cells type 2 *see* T-helper cells type 2
(Th2)
tissue distribution, **I**.389
tolerance induction, **I**.396–7, **I**.397 (Tab.)
clonal anergy, **I**.396, **I**.397 (Tab.)
co-stimulation lack, **I**.396
CTLA-4, **I**.396–7
PD-1, **I**.397
viral infection, **V1**.275 (Fig.)
hepatitis B, **V1**.283
HIV infection *see* HIV infection
HSV, **V1**.284–5, **V1**.510
HTLV type 1 tropism, **V2**.1288
Human respiratory syncytial virus,
V1.795–6
influenza, **V1**.664, **V1**.665
LCMV, **V2**.1072, **V2**.1075
measles, **V1**.726, **I**.805, **V2**.1433
see also T-helper cell(s)
CD5
B-cell downregulation, **I**.348
T cell development, **I**.455–6
CD7, intraepithelial lymphocytes, **I**.525–6
CD8
T cell development, **I**.455–6
TCR structure, **I**.460
CD8+ T-cell(s), **V1**.275, **I.419–34**
activation, **I**.404, **I**.426–8
'afferent,' **I**.404
APC interactions, **I**.404, **I**.426–7
Bcl-2 expression, **I**.428
CD4 T cell role, **I**.426
CD28, **I**.428
co-stimulatory molecules, **I**.428
cytokines, **I**.426, **I**.427–8
dendritic cells, **I**.404
'efferent,' **I**.404

GM-CSF, **I**.427–8
IFN-γ, **I**.427–8
IL-2, **I**.427–8
IL-4, **I**.427–8
IL-12, **I**.427–8
antigen presentation to
MHC class I, **I**.877
see also Major histocompatibility
complex (MHC) class I
MHC restriction, **I**.375, **I**.426,
I.427 (Fig.)
bacterial immunity, **I**.420
chemokine effects, **I**.224
chemokines produced, **I**.422
ciral infection, HTLV-1-associated
myelopathy/tropical spastic paraparesis
(HAM/TSP), **V2**.1290, **V2**.1429–30
cytokines produced, **I**.421–2
IL-5, **I**.57
IL-16, **I**.289
cytotoxicity, **I**.422–3
Fas/Fas ligand mediated apoptosis,
I.422–3
granzymes, **I**.422–3
induced apoptosis, **I**.422–3
perforin, **I**.422–3
viral infection, **I**.419–20
DNA vaccine priming, **I**.914
functions, **I**.404
granulomas, **I**.709
in immunity, **V1**.276
infection
histoplasmosis capsulati, **M**.527–8
parasite immunity, **I**.420–1
viral infection *see below*
intracellular antigen recognition, **I**.375
MHC class I antigen presentation, **V1**.275
primary infection, kinetics, **I**.493–4,
I.494 (Fig.)
Qa-1 reactive/HLA-E reactive, **I**.443, **I**.445,
I.444 (Fig.)
immune response regulation, **I**.445
subacute sclerosing panencephalitis, **V1**.731
tumor immunity, **I**.421
viral infection, **I**.419–20, **V1**.618–19
hepatitis B, **V1**.283–4, **V2**.1250
HIV infection *see* HIV infection
HSV, **V1**.285, **V1**.510
HTLV type 2, **V2**.1288
Human respiratory syncytial virus,
V1.795–6
influenza, **V1**.664–5
LCMV, **V2**.1072
localization pathology, **V1**.248
measles, **V1**.726, **I**.805, **V2**.1433
see also Cytotoxic T cell(s)
CD11a *see* Leukocyte function antigen-1
(LFA-1: CD11a)
CD11b *see* Complement receptor 3 (CR3:
CD11b/CD18)
CD14, **I**.114 (Tab.)
discovery, **I**.110
ligand comparison, **I**.124 (Fig.)
microbial recognition, **I**.24 (Tab.)
pattern recognition, **I**.123
single nucleotide polymorphisms, **I**.124

soluble, **I**.114 (Tab.), **I**.115
CD14 gene, **I**.580
CD16 *see* FcγRIII (CD16)
CD18 *see* Leukocyte function antigen-1
(LFA-1: CD11a)
CD19
BCR signaling, **I**.345
genetic deficiencies, **I**.345
CD21 *see* Complement receptor 2
(CR2:CD21)
CD22, B-cell downregulation, **I**.348
CD23 *see* FcεRII (CD23)
CD24 (heat stable antigen), lymphocyte
migration, **I**.506–7
CD25, T cell development, **I**.455
CD27 ligand (CD27L), **I**.288 (Tab.)
CD28
antigen presentation, **I**.383–4
CD4 T cells, **I**.392 (Fig.), **I**.395, **I**.399, **I**.428
B7–1 (CD80) interactions *see* B7–1 (CD80)
B7–2 (CD86) interactions *see* B7–2 (CD86)
expression in HIV infection, **I**.791
TCR–superantigen binding, **I**.560
CD30 ligand (CD30L), **I**.288 (Tab.)
CD31 gene, malaria, **I**.600
CD32 *see* FcγRII (CD32)
CD34+ cells, foamy virus targeting, **V2**.1315
CD34, lymphocyte migration, **I**.508 (Tab.)
CD36
gene polymorphisms, malaria susceptibility,
P.485–6
immunogenetics, **I**.582–3
malaria, **I**.599–600
upregulation in malaria, **P**.496–7
CD40
antigen presentation, **I**.29
CD4 T cells/APC interactions, **I**.392 (Fig.)
cell expression, **I**.384
CpG stimulation, **I**.911
hyper-IgM syndrome, **I**.778
CD40–CD40L interactions, B cell activation,
I.326–7
CD40 ligand (CD40L: CD154), **I**.288 (Tab.)
B-cell activation, **I**.348–9
CD4 T cells, **I**.396
dendritic cell stimulation, **I**.288–9
DNA vaccine co-administration, **I**.909,
I.919 (Tab.)
germinal center reactions, **I**.349
CD43, lymphocyte migration, **I**.508 (Tab.)
CD44
lymphocyte migration, **I**.508 (Tab.)
T cell development, **I**.455
CD45 *see* Intracellular adhesion molecule 1
(ICAM-1: CD45)
CD46 *see* Membrane cofactor protein
(MCP:CD46)
CD48, CD4 T cells/APC interactions,
I.392 (Fig.)
CD56, NK cells, **I**.79–80, **I**.85, **V1**.271–2
CD59, **I**.150 (Tab.), **I**.151
CD62, **V2**.1410–11
CD62L (L-selectin) *see* L-selectin (CD62L)
CD63, basophil activation marker, **I**.63
CD64 *see* FcγRI (CD64)

CD69
  eosinophils, **I**.58
  T cell development, **I**.455–6
CD72, B-cell downregulation, **I**.348
CD79a *see* Igα (CD79a)
CD79b *see* Igβ (CD79b)
CD80 (B7.1) *see* B7–1 (CD80)
CD81, Hepatitis C virus receptor/co-receptor, **V2**.1195
CD86 *see* B7–2 (CD86)
CD89 *see* FcαRI (CD89)
CD95 *see* Fas (CD95)
CD99, diapedesis, **I**.512–13
CD150 (signal lymphocyte activation molecule: SLAM)
  measles, **I**.803, **I**.804–5
    downregulation, **V1**.725–6, **I**.805
    Measles virus hemagglutinin (H) protein binding, **V1**.718–20, **V1**.719 (Fig.), **V1**.719 (Tab.)
  measles, receptor, **V2**.1432
CD154 (CD40L) *see* CD40 ligand (CD40L: CD154)
CD161, CD1d-reactive αβ T cells, **I**.441
CD203c (E-NPP3), **I**.63
CD402, CD4 T cells/APC interactions, **I**.392 (Fig.)
CDC Coryneform group F-1 bacteria, **B2**.981 (Tab.), **B2**.982 (Tab.), **B2**.990
CDC Coryneform group G bacteria, **B2**.981 (Tab.), **B2**.982 (Tab.), **B2**.990
CDC group EF-4 (eugonic fermenter 4), **B2**.1678–9, **B2**.1679 (Tab.)
CDNA clones, type I interferon receptors, **I**.253
C domains, αβ TCRs, **I**.460–1
cea gene, **B1**.138
CEA-scan, licensing, **I**.355 (Tab.)
Cedecea, **B2**.1490–1
  antibacterial susceptibility/resistance, **B2**.1491
    intrinsic, **B2**.1352 (Tab.)
  biochemistry, **B2**.1491
  characteristics, **B2**.1490–1, **B2**.1491 (Tab.)
  culture, **B2**.1491
  definition, **B2**.1490–1
  habitats, **B2**.1491
  pathogenicity, **B2**.1491
  16S r-DNA sequencing, **B2**.1338
Cedecea davisae, **B2**.1490–1
  biochemical tests, **B2**.1319 (Tab.)
  characteristics, **B2**.1491, **B2**.1491 (Tab.)
  habitats, **B2**.1491
Cedecea lapagei, **B2**.1490–1
  biochemical tests, **B2**.1319 (Tab.)
  characteristics, **B2**.1491, **B2**.1491 (Tab.)
Cedecea neteri, **B2**.1490–1
  biochemical tests, **B2**.1319 (Tab.)
  characteristics, **B2**.1491 (Tab.)
  habitats, **B2**.1491
Cefaclor
  development of, **B1**.478
  Haemophilus, **B2**.1702 (Tab.)
  structure, **B1**.477 (Fig.)
Cefamandole
  pharmacology, **B1**.478

structure, **B1**.477 (Fig.)
Cefazolin, **B1**.477 (Fig.), **B1**.478
  Eikenella corrodens, **B2**.1668
  Pasteurella multocida, **B2**.1655
Cefbuperazone, development of, **B1**.476
Cefepime
  Enterobacter, **B2**.1484–5
  spectrum of activity, **B1**.499 (Tab.)
Cefixime
  development of, **B1**.478
  structure, **B1**.477 (Fig.)
Cefmetazole, **B1**.476
Cefminox, **B1**.476
Cefodizime, **B1**.477 (Fig.)
Cefoperazone
  pharmacology, **B1**.478
  spectrum of activity
    melioidosis, **B2**.1631 (Tab.)
    Pasteurella multocida, **B2**.1655
  structure, **B1**.477 (Fig.)
Cefoperazone-sulfabactam, melioidosis treatment, **B2**.1631
Cefotaxime
  development of, **B1**.476–8
  intracranial abscess, **B1**.588
  pharmacology, blood–brain barrier, **B1**.478
  spectrum of activity, **B1**.499 (Tab.)
    Borrelia, **B2**.1831 (Tab.)
    Enterobacter, **B2**.1484–5, **B2**.1485–6
    Haemophilus, **B2**.1702 (Tab.)
    Klebsiella, **B2**.1480
    Pasteurella multocida, **B2**.1655
    Vibrio, **B2**.1514
  structure, **B1**.477 (Fig.)
  typhoid fever treatment, **B2**.1416
Cefotetan
  development of, **B1**.476
  Klebsiella, **B2**.1480
  pharmacology, **B1**.478
Cefoxitin
  Eikenella corrodens, **B2**.1668
  Klebsiella, **B2**.1480
Cefpirome, *Enterobacter,* **B2**.1484–5
Cefpodoxime, **B1**.478
Cefriaxone, gonorrhea treatment, **B1**.661
Cefsulodin
  development of, **B1**.476–8
  structure, **B1**.477 (Fig.)
Cefsulodin-Irgasan-novobiocin (CIN) medium, **B2**.1463
Ceftazidime
  intracranial abscess, **B1**.588
  melioidosis treatment, **B2**.1631, **B2**.1631 (Tab.)
  spectrum of activity
    Enterobacter, **B2**.1484–6
    Klebsiella, **B2**.1480
    Pasteurella multocida, **B2**.1655
  structure, **B1**.477 (Fig.)
Ceftibuten, **B1**.478
Ceftiofur, *Pasteurella multocida,* **B2**.1655
Ceftizoxime
  Pasteurella multocida, **B2**.1655
  structure, **B1**.477 (Fig.)
Ceftoxitin, structure, **B1**.477 (Fig.)

Ceftriaxone
  osteomyelitis, **B1**.698–9
  pharmacology, **B1**.478
    blood–brain barrier, **B1**.478
  spectrum of activity
    Actinobacillus actinomycetemcomitans, **B2**.1664
    Bacillus anthracis, **B2**.937–8
    Borrelia, **B2**.1831 (Tab.)
    Haemophilus, **B2**.1702 (Tab.), **B2**.1710
    Nocardia, **B2**.1145, **B2**.1165–6
  structure, **B1**.477 (Fig.)
  in syphilis, **B2**.1857–8
  typhoid fever treatment, **B2**.1416
Cefuroxime
  development of, **B1**.476–8
  spectrum of activity, **B1**.499 (Tab.)
    Bacillus anthracis, **B2**.937–8
    Borrelia, **B2**.1831 (Tab.)
    Enterobacter, **B2**.1484–5
    Haemophilus, **B2**.1702 (Tab.), **B2**.1703 (Tab.)
    Klebsiella, **B2**.1480
    Pasteurella multocida, **B2**.1655
  structure, **B1**.477 (Fig.)
Celecoxib (Celebrex), **I**.186–7
C elements, TCR, **I**.451
Celery 'pink rot,' **B1**.281
Celiac disease, *CTLA-4* gene polymorphisms, **I**.752
Cell activation, bispecific antibodies, **I**.361
Cell adhesion *see* Adhesion molecules
'Cell anus', **P**.164
Cell-associated enveloped virus (CEV), poxviruses *see* Poxviruses
Cell attachment/entry of viruses, **V1**.206–12, **V1**.236–40
  antibody interference, **V1**.277
  antibody-mediated enhancement, **V1**.211, **V1**.287
  astrovirus replication, **V2**.893–4
  bunyaviruses, **V2**.1034–5
  CNS infection, **V2**.1404–5
    hematogenous, **V2**.1404–5
    neural, **V2**.1405
  entry accessory factors, **V1**.212
  enveloped viruses, **V1**.107–8
  flaviviruses, **V1**.108–9
  herpesviruses, **V1**.490–1
  influenza viruses, **V1**.642
  Measles virus fusion (F) protein, **V1**.713–15
  Nidovirales order, **V1**.395
  oncogenic viruses, **V1**.344
  receptor-mediated endocytosis, **V1**.206, **V1**.206 (Fig.)
  reovirus σ1 protein, **V2**.933, **V2**.936–7
  rhabdoviruses *see* Rhabdoviruses
  see also Attachment proteins (viral); Cellular receptors; Replication, viruses
Cell-cell fusion, **B1**.98
Cell clearance, macrophages, **I**.31
Cell compartment distribution, viral replication, **V1**.108–9
Cell counts, in virus cultures, **V1**.89

Cell culture, viruses, **V1**.5, **V1**.86–90,
    V2.1539–41
  astrovirus, **V2**.889, **V2**.906
  Avian pneumovirus, **V1**.790
  cell lines, **V1**.87, **V1**.88, **V1**.89,
    V2.1540 (Tab.)
    aneuploid cells, **V1**.87
    contamination, **V1**.88–9
    engineered, **V2**.1541
    euploid cells, **V1**.87
    insect, **V1**.87
    international repositories, **V1**.86
    safety issues, **V1**.86
    storage, **V1**.89–90
  Colorado tick fever virus, **V2**.943
  contamination, **V1**.88–9
    by viruses, **V1**.88
  continuous, **V1**.5, **V1**.87
  cytospinning (shell vials), **V2**.1540–1
  detection, **V2**.1539–40
    cytopathic effect (CPE), **V2**.1539–40
    hemadsorption, **V2**.1540
  difficult viruses, **V2**.1537 (Tab.)
  enteroviruses, **V2**.876
  Feline astrovirus, **V2**.906
  foamy viruses, **V2**.1306–7
  Hepatitis B virus, **V2**.1232–3
  HHV, **V2**.1539
  historical aspects, **V1**.5
  HIV, **V2**.1539
  Human astrovirus, **V2**.889, **V2**.906
  maintenance, **V1**.89
  Marburg virus, **V2**.1091–2
  Measles virus, **V1**.733
  media, **V1**.86–7
    maintenance, **V1**.89
  Metapneumovirus, **V1**.790
  mixed-cell, **V1**.88, **V2**.1541
  Newcastle disease virus, **V1**.816
  Ovine astrovirus, **V2**.889
  Peste-des-petits-ruminants virus, **V1**.811
  pH, **V1**.86–7
  Pneumovirus, **V1**.790
  Porcine astrovirus, **V2**.906
  primary, **V1**.87
  prion diseases, **V2**.1387
  purity and safety aspects, **V1**.88–9, **V1**.91
  quality control, **V1**.89
  quantitative methods, **V1**.5
  Reston ebolavirus, **V2**.1091–2
  Rinderpest virus, **V1**.810
  rotaviruses, **V2**.949–50
  safety, **V1**.86, **V1**.91
  shell vial, **V1**.87
  specialized systems for, **V1**.88
  subculturing, **V1**.89
  Sudan ebolavirus, **V2**.1091–2
  suspension, **V1**.86–8
  types, **V1**.87–8
  virulence after, **V1**.251
  virus isolation procedure, **V1**.93–100
  virus release from, **V1**.91
  Zaire ebolavirus, **V2**.1091–2
Cell cycle
  G$_2$ phase arrest, **V2**.1326–7

respirovirus effects, **V1**.773–4
S phase
  adeno-associated viruses, **V1**.428
  DNA viruses–host interactions, **V1**.169
  HHV-8, **V1**.555
  k-cyclin (cyclin D homologue), **V1**.548
  latent nuclear antigen (LANA-1),
    V1.546–7
  papillomaviruses, **V1**.155, **V1**.459–60
  parvoviruses, **V1**.408, **V1**.418
Cell death, tumor pathogenesis, **V1**.341
Cell(s), definition, **P**.159
Cell density-dependent gene expression, **B1**.72
Cell division
  in protozoa, **P**.181–5, **P**.183 (Fig.)
    'ameba-like' division, **P**.181, **P**.183 (Fig.)
    longitudinal, **P**.181, **P**.183 (Fig.)
    multiple, **P**.181–5, **P**.184 (Fig.)
    oblique, **P**.181, **P**.183 (Fig.)
  regulation, **B1**.48
  Trypanosoma brucei, **P**.362
  see also individual species
Cell entry (viruses) *see* Cell attachment/entry
Cell envelope, Enterobacteriaceae, **B2**.1340–1
Cell junctions, **P**.162
Cell-mediated immune response, **P**.68, **P**.68–9,
    P.69
  acute bronchiolitis pathogenesis, **V1**.776
  analysis, **V2**.1544–5, **V2**.1544 (Tab.)
    blastogenic responses, **V2**.1545
    radioactivity label release assays, **V2**.1545
  bacterial immune interference *see* Immune
    evasion, bacteria
  CNS infection, **V2**.1412, **V2**.1413–15
    autoimmune reactions, **V2**.1414–15
    against brain antigens, **V2**.1414–15
    mechanisms of antiviral activity, **V2**.1414
    role of CD4/CD8 cells, **V2**.1413–14
  defects/dysfunction, respiratory infection,
    B1.626
  delayed-type hypersensitivity *vs.,* **I**.724–5
  DNA vaccine modulation, **I**.917
  fungal infection
    allergic bronchopulmonary aspergillosis,
      M.708–9
    aspergilloma, **M**.709
    aspergillosis, **M**.707–9
    Candida infection *see* Candidiasis
    coccidioidomycosis, **M**.510
    cryptococcosis, **M**.645
    histoplasmosis capsulati, **M**.527, **M**.528–9
    invasive aspergillosis, **M**.709
    oropharyngeal candidiasis, **M**.262–3
    penicilliosis marneffei, **M**.568
    vulvovaginal candidiasis, **M**.264, **M**.265–6
  human brucellosis, **B2**.1737
  humoral immune response *vs.,* **I**.489,
    I.490 (Fig.), **I**.490 (Tab.)
    protective immunity, **I**.489
  ILs, **P**.70–2
  inactivated vaccines, **V2**.1556
  melioidosis, **B2**.1630
  mucosal vaccination, **I**.828
  parasitic infection, **P**.68–9
    amebiasis, **P**.209–10

cutaneous leishmaniasis, **P**.299
cysticercosis, **P**.690
echinococcosis, **P**.690
Old World leishmaniasis, **P**.299–300
onchocerciasis, **P**.795
primary infection, **I**.493–4, **I**.494 (Fig.)
'prime-boost immunization,' **I**.846
subacute sclerosing panencephalitis (SSPE),
  V2.1432–3
suppression, in LCMV infection, **V2**.1075
tests of, brucellosis diagnosis, **B1**.745,
  B2.1741
viral infection
  adenoviruses, **V1**.445–6
  arteriviruses, **V1**.840
  bunyavirus, **V2**.1041
  CNS *see above*
  coronaviruses, **V1**.840–1
  HCMV, **V1**.524–5
  hepatitis A, **V2**.1170–1
  hepatitis C, **V2**.1206
  HHV, **V1**.532
  HSV, **V1**.284–5
  Human respiratory syncytial virus,
    V1.795–6
  LCMV, **V2**.1072–3
  measles, **V1**.726
  measles inclusion body encephalitis
    (MIBE), **V2**.1431
  mumps, **V1**.751
  rabies, **V2**.1115–16, **V2**.1124–5
  VZV, **V1**.515–16
see also individual components; individual
  effector cells
Cell membrane metabolism, positive-strand
  RNA viruses, **V1**.142
Cell membranes
  function, **P**.162
  ion transport across, **P**.161–2
  'p' and 'e' faces, **P**.161
  pores, **P**.161–2
  protozoa, **P**.160–2
  types, **P**.162, **P**.163 (Tab.)
  structure, **P**.160–2, **P**.162 (Fig.), **P**.168
Cell morphology, viral infection effects,
  V1.202, **V1**.203 (Fig.)
Cellobiose fermentation
  Enterobacteriaceae identification,
    B2.1319 (Tab.)
  Porphyromonas identification, **B2**.1924 (Tab.)
  Prevotella identification, **B2**.1924 (Tab.)
Cell receptors, innate malaria resistance, **P**.485
Cell-to-cell contact, HTLV transmission,
  V2.1288
Cellular infiltrates, onchocerciasis, **P**.794
Cellular receptors, **V1**.208 (Fig.), **V1**.209,
  V1.245–7, **V1**.246 (Fig.)
  binding consequences, **V1**.211–12
    pH-dependency, **V1**.211–12, **V1**.212–13
  capsid attachment sites, **V1**.208–9
    antibody-blocking, **V1**.209
  CNS, **V2**.1405–6, **V2**.1405–7, **V2**.1406 (Tab.)
  coronavirus spike (S) protein, **V1**.838
  definition, **V1**.245–6
  heparan sulfate, **V1**.209
  influenza hemagglutinin, **V1**.642, **V1**.652–3

Cellular receptors (*Continued*)
  polarized cells, **V1**.209
  properties, **V1**.245–6
  sialic acids, **V1**.209
  viral release from, **V1**.206, **V1**.212
  viruses
    alphaviruses, **V2**.1015
    astroviruses, **V2**.893–4
    Ebola virus, **V2**.1092
    flaviviruses, **V2**.996
    Hepatitis C virus, **V2**.1195
    HTLVs, **V2**.1288
    Marburg virus, **V2**.1092
    Murine hepatitis virus, **V1**.838
    picornaviruses, **V2**.866
    polioviruses, **V2**.866
    polyomaviruses, **V1**.473–4
    Rabies virus, **V2**.1108
    respiroviruses, **V1**.765–6
    rotaviruses, **V2**.949–50
    Sendai virus, **V1**.765–6
    Sindbis virus, **V2**.1015
    Venezuelan equine encephalitis virus,
      V2.1015
    Vesicular stomatitis virus, **V2**.1108
    see also Cell attachment/entry; *specific
      types; specific viruses*
Cellulitis
  anaerobic, **B2**.1112
  clostridial, **B2**.1112
  Erysipelothrix rhusiopathiae causing, **B2**.971
Cellulomonas, **B2**.992
  biochemical characteristics, **B2**.993 (Tab.)
  chemotaxonomic characteristics,
    B2.978 (Tab.)
  disease associations, **B2**.981 (Tab.)
  habitats, **B2**.978
Cellulose cysticercus, *Taenia solium,* **P**.679–80,
  P.685–6
Cellulose-degrading enzyme systems,
  B1.199–200
Cellulosimicrobium
  biochemical characteristics, **B2**.993 (Tab.)
  chemotaxonomic characteristics,
    B2.978 (Tab.)
  habitats, **B2**.978
Cell–virus interactions, **V1**.202–35
  absorption *see* Cell attachment/entry
  apoptosis, **V1**.229–30
    viral evasion mechanisms, **V1**.229–30
  cellular responses, **V1**.226–30
    INFs *see* Interferon(s)
    stress proteins, **V1**.228–9
  cellular RNA metabolism, **V1**.220–1
    degradation, **V1**.221
    oncogene activation, **V1**.220–1
    processing/transport, **V1**.221
    synthesis, **V1**.220–1
  classification, **V1**.205 (Tab.)
  cytopathic effects
    cell morphology, **V1**.202, **V1**.203 (Fig.)
    cytoskeleton disruption, **V1**.202–3
  DNA metabolism, **V1**.217–9
    biosynthesis, **V1**.217–18, **V1**.218 (Fig.)
    degradation, **V1**.219

    maintenance/transfer, **V1**.219
    modification, **V1**.219
    replication, **V1**.218–19
    S-phase, **V1**.217
  membrane fusion, **V1**.213–5
    fusion protein stabilization, **V1**.214
    hydrophobic fusion peptides, **V1**.213–14
    mechanisms, **V1**.212–15, **V1**.213 (Fig.)
    see also Cell attachment/entry
  metabolism effects, **V1**.217–26
    see also specific metabolites
  non-cytolytic with tumor viruses, **V1**.345
  nonproductive infection, **V1**.205–6,
    V1.205 (Tab.)
    apoptosis, **V1**.205
    latency, **V1**.204, **V1**.206
    nonproductive transformations, **V1**.205–6
  nuclear transit, **V1**.216
  penetration, **V1**.212–17
    membrane fusion *see above*
    multinucleated syncytia formation, **V1**.213
    viral fusion proteins, **V1**.213–14
    see also Cell attachment/entry
  productive infection, **V1**.204–5,
    V1.205 (Tab.)
    cytocidal infection, **V1**.205
    persistence, **V1**.205
    productive transformation, **V1**.205
  protein degradation, **V1**.226
  protein metabolism, **V1**.221–6
  protein processing, **V1**.224–5
    cleavage, **V1**.225
    folding, **V1**.224–5
    glycosylation, **V1**.225
    oligomerization, **V1**.224–5
    phosphorylation, **V1**.225
  protein synthesis, **V1**.222–4, **V1**.222 (Fig.)
    alternative open reading frames, **V1**.224
    eIF2, **V1**.222
    eIF4F, **V1**.222–3
    host synthesis inhibition, **V1**.210 (Fig.),
      V1.223–4
    internal ribosome entry sites (IRES),
      V1.222–3
    viral mRNA preferential translation,
      V1.223–4
  protein transport, **V1**.225–6
  quantitative aspects, **V1**.203–4
    multiplicity of infection (MOI), **V1**.203
    physical particle: plaque-forming unit
      rations, **V1**.203–4
    Poisson distribution, **V1**.203, **V1**.204 (Tab.)
    single hit relationships, **V1**.204
  response to oncogenic viruses, **V1**.346–7
  type, **V1**.204–6
    see also specific types
  uncoating of nonenveloped viruses,
    V1.215 (Fig.)
    destabilization, **V1**.215
    membrane fusion mechanisms, **V1**.215–17
    poxviruses, **V1**.216–17
  viral RNA metabolism, **V1**.219–20
    enhancers, **V1**.220
    preferential synthesis, **V1**.219–20
    RNA polymerases, **V1**.220
    transcription factors, **V1**.220

  see also specific viruses
Cell walls, **M**.69, **M**.78
  antibacterial agents, **B1**.436
  archaea, **B1**.44
  Candida, **M**.590–1
  chemotaxonomy, **B1**.24
  chromoblastomycosis, **M**.362–3
  composition, **B1**.42–3
    peptidoglycans, **B1**.42–3
  fungal *vs.,* **B1**.444
  gram-negative bacteria, **B1**.442
    composition, **B1**.43–4
  gram-positive bacteria, **B1**.441–2
    composition, **B1**.43
  historical aspects, **B1**.12
  hyphal, **M**.71, **M**.73 (Fig.)
  mycetoma, **M**.387, **M**.392
  structure, periplasmic space, **B1**.43
  synthesis, **M**.70–1, **M**.74
  see also individual species
Celsus, **M**.5
Centers for Disease Control and Prevention
    (CDC), **B1**.29, **B1**.319
  bioterrorism categories, **B1**.364
  Borrelia detection, **B2**.1829
  emerging bacterial infection, **B1**.365
  vaccine adverse event monitoring, **V2**.1565
  vaccine information, **V2**.1583
Centipeda periodontii, **B1**.296 (Tab.)
Central European encephalitis (CEE),
    V2.1003–4, **V2**.1426
  clinical features, **V2**.1426
  transmission, **V1**.372 (Tab.)
'Central' memory T cells, **I**.495, **I**.496 (Fig.)
Central nervous system (CNS)
  African trypanosomiasis, **P**.364, **P**.365
  neurovirulence of viruses, **V2**.1407
  receptors for viruses, **V2**.1405–7,
    V2.1406 (Tab.)
  replication of viruses, **V2**.1405, **V2**.1412
  SCF effects, **I**.274
  trichinellosis, **P**.761
  tropism of viruses, **V2**.1405–6
  Whipple's disease, **B2**.999
Central nervous system (CNS) infection,
    V2.1403–42
  Acanthamoeba, **P**.226, **P**.229
  alphaherpesviruses, **V2**.1418, **V2**.1418–22
  alphaviruses, **V2**.1018
  antiviral mechanisms
    consequences, **V2**.1415
    immune response *see below*
  arenavirus, **V2**.1072
  aspergillosis, **M**.697, **M**.700, **M**.705
  Bipolaris, **M**.743
  blastomycosis, **M**.489–90
  Borna disease virus infection, **V2**.1149–50
    immune cell infiltrates, **V2**.1149
  candidiasis *see* Candidiasis
  cell-mediated immune response *see* Cell-
    mediated immune response
  Chaetomium, **M**.743–4
  chemokine responses, **V2**.1409–10
  children *see* Children
  Chlamydia pneumoniae, **B2**.2017

Central nervous system (CNS) infection
(*Continued*)
  chromoblastomycosis, **M**.361–2
  Clostridium tetani neurotoxin action,
    B2.1065
  congenitally acquired rubella, **V2**.974–5
  cryptococcosis *see* Cryptococcosis
  Eikenella corrodens, **B2**.1667
  enteroviruses, **V2**.1422–4
    Coxsackie viruses, **V2**.1423–4
    echoviruses, **V2**.1424
    enterovirus, **V2**.1423
    poliovirus, **V2**.1422–3
  Exserohilum, **M**.743
  factors affecting virus disease development,
    V2.1406–7
  flaviviruses, **V2**.1424–6
  Fonsecaea pedrosoi, **M**.743–4
  frequencies, **V2**.1415–16, **V2**.1416 (Tab.)
  future prospects, **V2**.1433
  HHV-6 infection, **V1**.531
  HIV *see* HIV infection
  HSV, **V1**.507, **V2**.1418–21
  human brucellosis, **B2**.1738
  immune response, **V2**.1411–15, **V2**.1413
    CD4+ T-cells, **V2**.1413–14
      Borna disease virus infection, **V2**.1149
    CD8+ T-cells, **V2**.1413–14
      Borna disease virus infection, **V2**.1149
    complement activation, **V2**.1413
    cytokines, **V1**.292–3, **V1**.303–4,
      V2.1409–10
    effector lymphocyte passage to CNS,
      V2.1410–11
    enhanced viral pathogenicity, **V2**.1413
    humoral response, **V2**.1411–13
    IL-6, **V1**.303–4
    inhibition of virus entry by antibodies,
      V2.1411–12
    spread inhibition, **V2**.1411–15, **V2**.1413
    TNF-α, **V1**.303–4
    virus escape from, **V2**.1412
    virus persistence, **V2**.1413
  intracranial abscess *see* Intracranial abscess
  intracranial epidural abscess *see* Subdural
    empyema
  Mycoplasma pneumoniae pneumonia,
    B1.634
  Nocardia farcinica, **B2**.1161–2
  Ochroconis gallopavum, **M**.743
  Paracoccidioides brasiliensis, **M**.548–9
  paramyxoviruses, **V2**.1430, **V2**.1430–2,
    V2.1432–3, **V2**.1433
    measles virus, **V2**.1404–5, **V2**.1431–3
    mumps virus, **V2**.1430
  Pasteurella multocida, **B2**.1654–5
  pathology, virus infection-independent
    mechanisms, **V2**.1408
  pathways, **V2**.1403–5
    direct contact, **V2**.1403–4
    fecal-oral, **V2**.1403–4
    respiratory secretions, **V2**.1403–4
    routes, **V2**.1404–5
    vector-borne, **V2**.1403–4
  persistent infection, **V2**.1408
    humoral immune response, **V2**.1413

  phaeohyphomycosis, **M**.743, **M**.744 (Tab.),
    M.745, **M**.746–7
  polyomaviruses, **V2**.1416–18
  prion diseases *see* Prion diseases
  rabies *see* Rabies
  Ramichloridium obovoideum, **M**.743–4, **M**.745
  reovirus, **V2**.937
  retroviruses, **V2**.1426–30
  rhinocerebral zygomycosis, **M**.20–1,
    M.673–4, **M**.674 (Tab.), **M**.678
  rhinosporidiosis, **M**.462
  Scedosporium prolificans, **M**.743–4
  specimens, **M**.83 (Tab.), **M**.84, **M**.86 (Tab.)
  spinal epidural abscess *see* Spinal epidural
    abscess
  sporotrichosis, **M**.371, **M**.377, **M**.380
  subdural empyema *see* Subdural empyema
  systemic zygomycosis, **M**.673–5
  virus entry, **V2**.1404–5
    hematogenous, **V2**.1404–5
    inhibition by immune response,
      V2.1411–12
    neural, **V2**.1405
  virus-host cell interactions, **V2**.1403–15,
    V2.1407–8
    acute infection, **V2**.1407–8
    chemokine induction, **V2**.1409–10
    cytokines induction, **V2**.1409–10
    infection-independent mechanisms,
      V2.1408
    MHC CNS expression, **V2**.1410, **V2**.1415
    neural cell functions, **V2**.1409
    persistent, **V2**.1408
  VZV *see* Varicella-zoster virus infection
  Wangiella dermatitidis, **M**.743, **M**.744
Central pore, parvovirus capsids, **V1**.413
Central venous lines
  contamination, **B1**.393
  see also Catheter(s)
Centrifuges/centrifugation
  laboratory safety, **V2**.1520–3
  purification of viruses, **V1**.5–6
Centromeric instability and facial anomalies,
  I.777
Cephalexin
  development of, **B1**.478
  spectrum of activity, **B1**.499 (Tab.)
    Bacillus anthracis, **B2**.937–8
  structure, **B1**.477 (Fig.)
Cephaliophora, oculomycoses, **M**.275 (Tab.)
Cephaloridine, **B1**.476
  Citrobacter, **B2**.1476
  Leclercia, **B2**.1495
Cephalosporins, **B1**.476–8
  antibiotic-associated diarrhea due to,
    B2.1120
  classification, **B1**.476, **B1**.476 (Tab.)
  CNS infection
    intracranial abscess, **B1**.588,
      B1.589 (Tab.)
    subdural empyema, **B1**.591 (Tab.)
  development of, **B1**.476–8
  gonorrhea treatment, **B1**.661
  Haemophilus influenzae type b (Hib)
    meningitis, **B1**.573–4
  mode of action, **B1**.476

  oral, **B1**.478
  parenteral, **B1**.476–8
  pharmacology, **B1**.478
    blood–brain barrier, **B1**.478
    excretion, **B1**.478
  pharyngitis treatment, **B1**.611
  in pneumococcal meningitis, **B1**.571
  resistance
    Brucella, **B2**.1742
    Neisseria gonorrhoeae, **B1**.661
  spectrum of activity
    Actinobacillus actinomycetemcomitans,
      B2.1664
    Aeromonas, **B2**.1532–4
    Bacillus anthracis, **B2**.937–8
    Borrelia, **B2**.1830
    Campylobacter, **B2**.1548
    Cardiobacterium hominis, **B2**.1672–3
    Citrobacter, **B2**.1476
    Eikenella corrodens, **B2**.1668
    Enterobacter, **B2**.1484–5
    Hafnia, **B2**.1493
    Klebsiella, **B2**.1480
    Listeria, **B2**.957–8
    Pasteurella multocida, **B2**.1655
    Proteus, **B2**.1441–3
    Serratia, **B2**.1488–9
  structure, **B1**.476, **B1**.477 (Fig.)
  third generation, epiglottitis treatment,
    B1.613
  see also specific types
Cephalosporium, **M**.28 (Fig.)
Cephalothin, **B1**.476
  Kluyvera, **B2**.1494
  Leminorella, **B2**.1496
  Moellerella, **B2**.1496
  Pasteurella multocida, **B2**.1655
  structure, **B1**.477 (Fig.)
Cephamycin, **B1**.471 (Fig.)
Cephem, **B1**.471 (Fig.)
Cephradine, **B1**.477 (Fig.)
Ceramic filters, **B1**.453
Ceramide aminoethyl phosphonate (CAEP),
  P.205
Ceratopogonidae, Oropouche virus
  transmission, **V2**.1049
Cercariae, **P**.580
  Opisthorchis, **P**.581 (Fig.)
  Schistosoma, **P**.581 (Fig.), **P**.602–3,
    P.603 (Fig.)
  structure, **P**.581 (Fig.)
Cercarial dermatitis, **P**.582
Cereals, **B1**.283–6
  fungal spoilage, **B1**.284
  nutrients and spoilage, **B1**.267
Cerebellitis, VZV, **V2**.1422
Cerebellum development, Borna disease virus
  infection, **V2**.1147–8
Cerebral atrophy, in syphilis, **B2**.1843
Cerebral capillary endothelium, **B1**.557
Cerebral malaria *see* Malaria
Cerebral manifestations, infective endocarditis,
  B1.535
Cerebritis, histoplasmosis, **M**.523–4
Cerebrospinal fluid (CSF)
  aspergillosis, **M**.697

Cerebrospinal fluid (CSF) (*Continued*)
bacterial antigen detection, **B1**.559
bacterial cell counts, **B1**.558
bacterial meningitis
development/pathogenesis, **B1**.556–7
diagnosis, **B1**.557–9
biochemical analysis, **B1**.558–9
blood glucose ratio, **B1**.558–9
candidiasis, **M**.600
cryptococcosis, **M**.649, **M**.652, **M**.653
culture, **B1**.559
Aeromonas isolation, **B2**.1531
examination, **B1**.557–9
lumbar puncture, **B1**.557–8
microscopy, **B1**.559
mumps encephalitis/meningitis, **V2**.1430–1
Naegleria fowleri infection, **P**.236–7
normal microbiota, **B1**.305
pleocytosis, in mumps, **V2**.1430–1
protein, **B1**.558–9
shunts, infection, **B1**.392
specimens, **M**.83 (Tab.), **M**.84, **M**.86 (Tab.)
Cerinosterus cyanescens, **M**.371–2
Ceruloplasmin, **I**.205
Cervical cancer
Chlamydia trachomatis infection, **B2**.2013
diagnosis, cytology, **V2**.1533–4
high-risk HPVs, **V1**.448–9, **V1**.459
HPV infection, **V1**.448–9, **V1**.463 (Tab.)
epidemiological evidence, **V1**.373–4,
V1.466–7
Cervical intraepithelial neoplasia (CIN)
HIV infection, **V2**.1503–4
HPV infection, **V1**.465–6
Cervical lymphadenitis, *Mycobacterium avium*
complex causing, **B2**.1208
Cervicitis, *Chlamydia trachomatis* infection,
B2.2010
Cervix
'strawberry', **P**.259–60
trichomoniasis
edema, **P**.259–60
punctate hemorrhages, **P**.257–8
Cesarean section
HIV infection, **V2**.1473
HSV infection, **V2**.1466
Cestoda, **P**.575–6, **P**.677
Cestodaria, **P**.574–6
Cestodes (intestinal tapeworms), **P**.573, **P**.576,
I.682
classification, **P**.574–9
Pseudophyllidea, **P**.576–7
subclass Eucestoda, **P**.576
development, **P**.95–6
general biology, **P**.576
historical aspects, **P**.6, **P**.12–3
immune evasion
complement inhibition, **I**.685
protease inhibitors, **I**.687
immune response, **P**.95–6
immunoprophylaxis, **P**.96
life cycle, **P**.95, **P**.576, **I**.682
main features, **P**.575, **P**.575 (Fig.)
morphology/structure, **P**.575 (Fig.), **P**.576
see also Larval cestodes; *individual species*

Cestodiasis, historical aspects, **P**.12–3
Cestoidea, **P**.574–9
Cetacean morbillivirus
classification, **V1**.382–3
epizootiology, **V1**.814
seal mortality, **V1**.814
Cetuximab, licensing, **I**.355 (Tab.)
CFTR gene, **I**.593
Chabertiidae, **P**.594–5
Chaetomium, CNS infection, **M**.743–4
Chaetosphaeronema larense, **M**.391
Chagas, C., **P**.376, **P**.377 (Fig.)
Chagas disease, **P**.188, **P**.384–96
AIDS, **I**.678
cardiac disease, **P**.384–5
treatment, **P**.393
chronic disease, **P**.385
clinical features, **P**.385
myogenic form, **P**.386, **P**.387–8
neurogenic form, **P**.386
pathology, **P**.386
clinical features, **P**.384–5, **I**.678
acute phase symptoms, **P**.384–5
aneurysms, **P**.386, **P**.386 (Fig.)
cardiac disease *see above*
indeterminate phase, **P**.385
megacolon *see below*
megaesophagus *see below*
congenital, **P**.32, **P**.385
pathology, **P**.386
control, **P**.389, **P**.394–6
blood product contamination prevention,
P.395–6
chemotherapy/chemoprophylaxis,
P.144 (Tab.)
community-directed programs, **P**.122,
P.395
cost of, **P**.32–3
diagnosis, **P**.143 (Tab.)
monitoring by serology, **P**.395
social/economic development aspects,
P.32–3, **P**.396
Southern Core Initiative, **P**.116 (Fig.)
testing children, **P**.395
triatomine bug control, **P**.389, **P**.390,
P.394–5
vector/reservoir control, **P**.126,
P.145 (Tab.), **P**.389, **P**.390, **P**.394–5
diagnosis, **P**.388–9
blood culture, **P**.152–3
DNA, **P**.389
history-taking, **P**.389
microscopy, **P**.388
serological, **P**.389
tests, **P**.389
xenodiagnosis, **P**.388–9
epidemiology, **P**.30, **P**.46 (Tab.), **P**.389–92
immigrants, **P**.27–9
prevalence, **P**.30, **P**.31 (Tab.), **P**.32
public health aspects, **P**.105 (Tab.), **P**.389
socioeconomics, **P**.32
health importance, **P**.30–3
historical aspects, **P**.15–6
HLA association, **I**.597

immune response, **P**.86–7, **P**.385–6, **I**.680
autoimmunity, **P**.86–7
cytokines, **P**.86
eosinophils, **I**.70
Igs, **P**.385
immune evasion, **P**.86, **P**.87, **P**.385–6
immunodepression, **P**.86
macrophage role, **P**.86, **P**.385
T cells, **P**.385
incubation period, **P**.385
life expectancy, **P**.393
megacolon, **P**.386, **P**.388 (Fig.)
treatment, **P**.393, **P**.393 (Fig.)
megaesophagus, **P**.387 (Fig.)
treatment, **P**.393
mortality, **P**.28 (Tab.), **P**.29 (Tab.), **P**.32
outcome diversity, strain effects, **P**.382,
P.384
pathogenesis, **P**.387–8
autoimmunity, **P**.385–8, **P**.393–4
pathogen induced, **I**.753 (Tab.)
pathology, **P**.386–8
heart, **P**.386
intestine, **P**.386
neurological, **P**.386–7
in pregnancy, **P**.385
transfusion-acquired, **P**.27–9, **P**.32, **P**.379,
P.392, **P**.395–6
treatment, **P**.389–90, **P**.392–3
allopurinol, **P**.380, **P**.393
chemotherapy, **P**.392–3
cost of, **P**.32
cure rates, **P**.392–3
for heart disease, **P**.393
surgical, **P**.393
vaccination/vaccines, **P**.87, **P**.390, **P**.393–4
vectors, **P**.390
control, **P**.126, **P**.145 (Tab.), **P**.389, **P**.390,
P.394–5
see also Trypanosoma cruzi
Chagres virus infection, **V2**.1047
Chamberland, C, **V1**.3–4
Chancre, African trypanosomiasis, **P**.363–4
Chancroid, **B1**.663–4
causative agent, **B2**.1709, **B2**.1710–11
see also Haemophilus ducreyi
HIV-infection with, **B1**.663–4
therapy, **B1**.664–5
transmission, **B1**.663–4
vaccines, **I**.933 (Tab.)
Changeux, Jean-Pierre, **I**.11
Channel catfish *(Ictalurus punctatus), Bacillus
mycoides* infection, **B2**.944
Channel catfish virus (CCV), genome, **V1**.492,
V1.494 (Tab.)
Chaos, **B1**.17–8
Chaperones, **B1**.47
antigen processing, **I**.415
apoptosis functions, **I**.626
DNA vaccines, **I**.914, **I**.917
DNA viruses–host interactions, **V1**.169–70
influenza hemagglutinin assembly, **V1**.650
protein folding regulation, **B1**.47
protein secretion, **B1**.47

Characterization (of viruses), **V2**.1541–4
  immune response to *see* Immune response
  typing, **V2**.1541–2
    genotyping, **V2**.1542
    serotyping, **V2**.1542
    see also specific methods
  wild-type *vs.* attenuated strains, **V2**.1542–4
    see also Antiviral susceptibility testing
  see also Diagnosis, viral infection
Charcot–Leyden crystal proteins, **I**.57, **I**.66
Chédiak–Higashi syndrome, **I**.48–9, **I**.48 (Tab.),
    I.481, **I**.657–8, **I**.778
  granulocytes, **I**.481 (Fig.)
Cheese, **B1**.251–7
  defects and spoilage, **B1**.252
    bacterial toxins, **B1**.252
    fungal toxins, **B1**.252
  microbiological quality control, **B1**.256–7
  pathogenic bacteria in, **B1**.252–6
    see also individual species
Chelating agents, **B1**.428
Chemical agent susceptibility/resistance
  bacteria, **B1.421–65**
    see also individual species; specific agents
  viruses
    filoviruses, **V2**.1098
    picornaviruses, **V2**.869
Chemical pollutants, bioremediation, **B1**.201–2
Chemical preservatives, **B1**.267–8,
    B1.268 (Tab.)
Chemical treatment, virus release from culture,
    V1.91
Chemiosmotic driven transport systems, **B1**.49
Chemokine(s), **P**.70, **P**.72, **I**.273, **I.217–36**
  activity measurement, **I**.223
    two-well chambers, **I**.223
  CC type *see* CC chemokine(s)
  cell types
    basophils, **I**.58, **I**.60
    dendritic epidermal γδ T cells, **I**.437
  CNS expression, **V2**.1409–10
  C type, macrophage production, **I**.28–9
  CX3C type *see* CX3C chemokines
  CXC type *see* CXC chemokines
  in disease, **I**.227–30
    inflammatory disease models, **I**.228–9
    patient studies, **I**.229–30
    viral infection, **I**.227–8
  expression, TLR stimulus, **I**.697
  functions/roles
    airway hypersensitivity, **I**.734
    bacterial infection, **I**.651
    basophil histamine release, **I**.62
    granuloma formation *see below*
    lymphocyte effects *see below*
    neutrophil recruitment, **I**.37
    NK cell regulation, **I**.85–6
    phagocyte effects, **I**.223–4
  granuloma formation, **I**.708
    schistosomiasis, **I**.722–3
    tuberculosis, **I**.708, **I**.724–5
  HHV-8 coding, **V1**.550
  historical aspects/re-evaluation, **I**.11, **I**.217

HTLV-1-associated myelopathy/tropical
    spastic paraparesis (HAM/TSP),
    V2.1429–30
Human respiratory syncytial virus infection,
    V1.793–4
  immune evasion *see* Immune evasion
  immunological synapse, **I**.465
  induction, lymphotoxin, **I**.286–7
  inflammatory, **I**.224
  intracellular signaling, **I**.222–3
  lymphocyte effects, **I**.224–7, **I**.509–12
    lymphoid tissue homing, **I**.226–7
    memory/effector function, **I**.224–6
    nonlymphoid tissue homing, **I**.227
  mucosal immune response, **I**.522–4
  nomenclature, **I**.217
  production
    basophils, **I**.59 (Tab.)
    CD8 T cells, **I**.422
    eosinophils, **I**.59 (Tab.)
    intradermal DNA vaccine delivery,
      I.912–13
    keratinocytes, **I**.820–1
    macrophages, **I**.27–9
  receptor antagonists, **I**.230–2
    Molluscum contagiosum virus, **V1**.622
    natural chemokines, **I**.232
    synthetic, **I**.231–2
    Vaccinia virus, **V1**.622
  receptors, **I**.220–2, **I**.510 (Tab.)
    airway hypersensitivity, **I**.734
    binding domains, **I**.222 (Fig.)
    cell expression, **I**.220
    dendritic cell activation, **I**.393–4
    dendritic cells, **I**.377–8
    HHV-6 infection, **V1**.530–1
    lymphocyte expression, **I**.221 (Fig.)
    MF59 adjuvant, **I**.927
    phagocytes, **I**.223–4
    sequence recognition domains, **I**.221
    structure, **I**.219 (Fig.)
    T helper cell expression, **I**.511–12
    see also CC chemokine receptors
  release in CNS infection, **V2**.1409–10
  structure, **I**.217–20, **I**.219 (Fig.)
    activity relationships, **I**.221–2
    amino terminal region, **I**.221
    dimerization, **I**.217–19, **I**.220 (Fig.)
    ELR motif, **I**.221
  viral immune interference *see* Immune
    evasion, viruses
  see also specific types
Chemostats, **B1**.41–2
  cell populations, **B1**.41–2
  growth rates in, **B1**.41
Chemosterilants, **B1**.421–2
Chemotaxis
  assays, neutrophils, **I**.50 (Tab.), **I**.51
  basophils, **I**.58, **I**.60
  defensins, **I**.169
  eosinophils, **I**.60–1
  inhibition
    bacterial immune interference, **I**.648
    pertussis toxin, **I**.648
  prostaglandin E$_2$ effects, **I**.188

Proteus swarm cells, **B2**.1438–9
T cells, **I**.224
transforming growth factor-β, **I**.297
see also individual chemokines
Chemotaxonomy, **B1**.22 (Tab.), **B1**.24, **B1**.32–3
Chemotherapy/chemoprophylaxis, parasite
    control *see* Control of infection, parasitic
    disease
'Chemotypes,' *Salmonella* O antigen,
    B2.1401–2
Chick eggs, virus culture, **V1**.90
  inoculation route, **V1**.94
  isolation from, **V1**.94
Chick embryos, **V1**.90
  virus culture, **V1**.4–5
Chicken anemia virus, type species, **V1**.41
Chicken embryo culture, *Coxiella burnetii*,
    B2.2073
Chiclero's ear, **P**.323
Chiclero's ulcer, **P**.313, **P**.323, **P**.323 (Fig.)
Chikungunya, **V2**.1021–2
  clinical features, **V2**.1021–2
  dengue fever *vs.,* **V2**.1021–2
  distribution, **V2**.1021
  hemorrhagic fever, **V2**.1022
  history, **V2**.1021
  rubella *vs.,* **V2**.970
  SINV infection *vs.,* **V2**.1021–2
  transmission, **V1**.372 (Tab.), **V2**.1021
  West Nile virus infection *vs.,* **V2**.1021–2
Chikungunya virus (CHIKV), **V2**.1011 (Tab.)
  transmission, **V2**.1016–17
Child abuse, *Neisseria gonorrhoeae* typing,
    B1.662
Child care centers, bacterial infection, **B1**.361
Children
  adenovirus infection, **V1**.443–5
  ascariasis, malnutrition, **P**.727
  aspergillosis prophylaxis, itraconazole, **M**.729
  bacteremia, blood cultures, **B1**.513
  candidiasis, **M**.596, **M**.609
  CNS infection
    bacterial meningitis, **B1**.557–8, **B1**.567
    intracranial abscess, **B1**.582, **B1**.583
    spinal epidural abscess, **B1**.593
    subdural empyema, **B1**.590, **B1**.591
  cryptosporidiosis, **P**.409
  disease burdens, **P**.28 (Tab.)
  EBV infection, **V1**.566–9
  emerging bacterial infection, **B1**.361
  Enterobius vermicularis, **P**.731
  hepatitis A, **V2**.1171–2
  HSV-1 infection, **V1**.508
  Human respiratory syncytial virus infection,
    V1.783–4, **V1**.797–8
  influenza, **V1**.661
  Lassa fever, **V2**.1070
  malaria *see* Malaria
  nappy rash, **M**.596, **M**.609
  parasite control, **P**.124–5
    ascariasis, **P**.125
    schistosomiasis, **P**.125
    trichuriasis, **P**.125
  penicilliosis marneffei, **M**.562, **M**.564
  respiratory tract infection, **V1**.443–4

Children (*Continued*)
RSV infection, **B1**.400
sporotrichosis, **M**.368
testing for *Trypanosoma cruzi* infection,
P.395
toxocariasis, **P**.752
transcutaneous immunization, **I**.838
trichomoniasis (maternal), **P**.259
tuberculosis, **B2**.1200–1
urinary tract infection prevalence, **B1**.672
see also Infants; Neonatal infection
Chilling food, **B1**.269–70
crustacea, **B1**.279–80
microbial growth effect, **B1**.264
offal, **B1**.273
poultry carcass, **B1**.277
preservation, **B1**.268 (Tab.), **B1**.269–70
vegetables, **B1**.281
see also Freezing
Chilomastix, classification, **P**.196–7
Chilomastix mesnili, **P**.270–2
classification, **P**.270
epidemiology, **P**.272
infection, **P**.266
diagnosis, **P**.272
immune response, **P**.76
pathogenicitiy, **P**.272
structure/life cycle, **P**.266, **P**.270–2,
P.271 (Fig.)
animal reservoirs, **P**.272
cysts, **P**.271 (Fig.)
flagella, **P**.270–1
interhuman transmission, **P**.270
trophozoites, **P**.271 (Fig.)
Chimerisation, monoclonal antibody therapy,
I.365, **I**.366 (Fig.)
Chimpanzee cytomegalovirus, **V1**.494 (Tab.)
Chimpanzee, hepatitis C model, **V2**.1194
China
food-borne botulism, **B2**.1067
parasitic disease importance, **P**.27 (Fig.)
schistosomiasis control programs, **P**.628,
P.635–6
Chionyphe carteri, **M**.386
CHITI gene, **I**.600–1
Chitin, **M**.70–1
Paracoccidioides brasiliensis, **M**.542
Trichuris trichiuria eggs, **P**.717–18
Chitinase, *Coccidioides immitis*, **M**.504,
M.506 (Fig.)
Chitin synthase, **M**.71, **M**.80
Candida gene, **M**.608
Chitosan nanoparticles
DNA vaccines, **I**.825
intranasal vaccine delivery, **I**.831
Chitosomes, **M**.71
Chlamydia, **B2**.**2006–25**
antibacterial susceptibility/resistance,
B2.2020
erythromycin, **B2**.2020
in vitro tests, **B2**.2020
macrolides, **B1**.486–7
quinolones, **B1**.492
tetracycline, **B2**.2020
genetics, **B2**.2008–9

historical perspectives, **B2**.2006–7
assays, **B2**.2006–7
cell culture, **B2**.2006–7
discovery, **B2**.2006
immune evasion, **I**.659
lysosomal killing resistance, **I**.651
lysosome fusion inhibition, **I**.650
infection *see below*
reproductive cycle, **B2**.2007–8, **B2**.2008 (Fig.)
elementary body, **B2**.2007–9, **B2**.2008 (Fig.)
reticulate body, **B2**.2007–8
structure
LPS, **B2**.2008–9, **B2**.2019
major outer membrane protein, **B2**.2008–9
taxonomy, **B2**.2007, **B2**.2007 (Tab.)
see also individual species
Chlamydiaceae, **B2**.2007
Chlamydia infection
body fluid antichlamydial activity, **B2**.2020
conjunctivitis, **B1**.600
cystitis, **B1**.678
diagnosis, **B2**.2017–20
antibody detection, **B1**.753
culture, **B2**.2017–18
Doctor's office tests, **B2**.2019
ELISA, **B2**.2006–7, **B2**.2018
genotyping, **B2**.2018
microscopy, **B2**.2017
nucleic acid tests, **B2**.2018–19
see also Polymerase chain reaction
(PCR)
ribosomal tests, **B2**.2018–19
serology, **B1**.753, **B2**.2019–20
serotyping, **B2**.2018
endocarditis, **B1**.533–4, **B1**.537
immune response, **B2**.2009
anti-heat shock protein antibodies,
B2.2009
mucosal immune response, **I**.522–3
NK cell actions, **I**.100
proinflammatory cytokines, **B2**.2009
T-cell response, **B2**.2009
keratitis, **B1**.601–2
pathogenesis, **B2**.2009
serovar differences, **B2**.2009
screening, **B2**.2021–2
asymptomatic individuals, **B2**.2021
partner notification, **B2**.2021
samples, **B2**.2021
therapy, **B2**.2020–1
Chlamydiales, **B2**.2007
Chlamydia pneumoniae
genetics, **B2**.2009
immune evasion, **I**.659–60
infection *see below*
in vitro culture, **B2**.2017 (Fig.), **B2**.2018
taxonomy, **B2**.2007, **B2**.2007 (Tab.)
Chlamydia pneumoniae infection, **B2**.2015–17
apoptosis prevention, **B2**.2009
clinical conditions, **B2**.2015–17,
B2.2015 (Tab.), **B2**.2016 (Tab.)
aortic stenosis, **B2**.2016
arteriosclerosis, **B2**.2016–17
asthma, **B2**.2016
atherosclerosis, **B1**.365

carotid artery stenosis, **B2**.2016
chronic bronchitis, **B2**.2015–16
chronic obstructive lung disease, **B2**.2016
CNS infection, **B2**.2017
coronary heart disease, **B2**.2016
endocarditis, **B1**.533
inflammatory bowel disease, **B2**.2017
myocardial infarctions, **B2**.2016
pneumonia, **B2**.2016
PNS infection, **B2**.2017
respiratory tract infection, **B2**.2015–16
epidemiology, **B2**.2015
developing countries, **B2**.2015
differences by country, **B2**.2015
historical perspectives, **B2**.2006, **B2**.2015
serology, **B1**.753
therapy, **B2**.2021
roxithromycin, **B2**.2021
salicylic acid, **B2**.2021
vaccines
development status, **I**.933 (Tab.)
subunit vaccine development, **I**.940
Chlamydia psittaci
historical perspectives, **B2**.2006
infection *see below*
in vitro culture, **B2**.2018
taxonomy, **B2**.2007, **B2**.2007 (Tab.)
Chlamydia psittaci infection, **B2**.2014–15
in animals, **B2**.2015
avian, **B2**.2014
non-avian, **B2**.2014
clinical conditions, **B2**.2014–15,
B2.2014 (Tab.)
abortion, **B2**.2015
conjunctivitis, **B2**.2015
endocarditis, **B1**.533, **B1**.536
placentitis, **B2**.2015
pneumonia, **B2**.2014–15
epidemiology, **B2**.2014
risks in culture, **B2**.2008
serology, **B1**.753, **B2**.2020
therapy, **B2**.2021
Chlamydia trachomatis
antibacterial susceptibility/resistance,
B1.499 (Tab.), **B2**.2020
genetics, **B2**.2009
cryptic plasmid, **B2**.2009
historical perspectives, **B2**.2006
infection *see below*
in vitro culture, **B2**.2017–18, **B2**.2017 (Fig.)
major outer membrane protein, **B2**.2007
molecular detection, **B1**.723 (Tab.)
hybrid capture assay, **B1**.731
probe hybridization, **B1**.725
transcription-mediated amplification,
B1.729–30
serovars, **B2**.2007
infectivity differences, **B2**.2009
major outer membrane protein
differences, **B2**.2018
taxonomy, **B2**.2007, **B2**.2007 (Tab.)
Chlamydia trachomatis infection, **B2**.2009–14
clinical syndromes, **B2**.2010–14,
B2.2010 (Tab.)
adverse pregnancy outcomes, **B2**.2011

Chlamydia trachomatis infection
  clinical syndromes (*Continued*)
    arthritis, **B2**.2013
    cervical cancer, **B2**.2013
    cervicitis, **B2**.2010
    conjunctivitis, **B1**.599, **B2**.2012,
      B2.2012 (Fig.), **B2**.2013, **B2**.2013 (Fig.)
    ectopic pregnancy, **B2**.2011, **B2**.2019–20
    endometritis, **B2**.2010–11, **B2**.2011 (Fig.)
    epididymitis, **B2**.2012–13
    in vitro fertilization effects, **B2**.2012
    keratitis, **B1**.601, **B1**.602
    lymphogranuloma venereum *see below*
    neonatal infection, **B2**.2013
    neonatal pneumonia, **B2**.2012 (Fig.),
      B2.2013, **B2**.2019–20
    nongonococcal urethritis, **B2**.2011
    perihepatitis, **B2**.2010–11, **B2**.2011 (Fig.)
    post-abortion pelvic inflammatory disease,
      B2.2012
    postgonococcal urethritis, **B2**.2011
    proctitis, **B2**.2012–13
    salpingitis, **B2**.2010–11, **B2**.2011 (Fig.)
    tubal factor infertility, **B2**.2010–11
    uveitis, **B2**.2013
    vaseitis, **B2**.2012–13
  dendritic cell infection, **I**.656
  epidemiology, **B2**.2009–10
    asymptomatic carriers, **B2**.2009–10
    by country, **B2**.2009–10
    prevalence, **B2**.2009–10
    risk factors, **B2**.2010
    youth, **B2**.2010
  IL-10 induction, **I**.653
  immunogenetics, **I**.594–5
  lymphogranuloma venereum, **B2**.2006,
    B2.2012
    serology, **B1**.753
  reactive arthritis, **I**.594–5
  serology, **B1**.753, **B2**.2019–20
  therapy, **B2**.2020–1
    amoxicillin, **B2**.2021
    azithromycin, **B2**.2018
    clindamycin, **B2**.2021
    guidelines, **B2**.2021
    protein inhibitors, **B2**.2020
    quinolones, **B2**.2021
  vaccines
    development status, **I**.933 (Tab.)
    ISCOMs adjuvant, **I**.930–1
    live virus vectors, **I**.903
  see also Trachoma
Chlamydiazyme®, **B2**.2006–7, **B2**.2018
Chlamydoabsidia padenii, **M**.281 (Tab.)
Chlamydoconidia
  Candida albicans, **M**.74, **M**.604–5
  Candida dubliniensis, **M**.604–5
  zygomycete, **M**.659–60
Chlamydophila pneumoniae, pharyngitis,
  B1.611–12
Chlamydophila psittaci, pharyngitis, **B1**.611–12
Chloramine, **B1**.424
Chloramphenicol, **B1**.482–5
  intracranial abscess, **B1**.588
  melioidosis treatment, **B2**.1631

mode of action, **B1**.484
Oroya fever treatment, **B2**.1891
pharmacology, **B1**.484
plague, **B2**.1466
resistance, **B1**.484
  Bacteroides, **B2**.1930–1, **B2**.1935
  Coxiella burnetii, **B2**.2077–8
  Enterococcus, **B2**.891–2, **B2**.892 (Tab.)
  Porphyromonas, **B2**.1930–1, **B2**.1935
  Prevotella, **B2**.1930–1, **B2**.1935
spectrum of activity, **B1**.482–4, **B1**.499 (Tab.)
  Actinomyces, **B2**.1011
  Burkholderia cepacia complex, **B2**.1610
  Campylobacter, **B2**.1548
  Cardiobacterium hominis, **B2**.1672–3
  Citrobacter, **B2**.1476
  Enterobacter, **B2**.1484–5
  Ewingella, **B2**.1493
  Haemophilus, **B2**.1702 (Tab.), **B2**.1703,
    B2.1704
  Klebsiella, **B2**.1480
  Leclercia, **B2**.1495
  Listeria, **B2**.956, **B2**.957–8
  Moellerella, **B2**.1496
  Pasteurella multocida, **B2**.1655
  Staphylococcus, **B2**.794 (Tab.)
  Streptococcus, **B2**.861–2
  Vibrio, **B2**.1514
  Yokenella, **B2**.1498
structure, **B1**.482–4, **B1**.484 (Fig.)
toxicity/adverse effects, **B1**.484–5
  'gray baby' syndrome, **B1**.485
  irreversible aplastic anemia, **B1**.484–5
  typhoid fever, **B2**.1415–16
Chlorbutanol, **B1**.427
Chlorella, **M**.396
  experimental infection, **M**.401
  histopathology, **M**.407–8
  identification, **M**.405–6
  morphology, **M**.403
  starch granules, **M**.407–8
Chlorella protothecoides, **M**.396
  ecology, **M**.396
  identification, **M**.405–6
Chlorhexidine, **B1**.426
  fungal infection, **B1**.439
  handwash, **B1**.378, **B1**.766
    Actinetobacter contamination, **B2**.1303
  irrigations, catheter insertion into bladder,
    B1.388
  Klebsiella, **B2**.1480
  membrane permeability, **B1**.438
  mycotic keratitis therapy, **M**.307
  resistance, **B1**.442, **B1**.443, **B1**.444
  Serratia, **B2**.1489
Chlorine dioxide, **B1**.424
Chlorine gas, **B1**.430
Chlorine-releasing agents (CRAs),
  B1.423 (Tab.), **B1**.424
  action, **B1**.437 (Tab.), **B1**.440
N-Chloro compounds, **B1**.424
Chloroform-methanol residue vaccines, Q
  fever, **B2**.2075
5-Chloro-*N*-methylisothiazol-3-one (CMIT),
  B1.427

Chloroquine
  babesiosis, **P**.459
  malaria therapy, **P**.506
  mechanism of action, **P**.479, **P**.509
  resistance, **P**.34
    pfcrt gene, **P**.509
    Plasmodium see Plasmodium
  viral cell entry, **V1**.213
Chlorotetracycline
  Coxiella burnetii resistance, **B2**.2077–8
  structure, **B1**.485 (Fig.)
Choclo virus, **V2**.1666 (Tab.)
CHOHR genes, poxvirus host range control,
  V1.624
Cholangiosarcoma
  liver fluke infection, **P**.649
  opisthorchiasis, **P**.649–50
Cholangitis
  chronic, **I**.776
  microsporidiosis, **P**.539
  sclerosing, in AIDS, **P**.405
Cholecystectomy, bacteremia after, **B2**.1112
Cholecystitis
  acalculous, **P**.539
  clonorchiasis, **P**.651
  microsporidiosis, **P**.539
  opisthorchiasis, **P**.651
Cholecystokinin, Borna disease virus infection,
  V2.1147
Cholera
  bottled water, **B1**.216
  as emerging bacterial infection
    ecological changes encouraging, **B1**.362
    human migration, **B1**.360
    public health infrastructure breakdown,
      B1.364
  epidemics, London (1854), **B1**.335,
    B1.336 (Fig.)
  historical perspective, **B2**.1318–31
    transmission, **B1**.335, **B1**.336 (Fig.)
  mucosal immune response, **I**.528–9
  'rice water' stools, **B2**.1516–17
  toxins, *Escherichia coli* enterotoxin *vs.*,
    B2.1375
  vaccine development, **B1**.335, **I**.933 (Tab.)
Cholera toxin (CT), **B2**.1517–20
  as adjuvant, **I**.931–2, **I**.937–8
    bare skin immunization, **I**.823, **I**.824, **I**.826,
      I.826 (Fig.)
    intranasal vaccine delivery, **I**.831
    mucosal administration, **I**.926–7
    as mucosal vaccines, **I**.530
    transcutaneous immunization, **I**.837
  animal models, **B2**.1518
  bacteriophage-encoded, **B2**.1511–2,
    B2.1518
  genes, **B2**.1518
  IL-12 suppression, **I**.652
  MHC class II presentation interference,
    I.659
  secretory effect, **B2**.1518
  structure, **B2**.1517–18
  T cell apoptosis, **I**.655
  TNF-α suppression, **I**.652
Cholestasis
  ascending, liver fluke infection, **P**.649

Cholestasis (*Continued*)
  hepatitis A, **V2**.1172
  hepatitis E, **V2**.1179
Cholesterol
  mycoplasmas, **B2**.1969–70, **B2**.1975–6
  Pneumocystis, **M**.772, **M**.780, **M**.781
Choline binding protein Am (CbpA), **B1**.627
Chondroitin sulfate, upregulation in malaria,
  P.496–7
Chordopoxvirinae
  characteristics, **V1**.177 (Tab.)
  classification, **V1**.42–4, **V1**.43 (Tab.),
    V1.579 (Tab.), **V1**.582, **V1**.594
  phylogenetic comparison, **V1**.583,
    V1.584 (Fig.), **V1**.585 (Fig.)
  taxonomy, **V1**.595 (Tab.)
Chordopoxviruses *see Chordopoxvirinae*
Chorioallantoic membrane (CAM), **V1**.90,
  V1.94
Chorionic villus sampling, **V2**.1445
Chorioretinitis, **M**.317, **M**.318
  candidiasis, **M**.320–1
  congenital HCMV infection, **V2**.1449
  subacute sclerosing panencephalitis (SSPE),
    V1.725, **V2**.1432
Choroid plexus
  virus dissemination, **V1**.242–3
  virus entry route, **V2**.1404–5
Christie–Atkins–Munch-Petersen (CAMP)
  test, **B1**.668
CHROMagar system, **M**.604, **M**.604 (Fig.)
Chromatin organization
  somatic recombination, Igs, **I**.328–9
  TCR gene assembly, **I**.458
Chromatin remodeling, *Trypanosoma brucei*,
  P.361
Chromista, classification, **P**.195–6
Chromobacterium
  habitats, **B2**.1649–50
  waterborne, **B1**.211
Chromobacterium violaceum, **B2**.1679–81
  antibacterial susceptibility/resistance,
    B2.1680–1
  characteristics, **B2**.1680, **B2**.1680 (Tab.)
  geographical distribution, **B2**.1679–80
  infection, **B2**.1680
Chromoblastomycosis
  causative agents, **M**.22, **M**.29–30, **M**.30 (Fig.)
    Botryomyces caespitosus, **M**.357
    Cladophialophora arxii, **M**.357
    classification, **M**.359
    ecology, **M**.357
    Exophiala spinifera, **M**.357
    Fonsecaea compacta, **M**.29–30, **M**.357
    identification, **M**.83 (Tab.), **M**.360
    morphology, **M**.29–30, **M**.30 (Fig.), **M**.356,
      M.357 (Fig.), **M**.359–60, **M**.362–3,
      M.363–4
    Phaeosclera dematioides, **M**.357
    Phialophora verrucosa, **M**.29–30,
      M.30 (Fig.), **M**.356, **M**.357
    Rhinocladiella aquaspersa, **M**.29–30, **M**.357
    Sporothrix schenckii var. *luriei*, **M**.357
    Wangiella dermatitidis, **M**.357
    see also individual species

clinical presentation, **M**.360–2, **M**.362 (Fig.),
  M.363 (Fig.)
  CNS, **M**.361–2
  foot, **M**.361–2
  legs, **M**.361–2
  lungs, **M**.361–2
conceptual basis, **M**.29
diagnosis, **M**.83 (Tab.), **M**.358–9, **M**.363–4
  histopathology, **M**.128 (Tab.), **M**.139 (Fig.),
    M.362–3
  serology, **M**.363
  skin testing, **M**.363–4
  specimen site selection, **M**.83 (Tab.)
epidemiology, **M**.356, **M**.357–9
  animal infection, **M**.359
  nosocomial infection, **M**.359
  transplantation recipients, **M**.359
genetic susceptibility, **M**.359
history, **M**.29, **M**.356–7
immune response, **M**.363
  HLA, **M**.359
  transforming growth factor β -activated
    fibroblasts, **M**.361
immunosuppression, **M**.359
nomenclature, **M**.356–7
progression, **M**.361–2
therapy, **M**.364
  corticosteroids, **M**.359
  flucytosine, **M**.364
  itraconazole, **M**.364
  terbinafine, **M**.364
  thiabendazole, **M**.364
Chromopeptides, *Pseudomonas*, **B2**.1596
Chromophores, agglutination tests, **B1**.748–9
Chromosomal separation, microsporidians,
  P.533
Chromosomal translocations, Burkitt
  lymphoma (BL), **V1**.570
Chromosome(s)
  multiple, **B1**.46
  mutation, quinolones resistance, **B1**.492–3
  rearrangements, mycoplasmas, **B2**.1982
  replication, **B1**.46
  Salmonella molecular typing, **B2**.1410–11
  see also Genetics
Chromosome 5 gene cluster, immunogenetics,
  I.580–2, **I**.581 (Fig.)
Chromosome 17, immunogenetics, **I**.582,
  I.583 (Fig.)
Chromosome mobilizing ability (cma),
  conjugation, **B1**.101
Chromotrope 2R, microsporidiosis diagnosis,
  P.546
Chronic adult T-cell leukemia, **V2**.1289–90
Chronic asthma *see* Asthma
Chronic asymptomatic phase, HIV infection,
  I.790
Chronic atrophic candidiasis, **M**.598
Chronic bronchitis *see* Bronchitis
Chronic bronchopneumonitis, TAP deficiency,
  I.776
Chronic cavitary pulmonary aspergillosis
  (CCPA), **M**.697
Chronic cholangitis, cryptosporidiosis, **I**.776
Chronic fibrosing pulmonary aspergillosis
  (CFPA), **M**.697

Chronic gastritis, *Helicobacter pylori* infection,
  B2.1564–5, **B2**.1578, **B2**.1579
Chronic granulomatous disease (CGD), **I**.35,
  I.48, **I**.48 (Tab.), **B1**.741, **I**.768 (Fig.),
  I.769–70
  diagnosis, nitroblue tetrazolium assay,
    I.51 (Fig.), **I**.52
  genetics, **I**.48
    gene defects, **I**.769
    gp22 deficiency, **I**.769
    gp91 deficiency, **I**.769
  infection, **I**.770
    aspergillosis, **I**.48, **I**.770
    Burkholderia cepacia, **I**.770
    Nocardia, **I**.48
    recurrent, **I**.26
    Serrata marcescens, **I**.770
    Serratia burkholderia, **I**.48
    Staphylococcus aureus, **I**.48, **I**.770
  signs/symptoms, **I**.48
  therapy, **I**.50
    bone marrow transplants, **I**.50
Chronic hepatitis B *see* Hepatitis B
Chronic hyperplastic candidiasis, **M**.598
Chronic infection, **V1**.373–4
Chronic inflammatory arthropathy, HTLV
  infection, **I**.801
Chronic lead poisoning, EDTA, **B1**.428
Chronic lymphocytic leukemia (CLL),
  I.788 (Tab.)
Chronic mucocutaneous candidiasis, **M**.13,
  M.597, **M**.610–11, **I**.779
Chronic myelogenous leukemia, **I**.865 (Tab.)
Chronic myeloid leukemia, **I**.258
Chronic necrotizing pulmonary aspergillosis
  (CNPA), **M**.697
Chronic obstructive pulmonary disease
  (COPD), **B1**.647–9, **I**.734–5
  Chlamydia pneumoniae infection, **B2**.2016
  Chlamydia trachomatis infection, **B2**.2013
  pathogenesis, **B1**.648
  therapy of bacterial infection, **B1**.649
Chronic schistosomiasis, **I**.718–19
Chronic sinusitis, **B1**.615
Chronic suppurative otitis media, **B1**.617
Chronic wasting disease (CWD) of deer and
  elk, **V2**.1347, **V2**.1363–4
  bovine spongiform encephalopathy *vs.*,
    V2.1363
  clinical signs, **V2**.1364
  cross-species transmission, **V2**.1364
    to humans, **V2**.1371
  emerging viral infection, **V2**.1651 (Tab.)
Chrysonilia, oculomycoses, **M**.275 (Tab.)
Chrysosporium, **M**.811
  oculomycoses, **M**.275 (Tab.)
Chrysosporium parvum, **M**.811, **M**.815
  var. *crescens*
    histopathology, **M**.127 (Tab.),
      M.128 (Tab.), **M**.135 (Fig.)
    morphology, **M**.127 (Tab.)
Chrysoviridae
  classification, **V1**.27 (Tab.), **V1**.47 (Tab.)
  see also specific viruses
CHS1/LYST gene, **I**.481

Chyluria, **P**.152
  lymphatic filariasis, **P**.774
Chymotrypsin, **B2**.1924 (Tab.)
Chytridiales, **M**.51, **M**.53
Chytridiomycota, **M**.44 (Fig.), **M**.49–53
c-IAP1, **I**.135
c-IAP2, **I**.135
Ciclopirox, **M**.183 (Tab.), **M**.184–5, **M**.233–4
  mechanism of action, **M**.184–5
  therapy
    dermatophytoses therapy, **M**.184–5
    onychomycosis, **M**.187
    piedra, **M**.186
    seborrheic dermatitis, **M**.185
    tinea capitis, **M**.188–9
    tinea corporis, **M**.186
    tinea cruris, **M**.186
    tinea nigra, **M**.186
    tinea pedis, **M**.186–7
Ciclosporine, immunodeficiency, **I**.788 (Tab.)
Cidofovir, **V2**.1616
  HCMV infection, **V1**.527
    in AIDS/HIV infection, **V2**.1503, **V2**.1505
  hepatitis B therapy, **V2**.1616
  herpesvirus infection, **V2**.1616
  HPV infection, **V2**.1616
  HSV infection therapy, **V2**.1616
  mechanism of action, **V1**.590
  poxvirus infection, **V2**.1616
  progressive multifocal leucoencephalopathy, **V2**.1418
  smallpox therapy, **V1**.590
  structure, **V2**.1617 (Fig.)
Ciguatera fish poisoning, **B1**.280
Cilastatin, structure, **B1**.479 (Fig.)
Cilia
  Balantidium coli, **P**.276, **P**.277 (Fig.)
  dyskinesia, **B1**.626
  epithelial cells, **B1**.176
  protozoa, **P**.179, **P**.179 (Fig.), **P**.180 (Fig.)
Ciliated epithelia, rhinovirus pathogenesis, **V2**.873–4
Ciliates
  immune response, **P**.76
  nuclei, **P**.173
  pellicle, **P**.162, **P**.164
Cilo-inhibitory proteins, *Aspergillus fumigatus*, **M**.707
Cimetidine, **M**.184
Cinnamon, **B1**.287
Cinoxacin, structure, **B1**.494 (Fig.)
Ciprofloxacin
  cat-scratch disease treatment, **B2**.1898–9
  cyclosporiasis, **P**.415–16
  formulations, **B1**.493
  osteomyelitis, **B1**.699
  resistance, **B1**.444
    Neisseria gonorrhoeae, **B1**.661, **B2**.1292 (Fig.)
    Salmonella Typhi, **B2**.1416
  spectrum of activity, **B1**.492, **B1**.499 (Tab.)
    Bacillus anthracis, **B2**.938
    Borrelia, **B2**.1831 (Tab.)
    Enterobacter, **B2**.1484–5

Haemophilus, **B2**.1702 (Tab.), **B2**.1703 (Tab.), **B2**.1710
    Listeria, **B2**.957–8
    Nocardia, **B2**.1145, **B2**.1165–6
    Rahnella, **B2**.1497
    Salmonella Paratyphi A, **B2**.1421
  structure, **B1**.494 (Fig.)
  tularemia treatment, **B2**.1755
  typhoid fever, **B2**.1416
Circoviridae
  ambisense coding, **V1**.181
  characteristics, **V1**.177 (Tab.)
  classification, **V1**.27 (Tab.), **V1**.41–2, **V1**.41 (Tab.)
  see also specific viruses
Circovirus, **V1**.41
Circular dichroism (CD) spectroscopy, **V2**.1352, **V2**.1353 (Fig.)
Circulating anodic antigen (CAA), schistosomiasis, **P**.621–2
Circulating cathodic antigen (CCA), schistosomiasis, **P**.621–2
Circulating recombinant forms (CRFs), HIV-1, **V2**.1330–1
Circulatory failure, septic shock, **I**.699–701
Circum oval precipitin (COP) test, **P**.606, **P**.607 (Fig.)
Circumsporozoite-like antigen (CSL), *Cryptosporidium parvum*, **P**.402
Circumsporozoite protein (CSP) *see* Malaria
Circumsporozoite protein (CP), *Plasmodium*, **P**.82
Cirrhosis
  hepatitis B *see* Hepatitis B
  hepatitis C, **V2**.1205
  hepatocellular carcinoma, **V2**.1249
  Pasteurella multocida infection, **B2**.1654–5
cis-acting elements, TCR gene assembly, **I**.458
Cistern waters, **B1**.215, **B1**.216 (Tab.)
Citric acid, **B1**.422
Citrobacter, **B2**.1474–6
  antibacterial susceptibility/resistance, **B2**.1476
  biochemistry, **B2**.1475–6
  characteristics, **B2**.1474
  classification, **B2**.1474–5
    DNA–DNA analysis, **B2**.1338
  culture, **B2**.1475
  definition, **B2**.1474
  habitats, **B2**.1476
  H antigen, *Salmonella vs.*, **B2**.1402
  infection
    intestinal, **B2**.1347
    keratitis, **B1**.601
    nosocomial infection, **B1**.398 (Tab.)
  isolation/identification
    historical perspective, **B2**.1351
    screening tests, **B2**.1349 (Tab.)
    typing methods, **B2**.1476
  morphology, **B2**.1475
  as normal microbiota, **B1**.296 (Tab.)
  pathogenicity, **B2**.1476
  species, **B2**.1474–5, **B2**.1475 (Tab.)
    species 9 *see Citrobacter rodentium*
    species 10 *see Citrobacter gillenii*

    species 11 *see Citrobacter murliniae*
  waterborne, **B1**.221, **B1**.222–3
Citrobacter amalonaticus, **B2**.1475
  antibacterial susceptibility/resistance, **B2**.1476
    intrinsic, **B2**.1352 (Tab.)
  biochemical tests, **B2**.1319 (Tab.)
  biogroup 1 *see Citrobacter farmeri*
  characteristics, **B2**.1475–6, **B2**.1475 (Tab.)
  classification, **B2**.1475
  typing methods, **B2**.1476
Citrobacter braakii, **B2**.1475
  biochemical tests, **B2**.1319 (Tab.)
  characteristics, **B2**.1475–6, **B2**.1475 (Tab.)
  classification, **B2**.1475
Citrobacter diversus, **B2**.1475
  antibacterial susceptibility/resistance, **B2**.1476
    intrinsic, **B2**.1352 (Tab.)
  biochemical tests, **B2**.1319 (Tab.)
  characteristics, **B2**.1475 (Tab.)
  classification/nomenclature, **B2**.1337–8, **B2**.1475
  nosocomial infection, **B1**.398 (Tab.)
  pathogenicity, **B2**.1476
  typing methods, **B2**.1476
Citrobacter farmeri, **B2**.1475
  biochemical tests, **B2**.1319 (Tab.)
  characteristics, **B2**.1475 (Tab.)
  classification, **B2**.1475
Citrobacter freundii, **B2**.1474
  antibacterial susceptibility/resistance, **B2**.1476
    intrinsic, **B2**.1352 (Tab.)
  biochemical tests, **B2**.1319 (Tab.)
  characteristics, **B2**.1475–6, **B2**.1475 (Tab.)
  infection, **B1**.250
    intracranial abscess, **B1**.585
    nosocomial infection, **B1**.398 (Tab.)
  pathogenicity, **B2**.1476
  typing methods, **B2**.1476
  waterborne, **B1**.220
Citrobacter gillenii
  biochemical tests, **B2**.1319 (Tab.)
  characteristics, **B2**.1475 (Tab.)
  classification, **B2**.1475
Citrobacter intermedius
  biogroup a *see Citrobacter amalonaticus*
  biogroup b *see Citrobacter diversus*
Citrobacter koseri see Citrobacter diversus
Citrobacter murliniae
  biochemical tests, **B2**.1319 (Tab.)
  characteristics, **B2**.1475 (Tab.)
  classification, **B2**.1475
Citrobacter rodentium
  biochemical tests, **B2**.1319 (Tab.)
  characteristics, **B2**.1475 (Tab.)
  classification, **B2**.1475
Citrobacter sedlakii, **B2**.1475
  biochemical tests, **B2**.1319 (Tab.)
  characteristics, **B2**.1475 (Tab.)
  classification, **B2**.1475
Citrobacter werkmanii, **B2**.1475
  biochemical tests, **B2**.1319 (Tab.)
  characteristics, **B2**.1475–6, **B2**.1475 (Tab.)

Citrobacter werkmanii, (Continued)
classification, **B2**.1475
Citrobacter youngae, **B2**.1475
biochemical tests, **B2**.1319 (Tab.)
characteristics, **B2**.1475–6, **B2**.1475 (Tab.)
classification, **B2**.1475
Citrus stubborn, **B2**.1965–6
Civil unrest
epidemics, **P**.117
malaria epidemiology, **P**.513–14
parasite control effects, **P**.103–6, **P**.107 (Tab.)
African trypanosomiasis, **P**.107 (Tab.)
cutaneous leishmaniasis, **P**.107 (Tab.)
dracunculiasis, **P**.107 (Tab.), **P**.123–4
malaria, **P**.107 (Tab.)
onchocerciasis, **P**.107 (Tab.)
visceral leishmaniasis, **P**.107 (Tab.)
parasite infection burden, **P**.25–6
malaria, **P**.34
cJun NH$_2$-terminal kinase (JNK), **I**.43
c-Jun transcription factor, JC virus, **V1**.476–7
Ckβ8 (CCL23), **I**.218 (Tab.)
c-kit see Stem cell factor (SCF: *c-kit*)
Clades, papillomaviruses, **V1**.449–50
Cladograms, fungal classification, **M**.48
Cladophialophora, **M**.61–3
Cladophialophora arxii, chromoblastomycosis, **M**.357
Cladophialophora bantiana
histopathology, **M**.89 (Tab.), **M**.128 (Tab.), **M**.139 (Fig.)
infection
CNS, **M**.744, **M**.745
therapy, **M**.745
Cladophialophora carrionii
chromoblastomycosis, **M**.29–30, **M**.30 (Fig.), **M**.356
therapy, **M**.364
ecology, **M**.357–8, **M**.358 (Tab.)
histopathology, **M**.89 (Tab.), **M**.128 (Tab.)
morphology, **M**.30 (Fig.), **M**.360, **M**.362 (Fig.)
Cladorrhinum bulbillosum, oculomycoses, **M**.278 (Tab.)
Cladosporium
CNS infection, **M**.743
contact lens contamination, **M**.330–1
Cladosporium, in cereals, **B1**.284
Clams, microbiology, **B1**.280
Clarithromycin
pharmacology, **B1**.487
resistance, *Helicobacter pylori,* **B2**.1575
spectrum of activity
Bordetella, **B2**.1793–4
Borrelia, **B2**.1830
gram-positive anaerobic cocci, **B2**.912
Haemophilus, **B2**.1702 (Tab.), **B2**.1703 (Tab.), **B2**.1710
Helicobacter pylori, **B2**.1574–5
Mycobacterium, **B2**.1222–3
Mycoplasma pneumoniae, **B1**.634
Nocardia, **B2**.1145
Pasteurella multocida, **B2**.1655
structure, **B1**.486
Clarithromycin, toxoplasmosis, **P**.437

Classical swine fever (hog cholera), **V2**.993
Pestivirus infection, **V2**.1005
Classification
bacteria, **B1.15–36**
academic, **B1**.16, **B1**.17
attitudes to, **B1**.16
bacteriology, **B1**.17
characterization tests, **B1**.22–6
see also specific tests
classification process, **B1**.18–9, **B1**.19 (Fig.)
context-specificity, **B1**.16–7
evolution, **B1**.30
formal classification, **B1**.16–8
historical aspects, **B1**.17–8
operation, **B1**.17–8
rules, **B1**.18
future prospects, **B1**.33
GC ratios, **B1**.13
hierarchical, **B1**.17
historical aspects, **B1**.11, **B1**.13, **B1**.17–8
identification approaches, **B1**.19–22
Lockean *vs.* Aristotelian views, **B1**.13
mycoplasmas, **B2**.1966–70, **B2**.1966 (Fig.)
numerical, **B1**.11
polyphasic, **B1**.22 (Tab.), **B1**.26, **B1**.30, **B1**.33
process, **B1**.18–9
results, **B1**.26–7
presentation of, **B1**.26–8, **B1**.27 (Fig.)
service culture collections, **B1**.28–9
single-tier classification, **B1**.17
speciation, **B1**.30
species concept, **B1**.17, **B1**.20–2, **B1**.29–30
systems, **B1**.16–7
taxon concept, **B1**.17
type concept, **B1**.28–9
'type' concept, **B1**.28–9
vernacular/trivial classifications, **B1**.16
'weighting' of characters, **B1**.11
see also Nomenclature
fungi, **M**.4, **M**.43–4, **M**.49–51, **M**.50–51 (Tab.)
biological, **M**.44–5
future aspects of, **M**.51
genomics and bioinformatics, **M**.49
medically important fungi, **M**.46, **M**.51, **M**.53, **M**.63–6
mitosporic fungi, **M**.49, **M**.51
molecular markers, **M**.47
molecular methodology, **M**.46, **M**.46–7, **M**.47 (Tab.), **M**.49, **M**.63
morphological, **M**.45, **M**.46 (Tab.), **M**.49, **M**.51
phenotypic, **M**.46–7, **M**.46 (Tab.), **M**.49
phyla, **M**.44, **M**.44 (Fig.)
phylogenetic methods, **M**.44–9, **M**.47 (Tab.)
algorithms, **M**.47–8
cladograms, **M**.48
clinical significance, **M**.63
concept, **M**.47–9
phylograms, **M**.48, **M**.52 (Fig.), **M**.62 (Fig.)
statistical testing, **M**.48
tree formation, **M**.48, **M**.52 (Fig.)
problems, **M**.49
species, **M**.44

see also individual species
viruses, **V1.24–37**, **V1**.26, **V1**.176–80, **V1**.177 (Tab.), **V1.38–56**
Baltimore scheme, **V1**.109, **V1**.109 (Fig.), **V1**.180
binomial nomenclature, **V1**.35–6
definition, **V1**.25–6
biochemistry, **V1**.25
living matter, **V1**.25
negative features, **V1**.25
protein role, **V1**.25–6, **V1**.25 (Fig.)
virions *vs.,* **V1**.26
virus particles *vs.,* **V1**.26
by disease status, **V1**.26
double-stranded DNA viruses, **V1**.40–5, **V1**.43 (Tab.)
double-stranded RNA viruses, **V1**.40–1, **V1**.47–8, **V1**.47 (Tab.)
families, **V1**.26, **V1**.27 (Tab.), **V1**.29, **V1**.35, **V1**.39, **V1**.378
filtration, **V1**.24–5
genera, **V1**.26, **V1**.27 (Tab.), **V1**.29, **V1**.35, **V1**.39
definition, **V1**.582
hierarchical system, **V1**.26, **V1**.38–9
historical aspects, **V1**.7–8, **V1**.24–5, **V1**.38–9
orders, **V1**.26, **V1**.35, **V1**.39, **V1**.378
phylogenetic analysis *see* Phylogenetic analysis
reverse-transcribing viruses, **V1**.45–7, **V1**.46 (Tab.)
single-stranded DNA viruses, **V1**.40–1, **V1**.41–2, **V1**.41 (Tab.)
species, **V1**.29–35, **V1**.39–40, **V1**.54–5
classical definitions, **V1**.30
definition, **V1**.29, **V1**.31, **V1**.39–40
demarcation, **V1**.33–4
ecological niche occupancy, **V1**.32
evolutionary species, **V1**.30
as fuzzy sets, **V1**.30–1
as polythetic class, **V1**.31–2, **V1**.32 (Fig.)
polythetic definition, **V1**.55
as replicating lineages, **V1**.32
subfamilies, **V1**.35, **V1**.39
type species, definition, **V1**.32–3
see also Universal System of Virus Taxonomy; *specific viruses*
see also Identification
Class switching, **I**.327–8, **I**.330–2, **I**.331 (Fig.)
basophil effects, **I**.66
B cell development, **I**.491
IFN-γ effects, **I**.327
IgA *see* Immunoglobulin A (IgA)
IgE, **I**.327, **I**.331
IgG2, **I**.327
IgG3, **I**.327
IL-4 effects, **I**.280, **I**.327, **I**.331
junction region analysis, **I**.332
memory B cell development, **I**.327–8
plasma cell development, **I**.327–8
'switch' recombination regions, **I**.331, **I**.332
transforming growth factor-β effects, **I**.331
V(D)J recombination, **I**.330
Clathrin-coated pits, **P**.162
Clavam, structure, **B1**.471 (Fig.)

Clavibacter pyli, European corn borer protection, **B1**.203–4

Clavispora lusitaniae, **M**.583, **M**.586
　nosocomial infection, **M**.586

Clavispora obtusa, **M**.583

Clavulanate-sensitive β-lactamase, *Burkholderia pseudomallei,* **B2**.1620

Clavulanic acid
　Nocardia, **B2**.1165–6
　resistant enzymes, **B1**.472–3
　structure, **B1**.479 (Fig.)

Clay soils, **B1**.196

Clean Drinking Water Supply and Sanitation Decade (1981–90), **P**.832

Cleaners
　hospital, **M**.706
　wig, **M**.18–9

Clean rooms, airborne bacteria, **B1**.186 (Tab.)

Clearview®, *Chlamydia* diagnosis, **B2**.2019

Cleistothecia
　Aspergillus, **M**.692
　Histoplasma capsulatum, **M**.520

Climate change
　epidemics, **P**.117
　malaria, **P**.103–6, **P**.512–13
　parasite control, **P**.103–6

Climate, enteroviruses, **V2**.874

Clindamycin, **M**.789
　antimalarial action, **P**.479
　Babesia microti infection treatment, **P**.459
　bacterial vaginosis treatment, **B1**.666–8
　colitis associated, **B2**.1119
　mechanism of action, **P**.479
　resistance, *Bacteroides/Prevotella/Porphyromonas,* **B2**.1931, **B2**.1935
　spectrum of activity, **B1**.487
　　Chlamydia trachomatis, **B2**.2021
　　gram-positive anaerobic cocci, **B2**.912
　　Listeria, **B2**.957–8
　　Pasteurella multocida, **B2**.1655
　structure, **B1**.488 (Fig.)
　toxoplasmosis, **P**.437

Clinical Laboratory Improvement Act (1992), **V2**.1547–8

Clinical trials
　attenuated viral vaccine vectors, **I**.898–9
　gene therapy, **V2**.1590–1
　randomized, **B1**.313
　type I INFs, **I**.258–9, **I**.261
　vaccine efficacy, **V2**.1558
　virus-like particles, **I**.840–1

Clinico-epidemiological approach, malaria epidemiology, **P**.513

Cliofungin, **M**.154

CLIP®, applications, **B1**.733

Clofazimine
　leprosy treatment, **B2**.1203
　lobomycosis, **M**.434

Clonal anergy
　CD4 T cell tolerance induction, **I**.396, **I**.397 (Tab.)
　oral tolerance, **I**.543
　peripheral tolerance, **I**.749

Clonal deletion
　CD4 T cell tolerance induction, **I**.397 (Tab.)
　oral tolerance, **I**.543
　　　T cells, **I**.749

Clonal ignorance, CD4 T cell tolerance induction, **I**.397 (Tab.)

Clonal selection theory, antibody production, **I**.321–2

Cloning, type I interferon receptors, **I**.247

Clonorchiasis
　clinical manifestations, **P**.649–50
　　acute disease, **P**.649
　　bile duct cancer, **P**.641, **P**.648–9, **P**.651
　　hepatolithiasis, **P**.649
　control, **P**.40, **P**.654
　　reinfection, **P**.654
　diagnosis
　　antigen detection, **P**.653
　　egg morphology, **P**.652–3
　　PCR, **P**.653
　epidemiology, **P**.40, **P**.46 (Tab.)
　　geographical distribution, **P**.40, **P**.41 (Fig.)
　immune response, **P**.652
　pathogenesis/pathology, **P**.651
　　acute inflammatory reactions, **P**.651
　　carcinogenesis, **P**.651
　　cholecystitis, **P**.651
　public health importance, **P**.105 (Tab.)
　transmission, **P**.645

Clonorchis, **I**.682
　infection *see* Clonorchiasis
　life cycle
　　life span, **P**.646
　　primary intermediate hosts, **P**.646
　　secondary intermediate hosts, **P**.646
　prevalence, **P**.646–7
　transmission/epidemiology
　　age-related patterns, **P**.648
　　location in host, **P**.648
　　raw/undercooked food, **P**.647

Clonorchis sinensis, **P**.584, **P**.640
　classification, **P**.641–2
　historical aspects, **P**.11, **P**.641
　infection *see* Clonorchiasis
　life cycle, **P**.644 (Fig.)
　　animal reservoirs, **P**.646
　　in definitive host, **P**.645
　morphology, **P**.642–3
　　adult, **P**.642 (Fig.)
　movement, **P**.644
　nutrition, **P**.644

'Close contact,' definition, **I**.951 (Tab.)

Closteroviridae
　classification, **V1**.27 (Tab.), **V1**.51 (Tab.)
　see also specific viruses

Clostridial myonecrosis, in humans *see* gas gangrene

Clostridium, **B2**.1089
　antigens, **B2**.1047, **B2**.1097–111
　bacteriocins, **B2**.1046–7, **B2**.1093
　bacteriophages, **B2**.1046, **B2**.1093
　biochemistry
　　anaerobic growth, **B2**.1112, **B2**.1113
　　butyrate/butanol fermentation, **B1**.56
　　carbohydrate metabolism, **B2**.1095
　　formic acid fermentation, **B1**.55
　　lecithinases, **B2**.1094
　　lipases, **B2**.1094

　　nucleotide metabolism, **B2**.1095
　　oxidation-reduction potential, **B2**.1112, **B2**.1113
　　protein metabolism, **B2**.1095
　　proteolysis, **B2**.1094, **B2**.1095
　cell walls, **B2**.1045, **B2**.1092
　classification, **B2**.1035–6, **B2**.1042–3, **B2**.1090, **B2**.1091 (Fig.)
　conjugation, **B1**.103
　culture, **B2**.1093–4, **B2**.1113
　　agar plates, **B2**.1093
　　blood agar plates, **B2**.1093–4
　　colonies, **B2**.1093–4
　　cooked meat medium, **B2**.1094
　　egg yolk agar media, **B2**.1094
　　Macconkey's agar, **B2**.1094
　　selective media, **B2**.1094
　definition, **B2**.1035–6
　habitats, **B2**.1037, **B2**.1043, **B2**.1090
　hemolysis, **B2**.1093–4
　infection
　　antibody detection, **B1**.751
　　bacteremia, **B1**.523, **B2**.1116–17
　　cellulitis, **B2**.1112
　　endocarditis, **B1**.533
　　food poisoning and other diarrhea, **B2**.1117–18
　　intracranial abscess, **B1**.585
　　necrotizing jejunitis, **B2**.1118–19
　　spreading factors, **B1**.153 (Tab.)
　　types of diseases, **B2**.1089, **B2**.1116–19
　　wounds, **B2**.1112
　　see also Gas gangrene
　　see also Botulism; *Clostridium perfringens,* infection
　isolation/identification, **B2**.1095–6
　　differential characterization, **B2**.1096–7
　　EIAs, **B1**.756
　　immunoserology, **B1**.756–7
　　Nagler reaction, **B1**.756–7
　　staining reactions, **B2**.1090–1
　metabolism, **B2**.1043–7, **B2**.1094–6
　　anaeobiosis, **B2**.1094–5
　morphology, **B2**.1090, **B2**.1093–4
　　capsules, **B2**.1045, **B2**.1092
　　flagella, **B2**.1092
　　spores, **B2**.1044–5, **B2**.1091–2
　as normal microbiota, **B1**.296 (Tab.)
　pasteurization, **B1**.232–3
　pathogenic species, **B1**.203, **B2**.1035–7
　　historical background, **B2**.1036–7
　physical/chemical agent susceptibility/resistance, **B2**.1095
　physical features, **B2**.1043–7, **B2**.1090–3
　plasmids, **B2**.1045–6, **B2**.1092–3
　potatoes, **B1**.281
　species, **B2**.1091 (Fig.), **B2**.1098 (Tab.)
　　subtyping, **B2**.1096–7
　　toxin producing, **B2**.1097–111
　sterilization
　　heat, **B1**.446 (Tab.)
　　ionizing radiation, **B1**.450
　toxins, **B2**.1036, **B2**.1097–111
　　genetics, **B2**.1097–111

Clostridium, (Continued)
  virulence factors
    hemolysin, **B1**.153 (Tab.)
    hyaluronidase, **B1**.153 (Tab.)
    spreading determinants, **B1**.153 (Tab.)
  waterborne, **B1**.212
Clostridium acetobutylicum, **B2**.1063–4
Clostridium argentinense, **B2**.1051 (Fig.),
    B2.1059
  plasmids, **B2**.1045–6
  toxins, **B2**.1098 (Tab.)
Clostridium baratii, **B2**.1060
  bacteriophages, **B2**.1046
  botulism, **B2**.1039–40, **B2**.1042–3, **B2**.1062,
    B2.1070
  isolation/identification, **B2**.1096
  toxins, **B2**.1098 (Tab.)
Clostridium bifermentans, **B2**.1090, **B2**.1105–6,
    B2.1112
  culture, **B2**.1094
  habitats, **B2**.1090
  infection, **B2**.1117
  toxins, **B2**.1098 (Tab.), **B2**.1105–6
Clostridium botulinum, **B2**.1035–6
  antibacterial susceptibility/resistance,
    B2.1064–5
  antigens, **B2**.1047
  antitoxin, **B2**.1049, **B2**.1062–3
  bacteriocins, **B2**.1046–7
  bacteriophages, **B2**.1046– 58, **B2**.1093
  bioterrorism, **B1**.364
  cell walls, **B2**.1045
  classification, **B2**.1042–3
  culture, **B2**.1047–9, **B2**.1056–9, **B2**.1094
    colonies, **B2**.1048–9
  description, **B2**.1054
  flagella, **B2**.1045
  food
    canning, **B1**.265–6, **B1**.270–1, **B1**.275,
      B1.283
    fish, **B1**.279
    fruit, **B1**.283
    hazard analysis, **B1**.288
    heating, **B1**.265–6, **B1**.265 (Fig.)
    nuts, **B1**.287
    vegetables, **B1**.282, **B1**.283
    wheat, **B1**.284–5
  genomics, **B2**.1063–4
    C. histolyticum vs., **B2**.1108,
      B2.1109 (Tab.)
    C. novyi vs., **B2**.1108, **B2**.1109 (Tab.)
  grouping, **B2**.1039, **B2**.1039 (Tab.)
    group I (type A and proteolytic strains of
      types B and F), **B2**.1054–6
    group II (type E and nonproteolytic types
      E, B and F), **B2**.1056–7
    group III (types C and D), **B2**.1057–8
    group IV, **B2**.1059
  growth, **B2**.1047–9
  habitats, **B2**.1043
  infection
    vaccines, **I**.933 (Tab.)
    wounds, **B2**.1112, **B2**.1113
    yogurt, **B1**.249
    see also Botulism

isolation/identification, **B2**.1096
  EIAs, **B1**.751
  neurotoxin-antitoxin neutralization test,
    B2.1049
  staining reactions, **B2**.1043–4
metabolism, **B2**.1052
morphology, **B2**.1049, **B2**.1051 (Fig.)
motility, **B2**.1045
neurotoxins
  types, **B2**.1038–9, **B2**.1039 (Tab.), **B2**.1040
  see also Botulinum toxin
as pathogen, **B1**.203
phenotypic characteristics, **B2**.1049
physical and metabolic properties, **B2**.1043–7
physical/chemical agent susceptibility/
  resistance, **B2**.1095
physiology, **B2**.1049–52
plasmids, **B2**.1045–6
safety precautions for laboratory workers,
  B2.1076
in soil, **B2**.1043
spores, **B2**.1044
  distribution, **B2**.1043, **B2**.1054–5
  production in media, **B2**.1044
  resistance to physical and chemical agents,
    B2.1044, **B2**.1056, **B2**.1064–5
  staining, **B2**.1043–4
sterilization
  heat, **B1**.446 (Tab.)
  ionizing radiation, **B1**.271, **B1**.446 (Tab.),
    B1.450, **B1**.451
  thermoradiation, **B1**.454
toxins, **B2**.1098 (Tab.)
  genetics, **B2**.1097
  see also Botulinum toxin
Clostridium butyricum, **B2**.1059–60
  bacteriophages, **B2**.1046
  botulism, **B2**.1039–40, **B2**.1042–3, **B2**.1062,
    B2.1070
  capsules, **B2**.1045, **B2**.1092
  growth, **B2**.1051–2
  toxins, **B2**.1098 (Tab.)
Clostridium cadaveris, **B2**.1090
Clostridium carnis, **B2**.1090
  metabolism, **B2**.1094–5
Clostridium chauvoei, **B2**.1051 (Fig.)
  characteristics, **B2**.1108
  culture, **B2**.1093
  as pathogen, **B1**.203
  subtyping, **B2**.1096–7
  toxins, **B2**.1098 (Tab.)
Clostridium cochlearium, **B2**.1090
Clostridium difficile, **B1**.293–4, **B2**.1090,
    B2.1101–5
  bacteriocins, **B2**.1093
  capsules, **B2**.1092
  culture, **B2**.1093, **B2**.1094
    colonies, **B2**.1093
  infection *see below*
  isolate lacking toxin A gene, **B2**.1120
  isolation/identification, **B2**.1122
    subtyping, **B2**.1096
  metabolism, **B2**.1096
  non-toxigenic strains, **B2**.1120
  plasmids, **B2**.1092–3
  spores, **B2**.1122

superoxidise water, **B1**.425
toxins, **B2**.1098 (Tab.), **B2**.1101–5,
  B2.1103 (Fig.), **B2**.1120–1
  ADP-ribosyltransferase (CDT), **B2**.1105
  A and B, **B2**.1101–5, **B2**.1103 (Fig.),
    B2.1104 (Tab.)
  detection, **B2**.1122
  genetics, **B2**.1097
  pathogenic mechanism, **B2**.1120–1
  receptors, **B2**.1121
  synergistic actions, **B2**.1120
  variants, **B2**.1105
Clostridium difficile infection, **B2**.1119–23
  animal models, **B2**.1120
  antibiotics associated, **B1**.176, **B2**.1119
  bacteremia, **B1**.523
  bone and joint infection, **B1**.690–1
  clinical features, **B2**.1121–2
  community-acquired, **B2**.1122
  diagnosis, **B1**.757, **B2**.1122
  elderly/immunocompromised patients,
    B1.397
  epidemiology and control, **B2**.1122–3
  gas gangrene, **B2**.1112
  historical aspects, **B2**.1119
  nosocomial, **B1**.372, **B1**.396–7
    from equipment, **B1**.379–80
    prevalence, **B1**.396–7
    prevention, **B1**.397
    spread by contact with staff, **B1**.378
  pathogenesis, **B2**.1120–1
  pathology, **B2**.1119–20
  synonyms, **B2**.1119
  treatment, **B2**.1123
  vaccines
    development status, **I**.933 (Tab.)
    Salmonella vectors, **I**.847
    Vibrio cholerae vectors, **I**.844
Clostridium fallax, **B2**.1090, **B2**.1111
Clostridium haemolyticum, **B2**.1106–8
  metabolism, **B2**.1094–5
  as pathogen, **B1**.203
  staining reaction, **B2**.1090–1
  toxins, **B2**.1098 (Tab.), **B2**.1106,
    B2.1107 (Tab.), **B2**.1108
Clostridium hastiforme, **B2**.1059, **B2**.1929
Clostridium histolyticum, **B2**.1090, **B2**.1108–10
  classification, **B2**.1090
  colonies, **B2**.1093
  culture, **B2**.1093
  genetic relatedness to *C novyi* and *C.
    botulinum,* **B2**.1108, **B2**.1109 (Tab.)
  metabolism, **B2**.1094–6
  toxins, **B2**.1098 (Tab.), **B2**.1109–10
    β-toxin, **B2**.1109–10
    δ-toxin, **B2**.1110
    γ-toxin, **B2**.1110
    ∈-toxin, **B2**.1110
    α-toxin, **B2**.1109
  virulence factors, collagenase, **B1**.153 (Tab.)
Clostridium innocuum, **B2**.1051 (Fig.),
  B2.1966–7, **B2**.1966 (Fig.), **B2**.1980
Clostridium kluyveri, **B1**.56
Clostridium novyi, **B2**.1106–8
  bacteriophages, **B2**.1093

Clostridium novyi, (Continued)
  classification, **B2**.1090
  culture, **B2**.1094
  genetic relatedness to other species, **B2**.1108,
      B2.1109 (Tab.)
  infection
    bacteremia, **B1**.523
    gas gangrene, **B2**.1112, **B2**.1114
  isolation/identification, **B2**.1096
    staining reaction, **B2**.1090–1
  metabolism, **B2**.1094–5
  physical/chemical agent susceptibility/
      resistance, **B2**.1064, **B2**.1095
  spores, **B2**.1064
  toxins, **B2**.1098 (Tab.), **B2**.1106–8,
      B2.1107 (Tab.), **B2**.1114
    β-toxin, **B2**.1108
    δ-toxin, **B2**.1108
    γ-toxin, **B2**.1108
    η-toxin, **B2**.1108
    ∈-toxin, **B2**.1108
    θ-toxin, **B2**.1108
    α-toxin, **B2**.1107
    ξ-toxin, **B2**.1108
Clostridium perfringens, **B2**.1089–90, **B2**.
    1097–101
  antibacterial susceptibility/resistance,
      B2.1116
  bacteriocins, **B2**.1093
  capsules, **B2**.1045, **B2**.1092
  collagenase, **B2**.1113
  colonies, **B2**.1094
  culture, **B2**.1094
    non-toxic antigen in, **B2**.1113
  enterotoxin, **I**.556 (Tab.), **I**.565–6, **B2**.1100–1
    detection, **B2**.1101
    mechanism of action, **B2**.1101
    purification, **B2**.1101
  in foods
    cream, **B1**.248
    hazard analysis, **B1**.288
    herbs and spices, **B1**.288
    meat and meat products, **B1**.273–4
    milk, **B1**.231
    poultry, **B1**.276
    vegetables, **B1**.282
    wheat, **B1**.284–5
  genomics, **B2**.1063–4
  habitats, **B2**.1090
  hyaluronidase, **B2**.1113
  immune evasion
    pore-forming toxins, **I**.654–5
    superantigens, **I**.668
  infection
    bacteremia, **B1**.523, **B2**.1114, **B2**.1116–17
    β toxoid vaccination, **B2**.1119
    cellulitis, **B2**.1112
    food poisoning and other diarrhea,
        B2.1117–18
    gas gangrene *see* Gas gangrene
    mastitis, **B1**.230
    nosocomial, **B1**.401 (Tab.)
    types, **B2**.1116–19
  isolation/identification, **B1**.224, **B2**.1096
  morphology, **B2**.1051 (Fig.)

  pathogenicity, **B1**.203
    phagocytosis inhibition, **B2**.1113
  physical/chemical agent susceptibility/
      resistance, **B2**.1095
  plasmids, **B2**.1045–6, **B2**.1092–3
  skin colonization, **B1**.304
  spores, **B2**.1091–2
  subtyping, **B2**.1096
  toxins, **B2**.1097–101, **B2**.1098 (Tab.),
      B2.1099 (Tab.), **B2**.1113
    α-toxin (lecithinase), **B2**.1099, **B2**.1113–14
    β-toxin, **B2**.1099, **B2**.1118–19
    genetics, **B2**.1097
    ∈-toxin, **B2**.1099
    minor, **B2**.1100
    role in gas gangrene, **B2**.1099, **B2**.1113–14
    ι-toxin, **B2**.1099–100
  type A
    antitoxins, **B2**.1114
    pathogenicity, **B2**.1113
  type C, bowel disease, **B2**.1118–19
  virulence factors, **B2**.1113–14
    collagenase, **B1**.153 (Tab.)
    lecithinases, **B1**.153 (Tab.)
    phospholipases, **B1**.153 (Tab.)
Clostridium propionicum, **B1**.56
Clostridium putrificum
  colonies, **B2**.1093
  culture, **B2**.1093
Clostridium ramosum, **B2**.1966–7,
    B2.1966 (Fig.), **B2**.1980
  infection, **B2**.1117
Clostridium septicum, **B2**.1051 (Fig.)
  antibacterial susceptibility/resistance,
      B2.1116
  characteristics, **B2**.1108
  culture, **B2**.1093
  infection
    bacteremia, **B1**.523
    gas gangrene, **B2**.1112, **B2**.1114
  subtyping, **B2**.1096–7
  toxins, **B2**.1098 (Tab.), **B2**.1114
Clostridium sordellii, **B2**.1090, **B2**.1105–6
  antitoxin, **B2**.1119
  culture, **B2**.1094
  infection, **B2**.1117
  isolation/identification, **B2**.1096
  toxins, **B2**.1098 (Tab.), **B2**.1104 (Tab.),
      B2.1105–6
Clostridium sphenoides, **B2**.1090
Clostridium spiroforme, **B2**.1110–11
  toxins, **B2**.1098 (Tab.)
    ι-toxin, **B2**.1110–11
Clostridium sporogenes, **B2**.1055, **B2**.1060,
    B2.1090
  bacteriophages, **B2**.1093
  bioremediation, **B1**.212
  colonies, **B2**.1093
  culture, **B2**.1093, **B2**.1094
  habitats, **B2**.1090
  infection, **B2**.1114
  physical/chemical agent susceptibility/
      resistance, **B2**.1095
  spores, **B2**.1091–2
  sterilization
    heat, **B1**.270–1, **B1**.446 (Tab.)

  ionizing radiation, **B1**.446 (Tab.)
  test organism strain PA3679, **B1**.270–1
Clostridium subterminale, **B2**.1051 (Fig.),
    B2.1059, **B2**.1060
Clostridium tertium, **B2**.1094–5
Clostridium tetani, **B2**.1035–6
  biochemistry, **B2**.1052–3
  cell walls, **B2**.1045
  classification, **B2**.1042–3
  culture, **B2**.1047–9, **B2**.1053
  colonies, **B2**.1052
  description, **B2**.1052–3
  genetics of toxigenesis, **B2**.1097
  genomics, **B2**.1063–4
  infection *see* Tetanus
  isolation/identification, EIAs, **B1**.751
  morphology, **B2**.1049, **B2**.1051 (Fig.),
      B2.1090
  neurotoxin (tetanospasmin), **B2**.1053–4,
      B2.1098 (Tab.)
    botulinum type B toxin *vs.,* **B2**.1061
    detection, **B2**.1062–3
    domains, **B2**.1061–2
    experimental studies, **B2**.1042, **B2**.1053–4
    flagella, **B2**.1045
    genes, **B2**.1053–4
    growth, **B2**.1047–9, **B2**.1052
    habitats, **B2**.1042, **B2**.1043, **B2**.1053
    hemolysin (tetanolysin), **B2**.1053–4
    isolation, **B2**.1053
    lethal dose, **B2**.1036, **B2**.1053–4
    mechanism of action, **B1**.156 (Tab.),
        B2.1042, **B2**.1061–2, **B2**.1065
    membrane translocation, **B2**.1061–2
    metabolism, **B2**.1049–52
    molecular weight, **B2**.1061
    motility, **B2**.1045, **B2**.1047–8, **B2**.1052
    production control, **B2**.1062
    receptors, **B2**.1042
    spastic/rigid paralysis due to, **B2**.1053–4,
        B2.1061–2
    structure, **B2**.1042
    transmission to CNS, **B2**.1042, **B2**.1061–2
  physical/chemical agent susceptibility/
      resistance, **B2**.1064
  physiology, **B2**.1049–52
  plasmids, **B2**.1053–4
  safety precautions for laboratory workers,
      B2.1076
  in soil, **B2**.1043, **B2**.1053
  spores, **B2**.1044, **B2**.1064
Clostridium thermosaccharolyticum, **B1**.283
Clothing, decontamination, **B1**.378
Clotrimazole, **M**.147, **M**.183 (Tab.)
  candidiasis, **M**.609–10
  keratitis, **M**.309
  oropharyngeal candidiasis, **M**.189
  white piedra, **M**.197
Cloves, **B1**.287
Cloxacillin, **B1**.474 (Fig.)
ClpA, protein degradation, **B1**.47–8
ClpP, protein degradation, **B1**.47–8
Clusterin, **I**.150 (Tab.), **I**.151
  deficiency, **I**.154
Clustering hypothesis, BCR, **I**.342
'Cluster peptides,' HIV vaccines, **I**.871

CM2 protein *see* Influenza virus C

CMI/AAB Descriptions of Plant Viruses, **V1**.31

Cmv1 gene, **I**.588–9

Cmv2 gene, **I**.588–9

c-*myc* oncogene
  avian B cell lymphomas, **V1**.340
  Burkitt lymphoma, **V1**.570

Coagglutination assays, **B1**.755

Coagulation pathways, septic shock, **I**.699

Coal miners, **M**.228

Coal tar, phenol production, **B1**.422

Co-amoxiclav
  Haemophilus, **B2**.1703 (Tab.), **B2**.1710
  melioidosis treatment, **B2**.1631,
    B2.1631 (Tab.)

Coastal waters, **B1**.217, **B1**.220, **B1**.224

Cobalamin absorption, *Diphyllobothrium
  latum,* **P**.663

Cobas Amplicor, **B2**.2018–19

Cobra venom factor, **P**.209

Coccidia, **P**.464

Coccidia, **P**.188, **P**.422
  classification, **P**.190–1, **P**.197, **P**.422
  cyst types (oocysts and sporocysts), **P**.166,
    P.423
  intestinal, **P.399–421**
    immune response, **P**.76
    see also individual species
  merozoites
    apical pole and conoid, **P**.166 (Fig.), **P**.172,
      P.423
    structure, **P**.164, **P**.166 (Fig.), **P**.173,
      P.175 (Fig.)
  microgametes, **P**.170 (Fig.)
  motile forms, **P**.164
  storage materials, **P**.176 (Fig.)
  structure
    cyst wall, **P**.166
    pellicle, **P**.164, **P**.164 (Fig.)

Coccidioides
  growth pattern, **M**.70
  PCR detection, **M**.94

Coccidioides immitis, **M**.502, **M**.503,
    M.503 (Fig.), **M**.506–7, **M**.509
  chitinase, **M**.504, **M**.506 (Fig.)
  classification, **M**.503
    Emmonsia, **M**.809, **M**.810 (Tab.), **M**.811,
      M.820
  epidemiology, **M**.505
    geographical distribution, **M**.505,
      M.506 (Fig.)
  genetic analysis, **M**.503–4, **M**.514
  glucanase, **M**.504
  groups, **M**.503–4
  histopathology, **M**.89 (Tab.), **M**.127 (Tab.),
    M.128 (Tab.), **M**.135 (Fig.), **M**.510–11,
    M.516
    stains, **M**.122, **M**.124
  Histoplasma capsulatum var. *capsulatum vs.,*
    M.531–2, **M**.534
  history, **M**.4, **M**.21–6
  identification, **M**.513–16
    calcofluor white, **M**.513
    culture, **M**.513
    dermatophyte test medium, **M**.236
    exoantigen test, **M**.514

hematoxylin and eosin stain, **M**.513, **M**.516
  histopathology *see above*
  immunodiffusion, **M**.514–15
  methenamine silver stain, **M**.516
  nucleic acid probes, **M**.91
  periodic acid-Schiff stain, **M**.513
  serology, **M**.113, **M**.514
  specimens, **M**.513, **M**.515–16
metabolism, **M**.504–5
morphology, **M**.74, **M**.127 (Tab.), **M**.502,
    M.503, **M**.514
  arthroconidia, **M**.503–4, **M**.504 (Fig.),
    M.509
  degenerating ('disjunctor') cells, **M**.504,
    M.504 (Fig.)
  hyphae, **M**.503, **M**.504
  multimorphism, **M**.24–6, **M**.25 (Fig.),
    M.503 (Fig.)
  spherule-endospores, **M**.504, **M**.505 (Fig.),
    M.509, **M**.513, **M**.514
  proteases, **M**.504, **M**.506 (Fig.), **M**.509,
    M.514
resistance, **M**.510
Splendore–Hoeppli phenomenon, **M**.516
vaccines, **M**.510, **I**.933 (Tab.)

Coccidioides posadasii, **M**.502
  classification, **M**.44–5

Coccidioidin, **M**.93 (Tab.)

Coccidioidomycosis
  AIDS, **M**.113, **M**.508–10, **M**.516
  causative agents *see Coccidioides immitis*
  clinical presentation, **M**.507–13,
    M.508 (Fig.)
    disseminated disease, **M**.508, **M**.510
    endophthalmitis, **M**.317
    fungemia, **M**.513
    meningitis, **M**.508
    oculomycoses, **M**.275 (Tab.), **M**.288,
      M.295, **M**.299, **M**.317–8, **M**.324
    otitis externa, **M**.247–8
    reactivation, **M**.510–11
  diagnosis, **M**.125–7, **M**.508–9, **M**.513–16
    EIAs, **M**.113, **M**.514–15
    histopathology, **M**.510–11, **M**.516
    serology, **M**.92, **M**.93 (Tab.), **M**.113, **M**.514
    skin testing, **M**.509–10
    specimens, **M**.83 (Tab.), **M**.513, **M**.515–16
  epidemiology, **M**.505
    animal infection, **M**.506–7, **M**.507 (Tab.)
    geographical distribution, **M**.505,
      M.506 (Fig.)
    transplantation recipients, **M**.507–8,
      M.508–9, **M**.510, **M**.516
    travelers, **M**.506
  histopathology, **M**.128 (Tab.), **M**.135 (Fig.),
    M.510–11, **M**.516
  history, **M**.24–6
  immune response, **M**.509, **M**.514–15,
    M.515 (Fig.)
    ILs, **M**.510
    T cells, **M**.510
  immunosuppression, **M**.508–10, **M**.516
  pregnancy, **M**.508–9
  therapy, **M**.511
    amphotericin B, **M**.511
    echinocandins, **M**.154

fluconazole, **M**.511
itraconazole, **M**.511
ketoconazole, **M**.511
nikkomycin Z, **M**.511, **M**.512 (Fig.)
voriconazole, **M**.511
vaccine, **M**.510

Coccidiosis, **P**.188, **P**.422

Cochrane Collaboration, **P**.129

Cockles, microbiology, **B1**.280

'cocktail' vaccines, malaria vaccination,
    P.516–17

Coconuts, contamination, **B1**.287

Coding joints, somatic recombination, **I**.328

Codon 129, prion protein (PrP)
    polymorphisms, **V2**.1371–2

Codon 219, prion protein (PrP)
    polymorphisms, **V2**.1371–2

Codon optimization, DNA vaccines, **I**.916–17

Codons, **B1**.46
  mycoplasmas, **B2**.1980
  nonsense, **B1**.46
  termination, **B1**.47

Coenzyme(s), **B1**.45

Coenzyme A-linked alcohol dehydrogenase,
    B1.55

Coenzyme M, methanogenesis, **B1**.68–9

Coenzyme Q
  Candida, **M**.580
  homologues, *Pneumocystis,* **M**.781

Coevolution, viral evolution, **V1**.12

Cofactors, **B1**.45

Coffee plantation workers,
    paracoccidioidomycosis, **M**.545

Cognitive abnormalities
  neuro-AIDS, **V2**.1427–8
  progressive multifocal leucoencephalopathy
    (PML), **V2**.1417

Cognitive performance, hookworm infection,
    P.728

Cohort studies, **B1**.314–15, **V1**.363
  advantages/disadvantages, **V1**.362 (Tab.)
  association likelihood, **V1**.363
  bias in, **B1**.315
    loss to follow-up, **B1**.315
  case–control studies *vs.,* **V1**.361–2
  comparison cohort, **V1**.363
  design, **V1**.363
  exposure cohort, **V1**.363
  misclassification of cases, **B1**.315
  prospective, **B1**.314
  retrospective/historical, **B1**.315
  rubella epidemiology, **V1**.363
  statistical analysis, **B1**.316

Coiling phagocytosis, **I**.25

Cointegrate resolution, **B1**.96

Cokeromyces, **M**.660 (Tab.)

Cokeromyces recurvatus, **M**.663

Cold agglutinins, in *Mycoplasma pneumoniae*
    infection, **B1**.634

Cold shock, **B1**.450

Cold sores, recurrent HSV infection, **V1**.507,
    V1.507 (Fig.)

Cold, sterilization, **B1**.449–50

ColE1 origin of replication (ori), **I**.910–11

Coleopteran (beetle), bacterial pathogens,
    B1.203–4

Colicins, **B1**.136–8
  gene expression, **B1**.138
  immunity to, **B1**.139
  receptors, **B1**.138–9
  role of, **B1**.139
'Coliform bacteria,' **B2**.1335
  airborne concentrations in facilities, **B1**.186 (Tab.)
  fecal, **B1**.223
  meat and meat products, **B1**.273–4
  milk test, **B1**.234
  vegetables, **B1**.281–2
  water test, **B1**.223
Colistin (polymyxin E)
  spectrum of activity, **B1**.496
    Edwardsiella, **B2**.1491–2
    Ewingella, **B2**.1493
    Leclercia, **B2**.1495
    Leminorella, **B2**.1496
    Moellerella, **B2**.1496
    Yokenella, **B2**.1498
  structure, **B1**.497 (Fig.)
Collagen
  Ascaris lumbricoides cuticle, **P**.717
  schistosomiasis granulomas, **I**.722
  tuberculosis granulomas, **I**.717
Collagenases
  Clostridium perfringens, **B2**.1113
  functions, **B1**.153 (Tab.)
Collagen-vascular disease, **M**.232
Collectins, **V1**.273
  Human respiratory syncytial virus infection, **V1**.793–4
  macrophage pathogen recognition, **I**.22
  microbial recognition, **I**.24 (Tab.)
Colletotrichum
  morphology, **M**.286 (Fig.)
  oculomycoses, **M**.278 (Tab.), **M**.284, **M**.285
Collinsella, **B2**.1028–9
Collinsella aerofaciens
  differential characteristics, **B2**.1029 (Tab.)
  pathogenicity, **B2**.1029–30
Colon cancer
  Streptococcus bovis and endocarditis link, **B1**.529–30
  TCE peptide vaccines, **I**.865 (Tab.)
Colonization
  gram-positive/-negative bacteria, **B1**.294
  normal bacterial flora, **B1**.294–5
  prevalence estimation, **B1**.295
  prolonged, **B1**.294
  see also Adherence; Pathogenicity
Colon, normal microbiota, **B1**.302–3
  disruption by antibiotics, **B2**.1119–20
Colony-forming units (CFUs), **B1**.38
  rhizosphere soil population estimates, **B1**.204
Colony morphology, **B1**.19, **B1**.22–3, **B1**.22 (Tab.), **B1**.24, **B1**.32–3
Colony-stimulating factor(s) (CSFs), **I**.274 (Tab.), **I**.275–9
  aspergillosis, **M**.709, **M**.724
  candidiasis, **M**.259–60, **M**.593, **M**.613
  cryptococcosis, **M**.652–3
  keratinocyte production, **I**.820–1
  M-CSF, cryptococcosis therapy, **M**.652–3

  see also Granulocyte colony-stimulating factor (G-CSF); Granulocyte-macrophage colony-stimulating factor (GM-CSF); *individual types*
Colony stimulating factor-1 (CSF-1) *see* Macrophage-colony stimulating factor (M-CSF)
Colorado potato beetle, Bt resistance, **B1**.203–4
Colorado tick fever virus (CTFV), **V2**.942
  animal reservoirs, **V2**.942
  cell culture, **V2**.943
  detection, **V2**.943
  epidemiology, **V2**.942
  infection
    clinical manifestations, **V2**.942–3
    incubation period, **V2**.942–3
    treatment, **V2**.943
Colorimetric methods, antifungal susceptibility testing, **M**.157
Colostral antibodies, cryptosporidiosis, **P**.410
Coltivirus, **V1**.47–8, **V2**.932
Coltiviruses, **V2**.942–3
Columnar epithelial cells, influenza pathogenesis, **V1**.661–2
Coma, cerebral malaria, **P**.498
Comamonas acidovorans see Delftia (Comamonas) acidovorans
Comamonas testosteroni (Pseudomonas testosteroni), **B1**.224–5
Combination therapy, malaria, **P**.506–8
Combinatorial diversity, TCR, **I**.454
Combined Antiretroviral Therapy (CART), **V2**.1330, **V2**.1333–4, **V2**.1336
Commensal bacteria, **I**.111
Commerce, emerging bacterial infection, **B1**.360
Commercial assays
  Actinomyces identification, **B2**.1013–17
  Aeromonas identification, **B2**.1532
  Enterobacteriaceae identification, **B2**.1348, **B2**.1351–2
Commercial kits, nucleic acid amplification, **V2**.1538–9
Common cold *see* Rhinoviruses; Rhinovirus infection
Common Cold Research Unit (UK), **V2**.857–8
Common leader sequence, **V1**.395
Common mucosal immune system (CMIS), **I**.529 (Fig.)
  antigen processing/presentation, **I**.534–5
  cellular characteristics, **I**.535 (Fig.)
  CTLs, **I**.534
  definition, **I**.534
  IgA, **I**.534
  Langerhan's cells, **I**.534–5
  structure, **I**.535 (Fig.)
  Th1/Th2 cells, **I**.534–5, **I**.539 (Fig.)
  see also Mucosal immune response
Common pattern recognition, host resistance, **B1**.176–7
Common-source outbreaks, **V1**.357
  definition, **V1**.358
  emerging viral infection, **V2**.1662
  norovirus infection, **V2**.922

Common variable hypogammaglobulinemia, *Dysgonomonas* infection, **B2**.1677–8
Common variable immunodeficiency (CVID), **I**.781
  X-linked agammaglobulinemia *vs.,* **I**.781
Communicability of infection, **B1**.310
  period of, **B1**.310
Communicable Disease Control, Consultant (CCDC), **B1**.318, **B1**.319, **B1**.326, **B1**.327, **B1**.330, **B1**.407
Communicable disease, historical aspects, **B1**.4
Communicable Disease Report (CDR), **B1**.319, **B1**.322
Communicable Disease Surveillance Centre (CDSC), **B1**.318, **B1**.319, **B1**.322, **B1**.327
Community-acquired infection
  Clostridium difficile, **B2**.1122
  methicillin-resistant *Staphylococcus aureus,* **B1**.517–18
Community-based programs, parasite control *see* Control of infection, parasitic disease
Community-directed treatment with ivermectin (CDTI), **P**.121–2, **P**.127, **P**.787, **P**.788–9
  economics, **P**.40
  management, **P**.121
  sociopolitical problems, **P**.121–2
  technical problems, **P**.121–2
Community immunity, **I**.957–8, **I**.959 (Fig.)
Comomonas, endophthalmitis, **B1**.603
Comoviridae, **V1**.27 (Tab.), **V1**.51 (Tab.), **V1**.52
Comparison cohort, cohort studies, **V1**.363
Competence
  artificial *see* Artificial competence
  natural, **B1**.99–100
'Competitive' model, αβ/γδ T-cell separation, **I**.457
Complement, **I**.142 (Fig.), **I**.697–9, **I**.698 (Fig.), **I**.141–63, **V1**.273
  activation
    Burkholderia thailandensis infection, **B2**.1625
    CNS infection, **V2**.1413
    C-reactive protein, **I**.199–200
    multiple organ failure, **I**.698–9
  in adaptive immune response, **I**.141, **I**.148
    B-cell response, **I**.148, **I**.148 (Fig.)
  airway hypersensitivity, **I**.738
  alternative pathway, **I**.141, **I**.145 (Fig.), **V1**.274 (Fig.), **I**.698 (Fig.), **I**.771 (Fig.)
    activation, **I**.144–5, **I**.145 (Fig.)
    bacterial infection, **I**.645
    components, **I**.143 (Tab.)
    deficiencies, **I**.152, **I**.152 (Fig.)
    historical aspects, **I**.141
    regulation, **I**.150 (Fig.), **I**.151
    septic shock, **I**.697–8
  amebiasis, **P**.209
  apoptotic bodies clearance, **I**.148–9, **I**.354
    cell debris opsonization, **I**.148–9
  bacterial infection, **I**.662
    immune interference *see* Immune evasion, bacteria
  blocking, helminths, **I**.685–6
  classical pathway *see* Complement classical pathway

Complement (*Continued*)
  components, **I**.142–9, **I**.142 (Fig.),
    I.143 (Tab.), **I**.200
    active products, **I**.146
    anaphylactic fragments, **I**.147
    chemotactic fragments, **I**.147
    opsonic fragments, **I**.146–7
    perforin homology, **I**.475
    see also individual components
  deficiencies, **I**.151–4, **I**.152 (Fig.), **I**.770–1
    autoimmune disease associations, **I**.771
    meningococcal disease, **I**.154, **B1**.564
    meningococcal meningitis, **I**.594
    see also individual components
  discovery, **V1**.4
  in disease, **I**.154–7, **I**.155 (Tab.)
    Alzheimer's disease, **I**.155 (Tab.), **I**.156
    Guillain–Barré syndrome, **I**.156
    iatrogenic syndromes, **I**.155 (Tab.), **I**.157
    ischemia–reperfusion injury, **I**.155–6,
      I.155 (Tab.)
    membranoproliferative
      glomuleronephritis, **I**.155 (Tab.)
    multiple sclerosis, **I**.155 (Tab.), **I**.156
    myasthenia gravis, **I**.155 (Tab.)
    myocardial infarction, **I**.155–6, **I**.155 (Tab.)
    neurological disease, **I**.155 (Tab.), **I**.156
    rheumatoid arthritis, **I**.155 (Tab.)
    SLE, **I**.155
    stroke, **I**.155–6, **I**.155 (Tab.)
    transplant rejection, **I**.155–6
  fixation
    Ig, **I**.312
    IgG, **I**.312
    IgG1, **I**.307
    IgG3, **I**.307
    IgM, **I**.307, **I**.312
  histamine release, **I**.62
  historical aspects, **I**.141–2
  as host defence mechanism in lung, **B1**.624
  HSV infection, **V1**.284
  immune complex clearance, **I**.147, **I**.354
    SLE, **I**.147
  immune evasion
    C3b receptor, on HSV, **V1**.257–8
    C4-binding protein, **V1**.257–8
    cestodes, **I**.685
    Echinococcus, **I**.685
    Schistosoma, **I**.685
    Taenia, **I**.685
    see also Immune evasion
  immunogenetics, **I**.579–80
  innate immunity, **I**.141
  intracellular bacteria, **I**.649
  lectin pathway *see* Complement lectin
    pathway
  macrophage pathogen recognition, **I**.22–3
  measles, **V1**.725–6
  membrane attack complex *see* Membrane
    attack complex (MAC)
  microbial recognition, **I**.24 (Tab.)
  prion diseases, **V2**.1383–4
  production, macrophages, **I**.27
  receptors *see* Complement receptor(s)

  regulation, **I**.149–51, **I**.150 (Fig.), **I**.150 (Tab.)
    activation pathways, **I**.149–51
    deficiencies, **I**.153–4
    gene structure, **I**.151
    membrane attack pathway, **I**.151
  therapies, **I**.157–9, **I**.158 (Tab.)
    antibody-based, **I**.158, **I**.158 (Tab.)
    recombinant soluble forms, **I**.157–8,
      I.158 (Tab.)
    small molecule inhibitors, **I**.158–9
Vaccinia virus, **V1**.619–20
Vaccinia virus control protein (VCP), **V1**.257
Variola virus, **V1**.619–20
Complementarity-determining regions (CDRs)
  antibodies *see* Immunoglobulin(s)
  TCR–MHC–peptide interactions, **I**.461,
    I.462–3
  see also Hypervariable regions
Complementary DNA (cDNA) gene cloning,
  B1.126–7
Complementation *see* Genetics, of vertebrate
  viruses
Complementation group A deficiencies, **I**.575
Complementation group B deficiencies, **I**.575
Complementation group C deficiencies, **I**.575
Complement classical pathway, **I**.141,
    I.145 (Fig.), **V1**.274 (Fig.), **I**.698 (Fig.),
    I.771 (Fig.)
  activation, **I**.142–4, **I**.144 (Fig.)
    antibodies, **I**.142–3
    C1 complement protein, **I**.142–3,
      I.145 (Fig.)
    C1q, **I**.145 (Fig.)
    C1s, **I**.145 (Fig.)
    C2 complement protein, **I**.144, **I**.145 (Fig.)
    C3 complement protein, **I**.144, **I**.145 (Fig.)
    C4b2a3b complex, **I**.144
    C4b2a complex, **I**.144
    C4 complement protein, **I**.143–4,
      I.145 (Fig.)
    C5 complement protein, **I**.144
    C-reactive protein, **I**.142
    LPS, **I**.142
    nucleic acids, **I**.142
  C1r, **I**.145 (Fig.)
  components, **I**.143 (Tab.)
  deficiencies, **I**.151–2, **I**.152 (Fig.)
  historical aspects, **I**.141–2
  mannose-binding lectin activation, **V1**.273
  regulation, **I**.149–51, **I**.150 (Fig.)
  septic shock, **I**.697–8
Complement control protein domain (CCP),
  I.476 (Fig.)
Complement fixation tests (CFTs), **B1**.719,
    B1.749, **V2**.1545
  African trypanosomiasis diagnosis, **P**.367
  arenaviruses, **V2**.1068–9
  brucellosis diagnosis, **B1**.745
  Chagas disease, **P**.389
  Chlamydia detection, **B2**.2019
  glanders diagnosis, **B2**.1634
  histoplasmosis diagnosis, **M**.532
  human brucellosis diagnosis, **B2**.1740
  influenza diagnosis, **V1**.675
  Leptospira detection, **B1**.753
  mumps diagnosis, **V1**.754

  Mycoplasma pneumoniae detection, **B1**.752
  Mycoplasma pneumoniae diagnosis, **B2**.1995
Complement lectin pathway, **I**.141, **I**.145–6,
    I.145 (Fig.), **I**.698 (Fig.), **I**.771 (Fig.)
  activation, **I**.144 (Fig.)
    C2 complement protein, **I**.146, **I**.145 (Fig.)
    C3 complement protein, **I**.145 (Fig.)
    C4 complement protein, **I**.145 (Fig.)
    mannan-binding lectin, **I**.144 (Fig.),
      I.145–6, **I**.145 (Fig.)
    MBL-associated serine proteases,
      I.144 (Fig.), **I**.146, **I**.145 (Fig.)
  components, **I**.143 (Tab.)
  deficiencies, **I**.152–3
    recurrent bacterial infection, **I**.152
  regulation, **I**.149–51, **I**.150 (Fig.)
  septic shock, **I**.697–8
Complement-mediated lysis, **V1**.278
Complement membrane attack pathway,
    I.141, **I**.145 (Fig.), **I**.146
  components, **I**.143 (Tab.)
  deficiencies, **I**.153
  regulation, **I**.151
Complement receptor(s)
  B cells, **I**.147
  Candida albicans, **M**.593
  macrophages, **I**.25
  neutrophils, **I**.39, **I**.43
  pathogen binding, **I**.579–80
  phagocytes, **I**.146–7
  T cells, **I**.147
  see also individual types
Complement receptor 1 (CR1: CD35),
    I.146–7
  cell expression, **I**.151
    erythrocytes, **I**.147, **I**.151
    neutrophils, **I**.39
    polymorphonuclear leukocytes, **I**.151
  SLE, **I**.147
  soluble form as therapy
    sialyl Lewis antigen derivatization, **I**.157–8,
      I.158 (Tab.)
    TP10, **I**.157–8, **I**.158 (Tab.)
    truncated form (APT070), **I**.158,
      I.158 (Tab.)
Complement receptor 2 (CR2:CD21), **I**.146–7
  on B cells, **I**.148
  BCR signaling, **I**.347
Complement receptor 3 (CR3: CD11b/CD18),
    I.114, **I**.114 (Tab.), **I**.146–7
  eosinophils, **I**.60
  microbial recognition, **I**.24 (Tab.)
  neutrophils, **I**.39
  pathogen binding, **I**.579–80
Complement receptor 4 (CR4:CD11c/CD18),
    I.146–7
  microbial recognition, **I**.24 (Tab.)
  neutrophils, **I**.39
Complex transposons *see* Transposons
Composite transposons *see* Transposons
Composting, airborne bacteria generation,
    B1.186 (Tab.)
Compressed diatomaceous earth filters, **B1**.453
Computed tomography (CT), **B1**.723 (Tab.)
  amebiasis, **P**.211
  congenital HCMV infection, **V2**.1449

Computed tomography (CT) (*Continued*)
    cryptococcal meningoencephalitis, **M**.649
    in diagnosis, **P**.153
    echinococcosis, **P**.694
        alveolar echinococcosis, **P**.694
        cystic echinococcosis, **P**.695 (Fig.)
        intracranial abscess diagnosis, **B1**.586–7,
            B1.587 (Fig.)
        neurocysticercosis, **P**.692–3, **P**.693 (Fig.)
Computer analysis, Enterobacteriaceae
    identification, **B2**.1348
Computers, world-wide web, **B1**.32
Computer technology, **I**.9
Conalbumin, food, **B1**.267
Conant, N F, **M**.10, **M**.22–3, **M**.29–30, **M**.32
Concanavalin A, *Entamoeba histolytica*
    binding, **P**.202
Concatemeric intermediates, poxviruses,
    V1.169, **V1**.600, **V1**.602, **V1**.605 (Fig.)
Concentration exponent, **B1**.430–1,
    B1.431 (Tab.)
Conceptual diagrams, malaria epidemiology,
    P.513, **P**.515 (Fig.)
Concomitant immunity (premunition), **P**.94
    cestodes, **P**.95–6
    Hymenolepis diminuta, **P**.663
    malaria, **P**.493
    onchocerciasis, **P**.795
    schistosomiasis, **P**.94, **P**.605–6
    tapeworms, **P**.663
Concomitant immunity, helminth infection,
    I.683
Condidiobolus, antifungal resistance, **M**.352
Conditional lethal mutants, genetic analysis,
    V1.182–3
Condyloma acuminata, HPV infection,
    V1.463 (Tab.), **V1**.464–5, **V1**.466 (Fig.)
Confidence intervals, **B1**.316
Conflicts *see* Civil unrest
Confluent and reticulate papillomatosis of,
    Pityrosporum orbiculare, **M**.213–14
Conformational change, rhabdovirus
    glycoprotein (G), **V2**.1108
Congenital asplenia, **I**.771
Congenital heart disease
    endocarditis in, **B1**.525–6
    intracranial abscess complication, **B1**.583,
        B1.584 (Tab.)
Congenital infection
    congenitally acquired rubella (CAR) *see*
        Rubella
    enterovirus infection, **V2**.871
    oncogenic viruses, **V1**.343–4
    transmission, **V2**.1443
    see also Fetal infection; Neonatal infection
Congenital varicella syndrome (CVS),
    V2.1454–6, **V2**.1455 (Tab.)
    clinical manifestations, **V2**.1455,
        V2.1455 (Tab.)
    incidence, **V2**.1456
    pathogenesis, **V2**.1455
        gestational age, **V2**.1455
    reinfection, **V2**.1456
    risk, **V2**.1455–6
Congestive heart failure, infective endocarditis,
    B1.535
Conglutinin, **V1**.273

Conidia, **M**.77, **M**.77–9
    Aspergillus, **M**.687, **M**.691
    germination, **M**.77–9
    hydrophobic rodlets, **M**.78
    production, **M**.77, **M**.78 (Fig.), **M**.79 (Fig.)
Conidial head, *Aspergillus*, **M**.689–91,
    M.690 (Fig.), **M**.691 (Fig.)
Conidiobolus, **M**.347, **M**.348 (Tab.), **M**.349
    classification, **M**.53
    culture, **M**.352
    subcutaneous infection, **M**.349, **M**.350, **M**.351
        diagnosis, **M**.351–2
        histopathology, **M**.351–2
        immune response, **M**.350–2
        microscopy, **M**.351–2
Conidiobolus coronatus, **M**.347, **M**.349
    histopathology, **M**.128 (Tab.)
    morphology, **M**.349, **M**.350 (Fig.)
    subcutaneous infection, **M**.349, **M**.351
        immune response, **M**.351
Conidiobolus incongruus, **M**.347, **M**.349–50
    subcutaneous infection, **M**.349–50
    therapy, **M**.352
Conidiobolus lamprauges, **M**.347–50
Conidiogenesis
    blastic, **M**.77, **M**.78 (Fig.)
    thallic, **M**.77, **M**.79 (Fig.)
Conidiophore(s), **M**.77, **M**.78 (Fig.), **M**.79 (Fig.)
    Aspergillus, **M**.687, **M**.689–90, **M**.691–2
    Scopulariopsis brevicaulis, **M**.78 (Fig.)
Conjugate vaccines *see* Subunit vaccines
Conjugation, bacterial, **B1**.98, **B1**.100–4
    antibacterial resistance genes, **B1**.103–4
    chromosome mobilizing ability, **B1**.101
    discovery, **B1**.13
    F' formation, **B1**.102–3
    F plasmid, **B1**.100–1
        chromosomal insertion, **B1**.102–3,
            B1.102 (Fig.)
        high frequency transfer, **B1**.104
        transposable elements, **B1**.102
    Gram-positive *vs.* Gram-negative, **B1**.104
    high frequency of recombination, **B1**.102–3
    historical perspective, **B1**.100–1
    interrupted mating experiments, **B1**.102–3,
        B1.102 (Fig.)
    mating pair formation, **B1**.102
    pili, **B1**.101–2, **B1**.101 (Fig.)
        bacteriophage receptors, **B1**.102
        pilin, **B1**.101–2
    species, **B1**.103
        Brucella, **B2**.1730
        Enterococcus faecalis, **B1**.104
        Staphylococcus aureus, **B1**.104
        see also individual species
    transfer gene repression, **B1**.104
Conjugative transposons, **B1**.99
Conjunctivitis, **M**.299–300, **B1**.598–600
    acute hemorrhagic, **V1**.444 (Tab.)T
    adenoviruses infection, **V1**.160
    adults, **B1**.599
    amphotericin B therapy, **M**.299
    candidiasis, **M**.257, **M**.258 (Tab.), **M**.299,
        M.601

    causative organisms, **B1**.599–600
        Chlamydia psittaci, **B2**.2015
        Chlamydia trachomatis, **B2**.2012,
            B2.2012 (Fig.), **B2**.2013, **B2**.2013 (Fig.)
    clinical manifestations, **B1**.598–9
    diagnosis, **B1**.600
    HPV associations, **V1**.463 (Tab.)
    Malassezia infection, **M**.299
    neonatal, **B1**.599, **B1**.600
    nosocomial, **B1**.386
    oculomycoses, **M**.299–300
    predisposing factors, **B1**.598
    rhinosporidiosis, **M**.299–300
    treatment, **B1**.600
    trichinellosis, **P**.766 (Fig.)
    viral, **V1**.236
Connective tissue-activating peptide III
    (CTAPIII), basophil histamine release,
    I.62
Connective tissue capsules, **I**.685
Connectorless capsids, isocahedral viruses,
    V1.63
Connexin 43 gene mutation, asplenia, **I**.771
Conoid, **P**.166 (Fig.), **P**.172, **P**.423
Consensus sequences, bunyavirus genome,
    V2.1031 (Tab.)
Conservative (cut-and-paste) transposition,
    B1.93 (Fig.), **B1**.95
Conserved architecture, isocahedral viruses,
    V1.67–9, **V1**.68 (Fig.)
Conserved genes
    evolution (of viruses), **V1**.175
    poxviruses, **V1**.583–5
Conserved sequence element (CSE),
    alphaviruses, **V2**.1014
Constant (C) domains
    αβ TCRs, **I**.458, **I**.460
    γδ TCRs, **I**.458, **I**.460
    Ig heavy chains, **I**.305
    Ig light chains, **I**.304
    interactions, **I**.305
Constitutive mutants, **B1**.70
Construction work, aspergillosis, **M**.692, **M**.729
Consultant in Communicable Disease Control
    (CCDC), **B1**.318, **B1**.319, **B1**.326,
        B1.327, **B1**.330, **B1**.407
Contact amount, epidemiology, **I**.952,
    I.953 (Fig.)
Contact lenses
    Acanthamoeba keratitis, **P**.231–2
        prevention, **P**.238
    bacterial infection, **B1**.386
    fungal infection, **M**.329–30
        Alternaria, **M**.330–1
        aspergillosis, **M**.330–1
        candidiasis, **M**.331–2
        Cladosporium, **M**.330–1
        Curvularia, **M**.330–1
        Fusarium, **M**.330–1
        keratitis, **M**.330–1
        oculomycoses, **M**.329–32
    Fusarium
        F. dimerum, **M**.331
        F. oxysporum, **M**.331
        F. solani, **M**.330–1

Contact management, pneumococcal meningitis treatment, **B1**.571

Contact variables, epidemiology, **I**.952

Contagion, concept, **B1**.4

Contagious caprine pleuropneumonia, Peste-des-petits-ruminants virus *vs.,* **V1**.810

Contagious diseases, definition, **V1**.354–5

Contagious pustular dermatitis (Orf) *see* Orf virus (Contagious pustular dermatitis)

Contagium vivum fluidum, **V1**.3–4

Containment, control of disease by, **B1**.344–5

Containment levels, laboratory safety, **V2**.1520

Contamination
  control, clinical molecular diagnostics, **B1**.727
  specimens, site and source, **B1**.711–12, **B1**.712 (Tab.)

Contingency table, **B1**.316, **B1**.316 (Tab.)

Continuous ambulatory peritoneal dialysis (CAPD)
  associated peritonitis, *Fusarium,* **M**.754
  infection associated, **B1**.386–7
  infection prevention, **B1**.386–7

Continuous monitoring blood culture systems (CMBCS), **B1**.515, **B1**.515 (Tab.)

Continuous passage, virus attenuation, **V1**.197

Contour-clamped homogeneous electric field, candidiasis diagnosis, **M**.257

Contraceptive vaccines, BCE peptide vaccines, **I**.855 (Tab.), **I**.875

Contractile vacuoles, *Balantidium coli,* **P**.276, **P**.277 (Fig.)

Controlled atmospheric packaging, **B1**.268 (Tab.)

Controlled trials, **V1**.365

Controlling Inverted Repeat of Chaperone Expression (CIRCE element), **B2**.1874–5

Control of Communicable Diseases in Man, **V2**.1583

Control of infection
  bacterial disease, **B1**.344–8
    aims of programs, **B1**.344–5
    case-finding and screening, **B1**.347
    containment, **B1**.344–5
    elimination, **B1**.345
    eradication, **B1**.345
    hygiene role, **B1**.353–4
    outbreak control, **B1**.346–7
    quarantine and isolation, **B1**.347
    vaccination *see* Vaccination; Vaccine(s)
  parasitic disease, **P**.103–47
    affecting parameters, **P**.106 (Fig.)
    animal parasitic diseases, **P**.115–16
    basic reproductive number of infection effects, **P**.53
    chemotherapy/chemoprophylaxis, **P**.112, **P**.127–9, **P**.144 (Tab.)
      African trypanosomiasis, **P**.144 (Tab.)
      availability, **P**.128
      Chagas disease, **P**.144 (Tab.)
      community-based programs, **P**.64–5, **P**.121, **P**.789
      cysticercosis, **P**.144 (Tab.)
      dracunculiasis, **P**.144 (Tab.)
      drug resistance problems, **P**.128

economics, **P**.129
      leishmaniasis, **P**.144 (Tab.)
      lymphatic filariasis, **P**.144 (Tab.)
      malaria, **P**.144 (Tab.)
      neurocysticercosis, **P**.144 (Tab.)
      onchocerciasis, **P**.144 (Tab.)
      quality control, **P**.128
      schistosomiasis, **P**.127, **P**.144 (Tab.)
    community-based programs, **P**.120–5
      Chagas disease, **P**.122
      chemotherapy-based control, **P**.64–5, **P**.121, **P**.789
      filariasis control, **P**.122–3
      lymphatic filariasis control, **P**.122
      malaria control, **P**.124, **P**.517
      national scale-up, **P**.120–1
      onchocerciasis *see* Community-directed treatment with ivermectin (CDTI)
      schistosomiasis studies, **P**.604, **P**.604 (Fig.)
      vector control, **P**.121
      volunteers, **P**.121
    components/framework, **P**.108 (Fig.), **P**.110–15
      evaluation/monitoring, **P**.112
      objective definitions, **P**.111
      planning/resourcing, **P**.111–12
      situation analysis, **P**.110–11
    concepts, **P**.108–10
      control definition, **P**.108–9
      economics, **P**.110
      elimination of disease, **P**.108–9
      elimination of infection, **P**.108–9
      eradication, **P**.108–9
      eradication feasibility, **P**.109 (Tab.)
      eradication *vs.* control, **P**.108–9
      extinction, **P**.108–9
      isolated environments, **P**.110
      local control, **P**.109
    conflicts, **P**.103–6, **P**.107 (Tab.)
    diagnosis, **P**.129–30, **P**.143 (Tab.)
      dracunculiasis, **P**.143 (Tab.)
      serology, **P**.129–30
    Dientamoeba fragilis infection, **P**.269
    economics, **P**.103–6
    epidemiology *see* Epidemiology of infection, parasitic infection
    initiatives, **P**.103–8
    methods, **P**.112, **P**.115, **P**.115–30
      environmental management, **P**.112
      epidemics, **P**.115–16
      health education/social mobilization, **P**.115
      health system components, **P**.111 (Tab.)
      immunoprophylaxis, **P**.112–15
      large scale *vs.* small-scale, **P**.115–16
      mass treatment strategies, **P**.128
      school-age children, **P**.124–5
      vector/reservoir control, **P**.112, **P**.118–20, **P**.125–7, **P**.145 (Tab.)
    nongovernmental development organizations, **P**.103–6
    public–private partnerships, **P**.103–6, **P**.110
    sector-wide approaches to financing, **P**.103–6
    stratification of disease, **P**.115

integrated control, **P**.115
      leishmaniasis, **P**.134 (Tab.)
      lymphatic filariasis, **P**.139 (Tab.)
      malaria, **P**.131 (Tab.)
      onchocerciasis, **P**.137 (Tab.)
      schistosomiasis, **P**.141 (Tab.)
      trypanosomiasis, **P**.133 (Tab.)
    see also individual parasites; specific diseases/infection
    see also Vaccination; Vaccine(s)

Control of Substances Hazardous to Health (COSHH: 2002), **V2**.1515

Convulsions, Japanese encephalitis, **V2**.1424–5

Cook-chill foods, nosocomial infection, **B1**.377

Cooling towers, Legionnaires' disease, **B1**.375–6

Coombs antiglobulin test, human brucellosis diagnosis, **B2**.1739–40

Copper, acute phase response, **I**.208

Copper derivatives, **B1**.428
  action of, **B1**.437 (Tab.)

Copper, resistance to, **B1**.114

Copper/zinc-containing superoxide (Cu/Zn SOD), *Candida albicans* virulence factor, **M**.259

Coprinus cinereus, **M**.77

Coproantibodies, **P**.208

Coprococcus, **B2**.903–4, **B2**.917
  classification, **B2**.903–4, **B2**.905 (Tab.)
  definition/characteristics, **B2**.917
  growth requirements, **B2**.906
  identification, **B2**.906–7
  normal microbiota, **B2**.910

Coracidium, **P**.576

Corda's phenomenon, **M**.564

Cordocentesis, fetal infection diagnosis, **V2**.1445 (Tab.)

Core antigen (GAG) *see* Foamy viruses

Co-receptors, rotaviruses, **V2**.949–50

'Core groups,' epidemiology, **I**.952

Core-like particles (CLPs)
  Bluetongue virus, **V2**.941 (Fig.)
  orbiviruses, **V2**.941, **V2**.941 (Fig.)

Core (C) protein
  flaviviruses *see* Flaviviruses
  Hendra virus, **V1**.816
  henipaviruses, **V1**.816
  Hepatitis C virus *see* Hepatitis C virus (HCV)
  Human parainfluenza virus 3, **V1**.771
  Measles virus, **V1**.715–16, **V1**.717
  Nipah virus, **V1**.816
  paramyxoviruses, **V1**.704–5
  pestiviruses, **V2**.995–6
  respiroviruses, **V1**.763–4, **V1**.771
  Sendai virus *see* Sendai virus

Coriobacteriaceae, **B2**.1028–9

Corliss' classification of protozoa (1994), **P**.189–90, **P**.194–5

Cornea
  fusariosis, **M**.141 (Fig.)
  microsporidiosis, **P**.539–40
  specimens, **M**.84
  stains for *Acanthamoeba,* **P**.235
  ulceration, *Nocardia asteroides* infection, **B2**.1158–9

Cornea (*Continued*)
see also Keratitis
Corn-meal agar (CMA), **M**.604
Corn stunt, **B2**.1965–6
Coronary artery bypass surgery, infection after, **B1**.385
 Gordonia bronchialis, **B2**.1151–2
 Gordonia sputi, **B2**.1152
Coronary heart disease (CHD), *Chlamydia pneumoniae* infection, **B2**.2016
Coronaviridae, **V1**.26, **V1**.378
 characteristics, **V1**.139 (Tab.), **V1**.177 (Tab.)
 classification, **V1**.27 (Tab.), **V1**.51 (Tab.), **V1**.53, **V1**.390, **V1**.392, **V1**.824–5
 see also Coronaviruses; *Totiviridae; specific viruses*
Coronavirus
 classification, **V1**.53, **V1**.390, **V1**.392
 morphology, **V1**.391 (Fig.)
 type species, **V1**.824–5
 see also Coronaviruses
Coronaviruses
 'accessory proteins,' **V1**.395, **V1**.835–6
 ADP-ribose 1'-phosphotase, **V1**.832–3
 cell entry
  esterase, **V1**.212
  ligand conformational change, **V1**.139
  receptors, **V1**.207 (Tab.)
 classification, **V1**.824–5, **V1**.824 (Tab.)
  characteristics, **V1**.823
 cyclic phosphodiesterase, **V1**.832–3
 envelope (E) protein, **V1**.827, **V1**.836 (Tab.), **V1**.837
 gene expression, **V1**.119
 'genetic cassettes,' **V1**.835–6
 genome, **V1**.136, **V1**.136 (Fig.), **V1**.825
  common leader sequence, **V1**.395
  expression strategies, **V1**.829 (Fig.)
  non-translated region, **V1**.825–7
  open reading frames, **V1**.827
  organization, **V1**.136, **V1**.136 (Fig.)
  overlaps, **V1**.827–8
  packaging, **V1**.827
  pseudoknot, **V1**.827–8
  regulatory elements, **V1**.825–6
  structure, **V1**.828 (Fig.)
  transcription-regulating sequence, **V1**.826–7
 helicases, **V1**.834
 hemagglutinin-esterase (HE), **V1**.827, **V1**.836 (Tab.), **V1**.838–9
 infection *see* Coronavirus infection
 isolation/propagation and identification, **V1**.95–8, **V1**.96 (Tab.)
 membrane (M) protein, **V1**.827, **V1**.836 (Tab.), **V1**.837
  budding, **V1**.837
  cell-mediated immunity, **V1**.840
 molecular mass, **V1**.825
 morphology/structure, **V1**.76–7, **V1**.76 (Fig.), **V1**.138, **V1**.395, **V1**.825, **V1**.826 (Fig.)
  glycoproteins, **V1**.76
  M protein, **V1**.76
  nucleocapsid, **V1**.76
  replication component, **V1**.76
  transport component, **V1**.76

mRNA structure, **V1**.139, **V1**.140 (Tab.)
 nonstructural proteins, **V1**.827–8, **V1**.832–6
  see also specific types
 nucleocapsid (N) protein, **V1**.76, **V1**.827, **V1**.832, **V1**.836–7, **V1**.836 (Tab.)
  cell-mediated immunity, **V1**.840
 particle assembly/release, **V1**.144
 physical stability, **V1**.825
 protein processing, **V1**.141
 receptors, **V1**.246 (Fig.)
 recombination, **V1**.15, **V1**.188
 replicase (RNA polymerase), **V1**.827–8, **V1**.832–5, **V1**.833 (Fig.)
  intracellular localization, **V1**.835
  nsp13, **V1**.834
  post-translational modification, **V1**.832, **V1**.834
  proteinase domain, **V1**.832
  ribosomal frameshifting, **V1**.832
  RNA-dependent RNA polymerase activity, **V1**.833–4
  sequence analysis, **V1**.832
 replication, **V1**.828–9
  cell-specific factors, **V1**.136 (Fig.)
  errors, **V1**.132–3
  replicase *see above*
  RNA synthesis, **V1**.396
 reverse genetics, **V1**.830–1
 spike (S) protein, **V1**.827, **V1**.836 (Tab.), **V1**.837–8
  cell-mediated immunity, **V1**.840
  cell receptor, **V1**.838
  neutralizing antibodies, **V1**.840
 structural proteins, **V1**.836 (Tab.)
  see also specific types
 subgenomic RNAs, **V1**.828–30
  'discontinuous minus strand synthesis,' **V1**.401
 transcription, **V1**.829–30
 translation, **V1**.831–2
  ribosome scanning, **V1**.831
 see also Arteriviruses; *Coronaviridae; Coronavirus;* Toroviruses
Coronavirus infection, **V1**.823, **V1**.841 (Tab.), **V1**.845
 animal infection, **V1**.392
 immune response, **V1**.840–1
  cell-mediated, **V1**.840–1
  humoral, **V1**.840
  IFN activity, **I**.260 (Tab.)
  lymphokines, **V1**.840–1
 infection process, **V1**.241 (Tab.)
 neural spread, **V1**.244 (Tab.)
 respiratory tract infection, **V1**.366
Coronavirus N, **V1**.77
Corticosteroids, **M**.232
 acute bronchiolitis therapy, **V1**.777
 Angiostrongylus costaricensis infection, **P**.807–8
 HTLV-associated myelopathy(HAM)/ tropical spastic paraparesis (TSP), **V2**.1290
 prototheosis predisposition, **M**.401
 therapy
  aspergillosis, **M**.695, **M**.698, **M**.707
  chromoblastomycosis, **M**.359

endophthalmitis, **M**.320
 mycotic keratitis, **M**.315
 opportunistic infection, **M**.12
 PCP, **M**.789–90
 penicilliosis marneffei, **M**.562
 Pneumocystis carinii infection, **M**.784, **M**.789–91
 seborrheic dermatitis, **M**.185
 septic shock, **I**.702
 toxocariasis therapy, **P**.755
Corticotropin-releasing factor (CRF), **I**.208
Corticoviridae
 classification, **V1**.27 (Tab.), **V1**.43 (Tab.)
 see also specific viruses
Corynebacterium
 biochemistry, species, **B2**.982 (Tab.)
 cell wall composition, **B2**.1010 (Tab.)
 classification, **B2**.1137–8
  chemotaxonomic characteristics, **B2**.978 (Tab.), **B2**.980
 corynemycolic acids, **B2**.1145–6
 habitats, **B2**.977–8
  vegetables, **B1**.281
 infection
  antibody detection, **B1**.751
  disease associations, **B2**.981 (Tab.)
  keratitis, **B1**.601
  urinary tract, **B1**.678
 isolation/identification, **B2**.978–9, **B2**.1013
  double diffusion, **B1**.756
  EIAs, **B1**.751, **B1**.756
  immunoserology, **B1**.756
  staining properties, **B2**.1139–40
  typing systems, **B2**.978–9
 lipophilic, **B2**.981 (Tab.), **B2**.989
 morphology, **B2**.977 (Fig.), **B2**.980
  species, **B2**.982 (Tab.)
 non-lipophilic, **B2**.981 (Tab.), **B2**.986–9
 as normal microbiota, **B1**.296 (Tab.)
  oral, **B1**.609
  skin colonization, **B1**.304
 pasteurization, **B1**.232–3
 phytopathogenicity, **B1**.202
 species, **B2**.980, **B2**.982 (Tab.)
  see also individual species
 Staphylococcus aureus carriage inhibition, **B2**.778–9
Corynebacterium accolens, **B2**.982 (Tab.), **B2**.989
Corynebacterium afermentans
 subspecies *afermentans*, **B2**.982 (Tab.), **B2**.986
 subspecies *lipophilum*, **B2**.982 (Tab.), **B2**.989
Corynebacterium amycolatum, **B2**.980, **B2**.982 (Tab.), **B2**.986
 disease associations, **B2**.981 (Tab.)
  endocarditis, **B1**.532–3
 habitats, **B2**.977–8
 identification, **B2**.979
Corynebacterium appendicis, **B2**.982 (Tab.), **B2**.989
Corynebacterium argentoratense, **B2**.982 (Tab.), **B2**.986
Corynebacterium atypicum, **B2**.980, **B2**.982 (Tab.), **B2**.986
 identification, **B2**.979

Corynebacterium aurimucosum, **B2**.982 (Tab.), **B2**.986

Corynebacterium auris, **B2**.982 (Tab.), **B2**.986
  habitats, **B2**.977–8

Corynebacterium confusum, **B2**.980, **B2**.982 (Tab.), **B2**.987

Corynebacterium coyleae, **B2**.982 (Tab.), **B2**.987

Corynebacterium diphtheriae, **B2**.980–6, **B2**.982 (Tab.)
  antibacterial susceptibility/resistance, **B2**.985
    fusidic acid, **B1**.488
  biochemistry, **B2**.980, **B2**.982 (Tab.)
    nitrate reduction, **B1**.66
  biotypes, **B2**.980
    belfanti, **B1**.612 (Tab.), **B2**.982 (Tab.)
    gravis, **B1**.612 (Tab.), **B2**.980, **B2**.982 (Tab.)
    intermedius, **B1**.612 (Tab.), **B2**.980
    mitis, **B1**.612 (Tab.), **B2**.980
  cellular morphology, **B2**.980
  colony morphology, **B2**.980
  conjunctivitis, **B1**.598–9
  disease associations, **B2**.981 (Tab.)
  genome, **B2**.984
  habitats, **B2**.977–8
  immune evasion, **I**.655
  infection *see* Diphtheria
  iron-dependent repression, **B1**.165–6
  isolation/identification, **B1**.612 (Tab.)
    typing, **B2**.984
  metachromatic granules, **B2**.981 (Fig.)
  pathogenesis, **B1**.608–9
  physical/chemical agent susceptibility/resistance, **B2**.980
  polyphosphate granules, **B2**.980
  tox+ bacteriophage, **B2**.984
  tox gene, **B2**.984
  toxigenic, **B2**.984
    isolation rare after vaccination, **B1**.348–9
    screening by PCR, **B2**.984
  toxin *see* Diphtheria toxin

Corynebacterium durum, **B2**.980, **B2**.982 (Tab.), **B2**.987
  habitats, **B2**.977–8

Corynebacterium falsenii, **B2**.982 (Tab.), **B2**.987

Corynebacterium freneyi, **B2**.982 (Tab.), **B2**.987

Corynebacterium glucuronolyticum, **B2**.982 (Tab.), **B2**.987
  disease associations, **B2**.981 (Tab.)
  habitats, **B2**.977–8

Corynebacterium imitans, **B2**.982 (Tab.), **B2**.987

Corynebacterium jeikeium, **B2**.982 (Tab.), **B2**.990
  disease association, endocarditis, **B1**.532–3
  disease associations, **B2**.981 (Tab.)
  habitats, **B2**.977–8
  nosocomial infection, **B1**.401 (Tab.)
  skin colonization, **B1**.304

Corynebacterium kroppenstedtii, **B2**.980, **B2**.982 (Tab.), **B2**.990
  identification, **B2**.979

Corynebacterium lipophiloflavum, **B2**.982 (Tab.), **B2**.990

Corynebacterium macginleyi, **B2**.982 (Tab.), **B2**.990
  disease associations, **B2**.981 (Tab.)
  habitats, **B2**.977–8

Corynebacterium matruchotii, **B2**.980, **B2**.982 (Tab.), **B2**.987–8

Corynebacterium matruchotii-like strain, **B2**.988

Corynebacterium minutissimum, **B2**.982 (Tab.), **B2**.988
  disease associations, **B2**.981 (Tab.)

Corynebacterium mucifaciens, **B2**.982 (Tab.), **B2**.988

Corynebacterium 'nigricans,' **B2**.982 (Tab.), **B2**.988
  disease associations, **B2**.981 (Tab.)

Corynebacterium propinquum, **B2**.982 (Tab.), **B2**.988

Corynebacterium pseudodiphtheriticum, **B2**.982 (Tab.), **B2**.988
  disease associations, **B2**.981 (Tab.)
  identification, **B1**.612 (Tab.)

Corynebacterium pseudotuberculosis, **B2**.982 (Tab.), **B2**.988
  disease associations, **B2**.981 (Tab.)

Corynebacterium riegelii, **B2**.982 (Tab.), **B2**.988
  disease associations, **B2**.981 (Tab.)

Corynebacterium simulans, **B2**.982 (Tab.), **B2**.988–9

Corynebacterium singulare, **B2**.982 (Tab.), **B2**.989

Corynebacterium striatum, **B2**.982 (Tab.), **B2**.989
  disease associations, **B2**.981 (Tab.)
  endocarditis, **B1**.532–3
  habitats, **B2**.977–8

Corynebacterium sundsvallense, **B2**.980, **B2**.982 (Tab.), **B2**.989

Corynebacterium thomssenii, **B2**.982 (Tab.), **B2**.989

Corynebacterium ulcerans, **B2**.982 (Tab.), **B2**.989
  disease associations, **B2**.981 (Tab.)
  identification, **B1**.612 (Tab.)
  infection
    mastitis, **B1**.230
    milk-borne, **B1**.231, **B1**.235, **B1**.242
  in milk, **B1**.242

Corynebacterium urealyticum, **B2**.980, **B2**.982 (Tab.), **B2**.990
  disease associations, **B2**.981 (Tab.)
  habitats, **B2**.977–8
  skin colonization, **B1**.304

Corynebacterium xerosis, **B2**.982 (Tab.), **B2**.989
  endocarditis, **B1**.532–3

Coryneform bacteria, **B2**.977
  characteristics, **B2**.977
  common features, **B2**.977
  disease associations, **B2**.981 (Tab.)
  morphology, **B2**.977 (Fig.)
  see also individual species

Corynespora cassiicola, **M**.391

Corynosoma, **P**.598
  structure, **P**.596 (Fig.)

Cosmid cloning vectors, **B1**.120–1
  Trypanosoma cruzi, **P**.382

Costa, filaments, **P**.170–2

Costa Rica, New World leishmaniasis incidence, **P**.313–14

Cote d'Ivoire ebolavirus (CIEBOV), **V1**.382
  classification, **V2**.1086
  historical aspects, **V2**.1085
  outbreaks, **V2**.1087 (Tab.)

Co-trimoxazole (trimethoprim-sulfamethoxazole)
  intracranial abscess, **B1**.588
  PCP, **M**.764, **M**.789
    AIDS, **M**.764, **M**.783–4, **M**.789, **M**.790
    resistance, **M**.764, **M**.790, **M**.791–2, **M**.796
  spectrum of activity
    Actinobacillus actinomycetemcomitans, **B2**.1664
    Blastocystis hominis, **P**.567
    Bordetella, **B2**.1793–4
    Burkholderia cepacia complex, **B2**.1610
    Haemophilus, **B2**.1702–3, **B2**.1702 (Tab.), **B2**.1703 (Tab.), **B2**.1710
    Klebsiella, **B2**.1480
    Nocardia, **B2**.1145, **B2**.1165–6
    Tropheryma whippelii, **B2**.1002
  therapy
    cyclosporiasis, **P**.415–16
    gonorrhea, **B1**.662
    human brucellosis, **B2**.1743
    isosporiasis, **P**.414
    melioidosis, **B2**.1631, **B2**.1631 (Tab.)
    paracoccidioidomycosis, **M**.551
    urinary tract infection, **B1**.679
    zygomycosis, **M**.352

Cottonrat *(Sigmodon hispidus),* arenaviruses association, **V2**.1060 (Tab.), **V2**.1061

Cottontail rabbit papillomavirus (CRPV)
  genome organization, **V1**.451 (Fig.)
  historical aspects, **V1**.448
  infection
    latent infection, **V1**.453
    temporal/spatial expression patterns, **V1**.453
  type species, **V1**.45

Coughing, mechanical removal of bacteria, **B1**.176

Coumermycin, *Listeria,* **B2**.957–8

Counseling, Kaposi's sarcoma, **V2**.1503

Counter-clamped homogeneous electric field, *Enterococcus,* **B2**.894

Countercurrent immunoelectrophoresis (CIE)
  amebiasis, **P**.211–12
  bacterial infection, **B1**.749
    Streptococcus pneumoniae polysaccharides, **B1**.632
  mycology, **M**.34
  trichinellosis diagnosis, **P**.765, **P**.766 (Fig.)

Country-cured hams, **B1**.274

Covalent coupling, as carrier protein, **I**.863

Covalently closed circle DNA, artificial competence, **B1**.100

Covalent modification, **B1**.76

Cover of Vaccination Evaluated Rapidly (COVER) program, **B1**.326

Cowdria, **B2**.2026, **B2**.2049–50, **B2**.2053

Cowdry bodies
 in HSV infection, **V1**.508–9
 subacute sclerosing panencephalitis, **V1**.725
Cowen, David, **P**.17–8
Cowpea mosaic virus
 cellular entry, **V1**.215
 phylogenetics, **V1**.174
Cowpox virus (CPXV), **V1**.587
 classification, **V1**.583
 cytokine response modifier A (CrmA),
  V1.287
 immune evasion
  caspase inhibition, **V1**.324
  chemokine binding proteins, **V1**.320,
   I.622–3
  complement interference, **V1**.313, **I**.639
  cytokine expression/activation, **V1**.316,
   I.623
  IFN receptors, **V1**.315, **I**.619
  receptor homologues, **I**.620–1
  secreted cytokine receptors, **V1**.318,
   V1.585–6
  serpins, **V1**.623
  TNF analogue secretion, **V1**.621–2
 phylogenetics, **V1**.585
 smallpox eradication, **V1**.579–80
 transmission, **V1**.371 (Tab.)
 viral complement control protein, **V1**.313
 virion maturation, **V1**.614, **V1**.614 (Fig.)
Coxiella burnetii, **B2.2072–80**
 antibacterial susceptibility/resistance,
  B2.2077
  chloramphenicol, **B2**.2077–8
  chlorotetracyline, **B2**.2077–8
  erythromycin, **B2**.2077–8
  evaluation, **B2**.2078
  streptomycin, **B2**.2077–8
 antigens, **B1**.748, **B2**.2076
  GroEL, **B2**.2076
 cell wall composition, **B2**.2075–6
  LPS, **B2**.2073, **B2**.2075
 classification, **B2**.2026, **B2**.2027,
  B2.2027 (Fig.), **B2**.2072–3
  DNA sequencing, **B2**.2072–3
  16S rDNA, **B2**.2072–3
  23S rDNA, **B2**.2072–3
 genome, **B2**.2074–5
  characterized genes, **B2**.2075
  genomic groups, **B2**.2074
  open reading frames, **B2**.2074
  restriction fragment length polymorphisms,
   B2.2074
  rRNA operon, **B2**.2074–5
 habitats, **B2**.2073
 history, **B2**.2072
 immune evasion, **I**.651
  complement surface masking, **I**.662–3
  IL-10 induction, **I**.653
  MHC class II antigen presentation, **I**.657–8
 infection *see* Q fever
 isolation, **B2**.2073–4
  cell culture, **B2**.2073
  chicken embryo culture, **B2**.2073
  mass culture, **B2**.2074
  plaque formation, **B2**.2073–4
 laboratory worker immunization, **B1**.767

 macrophage infection, **I**.30
 microenvironment, **B2**.2073
  phagolysosome, **B2**.2073
  phagolysosomes, **B2**.2077
 in milk, **B1**.230, **B1**.231–2
 morphology, **B2**.2073, **B2**.2074 (Fig.),
  B2.2076 (Fig.)
 pasteurization, **B1**.232–3
 plasmids, **B2**.2074–5
Coxsackie-adenovirus receptor (CAR), **V1**.441
Coxsackie virus
 antigenic variation, **V2**.876–7
 historical aspects, **V2**.857
 isolation/propagation and identification,
  V1.96 (Tab.), **V1**.100, **V2**.877 (Tab.)
 molecular mimicry, **V1**.283
 post-translational protein modification,
  V1.140, **V2**.867
Coxsackievirus A infection, nosocomial,
 B1.400
Coxsackievirus B infection, nosocomial, **B1**.400
Coxsackie virus infection, **V2**.870,
 V2.875 (Tab.), **V2**.1482–3
 age-related prevalence, **V2**.876 (Tab.)
 clinical aspects
  acute epidemic hemorrhagic conjunctivitis
   (AHC), **V2**.872
  cardiac disease, **V2**.871
  diabetes mellitus association, **V1**.283,
   V2.872
  enteroviral meningoencephalitis, **V2**.1509
  exanthems, **V2**.872
  hand-foot-and-mouth disease (HFMD),
   V2.871–2
  herpangina, **V2**.871
  meningitis, **V2**.1423–4
  myocarditis association, **V1**.283
  paralysis, **V2**.871, **V2**.1423–4
  pleurodynia (Bornholm disease), **V2**.871
 CNS, **V2**.1423–4
 congenital infection, **V2**.1483
 fetal infection, **V2**.1482–3
 immune response, **V1**.283
  NK cells, **I**.96
 immunopathology, **V1**.283
 neonatal infection, **V2**.871, **V2**.1444 (Tab.),
  V2.1483
 perinatal infection, **V2**.1444 (Tab.), **V2**.1483
 persistent infection, **V2**.869
 in pregnancy, **V2**.1444 (Tab.), **V2**.1483
CpG motifs
 actions
  B7–1 (CD80) upregulation, **I**.911
  B7–2 (CD86) upregulation, **I**.911
  CD40 upregulation, **I**.911
  IFN-α production, **I**.911
  IFN-γ production, **I**.911
  IL-6 production, **I**.911–12
  IL-10 production, **I**.911
  IL-12 production, **I**.911
  IL-18 production, **I**.911
  Th1 cell stimulation, **I**.911
  TNF-α production, **I**.911
 as adjuvant, **I**.931
  cytokine stimulation, **I**.931
  DNA vaccines *see* DNA vaccines

  hepatitis B vaccine, **I**.937
  intranasal vaccine delivery, **I**.831–2, **I**.864
  mechanism of action, **I**.926, **I**.931
  Th1 cell responses, **I**.926, **I**.931
  vaccine models, **I**.931
 bare skin immunization, **I**.824, **I**.825
 binding/signal transduction, **I**.911
 CR2/CD19/CD81 complex, BCR signaling,
  I.347
Crabs, microbiology, **B1**.279–80
Cranial nerve palsy, enterovirus 70, **V2**.1423
Crayfish, *Paragonimus* intermediate host,
 P.646
C-reactive protein (CRP), **I**.114 (Tab.),
 I.199–200
 acute phase response, **I**.195 (Fig.), **B1**.739
 complement activation, **I**.199–200
  classical pathway, **I**.142
 heart disease predictor, **I**.200, **I**.206
 inflammation marker, **I**.199, **I**.206
 Leishmania donovani infection, **I**.199–200
 malaria immunity, **P**.490
 as marker, **I**.194
 microbial recognition, **I**.24 (Tab.)
 phosphorylcholine binding, **I**.199
 phosphorylethanolamine binding, **I**.199
 production, **I**.196 (Fig.)
  IL-6, **I**.285
 structure, **I**.199, **I**.199 (Fig.)
Cream, **B1**.248
 associated infection, **B1**.248
Cresols, **B1**.422, **B1**.423 (Tab.)
Cresyl echt violet, *Pneumocystis,* **M**.787
Cresylic acid, **B1**.422
Creutzfeldt–Jakob disease (CJD), **V2**.1347
 amyloid plaques, **V2**.1365
 incidence, **V2**.1347, **V2**.1366–7
 see also Iatrogenic Creutzfeldt–Jakob disease
  (iCJD); Sporadic Creutzfeldt–Jakob
  disease (sCJD); Variant
  Creutzfeld–Jakob disease (vCJD)
Creutzfeldt-Jakob disease (CJD), transmission,
 B1.380–1
Cricetidae, arenaviruses associated, **V2**.1061
Crick, F H C, **B1**.13
Crimean–Congo hemorrhagic fever (CCHF),
 V2.1045–6
 emerging infection, **V2**.1648 (Tab.)
 epidemiology, **V2**.1049–50
 pathogenesis, **V2**.1050
 transmission, **V1**.372 (Tab.)
Crimean–Congo hemorrhagic fever virus
 classification, biosafety level 4, **V2**.1526
 G1 glycoprotein, **V2**.1034
 genome structure, **V2**.1034
 transmission, **V2**.1049–50
Crithidia, nucleus, **P**.172 (Fig.)
Critical control point, hazard analysis critical
  control point system, **B1**.288
Critical limits, hazard analysis critical control
  point system, **B1**.288
Critical micelle concentration (CMC), **B1**.432
Crixivan *see* Indinavir
CRKOL gene, **I**.774–5
CRM197, *Streptococcus pneumoniae* vaccine,
 I.936

Crohn's disease
  HLA association, **I.**577
  IBD5 gene association, **I.**581
  IL-15, **I.**282
  Mycobacterium paratuberculosis association, **B2.**1182
  nucleotide-binding oligomerization domains, **I.**115, **I.**125
  Pseudomonas fluorescens role, **B2.**1603
  Th1/Th2 balance, **I.**755–6
  therapy
    anti-inflammatory drugs, **I.**209
    monoclonal antibody therapy, **I.**357
Crops
  GMO's application, **B1.**198
  see also specific crops
Cross-challenge studies, noroviruses, **V2.**918
Cross-neutralization, arenaviruses, **V2.**1069
Cross-placenta infection
  Ancylostoma duodenale, **P.**720–1
  Parvovirus B19 virus infection, **V2.**1468
'Crosspriming,' **I.**404
  DNA vaccines, **I.**914, **I.**915 (Fig.)
Crossreacting material (CRM), conjugate vaccine carrier, **I.**935
Cross-sectional surveys *see* Transmission dynamics
Crotonase, **B1.**56
Croup (laryngotracheobronchitis), **V1.**774–6
  clinical manifestations, **V1.**775
  diagnosis, **V1.**775
  disease importance, **V1.**774
  epidemiology, **V1.**365–6, **V1.**774
  etiology, **V1.**774
  pathogenesis, **V1.**774–5
  prevention, **V1.**775–6
  treatment, **V1.**775
Crown gall disease, **B1.**202
Crude oil, bioremediation, **B1.**201
Crustacea
  chilling, **B1.**279–80
  commercial importance, **B1.**279
  food-borne illness, **B1.**279–80
  harvesting, **B1.**279
  microbiology, **B1.**279–80
  polluted water, **B1.**279–80
Cryoelectron microscopy
  astrovirus morphology, **V2.**891–2, **V2.**892 (Fig.)
  hepatitis E virus structure, **V2.**1175
  herpesviruses morphology/structure, **V1.**490
  noroviruses, **V2.**913
Cryopreservation, cell cultures, **V1.**89
Crypt cell hyperplasia
  ascariasis, **P.**727
  microsporidiosis, **P.**537
  rotavirus infection, **V2.**950
Cryptic infection, parvovirus infection, **V1.**423–4
Cryptic plasmid, *Chlamydia trachomatis,* **B2.**2009
Cryptidins *see* α-Defensins
Cryptobacterium, **B2.**1028–9
Cryptococcal antigen test, **M.**35, **M.**93 (Tab.), **M.**109, **M.**641, **M.**649
  prognosis, **M.**653

Cryptococcal meningitis, HTLV infection, **I.**802–3
Cryptococcosis, **I.**290–2, **M.637–58**
  in AIDS *see* AIDS, concomitant infection
  blepharitis, **M.**296, **M.**297
  causative agents *see Cryptococcus neoformans*
  clinical presentation, **M.**645–8
    CNS infection, **M.**140 (Fig.), **M.**645–6, **M.**648, **M.**650–1
    cutaneous, **M.**647–8
    endophthalmitis, **M.**648
    genitourinary tract infection, **M.**648
    granulomas, **M.**534
    meningoencephalitis *see* Meningoencephalitis, cryptococcosis
    oculomycoses, **M.**280 (Tab.), **M.**287, **M.**324–5, **M.**648
    ophthalmic, **M.**648
    prostate, **M.**648
    pulmonary *see below*
  diagnosis, **M.**125–7, **M.**648–50
    cerebrospinal fluid, **M.**649, **M.**652, **M.**653
    EIAs, **M.**110
    histopathology, **M.**128 (Tab.), **M.**132 (Fig.), **M.**133 (Fig.), **M.**140 (Fig.)
    Pastorex test, **M.**109–10
    PCR, **M.**94, **M.**110
    reverse passive latex agglutination, **M.**109–10
    serology, **M.**16, **M.**92, **M.**93 (Tab.), **M.**109–10
    specimen site selection, **M.**83 (Tab.)
  endophthalmitis, **M.**317
  epidemiology, **M.**11, **M.**12, **M.**18, **M.**643–4
    AIDS *see* AIDS
    birds, **M.**643
    HAART, **M.**644, **M.**651, **M.**652, **M.**653
  histoplasmosis capsulati *vs,* **M.**534
  history, **M.**16–8, **M.**17 (Fig.), **M.**18 (Fig.), **M.**637–8
  immune response, **M.**16, **M.**644–5
    CD4 cells, **M.**645
    cell-mediated, **M.**645
    colony-stimulating factors, **M.**652–3
    humoral, **M.**645
  immunosuppression, **M.**644, **M.**645–9
    therapy, **M.**652
    see also AIDS
  mastitis, **B1.**230
  nosocomial infection, **B1.**374, **B1.**403
  pathophysiology, **M.**644–5
  prognosis, **M.**653
  prophylaxis, **M.**653
    fluconazole, **M.**653
  pulmonary, **M.**646–7, **M.**649–50, **M.**650 (Fig.)
    AIDS, **M.**647, **M.**650
  therapy, **M.**149–50, **M.**650–3
    amphotericin B, **M.**651–2
    amphotericinB/flucytosine combination, **M.**651–2
    cytokines, **M.**652–3
    echinocandins therapy, **M.**651
    fluconazole, **M.**651–2
    flucytosine, **M.**651
    GM-CSF, **M.**652–3

immunosuppressive therapy withdrawal, **M.**652
intracranial pressure, **M.**652
vaccines, **M.**653, **I.**933 (Tab.)
  peptides, **I.**861 (Tab.)
Cryptococcus, **M.**638
  cell walls, **M.**124
    staining, **M.**124
  classification, **M.**63, **M.**65 (Tab.)
  environmental source identification, **M.**95
  histopathology, **M.**125
  identification
    Pastorex test, **M.**109–10
    PCR, **M.**94, **M.**110
    reverse passive latex agglutination, **M.**109–10
    urease, **M.**640–1
Cryptococcus albidus, **M.**638
Cryptococcus bacillospora, **M.**638
Cryptococcus laurentii, **M.**638
  oculomycoses, **M.**287
Cryptococcus neoformans, **M.637–58**
  biochemistry
    catecholamine degradation, **M.**642
    glucuronoxylomannan *see below*
    glycine metabolism, **M.**638
    iron receptors, **M.**641–2
    melanin production, **M.**642
    phenol oxidase, **M.**16–7, **M.**640–2
  ecology, **M.**643
    eucalyptus trees, **M.**643
    guano, **M.**643
  genetic analysis, PCR, **M.**110
  geographical distribution, **M.**644
  glucuronoxylomannan, **M.**16, **M.**641
    antigen test, **M.**35, **M.**641, **M.**649, **M.**650, **M.**653
  growth, **M.**73, **M.**640–3
  histopathology, **M.**89 (Tab.), **M.**126 (Tab.), **M.**128 (Tab.), **M.**130, **M.**132 (Fig.), **M.**133 (Fig.), **M.**640–1, **M.**641 (Fig.)
    stains, **M.**123 (Tab.), **M.**124
  history, **M.**16–8, **M.**17 (Fig.), **M.**18 (Fig.), **M.**637–8
  identification, **M.**640–1
    biochemical tests, **M.**640–1
    blood cultures, **M.**86–7, **M.**649–50
    histopathology *see above*
    PCR, **M.**110
    serology, **M.**638–41, **M.**644
  infection *see* Cryptococcosis
  life cycle, **M.**639–40
  morphology, **M.**75, **M.**126 (Tab.), **M.**638–40
    basidiospores, **M.**639, **M.**640 (Fig.), **M.**644–5
    capsule, **M.**93 (Tab.), **M.**639 (Fig.), **M.**641–2
    teleomorphs, **M.**18, **M.**639, **M.**640 (Fig.)
  neurotrophism, **M.**645
  nomenclature, **M.**637–8
  phenotypic switching, **M.**76
  reproduction
    asexual, **M.**639, **M.**639 (Fig.)
    pheromones, **M.**639
    sexual, **M.**18, **M.**639–40, **M.**640 (Fig.)

Cryptococcus neoformans, (Continued)
  resistance
    canavanine, **M**.638, **M**.638 (Tab.)
    echinocandin, **M**.154, **M**.176
    flucytosine, **M**.176
  serotypes, **M**.638–41, **M**.644
    genetic analyses, **M**.639
    nomenclature, **M**.639
  susceptibility testing, **M**.169–70
  var. *gattii*, **M**.638
    asexual reproduction, **M**.639
    differentiation, **M**.638, **M**.638 (Tab.)
    ecology, **M**.643
    geographical distribution, **M**.644
    growth, **M**.642–3
    histopathology, **M**.140 (Fig.)
    meningoencephalitis, **M**.646
  var. *grubii*, **M**.639
    geographical variation, **M**.644
    growth, **M**.642–3
    meningoencephalitis, **M**.646
    rotting vegetation, **M**.643
  var. *neoformans*, **M**.638, **M**.639
    asexual reproduction, **M**.639
    blepharitis, **M**.297
    differentiation, **M**.638, **M**.638 (Tab.)
    ecology, **M**.643
    geographical distribution, **M**.644
    growth, **M**.642–3
    meningoencephalitis, **M**.646
    noncapsular antigens, **M**.110
    rotting vegetation, **M**.643
    skin infection, **M**.647–8
  virulence factors, **M**.79, **M**.641–2, **M**.646
'Cryptogenes,' trypanosomes, **P**.362
Cryptogenic abscess, **B1**.583
Crypto-LA test, **M**.109–10
Cryptosporidial oocyst wall protein (COWP)
  Cryptosporidium parvum classification, **P**.400
  structure, **P**.401–2
Cryptosporidiosis, **P**.399–410
  in AIDS/HIV infection *see* AIDS,
    concomitant infection
  cell invasion/establishment, **P**.402
    apical complex, **P**.402
    circumsporozoite-like antigen, **P**.402
    glycoproteins, **P**.402
    host cell cytoskeleton, **P**.402
  chemotherapy, **P**.410
  clinical aspects, **P**.404–5, **I**.677
    in AIDS, **P**.404–5
    biliary disease, **P**.405
    chronic cholangitis, **I**.776
    diarrhea, **P**.404–5, **P**.408
    disaccharide malabsorption, **P**.408
    'enterocyte immaturity hypothesis,' **P**.408
    nutritional impairment, **P**.405
    severe combined immunodeficiency,
      P.404–5
    villous atrophy, **P**.407, **P**.408
  diagnosis, **P**.408–9, **P**.408 (Fig.)
    fecal samples, **P**.151
    immunoassays, **P**.154
    string test, **P**.151

epidemiology, **P**.409–10
  in children, **P**.409
  developed countries, **P**.409
  developing countries, **P**.409
  HLA class II expression deficiency, **I**.776
  immunocompetent, **P**.409
  immunocompromised, **P**.399, **P**.409–10
  isosporiasis *vs.*, **P**.414
  transmission, **P**.409
  X-linked hyper-IgM-CD40 ligand
    deficiency, **I**.778
immunology, **P**.76, **P**.405–7
  animal models, **P**.405–7
  CD4 T cells, **P**.406
  human models, **P**.407
  humoral immunity, **P**.406–7
  IFN-γ, **P**.407
  secretory IgA, **P**.407
  T helper cells, **P**.406
  transforming growth factor-β, **P**.407
immunotherapy, **P**.410
  IFN-γ, **P**.406, **P**.407
microsporidiosis co-infection, **P**.546–7
milk-borne, **B1**.242
nosocomial, **B1**.403
pathology, **P**.407–8
  host-specificity, **P**.409
  infection distribution, **P**.407
  mucosal abnormalities, **P**.407–8
  physiological disturbances, **P**.408
public health importance, **P**.44, **P**.45
Cryptosporidium, **P**.188
  antibacterial susceptibility/resistance, **B1**.434
  cell biology, **P**.401–2
  classification, **P**.190–1, **P**.399–400
    genomic analysis, **P**.399
  genetics, **P**.403–4
  historical aspects, **P**.399
  infection *see* Cryptosporidiosis
  metabolism, **P**.402–3
  molecular studies, **P**.400–4
  waterborne, **B1**.214, **B1**.218–19
  see also individual species
Cryptosporidium baileyi, **P**.400
Cryptosporidium felis, **P**.400
Cryptosporidium meleagridis, **P**.400
Cryptosporidium muris, **P**.400
Cryptosporidium nasorum, **P**.400
Cryptosporidium parvum, **P**.188, **P**.400,
  P.401 (Fig.), **I**.677
  AIDS, **P**.97
  cell biology, **P**.401–2
  classification, **P**.400, **I**.675–6
  genetics, **P**.403–4
    gene sequencing/characterization, **P**.403–4
    genomic maps, **P**.404
    microsatellite analysis, **P**.404
    pulsed field gel electrophoresis, **P**.403
    species differentiation, **P**.404
    strain differences, **P**.404
    taxonomic evaluation, **P**.404
  historical aspects, **P**.18
  immune response, **P**.76
  infection *see* Cryptosporidiosis
  in vitro culture, **P**.400–1, **P**.406

life cycle, **P**.400, **I**.677
  merogony (schizogony), **P**.400
  merozoites, **P**.400
  sporozoites, **P**.400
  trophozoites, **P**.400
metabolism, **P**.403
  glycolytic pathway, **P**.403
  mannitol cycle, **P**.403
  protein synthesis, **P**.403
  shikimate pathway, **P**.403
morphology, eggs, **P**.413 (Fig.)
structure
  apical complex organelles, **P**.402
  oocyst wall, **P**.401–2
transmission, **I**.677
Cryptosporidium parvum, in milk, **B1**.235
Cryptosporidium serpentis, **P**.400
Cryptosporidium wrairi, **P**.400
Crystallographic analysis, TCR, **I**.460–1
  αβ TCRs, **I**.460–1
  γδ TCRs, **I**.461
  MHC–peptide interactions, **I**.461–3
Crytobacterium curtum, differential
  characteristics, **B2**.1029 (Tab.)
CSF1R gene, **I**.580
CSF2 gene, **I**.580
Csk-binding protein (CBP), **I**.343
Csk tyrosine kinase
  BCR signaling, **I**.343
  structure, **I**.343 (Fig.)
CTACK *see* Cutaneous T-cell attracting
  chemokine (CTACK:CCL27)
Ctenocephalides canis, **B2**.2037
Ctenocephalides felis, **B2**.2037, **B2**.2040
CTLA-4
  CD4 T cells, **I**.399
    tolerance induction, **I**.396–7
  deficiency, **I**.749
  DNA vaccine co-administration, **I**.909,
    I.919 (Tab.)
  IL-2 effects, **I**.279–80
  immunogenetics, **I**.582–3
CTLA-4 gene, **I**.582–3
  polymorphisms
    diabetes mellitus type I, **I**.752
    Graves' disease, **I**.752
    hepatitis C, **I**.588
CTLs *see* Cytotoxic T cell(s) (CTLs)
C-type lectins, **I**.114, **I**.114 (Tab.)
  macrophage pathogen recognition, **I**.23
  microbial recognition, **I**.24 (Tab.)
Cubic viruses, **V1**.6
Culex
  Barmah Forest virus transmission, **V2**.1023
  Eastern equine encephalitis virus
    transmission, **V2**.1019
  Getah virus transmission, **V2**.1023
  Japanese encephalitis virus transmission,
    V2.1001
  Murray Valley encephalitis transmission,
    V2.1003
  Sindbis virus transmission, **V2**.1023
  St Louis encephalitis virus transmission,
    V2.1001–2
  West Nile virus transmission, **V2**.1002
Culicoides, Onchocerca vector, **P**.781

Culiseta
  Eastern equine encephalitis virus
    transmission, **V2**.1019
  Sindbis virus transmission, **V2**.1023
Culture
  bacteria
    cat-scratch disease diagnosis, **B2**.1895
    cerebrospinal fluid, **B1**.559
    Chlamydia infection diagnosis, **B2**.2017–18
    glanders diagnosis, **B2**.1634
    human brucellosis diagnosis, **B2**.1739
    limitations for monitoring airborne
      organisms, **B1**.190–1
    media, **B1**.37–8, **B1**.714–15
      chemically defined, **B1**.37
      classification, **B1**.715
      complex media, **B1**.37
      enrichment, **B1**.37–8
      minimal medium, **B1**.37
    melioidosis diagnosis, **B2**.1630
    pharyngitis diagnosis, **B1**.611
    reference cultures, **B1**.28–9
    syphilis diagnosis, **B1**.745–6
    see also individual species
  mycology, **M**.85–7
    diagnosis
      dermatophytes, **M**.10, **M**.91 (Tab.),
        M.236
      histoplasmosis, **M**.532
      hyalohyphomycosis, **M**.751
      Malassezia dermatis, **M**.206–7
      mycetoma, **M**.389–90
      Paracoccidioides brasiliensis, **M**.552–3
    history, **M**.10, **M**.33–4
    incubation, **M**.85–6, **M**.91
    media, **M**.33–4, **M**.85, **M**.86, **M**.86 (Tab.)
      morphological, **M**.90–1, **M**.91 (Tab.)
      Mycetoma culture, **M**.389–90
      see also specific types
    safety principles, **M**.92
    see also specific infection
  parasites
    Acanthamoeba, **P**.235
    Blastocystis hominis, **P**.564, **P**.565–6
    Brachiola algerae, **P**.548
    Cryptosporidium parvum, **P**.400–1, **P**.406
    Dientamoeba fragilis, **P**.268
    hookworm, **P**.151
    Leishmania, **P**.301
    microsporidians, **P**.547, **P**.548
    Naegleria fowleri, **P**.232
    Schistosoma, **P**.151
    Toxoplasma gondii, **P**.428–9
    Trachipleistophora hominis, **P**.548
    Trichomonas vaginalis, **P**.260–1
    Trypanosoma, **P**.358–9, **P**.367, **P**.379
Culture filter antigen (CFA), pythiosis, **M**.422
Culture media
  sterilization, **V1**.87
  viruses, **V1**.86–8
  see also Culture
Cumulative incidence, definition, **B1**.310
Cunninghamella, **M**.20, **M**.660 (Tab.), **M**.663
  oculomycoses, **M**.287
    rhino-orbital-cerebral zygomycosis, **M**.290

Cunninghamella bertholletiae, **M**.663,
    M.664 (Fig.)
  infection, **M**.21, **M**.663, **M**.674–5
Cunninghamella elegans, **M**.663
Cured meat, pH, **B1**.272
Curli, **B1**.148–9
Curtis, F, **M**.16
Curtobacterium, **B2**.992
  biochemical characteristics, **B2**.993 (Tab.)
Curvularia
  allergic fungal sinusitis, **M**.675
  histopathology, **M**.89 (Tab.)
  infection
    CNS, **M**.743
    contact lens contamination, **M**.330–1
    keratitis, **M**.301–2, **M**.307–9, **M**.313,
      M.313 (Fig.), **M**.327–8
    oculomycoses, **M**.278 (Tab.), **M**.283–4,
      M.284 (Fig.)
Curvularia geniculata, **M**.89 (Tab.),
    M.128 (Tab.), **M**.139 (Fig.)
Curvularia lunata, **M**.89 (Tab.)
  contact lens contamination, **M**.330–1
  endophthalmitis, **M**.323
Cushing's disease, **M**.232
Cutaneous blastomycosis, **M**.488, **M**.489 (Fig.),
    M.492
Cutaneous candidiasis *see* Candidiasis,
    cutaneous/mucocutaneous
Cutaneous cryptococcosis, **M**.647–8
Cutaneous granulomas, pythiosis, **M**.418–19,
    M.419 (Fig.), **M**.421
Cutaneous hyalohyphomycosis, **M**.138 (Fig.)
Cutaneous invasive aspergillosis, **M**.701, **M**.719
Cutaneous leishmaniasis *see* Leishmaniasis,
    New World; Leishmaniasis, Old World
Cutaneous lymphocyte-associated antigen
    (CLA)
  lymphocyte migration, **I**.507, **I**.508 (Tab.)
  memory T cells, **I**.227
Cutaneous penicilliosis marneffei, **M**.567,
    M.567 (Fig.), **M**.569
Cutaneous T-cell attracting chemokine
    (CTACK:CCL27), **I**.218 (Tab.)
  CCR10 binding, **I**.227
Cuticles
  Ascaris lumbricoides, **P**.717
  Onchocerca volvulus, **P**.782
CX3C chemokines, **I**.217
  macrophage production, **I**.28–9
  receptors, **I**.510 (Tab.)
CX3CL1 (neurotacin:fractalkine), **I**.220
CXC3 chemokine receptor binding, Human
    respiratory syncytial virus glycoprotein
    (G), **V1**.786, **V1**.789
CXC chemokine receptors, **I**.220,
    I.510 (Tab.)
  cell expression, **I**.220
  CXCR1, **I**.223–4
    antagonists, **I**.230
    bacterial infection, **I**.227
    ligands, **I**.224
  CXCR2
    antagonists, **I**.230
    bacterial infection, **I**.227
    ligands, **I**.224
    neutrophils, **I**.223–4

CXCR3, **I**.510 (Tab.)
  inflammatory disease, **I**.227
  memory lymphocytes, **I**.225
  NK cells, **I**.224
  synthetic antagonists, **I**.231–2
  T cells, **I**.224
  Th1 cells, **I**.225
CXCR4, **I**.510 (Tab.)
  B cell homing, **I**.226
  cell expression, **I**.223–4
  HIV infection, **I**.227–8, **I**.584–5
  neutrophils, **I**.223–4
  synthetic antagonists, **I**.231
CXCR5, **I**.225–6, **I**.510 (Tab.)
  lymphoid tissue homing, **I**.226
  naive B cells, **I**.400
CXCR6, **I**.510 (Tab.)
  neutrophils, **I**.223–4
  phagocytes, **I**.223–4
CXC chemokines, **I**.217, **I**.218 (Tab.)
  basophil chemotaxis, **I**.58, **I**.60
  macrophages, **I**.28–9
  receptors *see above*
  structure, **I**.217–19
CXCL1 *see* GROα (CXCL1)
CXCL2 (GROβ), **I**.218 (Tab.)
CXCL3 (GROγ), **I**.218 (Tab.)
CXCL4, **I**.218 (Tab.)
CXCL5 (ENA-78), **I**.218 (Tab.)
  ELR motif, **I**.221
CXCL6 *see* Granulocyte chemoattractant
    protein 2 (GCP-2:CXCL6)
CXCL7 *see* Neutrophil-activating peptide-2
    (NAP-2:CXCL7)
CXCL8 *see* Interleukin-8 (IL-8)
CXCL9 (Mig), **I**.218 (Tab.)
CXCL10 *see* Interferon-inducible protein 10
    (IP-10:CXCL10)
CXCL11, **I**.218 (Tab.)
  granuloma formation, **I**.708
CXCL12 *see* Stromal-derived factor 1α
    (SDF-1α:CXCL12)
CXCL13 *see* B-cell-attracting chemokine
    (BCA-1:CXCL13)
CXCL14 (BRAK), **I**.218 (Tab.)
CXCL16, **I**.218 (Tab.)
CXCR1 *see* CXC chemokine receptors
CXCR2 *see* CXC chemokine receptors
CXCR3 *see* CXC chemokine receptors
CXCR4 *see* CXC chemokine receptors
CXCR4, HIV coreceptor, **V1**.106, **V1**.253,
    V2.1323
CXCR5 *see* CXC chemokine receptors
Cyanobacteria
  carbon cycling, **B1**.199
  foliar surface nutrient fixation, **B1**.198
  lichen formation, **B1**.201
  nitrogen fixation, **B1**.201
  oxygenic photosynthesis evolution, **B1**.195
  photosynthesis, **B1**.68
  phylogeny, **B1**.30–1
  substrate changes and colonization,
    B1.199–200
Cyclical reproductive pattern, *Onchocerca
    volvulus,* **P**.783

Cyclic AMP (cAMP)
  catabolite gene activator protein complex,
    B1.73
  role in catabolite repression, **B1**.73
Cyclic neutropenia, **I**.765
Cyclic phosphodiesterase
  coronaviruses, **V1**.832–3
  toroviruses, **V1**.832–3
Cyclic photosynthesis, **B1**.68
Cycling probe technology, **B1**.731–2,
  B1.734 (Fig.)
Cycloheximide, **M**.245
Cycloheximide, *Chlamydia* culture,
  B2.2017–18, **B2**.2017 (Fig.)
Cyclooxygenases (COX), **I**.186–7
  arachidonic acid production, **I**.181–4
  eosinophils, **I**.57
  neutrophil priming, **I**.44
  neutrophil production, **I**.46
  structures, **I**.186
  type 1 (COX1), **I**.186
  type 2 (COX2), **I**.186
    IL-17 effects, **I**.290
    selective inhibitors, **I**.186–7
Cyclopharynx, *Balantidium coli,* **P**.275–6
Cyclophilin A (CypA), HIV replication,
  V2.1324–5
Cyclophosphamide
  in Burkitt lymphoma (BL), **V1**.570
  immunodeficiency, **I**.788 (Tab.)
Cyclophyllidea, **P**.575–6, **P**.677
  Anoplocephalidae, **P**.577
  Davaineidae, **P**.577–8
  Dipylididae, **P**.578
  Hymenolepididae, **P**.578
  Mesocestoididae, **P**.578
  structure/life cycles, **P**.577–9
  Taeniidae, **P**.579
Cyclops, Dracunculus life cycle, **P**.830
Cycloserine, **B1**.481
Cyclospora, **P**.188
  classification, **P**.190–1
  infection *see* Cyclosporiasis
Cyclospora cayetanensis, **P**.188
  classification, **P**.414–15
  historical aspects, **P**.18, **P**.414
  infection *see* Cyclosporiasis
  life cycle, **P**.415
  morphology, **P**.416 (Fig.)
Cyclosporiasis, **P**.414–16
  in AIDS/HIV infection, **P**.45, **P**.97, **P**.414
    relapse, **P**.415–16
  chemotherapy, **P**.415–16
  clinical aspects, **P**.415
    diarrhea, **P**.415
  diagnosis, **P**.415
  epidemiology, **P**.415
    immunocompromised, **P**.415
    outbreaks, **P**.415
    travelers, **P**.415
  immune response, **P**.76
  pathology, **P**.415
  public health importance, **P**.44, **P**.45
Cyclosporin A
  aspergillosis, **M**.708

Aspergillus fumigatus, **M**.708
Cyclosporin A, cystic echinococcosis
  treatment, **P**.698–9
Cylindrocarpon
  histopathology, **M**.128 (Tab.)
  oculomycoses, **M**.275 (Tab.), **M**.283
Cylindrocarpon (Phialophora) cyanescens,
  M.238 (Fig.), **M**.391
Cymevene *see* Ganciclovir
CYP1A1 gene polymorphisms, **I**.587
Cypovirus, **V1**.47–8, **V2**.932
Cyprinoid fish, fluke intermediate hosts, **P**.646
Cys-scanning mutagenesis, LacY interactions,
  B1.49
Cystacanth, **P**.596
Cystatin
  Brugia malayi immune evasion, **I**.687
  helminths, **I**.687
  Onchocerca, **I**.687
Cysteine proteases
  Entamoeba histolytica, **P**.205
  liver/lung flukes, **P**.652
Cysteine, *Trypanosoma brucei in vitro*
  cultivation, **P**.358
Cysticercoids, **P**.576, **P**.577
Cysticercosis
  AIDS, **P**.691
  control, **P**.119, **P**.700–1
    animal reservoir hosts, **P**.119, **P**.119–20,
      P.122
    case management, **P**.119
    chemotherapy/chemoprophylaxis,
      P.144 (Tab.)
    diagnosis, **P**.143 (Tab.)
    health education, **P**.700–1
    individual treatment, **P**.119
    targeted treatment, **P**.700–1
    universal treatment, **P**.119
    vaccine/vaccination, **P**.691–2, **P**.700–1,
      I.855 (Tab.), **I**.874–5
  diagnosis, **P**.690
  epidemiology, **P**.699–700
    asymptomatic carriers, **P**.700
    control measure evaluations, **P**.700–1
  as erradicable disease, **P**.120
    International Task Force for Disease
      Eradication, **P**.120
  geographic distribution, **P**.677, **P**.699
  historical aspects, **P**.677–8
  immune evasion mechanisms, **P**.691
    immune-privileged sites, **P**.691
  immune response, **P**.95
    anti-antigen B (paramyosin) antibodies,
      P.689–90
    cellular immune response, **P**.690
  KETc antigens, **I**.874–5
  ocular, **P**.687–8
    diagnosis, **P**.692–3
    treatment, **P**.696
  poverty, **P**.119
  as public health problem, **P**.105 (Tab.), **P**.677
  treatment
    albendazole, **P**.697–8
    praziquantal, **P**.119–20, **P**.697–8
    steroids, **P**.697–8
  see also Neurocysticercosis

Cysticercus larva, **P**.579
  Taenia solium see Taenia solium
Cystic fibrosis, **B1**.623, **B1**.649–51
  allergic bronchopulmonary aspergillosis,
    M.693–4, **M**.712
  antibiotic use, **B1**.650–1
  aspergillosis, **M**.693–4, **M**.712
  clinical features, **B1**.650
  defensins, **I**.520–1
  gene therapy, **B1**.651
    animal models, **V2**.1600
    clinical trials, **V2**.1601
  infection, **B1**.650
    Burkolderia infection *see Burkholderia*
      cepacia complex
    organisms, **B1**.650
    Pseudomonas aeruginosa infection, **B1**.399,
      B1.650
    rapidly growing mycobacteria, **B2**.1250,
      B2.1252, **B2**.1256
    Staphylococcus aureus, **B1**.650
    Stenotrophomonas maltophilia infection,
      B2.1637
    therapy, **B1**.650–1
  lung transplantation, **B1**.651
  mucociliary clearance defects, **B1**.626,
    B1.650
Cystic fibrosis transmembrane conductance
  regulatory (CTFR) gene mutations,
  M.672
Cystitis
  acute, **B1**.673, **B1**.676, **B1**.678
    clinical features, **B1**.673
    treatment, **B1**.679
  Escherichia coli, uropathogenic adherence
    specificity, **B1**.147–8
  hemorrhagic, **V1**.444
Cystosomes, *Balantidium coli,* **P**.275–6
Cystoviridae
  classification, **V1**.27 (Tab.), **V1**.47 (Tab.),
    V1.48
  see also specific viruses
Cysts
  Balantidium coli, **P**.277, **P**.278 (Fig.),
    P.279 (Fig.)
  Blastocystis hominis, **P**.557, **P**.559,
    P.559 (Fig.), **P**.560–1
  Chilomastix mesnili, **P**.271 (Fig.)
  Endolimax nana, **P**.223, **P**.223 (Fig.)
  Entamoeba chattoni, **P**.223 (Fig.)
  Entamoeba coli, **P**.220 (Fig.)
  Entamoeba moshkovskii, **P**.222
  Entamoeba polecki, **P**.222 (Fig.)
  Iodamoeba bütschlii, **P**.223–4, **P**.224 (Fig.)
  Isospora belli, **P**.411–12
  Retortamonas intestinalis, **P**.271 (Fig.)
  walls
    composition, **P**.166
    protozoa, **P**.165–8, **P**.178–9
Cytidime-5′-monophospho-*N*-acetylneuraminic
  acid (CMP-NANA), **B2**.1288
Cytoadherence
  malaria pathology/pathophysiology, **P**.496–7
  Plasmodium, **P**.472, **P**.473–4
  Plasmodium falciparum, **P**.472, **P**.473–4
Cytochalasin D, microsporidians, **P**.550

Cytochalasin(s), LCMV entry, **V2**.1065

Cytochrome(s), **B1**.63

  chemotaxonomy, **B1**.24

Cytochrome *b, Pneumocystis jirovecii,* **M**.764, **M**.790–1, **M**.796

Cytochrome *c,* **B1**.64

  apoptosome assembly, **I**.135

  mitochondrial apoptosis, **I**.132, **I**.624

Cytochrome *d* oxidase, **B1**.64

Cytochrome oxidases, testing for presence of, **B1**.223

Cytochrome P450 14α-demethylase, *Candida* gene, **M**.608

Cytocidal infection, cell–virus interactions, **V1**.205

Cytoecetes microti, **B2**.2049–50

Cytofectins, DNA vaccines, **I**.913, **I**.917

Cytokine(s), **I.273–99, P.70–3, V1.292–310**

  actions

    antigen presentation, **I**.384

    basophil histamine release, **I**.62

    CD8 T cell activation, **I**.426, **I**.427–8

    dendritic cell stimulation, **I**.378

    HIV infection, **I**.791, **I**.797

    IgA synthesis, **I**.536–7, **I**.537 (Fig.)

    macrophage development, **I**.21–2

    monoclonal antibody blocking, **I**.357

    neutrophil priming, **I**.43

    Th1/Th2 differentiation, **I**.398, **I**.399

  as adjuvants, **I**.928 (Tab.)

    bare skin immunization, **I**.824

    HIV vaccines, **I**.832, **I**.871

    intranasal vaccines, **I**.832

  AIDS-dementia complex (ADC), **V1**.304

  anti-inflammatory, **I**.274 (Tab.), **I**.292–7

  classification, **I**.274 (Tab.)

  counter- inflammatory, **P**.72 (Tab.)

  definition, **P**.70

  destruction, **I**.686

  granuloma formation, **I**.707

    tuberculosis, **I**.713

  historical aspects/re-evaluation, **I**.10–11

  hormones *vs.,* **I**.273, **I**.274 (Fig.)

  immune response, **V1**.276

    innate immune response, **I**.403

    mucosal immune response, **I**.522–4, **I**.535–7

    regulation, **P**.72 (Fig.)

  induction, **V1**.293–8

    Burkholderia thailandensis, **B2**.1625–6

  in infection

    adenovirus immune evasion, **V2**.1596–7

    African trypanosomiasis, **P**.81 (Fig.)

    bacterial infection, **I**.651

      see also Immune evasion, bacteria

    Borna disease virus infection, **V2**.1149–50

    candidiasis, **M**.259–60, **M**.589–90

    CNS infection, **V1**.292–3, **V1**.303–4, **V2**.1409–10

    coronavirus infection, **V1**.840–1

    cryptococcosis therapy, **M**.652–3

    helminth homologues, **I**.687

    helminth infection, **P**.88

    hepatitis B, **V2**.1250

    HHV-6 infection, **V1**.530–2

    histoplasmosis capsulati, **M**.527–8

HTLV-1-associated myelopathy/tropical spastic paraparesis (HAM/TSP), **V2**.1429–30

  Human respiratory syncytial virus infection, **V1**.793–4

  malaria, **P**.490–1

    pathology/pathophysiology, **P**.496

  measles, **V1**.727

  in measles, **I**.806

  parasitic infection, **P**.70, **P**.72–3, **P**.72 (Tab.), **I**.679–80

  severe acute respiratory syndrome (SARS), **V1**.840–1

  viral infection, **I**.620

lymphoid cell growth factors, **I**.274 (Tab.), **I**.279–84

myeloid cell growth factors, **I**.273–9, **I**.274 (Tab.)

  paracrine *vs.* autocrine, **I**.273

  production, **P**.70–2, **P**.72 (Tab.)

    basophils, **I**.59 (Tab.), **I**.399

    CD1d-reactive αβ T cells, **I**.442

    CD4 T cells, **I**.395

    CpG adjuvant, **I**.931

    dendritic cells, **I**.28 (Tab.)

    eosinophils, **I**.59 (Tab.)

    intraepithelial lymphocytes, **I**.527

    macrophages, **I**.27–8, **V1**.272–3, **I**.378, **B1**.624

    mast cells, **I**.399

    monophosphoryl lipid adjuvant, **I**.929

    NK cells, **I**.81–2, **V1**.271–2

    prostaglandin E$_2$ effects, **I**.188

    superantigen stimulation, **I**.561

    T cells, **P**.68, **P**.70–3

    TLR stimulus, **I**.697

  proinflammatory *see* Proinflammatory cytokines

  receptors

    eosinophils, **I**.64

    NK cells, **V1**.272

    type 2 family, **I**.256

    viral analogues, **V1**.229–30

  recombinant virus use, **V1**.304–5

  regulatory, **I**.274 (Tab.), **I**.292–7

  skin, **I**.820

  thrombocyte growth factors, **I**.273–9, **I**.274 (Tab.)

  upregulation, DNA vaccines, **I**.896

  see also individual types; specific cytokines; specific types

'Cytokine model,' HHV-8 pathogenesis, **V1**.554–5

Cytolethal distending toxin (CDT), **I**.655

  Campylobacter, **B2**.1551

Cytolysins, **I**.654

Cytolysis, **V1**.345

Cytomegalic inclusion disease (CID), HCMV infection, **V1**.521

  congenital, **V2**.1449

Cytomegalovirus (CMV) *see* Human cytomegalovirus (HCMV)

Cytomeres, uninuclear, **P**.184 (Fig.), **P**.185

Cytopathic effect (CPE), **V1**.87, **V1**.93–4, **V1**.94 (Fig.)

  absence, hepatitis A, **V2**.1166–7

  arboviruses, **V1**.95

  cell culture, **V2**.1539–40

Cytopathic inhibition assay, interferon-α, **I**.238

Cytopathology, **V2**.1533–4, **V2**.1534 (Tab.)

  HCMV infection diagnosis, **V2**.1534 (Tab.)

  HPV infection diagnosis, **V2**.1533–4, **V2**.1534 (Tab.)

  HSV infection diagnosis, **V2**.1534 (Tab.)

  measles diagnosis, **V2**.1534 (Tab.)

  Molluscum contagiosum virus infection diagnosis, **V2**.1534 (Tab.)

  parainfluenza virus infection diagnosis, **V2**.1534 (Tab.)

  Respiratory syncytial virus infection diagnosis, **V2**.1534 (Tab.)

  stains, **V2**.1533

  VZV infection diagnosis, **V2**.1534 (Tab.)

Cytophaga, **B2**.1930

Cytoplasm

  composition, **B1**.45–6

  protozoa, **P**.169–72

Cytoplasmic domains, FcγRII (CD32), **I**.314

Cytoplasmic membrane

  composition, **B1**.44–5

  electric potential across, **B1**.64

  transport of solutes into *see* Transport

Cytopyge, **P**.164

  Balantidium coli, **P**.277 (Fig.)

Cytorhabdovirus, **V2**.1104–5

  characteristics, **V1**.129 (Tab.)

  classification, **V1**.385

  genome structure, **V1**.387 (Tab.), **V2**.1112 (Fig.)

  members, **V1**.385–6

Cytoskeleton, **M**.70–1, **P**.169–70

  actin, **I**.37

  apoptosis, **I**.136

  cell–virus interactions, **V1**.202–3

  microfilaments, **I**.37–8

  microtubules, **I**.37–8

  neutrophil recruitment, **I**.37–8

  respirovirus interactions, **V1**.774

  Trypanosoma brucei, **P**.356 (Fig.)

Cytospinning (shell vials), **V2**.1540–1

Cytostomes, **P**.162

  definition, **P**.164

  structure, **P**.164, **P**.166 (Fig.)

Cytotonic enterotoxins, *Aeromonas* pathogenicity, **B2**.1536

Cytotoxic granules *see* Cytotoxic T cell(s) (CTLs); Lymphocyte-mediated cytotoxicity; Natural killer (NK) cells

Cytotoxicity assays, NK cells, **I**.82

Cytotoxic T cell(s) (CTLs), **P**.68

  activation, perforin, **I**.478

  chemokine receptors, **I**.225

  common mucosal immune system, **I**.534

  cytotoxic granules, **I**.474–7

    Fas ligand, **I**.477

    see also Fas ligand (Fas-L)

    granulysin, **I**.477

    granzymes *see* Granzyme(s)

    killing mechanisms, **I**.479 (Fig.)

    perforin *see* Perforin

    serglycine, **I**.475

  IFN-γ production, **I**.478

  infection

    adenovirus infection, **V1**.445–6

Cytotoxic T cell(s) (CTLs)
  infection (*Continued*)
    candidiasis, **M**.261
    malaria, **P**.82, **P**.490
    oropharyngeal candidiasis, **M**.263
    parasitic infection, **P**.68–9
    picornavirus infection, **V1**.283
  intraepithelial lymphocytes, **I**.525–6
  killing mechanisms, **I**.479 (Fig.)
    adhesion ring, **I**.474, **I**.474 (Fig.)
    binding, **I**.472
    lymphocyte-mediated cytotoxicity 1, **I**.474
  knockout mice, babesiosis, **P**.456
  LCMV infection, **V2**.1072
    CNS pathology, **V2**.1073–4
    immunopathology, **V2**.1073
    immunosuppression, **V2**.1075
  live virus vaccine response, **I**.902
  localization of viral pathology and, **V1**.248
  memory cells, **I**.471
  morphology and function, **I**.472–3,
    I.473 (Fig.), **I**.474 (Fig.)
  perforin deficiency, **I**.480–1
  priming, DNA vaccines, **I**.896
  responses, virosome vaccines, **I**.838
  TCR, **I**.474
  see also CD8+ T-cell(s)
Cytovene see Ganciclovir
Czapek Dox agar, **M**.662

D1R/D12L capping enzyme, poxviruses,
  V1.610–11
D1R gene, poxvirus mRNA capping, **V1**.609
D4 protein, poxvirus replication, **V1**.169 (Tab.)
D5 protein, poxvirus replication, **V1**.168–9,
  V1.169 (Tab.)
D12L gene, poxvirus mRNA capping, **V1**.609
Dacliuzumab, **I**.333
Dacryoadenitis, **M**.299
Dacryocanaliculitis, **M**.298
  causative agents, **M**.298
  therapy, **M**.298
Dacryocystitis, **M**.298–9
  causative agents, **M**.298, **M**.299
Dahi (Indian yogurt), **B1**.249
Dairy farming, prototothecosis, **M**.396–7,
  M.399–400
Dairy products, **B1**.229–62
  Bacillus spoilage, **B2**.923–4
  Brucella melitensis infection, **B2**.1722
  human brucellosis, **B2**.1722
  Propionibacterium, **B2**.1030–1
  see also individual products; individual
    species
Dakar bat virus (DBV), **V2**.997–9,
  V2.998 (Tab.)
Dalfopristin, **B1**.489
  spectrum of activity, **B1**.499 (Tab.)
  structure, **B1**.489 (Fig.)
Damped oscillations, infection models, **I**.956
Danazol, **V2**.1290
Dandruff (pityriasis capitis), **M**.14–5
  seborrheic dermatitis, **M**.211–12
Dapaong tumor, **P**.811–12, **P**.812 (Fig.)

Dapsone
  leprosy therapy, **B2**.1203, **B2**.1219–20
  Mycobacterium leprae, **M**.454
  resistance, **B2**.1220
  rhinosporidiosis, **M**.454, **M**.471–2
  structure, **B1**.490 (Fig.)
  toxoplasmosis, **P**.437, **P**.438–9
Dark-field microscopy, **B1**.714
  Borrelia morphology, **B2**.1819
Dark, firm and dry (DFD) meat, **B1**.272
Dark repair, repair of UV-induced DNA
  damage, **B1**.451–2
Darling, S T A, **M**.22 (Fig.), **M**.23
'Darmbrand' (enteritis necroticans),
  B2.1118–19
Data analysis
  nosocomial infection surveillance, **B1**.405
  outbreak investigation, **B1**.327–8
Data-collection systems, **B1**.318–22,
  B1.321 (Tab.)
  active, **B1**.318–19
  general practice reporting, **B1**.320
  hospital data, **B1**.321
  laboratory reporting system, **B1**.319–20
  miscellaneous, **B1**.322
  mortality data, **B1**.319
  outbreak investigation, **B1**.327–8
  passive, **B1**.318, **B1**.325
  routine, **B1**.321 (Tab.)
    vaccine efficacy studies, **B1**.324–5
  routine serological surveillance, **B1**.321–2
  sexually transmitted diseases, **B1**.320–1
  statutory notification, **B1**.319
Davaineidae, **P**.577–8
Day care centers
  airborne bacteria, **B1**.186 (Tab.)
  emerging viral infection, **V2**.1659
DC-CK1 (CCL18), **I**.218 (Tab.)
DC-SIGN
  HIV infection, **I**.794
  microbial recognition, **I**.24 (Tab.)
DDT
  malaria control, **P**.517
  resistance, mosquitoes, **P**.126
Deafness
  congenitally acquired rubella, **V2**.973–4
  mumps, **V1**.750
Deaminases, **B2**.1435
Deaminating agents, mutagens, **V1**.183
Death certificates, **B1**.319, **B1**.321 (Tab.)
Death domain (DD), caspases, **I**.134
Death effect or domain (DED), caspases, **I**.134
Death-inducing signal complex (DISC)
  apoptosis, **I**.623–4
  assembly, **I**.134
  caspase-8 activation, **I**.134
Death-receptor inhibitors, virus infection,
  I.625 (Fig.), **I**.626–7
Death receptors, apoptosis induction, **I**.131,
  I.623–4
Decay-accelerating factor (DAF), **B1**.148–9,
  I.150 (Tab.), **I**.151
  deficiency, **I**.154
  diffusely adhering *Escherichia coli* receptor
    usage, **B1**.148–9
Decompensated cirrhosis, hepatitis B, **V2**.1248

Decontamination
  digestive tract, **B1**.390
  hands, **B1**.378
  hepatitis B/C and HIV, **B1**.383
  hospital equipment, **B1**.380
Decoy proteins, apoptosis, **I**.135
'Decreasing potential' hypothesis, memory T
  cell persistence, **I**.495, **I**.496 (Fig.)
Dectin-1, **I**.24 (Tab.)
Deep dermatophytic granulomas,
  Microsporum canis, **M**.138 (Fig.)
Defective interfering particles, **V1**.186–7
  persistent infection, **V1**.186–7
  physical particle:plaque-forming unit rations,
    V1.204
  rhabdoviruses, **V2**.1103
  Rubella virus, **V2**.964
  subacute sclerosing panencephalitis (SSPE),
    V1.186–7
  Vesicular stomatitis virus, **V1**.186
Defective ribosomal products (DRP), **I**.410
Defensin(s), **I**.166–71, **I**.520–1
  α_2-macroglobulin binding, **I**.168
  adenovirus infection, **V1**.445
  adrenocorticotrophic hormone antagonism,
    I.169–70
  antiviral properties, **I**.168
  aspergillosis, **M**.708
  biosynthesis, **I**.170
  calcium channel activation, **I**.170
  in chemotaxis, **I**.169
  cystic fibrosis, **I**.520–1
  evolution, **I**.166–7
  expression, **I**.167–8, **I**.520
    cell types, **I**.168
    neutrophils, **I**.40–1
    species differences, **I**.167
  induction, **I**.520–1
  inflammation, **I**.520–1
  mechanism of action, **I**.168–9, **I**.520–1
  microbial resistance, **I**.169
    Brucella, **I**.168
    Burkholderia, **I**.168
  monocyte chemotaxis, **I**.169
  Paneth cells, **I**.168
  skin keratinocytes, **I**.168
  storage/delivery, **I**.167, **I**.170–1
  structure, **I**.166, **I**.167 (Fig.), **I**.170–1, **I**.520
    β-sheet, **I**.166
    function relationship, **I**.171
    nonhuman, **I**.166, **I**.167 (Fig.)
α-Defensins, **I**.520
  anti-HIV properties, **I**.168
  biosynthesis, **I**.170, **I**.171 (Fig.)
    matrix metalloproteinase-7, **I**.170
  evolution, **I**.166–7
  species differences, **I**.167
    mice, **I**.168
  storage/secretion, **I**.170
    Paneth cells, **I**.168
  structure, **I**.166 (Fig.), **I**.167 (Fig.)
β-Defensins, **I**.520
  biosynthesis, **I**.171 (Fig.)
  evolution, **I**.166–7
  expression, **I**.520

β-Defensins (*Continued*)
  skin keratinocytes, **I**.168
  species differences, **I**.167
    mice, **I**.168
    snake venom, **I**.166
  storage/secretion, **I**.170–1
  structure, **I**.166 (Fig.), **I**.167 (Fig.)
θ-Defensins
  biosynthesis, **I**.167 (Fig.)
  discovery, **I**.166
  evolution, **I**.167
  structure, **I**.167 (Fig.)
Definitive hosts
  Echinococcus, **P**.684
  Echinococcus granulosus, **P**.119
  Echinococcus multilocularis, **P**.119, **P**.684
  Echinococcus vogeli, **P**.684–5
  liver flukes, **P**.645–6
  lung flukes, **P**.645–6
  Taenia solium, **P**.684
Deforestation, malaria epidemiology, **P**.34,
  P.512–13
Deformin, *Bartonella bacilliformis,* **B2**.1891
Dehydration of foods
  milk powder, **B1**.245–8
  rice, **B1**.285–6
  wheat, **B1**.284
Dehydroacetic acid, pH, **B1**.432
Deinococcus radiodurans
  chromosomes, **B1**.46
  sterilization
    ionizing radiation, **B1**.451
    moist heat, **B1**.448
    ultraviolet radiation, **B1**.451
    unsuitability as a BI, **B1**.454
Delavirdine, **V2**.1622–3
  HIV infection, **V2**.1336
  resistance, **V2**.1623
  structure, **V2**.1622 (Fig.)
Delayed-type hypersensitivity (DTH), **I**.375–6,
  I.705–29
  cell-mediated immunity *vs.,* **I**.724–5
  definition, **I**.705
  disease pathology, **I**.709–10
    Koch phenomenon, **I**.709–10
    organ function effects, **I**.709
  granulomatous inflammation, **I**.706–9,
    I.707 (Fig.)
    amplification, **I**.707–8
    Th1 cells *see* T-helper cells type 1 (Th1)
    Th1/Th2 cell balance, **I**.706, **I**.708–9
    see also Granuloma(s)
  histoplasmin, **M**.529
  infection
    candidiasis, **M**.261
    cutaneous leishmaniasis, **P**.299
    histoplasmosis capsulati, **M**.527, **M**.529
    leishmaniasis, **P**.78
    measles, **V1**.727–9, **I**.804
    Old World leishmaniasis, **P**.302
    trichomoniasis, **P**.259
  skin reaction, **I**.706 (Fig.)
  T-cell-mediated immunopathology, **V1**.280
Delbrück, Max, **V1**.25
D elements, TCR, **I**.450–1

Deletion mutants, genetic analysis, **V1**.184
Delftia (Comamonas) acidovorans, **B2**.1635–6
  waterborne, **B1**.224–5
Delta antigen
  filoviruses, **V2**.1091
  Hepatitis delta virus, **V2**.1270
DELTA Computer System, **V1**.35
ΔTas virus, foamy viruses, **V2**.1309, **V2**.1313
Deltaretrovirus
  classification, **V1**.46, **V2**.1286 (Tab.)
  human disease, **V2**.1285
Deltaretroviruses
  characteristics, **V2**.1284
  transformation, **V1**.336
  tumors associated, **V1**.331 (Tab.)
DELTA study, **V2**.1334
Deltavirus
  characteristics, **V1**.129 (Tab.)
  classification, **V1**.27 (Tab.), **V1**.48, **V1**.127–8,
    V2.1269
Dematiaceae, **M**.359
Demecolcine, microsporidians, **P**.550
Dementia
  in progressive multifocal
    leucoencephalopathy (PML), **V2**.1417
  Whipple's disease, **B2**.999
Demography
  emerging bacterial infection, **B1**.359–60
  global population estimates, **B1**.360 (Fig.)
DeMonbreun, W A, **M**.23
Demyelination
  multiple sclerosis, **I**.757
  progressive multifocal leucoencephalopathy
    (JC virus infection), **V2**.1417,
    V2.1417 (Fig.)
  progressive multifocal leucoencephalopathy
    (PML), **V1**.477
Dendritic cells (DCs), **V1**.273, **I**.656
  activation, **I**.393–4, **I**.394 (Tab.)
    adjuvants, **I**.926
    cytokine stimulation, **I**.378
    ELC, **I**.393–4
    flagellins, **I**.393–4
    IL-1, **I**.393–4
    IL-6, **I**.393–4
    LPS, **I**.393–4
    TLRs, **I**.393–4
    TNF-α, **I**.393–4
  airway hypersensitivity, **I**.736–7
  as APCs, **I**.29, **I**.112, **I**.376, **I**.656, **I**.903
    CD1a/b/c-reactive αβ T cells interactions,
      I.442
    CD4 T cells, **I**.392, **I**.393
      see also CD4+ T-cell(s)
    CD8 T-cells, **I**.404
    crosspresentation, **I**.630–1, **I**.631 (Fig.)
    MHC class I antigen presentation, **I**.630–1
    T cells, **I**.378
    Th1 cells, **I**.903
  bacterial infection, **I**.656
    immune interference, **I**.656, **I**.667–8
  biological activity, **I**.630–1
  candidiasis, **M**.260
  CD1 expression, **I**.442

chemokine receptors, **I**.224, **I**.377–8, **I**.393–4
  CCR1, **I**.224, **I**.393–4
  CCR2, **I**.224, **I**.393–4
  CCR3, **I**.224
  CCR5, **I**.224, **I**.393–4
  CCR6, **I**.393–4
  CCR7, **I**.393–4
chemotaxis, defensins, **I**.169
CpG binding/signal transduction, **I**.911, **I**.931
cytokines produced, **I**.28 (Tab.)
  IL-12, **I**.288–9
  IL-18, **I**.290
  INFs, **I**.123
  Th1/Th2 differentiation, **I**.399
development, **I**.22, **I**.113, **I**.113 (Fig.),
  I.377–8, **I**.393 (Fig.)
  IL-10, **I**.750
DNA vaccines, **I**.914–16
  bare skin routes, **I**.825
  intradermal delivery, **I**.912–13
Fas-mediated apoptosis, **I**.903
functions, **I**.22
historical aspects/re-evaluation, **I**.8
immune evasion, **V1**.323
mobilization, **I**.377–8
mucosal immune response, **I**.538
  nasal-associated lymphoid tissue, **I**.533
pattern-recognition receptors, **I**.750–1
peripheral tolerance, **I**.750–1, **I**.750 (Fig.)
Peyer's patches, **I**.538
stratified epithelium, **I**.827
in thymus, **I**.377–8
TLRs, **I**.750–1
tolerance induction, **I**.737
vaccines
  DNA vaccines *see above*
  live vaccines, **I**.903
  TCE peptide vaccines, **I**.879
viral infection
  HIV infection, **I**.794
  HSV infection, **V1**.284
  measles, **V1**.727, **V1**.728 (Fig.), **I**.805
  viral immune interference, **I**.630–2,
    I.632 (Fig.)
Dendritic cell (DC)-specific intracellular
  adhesion molecule-3 grabbing
  nonintegrin (SIGN), **B2**.1184
Dendritic epidermal γδ T cells *see* γδ T-cells
Dendrograms, **B1**.27–8, **B1**.27 (Fig.)
Dengue fever, **V2**.1000–1
  chikungunya *vs.,* **V2**.1021–2
  clinical signs, **V1**.372–3
  emerging infection, **I**.6, **V2**.1663
  epidemiology, **V1**.372–3
  IL-6, **V1**.297
  immunogenetics, **I**.588
  immunopathology, **V1**.279 (Tab.)
  medical importance, **V1**.372–3
  TNF-α induction, **V1**.296
  transmission, **V1**.372 (Tab.)
  vaccines, **I**.899, **I**.933 (Tab.)
Dengue hemorrhagic fever (DHF), **V1**.372–3,
  V2.1000–1
  immunopathology, **V2**.999

Dengue shock syndrome (DSS), **V1**.372–3
immunopathology, **V2**.999
Dengue virus, **V2**.998 (Tab.), **V2**.1000–1
cell receptors, **V1**.211
emerging infection, **V2**.1648 (Tab.)
epidemiology, **V2**.997
laboratory-acquired infection, **V2**.1517,
V2.1517 (Tab.)
molecular epidemiology, **V1**.198
viremia, **V1**.242
virion structure, **V2**.993
Denitrification, **B1**.65, **B1**.66
environmental problem, **B1**.200
Dense bodies, **P**.178
Densoviridae
classification, **V1**.41 (Tab.), **V1**.408–9,
V1.409 (Tab.)
see also specific viruses
Densovirinae, **V1**.42
Densovirus
classification, **V1**.42
genome structure, **V1**.413–14
Dental caries, *Veillonella*, **B2**.1314
Dental (odontogenic) infection, intracranial
abscess complication, **B1**.582–3,
B1.584 (Tab.)
Dental plaque, **B1**.294–5
Fusobacterium, **B2**.1950
gram-positive anaerobic cocci, **B2**.910
Leptotrichia, **B2**.1952
normal microbiota, **B1**.609 (Tab.)
pathogen-related oral spirochetes,
B2.1859–60
Dentistry
endocarditis after, **B1**.527
HIV transmission, **B1**.382
Dentists, Hepatitis B virus status, **V2**.1256
Denture stomatitis, **M**.598
Deoxyribonuclease production, **B2**.1351
Deoxyuridine triphosphatase (dUTPase)
herpesviruses, **V1**.500
HSV type 1 (HSV-1), **V1**.500
Department of Environment, Food and Rural
Affairs (DEFRA), **B1**.330
viricides, regulations for veterinary use,
B1.434
Dependovirus, **V1**.409–10
classification, **V1**.157, **V1**.410
gene therapy vectors, **V1**.428–9
gene transcription, **V1**.414 (Fig.)
genome structure, **V1**.409–10, **V1**.414 (Fig.),
V1.415
inverted terminal repeats, **V1**.409–10
Rep68 proteins, **V1**.415
Rep78 proteins, **V1**.415
infection *see Dependovirus* infection
members, **V1**.411 (Tab.)
see also Adeno-associated viruses (AAV);
Dependoviruses
Dependoviruses, **V1**.440, **V1**.441 (Fig.)
infection *see Dependovirus* infection
see also Dependovirus
Dependovirus infection, **V1**.427–9
epidemiology, **V1**.427–8
pathogenesis, **V1**.428

Depigmentation
onchocerciasis, **P**.793, **P**.794 (Fig.)
post kala-azar leishmaniasis, **P**.298
Depot effects, **I**.926
MF59 adjuvant, **I**.927
Dequalinium chloride, **B1**.428
Dermabacter, **B2**.991
chemotaxonomic characteristics,
B2.978 (Tab.)
identification, **B2**.979
Dermabacter hominis, **B1**.296 (Tab.), **B2**.991
biochemical characteristics, **B2**.993 (Tab.)
disease associations, **B2**.981 (Tab.)
habitats, **B2**.977–8
Dermacentor andersoni, **B2**.1753
Dermacentor, *Rickettsia* transmission,
B2.2037–8
Dermacoccus nishinomiyaensis, **B1**.296 (Tab.),
B1.304
Dermatitis
atopic *see* Atopic dermatitis
cercarial, **P**.582
dermatophytic pseudomycetoma, **M**.232,
M.238
seborrheic, **M**.14–5, **M**.18 (Fig.)
topical corticosteroids, **M**.185
Dermatomycoses, **M.244–54**
amorofine therapy, **M**.252
causative agents, **M**.248–52
therapy, **M**.252–3
fluconazole, **M**.253
Dermatomycotic molds, **M.244–54**
onychomycosis, **M**.244–6
Aphanoascus fulvescens, **M**.247
clinical features, **M**.244–5
diagnosis, **M**.245
etiology, **M**.245–6
Onychocola canadensis, **M**.247
Scytalidium, **M**.246–7
specific fungi, **M**.248–52
therapy, **M**.252–3
otitis externa, **M**.247–8
Dermatophilosis, **B2**.1150–1
Dermatophilus, **B2**.1137–8, **B2**.1150–1
diaminopimelic acid and sugars, **B2**.1145
Dermatophilus chelonae, **B2**.1150–1
Dermatophilus congolensis, **B2**.1150–1
Dermatophytes, **M**.220–1, **M**.244
anamorphs, **M**.45–6, **M**.221 (Tab.)
anthropophilic infectious fungi, **M**.223,
M.227–8, **M**.227 (Tab.)
classification, **M**.10, **M**.45–6, **M**.61, **M**.220,
M.221, **M**.227 (Tab.), **M**.229–31
anthropophilic, **M**.45–6, **M**.223, **M**.225,
M.227–8, **M**.227 (Tab.)
geophilic, **M**.45–6, **M**.222–3, **M**.223,
M.227 (Tab.)
zoophilic, **M**.45–6, **M**.223, **M**.225, **M**.227,
M.227 (Tab.), **M**.239
ecology, **M**.222–5, **M**.227 (Tab.)
evolution, **M**.45–6, **M**.223
geographical distribution, **M**.228–9,
M.229 (Tab.)
granule formation, **M**.385–6, **M**.392, **M**.394
griseofulvin resistance, **M**.177

history, **M**.4, **M**.5, **M**.9, **M**.10, **M**.10 (Fig.),
M.220–1
identification, **M**.221, **M**.235–8
culture, **M**.10, **M**.91 (Tab.), **M**.236
histopathology, **M**.89 (Tab.), **M**.128 (Tab.),
M.238
microscopic examination, **M**.235
physiological tests, **M**.237
specimen site selection, **M**.83 (Tab.),
M.238
immune response, **M**.232–3
infection *see* Dermatophytoses
molecular taxonomy, **M**.229–31
morphology, **M**.223
microscopic, **M**.236
phylogeny, **M**.229–31
teleomorphs, **M**.10, **M**.45–6, **M**.77, **M**.78–9,
M.221, **M**.221 (Tab.)
transmission, **M**.222–3, **M**.225, **M**.227, **M**.238
Dermatophyte test medium (DTM), **M**.33–4,
M.236
Dermatophytoses, **M**.221, **M**.238
causative agents, **M**.221–2, **M**.222 (Tab.),
M.224 (Tab.), **M**.226 (Tab.)
see also individual species
clinical presentation, **M**.231–2
epidemiology, **M**.225–8
hair, **M**.221, **M**.238
histopathology, **M**.89 (Tab.), **M**.128 (Tab.),
M.138 (Fig.), **M**.238
history, **M**.10
immune response, **M**.232–3
inflammatory response, **M**.232–3
nomenclature, **M**.228–9
oculomycoses
blepharitis, **M**.297
dacryocanaliculitis, **M**.298
dacryocystitis, **M**.298
prevention, **M**.186, **M**.187, **M**.188, **M**.238–9
pseudomycetoma, **M**.232, **M**.238
dermatitis, **M**.232, **M**.238
spread, **M**.222–3, **M**.225, **M**.238
susceptibility to, **M**.232
therapy, **M**.11, **M**.186, **M**.233–5
allylamines/butenafine, **M**.184
azoles, **M**.182–3, **M**.183 (Tab.)
ciclopirox, **M**.184–5
griseofulvin, **M**.11, **M**.184
tolnaftate, **M**.185
travelers, **M**.228–9
see also specific infection
Dermatotolymphangitis, acute, lymphatic
filariasis, **P**.773
Dermis, anatomy, **I**.820
Dermonecrotic toxin (DNT), *Bordetella*,
B2.1789 (Tab.), **B2**.1795–6
Dermosporidium, **M**.456–7
Descriptive analysis, epidemiological,
B1.311–12
Desferrioxamine, **M**.13, **M**.21, **M**.672–3, **M**.675
Plasmodium inhibition, **P**.478
Desmosomes, **P**.179–80
'Destruens equi,' **M**.412
Desulfitobacterium dehalogenans, **B1**.67
Desulfomonas, **B1**.201
Desulfomonas pigra, **B1**.296 (Tab.)

Desulfotomaculum, **B1**.201

Desulfotomaculum nigrificans, canning process, **B1**.283

Desulfovibrio, **B1**.66, **B1**.201

Desulfovibrio desulfuricans, **B1**.66

Detergents, virus inactivation, **V1**.91

Deterministic models, **B1**.344

Deuteromycetes (Fungi Imperfecti), **M**.49, **M**.51

Deuteromycotina (Deuteromycetes), **M**.359, **M**.371–2

Developed countries
  Blastocystis hominis, **P**.566
  cryptosporidiosis, **P**.409

Developing countries
  Blastocystis hominis, **P**.566
  campylobacter enteritis, **B2**.1550
  Chlamydia pneumoniae infection, **B2**.2015
  cholera, **B2**.1508–9
  cryptosporidiosis, **P**.409
  rubella epidemiology, **V2**.970–1
  shigellosis, **B2**.1387–8

Development projects, epidemics, **P**.117

Dexamethasone, endophthalmitis, **M**.320

DFMO (difluormethylornithine: eflornithine: Ornidyl) *see* Eflornithine (difluormethylornithine: DFMO: Ornidyl)

d'Herelle, F H, **B1**.9

dhfr gene, drug resistance, **P**.480

dhfr-ts gene, pyrimethamine resistance, **P**.480

dhps gene, drug resistance, **P**.480

Diabetes mellitus, **M**.11, **M**.232
  aspergillosis, **M**.694–5
  Burkholderia thailandensis infection, **B2**.1626
  congenitally acquired rubella, **V2**.975
  Coxsackie virus association, **V1**.283, **V2**.872
  development, IL-4 therapy, **I**.280–1
  diabetic foot ulcers *see* Osteomyelitis
  enterovirus infection association, **V2**.872
  immunodeficiency, **I**.788 (Tab.)
  melioidosis, **B2**.1629
  NK cells, **I**.103
  systemic zygomycosis, **M**.674–5, **M**.677–8
  urinary tract infection, **B1**.673, **B1**.679
  zygomycosis, **M**.20–1

Diabetes mellitus type I
  etiology, **I**.758
  genetics
    CTLA-4 gene, **I**.752
    HLA-DQ association, **I**.577, **I**.752, **I**.758
    HLA-DR association, **I**.577, **I**.752, **I**.752 (Tab.)
  IL-18, **I**.290–2
  NOD mouse model, **I**.758
  pathogen induced, **I**.753 (Tab.)
  prevalence, **I**.748 (Tab.)
  Th1/Th2 balance, **I**.755–6

Diagnosis
  bacterial infection, **B1**.711, **B1**.712–20
  fungal infection, **M**.82–96
    methods of identification, **M**.87–91, **M**.88 (Tab.), **M**.89 (Tab.)
    microscopic examination, **M**.87
    see also individual species

parasitic infection, **P**.148–55
  biopsy *see* Biopsy
  blood *see* Serology/serological diagnosis
  endemic areas, **P**.149
  immunological diagnosis *see* Immunoassays
  life cycle effects, **P**.148–9
  molecular diagnostics, **P**.154
    see also individual methods
  natural history effects, **P**.148–9
  non-endemic areas, **P**.149
  parasite control *see* Control of infection, parasitic disease
  public health effects, **P**.149–50
  research, **P**.150
  resource effects, **P**.149
    economics, **P**.149
    technology, **P**.149
  specimens, **P**.150–3
  stool samples *see* Fecal analysis
  urogenital samples, **P**.152
    culture, **P**.152
    macroscopic examination, **P**.152
    microscopic examination, **P**.152
  see also specific infection

viral infection, **V2**.1532–50
  infectivity, **V2**.1539–41
    animal inoculation, **V2**.1539
    embryonated eggs, **V2**.1539
  interpretation, **V2**.1548
    serology, **V2**.1547 (Tab.), **V2**.1548
  principles, **V2**.1532–3
  quality assurance/control, **V2**.1547–8
  specimens, **V2**.1533
  viral identification, **V1**.34
  virion detection, **V2**.1533–9
    nucleic acids, **V2**.1535–9
    viral antigens, **V2**.1535
  see also Characterization (of viruses); *specific assays/tests; specific infection; specific viruses*
  see also Immunoserology; Serology/serological diagnosis; *individual species; specific assays*

Diagnostic puncture, alveolar echinococcosis diagnosis, **P**.694

Dialister (Bacteroides), **B2**.1913–14

Dialister (Bacteroides) pneumosintes, **B2**.1913–14, **B2**.1929–30

Dialysis centers, hepatitis B transmission, **V2**.1256–7

Diamidines, **B1**.423 (Tab.), **B1**.426
  Old World leishmaniasis, **P**.306–7

Diaminodiphenylsulfone *see* Dapsone

Diaminopimelic acid (DAP), **B2**.1948, **B2**.1953
  Actinomycetes, aerobic, **B2**.1145
  Clostridium, **B2**.1092

Diaminopyrimidines, **B1**.491–2
  mode of action, **B1**.492
    dihydrofolate reductase inhibition, **B1**.492
  pharmacology, **B1**.492
  resistance, **B1**.492
  spectrum of activity, **B1**.491
  structure, **B1**.491
  toxicity/adverse effects, **B1**.492
  see also specific types

Diapedesis, **I**.503, **I**.512–13
  CD99, **I**.512–13
  definition, **I**.505
  high endothelial venules, **I**.503
  neutrophils, **I**.37, **I**.38
  platelet endothelial cell adhesion molecule-1, **I**.38
  VE-cadherin, **I**.512–13
  see also Lymphocyte(s), migration/homing

Diarrhea
  adenovirus infection, **V1**.444
  Balantidium coli infection, **P**.279
  bloody, **B2**.1377, **B2**.1378–9
  bloody, amebic dysentery, **P**.207
  causative organisms
    Arcobacter, **B2**.1557
    Campylobacter, **B2**.1550
    Clostridium perfringens, **B2**.1117–19
    Escherichia coli, diffusely adherent, **B2**.1379
    Escherichia coli, enteroaggregative, **B2**.1378–9
    Escherichia coli, enteropathogenic, **B2**.1373–4
    Escherichia coli, enterotoxigenic, **B2**.1375
    Escherichia coli, vero-cytotoxic-producing, **B2**.1377
    Providencia alcalifaciens, **B2**.1451
    Salmonella, **B2**.1426
    Shigella, **B2**.1387
  child care centers, **B1**.361
  cryptosporidiosis, **P**.404–5, **P**.408
  cyclosporiasis, **P**.415
  giardiasis, **P**.245–7
  infantile, **B2**.1373–5, **B2**.1378–9
  microsporidiosis, **P**.537
  morbidity, **P**.26 (Fig.)
  mortality, **P**.26 (Fig.), **P**.28 (Tab.), **P**.29 (Tab.)
  Prototheca, **M**.398–9
  salmonellosis, **B2**.1426
  self-limiting, isosporiasis, **P**.412
  watery, **B2**.1387

Diarrheal disease, **V2**.911–12
  see also specific viral infection

Diarrhetic shellfish poisoning (DSP), **B1**.280

Diazonium Blue B, **M**.202–3

Dibromopropamidine, **B1**.426

Dichelobacter, **B2**.1930

Dichelobacter nodosus, **B2**.1930

Dichloramine, **B1**.424

Dichloroflavan, rhinovirus infection therapy, **V2**.879

Dichloroisocyanuric acid (NaDCC), sodium salts, **B1**.424

Dichotomophthora, oculomycoses, **M**.278 (Tab.), **M**.283–4

Dicistroviridae
  classification, **V1**.27 (Tab.), **V1**.51 (Tab.)
  see also specific viruses

Dick test, **B2**.856

Dicrocoeliidae, **P**.585

Dicrocoelioidea, **P**.585

Dicrocoelium, **P**.585
  as zoonosis, **P**.642

Dictyosomes, **P**.176–7

Didanosine, **V2**.1620
  HIV infection, **V2**.1334
    point mutation resistance, **V2**.1337 (Fig.)
    structure, **V2**.1620 (Fig.)
Didehydrodideoxyuridine *see* Stavudine
Didelphis (opossum)
  control, **P**.119
  Leishmania braziliensis, **P**.326
  Leishmania infantum chagasi, **P**.320
  Trypanosoma cruzi, **P**.382, **P**.391
Dideoxycytosine *see* Zalcitabine
Dideoxyinosine *see* Didanosine
Dienes typing, **B2**.1445, **B2**.1445 (Fig.),
  B2.1446
Dientamoeba, classification, **P**.196–7
Dientamoeba fragilis, **P**.187–8, **P**.266–70
  biochemistry/molecular biology, **P**.267
    ferridoxin-mediated electron transport,
      P.267
    pyruvate metabolism, **P**.267
    small subunit ribosomal RNA, **P**.267
  classification, **P**.266
    Histomonas meleagridis vs., **P**.266
  differential diagnosis, *Blastocystis hominis*
    vs., **P**.565
  epidemiology, **P**.269
    distribution, **P**.269
    transmission, **P**.269
  infection *see Dientamoeba fragilis* infection
  structure/life cycle, **P**.266–7, **P**.267 (Fig.)
    binucleate forms, **P**.267
    Enterobius vermicularis vector, **P**.267,
      P.269
    nutrition, **P**.267
    trichomonad cell type, **P**.267
    trophozoites, **P**.267, **P**.269
  as trichomonad, **P**.200
Dientamoeba fragilis infection, **P**.266
  in AIDS, **P**.267–8
  asymptomatic infection, **P**.267–8
  chemotherapy, **P**.269
  clinical aspects, **P**.267–8
  diagnosis, **P**.268
    cultivation, **P**.268
    fecal examination, **P**.268
    preservatives/fixatives, **P**.268
  immunology, **P**.76, **P**.268
  pathology, **P**.268
    intestinal wall changes, **P**.268
  peripheral eosinophilia, **P**.267–8
Diesel, bioremediation, **B1**.201
Dietary changes, emerging bacterial infection,
  B1.360–1
Diethylcarbamazine (DEC)
  Angiostrongylus costaricensis therapy, **P**.810
  lymphatic filariasis prophylaxis/treatment,
    P.777
  onchocerciasis therapy, **P**.789
  toxocariasis therapy, **P**.755
Dietzia, **B2**.1151
  isolation/identification, **B2**.1144–5
    staining properties, **B2**.1139–40
  mycolic acids, **B2**.1146
Dietzia maris, **B2**.1151
Differential stains, **B1**.713 (Tab.)

Diffuse cutaneous leishmaniasis (DCL) *see*
  Leishmaniasis, Old World
Diffusely adherent *Escherichia coli* (DAEC)
  see Escherichia coli, diffusely adherent
  (DAEC)
Diffusion of solutes, simple (passive), **B1**.48–9
Difluormethylornithine (DFMO: eflornithine:
  Ornidyl) *see* Eflornithine
  (difluormethylornithine: DFMO:
  Ornidyl)
Digenea, **P**.580–6
diGeorge syndrome, **I**.774–5
Dihydrofolate reductase (DHFR)
  antimalarial target, **P**.477, **P**.509
  herpesviruses, **V1**.500
  inhibition
    diaminopyrimidines, **B1**.492
    trimethoprim, **B1**.492
  Pneumocystis, **M**.790
Dihydrolase reactions, *Aeromonas*
  identification, **B2**.1532
Dihydropteroate synthase (DHPS)
  antimalarial target, **P**.477, **P**.509
    mechanism of action, **P**.480
  Pneumocystis jirovecii, **M**.764, **M**.790,
    M.791–2, **M**.796
Dihydroxyeicosatetraenoic acid, **I**.185–6
Dihydroxyfolate reductase (DHFR)–
  thymidylate synthase (TS),
  Cryptosporidium parvum, **P**.403–4
Di-iodohydroxyquin, amebiasis chemotherapy,
  P.213
Diloxanide furoate, amebiasis chemotherapy,
  P.213
Dilution plate count, **B1**.205
Dimerization, pyrogenic exotoxins, **I**.559
Dimethyl sulfoxide, skin immunization, **I**.822
Dimorphic species, **M**.21–2, **M**.74–6,
  M.74 (Tab.)
  Blastomyces dermatitidis, **M**.25 (Fig.), **M**.480,
    M.485, **M**.487 (Fig.), **M**.488, **M**.492–3,
    M.495–6
  blepharitis, **M**.287–8
  Candida, **M**.74, **M**.583
  Candida albicans, **M**.74, **M**.75–6, **M**.75 (Fig.)
  Candida glabrata, **M**.75
  capacity of, **M**.75
  Coccidiodes immitis see Coccidioides immitis
  Cokeromyces recurvatus, **M**.663
  Histoplasma capsulatum, **M**.22–3, **M**.22 (Fig.),
    M.74
  Histoplasma capsulatum var. *capsulatum,*
    M.22–3
  identification
    exoantigen test, **M**.91
    nucleic acid probes, **M**.91
  Malassezia furfur, **M**.74
  Paracoccidioides brasiliensis see
    Paracoccidioides brasiliensis
  Penicillium marneffei, **M**.565, **M**.566,
    M.569–70
  Sporothrix schenckii, **M**.22–3, **M**.28,
    M.29 (Fig.)
  see also individual species
Dinger's discs, **B2**.1871–2
Dinitrogenase reductase-activating
  glycohydrolase (DRAG), **B1**.63

Dinitrogenase reductase ADP-
  ribosyltransferase (DRAT), **B1**.63
2,4-Dinitrophenol (DNP), **B1**.438
Dinoflagellates, toxins, **B1**.280
Dipetalonema, **P**.591
Diphasic variation, *Salmonella* H antigen,
  B2.1404
Diphosphatidylglycerol (DPG)
  Brucella, **B2**.1724
  Burkholderia, **B2**.1613
Diphtheria, **B1**.612–13
  clinical manifestations, **B2**.984–5
    'bullneck appearance,' **B2**.984–5
    cardiac toxicity, **B2**.985
    laryngeal, **B2**.984–5
    neurologic toxicity, **B2**.985
    pharyngitis, **B1**.611–12, **B2**.984–5
  control, **B1**.348–9
  cutaneous, **B2**.985
    role in spread of infection, **B2**.985
    transmission, **B2**.985
  diagnosis, **B1**.612
    Elek immunoprecipitation test, **B1**.612–13
    screening tests, **B1**.612
    toxigenicity tests, **B1**.612–13
  emerging bacterial infection, **B1**.364,
    B1.364 (Fig.)
  epidemiology, **B1**.612
    age-specific incidence, **B1**.348, **B1**.348 (Fig.)
    Russia, **B1**.364 (Fig.)
  immunity, **B1**.348
    herd, **B1**.348
  invasive disease, **B2**.985
  laboratory worker immunization, **B1**.767
  pathogenesis, **B1**.612
  pathogenicity, **B2**.984
  respiratory, **B2**.984–5
  toxin *see* Diphtheria toxin
  transmission, **B1**.348
    nosocomial spread, **B1**.378
    theories, **B1**.337
    vaccine effect on, **B1**.348–9
  treatment, **B2**.985
  vaccines/vaccination, **I**.855 (Tab.), **B2**.985–6
    diphtheria toxoid, **B1**.348, **B2**.986
    effect on incidence/outbreaks, **B1**.348
    USA schedules, **V2**.1560 (Fig.)
Diphtheria antitoxin, **B2**.985
Diphtheria–tetanus–pertussis (DTP) vaccine,
  B1.646–7
Diphtheria toxin, **I**.655, **B2**.980–1
  as adjuvant, **I**.925
  DNA damage, **I**.655
  fragments A and B, **B2**.980–1
  iron effect, **B2**.981
  mechanism of action, **B1**.156 (Tab.)
  production, **B2**.980–1
  testing, **B2**.984
  translation and elongation factor role,
    B2.980–1
  vaccine, virosomes adjuvant, **I**.929
Diphtheria toxoid (DTx), as adjuvant/carrier,
  I.862–3
  conjugate vaccines, **I**.935
  subunit vaccines, **I**.935

Diphtheria toxoid (DTx) (*Continued*)
transcutaneous immunization, **I**.837
Diphyllobothriidae, **P**.576–7
structure/life cycle, **P**.577
Diphyllobothrium, **P**.576, **P**.674, **P**.677
discovery, **P**.658
geographical distribution, **P**.658
location in host, **P**.662
reproductive system, **P**.661
see also individual species
Diphyllobothrium cordatum, **P**.674
Diphyllobothrium dendriticum, **P**.673
Diphyllobothrium hians, **P**.674
Diphyllobothrium houghtoni, **P**.674
Diphyllobothrium latum, **P**.671–3
geographical distribution, **P**.671
historical aspects, **P**.12
infection *see Diphyllobothrium latum*
infection
life cycle, **P**.671–2, **P**.672 (Fig.)
intermediate hosts, **P**.671–2
pseudoapolysis, **P**.671–2
location in host, **P**.672
morphology/structure, **P**.671
transmission/epidemiology, **P**.672
prevalence, **P**.672
Diphyllobothrium latum infection
clinical manifestations, **P**.672
cobalamin absorption, **P**.663
pernicious anemia, **P**.672, **P**.673
vitamin B$_{12}$ absorption, **P**.663, **P**.672
control, **P**.673
chemotherapy, **P**.673
prophylaxis, **P**.673
transmission, **P**.673
diagnosis, **P**.673
immunity, **P**.673
pathogenesis/pathology, **P**.673
public health importance, **P**.44
Diphyllobothrium nihonkaiense, **P**.673–4
Diphyllobothrium orcini, **P**.674
Diphyllobothrium pacificum, **P**.674
Diphyllobothrium scotium, **P**.674
Diphyllobothrium ursi, **P**.674
Diphyllobothrium yonagoense, **P**.674
Diphylobothriidae, **P**.677
Diplococci, **B2**.1270
Diplodia, fruit, **B1**.282
Diplogonoporus, **P**.576–7
Diplomomnadida, **I**.675–6
Diplostomidae, **P**.580, **P**.582
Diplostomoidea, **P**.580, **P**.582
Dipylididae, **P**.578
Dipylidium, **P**.578
Dipylidium caninum, **P**.674
Direct agglutination test (DAT)
Old World leishmaniasis, **P**.302
visceral leishmaniasis control, **P**.129–30
Directed mutagenesis *see* Genetic analysis
Direct fluorescent antibody (DFA) test, **M**.491,
M.492, **M**.496
Legionella, **B2**.1773
Direct immunofluorescence, **V2**.1535
measles diagnosis, **V1**.732
microsporidiosis, **P**.151

Q fever diagnosis, **B2**.2077
syphilis diagnosis, **B2**.1843, **B2**.1844–5
Dirithromycin
Pasteurella multocida, **B2**.1655
structure, **B1**.486
Dirofilaria, **P**.591
structure/life cycle, **P**.591
Dirofilaria immitis vaccines, **I**.823
Disability adjusted life year (DALY), parasitic
disease effects, **P**.25, **P**.25 (Fig.),
P.27 (Fig.), **P**.28 (Tab.)
Disaccharide malabsorption, cryptosporidiosis,
P.408
Disasters, emerging bacterial infection, **B1**.360
Discontinuous DNA synthesis, **V1**.149–50,
V1.150 (Fig.)
Discontinuous ('split') genes, gene cloning,
B1.126–7
'Discontinuous minus strand synthesis,'
V1.399–401
Disease, infection *vs.*, **I**.948
Disease status, viral classification, **V1**.26
Disease transmission *see* Transmission of
infection(s)
Dishwashers, candidiasis, **M**.597
Disinfectants/disinfection
aerial, **B1**.430
definition, **B1**.421
hands, **B1**.378
hepatitis B control, **V2**.1257
microsporidians, **P**.550
mode of action, **B1**.497
Q fever control, **B2**.2079
susceptibility/resistance
Brucella, **B2**.1733
Campylobacter, **B2**.1545
Clostridium, **B2**.1095
Enterobacteriaceae, **B2**.1346
Legionella, **B2**.1777
Mycobacterium, **B2**.1216–17
Proteus, **B2**.1441
Disk diffusion, **B1**.717
antibacterial susceptibility testing, **B1**.498
antifungal testing, **M**.158
Disoxaril, rhinovirus infection therapy, **V2**.879
Disposable screens, African trypanosomiasis
vector control, **P**.369, **P**.370 (Fig.)
Disseminated aspergillosis, **M**.137 (Fig.)
Disseminated candidiasis, **M**.601, **M**.612
Disseminated fusariosis, **M**.754
Disseminated intravascular coagulation (DIC),
I.700
filovirus infection, **V2**.1095
septic shock, **I**.701
Disseminated nocardiosis, **M**.140 (Fig.)
Disseminated rhinosporidiosis, **M**.461, **M**.463,
M.464, **M**.465 (Fig.), **M**.466 (Fig.)
Disulfide bonds, Ig structure, **I**.305, **I**.306
Disulfide-stabilized Fv (dsFv), **I**.367–8,
I.368 (Fig.)
Diversity (of fungi), **M**.69
Dizziness, onchocerciasis, **P**.794
DNA, **B1**.42
antibacterial agents, intercalation, **B1**.438
bacteriocins, **B1**.137, **B1**.138

base ratios, **B1**.13, **B1**.22 (Tab.), **B1**.25,
B1.32–3
bacterial classification, **B1**.13
GC ratios, **B1**.13
biosynthesis, **B1**.46–8
Brucella classification, **B2**.1721
cell–virus interactions *see* Cell–virus
interactions
E2 protein binding, papillomaviruses, **V1**.458
Haemophilus, **B2**.1693, **B2**.1697–8, **B2**.1704,
B2.1705–6, **B2**.1706 (Fig.)
Hepatitis B virus structure, **V2**.1230
historical aspects, **V1**.6
hybridization, **B1**.22 (Tab.), **B1**.25, **B1**.32–3
discovery, **B1**.13
Legionella, **B2**.1771
hybridization assays *see* Hybridization assays
integration, tumor viruses, **V1**.345
Listeria, **B2**.955, **B2**.962
Mycobacterium, **B2**.1186–9, **B2**.1193–4
repair
ionizing radiation, **B1**.271, **B1**.451
ultraviolet radiation, **B1**.451–2
replication, **B1**.46
herpesviruses *see* Herpesviruses
HSV type 1 (HSV-1) *see* Herpes simplex
virus type 1 (HSV-1)
origin (*oriC*), **B1**.46
regulation, **B1**.46–8
sequencing, **B1**.732–4
Coxiella burnetii, **B2**.2072–3
Mycobacterium, **B2**.1193–4
slow growing mycobacteria identification,
B2.1193–4
see also Polymerase chain reaction
soil bacteria
analysis, **B1**.206
metabolism quantification, **B1**.206
Staphylococcus, **B2**.771–2
sterilization
dry heat, **B1**.449
freeze-drying, **B1**.450
ionizing radiation, **B1**.450–1
moist heat, **B1**.448–9
ultraviolet radiation, **B1**.451, **B1**.452 (Fig.)
transduction, **B1**.142
DNA analysis
Burkholderia cepacia typing, **B2**.1614–15
Burkholderia thailandensis typing, **B2**.1623–4
pharyngitis diagnosis, **B1**.611
DNA assays
HCMV infection, **V1**.526
hepatitis B, **V2**.1251–5
DNA bacteriophages, mutation rates, **V1**.16–7
DNA-based assays
aspergillosis diagnosis, **M**.718
Aspergillus fumigatus, **M**.692
candidiasis diagnosis, **M**.257
pythiosis diagnosis, **M**.423
DNA-binding protein (DBP)
adenoviruses replication, **V1**.160, **V1**.161,
V1.162
EBV immediate early gene product, **V1**.564
DNA deletions, **B1**.87
mobile elements, **B1**.95–6

DNA deletions (*Continued*)
transposable elements, **B1**.94
DNA-dependent DNA polymerases
DNA virus replication, **V1**.147–8
mistake rate, **V1**.57
proofreading, **V1**.57
sequence analysis, **V1**.113–14
DNA duplications, **B1**.87
transposable elements, **B1**.94
DNA endonucleases (restriction enzymes),
B1.81, **B1**.119, **B1**.119 (Fig.)
plasmid genes, **B1**.115
DNA fingerprinting
characterization testing, **B1**.22 (Tab.), **B1**.25
epidemiological typing, **B1**.405
DNA gyrase (topoisomerase II), quinolones,
B1.492
DNA hybridization
mycoses, **M**.34
in viral diagnosis, **V2**.1536–7
DNA-hybridization groups, *Salmonella*
nomenclature, **B2**.1398–9
DNA inversions, **B1**.87
transposable elements, **B1**.94
Dna J chaperones, function, **B1**.47
Dna K chaperones, function, **B1**.47
DNA ligase I, SV40 replication, **V1**.154 (Tab.)
DNA ligase 4 deficiency, **I**.776
DNA ligases, poxviruses, **V1**.168, **V1**.605–6
DNA, maxicircles and minicircles, **P**.296
DNA methyl transferase, **I**.777
DNA microarrays
Borrelia, **B2**.1826
Escherichia, **B2**.1371–2
influenza diagnosis, **V1**.677
DNA polymerase(s)
adenoviruses, **V1**.147–8, **V1**.149 (Tab.),
V1.160, **V1**.162
DNA-directed, **B1**.46
herpesviruses, **V1**.500
poxviruses, **V1**.147–8, **V1**.168, **V1**.169 (Tab.),
V1.603–4
SV40 replication, **V1**.154 (Tab.)
DNA polymerase δ
HPV replication, **V1**.457
parvovirus replication, **V1**.418
DNA polymerase α-primase
HPV replication, **V1**.457
SV40 replication, **V1**.153, **V1**.154 (Tab.)
DNA probes, **B1**.725
antibacterial susceptibility testing,
B1.498–500
arenavirus infection, **V2**.1075–6
Blastomyces dermatitidis, **M**.496
Burkholderia thailandensis typing, **B2**.1623
Candida, **M**.605–6, **M**.608
Enterococcus, **B2**.887
fungi classification, **M**.47
Fusobacterium, **B2**.1950
gram-positive anaerobic cocci, **B2**.907
Legionella pneumophila, **B2**.1773
syphilis diagnosis, **B2**.1852
DNA provirus, **V1**.7, **V1**.338, **V1**.345
DNA regulatory sequences, polyomaviruses,
V1.474

DNase, Enterobacteriaceae identification,
B2.1319 (Tab.)
DNA technology, **P**.150
echinococcosis diagnosis, **P**.690
malaria diagnosis, **P**.504
protozoa classification, **P**.193
DNA tumor viruses, **V1**.330–3, **V1**.332 (Tab.)
large, tumors associated, **V1**.332 (Tab.)
oncogenes, **V1**.336–8
small, tumors associated, **V1**.332 (Tab.)
DNA vaccines, **I**.488, **I**.488 (Tab.), **I**.489 (Tab.),
V2.1553–4, **I.909–24**
advantages, **I**.909
clinical trials, **I**.920–1
Hepatitis B virus vaccine, **I**.825
HIV vaccine, **I**.920–1
malaria vaccine, **I**.920–1
Salmonella, **I**.901
CpG motifs, **I**.911–12
immune recognition, **I**.911–12
immunostimulation, **I**.911–12, **I**.916
immunosuppression, **I**.912
proinflammatory sequences, **I**.911
signal transduction, **I**.911
TLRs 9 binding, **I**.911
CTL priming, **I**.896
cytokine upregulation, **I**.896
delivery routes, **I**.912–13
attenuated bacterial vectors, **I**.913
bare skin routes, **I**.825
cytofectins, **I**.917
electroporation, **I**.917
encapsulation, **I**.913
intradermal/ballistic, **I**.912–13
intramuscular, **I**.912
liposomes, **I**.917
mucosal, **I**.913
polymeric bioparticles, **I**.918
disadvantages, **I**.909
expression vectors, **I**.910–12
helper-T cell response, **V2**.1553–4
historical aspects/re-evaluation, **I**.14–5,
I.909–10
IFN-γ production, **I**.896
IL-6 production, **I**.896
IL-12 production, **I**.896
immunogenicity augmentation, **I**.916–19
adjuvants, **I**.918–19, **I**.918 (Tab.)
codon optimization, **I**.916–17
delivery, **I**.917–18
inserted gene modification, **I**.917
'prime boosting' *see* 'Prime-boost
immunization'
promoters, **I**.916
mechanism of action, **I**.896
multivalent vaccines, **V2**.1553–4
peptide vaccines, **I**.879
plasmids, **I**.910–11, **I**.910 (Fig.)
APC transfection, **I**.914–16, **I**.915 (Fig.)
ColE1 origin of replication (ori), **I**.910–11
crosspriming, **I**.914, **I**.915 (Fig.)
HCMV immediate/early promoter, **I**.910
processing/presentation, **I**.913 (Fig.),
I.914–6
promotor/enhancer, **I**.910

Rous sarcoma virus long terminal repeat,
I.910
somatic cell priming, **I**.914
SV40 early promoter, **I**.910
transcriptional termination sequence, **I**.910
uptake of, **I**.913
'prime-boost immunization,' **I**.846
safety, **I**.919–20
anti-DNA antibody induction, **I**.920
autoimmunity, **I**.920
integration potential, **I**.919–20
tolerance induction, **I**.920
sequential schedule, **V2**.1554
Shigella vector, **I**.901
specific infection
bunyaviruses, **V2**.1050–1
hepatitis B, **V2**.1554
hepatitis C, **V2**.1554
HIV, **V2**.1333, **V2**.1554
HPV, **V2**.1554
HSV, **V2**.1554
influenza, **V2**.1554
mycoplasma, **B2**.1993–4
rabies, **V2**.1116, **V2**.1554
tuberculosis, **I**.717
transcriptional silencing, **I**.916
virosome vaccines, **I**.839
DNA viruses
attenuation, continuous passage, **V1**.197
characteristics, **V1**.177 (Tab.)
double-stranded *see* DNA viruses, double-
stranded
evolution
genome mutation, **V1**.16–7
recombination, **V1**.14
gene expression, **V1**.110
temporal control, **V1**.118–19
genome replication, **V1**.122–3, **V1**.147–50,
V1.148 (Tab.)
auxillary regions, **V1**.148
discontinuous DNA synthesis, **V1**.149–50,
V1.150 (Fig.)
DNA-dependent DNA polymerase,
V1.147–8
helicase, **V1**.149
initiation, **V1**.150 (Fig.)
lagging-strand DNA replication,
V1.149–50, **V1**.150 (Fig.)
leading-strand DNA replication,
V1.149–50, **V1**.150 (Fig.)
origin recognition proteins, **V1**.148,
V1.149 (Tab.)
origins of replication, **V1**.147–50
priming, **V1**.147–50
replication compartments/centers,
V1.170–1
transcription factors, **V1**.148
viral proteins, **V1**.149 (Tab.)
genome size, **V1**.176
host–virus interactions, **V1**.169–72
chaperones, **V1**.169–70
proteins, **V1**.169–70
repair/recombination machinery, **V1**.171
S-phase induction, **V1**.169
transformation, **V1**.171

DNA viruses (*Continued*)
immune evasion, **V1**.286
MHC class II interference, **V1**.287
infection
IL-6, **V1**.297
TNF-α induction, **V1**.296
infectious DNA, **V1**.182
mobile replicons, **V1**.12
mRNA transcription, **V1**.110
origins, **V1**.12
RNA viruses *vs.*, **V1**.12
recombination, **V1**.187–8
replication, **V1**.217, **V1.147–73**
proofreading, **V1**.17
replicative elements *vs.*, **V1**.12
see also specific viruses
DNA viruses, double-stranded
classification, **V1**.27 (Tab.), **V1**.40–5,
V1.43 (Tab.)
genome packaging, **V1**.67
expansion transition, **V1**.67
genome replication, **V1**.123 (Fig.)
see also specific viruses
DNA viruses, single-stranded
classification, **V1**.27 (Tab.), **V1**.40–1,
V1.41–2, **V1**.41 (Tab.)
replication, **V1**.110
see also specific viruses
DNMT3B gene, **I**.777
Dobell and Laidlaw medium
Chilomastix mesnili cultivation, **P**.272
Dientamoeba fragilis cultivation, **P**.268
Enteromonas hominis cultivation, **P**.270
Dobrava-Belgrade virus (DOBV),
V2.1666 (Tab.)
Dobrava virus, **V2**.1045
Doctor's office tests, *Chlamydia* infection
diagnosis, **B2**.2019
Dogs
airborne endotoxin exposure, **B1**.189
bites *see* Bites
blastomycosis, **M**.480–1, **M**.483–4, **M**.488
kennel cough and tracheobronchitis, **B2**.1810
otitis, **M**.214
Paracoccidioides brasiliensis, **M**.544
prototothecosis, **M**.398, **M**.400, **M**.407
pythiosis, **M**.419–20, **M**.420 (Fig.)
rabies, **V2**.1119
rhinosporidiosis, **M**.458
Dolipores, **M**.72, **M**.73 (Fig.)
septa, **M**.73 (Fig.)
Dolphin morbillivirus, **V1**.712–13
emerging infection, **V2**.1651 (Tab.)
Dolphins
lobomycosis, **M**.430, **M**.431, **M**.432, **M**.433
sporotrichosis, **M**.371
Domestic animals
emerging viral infection, **V2**.1659–60
gastrointestinal nematodes, **P**.713–14
Leishmania braziliensis, **P**.326–7
rabies vaccination, **V1**.370
Domoic acid poisoning, **B1**.280
Donath, Julius, **I**.748
Donovan bodies, **B1**.665

*Donovania granulomatosis see Klebsiella
granulomatis*
Donovanosis, **B1**.665
Dopamine circuits, Borna disease virus
infection, **V2**.1146–7
Doratomyces, oculomycoses, **M**.278 (Tab.)
Dorsal root ganglia, VZV infection, **V1**.513,
V1.515
Dose-dependency, aminoglycosides, **B1**.469–70
Dose–response, **B1**.316
Dose variation, antibacterial
pharmacodynamics, **B1**.469–70
Dosing interval, antibacterial
pharmacodynamics, **B1**.469–70
Dot-blot hybridization, **V2**.1536
astrovirus detection, **V2**.906–7
Dothideales, **M**.199
Double diffusion immunoprecipitation, **M**.34
Corynebacterium detection, **B1**.756
Double membrane vesicles, **V1**.835
'Double-negative' cells, T cell development,
I.455
'Double-positive' cells, T cell development,
I.455
Double-strand break repair mechanisms,
V1.169–70
Double-stranded RNA (dsRNA)
as pathogen-associated molecular patterns,
I.896
TLR-3 binding, **I**.119
'Double-walled organelle', **P**.174, **P**.175 (Fig.)
Downstream transcription factors, BCR
signaling, **I**.346–7
Doxorubicin, Kaposi's sarcoma therapy,
V1.553
Doxycycline
human brucellosis treatment, **B2**.1742–3
isolation/identification, *Bacillus anthracis*,
B2.938
mechanism of action, **P**.479
melioidosis treatment, **B2**.1631
Q fever treatment, **B2**.2078
spectrum of activity, **B1**.499 (Tab.)
Actinobacillus actinomycetemcomitans,
B2.1664
Borrelia, **B2**.1831 (Tab.)
Edwardsiella, **B2**.1491–2
Listeria, **B2**.957–8
structure, **B1**.485 (Fig.)
in syphilis, **B2**.1857–8
Dracunculiasis, **P.830–4**
clinical features, **P**.39, **P**.831–2
sites, **P**.831–2
control, **P**.123–4
chemotherapy/chemoprophylaxis,
P.144 (Tab.)
conflict effects, **P**.107 (Tab.), **P**.123–4
diagnosis, **P**.143 (Tab.)
trends, **P**.117 (Fig.)
vector/reservoir control, **P**.145 (Tab.)
see also below
diagnosis, **P**.832
immunodiagnosis, **P**.832
epidemiology, **P**.46 (Tab.), **P**.830–1
geographical distribution, **P**.39, **P**.830
incidence, **P**.831–2, **P**.833 (Fig.)
seasonal incidence, **P**.830

eradication campaigns, **P**.39, **P**.832–4
active surveillance, **P**.832
containment, **P**.833–4
Guinea Worm Eradication Programme,
P.110
health education, **P**.832
International Commission for the
Certification of the Eradication of
Dracunculiasis, **P**.123–4
International Water Decade, **P**.123–4
water treatment, **P**.833–4
historical aspects, **P**.10–1
public health importance, **P**.39, **P**.105 (Tab.)
transmission, **P**.830–1, **P**.831 (Fig.)
treatment, **P**.832
chemotherapy, **P**.832
surgery/removal, **P**.831 (Fig.), **P**.832
zoonotic aspects, **P**.834
Dracunculidae, **P**.591
features, **P**.591
Dracunculoidea, **P**.591
Dracunculus, **P**.591
classification, **P**.591
Onchocerca volvulus vs., **P**.782
historical aspects, **P**.10–1
infection *see* Dracunculiasis
structure/life cycle, **P**.591
Dracunculus medinensis
infection *see* Dracunculiasis
life cycle, **P**.830
structure, **P**.591, **P**.830
DRADA, **V2**.1433, **V2**.1435 (Fig.)
Drechslera, in cereals, **B1**.284
Drepanidotaenia, **P**.578
Dreschlera, allergic fungal sinusitis, **M**.675
Dried blood spots (DBS), neonatal HCMV
infection, **V2**.1452
Dried food, **B1**.268–9, **B1**.268 (Tab.)
herbs and spices, **B1**.287–8
processes, **B1**.268–9
ingredients, **B1**.269
microbial numbers, **B1**.269
product integrity, **B1**.269
Drinking water
filtration, **P**.833–4
nitrate levels excess, **B1**.200
treatment
dracunculiasis eradication, **P**.833–4
giardiasis prevention, **P**.251–2
Naegleria fowleri prevention, **P**.237–8
UV radiation disinfection use, **B1**.452
Drinks, bacterial infection transmission, **B1**.310
DRM, rhabdoviruses, **V1**.73–4
Droplet transmission, **V1**.239–40, **V1**.354,
V1.355, **V2**.1403–4
filovirus, **V2**.1093–4
rhinoviruses, **V1**.354
Drosophila X virus, type species, **V1**.48
Drug efflux, antibiotic resistance mechanism,
B1.440
Drug(s), liposome formulations, **P**.307
Drug resistance
African trypanosomiasis strains, **P**.371
chemotherapy/chemoprophylaxis control
methods, **P**.128
control strategies, **P**.128

Drug resistance (*Continued*)
diagnosis, **P**.154
disease control effects, **P**.64
malaria diagnosis, **P**.150, **P**.154
parasite control measures, **P**.127–8
Plasmodium see Plasmodium
see also specific diseases; specific drugs
Dry heat, **B1**.449
time-temperature relationships, **B1**.448 (Tab.)
uses, **B1**.445 (Tab.)
validation and monitoring, **B1**.454 (Tab.)
Drying, *Campylobacter* susceptibility/
resistance, **B2**.1545
dsRNA adenosine deaminase activity
(DRADA), **V2**.1433, **V2**.1435 (Fig.)
Dubois, A, **M**.24
Duck adenovirus (EDS'76), **V1**.444–5
Duck astrovirus, **V2**.890 (Tab.)
Duck Hepatitis B virus (DHBV)
discovery, **V2**.1227
Hepatitis delta virus interactions, **V2**.1271
type species, **V1**.46–7
uptake, **V2**.1233
Duck parvovirus, **V1**.410
Duclaux, E, **M**.4, **M**.9
Duffy blood group determinants
malaria association, **I**.599
Plasmodium cell invasion, **P**.472, **P**.474–5
polymorphisms, malaria epidemiology, **P**.512
Dugbe virus
G1 glycoprotein, **V2**.1034
post-translational modification, **V2**.1038
G2 glycoprotein, **V2**.1034
genome structure, **V2**.1034
consensus sequences, **V2**.1031 (Tab.)
M (medium) segment, **V2**.1034
transcription, **V2**.1035
Duhamel-Haddad procedure, **P**.393 (Fig.)
Duke criteria, **B1**.536, **B1**.538
Dulcitol fermentation, Enterobacteriaceae
identification, **B2**.1319 (Tab.)
Duncan syndrome, **V1**.568
Duodenal aspirates, *Strongyloides* diagnosis,
P.741
Duodenal ulcers, *Helicobacter pylori*, **B1**.365,
B2.1564
Duplications, mobile elements, **B1**.95–6
Dural tears, recurrent pneumococcal
meningitis, **B1**.571, **B1**.572
van Durme, Paul, **P**.9
dUTPase
HSV-1 replication, **V1**.165 (Tab.)
poxvirus replication, **V1**.169 (Tab.)
Duttonella, **P**.351
Duvenhage virus, **V2**.1103–4
D value
heat, **B1**.265–6, **B1**.265 (Fig.), **B1**.446,
B1.446 (Tab.), **B1**.449
ionizing radiation, **B1**.271, **B1**.446 (Tab.)
Dyes
antibacterial, **B1**.427–8
Brucella culture, **B2**.1735
Dye test (DT), toxoplasmosis, **P**.435
Dynamic equilibria, infection *see* Infection(s),
mathematical models

Dysarthria, in progressive multifocal
leucoencephalopathy, **V2**.1417
Dysentery
bacillary
drug-resistance, **B2**.1392–4
treatment, **B2**.1392–4
see also Shigella dysenteriae; Shigellosis
clinical manifestations, **B2**.1387
Dyserythropoiesis, anemia in malaria, **P**.499
Dysgammaglobulinemia, respiratory tract
infection, **B1**.626
Dysgonomonas
characteristics, **B2**.1679 (Tab.)
habitats, **B2**.1649–50
as normal microbiota, **B1**.296 (Tab.)
see also individual species
Dysgonomonas capnocytophagoides
antibacterial susceptibility/resistance,
B2.1678
characteristics, **B2**.1678, **B2**.1679 (Tab.)
habitats, **B2**.1649–50
identification, **B2**.1678
infection in humans, **B2**.1677–8
Dysgonomonas gadei, **B2**.1679 (Tab.)
Dysgonomonas rossii, **B2**.1679 (Tab.)
Dyspepsia, *Helicobacter pylori* infection,
B2.1580
Dyspnea, trichinellosis, **P**.762
Dystonia, in progressive multifocal
leucoencephalopathy, **V2**.1417

E1A protein, protein synthesis control, **V1**.118
E1 glycoprotein, alphaviruses *see* Alphaviruses
E1L gene, **V1**.609
E1 protein
Hepatitis C virus *see* Hepatitis C virus
(HCV)
HPV replication, **V1**.457
papillomaviruses *see* Papillomaviruses
pestiviruses, **V2**.995–6
Rubella virus *see* Rubella virus (RV)
E2A gene, B cell development, **I**.325
E2 envelope protein, hepatitis C virus, **I**.870–1
E2 glycoprotein, alphaviruses *see* Alphaviruses
E2 protein
Hepatitis C virus *see* Hepatitis C virus
(HCV)
HPV replication, **V1**.457
papillomaviruses *see* Papillomaviruses
pestiviruses *see* Pestiviruses
Rubella virus *see* Rubella virus (RV)
E3L gene, poxvirus host range control, **V1**.620,
V1.624
E3 protein, alphaviruses, **V2**.1014
E4 protein, papillomaviruses, **V1**.458
E5 protein, papillomaviruses, **V1**.458–9
E6 protein
high-risk HPVs, **V1**.455–6, **V1**.459
low-risk HPVs, **V1**.455–6, **V1**.459
papillomaviruses *see* Papillomaviruses
E6 protein, papillomaviruses, **V1**.460
E7 protein
high-risk HPVs, **V1**.455–6, **V1**.459, **V1**.461
low-risk HPVs, **V1**.455–6, **V1**.459, **V1**.461
papillomaviruses *see* Papillomaviruses

E9 protein, poxvirus replication, **V1**.168–9
E12 protein, B cell development, **I**.325
E47 protein, B cell development, **I**.325
E200K mutation, prion protein (PrP), **V2**.1368
Ear
anatomy, **B1**.607
external auditory meatus, *Staphylococcus,*
B2.777
infection, **B1**.617–18
intracranial abscess, **B1**.582, **B1**.584–5,
B1.584 (Tab.)
subdural empyema, **B1**.590, **B1**.591 (Tab.)
see also Otitis media; Otomycoses;
*individual species; specific diseases/
infection*
skin biopsies, *Borrelia* infection, **B2**.1828
Early termination factors, poxviruses,
V1.599 (Tab.)
Early transcription factors, poxviruses,
V1.599 (Tab.)
East African Network for Monitoring
Antimalarial Treatment (EANMAT),
P.480
Eastern equine encephalitis virus (EEEV),
V1.372 (Tab.), **V2**.998 (Tab.), **V2**.1010,
V2.1011 (Tab.)
biological warfare agent, **V2**.1018
epidemiology, **V1**.373
evolution, **V1**.13
genetic conservation, **V2**.1019–20
transmission, **V1**.372 (Tab.), **V2**.1016–17,
V2.1016 (Fig.), **V2**.1019
reservoir hosts, **V2**.1017
Eastern equine encephalomyelitis, **V2**.1019–20
clinical features, **V2**.1019
distribution, **V2**.1019
history, **V2**.1019
EBF (early B-cell factor), B cell development,
I.325
Ebola virus (EBOV)
artificial replication systems, **V2**.1093
cellular receptor, **V2**.1092
classification, **V1**.48, **V1**.382, **V2**.1086
biosafety level 4, **V2**.1526
disease importance, **V1**.382
as emerging infection, **V2**.1648 (Tab.)
epidemiology, **V2**.1093
laboratory-acquired infection,
V2.1517 (Tab.)
outbreaks, **V2**.1085–6, **V2**.1087 (Tab.)
transmission, **V1**.371 (Tab.)
genome structure, **V1**.387 (Tab.),
V2.1088 (Fig.)
glycoprotein (GP), **V2**.1089–90
transcription, **V2**.1093
historical aspects, **V2**.1085
infection *see* Ebola virus (EBOV) infection
infectivity, particle size, **V2**.1086
morphology/structure, **V2**.1088 (Fig.)
M proteins, **V1**.69–70
protein structures, **V1**.70 (Tab.)
non structural glycoproteins, **V2**.1091
nucleoprotein (NP), **V2**.1086–8
small secreted glycoprotein (ssGP), **V2**.1091
immune evasion, **V2**.1096
VP30 (minor nucleoprotein), **V2**.1090–1
VP35 (polymerase cofactor), **V2**.1089

Ebola virus (EBOV) infection, **B1**.400
  risk categorization, **B1**.762
  vaccines, **I**.933 (Tab.)
Echinocandins, **M**.154–5, **M**.169 (Tab.)
  activity, **M**.154, **M**.155
  characteristics, **M**.155 (Tab.)
  mechanism of action, **M**.70–1, **M**.154
  pharmacokinetics, **M**.154
  resistance, **M**.176
    Cryptococcus neoformans, **M**.154, **M**.176
    Fusarium, **M**.176
    Histoplasma capsulatum, **M**.154
  therapy
    aspergillosis, **M**.155
    candidiasis, **M**.154, **M**.155
    coccidiomycosis, **M**.154
    cryptococcosis, **M**.651
    phaeohyphomycosis, **M**.745
Echinochasmus, **P**.582–3
Echinococcosis
  AIDS, **P**.691
  alveolar *see below*
  cellular immune response, **P**.690
  control
    animal reservoir hosts, **P**.119
    vector elimination, **P**.109
  diagnosis, **P**.694–6
    brain biopsies, **P**.153
    computed tomography, **P**.694
    EIAs, **P**.154
    magnetic resonance imaging, **P**.694
    serology, **P**.694
    ultrasound, **P**.694
  differential diagnosis, **P**.694
  humoral immune response, **P**.689
  immune evasion mechanisms, **P**.691
  treatment
    ivermectin, **P**.698–9
    percutaneous aspiration–injection–
      re-aspiration, **P**.699
  vaccine development, **P**.691–2
Echinococcosis, alveolar, **P**.677
  AIDS, **P**.691
  anti-antigen 5 antibodies, **P**.689
  clinical manifestations, **P**.688–9
  control, **P**.702
    hygiene, **P**.702
    reservoir hosts, **P**.119
    sanitation, **P**.702
  diagnosis, **P**.694
    computed tomography, **P**.694
    diagnostic puncture, **P**.694
    immunoassays, **P**.694
    magnetic resonance imaging, **P**.694
    radiographic screening, **P**.688–9
    serology, **P**.694
    ultrasound, **P**.694
  differential diagnosis, **P**.688–9
  epidemiology, **P**.702
  genetic susceptibility, **P**.691
  geographical distribution, **P**.677, **P**.702
  IgE, **P**.689
  location in host, **P**.686
  pathogenesis, **P**.680

treatment
  albendazole, **P**.696–7, **P**.699
  bile shunts, **P**.696
  liver transplantation, **P**.699
  mebendazole, **P**.699
Echinococcosis, cystic, **P**.677
  allergic reactions, **P**.688
  anti-antigen 5 antibodies, **P**.689
  anti-antigen B antibodies, **P**.689–90
  asymptomatic, **P**.688
  clinical manifestations, **P**.688
    eosinophilia, **P**.694–6
    hypergammaglobulinemia, **P**.694–6
  control, **P**.701–2
  diagnosis, **P**.690
    computed tomography, **P**.695 (Fig.)
    immunoassays, **P**.694–6
    serology, **P**.694–6
  geographical distribution, **P**.677, **P**.701
  IgE, **P**.689
  location in host, **P**.686
  mass screening programs, **P**.688
  pulmonary complications, **P**.688
  treatment
    albendazole, **P**.698–9
    bile shunts, **P**.696
    cyclosporin A, **P**.698–9
    mebendazole, **P**.698–9
    pericystectomy, **P**.696–7
    praziquantal, **P**.698–9
    surgery, **P**.696–7
Echinococcosis, polycystic, **P**.677
  clinical manifestations, **P**.689
  epidemiology, **P**.702
  geographical distribution, **P**.677
  location in host, **P**.686
  treatment, **P**.699
Echinococcus, **P**.579, **P**.677, **I**.682
  historical aspects, **P**.678
  immune evasion
    complement inhibition, **I**.685
    host molecule incorporation, **I**.684
  infection *see* Echinococcosis
  life cycle, **P**.579, **P**.678–80, **P**.685 (Fig.)
    definitive host, **P**.684
    development in host, **P**.679
  morphology/structure, **P**.579
    eggs, **P**.678–9
    hydatid cysts, **P**.679
    proglottids, **P**.678
    strobila, **P**.678
  see also individual species
Echinococcus granulosus, **P**.677
  European biotype, **P**.701
    intermediate hosts, **P**.684
  genetic heterogeneity, **P**.701
  glutathione-S-transferase, **P**.682–3
  historical aspects, **P**.12–3
  host strains/isolates, **P**.683
  infection *see* Echinococcosis, cystic
  life cycle
    definitive hosts, **P**.119
    intermediate host, **P**.684, **P**.701
    intermediate hosts, **P**.684
    protoscolices development, **P**.679

morphology, **P**.679 (Fig.)
  hydatid cyst, **P**.680, **P**.681, **P**.681 (Fig.)
  protoscolices, **P**.681 (Fig.)
northern biotype, **P**.701
  intermediate host, **P**.684, **P**.701
paramyosin, **P**.682–3
Echinococcus multilocularis, **P**.677
  alveolar cyst development, **P**.681
  calcareous corpuscles, **P**.681–2
  genetic heterogeneity, **P**.701
  hydatid cyst development, **P**.680, **P**.682 (Fig.)
  infection *see* Echinococcosis, alveolar
  life cycle, **P**.679, **P**.702
    definitive host, **P**.119, **P**.684
    intermediate hosts, **P**.701, **P**.702
Echinococcus oligarthrus, **P**.677
  infection *see* Echinococcosis, polycystic
  life cycle, **P**.684–5
Echinococcus vogeli, **P**.677
  definitive host, **P**.684–5
  infection *see* Echinococcosis, polycystic
  intermediate host, **P**.684–5
  metacestode, **P**.680–1
Echinoparyphium, **P**.582–3
Echinorhynchida, **P**.597–8
Echinorhynchidae, **P**.597–8
Echinostoma, **P**.582–3
  classification, **P**.641–2
  structure/life cycle, **P**.583
Echinostomatidae, **P**.582–3
  features, **P**.582
Echinostomatoidae, **P**.582–3
  Echinostomatidae, **P**.582–3
  Fasciolidae, **P**.583
Echinostomida, **P**.579–80
Echoviruses
  antibacterial agents, **B1**.440
  antigenic variation, **V2**.876–7
  infection *see* Echovirus infection
  isolation/propagation and identification,
    V1.100, **V2**.877 (Tab.)
Echovirus infection, **V2**.875 (Tab.), **V2**.1482–3
  aseptic meningitis, **V2**.863
  CNS infection, **V2**.1424
  congenital infection, **V2**.1483
  enteroviral meningoencephalitis, **V2**.1509
  exanthems, **V2**.872
  fetal infection, **V2**.1482–3
  herpangina, **V2**.871
  neonatal infection, **V2**.1424, **V2**.1444 (Tab.),
    V2.1483
  nosocomial infection, **B1**.400
  perinatal infection, **V2**.1483
  in pregnancy, **V2**.1444 (Tab.), **V2**.1483
  prevalence, age-related, **V2**.876 (Tab.)
Echovirus-1, CNS receptors, **V2**.1406 (Tab.)
Echovirus-3 infection, **V2**.871
Echovirus-6 infection, **V2**.869–70
  persistent infection, **V2**.869
Echovirus-7, CNS receptors, **V2**.1406 (Tab.)
Echovirus-8, CNS receptors, **V2**.1406 (Tab.)
Echovirus-9 infection, **V2**.869–70
Echovirus-22, CNS receptors, **V2**.1406 (Tab.)
Ecological classification, malaria epidemiology,
  P.513

Ecological factors, emerging bacterial infection, **B1**.362

Ecological niche occupancy, viral species, **V1**.32

Econazole, **M**.183 (Tab.)
  Aspergillus otomycosis, **M**.700–1
  keratitis, **M**.309
  tinea capitis, **M**.234
  tinea corporis, **M**.186
  tinea cruris, **M**.186
  tinea manuum, **M**.186–7
  tinea nigra, **M**.186
  tinea pedis, **M**.186–7

Economic immigrants, parasitic disease spread, **P**.26–7

Economics
  African trypanosomiasis control, **P**.370
  chemotherapy/chemoprophylaxis control methods, **P**.129
  cysticercosis, **P**.119
  edible vaccines, **I**.828
  parasite control, **P**.110
  vaccination models, **I**.962, **I**.964

ECP, eosinophils, **I**.65–6

Ectoparasites, *Bartonella* transmission, **B2**.1887

Ectopic infection, paragonimiasis, **P**.650

Ectopic murine leukemia virus, **V1**.207 (Tab.)

Ectopic pregnancy, *Chlamydia trachomatis* infection, **B2**.2011, **B2**.2019–20

Ectoplasm, **P**.169

Ectromelia virus (ECTV)
  classification, **V1**.583
  immune evasion
    cytokine analogues, **V1**.316–17, **I**.620
    cytokine receptor homologues, **V1**.318, **I**.620–1
  virion maturation, **V1**.614

Eczema herpeticum, **V1**.507

Eczematous reactions, bare skin immunization, **I**.826–7

Edema
  African trypanosomiasis, **P**.365
  tissue, trichinellosis, **P**.761–2

Edge Hill virus, **V2**.998 (Tab.)

Edible vaccines (transgenic plants) *see* Vaccination

Edmonston B strain, Measles virus vaccine, **V1**.734–5

Edmonston Enders strain, Measles virus vaccine, **V1**.735

Edmonston Zagreb strain, Measles virus vaccine, **V1**.735

Education
  antibacterial control, **B1**.468
  toxocariasis control, **P**.755

Edwardsiella, **B2**.1491–2
  antibacterial susceptibility/resistance, **B2**.1491–2
  antigens, **B2**.1492
  classification, **B2**.1491
  culture, **B2**.1491
  definition, **B2**.1491
  Group GA 7752 *see Edwardsiella ictaluri*
  habitats, **B2**.1492
  infection, **B2**.1492
    intestinal, **B2**.1347

pathogenicity, **B2**.1492
  typing methods, **B2**.1492
  see also individual species

Edwardsiella aerogenes, **B2**.1352 (Tab.)

Edwardsiella anguillimortifera see Edwardsiella tarda

Edwardsiella cloacae, **B2**.1352 (Tab.)

Edwardsiella hoshinae, **B2**.1491
  antibacterial susceptibility/resistance, **B2**.1491–2
  biochemical tests, **B2**.1319 (Tab.)
  pathogenicity, **B2**.1492

Edwardsiella ictaluri, **B2**.1491
  antibacterial susceptibility/resistance, **B2**.1491–2
  biochemical tests, **B2**.1319 (Tab.)
  pathogenicity, **B2**.1492

Edwardsiella tarda, **B2**.1491
  antibacterial susceptibility/resistance, **B2**.1491–2
    intrinsic, **B2**.1352 (Tab.)
  antigens, **B2**.1492
  biochemical tests, **B2**.1319 (Tab.)
  culture, **B2**.1491
  pathogenicity, **B2**.1492
  typing methods, **B2**.1492

Efavirenz, **V2**.1623
  HIV infection, **V2**.1336
  HIV resistance, **V2**.1336
    point mutations, **V2**.1337 (Fig.)
  resistance, **V2**.1623
  structure, **V2**.1622 (Fig.)

Effective concentration (EC$_{50}$), antiviral chemotherapy, **V2**.1608–9

Effective reproduction number *(R) see* Infection(s), mathematical models

Effector cell inhibition
  helminths, **I**.686
  Paragonimus, **I**.686

'Effector' memory T cells, **I**.495, **I**.496 (Fig.)

Effectors, **B1**.45–6
  negative, **B1**.45–6
  positive, **B1**.45–6, **B1**.58

'Efferent' activation, CD8 T cells, **I**.404

Effluent irrigation, airborne bacteria, **B1**.186 (Tab.)

Eflornithine (difluormethylornithine: DFMO: Ornidyl)
  African trypanosomiasis, **P**.371
  development of, **P**.128

Eggerthelia lenta, **B2**.1028–30
  differential characteristics, **B2**.1029 (Tab.)
  pathogenicity, **B2**.1029–30

Egg inoculation, influenza viruses, **V1**.636

Eggplant mottle dwarf virus, **V2**.1107 (Fig.)

Eggs, **B1**.251, **B1**.278–9
  ammonium sulfate, **B1**.279
  Ancylostoma duodenale, **P**.720
  Ascaris lumbricoides, **P**.715, **P**.716 (Fig.)
  consistency, **B1**.278–9
  contamination, **B1**.278–9
    transmission, **B1**.278
  Cryptosporidium parvum, **P**.413 (Fig.)
  Echinococcus, **P**.678–9
  Enterobius vermicularis, **P**.716 (Fig.), **P**.717
  Fasciola gigantica, **P**.642

Fasciola hepatica, **P**.640 (Fig.), **P**.642
  heat treatment, **B1**.279
  hookworm, **P**.716 (Fig.), **P**.717
  Isospora belli, **P**.413 (Fig.)
  morphology
    clonorchiasis diagnosis, **P**.652–3
    opisthorchiasis, **P**.652–3
  Necator americanus, **P**.716 (Fig.)
  Onchocerca volvulus, **P**.782
  Opisthorchis, **P**.643
  Opisthorchis viverrini, **P**.642 (Fig.)
  Paragonimus westermani, **P**.641 (Fig.)
  pasteurization, **B1**.269, **B1**.271, **B1**.279
  pH, **B1**.279
  refrigeration, **B1**.278
  Schistosoma japonicum, **P**.627 (Fig.)
  shell physical barrier, **B1**.278
  spoilage, **B1**.278–9
  spray drying, **B1**.269
  storage temperature, **B1**.278
  Taenia solium, **P**.678–9
  tapeworms, **P**.661, **P**.661 (Fig.)
  Toxocara, **P**.751 (Fig.)
  Trichuris trichiuria, **P**.716 (Fig.), **P**.717–18
  uses, **B1**.278–9
  washing, **B1**.278–9

Egr-1 transcription factor, **I**.347

Ehrenberg, C G, **B1**.10–11

Ehrlichia
  antibacterial susceptibility/resistance, **B2**.2065–6
    antibiotics, **B2**.2065–6
    physical stability and chemical inactivation, **B2**.2065
  antigens, **B2**.2055–7
    diversity, **B2**.2053–5
  classification, **B2**.2026, **B2**.2048–9, **B2**.2049–50, **B2**.2053
  culture, **B2**.2052
  genome, **B2**.2053–5
    gene cloning, **B2**.2053–5
  GroESL heat shock protein, **B2**.2055–6
  habitats, hosts and diseases, **B2**.2049 (Tab.), **B2**.2050–1
  infection *see* Ehrlichiosis
  isolation/identification, **B2**.2052, **B2**.2057
  lysosomal killing resistance, **I**.651
  metabolism, **B2**.2053
  microenvironment, **B2**.2051
  morphology, **B2**.2051
  replication, **B2**.2052
  staining procedures, **B2**.2051–2
  surface_Ag_2 proteins, **B2**.2055–6
  ticks transmission, **B2**.2066–7

Ehrlichia bovis, **B2**.2049–50

Ehrlichia canis
  antigens
    diversity, **B2**.2055
    genes, **B2**.2053–5
    MAP2, **B2**.2056
  classification, **B2**.2026, **B2**.2027 (Fig.), **B2**.2049–50
  habitats, hosts and diseases, **B2**.2049 (Tab.), **B2**.2050–1
  identification and typing methods, **B2**.2057

Ehrlichia canis (Continued)
  infection, **B2**.2059
Ehrlichia chaffeensis
  antibiotic sensitivity, **B2**.2065–6
  antigens, **B2**.2055–7
    diversity, **B2**.2055
    genes, **B2**.2053–5
    MAP2, **B2**.2056
  habitats, **B2**.2049 (Tab.)
  hosts, **B2**.2027 (Fig.)
  infection *see Ehrlichia chaffeensis* infection
  isolation/identification, **B2**.2057
  microenvironment and morphology, **B2**.2051,
    B2.2052 (Fig.)
Ehrlichia chaffeensis infection, **B1**.362,
    B2.2049 (Tab.), **B2**.2057–9
  characteristics, **B2**.2057–8, **B2**.2058 (Tab.)
  diagnosis, **B2**.2057–8, **B2**.2063–5
    culture-based assays, **B2**.2065
    molecular diagnostic assays, **B2**.2064–5
    patient samples, **B2**.2058–9
    serological assays, **B2**.2063–4
    specimen collection, **B2**.2063–5
  epidemiology and natural history, **B2**.2061–2
    immunocompromised patients, **B2**.2058
  hospitalization, **B2**.2058
  pathogenesis, **B2**.2058–9
  tick testing as a predictor of disease,
    B2.2066–7
  treatment, **B2**.2066
  see also Ehrlichiosis
Ehrlichia ewingii
  classification, **B2**.2027 (Fig.)
  habitats, **B2**.2049 (Tab.), **B2**.2050–1
  hosts, **B2**.2049 (Tab.), **B2**.2050–1
  infection, **B2**.2049 (Tab.), **B2**.2050–1,
    B2.2058 (Tab.), **B2**.2059
    epidemiology and natural history,
      B2.2061–2
    tick testing as a predictor of disease,
      B2.2066–7
    treatment, **B2**.2066
  isolation/identification, **B2**.2057
  surface antigen genes, **B2**.2053–5
Ehrlichia muris
  habitats, hosts and diseases, **B2**.2049 (Tab.)
  surface antigen genes, **B2**.2053–5
Ehrlichia phagocytophila see Anaplasma
    phagocytophilum (Ehrlichia
    phagocytophilia)
Ehrlichia risticii
  genome, **B2**.2053
  microenvironment and morphology, **B2**.2051,
    B2.2052 (Fig.)
Ehrlichia ruminantium
  antigens, **B2**.2056–7
    genes, **B2**.2053–5
    MAP2, **B2**.2056
  classification, **B2**.2027 (Fig.)
  habitats, hosts and diseases, **B2**.2049 (Tab.),
    B2.2050–1
  identification and typing methods, **B2**.2057
Ehrlichiosis, **B2**.2049 (Tab.), **B2**.2057–9,
    B2.2058 (Tab.)
  clinical features, **B2**.2058 (Tab.)
  epidemiology and natural history, **B2**.2061–3

"ewingii" *(Ehrlichia ewingi),* **B2**.2059
  human, **B1**.362
  human granulocytic *see Anaplasma*
    phagocytophilum (Ehrlichia
    phagocytophilia), infection (human
    anaplasmosis)
  prevention, **B2**.2066
  specimen collection and diagnosis, **B2**.2063–5
  transmission, pathogenesis, and clinical
    manifestations, **B2**.2057–61
Ehrlich, Paul, **B1**.6, **B1**.155
  autoimmune disease, **I**.748
  complement, **I**.141
Eichstedt, C, **M**.14–5
eIF2, protein synthesis, **V1**.222
eIF4E, **V1**.112
  viral interference, **V1**.120–1
eIF4F, protein synthesis, **V1**.222–3
eIF4G, protein synthesis, **V1**.140
Eikenella
  classification, **B2**.1271
  habitats, **B2**.1649–50
Eikenella corrodens, **B1**.296 (Tab.), **B2**.1666–8
  antibacterial susceptibility/resistance,
    B2.1668
  characteristics, **B2**.1668 (Tab.)
  culture, **B2**.1667–8
  infection, **B2**.1667
    clinical significance, **B2**.1667
    endocarditis, **B1**.532
    gingivitis, **B1**.614
  isolation/identification, **B2**.1667–8
  taxonomy, **B2**.1666
  virulence and pathogenicity, **B2**.1666
Eiken test, **M**.109
Eimeria
  flagellum, **P**.180 (Fig.)
  merozoites, **P**.177 (Fig.), **P**.178 (Fig.)
  oocysts, **P**.167 (Fig.)
  structure, **P**.177 (Fig.)
    membranes, **P**.163 (Tab.)
Eimeria maxima, macrogamete, **P**.167 (Fig.)
ELA-2 gene, severe combined neutropenia,
    I.765
Elastase
  Aspergillus, **M**.688, **M**.692, **M**.706, **M**.707
  Pseudomonas aeruginosa, **B2**.1600–1
Elastase-2 gene mutations, severe combined
    neutropenia, **I**.765
ELC *see* Epstein–Barr virus-induced receptor
    ligand chemokine (ELC:CCL19)
Elderly patients
  antibiotic-associated diarrhea, **B2**.1120
  bacteriuria, **B1**.394
  hematogenous infection of the spine,
    B1.684–5
  influenza, **V1**.661
  microsporidiosis, **P**.539
  nosocomial infection, **B1**.394–5
    pneumonia, **B1**.394
  susceptibility to viral infection, **V1**.264
  VZV infection, **V1**.514
  see also Age
Electrocardiography (ECG)
  Chagas disease, **P**.384–5
  mumps, **V1**.750

Electrochemical potential (δp), **B1**.64
Electroencephalography (EEG), subacute
    sclerosing panencephalitis (SSPE),
    V2.1432
Electron acceptors
  aerobic respiration, **B1**.64
  anaerobic respiration, **B1**.65, **B1**.66, **B1**.67
  carbon compounds, **B1**.67
  halocarbons, **B1**.67
  inorganic compounds, **B1**.65
  organic compounds, **B1**.54
  oxidized metals, **B1**.67
  oxygen, **B1**.65
  sulfur, **B1**.66
Electron carriers, in bacterial respiration,
    B1.63–4
Electron cryomicroscopy *see* Cryoelectron
    microscopy
Electron donors, anaerobic respiration, **B1**.66,
    B1.67
Electron microscopy, **B1**.714
  advantages, **V2**.1534–5
  Bartonella classification, **B2**.1887
  in diagnosis, **V2**.1534–5
  historical aspects, **V1**.6
  limitations, **V2**.1534
  negative contrast (staining), **V1**.6
  poxvirus intracellular mature virus, **V1**.597
  prion protein structure, **V2**.1354 (Fig.)
  progressive multifocal leucoencephalopathy
    (PML), **V2**.1418
  soil bacteria analysis, **B1**.207
  Tropheryma whippelii, **B2**.1002
  viruses
    astrovirus detection, **V2**.889, **V2**.905–6
    astroviruses, **V2**.890–1
    filoviruses, **V2**.1096–7, **V2**.1097 (Tab.)
    helical viruses, **V1**.59–60, **V1**.59 (Fig.),
      V1.60 (Fig.)
    Human astrovirus, **V2**.890–1
    isocahedral viruses, **V1**.62
    Mononegavirales, **V1**.380–1
    noroviruses, **V2**.912, **V2**.921
    rotaviruses, **V2**.952
    sapoviruses, **V2**.925
Electron transport
  chemotaxonomy, **B1**.24
  photosynthesis, **B1**.67–8
Electroporation
  artificial competence, **B1**.100
  DNA vaccine delivery, **I**.917
  skin immunization, **I**.822
Elek immunoprecipitation test, **B2**.984
  diphtheria diagnosis, **B1**.612–13
Elementary body (EB), *Chlamydia,* **B2**.2007–9,
    B2.2008 (Fig.)
Elephantiasis, **P**.774, **P**.774 (Fig.)
11-S regulators, proteasomes, **I**.411
Elford, William, **V1**.24–5
'Elimination of disease,' **P**.108–9
'Elimination of infection'
  bacteriology, **B1**.345
  parasitology, **P**.108–9
ELISAs *see* Enzyme-linked immunosorbent
    assay (ELISA)
ELISPOT, MHC class I–peptide binding, **I**.407

El Moro Canyon virus, **V2**.1666 (Tab.)

Elongation factor gene (EFG-α), *Blastocystis hominis*, **P**.562–3

ELR motif, chemokines, **I**.221

Embden–Meyerhoff pathway, *Schistosoma*, **P**.605–6

Embryonated eggs, **V1**.90
  infection diagnosis, **V2**.1539
  influenza diagnosis, **V1**.674
  virus culture, **V1**.4–5

Emerging infection
  bacterial, **B1**.317, **B1**.355, **B1.359–67**
    antibiotic resistance, **B1**.362–4
    bioterrorism, **B1**.364–5
    definitions, **B1**.359
    demographic changes causing, **B1**.359–60
    ecological changes causing, **B1**.362
    land use patterns, **B1**.362
    microbial adaptation/change causing, **B1**.362–4
    public health infrastructure, **B1**.364
    societal changes causing, **B1**.360–1
    technology changes causing, **B1**.361–2
    travel and commerce role, **B1**.360
    see also individual species/infection
  viral infection, **V2**.1648 (Tab.), **V2.1646–69**
    advanced medical care, **V2**.1660
    agricultural practices, **V2**.1660–1
    behavioral factors, **V2**.1658–62
      day care centers, **V2**.1659
      domestic pets, **V2**.1659–60
      epidemiology, **V2**.1661–2
      sexual behavior, **V2**.1659
      transportation, **V2**.1658–9
    bioterrorism, **V2**.1660
    common source epidemics, **V2**.1662
    environmental factors, **V2**.1662–5
      arthropod vectors, **V2**.1658
    host factors, **V2**.1655–8
      age, **V2**.1655
      immune response, **V2**.1655
      persistent infection, **V2**.1655–6
      resistance *vs.* virulence, **V2**.1656–7
      'species-jumping,' **V2**.1657–8
      spread in, **V2**.1658
    laboratory safety, **V2**.1515, **V2**.1518
    prevention/control, **V2**.1665–7
      interventional phase, **V2**.1667
      investigative phase, **V2**.1665
    propagated epidemics, **V2**.1661
    quasi-species, **V1**.193
    recognition, **V2**.1646–52, **V2**.1667 (Fig.)
      PCR, **V2**.1646–7
    virus factors, **V2**.1652–5
      epidemic potential, **V2**.1655
      mutations, **V2**.1652–4
      polygenic variation, **V2**.1652
      reassortment, **V2**.1654
      recombination, **V2**.1654
  see also specific organisms

Emetic syndrome, **B1**.285

Emmons, C W, **M**.16, **M**.23, **M**.26, **M**.32

Emmonsia, **M**.809, **M**.811–12, **M**.818, **M**.819 (Fig.)
  Blastomyces dermatitidis, **M**.810 (Tab.), **M**.811–12, **M**.817, **M**.818, **M**.819–20, **M**.819 (Fig.), **M**.821
    classification, **M**.811, **M**.819–20
  Coccidioides immitis, **M**.809, **M**.810 (Tab.), **M**.811, **M**.820
    ecology, **M**.810 (Tab.), **M**.812
  Histoplasma capsulatum, **M**.810 (Tab.), **M**.811, **M**.817, **M**.820
    history, **M**.26
    infection *see* Adiaspiromycosis
    mating studies, **M**.819–20
    meiotic stage, **M**.811–12
  Paracoccidioides brasiliensis, **M**.810 (Tab.), **M**.811, **M**.820
  see also Emmonsia crescens; Emmonsia parva

Emmonsia crescens, **M**.21–2, **M**.809
  adiaspores, **M**.809, **M**.811, **M**.815 (Fig.), **M**.816, **M**.817 (Fig.)
  classification, **M**.811
  ecology, **M**.810 (Tab.), **M**.812
  geographical distribution, **M**.810 (Tab.), **M**.812, **M**.820–1
  histopathology, **M**.815, **M**.815 (Fig.), **M**.816 (Fig.), **M**.817 (Fig.)
  history, **M**.26, **M**.811
  infection, **M**.813–14
    animals, **M**.812
    human, **M**.813–14
    immune response, **M**.816–17
    therapy, **M**.821
    see also Adiaspiromycosis
  meiotic stage, **M**.811–12, **M**.819–20, **M**.820 (Fig.), **M**.821 (Fig.)
  mycology, **M**.810 (Tab.), **M**.818, **M**.818 (Fig.), **M**.819 (Fig.), **M**.821

Emmonsia parva, **M**.21–2, **M**.809
  adiaspores, **M**.816
  classification, **M**.811
  ecology, **M**.810 (Tab.), **M**.812
  geographical distribution, **M**.810 (Tab.), **M**.812
  history, **M**.26, **M**.811
  infection
    AIDS, **M**.814–15
    bone, **M**.818
    immune response, **M**.817
    osteomyelitis, **M**.818
    osteomyelosis, **M**.818
    therapy, **M**.821
    unconfirmed reports, **M**.815
    see also Adiaspiromycosis
  morphology, **M**.74
  mycology, **M**.810 (Tab.), **M**.818, **M**.818 (Fig.), **M**.821

Emmonsia pasteuriana
  classification, **M**.811–12
  diagnosis, **M**.809
  ecology, **M**.809
  geographical distribution, **M**.809
  infection, AIDS, **M**.809, **M**.818
  mycology, **M**.809, **M**.818

Emmonsiella capsulata, **M**.520, **M**.521

Emotional disturbances, Japanese encephalitis, **V2**.1424–5

Emotional lability, babesiosis, **P**.454

Empyema
  diagnosis and treatment, **B1**.641–3
  pneumonia complication, **B1**.632, **B1**.641–3
  streptococcal, **B1**.244–5, **B1**.632

E^{ms} protein *see* Pestiviruses

Emtricitabine, **V2**.1621
  HIV infection, **V2**.1334
    point mutation resistance, **V2**.1337 (Fig.)
    structure, **V2**.1620 (Fig.)

Emtriva *see* Emtricitabine

Emulsions, as adjuvants, **I**.928 (Tab.)

ENA-78 (CXCL5) *see* CXCL5 (ENA-78)

Encapsidation signal ( ), Hepatitis B virus, **V2**.1235–6

Encapsulated bacteria *see* Infection(s), bacterial

Encapsulation, DNA vaccine delivery, **I**.913

Encephalitis
  Eastern equine encephalitis virus infection, **V2**.1019
  enterovirus infection, **V2**.871
    Enterovirus 70, **V2**.1423
  frequency in viral infection, **V2**.1416 (Tab.)
  measles, **V2**.1431
    measles inclusion body (MIBE), **V2**.1431
  mumps, **V2**.1430
  Murray Valley, **V2**.1424, **V2**.1426
  reovirus infection, **V2**.937
  Russian spring-summer, **V2**.1424, **V2**.1426
  toxoplasmosis, **P**.432
  viral tick-borne, **B1**.231
  VZV infection, **V2**.1422

Encephalitozoon
  classification, **P**.190–1, **P**.198, **P**.534
  historical aspects, **P**.535–6
  human infection
    disseminated infection, **P**.542
    transmission, **P**.543–4
    see also Microsporidiosis
  meront, **P**.534
  public health importance, **P**.45
  serology, **P**.536
  see also Microsporidians; *individual species*

Encephalitozoon cuniculi, **M**.69, **P**.189
  human infection
    AIDS, **P**.539, **P**.541
    disseminated infection, **P**.536, **P**.541, **P**.542
    enteric infection, **P**.538–9
    infection in AIDS, **M**.69
    renal failure, **P**.542
    transmission, **P**.544
    see also Microsporidiosis
  in vitro culture, **P**.546, **P**.548
    albendazole effects, **P**.548
    resistance to chemical agents, **P**.550

Encephalitozoon hellem, **P**.189
  avian infection, **P**.544
  classification, **P**.541
  disseminated infection, **P**.543
    albendazole treatment, **P**.550
    respiratory infection, **P**.542, **P**.543
    transmission, **P**.544

Encephalitozoon hellem,
 disseminated infection (*Continued*)
  see also Microsporidiosis
 in vitro culture, **P**.546, **P**.548
 ocular disease, **P**.541
 pH effects, **P**.550
 structure/life cycle
  spores, **P**.530 (Fig.), **P**.532–3, **P**.532 (Fig.),
   P.533 (Fig.)
  sporonts, **P**.532 (Fig.)
  sporoplasm, **P**.532 (Fig.)
Encephalitozoon intestinalis, **P**.189
 human infection
  disseminated infection, **P**.542
  rhinosinusitis, **P**.542
  transmission, **P**.544
  treatment, **P**.548–9
  see also Microsporidiosis
 in vitro culture, **P**.546, **P**.548
Encephalomyocarditis, **V1**.371 (Tab.)
 IL-18, **I**.290–2
 NK cells, **I**.96
Encephalomyocarditis virus, **V1**.50
Encephalopathy
 African trypanosomiasis, **P**.365
 cat-scratch disease, **B2**.1892
 hyperammonaemic, **B2**.1447
Encystation, **P**.165
Encystation-specific vesicles (ESVs), *Giardia,*
 P.243
Encystment, *Toxoplasma gondii,* **I**.677
Endemic infection
 basic reproductive number of infection (*R*₀),
  P.52
 definition, **B1**.310
 dynamic equilibria, **I**.956–7
Endemic outbreaks, definition, **V1**.358
Endocarditis
 aspergillosis, **M**.700, **M**.705, **M**.711, **M**.719
  invasive, **M**.700, **M**.705, **M**.711, **M**.719
 Blastoschizomyces capitatus, **M**.625
 candidiasis, **M**.98, **M**.595, **M**.600
Endocarditis, infective
 acute, **B1**.525
 Bartonella
  B. henselae infection, **B2**.1894
  B. quintana infection, **B2**.1894
  HIV infection, **B2**.1894
 blood cultures, **B1**.511–12, **B1**.537
  negative, **B1**.533, **B1**.537
 causative organisms, **B1**.528–33,
  B1.528 (Tab.)
  Actinobacillus actinomycetemcomitans,
   B2.1663
  Bartonella see above
  Cardiobacterium hominis, **B2**.1671–2
  Eikenella corrodens, **B2**.1667
  Enterococci, **B1**.528–31, **B1**.539
  Enterococcus, **B2**.896
  Erysipelothrix rhusiopathiae, **B2**.970–1,
   B2.974
  Gordonia sputi, **B2**.1152
  gram-negative bacilli, **B1**.532
  HACEK group, **B1**.532, **B1**.533, **B1**.537,
   B1.540
  human brucellosis, **B2**.1738

Kingella kingae, **B2**.1670
  Nocardia asteroides, **B2**.1158
  Propionibacterium acnes, **B2**.1032
  Q fever, **B1**.748, **B2**.2076
  rapidly growing mycobacteria, **B2**.1249–50,
   B2.1252, **B2**.1255, **B2**.1261
  Salmonella, **B1**.532
  *Staphyloccus aureus see Staphylococcus
   aureus* infection
  Staphylococci, **B1**.531–2, **B1**.535,
   B1.539–40
  Stenotrophomonas maltophilia, **B2**.1636–7
  streptococci, **B1**.244–5, **B1**.248, **B1**.528–31,
   B1.539
 chronic, **B1**.525
 classification, **B1**.525
 clinical features, **B1**.525, **B1**.534,
  B1.534 (Fig.), **B1**.534 (Tab.)
  peripheral manifestations, **B1**.528
 complications, **B1**.534
 'culture-negative', **B1**.533–41
  clinical complications, **B1**.534–5
  fastidious organisms, **B1**.533
  previous antibiotics, **B1**.533
  special isolation techniques, **B1**.533
  Tropheryma whippelii, **B2**.999
 definition, **B1**.524–5
 diagnosis, **B1**.535–8
  culture, **B1**.537
  echocardiography, **B1**.536–7
  medical history, **B1**.536
  molecular methods, **B1**.537–8
  serology, **B1**.537
 epidemiology, **B1**.525–6
  incidence, **B1**.525
  intravenous drug users, **B1**.526, **B1**.527,
   B1.531, **B1**.533
  mortality, **B1**.525
 intracranial abscess complication, **B1**.583,
  B1.585
 laboratory findings, **B1**.536
 'malignant', **B1**.526–7
 'marantic,' **B1**.526–7
 medical history, **B1**.536
 'mural,' **B1**.526–7
 native valve
  community-acquired, **B1**.531–2
  hospital-acquired, **B1**.525–6
 nosocomial, **B1**.526
 pathogenesis, **B1**.526–8
 predisposing conditions, **B1**.525–6, **B1**.536
 prevention, **B1**.541
 prosthetic valve, **B1**.392, **B1**.526, **B1**.528,
  B1.531–2, **B1**.538
  early, **B1**.538
  features, **B1**.538
  frequency, **B1**.538
  late, **B1**.538
  mortality, **B1**.538–9
  prevention, **B1**.541
 right-sided, **B1**.535
 subacute, **B1**.525, **B1**.529
 surgery, **B1**.540–1
 treatment, **B1**.539–41
  guidelines, **B1**.539
 vegetations, **B1**.526–8, **B1**.534, **B1**.536

Endocrine signals, development, **V1**.334
Endocrinology, *Taenia solium,* **P**.683
Endocytosis
 antigen uptake by APCs, **I**.382
 influenza virus, **V1**.107–8
 macrophages, **I**.25, **I**.26 (Fig.)
 Nidovirales order, **V1**.395
 parvoviruses, **V1**.417
 Trypanosoma brucei, **P**.355, **P**.357 (Fig.)
 viral replication, **V1**.107–8
Endodyogeny, **P**.181, **P**.183 (Fig.), **P**.425
 Blastocystis hominis, **P**.560–1
Endogenous avian virus (EAV), risk in vaccine
 production, **V2**.1297
Endogenous retroviruses, **V1**.182
Endogenous viruses, genomes, **V1**.181–2
Endolimax, classification, **P**.197, **P**.218
Endolimax nana, **P**.187, **P**.200, **P**.218, **P**.223
 Blastocystis hominis vs., **P**.565
 cysts, **P**.223, **P**.223 (Fig.)
 infection
  AIDS patients, **P**.223
  immune response, **P**.218–19
  treatment withholding, **P**.220
 life cycle, **P**.219
 trophozoites, **P**.223
Endolymphatic labyrinthitis, mumps, **V1**.750
Endometritis, *Chlamydia trachomatis* infection,
 B2.2010–11, **B2**.2011 (Fig.)
Endonuclease G, mitochondria apoptosis, **I**.132
Endonuclease, repair of UV-induced DNA
 damage, **B1**.451–2
Endonuclease restriction analysis, influenza
 diagnosis, **V1**.677
Endophagy (indoor feeding), mosquito
 (*Anopheles*), **P**.470
Endophthalmitis, **M**.317, **M**.317–27, **B1**.602–4
 after intraocular surgery, **B1**.386
 causative agents, **M**.317
  Acremonium, **M**.317, **M**.326
  Alternaria, **M**.323
  Aspergillus, **M**.317, **M**.318, **M**.320, **M**.322,
   M.700, **M**.719
  Aspergillus fumigatus, **M**.317, **M**.323,
   M.330 (Fig.)
  Aspergillus terreus, **M**.322
  Blastomyces dermatitidis, **M**.317, **M**.324
  Candida, **M**.317, **M**.318–19, **M**.319–20,
   M.320–1, **M**.329–30, **M**.586, **M**.601
  Coccidioides immitis, **M**.317
  Cryptococcus, **M**.317, **M**.648
  Curvularia lunata, **M**.323
  dematiaceous fungi, **M**.323
  Exophiala jeanselmei var. *jeanselmei*
   infection, **M**.323
  Fusarium, **M**.317, **M**.326
  histoplasmosis, **M**.317, **M**.325
  Lasiodiplopodia theobromae, **M**.323
  Microsphaeropsis olivacea, **M**.323
  Paecilomyces, **M**.317
  Paecilomyces lilacinus, **M**.326–7, **M**.330
  Pneumocystis carinii, **M**.317
  Scedosporium apiospermum, **M**.317,
   M.323–4
  sporotrichosis, **M**.317, **M**.325–6
  zygomycetes, **M**.326

Endophthalmitis (*Continued*)
  clinical manifestations, **B1**.603
  definitions, **M**.317–27
  diagnosis, **M**.318, **B1**.603
  Enterococcus faecalis, **B2**.896
  occurrence, **M**.317–18
  post-traumatic, *Bacillus cereus,* **B2**.940
  predisposing factors, **M**.318, **B1**.602–3
  therapy, **M**.319
    amphotericin B, **M**.319, **M**.320, **M**.321–4,
      M.326–7
    fluconazole, **M**.319, **M**.321–4, **M**.326–7
    intravitreal corticosteroids, **M**.320
    intravitreal dexamethasone, **M**.320
    itraconazole, **M**.319
    ketoconazole, **M**.319, **M**.320, **M**.326–7
    miconazole, **M**.319, **M**.320, **M**.326–7
    natamycin, **M**.320
  treatment, **B1**.604
Endoplasm, **P**.169
Endoplasmic reticulum (ER)
  MHC class I assembly, **I**.408
  MHC class II-peptide binding, **I**.382–3
  protozoa, **P**.174–5
  rough (rER), **P**.174–5
  smooth (sER), **P**.174–5
Endoplasmic reticulum-associated degradation
    (ERAD), **I**.414
Endopolygeny, **P**.185
Endoscopic retrograde
    cholangiopancreatography (ERCP)
  ascariasis diagnosis, **P**.730
  cryptosporidiosis, **P**.405
  fascioliasis, **P**.650
  paragonimiasis diagnosis, **P**.653
Endoscopy
  Anisakis diagnosis, **P**.817
  fibreoptic
    decontamination, **B1**.380
    nosocomial infection from, **B1**.380
    organisms transmitted by, **B1**.380
    Mycobacterium, **B2**.1217
  neurocysticercosis treatment, **P**.696
Endosomes
  antigen processing, **I**.414, **I**.415
  MHC class I–peptide interactions, **I**.415
Endospores, *Bacillus see Bacillus,* endospores
Endothelial cells
  G-CSF production, **I**.276
  GM-CSF production, **I**.277
  Histoplasma capsulatum var. *capsulatum*
    phagocytosis, **M**.526–7, **M**.528 (Fig.)
  MHC class I antigen presentation, **I**.426–7
  neutrophil interactions, **I**.38
  septic shock, **I**.700–1
  virus dissemination, **V1**.242–3
Endothelial leukocyte adhesion molecule 1
    (ELAM), **I**.697
Endothelium, lymphocyte trafficking into CNS,
    V2.1411, **V2**.1411 (Fig.)
Endotoxin(s), **B1**.157–60
  airborne dispersal, **B1**.189
  Bordetella, **B2**.1796
  Burkholderia cepacia complex, **B2**.1617
  Haemophilus influenzae type b (Hib), **B1**.557

  hygiene hypothesis, **I**.738–9
  see also Lipopolysaccharide (LPS)
δ-Endotoxin (crystalline protein), *B.*
    thuringiensis, **B1**.203–4
Endpoint determination, susceptibility testing,
    M.156
Energy metabolism
  tapeworms, **P**.662
  Trypanosoma brucei, **P**.359
Enfurvirtide, **V2**.1625
Engyododontium alba, oculomycoses,
    M.275 (Tab.)
Enhancers
  gene transcription, **V1**.113
  neurovirulence, **V2**.1407
  viral RNA metabolism, **V1**.220
Enolase, *Candida,* **M**.100, **M**.591, **M**.607
Enoxacin, *Listeria,* **B2**.957–8
Enoyl-ACP reductase, **B1**.436–8, **B1**.441,
    B1.443–4
E-NPP3 (CD203c), **I**.63
Enrichment media, **B1**.37–8
  Salmonella culture, **B2**.1400
Enrofloxacin, spectrum of activity, **B1**.492
Entamoeba
  Blastocystis hominis vs., **P**.565
  classification, **P**.197
  see also individual species
Entamoeba chattoni, **P**.200, **P**.218, **P**.222–3
  animal reservoirs, **P**.219, **P**.222
  cysts, **P**.223 (Fig.)
  epidemiology, **P**.222
Entamoeba coli, **P**.187, **P**.200, **P**.218, **P**.220–1
  cysts, **P**.220 (Fig.)
  incidence, **P**.220
  infection
    immune response, **P**.218–19
    pathogenicity, **P**.221
    treatment withholding, **P**.220
  life cycle, **P**.219
  trophozoites, **P**.220–1
Entamoeba dispar, **P**.200, **P**.201, **P**.206
  classification, **P**.191
  detection, **P**.211
  epidemiology, **P**.212
Entamoeba ecuadoriensis, **P**.222
Entamoeba gingivalis, **P**.187, **P**.218, **P**.221
  infection
    diagnosis, **P**.220
    HIV infection, **P**.221
    periodontal disease, **P**.221
    treatment, **P**.220
  transmission, **P**.221
  trophozoites, **P**.221, **P**.221 (Fig.)
Entamoeba hartmanni, **P**.200
  classification, **P**.191
Entamoeba histolytica, **P**.187, **P**.200–1, **I**.679
  biochemistry, **P**.204–6
    enzymes, **P**.204–5, **P**.205–6
    glycoproteins, **P**.202, **P**.205
    isoenzyme patterns (zymodemes), **P**.200–1,
      P.211
    lipid metabolism, **P**.204
    lytic factor, **P**.205–6
    metabolism, **P**.204–5

    nucleic acid metabolism, **P**.204
    plasma membrane, **P**.205
    protein metabolism, **P**.204
    pyruvate degradation, **P**.204
    surface molecules, **P**.205
  classification, **P**.191, **P**.201, **I**.675–6
  cysts, **P**.214
  Entamoeba dispar relationship, **P**.200–1
  galactose adhesin, **P**.205
  genetics/molecular biology, **P**.206
    DNA, **P**.206
    genes cloned, **P**.206
  historical aspects, **P**.13
  immune evasion, **P**.209
  immune response, **P**.75, **P**.208–10
    monoclonal antibodies, **P**.211
  infection *see* Amebiasis
  invasion/infection process, **P**.205–6
  life-cycle, **P**.204
  locomotory system, **P**.178 (Fig.)
  strains, **P**.200–1
    invasive (pathogenic), **P**.200–1
    noninvasive (nonpathogenic), **P**.201
  structure, **P**.201–4
    cell morphology, **P**.201–2, **P**.201 (Fig.)
    chromatoid bodies, **P**.202, **P**.203
    cylindrical particles in, **P**.203
    cyst, **P**.203, **P**.204 (Fig.)
    cyst wall, **P**.166
    cytoplasm, **P**.169 (Fig.), **P**.202–3
    cytoskeleton, **P**.202–3
    lobopodia, **P**.201–2
    mitochondria, **P**.202
    molecular chaperones, **P**.202
    nucleus, **P**.203
    plasma membrane, **P**.202
    pyridine nucleotide transhydrogenase,
      P.202
    ribosomes, **P**.202
    trophozoite, **P**.201–2, **P**.201 (Fig.),
      P.202 (Fig.), **P**.203 (Fig.)
    vacuoles/lysosomes, **P**.202
Entamoeba invadens, **P**.200, **P**.203
Entamoeba moshkovskii, **P**.200, **P**.218, **P**.221–2
  classification, **P**.191
  cysts, **P**.222
  genome sequencing, **P**.219
  isolates, **P**.221
  life cycle, **P**.219
  trophozoites, **P**.222, **P**.222 (Fig.)
Entamoeba polecki, **P**.218, **P**.222–3
  cysts, **P**.222 (Fig.)
  infection
    epidemiology, **P**.222
    treatment withholding, **P**.220
  life cycle, animal reservoirs, **P**.219
  trophozoites, **P**.222
Entamoebidea, **P**.201
Entecavir, **V2**.1625
  structure, **V2**.1621 (Fig.)
Enteric disease, edible vaccine, **I**.829
Enteric fever
  immune response, **B1**.744
  Salmonella infection, **B2**.1424
  Widal reaction, **B1**.744

Enteric group 1 *see Escherichia vulneris*
Enteric group 8 *see Kluyvera*
Enteric group 9 *see Enterobacter sakazakii*
Enteric group 10 *see Escherichia fergusonii*
Enteric group 11 *see Escherichia hermannii*
Enteric group 15 *see Cedecea*
Enteric group 17 *see Enterobacter asburiae*
Enteric group 19 *see Enterobacter cancerogenus*
Enteric group 40 *see Ewingella americana*
Enteric group 41 *see Leclercia adecarboxylata*
Enteric group 45 *see Yokenella regensburgei*
Enteric group 46 *see Moellerella wisconsensis*
Enteric group 47 *see Klebsiella*
Enteric group 57 *see Leminorella*
Enteric group 59, **B2**.1319 (Tab.)
Enteric group 63, **B2**.1319 (Tab.)
Enteric group 64, **B2**.1319 (Tab.)
Enteric group 75 *see Enterobacter hormaechei*
Enteric infection
   Dysgonomonas capnocytophagoides, **B2**.1677–8
  microsporidiosis *see* Microsporidiosis
Enteric RNA viruses *see* RNA viruses
Enteritis
  infantile, *Escherichia coli,* enteropathogenic, **B2**.1372–4
  sarcocystosis, **P**.448
Enteritis necroticans ('Darmbrand'), **B2**.1118–19
Enteroaggregative *Escherichia coli* (EAggEC) *see Escherichia coli,* enteroaggregative (EAggEC)
Enterobacter, **B2**.1483–7
  antibacterial susceptibility/resistance, **B2**.1484–6
  antigens, **B2**.1486
  biochemistry, **B2**.1484
  capsules, **B2**.1343
  characteristics, **B2**.1483–4, **B2**.1485 (Tab.)
  classification, **B2**.1483–4
  culture, **B2**.1484
    morphology, **B2**.1345 (Tab.)
    temperature, **B2**.1344
  definition, **B2**.1483
  fimbriae, **B2**.1342–3
  habitats, **B2**.1486–7
  infection
    bacteremia, **B1**.521
    intestinal, **B2**.1347
    intracranial abscess, **B1**.585
    keratitis, **B1**.601
    nosocomial infection, **B1**.398 (Tab.)
  isolation/identification
    biochemical tests, **B2**.1484
    gelatin liquefaction, **B2**.1351
    historical perspective, **B2**.1351
    screening tests, **B2**.1349 (Tab.)
    typing methods, **B2**.1486
  morphology, **B2**.1484
  normal microbiota, **B1**.296 (Tab.)
  pathogenicity, **B2**.1486–7
  soil pathogens, **B1**.203
  waterborne, **B1**.221, **B1**.222–3

Enterobacter aerogenes, **B2**.1483
  antibacterial susceptibility/resistance, **B2**.1486
  antigens, **B2**.1486
  biochemical tests, **B2**.1319 (Tab.), **B2**.1484
  characteristics, **B2**.1485 (Tab.)
  infection
    extraintestinal, **B2**.1346–7
    nosocomial, **B1**.398 (Tab.)
  pathogenicity, **B2**.1486–7
  typing methods, **B2**.1486
  waterborne, **B1**.211–12
Enterobacter agglomerans complex, **B2**.1483–4
  biochemical tests, **B2**.1319 (Tab.)
  classification/nomenclature, **B2**.1337
    DNA–DNA hybridization, **B2**.1337
  culture, pigment production, **B2**.1345
  DNA 3, **B2**.1319 (Tab.)
  DNA 13 *see Pantoea agglomerans*
Enterobacter amnigenus, **B2**.1483
  biochemical tests, **B2**.1319 (Tab.)
  characteristics, **B2**.1485 (Tab.)
Enterobacter asburiae, **B2**.1483–4
  biochemical tests, **B2**.1319 (Tab.), **B2**.1484
  characteristics, **B2**.1485 (Tab.)
Enterobacter cancerogena see Enterobacter cancerogenus
Enterobacter cancerogenus, **B2**.1483
  biochemical tests, **B2**.1319 (Tab.), **B2**.1484
  characteristics, **B2**.1485 (Tab.)
  classification/nomenclature, **B2**.1337–8
  pathogenicity, **B2**.1487
Enterobacter cloacae, **B2**.1483
  antibacterial susceptibility/resistance, **B2**.1485
  antigens, **B2**.1486
  biochemical tests, **B2**.1319 (Tab.), **B2**.1484
  characteristics, **B2**.1485 (Tab.)
  DNA–DNA analysis, **B2**.1338
  infection
    extraintestinal, **B2**.1346–7
    nosocomial infection, **B1**.398 (Tab.)
  pathogenicity, **B2**.1486–7
  typing methods, **B2**.1486
  waterborne, **B1**.211–12, **B1**.220
Enterobacter dissolvens, **B2**.1483–4
  biochemical tests, **B2**.1319 (Tab.)
Enterobacter gergoviae, **B2**.1483–4
  biochemical tests, **B2**.1319 (Tab.), **B2**.1484
  characteristics, **B2**.1485 (Tab.)
Enterobacter hormaechei, **B2**.1483, **B2**.1484
  biochemical tests, **B2**.1319 (Tab.), **B2**.1484
  characteristics, **B2**.1485 (Tab.)
Enterobacteriaceae, **B2**.1317–59, **B2**.1474–506
  antibacterial susceptibility/resistance, **B1**.442, **B2**.1352–4
    acquired, **B2**.1352
    epidemiology, **B2**.1354
    identification, **B2**.1354
    intrinsic, **B2**.1352, **B2**.1352 (Tab.)
  antibiotic susceptibility testing, **B2**.1352–4
  antigens, **B2**.1339–44
    cell envelope, **B2**.1340–1
    cell wall, **B2**.1340–1

enterobacterial common antigen, **B2**.1343–4
  F antigen, **B2**.1339–40
  H antigens, **B2**.1339–40, **B2**.1342
  K antigen, **B2**.1339–40, **B2**.1343
  nomenclature, **B2**.1339–40
  O antigen *see below*
  virulence effects, **B2**.1340
cell structure, **B2**.1339–44
  capsules, **B2**.1339–40, **B2**.1343
  cell walls, **B2**.1340–1
  fimbriae *see below*
  flagella, **B2**.1339–40, **B2**.1342
  morphology, **B2**.1339
characteristics, **B2**.1513 (Tab.)
culture, **B2**.1344–6
  amino acid requirements, **B2**.1345
  bile salts, **B2**.1345
  liquid media, **B2**.1345
  morphology, **B2**.1344–5, **B2**.1345 (Tab.)
  pigment production, **B2**.1345
  preservation, **B2**.1346
  solid media, **B2**.1344–5
  temperature, **B2**.1344
  vitamin requirements, **B2**.1345
  'working cultures,' **B2**.1346
fimbriae, **B2**.1339–40, **B2**.1342–3
  classification, **B2**.1342–3
  functions, **B2**.1343
  sex pili, **B2**.1342–3
genetic organization, **B2**.1344
  bacteriophages, **B2**.1344
  plasmids, **B2**.1344
habitats, **B2**.1346
historical perspective, **B2**.1318–31
infection, **B2**.1346–7
  antibody detection, **B1**.751–2
  bacteremia, **B1**.520–1
  extraintestinal infection, **B2**.1346–7
  hemolytic–uremic syndrome, **B2**.1347
  intestinal infection, **B2**.1347
  nosocomial infection, **B1**.397
  otitis media, **B1**.617
  risk categorization, **B1**.762
  urinary tract infection, **B2**.1346–7
  vaccine development, **B2**.1344
information resources, **B2**.1354–5
isolation/identification, **B2**.1347–52
  biochemical tests, **B2**.1319 (Tab.), **B2**.1330 (Tab.), **B2**.1348
  commercial kits, **B2**.1348, **B2**.1351–2
  computer analysis, **B2**.1348
  DNA hybridization, **B1**.25
  extraintestinal specimens, **B2**.1347
  genetic definition, **B2**.1318
  historical perspective, **B2**.1350–1
  immunoserology, **B1**.757
  intestinal specimens, **B2**.1347
  microscopy, **B2**.1347
  molecular definition *see below*
  phenotypic definition, **B2**.1318
  problem strains, **B2**.1348–50
  screening tests, **B2**.1348, **B2**.1349 (Tab.)
  typing, **B2**.1352

Enterobacteriaceae (*Continued*)
  LPS, **B2**.1340–1
    as exotoxin, **B2**.1340–1
    2-keto-3-deoxyoctonic acid, **B2**.1340
    lipid A, **B2**.1340–1
  molecular definition, **B2**.1318, **B2**.1351
    DNA–DNA hybridization, **B2**.1318,
      B2.1338–9
    16S r-DNA sequencing, **B2**.1318, **B2**.1338
  motility, **B2**.1342
    temperature limits, **B2**.1342
  nomenclature/classification, **B2**.1331–9
    antigenic analysis, **B2**.1332
    biochemistry, **B2**.1332
    'coliform bacteria,' **B2**.1335
    control of, **B2**.1335–6
    current status, **B2**.1335
    decision by usage, **B2**.1335–6
    evolutionary relationships, **B2**.1333 (Fig.),
      B2.1334 (Fig.)
    evolution of, **B2**.1333–5
    International Committee on Systematic
      Bacteriology, **B2**.1335–6
    lactose fermenters, **B2**.1335
    new species, **B2**.1339
    nucleic acid hybridization, **B2**.1332,
      B2.1334 (Fig.)
    proposed changes, **B2**.1336–8
    species, **B2**.1317, **B2**.1338–9
  normal nasopharyngeal flora, **B1**.609
  nutrition, **B2**.1344–6
  O antigen, **B2**.1339–42
    bacteriophage receptor, **B2**.1341
    rough variants, **B2**.1341–2
    species relationships, **B2**.1341
    structure, **B2**.1341
    virulence effects, **B2**.1341–2
  physical/chemical agent susceptibility/
    resistance, **B2**.1345–6
    disinfectants, **B2**.1346
    temperatures, **B2**.1345–6
  'unculturable,' **B2**.1330 (Tab.), **B2**.1337
  as vaccine vector, **I**.899
  see also individual genera; individual species
Enterobacterial common antigen
  Enterobacteriaceae, **B2**.1343–4
  Erwinia chrysanthemi, **B2**.1343–4
  Plesiomonas, **B2**.1343–4
Enterobacterial repetitive intergenic consensus
    (ERIC-PCR)
  Aeromonas typing, **B2**.1535
  Salmonella molecular typing, **B2**.1409,
    B2.1411
Enterobacteria phage λ, renaming, **V1**.40
Enterobacter intermedium, classification,
    B2.1336
Enterobacter intermedius, **B2**.1483–4
  biochemical tests, **B2**.1319 (Tab.)
  characteristics, **B2**.1485 (Tab.)
Enterobacter nimipressuralis, **B2**.1483–4
  biochemical tests, **B2**.1319 (Tab.)
Enterobacter pyrinus, **B2**.1483–4
  biochemical tests, **B2**.1319 (Tab.)
Enterobacter sakazakii, **B2**.1483
  biochemical tests, **B2**.1319 (Tab.), **B2**.1484
  characteristics, **B2**.1485 (Tab.)

  culture, pigment production, **B2**.1345
  infection, milk powder, **B1**.247
  pathogenicity, **B2**.1487
Enterobactin, **B1**.151
Enterobius, **P**.593
  life cycle, **P**.593
  structure, **P**.593
Enterobius vermicularis, **P**.713, **P**.730–1
  biology, **P**.730–1
  Dientamoeba fragilis vector, **P**.267, **P**.269
  epidemiology/population biology, **P**.731
    children, **P**.731
    infection predisposition, **P**.724
  infection *see below*
  life expectancy, **P**.60 (Tab.)
  morphology, **P**.717
    eggs, **P**.716 (Fig.), **P**.717
  transmission, **P**.731
    within families, **P**.731
Enterobius vermicularis infection
  biology, **P**.730–1
  clinical manifestations, **P**.731
    appendix infection, **P**.731
    local irritation/itching, **P**.731
    urinary tract infection, **P**.731
  control, **P**.731–2
    anthelmintics, **P**.732
    personal hygiene, **P**.732
    reinfection, **P**.732
  diagnosis, **P**.151, **P**.731–2
  epidemiology, **P**.46 (Tab.)
  public health importance, **P**.44
Enterococci
  canned cured meats, **B1**.275
  glycopeptide antibiotic effects, **B1**.480–1
  infection
    endocarditis, **B1**.527, **B1**.539
    nosocomial, **B1**.396, **B2**.893–4, **B2**.896
    opportunistic, **B2**.895
    urinary tract, **B2**.896
Enterococcus, **B2**.833–5, **B2**.882–97
  antibacterial susceptibility/resistance, **B1**.433,
    B2.886, **B2**.891–3, **B2**.892 (Tab.)
    acquired, **B2**.891, **B2**.892
    aminoglycosides, **B2**.891–2, **B2**.892 (Tab.),
      B2.893
    detection problems, **B2**.893–4
    high-level, **B2**.892–3
    intrinsic, **B2**.891
    patterns and mechanisms, **B2**.892 (Tab.)
    vancomycin *see* Vancomycin-resistant
      enterococci (VRE)
  antigens, **B2**.886–7
  bacteremia, **B1**.518, **B2**.896
  bacteriocins, **B2**.894–5
  bacteriophage, **B2**.894–5
  cell wall structure, **B2**.886–7
  classification, **B2**.882–5, **B2**.887–90
    genus definition, **B2**.882–5
    groups I-V, **B2**.888 (Tab.), **B2**.889
    phenotypic characteristics, **B2**.883 (Tab.),
      B2.888 (Tab.)
    phylogenetic relationships, **B2**.882,
      B2.884 (Fig.)

  species, **B2**.884–5, **B2**.885 (Tab.), **B2**.887,
    B2.888 (Tab.)
  culture and morphology, **B2**.882, **B2**.885–6
  genetic mechanisms, **B2**.886
    conjugative transposons, **B2**.886
    plasmid exchange (pheromone-induced),
      B2.886, **B2**.896
  habitats, **B2**.885
  historical perspective, **B2**.882–5
  identification, **B2**.887–90
    16S rRNA gene sequence analysis,
      B2.884–5, **B2**.890
    API system, **B2**.889–90
    DNA-DNA reassociation experiments,
      B2.884–5, **B2**.887, **B2**.890
    DNA probes, **B2**.887
    molecular methods, **B2**.890
    SDS-PAGE analysis of WCP profiles,
      B2.890, **B2**.890 (Fig.)
  infection, nosocomial infection, **B1**.396
  isolation, **B2**.890–1
  metabolism and growth requirements,
    B2.886
  as normal microbiota, **B1**.296 (Tab.), **B1**.303,
    B2.885, **B2**.895
  pathogenicity, **B2**.895–7
    invasive properties, **B2**.897
    translocation across intestine, **B2**.897
  typing, **B1**.396
    methods, **B2**.893–4
  virulence, **B2**.895–7
    adhesins, **B2**.897
    aggregation substance, **B2**.886, **B2**.896–7
    hemolysin, **B2**.894–7
    neutrophil-resistance, **B2**.897
Enterococcus asini, **B2**.888 (Tab.), **B2**.889
Enterococcus avium
  endocarditis, **B1**.530–1
  phenotypic characteristics, **B2**.888 (Tab.),
    B2.889
Enterococcus canis, **B2**.888 (Tab.), **B2**.889
Enterococcus casseliflavus, **B2**.885–6
  infection, **B2**.895
    bacteremia, **B1**.518
  phenotypic characteristics, **B2**.888 (Tab.),
    B2.889
Enterococcus cecorum, **B2**.888 (Tab.), **B2**.889
Enterococcus columbae, **B2**.888 (Tab.), **B2**.889
Enterococcus dispar, **B2**.888 (Tab.), **B2**.889
Enterococcus durans
  endocarditis, **B1**.530–1
  isolation, **B2**.890–1
  phenotypic characteristics, **B2**.888 (Tab.),
    B2.889
Enterococcus faecalis
  antibacterial susceptibility/resistance, **B1**.433,
    B1.438
    antibiotic resistance, **B2**.891, **B2**.892–3
    quinolone resistance, **B1**.493 (Tab.)
  classification, **B2**.882–3, **B2**.888 (Tab.)
  conjugation, **B1**.104
  habitats, **B2**.885
  identification systems, **B2**.889–90
    mannitol-negative variants, **B2**.889
    phenotypic characteristics, **B2**.888 (Tab.),
      B2.889

Enterococcus faecalis (*Continued*)
infection, **B2**.895
bacteremia, **B1**.518
endocarditis, **B1**.530–1
endophthalmitis, **B1**.603
nosocomial, **B1**.396
isolation, **B2**.884–5
metabolism and growth requirements,
B2.886
quorum sensing, **B1**.172
reclassification, **B2**.882–3
virulence, **B2**.896–7
hemolysin, **B2**.896, **B2**.897
waterborne, **B1**.223–4
Enterococcus faecium
antibacterial susceptibility/resistance,
B1.433
antibiotic resistance, **B2**.891, **B2**.892–3
classification change, **B2**.882–3
habitats, **B2**.885
identification systems, **B2**.889–90
infection, **B2**.895
bacteremia, **B1**.518
endocarditis, **B1**.530–1, **B1**.539
nosocomial, **B1**.393, **B1**.396
neutrophil-resistance, **B2**.897
phenotypic characteristics, **B2**.888 (Tab.),
B2.889
reclassification, **B2**.882–3
Enterococcus gallinarum
bacteremia, **B1**.518
endocarditis, **B1**.530–1
phenotypic characteristics, **B2**.888 (Tab.),
B2.889
Enterococcus gilvus, **B2**.888 (Tab.), **B2**.889
Enterococcus haemoperoxidus, **B2**.888 (Tab.),
B2.889
Enterococcus hirae, **B2**.888 (Tab.), **B2**.889
Enterococcus malodoratus, **B2**.888 (Tab.),
B2.889
Enterococcus moranviensis, **B2**.889
phenotypic characteristics, **B2**.888 (Tab.),
B2.889
Enterococcus mundtii, **B2**.885–6
phenotypic characteristics, **B2**.888 (Tab.),
B2.889
Enterococcus pallens, **B2**.888 (Tab.), **B2**.889
Enterococcus phoeniculicola, **B2**.888 (Tab.),
B2.889
Enterococcus pseudoavium, **B2**.888 (Tab.),
B2.889
Enterococcus raffinosus
bacteremia, **B1**.518
infection, **B2**.895
phenotypic characteristics, **B2**.888 (Tab.),
B2.889
Enterococcus ratti, **B2**.888 (Tab.), **B2**.889
Enterococcus saccharolyticus, **B2**.888 (Tab.),
B2.889
Enterococcus sulfureus, **B2**.885–6
phenotypic characteristics, **B2**.888 (Tab.),
B2.889
Enterococcus villorum, **B2**.888 (Tab.), **B2**.889
Enterocolitis
necrotizing, **B1**.395
postoperative, **B2**.1119

staphylococcal, **B2**.1119
'Enterocyte immaturity hypothesis,'
cryptosporidiosis, **P**.408
Enterocytozoon
classification, **P**.190–1, **P**.198, **P**.534
human infection
albendazole treatment, **P**.550
transmission, **P**.543–4
see also Microsporidiosis
public health importance, **P**.45
structure/life cycle
meronts, **P**.531–2, **P**.534
sporogenic stage, **P**.534
see also Microsporidians; *individual species*
Enterocytozoon bieneusi, **P**.189
classification, **P**.537
enteric infection, **P**.537–8
acalculous cholecystitis, **P**.539
in Africa, **P**.538
AIDS indicator, **P**.538
crypt hyperplasia, **P**.537
diarrhea, **P**.537
elderly, **P**.539
HIV infection, **P**.537, **P**.539
organ transplant patients, **P**.539
travelers' diarrhea, **P**.539
treatment, **P**.548, **P**.549
see also Microsporidiosis
Enterocytozoon intestinalis co-infection,
P.538–9
geographical distribution, **P**.537
historical aspects, **P**.18
host cell penetration, **P**.531
resistance to chemical agents, **P**.550
structure/life cycle
meronts, **P**.531–2, **P**.532 (Fig.),
P.534 (Fig.)
spores, **P**.533 (Fig.)
sporogonal plasmodium, **P**.533 (Fig.)
sporogonic stage, **P**.532 (Fig.)
as zoonosis, **P**.544–5
see also Microsporidians
Enterocytozoon intestinalis
classification, **P**.538
disseminated infection, **P**.542, **P**.543
see also Microsporidiosis
Entercytozoon bieneusi co-infection, **P**.538–9
enteric infection, **P**.538–9
cholangitis, **P**.539
cholecystitis, **P**.539
lamina propria, **P**.538
travelers' diarrhea, **P**.539
treatment, **P**.548
see also Microsporidiosis
morphology, **P**.538 (Fig.)
see also Microsporidians
Enterohemorrhagic *Escherichia coli* (EHEC)
see Escherichia coli, enterhemorrhagic
(EHEC)
Enteroinvasive *Escherichia coli* (EIEC) *see*
Escherichia coli, enteroinvasive (EIEC)
Enteromonas, classification, **P**.196–7
Enteromonas hominis, **P**.270
classification, **P**.270
distribution, **P**.270

infection, **P**.266
diagnosis, **P**.270
pathogenicity, **P**.270
treatment, **P**.270
structure/life cycle, **P**.266, **P**.270
nutrition, **P**.270
recurrent flagellum, **P**.270
trophozoites, **P**.270, **P**.271 (Fig.)
Enteropathogenic *Escherichia coli* (EPEC) *see*
Escherichia coli, enteropathogenic
(EPEC)
Entero-test, **P**.247–8
microsporidiosis diagnosis, **P**.546
Enterotest, *Helicobacter* identification, **B2**.1574
Enterotoxigenic *Escherichia coli* (ETEC) *see*
Escherichia coli, enterotoxigenic
(ETEC)
Enterotoxins
Aeromonas pathogenicity, **B2**.1535–6
microorganisms, **I**.565–6
rotavirus NSP4 protein, **V2**.951, **V2**.953 (Fig.)
Shigella flexneri, **B2**.1390
superantigens, **I**.562
Enteroviruses
antigenic variation, **V2**.877 (Tab.)
characteristics, **V2**.861 (Tab.)
classification, **V2**.858, **V2**.859 (Fig.)
genus clustering, **V2**.860 (Fig.)
detection/isolation, **V2**.877 (Tab.)
cytospinning, **V2**.1540–1
mixed cell culture, **V1**.88
sample type, **V2**.1532–3
fecal excretion, **V2**.876
genome structure, **V2**.864 (Fig.)
historical aspects, **V2**.857–8
host cell effects, **V2**.869
host range, **V2**.869
infection *see* Enterovirus infection
mollusks, **B1**.280
pathogenesis, **V2**.869–70
properties, **V2**.1162 (Tab.)
protein synthesis, **V1**.115–16
receptors, **V2**.867 (Tab.)
serotypes/groups, **V2**.857 (Tab.), **V2**.1423
size, **V2**.859
transmission, **V2**.1422–3
Enterovirus infection, **V2**.869–72
clinical features, **V2**.870–2, **V2**.876 (Tab.)
agammaglobulinemia, **I**.780
aseptic meningitis, **V2**.870
cardiac disease, **V2**.871
congenital infection, **V2**.871
diabetes mellitus, **V2**.872
encephalitis, **V2**.871
exanthems, **V2**.872
eye infection, **V2**.875
gastroenteritis, **V2**.872
hepatitis, **V2**.872
herpangina, **V2**.871
meningoencephalitis *see below*
mucocutaneous syndromes, **V2**.871–2
neonatal infection, **V2**.871
paralytic disease, **V2**.870–1
respiratory disease, **V2**.872

Enterovirus infection (*Continued*)
  of CNS *see* Central nervous system (CNS) infection
  control, **V2**.878–83
    intravenous Ig, **V2**.878
    pleconaril, **V2**.878
  diagnosis, **V2**.876–7
    antibody detection, **V2**.877
    antigenic variation, **V2**.876–7
    isolation in cell culture, **V2**.876
    isolation in murine neonates, **V2**.877
    molecular biology, **V2**.877
    serotype identification, **V2**.876
    specimen collection, **V2**.876
  epidemiology, **V1**.368–9, **V2**.874–5
    age-related prevalence, **V2**.876 (Tab.)
    climate, **V2**.874
    surveillance, **V2**.874–5
    transmission, **V2**.874
  fetal infection, **V2**.1482–3
  host factors, **V2**.870
    age, **V2**.870
    malnutrition, **V2**.870
    pregnancy, **V2**.870
  meningoencephalitis, **V2**.1509
    Coxsackie virus infection, **V2**.1509
    echovirus infection, **V2**.1509
  nosocomial infection, **B1**.400
  rubella *vs.*, **V2**.970
Enterovirus 70 infection, **V2**.870, **V2**.1423
  acute epidemic hemorrhagic conjunctivitis (AHC), **V2**.872
  clinical features, **V2**.1423
  CNS, **V2**.1423
  meningitis, **V2**.1423
  paralysis, **V2**.871
Enterovirus 71 infection, **V2**.1423
  encephalitis, **V2**.871
  hand-foot-and-mouth disease (HFMD), **V2**.871–2
  paralysis, **V2**.871
Enterovirus, classification, **V1**.50–2
Entner–Doudoroff pathway *see* KDPG pathway (Entner–Doudoroff pathway)
Entomobirnavirus, **V1**.48
Entomophthora, **M**.347
Entomophthorales, **M**.347
  classification, **M**.53, **M**.54 (Tab.)
  see also individual species
Entomophthoromycosis (entomophthoramycosis), **M**.347, **M**.350
  definition, **M**.347
  immune response, **M**.350–1
  see also Zygomycosis, subcutaneous
Entomoplasma
  characteristics, **B2**.1958 (Tab.)
  classification, **B2**.1967
  metabolism, **B2**.1969
Entomopoxvirinae, **V1**.42–4, **V1**.579 (Tab.), **V1**.582
  classification, **V1**.43 (Tab.), **V1**.594
  taxonomy, **V1**.595 (Tab.)
Entomopoxvirus A, **V1**.595 (Tab.)
Entomopoxvirus B, **V1**.595 (Tab.)
Entomopoxvirus C, **V1**.595 (Tab.)

Entopolypoides, **P**.459
Envelope antigens (ENV), foamy viruses *see* Foamy viruses
Enveloped viruses, cellular entry, **V1**.108 (Fig.)
Envelope (E) proteins
  arteriviruses, **V1**.827, **V1**.836 (Tab.), **V1**.837, **V1**.840
  coronaviruses, **V1**.827, **V1**.836 (Tab.), **V1**.837
  flaviviruses *see* Flaviviruses
  Infectious bronchitis virus, **V1**.831–2, **V1**.837
  Murine hepatitis virus, **V1**.831–2, **V1**.837
  retroviruses, **V2**.1322–3, **V2**.1591
  Severe acute respiratory syndrome coronavirus, **V1**.837
  Transmissible gastroenteritis virus, **V1**.837
env gene
  foamy viruses, **V2**.1308
  HTLVs, **V2**.1285–7
Env glycoproteins, HIV *see* HIV
Environment
  airborne bacterial survival, **B1**.188
  antibacterial therapy, **B1**.466
  astrovirus transmission, **V2**.901
  Candida albicans as pathogen, **M**.258–9
  leprosy epidemiology, **B2**.1203
  malaria epidemiology, **P**.512–13
  management
    Old World leishmaniasis control, **P**.308
    parasite control, **P**.112
  nitrates, **B1**.200
  population immunity effects, **B1**.353–5
  respiratory tract infection, **B1**.626
  source of bacterial infection, **B1**.329
  specimens, leptospires, **B2**.1879
  virus survival, **V1**.249
Environmental contamination, definition, **I**.951 (Tab.)
Enviroxime, structure, **V2**.1626 (Fig.)
Enzyme(s), **B1**.45–6
  antibacterial interaction with, **B1**.438
  characterization testing, **B1**.22 (Tab.), **B1**.24
  constitutive expression, **B1**.70
  coordinate induction, **B1**.70
  effectors, **B1**.45–6
  feedback inhibition *see* Feedback inhibition
  inducible, **B1**.70
  periplasmic, **B1**.45–6
  reactions, **B1**.45–6
    catabolic and anabolic, **B1**.45
    kinetics, **B1**.45
  see also specific enzymes
Enzyme antigens, liver flukes, **P**.652
Enzyme immunoassays (EIAs), **B1**.718–9, **B1**.749–50, **V2**.1535, **V2**.1545
  aspergillosis, **M**.106–7
  astrovirus detection, **V2**.906
  Bartonella, **B2**.1897
  Blastomyces dermatitidis, **M**.112–13
  Bordetella parapertussis, **B1**.752
  Borrelia, **B1**.753
  Campylobacter jejuni, **B1**.751–2
  candidiasis, **M**.99, **M**.103–4
  Clostridium, **B1**.756
    C. botulinum, **B1**.751
    C. tetani, **B1**.751

Coccidioides immitis, **M**.113, **M**.514–15
Corynebacterium, **B1**.751, **B1**.756
Cryptococcus neoformans, **M**.110
Escherichia coli O157, **B1**.751
HBsAg, **V2**.1253
HCMV infection, in pregnancy, **V2**.1450
histoplasmosis, **M**.532
HTLV, **V2**.1293
human brucellosis diagnosis, **B2**.1740–1
influenza diagnosis, **V1**.675
inhibition, anti-HBc, **V2**.1253
Legionella, **B1**.752, **B1**.758
  L. pneumophila, **B2**.1773, **B2**.1774
limitations, **V2**.1535
measles diagnosis, **V1**.732–3
mumps diagnosis, **V1**.755–6
Mycoplasma pneumoniae, **B1**.752, **B2**.1995
mycosis immunodiagnosis, **M**.35
Neisseria
  N. gonorrhoeae, **B1**.751
  N. meningitidis, **B1**.751
norovirus detection, **V2**.921
staphylococci, **B1**.750
syphilis diagnosis, **B1**.663, **B1**.746, **B2**.1849
tularemia diagnosis, **B1**.752
vaccine response, **V2**.1558
see also specific types
Enzyme-linked immunosorbent assay (ELISA), **M**.35, **B1**.718, **V2**.1535
  alphavirus infection diagnosis, **V2**.1018
  amebiasis, **P**.211–12
  American visceral leishmaniasis, **P**.335–6
  Angiostrongylus cantonensis infection, **P**.806–7
  Angiostrongylus costaricensis infection, **P**.810
  Anisakis infection, **P**.817
  arenavirus infection, **V2**.1076
  Aspergillus detection, **M**.712, **M**.713, **M**.714, **M**.715
    galactomannan, **M**.714
    PCR *vs.*, **M**.715
  Avian infectious bronchitis virus infection, **V1**.844
  Bartonella, **B2**.1898
  Blastocystis hominis infection, **P**.563–4
  Bordetella pertussis, **B2**.1792
  Borna disease virus infection, **V2**.1150
  Borrelia, **B2**.1829–30
  botulinum toxin, **B2**.1063
  Bovine torovirus, **V1**.846
  Burkholderia, **B2**.1613
    B. cepacia complex, **B2**.1613
    B. thailandensis, **B2**.1621
  Chagas disease, **P**.389
  Chlamydia infection diagnosis, **B2**.2006–7, **B2**.2018
  Colorado tick fever virus, **V2**.943
  cryptosporidiosis, **P**.408–9
  cystic echinococcosis, **P**.694–6
  Echinococcus granulosis infection, **P**.154
  Echinococcus multilocularis infection, **P**.154
  enteroviruses, **V2**.877
  fecal analysis, **P**.151
  Feline astrovirus detection, **V2**.899

Enzyme-linked immunosorbent assay (ELISA)
(*Continued*)
  filovirus infection diagnosis, **V2**.1096–7,
    V2.1097 (Tab.)
  giardiasis, **P**.248
  glanders diagnosis, **B2**.1633, **B2**.1634
  Gnathostoma spinigerum infection, **P**.821–2
  Haemophilus, **B2**.1710
  Helicobacter identification, **B2**.1573
  henipavirus infection, **V1**.818
  Hepatitis C virus, **V2**.1212–13
    core protein, **V2**.1211
    NS4 protein, **V2**.1210
  HIV
    HIV-1 *vs.* HIV-2 detection, **V2**.1331
    in neonate, **V2**.1472–3
    in pregnancy, **V2**.1472
  HSV infection, **V2**.1421
    in pregnancy, **V2**.1465
  human brucellosis diagnosis, **B2**.1739–40
  Human coronaviruses infection, **V1**.842
  Japanese encephalitis (JE) virus, **V2**.1425
  leptospires, **B2**.1867, **B2**.1879–80
  liver/lung fluke infection, **P**.653
  lymphatic filariasis, **P**.776–7
  malaria, **P**.488, **P**.503
    antigen detection, **P**.504
  melioidosis diagnosis, **B2**.1621, **B2**.1630
  microsporidiosis, **P**.536
  mumps diagnosis, **V1**.754
  neurocysticercosis, **P**.692, **P**.693–4
  Old World leishmaniasis, **P**.302
  parasite disease control, **P**.130
  Pneumocystis, **M**.793–4
  Porcine transmissible gastroenteritis virus
    infection, **V1**.844–5
  Prototheca zopfii, **M**.400
  Pythium insidiosum, **M**.424
  rotavirus infection diagnosis, **V2**.952
  rubella, **V2**.978
  sapoviruses, **V2**.924–5
  schistosomiasis, **P**.606, **P**.621–2, **P**.635
  Streptobacillus moniliformis, **B2**.1911
  Streptococcus pneumoniae antibodies, **B1**.631
  Strongyloides infection, **P**.741–2
  Taenia infection, **P**.664
  Taenia solium infection, **P**.154
  tapeworm infection, **P**.664
  toxocariasis, **P**.754–5
  toxoplasmosis, **P**.434–5
  trichinellosis, **P**.765
  tularemia diagnosis, **B2**.1754
  VZV infection
    infants, **V2**.1457–8
    in pregnancy, **V2**.1456–7
  West Nile virus, **V2**.1425
Enzyme-linked virus-inducible system
  (ELVIS), **V2**.1541
Eosinophil(s), **I**.55
  activation, **I**.64–5
    Ig mediated, **I**.64–5
    morphological changes, **I**.65
    non-Ig mediated, **I**.64
  adhesion molecules, **I**.59 (Tab.)

airway hypersensitivity *see* Airway
  hypersensitivity/hyperreactivity
  antigen presentation, **I**.67
  apoptosis, **I**.57–8
    macrophage clearance, **I**.58
  basic biology, **I**.55–8
  cell trafficking, **I**.58–61
    adhesion, **I**.60
    chemotaxis, **I**.60–1
    see also individual chemokines
  chemokine receptors, **I**.220
    CC chemokines, **I**.223–4
  chemokines, **I**.59 (Tab.)
    cytokines produced, **I**.59 (Tab.), **I**.67
      GM-CSF, **I**.67, **I**.277
      IL-1α, **I**.67
      IL-3, **I**.67, **I**.275
      IL-4, **I**.280
      IL-5, **I**.67
      leukotriene B₄, **I**.185
      lymphotoxin, **I**.67
      nerve growth factor, **I**.67
      neurotrophin-3, **I**.67
      platelet-activating factor, **I**.191
      TGF-β, **I**.67
      TNF-α, **I**.67
  degranulation, **I**.65
  effector molecules
    arachidonic acid, **I**.57
    Charcot–Leyden crystal proteins, **I**.57, **I**.66
    cyclooxygenase, **I**.57
    ECP, **I**.65–6
    eosinophil-derived neurotoxin, **I**.65–6
    EPO, **I**.65
    5-lipoxygenase, **I**.57
    major basic protein, **I**.65
    major granule proteins, **I**.65–6
    prostaglandin E₂, **I**.66
    reactive oxygen intermediates, **I**.66
  effector molecules/granules, **I**.65–6,
    I.65 (Tab.)
    granules, **I**.57
  functions, **I**.61–6
    immunomodulatory capabilities, **I**.67
  growth/differentiation, **I**.57
    CD40 engagement, **I**.58
    GM-CSF, **I**.57–8
    IL-3, **I**.55, **I**.57–8, **I**.275
    IL-5, **I**.55, **I**.57–8, **I**.278, **I**.278 (Fig.)
    IL-9, **I**.282
    IL-12, **I**.57
    IL-15, **I**.58
    nitric oxide, **I**.58
  in infectious disease, **I**.67–71, **I**.69 (Tab.)
    Angiostrongylus, **I**.57
    Brugia malayi, **I**.70
    Fasciola hepatica, **I**.70
    Helmgmosomoides polygrias, **I**.70
    helminth infection, **I**.55, **I**.68–70
    HIV, **I**.55, **I**.71
    Human respiratory syncytial virus
      infection, **V1**.793–4
    Hymenolepis diminuta, **I**.70
    Limosoides sigmoidontis, **I**.70
    lymphatic filariasis, **I**.68–9

    Mesocestoides corti, **I**.70
    Nippostrongylus, **I**.65
    Nippostrongylus brasiliensis, **I**.70
    Onchocerca, **I**.60, **I**.70
    pythiosis, **M**.421–2
    respiratory syncytial virus, **I**.71
    Schistosoma mansoni, **I**.69–70
    Strongyloides ratti, **I**.70
    Strongyloides venezuelensis, **I**.70
    Toxocara canis, **I**.70
    Trichinella spiralis, **I**.70
    Trichostrongylus, **I**.60, **I**.70
    Trypanosoma cruzi, **I**.70
    viral infection, **I**.71
    see also individual types
  integrins, **I**.59 (Tab.)
  5-lipoxygenase, **I**.184
  MHC class II, **I**.67
  morphology, **I**.56 (Fig.), **I**.57
  natural history, **I**.57–8
    lifespan, **I**.57–8
  receptors, **I**.64
    C3a receptor, **I**.146–7
    chemokine receptors *see above*
    FcεRI, **I**.64, **I**.316
    FcεRIII, **I**.64
    FcγRI, **I**.64–5
    FcγRII (CDw32), **I**.64–5
    FcγRIII, **I**.64–5
    FcγRIIIa, **I**.315
    FcγRIIIb, **I**.315
Eosinophil-derived neurotoxin (EDN), **I**.65–6
Eosinophilia, **I**.67
  Angiostrongylus cantonensis infection,
    P.805–6, **P**.806 (Fig.)
  cerebrospinal fluid, **P**.807
  cystic echinococcosis, **P**.694–6
  Dientamoeba fragilis infection, **P**.267–8
  IL-5, **I**.69, **I**.278, **I**.278 (Fig.)
  infectious diseases, **I**.69 (Tab.)
  intestinal nematode infection, **P**.90
  liver/lung fluke infection, **P**.653
  onchocerciasis, **P**.796
  opisthorchiasis, **P**.651
  paragonimiasis, **P**.650–1
  parasitic infection, **P**.69
  schistosomiasis, **P**.616, **P**.617–18
  tapeworm infection, **P**.663
  trichinellosis, **P**.765
Eosinophil peroxidase, **I**.521
Eotaxin(s), **I**.60–1
  airway hypersensitivity, **I**.736–7
  CCR3 binding, **I**.60
  effects
    basophils, **I**.60, **I**.66
    eosinophils, **I**.60–1, **I**.64
  genes, **I**.582
  knockout mice, **I**.61
  mechanism of action, **I**.60–1
  neurocysticercosis, **P**.690
  receptor *see* CC chemokine receptors, CCR3
    (eotaxin receptor)
  release
    IL-4, **I**.61
    lymphotoxin, **I**.61

Eotaxin(s) (*Continued*)
  signal transduction, **I**.60
  structure, **I**.60–1
Eotaxin-1 (CCL11), **I**.218 (Tab.)
Eotaxin-2 (CCL24), **I**.61, **I**.218 (Tab.)
  basophil cytokine production, **I**.66
Eotaxin-3 (CCL26), **I**.61, **I**.218 (Tab.)
EPEC *see Escherichia coli*, enteropathogenic
  (EPEC)
Eperythrozoon
  classification, **B2**.1964, **B2**.1968
  genome structure, **B2**.1973–4
Ephemerovirus
  characteristics, **V1**.129 (Tab.)
  classification, **V1**.385, **V2**.1104
  genome
    size, **V2**.1111
    structure, **V1**.387 (Tab.), **V2**.1112 (Fig.)
  members, **V1**.385–6
  type species, **V2**.1104
    see also Bovine ephemeral fever virus
      (BEFV)
Ephemeroviruses, replication, **V2**.1111
Epicoccum, in cereals, **B1**.284
Epidemic curve, **B1**.312–13, **B1**.312 (Fig.)
Epidemic hypochlorrhydia, *Helicobacter pylori*
  infection, **B2**.1579
Epidemic jaundice, **V2**.1160
Epidemic keratoconjunctivitis (shipyard eye),
  V1.444, **V1**.444 (Tab.)
Epidemic relapsing fever *(Borrelia)*, **B2**.1823
Epidemics
  African trypanosomiasis, **P**.142 (Tab.)
  causes, **P**.117, **P**.127
  definition, **B1**.310, **V1**.358, **V1**.667
  emerging viral infection potential, **V2**.1655
  Hamer's theory, **B1**.336–7, **B1**.342–3
  historical aspects, **B1**.336–8
  influenza, **V1**.635 (Tab.), **V1**.668
  malaria, **P**.513–14
  mathematical theories, **B1**.337–8
  migration, **P**.117, **P**.127
  parasite control, **P**.115–16
  recent, **P**.142 (Tab.)
  rubella epidemiology, **V2**.971 (Fig.)
  schistosomiasis, **P**.142 (Tab.)
  shape, **I**.950, **I**.950 (Fig.)
  theories, **B1**.336–8
  threshold value, **I**.956
  urbanization, **P**.117
  vegetation changes, **P**.117
Epidemiological surveillance, malaria
  diagnosis, **P**.505–6
Epidemiology of infection, **I**.950–7
  bacterial infection, **B1.309–34**, **B1**.117–19,
    B1.335–58
    analytical methods, **B1**.313–14
      case-control studies, **B1**.315–16,
        B1.315 (Fig.)
      cohort studies, **B1**.314–15
      experimental/intervention studies,
        B1.313, **B1**.314 (Fig.)
      prevalence/incidence studies, **B1**.313–14,
        B1.314 (Fig.)
      statistical analysis, **B1**.316
    basic principles, **B1**.338–53

chromosome analysis, **B1**.117–19
concepts, **B1**.309–10, **B1**.338–53
  communicability, **B1**.310
  host response, **B1**.310
  incubation period, **B1**.310
  infection reservoir, **B1**.309
  occurrence, **B1**.310
  source of infection, **B1**.309–10
  transmission mode, **B1**.310
data-collection systems *see* Data-collection
  systems
effective reproduction number, **B1**.340,
  B1.346
environmental and social effects, **B1**.353–5
historical perspectives, **B1**.336–8
in individuals, **B1**.338–9
  immunity development, **B1**.339
infection source, control, **B1**.328–9
mathematical models, **B1**.330–2, **B1**.341–4
  continuous time model, **B1**.337, **B1**.343
  deterministic model, **B1**.344
  developing and using a model,
    B1.331 (Fig.)
  dynamic behaviour, **B1**.342–3
  Hamer–Soper model, **B1**.337, **B1**.343
  Hamer's theory of epidemics, **B1**.336–7,
    B1.342–3, **B1**.343 (Fig.)
  herd immunity and vaccination effect,
    B1.348
  heterogeneity, **B1**.343–4
  history, **B1**.330
  mass action model/assumption, **B1**.337,
    B1.342
  model structure, **B1**.331
  model type, **B1**.331–2
  Reed–Frost model, **B1**.337, **B1**.343
  reproductive rate (R_0) (potential to
    spread), **B1**.330–1
  stochastic models, **B1**.344
  structure of model, **B1**.342 (Fig.)
methods, **B1**.311–16
  collection of observations, **B1**.311
  descriptive analysis, **B1**.311–3
  experimental study design, **B1**.313,
    B1.314 (Fig.)
  interviews/questionnaires, **B1**.311
  medical records, **B1**.311
  sources of data, **B1**.311
  surveys and analytical studies, **B1**.313–14
  time/place/person, **B1**.312–13
  variables, **B1**.311–12
molecular, **B1**.735–6
natural history, **I**.953
  gonorrhea, **I**.954 (Fig.)
outbreak control, **B1**.327, **B1**.328–30
persistence thresholds, **B1**.340–1
in populations, **B1**.339–41
  basic reproduction number *see* Basic
    reproduction number (R_0)
  effective reproductive number *see*
    Infection(s), mathematical models
  herd immunity *see* Herd immunity
  persistence thresholds, **B1**.340–1
specific bacterial infection
  diffusely adherent *Escherichia coli*,
    B2.1379

enteroaggregative *Escherichia coli*,
  B2.1378–9
enteroinvasive *Escherichia coli* EIEC),
  B2.1374–5
enteropathogenic *Escherichia coli*,
  B2.1372–4
enterotoxigenic *Escherichia coli*,
  B2.1375
legionellosis, **B2**.1764–6
vero-cytotoxin-producing *Escherichia
  coli*, **B2**.1377–8
spread of infection, control, **B1**.329
strategies for disease control *see* Control
  of infection
surveillance *see* Surveillance,
  epidemiological
natural history, **I**.953–5
  population classification, **I**.954–5
  susceptible, exposed, infectious, resistant
    (SEIR) model, **I**.954–5
  susceptible, infectious, resistant (SIR)
    model, **I**.954–5
  susceptible, infectious, susceptible (SIS)
    model, **I**.954–5
parasitic infection, **P.50–66**
  basic reproductive number of infection
    (R_0), **P**.52–4
    determining rate processes, **P**.60 (Tab.)
    effects on control programs, **P**.53
    endemic infection, **P**.52
    establishment, **P**.53
    genetic variability, **P**.53–4
    immunity development, **P**.53–4,
      P.54 (Fig.)
    oscillating equilibria, **P**.52
    serological surveys, **P**.53, **P**.53 (Fig.)
  control of disease, **P**.63–5
    community-based chemotherapy, **P**.64–5
    drug-resistance effects, **P**.64
    interventions, **P**.63–4
    program assessment, **P**.65
    treatment frequency, **P**.64–5
  definitions/basic concepts, **P**.50, **P**.50–1
    see also specific terms
  diagnostic techniques, **P**.150
  heterogeneity/infection predisposition,
    P.54–6
    frequency distribution of numbers/host,
      P.54
    host genetic factors, **P**.55, **P**.56–7
    human behavior, **P**.54–7
    parasite aggregation, **P**.54–5, **P**.55–6,
      P.55 (Fig.), **P**.56 (Fig.)
  macroparasites, **P**.52
    basic reproductive number of infection,
      P.52–3
    directly transmitted, **P**.59 (Fig.)
    generation times, **P**.52
    indirectly transmitted, **P**.59 (Fig.)
    infection/morbidity quantification, **P**.52
    numbers per host, **P**.52, **P**.52 (Fig.)
  microparasites, **P**.51–2, **P**.60 (Fig.)
    basic reproductive number of infection
      (R_0), **P**.52
    definition, **P**.51
    generation time, **P**.51
    host population stratification, **P**.51

Epidemiology of infection
  parasitic infection
    microparasites (*Continued*)
      infection *vs.* disease, **P**.51
      transmission rate, **P**.52
    molecular biology, **P**.50
      genome sequences, **P**.50
      linkage/segregation analysis, **P**.50
    prevalence *vs.* infection intensity, **P**.54,
      P.55 (Fig.)
      past infection effects, **P**.54, **P**.54 (Fig.)
    reproductive success effects, **P**.51
    statistical approaches, **P**.50–1
    transmission dynamics *see* Transmission
      dynamics
    transmission success effects, **P**.51
    see also individual species; specific diseases/
      infection
  pathogen heterogeneities, **I**.955
  quantification of transmission probability,
    I.951–2
    frequency *vs.* contact intimacy, **I**.952 (Fig.)
    transmission route effects, **I**.952
  social/environmental setting, **I**.952–3
    contact amount, **I**.952, **I**.953 (Fig.)
    contact variables, **I**.952
    'core groups,' **I**.952
    population definition, **I**.953
    'transmission coefficient,' **I**.952–3
  transmission routes, **I**.951
    classification, **I**.951, **I**.951 (Tab.)
    infection mode, **I**.951, **I**.951 (Tab.)
    source, **I**.951, **I**.951 (Tab.)
  viral infection, **I**.953, **I**.954 (Fig.), **V1.353–77**
    analytical studies, **V1**.361–4
      case–control studies *see* Case–control
        studies
      cohort studies *see* Cohort studies
      vaccine effectiveness, **V1**.363–4
    bloodborne transmission, **V1**.369–70
    case–control studies *see* Case–control
      studies
    chronic infection, **V1**.373–4
    cohort studies *see* Cohort studies
    common source outbreaks *see* Common-
      source outbreaks
    definition, **V1**.353
    emerging infection, **V2**.1661–2
    epidemic curve, **V1**.358, **V1**.358 (Fig.)
    experimental, **V1**.364–5
      controlled trials, **V1**.365
      simulations, **V1**.364–5
    gastrointestinal tract infection, **V1**.368–9
    incidence, **V1**.359–60
      definition, **V1**.359
      incidence rate (density), **V1**.359–60,
        V1.360 (Fig.)
      risk, **V1**.359
    intermediate hosts, **V1**.353–4
    monitoring/surveillance, **V1**.360–1,
      V1.361 (Fig.)
      examples, **V1**.360–1
      localized infection, **V1**.361
      national data, **V1**.360–1
    natural history, **I**.953, **I**.954 (Fig.)
      Hepatitis B virus, **I**.953–4, **I**.954 (Fig.)

measles, **I**.954 (Fig.)
    nosocomial transmission, **V1**.357
    observational, **V1**.356–64
      etiology confirmation, **V1**.364
      personal factors, **V1**.356–7, **V1**.357 (Tab.)
      place, **V1**.357
      temporal factors, **V1**.358
    outbreaks
      definitions, **V1**.358, **V1**.361
      see also specific types
    persistent infection, **V1**.353–4
    point source outbreaks *see* Point-source
      outbreaks
    prevalence, **V1**.360
      definition, **V1**.360
      serological surveys, **V1**.360
    respiratory infection, **V1**.365–7
      seasonality, **V1**.366
    seasonal outbreaks, **V1**.358, **V1**.359 (Fig.)
    zoonoses, **V1**.370–3
      arthropod transmission, **V1**.372–3,
        V1.372 (Tab.)
      non-arthropod transmission, **V1**.370–2,
        V1.371 (Tab.)
    see also Transmission of infection(s),
      viruses; *specific diseases/infection;*
      specific viruses
Epidermal growth factor (EGF)
  giardiasis exogenous application, **P**.246–7
  poxviruses, **V1**.257
Epidermis
  anatomy, **I**.820
  viral infection, **V1**.236
Epidermodysplasia verruciformis, **V1**.463–4,
  V1.463 (Tab.), **V1**.464 (Fig.), **V2**.1508
  oncogenesis, **V1**.463–4
Epidermophyton, **M**.220, **M**.221, **M**.222 (Tab.),
  M.223 (Tab.), **M**.224 (Tab.)
  histopathology, **M**.128 (Tab.)
  morphology, **M**.222, **M**.222 (Tab.)
Epidermophyton floccosum, **M**.9–10, **M**.222,
  M.224 (Tab.), **M**.227 (Tab.)
  classification, **M**.229–30
  epidemiology, **M**.228
  geographical distribution, **M**.229 (Tab.)
  infection, **M**.231, **M**.232
Epididymitis
  Chlamydia trachomatis infection, **B2**.2012–13
  mumps, **V1**.749
Epididymoorchitis, human brucellosis, **B2**.1738
Epiglottitis, **B1**.613
  causative organisms, **B1**.613
  clinical features, **B1**.613
  differential diagnosis, **B1**.613
  epidemiology, **B1**.613
  treatment, **B1**.613
Epi-Info, **B1**.326
Epilepsy, late-onset, neurocysticercosis,
  P.686–7
Epilythic growth patterns, **M**.195
Epimastigotes, *Trypanosoma brucei,* **P**.357–8
Epimerization reactions, **B1**.57
Epiphytic growth patterns, **M**.195
Episomes
  viral evolution, **V1**.14
  see also Plasmid(s)

Epithelial cells
  Bordetella invasion/survival, **B2**.1806
  candidiasis, **M**.260
  CD4 T cell antigen presentation, **I**.394
  γδ T-cell development, **I**.527
  intraepithelial lymphocyte interactions,
    I.527–9, **I**.528 (Fig.)
  LPS-binding protein, **I**.115–16
  MHC class I antigen presentation, **I**.426–7
Epithelia, mucosal vaccination, **I**.827,
  I.827 (Tab.)
Epithelium
  respiratory, **B1**.623
    failure, **B1**.626
  stratified, microfold (M) cells, **I**.827
Epitope analysis, **V1**.194
Epitope mapping, **V2**.1546
Epitope spreading, autoimmune disease, **I**.756
Epitope suppression, conjugate vaccines, **I**.935
Epivir *see* Lamivudine
Epizootic hemorrhagic disease virus (EDHV),
  V2.942
Epizootic lymphangitis, histoplasmosis, **M**.24
EPO, eosinophils, **I**.65
Epoxides, **B1**.438
Epsilometer test (E-test)
  antibacterial susceptibility testing, **B1**.498
  Helicobacter pylori antibacterial resistance,
    B2.1575–6
  mycology, **M**.609, **M**.610 (Fig.)
  antifungal susceptibility testing, **M**.158
Epsilonretrovirus, **V1**.46, **V2**.1286 (Tab.)
Epstein–Barr virus (EBV), **V1.559–77**
  B-cells, **V1**.248–9
  capsid proteins, **V1**.564
  cell culture systems, **V1**.88
    genetically-engineered cell culture, **V1**.88
  characteristics, **V1**.489 (Tab.)
  classification, **V1**.559
    biosafety level 2, **V2**.1525
  detection, cell culture, **V2**.1539
  discovery, **V1**.559
  EBV-encoded RNAs (EBERs 1 and 2),
    V1.560, **V1**.563
  episome maintenance, **V1**.260–1
    EBNA 1 role, **V1**.561
  gene expression, **V1**.566
    early, **V1**.564, **V1**.564 (Tab.)
    immediate early (Z and R), **V1**.563–4
    late, **V1**.564
    latent, **V1**.560 (Fig.), **V1**.561, **V1**.561 (Tab.)
    lytic, **V1**.563
    regulation, **V1**.499
    in tumors, **V1**.566, **V1**.566 (Tab.), **V1**.567
  genome, **V1**.494 (Tab.)
    circularization, **V1**.560
    open reading frames, **V1**.560, **V1**.561 (Tab.)
    organization, **V1**.560 (Fig.)
    structure, **V1**.492, **V1**.493, **V1**.493 (Fig.),
      V1.560
  glycoproteins, **V1**.564–5, **V1**.565 (Tab.)
    gp42, **V1**.565
    gp85, **V1**.564–5
    gp110, **V1**.565
    gp340/220, **V1**.564–5

Epstein–Barr virus (EBV) (*Continued*)
  host range, **V1**.559
  immortalization, **V1**.559, **V1**.565–6
    EBNA 2 role, **V1**.562
    peripheral blood lymphocytes, **V1**.345
  immune evasion, **V1**.298 (Tab.)
    antigen processing, **I**.633
    apoptosis mitochondrial pathways,
      V1.324–5
    complement, **V1**.287
    cytokine analogues, **V1**.288, **V1**.298 (Tab.),
      V1.303, **V1**.317–18, **I**.620, **I**.623, **I**.687
    cytokine binding proteins, **V1**.319, **I**.621
    cytokine signal transduction, **V1**.316–17
    EBNA 1 role, **V1**.561
    IFN interference, **V1**.230
    MHC interference, **V1**.287, **V1**.321
    superantigens, **I**.637–8
    TNF-α inhibition, **V1**.301–2
  infection *see* Epstein–Barr virus (EBV)
    infection
  latent membrane protein 1 (LMP1),
    V1.316–17, **V1**.336–7, **V1**.562–3
    functions, **V1**.562–3
  latent membrane protein 2 (LMP2),
    V1.336–7, **V1**.563
  latent membrane proteins (LMP), **V1**.560–1,
    I.623
    activation, **V1**.562
    see also specific types
  localization, **V1**.248–9, **V1**.248 (Fig.)
  lymphoma cells, **V1**.248–9
  lytic cycle, **V1**.563
  molecular biology, **V1**.560–6
  morphology and structure, **V1**.559–60
  nuclear antigens (EBNAs), **V1**.336–7,
    V1.560–2
    EBNA 1, **V1**.561, **V1**.566
    EBNA 2, **V1**.562, **V1**.565
    EBNA 3A, B, C, **V1**.562
    EBNA LP, **V1**.562
    EBNA mRNA synthesis, **V1**.566
    LP, **V1**.565
  oncogenes, **V1**.336–7, **V1**.561 (Tab.),
    V1.570
  proteins, **V1**.561–4
    genes encoding, **V1**.561 (Tab.)
    latent, **V1**.561
    lytic, **V1**.563, **V1**.564 (Tab.)
    see also specific types
  receptors, **V1**.207 (Tab.)
    B cell activation, **V1**.212
    C3d complement receptor, **V1**.212
    CD21, **V1**.564–5
  replication, **V1**.566
    early proteins, **V1**.564, **V1**.564 (Tab.)
    EBNA 1 role, **V1**.561
  shedding, **V1**.248 (Fig.)
  superantigens, **I**.563–4
  TP1 and TP2, **V1**.560–1
  transcription, latency types I and II, **V1**.567
  types A (1) and B (2), **V1**.560
Epstein–Barr virus-induced receptor ligand
  chemokine (ELC:CCL19), **I**.218 (Tab.),
    I.226
  B cell homing, **I**.226

dendritic cell activation, **I**.393–4
Epstein–Barr virus (EBV) infection,
  V1.248 (Fig.), **V1**.566–73
  conditions associated, **V1**.567–73,
    V1.567 (Tab.)
    Burkitt's lymphoma, **V1**.248 (Fig.)
    hemophagocytic syndrome, **I**.778
    Hodgkin's disease, **V1**.571
    lymphomas, **V1**.570–1, **I**.795–6, **V2**.1507–8
    lymphoproliferative disease, **V1**.570–1
    T cell lymphomas, **V1**.571
    tumors, **V1**.345, **V1**.566 (Tab.), **V1**.571–3
    X-linked proliferative syndrome, **I**.779
  diagnosis, serology, **V2**.1546, **V2**.1546 (Tab.)
  entry into host cells, **V1**.344–5
    B cells, **V1**.565
  epidemiology, **V1**.566–7
    in HIV infection, **V1**.336–7, **V1**.345,
      V2.1499 (Tab.), **V2**.1503
    in children, **V2**.1505
  immune response, **V1**.568–9
    antibodies, **V1**.568–9, **V1**.569 (Fig.),
      V1.570
    IFN-γ, **V1**.302–3
    IL-1, **V1**.296–7
    IL-2, **V1**.302–3
    IL-4, **V1**.302–3
    IL-5, **I**.277, **V1**.302–3
    IL-6, **V1**.302–3
    IL-10, **V1**.302–3
    IL-18, **I**.290–2
    NK cells, **I**.94–5
    TNF-α, **V1**.296, **V1**.302–3
  immunodeficient patients, **V1**.570–1
    bone marrow transplants, **V2**.1507
    HIV infection *see above*
    non-HIV, **V2**.1507–8
    T cell deficiency, **V1**.274
  immunogenetics, **I**.588
  immunopathology, **V1**.279 (Tab.), **V1**.280
  latent infection, **V1**.206, **V1**.260, **V1**.336–7,
    V1.345, **V1**.560
  medical importance, **V1**.162
  oncogenesis, **V1**.336–7
    mechanisms, **V1**.338 (Tab.), **V1**.342 (Tab.)
    multi-step process, **V1**.345
    tumors associated, **V1**.345, **V1**.566 (Tab.),
      V1.571–3
  primary effusion lymphoma, **V1**.553–4
  primary infection, **V1**.567
  transmission, **V1**.566–9
  vaccines, **V1**.573, **I**.933 (Tab.)
    gp340, **V1**.573
    trials, **V1**.573
  see also Infectious mononucleosis (IM)
Equine arteritis virus (EAV)
  accessory proteins, **V1**.835–6
  double membrane vesicles, **V1**.835
  genome
    expression strategies, **V1**.829 (Fig.)
    sequencing, **V1**.398
    structure, **V1**.828 (Fig.)
  glycoproteins, **V1**.827
    GP₂ glycoprotein, **V1**.839
    GP₃ glycoprotein, **V1**.839

GP₄ glycoprotein, **V1**.836 (Tab.)
  GP₅ glycoprotein, **V1**.840
  major surface glycoprotein (MSG), **V1**.838
  infection, **V1**.841 (Tab.)
    containment, **V1**.846–7
    diagnosis, **V1**.846–7
    neutralizing antibodies, **V1**.846
    vaccination, **V1**.846–7
  membrane (M) protein, antibodies, **V1**.840
  nucleocapsid (N) protein, antibodies, **V1**.840
  replicase (RNA polymerase), **V1**.833 (Fig.)
    intracellular localization, **V1**.835
  subgenomic RNAs, **V1**.830
  transmission, **V1**.846
  type species, **V1**.53, **V1**.392, **V1**.825
Equine foamy virus (EFV), **V2**.1304–5
Equine herpesvirus 1, **V1**.494 (Tab.)
Equine herpesvirus 2
  characteristics, **V1**.542 (Tab.)
  genome sequences, **V1**.494 (Tab.)
Equine herpesvirus 4, **V1**.494 (Tab.)
Equine immunodeficiency virus (EIV), gene
  therapy vector, **V2**.1592–3
Equine infectious anemia virus (EIAV)
  antigenic variation, **V1**.262
  infection, **V1**.282
Equine protozoal encephalomyelitis (EPM),
  P.446
Equine rhinitis B virus, **V1**.50–2
Equine torovirus (EToV: Berne virus)
  accessory proteins, **V1**.835–6
  classification, **V1**.392
  genome
    expression strategies, **V1**.829 (Fig.)
    sequencing, **V1**.398
    structure, **V1**.828 (Fig.)
  infection, **V1**.841 (Tab.)
  replicase (RNA polymerase), **V1**.833 (Fig.)
  type species, **V1**.824–5
Eradication, of bacterial disease, **B1**.345
Eradication, parasite control, **P**.108–9
Erbitux, licensing, **I**.355 (Tab.)
Erbovirus, **V1**.50–2
ERC-55, papillomavirus E6 protein binding,
  V1.460 (Tab.)
Ergosterol, **M**.70
  azole action, **M**.173
  polyene action, **M**.172
Eriocher, Paragonimus intermediate host,
  P.646
Erosio interdigitalis, **M**.597
ERp56, MHC class I assembly, **I**.408
Errantivirus, **V1**.47
Error catastrophe, antiviral chemotherapy,
  V1.19–20
Error frequency, RNA-dependent RNA
  polymerases, **V1**.132–3
Ertapenem, spectrum of activity, **B1**.478–80,
  B1.499 (Tab.)
Erwingella americana, biochemical tests,
  B2.1319 (Tab.)
Erwinia
  characteristics, **B2**.1330 (Tab.)
  phytopathogenicity, **B1**.202
  see also individual species
Erwinia carotovora, **B1**.281

Erwinia chrysanthemi, **B2**.1343–4
Erwinia dissolvens see Enterobacter dissolvens
Erwinia nimipressurlaris see Enterobacter nimipressuralis
Erysipelas
  swine, **B2**.970–3
  vaccine, **B2**.974
  see also Erysipelothrix rhusiopathiae, infection
Erysipeloid, **B2**.971
  see also Erysipelothrix rhusiopathiae, infection
Erysipelothrix
  classification, **B2**.970
  definition, **B2**.970
  habitats, **B2**.970
Erysipelothrix rhusiopathiae, **B2**.970–4
  antibacterial susceptibility/resistance, **B2**.974
  cell wall composition, **B2**.973
  characteristics, **B2**.970, **B2**.972 (Tab.)
  culture, **B2**.971–2
  distribution, **B2**.970
  habitats, **B2**.970
  infection, **B2**.970–4
    animals, **B2**.970–1
    diagnosis, **B2**.971–2, **B2**.972 (Tab.)
    endocarditis, **B1**.532–3, **B2**.970–1, **B2**.974
    epidemiology, **B2**.971
    human, **B2**.971
    prevention, **B2**.974
    transmission, **B2**.971
    treatment, **B2**.974
    see also Erysipelas; Erysipeloid
  isolation/identification, **B2**.971–2
    typing methods, **B2**.972
  metabolism, **B2**.972–3
  morphology, **B2**.973
  pathogenicity, **B2**.973–4
  virulence factors, **B2**.973–4
Erysipelothrix tonsillarum, **B2**.970, **B2**.973
Erythema infectiosum (EI), **V1**.411–12
Erythema migrans, Lyme borreliosis, **B2**.1821
Erythema nodosum leprosum (ENL), **B2**.1205
Erythema nodosum, *Yersinia pseudotuberculosis* infection, **I**.563
Erythritol fermentation, Enterobacteriaceae identification, **B2**.1319 (Tab.)
Erythroblasts, viruses replicating in, **V1**.243 (Tab.)
Erythrocyte(s)
  acute phase response, **I**.207
  Babesia infection, **P**.452
  complement receptor 1, **I**.147, **I**.151
  immune complex clearance, **I**.147
  membrane, **P**.162 (Fig.)
  Plasmodium development, **P**.467–8
  Plasmodium invasion, **P**.472
  Schistosoma ingestion, **P**.606
Erythrocyte-binding antigen (EBA), *Plasmodium,* **I**.676
Erythrocyte sedimentation rate (ESR), acute phase response, **I**.206
Erythroid cells, IL-3 effects, **I**.275
Erythroleukemia, murine leukemia virus, **V1**.339–40

Erythromycin
  BA treatment, **B2**.1899
  pelliosis hepatitis treatment, **B2**.1899
  resistance
    Chlamydia, **B2**.2020
    Coxiella burnetii, **B2**.2077–8
    Staphylococcus, **B2**.794 (Tab.), **B2**.803
    Treponema pallidum, **B2**.1858
  spectrum of activity, **B1**.485, **B1**.499 (Tab.)
    Actinomyces, **B2**.1011
    Bordetella, **B2**.1793–4
    Borrelia, **B2**.1831 (Tab.)
    Campylobacter, **B2**.1548
    gram-positive anaerobic cocci, **B2**.912
    Haemophilus, **B2**.1702 (Tab.), **B2**.1704
    Legionella, **B1**.635, **B2**.1776–7
    Listeria, **B2**.956, **B2**.957–8
    Mycoplasma, **B2**.1992
    Mycoplasma pneumoniae, **B1**.634
    Streptococcus, **B2**.861–2
  structure, **B1**.486
Erythromycin A, structure, **B1**.486 (Fig.)
Erythrophagocytosis
  anemia in malaria, **P**.499
  Entamoeba histolytica, **P**.209
Erythropoiesis, prostaglandin E$_2$ effects, **I**.188
Erythropoietin receptor, interferon-γ receptor *vs.,* **I**.250
Erythrotoxin B (SPEB), *Streptococcus pyogenes,* **I**.556 (Tab.), **I**.565
Erythrovirus, **V1**.411–12
  classification, **V1**.42
  genome structure, **V1**.414 (Fig.), **V1**.415–16
    NS1 site, **V1**.415–16
    VP1 site, **V1**.415–16
    VP2 site, **V1**.415–16
  infection, **V1**.429–33
  members, **V1**.411 (Tab.)
  non-human species, **V1**.412
Eschar, in anthrax, **B2**.932
Escherichia
  antibacterial susceptibility/resistance, **B2**.1369–70
  antigens, **B2**.1362–5
  cell wall structure, **B2**.1362–5
  culture, **B2**.1362, **B2**.1365–6
  definition, **B2**.1360
  fimbriae, **B2**.1342–3
  genetics, **B2**.1362
  habitats, **B2**.1361
  infection
    intestinal, **B2**.1347
    TLR-5, **I**.121
  isolation/identification, **B2**.1365–9
  metabolism, **B2**.1362
  morphology, **B2**.1361–2
  as normal microbiota, **B1**.296 (Tab.), **B2**.1372
  pathogenicity, **B2**.1369 (Tab.), **B2**.1372–80, **B2**.1373 (Tab.)
  species, **B2**.1360, **B2**.1361 (Tab.)
  typing methods, **B2**.1370–2
    conventional, **B2**.1370
    molecular, **B2**.1370–2
  waterborne, **B1**.221

Escherichia adecarboxylata see Leclercia adecarboxylata
Escherichia albertii, **B2**.1360
  characteristics, **B2**.1361 (Tab.)
Escherichia blattae, **B2**.1360
  biochemical tests, **B2**.1319 (Tab.)
  characteristics, **B2**.1361 (Tab.)
  habitats, **B2**.1361
Escherichia coli, **B2**.1360
  adhesins, **B1**.674–6
  aerobactin, **B1**.676
  as airborne bacteria, **B1**.189
  antibacterial susceptibility/resistance, **B1**.433, **B1**.436–8, **B1**.499 (Tab.), **B2**.1370
    antibiotics, **B1**.440, **B1**.444
    mechanisms of action, **B1**.472 (Fig.)
    phenol, **B1**.431 (Fig.)
    quinolone resistance, **B1**.493 (Tab.)
  antigens, **B2**.1363–5
    F antigens, **B2**.1365
    H antigens, **B2**.1365
    K antigens, **B2**.1364–5
    O antigens, **B2**.1364
  artificial competence, **B1**.99
  biochemistry/metabolism, **B2**.1362
    ABC transport, **B1**.49
    acetate as carbon source, **B1**.53–4
    catabolite repression, **B1**.73
    energy charge, **B1**.40
    glyoxylate bypass, **B1**.53
    inducible transport system, **B1**.50
    ion gradient-linked transport, **B1**.49
    KDPG pathway, **B1**.58–9
    lac operon, **B1**.70–1, **B1**.71 (Fig.)
    lactose, **B1**.24
    nitrate reduction, **B1**.66
    oxidative stress, **B1**.65
    pentose fermentation, **B1**.57
    phosphoenolpyruvate phosphotransferase system, **B1**.50
    proteins, **B1**.42
    pyruvate dehydrogenase complex, **B1**.52–4
    respiration, **B1**.64
    starvation, **B1**.75
    sugar fermentation, **B1**.115
    superoxide dismutase, **B1**.65
  capsules, **B2**.1343, **B2**.1361–2
  cell division regulation, **B1**.48
  cell wall, **B1**.43–4, **B2**.1362–5, **B2**.1363 (Fig.)
  characteristics, **B2**.1361 (Tab.)
  classification
    Pseudomonas vs., **B2**.1592–3
    Shigella relationships, **B2**.1318
  colicins *see* Colicins
  covalent modification, **B1**.76
  culture, **B2**.1365–6
    morphology, **B2**.1345 (Tab.)
  cytoplasmic membrane, **B1**.44–5
  cytotoxic necrotizing factor 1, **B1**.676
  facilitated diffusion, **B1**.48–9
  fimbriae, **B2**.1362
    F1C, **B1**.675
    P fimbriae/receptors, **B1**.674–5, **B1**.675 (Fig.)
    type 1 (mannose-sensitive), **B1**.674, **B1**.676

Escherichia coli,
 fimbriae (*Continued*)
  type 2 (mannose-resistant [MR]), **B1**.675–6
 fimbrial colonization factor CFa/I, **I**.829
 flagella, **B1**.148–9, **B1**.151–2, **B2**.1361
  type 1 (mannose-sensitive), **B1**.148–9
 foods
  in cheese, **B1**.255–6
  in cream, **B1**.248
  herbs and spices, **B1**.287
  meat and meat products, **B1**.273–5
  in milk, **B1**.239–42
  nuts, **B1**.287
  poultry, **B1**.276
 genetics, **B2**.1362
  L-arabinose operon, **B1**.71–2
  chromosomal replication, **B1**.46
  constitutive mutants, **B1**.70
  genome sequence, **B2**.1344
  glucose -6-phosphate isomerase negative
   mutants, **B1**.57
  lactic dehydrogenase mutants, **B1**.55
  plasmids, **B1**.115
  recombination discovery, **B1**.13
  R plasmids, **B2**.1276
  tryptophan operon regulation, **B1**.72
 growth curve, death phase, **B1**.40
 habitats, **B2**.1361
 heat shock response, **B1**.74
 hemolysin production, **B1**.48, **B1**.676
 historical perspective, **B2**.1360
 immune evasion
  complement shedding, **I**.663
  membrane attack complex inhibition, **I**.664
  MHC class II antigen presentation, **I**.659
  pore-forming toxins, **I**.654–5
 infection *see Escherichia coli* infection
 iron-dependent repression, **B1**.165–6
 iron scavenging, **B1**.151
 iron siderophores, **B1**.676
 isolation/identification, **B2**.1365–9
  biochemical tests, **B2**.1319 (Tab.)
  carcass testing, **B1**.289
  historical perspective, **B2**.1350
  problem strains, **B2**.1348–50
  screening tests, **B2**.1349 (Tab.)
  serology, **B1**.757
  typing methods, **B2**.1370–2
 LPS, **B1**.158
  genetic loci involved in biosynthesis,
   B1.160
  virulence, **B1**.158–9
 morphology, **B2**.1361–2
 motility, **B1**.151–2, **B2**.1342
 in normal microbiota, **B1**.296 (Tab.),
  B1.302–3, **B2**.1372
 pathogenicity, **B2**.1369 (Tab.), **B2**.1372–80,
  B2.1373 (Tab.), **B2**.1376 (Tab.)
 pili, **B1**.44, **B1**.101 (Fig.)
 porins, **B1**.43
 sigma factors, **B1**.74–5, **B1**.440, **B1**.448
 signal transduction, **B1**.168–9
 sterilization
  freezing and thawing, **B1**.450
  ionizing radiation, **B1**.271, **B1**.451

 moist heat, **B1**.448
 UV radiation, **B1**.451
 tritrpticin sensitivity, **I**.172
 as vaccine vector, **I**.899, **I**.902
  attenuated vaccines, **I**.830–1
 virulence factors
  K-antigens, **B1**.154
  LPSs, **B1**.158–9
  plasmid determination, **B1**.114
 waterborne, **B1**.212
  testing, **B1**.223, **B1**.225
 see also individual types
Escherichia coli, diffusely adherent (DAEC),
  B2.1379
 adhesins, **B1**.148–9
 identification, **B2**.1369
 infection, **B2**.1379
  inflammatory bowel diseases link,
   B1.148–9
Escherichia coli, enterhemorrhagic (EHEC)
 meat, **B1**.273–4
 Shiga-like toxin, **B1**.156 (Tab.)
  nomenclature, **B2**.1339
 vaccines, **I**.933 (Tab.)
 vegetables, **B1**.282
Escherichia coli, enteroaggregative (EAggEC),
  B2.1378–9
 identification, **B2**.1369
 infection, **B2**.1378–9
Escherichia coli, enteroinvasive (EIEC),
  B2.1374–5
 identification, **B2**.1367, **B2**.1367 (Fig.)
 infection, **B2**.1374–5
 vegetables, **B1**.282
Escherichia coli, enteropathogenic (EPEC),
  B2.1372–4
 adherence, host specificity, **B1**.147–8
 adhesins, **B1**.148–9
 curli synthesis, **B1**.148–9
 fimbriae, type IV, **B1**.148–9
 flagella, adhesive properties, **B1**.148–9
 identification, **B2**.1366–7, **B2**.1367 (Fig.)
 infection, **B2**.1372–4
 K-88 strain, **B1**.147–8
 K-99 strain, **B1**.147–8
 phagocytic uptake inhibition, **I**.649
 subversion of host cell signal transduction,
  B1.164–5, **B1**.166 (Fig.)
 vegetables, **B1**.282
 virulence factors, **B2**.1373 (Tab.), **B2**.1374
Escherichia coli, enterotoxigenic (ETEC),
  B2.1375–7
 heat-labile enterotoxin *see Escherichia coli*
  heat labile enterotoxin (LT)
 heat-stable enterotoxin, **B1**.157 (Tab.)
 identification, **B2**.1367, **B2**.1368 (Fig.)
 infection, **B2**.1375
 vaccines
  cholera enterotoxin adjuvants, **I**.932
  development status, **I**.933 (Tab.)
  LT adjuvants, **I**.932
 vegetables, **B1**.282
 virulence factors, **B2**.1373 (Tab.), **B2**.1375–7

Escherichia coli heat labile enterotoxin (LT),
  B1.156 (Tab.), **I**.538, **I**.931–2, **I**.937–8
 bare skin immunization, **I**.823, **I**.824, **I**.826,
  I.826 (Fig.)
 enterotoxigenic *Escherichia coli* (ETEC)
  vaccines, **I**.932
 IL-12 suppression, **I**.652
 intranasal vaccine delivery, **I**.831, **I**.864
 MHC class II presentation interference,
  I.659
 mucosal administration, **I**.926–7
 T cell apoptosis, **I**.655
 TNF-α suppression, **I**.652
 transcutaneous immunization, **I**.837
 transgenic plant expression, **I**.829
Escherichia coli infection, **B2**.1372–80
 acute phase response, **B1**.740
 avoidance of host immune defenses, **B1**.154
 bacteremia due to, **B1**.520
 bloody diarrhea
  egg products, **B1**.279
  meat, **B1**.273–4
 cheese, **B1**.255–6
 dendritic cell infection, **I**.656
 endophthalmitis, **B1**.603
 extraintestinal, **B2**.1346–7
 hospital-acquired bacteremia, **B1**.393
 intracranial abscess, **B1**.585
  animal models, **B1**.583–4
 mastitis, **B1**.230
 milk-borne, **B1**.239–42
 neonatal meningitis, **B1**.574–5
 nosocomial, **B1**.397, **B1**.398 (Tab.)
  bacteremia, **B1**.393
  food-borne, **B1**.377
 pneumonia, **B1**.637
 vaccines
  BCE peptide vaccines, **I**.855 (Tab.)
  Vibrio cholerae vectors, **I**.844
 yogurt, **B1**.249–50
Escherichia coli K-12
 capsule composition, **B1**.44
 protein synthesis, **B1**.47
Escherichia coli, O26:H11, **B1**.273–5
Escherichia coli, O103, **B1**.273–4
Escherichia coli, O104, **B1**.273–4
Escherichia coli, O111, **B1**.273–4
Escherichia coli, O157:H7
 antigens, virulence effects, **B2**.1340
 bioterrorism, **B1**.768
 case-control study, **B1**.315–16
 foods
  egg products, **B1**.279
  fruit, **B1**.283
  hazard analysis, **B1**.288
  meat, **B1**.273–4
  vegetables, **B1**.282
 isolation/identification
  EIAs, **B1**.751
  screening tests, **B2**.1349 (Tab.)
  serology, **B1**.757
 outbreaks
  childcare centers, **B1**.361
  hamburger contamination, **B1**.361

Escherichia coli, O157:H7 (*Continued*)
  Shig toxin/verotoxin production, nomenclature difficulties, **B2**.1339
  study on carriage, **B1**.320
  waterborne, **B1**.212, **B1**.218
Escherichia coli, uropathogenic (UPEC), **B1**.674, **B1**.674–7, **B2**.1379–80
  adherence, **B1**.147–8, **B1**.674–6
  adhesins, **B1**.147–8
  antibacterial susceptibility/resistance, **B1**.679
  colonization, **B1**.677
  pathogenesis, **B1**.674–7
  vaccine development, **B1**.680, **I**.933 (Tab.)
  virulence factors organization, **B1**.677
Escherichia coli, verotoxigenic (VTEC), **B1**.239–44, **B1**.255–6, **B2**.1377–8
  in foods
    cheese, **B1**.255–6
    meat, **B1**.273–5
    milk, **B1**.230, **B1**.231–2, **B1**.235 (Tab.), **B1**.239–42
    yogurt, **B1**.249–50
  infection, **B2**.1377–8
  isolation/identification, **B2**.1367–9
  nomenclature, **B2**.1339
  serogroup O157:H7 *see Escherichia coli,* O157:H7
  virulence factors, **B2**.1373 (Tab.), **B2**.1378
Escherichia fergusonii, **B2**.1360
  biochemical tests, **B2**.1319 (Tab.)
  characteristics, **B2**.1361 (Tab.)
  habitats, **B2**.1361
Escherichia hermannii, **B2**.1360
  antibacterial susceptibility/resistance, **B2**.1369–70
    intrinsic, **B2**.1352 (Tab.)
  biochemical tests, **B2**.1319 (Tab.)
  characteristics, **B2**.1361 (Tab.)
  habitats, **B2**.1361
Escherichia vulneris, **B2**.1360
  biochemical tests, **B2**.1319 (Tab.)
  characteristics, **B2**.1361 (Tab.)
  habitats, **B2**.1361
Esculin hydrolysis
  Enterobacteriaceae identification, **B2**.1319 (Tab.)
  Porphyromonas identification, **B2**.1924 (Tab.)
  Prevotella identification, **B2**.1924 (Tab.)
E-selectin, **I**.505–6
  cytokine stimulation, **I**.506–7
  lymphocyte migration, **I**.506–7, **I**.508 (Tab.)
  Th1 cells, **I**.400
  upregulation in malaria, **P**.496–7
E site, tRNA, **B1**.47
Esophageal cancer, HPV associations, **V1**.463 (Tab.)
Esophageal candidiasis *see* Candidiasis, gastrointestinal
Esophagus
  aspergillosis, **M**.701
  candidiasis *see* Candidiasis, gastrointestinal
  normal microbiota, **B1**.302
  zygomycosis, **M**.20–1
'Espundia,' **P**.327, **M**.412
'Essential mixed cryoglobulinemia,' hepatitis C, **V2**.1208

Essential oils, herbs and spices, **B1**.287
Esters, **B1**.422
  antibacterial, **B1**.423 (Tab.)
Estuarine areas, bacteriology of, **B1**.216
Etanercept, mechanism of action, **I**.357
E-test *see* Epsilometer test (E-test)
Ethambutol (EMB), **B1**.481
  Mycobacterium, **B2**.1218
  Mycobacterium tuberculosis, **B2**.1197, **B2**.1218
Ethanol, **B1**.427
  action of, **B1**.438
  fermentation, **B1**.56
  formation by bacteria, **B1**.54
  see also Alcohol(s)
Ethmoid sinus, respiratory tract, **B1**.606–7
Ethnic background, lobomycosis, **M**.430–1
Ethnicity, innate malaria resistance, **P**.485
Ethylamine, systemic $\gamma\delta$ T cell binding, **I**.440 (Fig.)
Ethylenediamine tetraacetic acid (EDTA), action of, **B1**.428, **B1**.436, **B1**.437 (Tab.)
Ethylene imine, **B1**.439
Ethylene oxide, **B1**.429, **B1**.438–9
  sterilization, **B1**.445 (Tab.)
    thermochemical treatment, **B1**.454
    validation and monitoring, **B1**.454 (Tab.), **B1**.455
Ethylene sulfide, **B1**.439
Ets transcription factors, **I**.347
Euascomycetes, **M**.55 (Tab.), **M**.62 (Fig.)
Eubacterium, **B2**.1027–30
  antibacterial susceptibility/resistance, **B2**.1028
  cell walls, **B1**.42–4, **B2**.1028
  classification, **B2**.904, **B2**.1028–9
    changes to, **B2**.1028, **B2**.1028 (Tab.)
    differential characteristics, **B2**.1029 (Tab.)
  culture, **B2**.1027–8
  genus definition, **B2**.1027
  habitats, **B2**.1027
  historical perspective, **B2**.1027
  infection
    intracranial abscess, **B1**.585
    periodontitis, **B2**.1029–30
  isolation, **B2**.1029
  metabolism, **B2**.1028
    fermentation, **B2**.1027, **B2**.1028
  morphology, **B2**.1027
  normal microbiota, **B1**.296 (Tab.), **B1**.301
  in normal microbiota, **B2**.1029
  pathogenicity, **B2**.1029–30
  virulence factors, **B2**.1029–30
Eubacterium brachy, **B2**.1029 (Tab.)
  pathogenicity, **B2**.1029–30
Eubacterium budayi, **B2**.1028
Eubacterium cellulosolvens, **B2**.1028
Eubacterium combesii, **B2**.1029 (Tab.)
  pathogenicity, **B2**.1029–30
Eubacterium contortum, **B2**.1029 (Tab.)
  pathogenicity, **B2**.1029–30
Eubacterium cylindroides, **B2**.1029 (Tab.)
  pathogenicity, **B2**.1029–30
Eubacterium limosum, **B2**.1030
  characteristics, **B2**.1029 (Tab.), **B2**.1030

  isolation, **B2**.1030
  metabolism, **B2**.1028
  pathogenicity, **B2**.1029–30
Eubacterium minutum, **B2**.1029 (Tab.)
Eubacterium moniliforme, **B2**.1029 (Tab.)
Eubacterium multiforme, **B2**.1029 (Tab.)
Eubacterium nodatum, **B2**.1029 (Tab.)
  pathogenicity, **B2**.1029–30
Eubacterium rectale
  differential characteristic, **B2**.1029 (Tab.)
  pathogenicity, **B2**.1029–30
Eubacterium saburreum, **B2**.1029 (Tab.)
  pathogenicity, **B2**.1029–30
Eubacterium saphenum, **B2**.1029 (Tab.)
Eubacterium sulci, **B2**.1029 (Tab.)
  reclassification, **B2**.1946
Eubacterium tenue, **B2**.1029 (Tab.)
  metabolism, **B2**.1028
  pathogenicity, **B2**.1029–30
Eubacterium uniforme, **B2**.1028
Eubacterium xylanophilium, **B2**.1028
EUCALB, *Borrelia* detection, **B2**.1829, **B2**.1830 (Tab.)
Eucalyptus trees, *Cryptococcus neoformans,* **M**.643
Eucestoda, **P**.576, **P**.677
Eucoleus, **P**.589
Euglenozoa, **P**.350
Euglobin, **I**.141
Eukarya, phylogeny, **B1**.30–1
Eukaryotes, **B1**.11, **P**.159
  cellular components and structure, **P**.160–72, **P**.160 (Tab.)
  prokaryotes *vs.,* **P**.160 (Tab.)
  unicellular, **P**.159–60
    evolution, **P**.159–60
Eukaryotic expression systems, **V1**.92
Eumycetoma, **M.385–95**
  causative agents, **M**.386 (Tab.)
    see also individual species
  clinical appearance, **M**.388
  diagnosis, **M**.388–92
  epidemiology, **M**.387–8
  history, **M**.27, **M**.386
  pathogenesis, **M**.386–7
  therapy, **M**.393
  surgery, **M**.393
Eumycotic black grain mycetoma, **M**.139 (Fig.)
Eumycotic white grain mycetoma, **M**.139 (Fig.)
Europe
  food-borne botulism, **B2**.1069
  general practitioner reporting system, **B1**.320
  nosocomial infection control, **B1**.406
European biotype *see Echinococcus granulosus*
European brown hare syndrome virus (EBHSV), **V2**.912
European Collection of Animal Cell Cultures, **V1**.86
European Confederation of Medical Mycology (ECMM), **M**.30
European corn borer, **B1**.203–4
European Respiratory Society, pneumonia treatment guidelines, **B1**.639 (Tab.)
European Working Group for Legionella Infections (EWGLI), **B2**.1776

Europe, rubella vaccination programs, **V2**.982–3

Eurotiales, **M**.55 (Tab.), **M**.61–3

Eurytrema, as zoonosis, **P**.642

Eutrophication, **B1**.200

Evaluation/monitoring, parasite control, **P**.112

Evan's blue test, **M**.453, **M**.453 (Fig.), **M**.455

EVER gene mutations, **I**.772

Everglades virus (EVEV), **V2**.1011 (Tab.)

human infection, **V2**.1020–1

Evoked interferon-γ assays (EGIA)

hypersensitivity measurement, **B1**.747

tuberculosis diagnosis, **B1**.747

Evolutionarily conserved signaling intermediate in Toll pathways (ECSIT), **I**.122

Evolutionary species, viral species, **V1**.30

Evolution/origin

bacteria, **B1**.30

controversy, **B1**.30–1

hierarchy for lineage, **B1**.31

speciation, **B1**.30

see also Phylogeny

fungi, **M**.43, **M**.222–3

viruses, **V1**.55–6, **V1**.175–6, **V1**.**11–23**

amino acid sequence comparisons, **V1**.175–6

antiviral chemotherapy resistance, **V1**.19–20, **V2**.1632

conserved genes, **V1**.175

genome reengineering, **V1**.56

mechanisms, **V1**.14–7

genome mutation, **V1**.16–7

mutations, **V1**.19

recombination, **V1**.14–6

see also Origin (of viruses); *specific viruses*

Ewingella, **B2**.1492–3

antibacterial susceptibility/resistance, **B2**.1493

biochemical tests, **B2**.1492

culture, **B2**.1492

definition, **B2**.1492

habitats, **B2**.1493

pathogenicity, **B2**.1493

Ewingella americana, **B2**.1492

antibacterial susceptibility/resistance, **B2**.1493

intrinsic, **B2**.1352 (Tab.)

biochemical tests, **B2**.1492

culture, **B2**.1492

habitats, **B2**.1493

as normal microbiota, **B1**.296 (Tab.)

pathogenicity, **B2**.1493

Exanthem *see* Rashes/exanthem

Exanthem subitum (roseola), **V1**.527–8

'Excess mortality,' influenza, **V1**.669, **V1**.671 (Tab.)

Excision repair

bacterial spores, **B1**.452

nonsporulating bacteria, **B1**.451–2

Exclusion controls, rabies control, **V1**.370–1

Excretory systems, larval cestodes, **P**.681–2

Excystation

Balantidium coli, **P**.277

Isospora belli, **P**.411

Executioners, caspases, **I**.133–4

Exflagellation, *Plasmodium,* **P**.468

Exiguobacterium, **B2**.991–2

chemotaxonomic characteristics, **B2**.978 (Tab.)

habitats, **B2**.978

Exiguobacterium acetylicum, **B2**.991–2

biochemical characteristics, **B2**.993 (Tab.)

Exoantigen test, **M**.34

Blastomyces dermatitidis, **M**.495–6

Coccidioides immitis, **M**.514

dimorphic fungi identification, **M**.91

Histoplasma capsulatum var. *capsulatum,* **M**.111

Penicillium marneffei, **M**.566

Exocervicitis, trichomoniasis, **P**.257–9

Exocytosis

protozoa, **P**.164

Trypanosoma brucei, **P**.355, **P**.357 (Fig.)

Exodus-1 (CCL20) *see* CCL20

Exodus-2 (CCL21) *see* Secondary lymphoid tissue chemokine (SLC:CCL21)

Exodus-3 (CCL19) *see* Epstein–Barr virus-induced receptor ligand chemokine (ELC:CCL19)

Exofoliative toxins, *Staphylococcus aureus,* **I**.556 (Tab.), **I**.564–5

Exogenous proteins, antigen processing, **I**.414–15

Exophiala

histopathology, **M**.89 (Tab.)

oculomycoses, **M**.278 (Tab.), **M**.283–4

Exophiala dermatitidis, keratitis, **M**.328

Exophiala jeanselmei

histopathology, **M**.89 (Tab.), **M**.128 (Tab.)

mycetoma, **M**.390, **M**.390 (Tab.), **M**.392 (Tab.)

Exophiala jeanselmei var. *jeanselmei,* endophthalmitis, **M**.323

Exophiala spinifera infection

chromoblastomycosis, **M**.357

disseminated, **M**.745

Exophila, **M**.61–3

Exopolysaccharides, **B1**.153–4

Burkholderia cepacia complex, **B2**.1614

Burkholderia thailandensis, **B2**.1622

Exosomes, MHC class I, **I**.415

Exotoxin(s), **B1**.155–7, **B1**.156 (Tab.)

attachment and entry into target cells, **B1**.155–7

A + B subunits, **B1**.155, **B1**.156 (Tab.)

definition, **B1**.147

genes for production, **B1**.157

Pseudomonas aeruginosa, **B2**.1600

superantigens, **B1**.157, **B1**.157 (Tab.)

see also specific toxins; specific types

Exotoxin A *see Pseudomonas aeruginosa*

Exotoxin A (ETA), *Pseudomonas aeruginosa,* **B2**.1600

Exotoxin S, *Pseudomonas aeruginosa,* **B2**.1600

Exotoxin Z (SMEZ), **I**.557

Experimental allergic encephalitis (EAE), **I**.759

candidate therapy identification, **I**.759

chemokine deletion effects, **I**.228

epitope spreading, **I**.756

IL-2 gene defects, **I**.752

IL-4 therapy, **I**.280–1

IL-18, **I**.290–2

molecular mimicry, **I**.753

superantigens, **I**.562, **I**.755, **I**.759

transforming growth factor-β, **I**.297

Exposure cohort, cohort studies, **V1**.363

Expressed sequence tags (EST), *Paracoccidioides brasiliensis,* **M**.543

Expression site associated genes (ESAG), trypanosomes, **P**.355

transferrin receptor variants, **P**.363

Expression vectors, DNA vaccines, **I**.910–12

Expulsion chemotherapy, gastrointestinal nematode infection intensity, **P**.723

Exserohilum infection

allergic fungal sinusitis, **M**.675

CNS, **M**.743

histopathology, **M**.89 (Tab.)

keratitis, **M**.301–2

Exserohilum rostratum, oculomycoses, **M**.278 (Tab.)

External auditory canal, *Aspergillus* otomycosis, **M**.700–1

Extinction, parasite control, **P**.108–9

Extracellular alarmones, **B1**.448

Extracellular enveloped virus (EEV)

poxviruses *see* Poxviruses

Vaccinia virus, **V1**.586

Extracellular enzymes, *Burkholderia thailandensis,* **B2**.1624

Extracellular induction components, **B1**.448

Extracellular matrix components (ECM), degradation by *Entamoeba histolytica,* **P**.205–6

Extracellular matrix deposition, airway hypersensitivity, **I**.731–2

Extracellular pathogens

CD4 T cells, **I**.390

protective immunity, **I**.489

see also individual species

Extracellular polysaccharide (EPS) production, **B1**.149–50, **B1**.150 (Fig.)

Extracellular sensing components (ESC), **B1**.448

Extracellular signal-regulated kinase (ERK), **I**.43

Extracellular slime, *Salmonella,* **B2**.1343

Extrachromosomal DNA, *Plasmodium,* **P**.479

Extrapyramidal disease, in progressive multifocal leucoencephalopathy (PML), **V2**.1417

Extravasation *see* Diapedesis

Extromelia virus infection, **I**.96

Eye(s)

normal microbiota, **B1**.598, **B1**.599 (Tab.)

specimens, **M**.83 (Tab.), **M**.84, **M**.86 (Tab.)

Eye infection, **B1**.598, **B1**.599 (Tab.)

Bacillus cereus in posttraumatic endophthalmitis, **B2**.940

Capnocytophaga canimorsus, **B2**.1674–5

enterovirus infection, **V2**.875

fungal infection *see* Oculomycoses

HSV, **V1**.507

Mycobacterium chelonae, **B2**.1252

nosocomial, **B1**.386

Pasteurella multocida infection, **B2**.1654–5

Eye infection (*Continued*)
 see also Conjunctivitis; Endophthalmitis;
  Keratitis
Eyelid, fungal infection see Blepharitis

F₁ protein
 Measles virus, **V1**.716 (Fig.)
 paramyxoviruses, **V1**.705–6
F(ab)₂ antibody fragments, **I**.367, **I**.367 (Fig.)
 Ig structure, **I**.304
F₂ protein
 Measles virus, **V1**.716 (Fig.)
 paramyxoviruses, **V1**.705, **V1**.706
Fab antibody fragments, **I**.367, **I**.367 (Fig.)
 Ig structure, **I**.304
FabI, FabK, FabL (enoyl-ACP reductases),
  B1.436–8, **B1**.441
Face, rhinosporidiosis, **M**.460, **M**.461 (Fig.)
Facial hair, **M**.196, **M**.227–8, **M**.231
 tinea barbae, **M**.228, **M**.231
 white piedra, **M**.196
Facilitated diffusion, **B1**.48–9
Factor VIII, HIV contamination, **B1**.380–1
Factor IX hemophilia, gene therapy, **V2**.1601
Factor B, **I**.143 (Tab.)
 alternate pathway activation, **I**.145,
  I.145 (Fig.)
 deficiency, **I**.152
Factor D, **I**.143 (Tab.)
 alternate pathway activation, **I**.145,
  I.145 (Fig.)
 deficiency, **I**.152
Factor H, **I**.150 (Tab.)
 alternate pathway activation, **I**.145
 deficiency, **I**.153, **I**.770–1
  membranoproliferative
   glomuleronephritis, **I**.154
Factor H-like 1 (fHL-1), **I**.150 (Tab.)
Factor I, **I**.150 (Tab.), **I**.151
 deficiency, **I**.153, **I**.770–1
Factor I domain, **I**.476 (Fig.)
Facultative anaerobes
 bacteria *see* Anaerobic bacteria
 Toxocara, **P**.750–1
FADD, death-inducing signaling complex
  assembly, **I**.134
'Failure rate,' vaccination models, **I**.961
Falciparum malaria *see* Malaria
Famciclovir (FCV), **V2**.1616
 biochemical properties, **V2**.1614 (Tab.)
 herpes encephalitis, **V2**.1421
 HSV infection, **V2**.1501
  latent infection, **V2**.1638
 structure, **V2**.1613 (Fig.)
 VZV infection, **V1**.517, **V2**.1507
  HIV infection, **V2**.1502
  in pregnancy, **V2**.1460
Familial clustering of disease, immunogenetics,
  I.572
Familial cold urticaria, **I**.125
Familial eosinophilia, *IFNGR1* gene, **I**.581
Familial hemophagocytic lymphohistiocytosis
  (FHL), **I**.481, **I**.778
Familial prion disease, **V2**.1367–9
 prion protein (PrP) mutations, **V2**.1367–9

Families, viral classification, **V1**.26,
  V1.27 (Tab.), **V1**.29, **V1**.35, **V1**.39,
  V1.378
Family studies, leprosy, **I**.590
F antigens
 Enterobacteriaceae, **B2**.1339–40
 Escherichia coli, **B2**.1365
Farcy *see* Glanders
Farmers/farm workers, **M**.368, **M**.458
 lobomycosis, **M**.431
 prototheosis, **M**.396–7, **M**.399–400
 rhinosporidiosis, **M**.458
 sporotrichosis, **M**.368
Farming *see* Agriculture/agricultural workers
  infection
Farr, W, **B1**.317
Fas (CD95)
 B cell maturation/activation, **I**.348–9
 eosinophil apoptosis, **I**.58
 homeostatic function, **I**.480
 mutations, autoimmune disease, **I**.756
 neutrophils, **I**.45
 see also Fas/Fas ligand mediated apoptosis
Fasciola, **P**.583, **I**.682
 classification, **P**.641–2
 immune evasion
  antibody destruction, **I**.685–6
  glutathione *S*-transferases, **I**.686
  glycocalix barrier, **I**.685
 infection *see* Fascioliasis
 life cycle, **P**.583
  definitive host, **P**.645–6
  life span, **P**.646
 morphology/structure, spines, **P**.642
 nutrition, **P**.644
 structure, **P**.583
 transmission/epidemiology
  distribution within communities, **P**.648
  location in host, **P**.648
 see also individual species
Fasciola gigantica, **P**.640
 geographical distribution, **P**.647
 historical aspects, **P**.640–1
 infection *see* Fascioliasis
 life cycle, intermediate hosts, **P**.646
 morphology, **P**.642
  eggs, **P**.642
 veterinary importance, **P**.641
Fasciola hepatica, **P**.640
 geographical distribution, **P**.647
 historical aspects, **P**.640–1
 infection *see* Fascioliasis
 life cycle, **P**.643 (Fig.)
  intermediate hosts, **P**.646
 morphology, **P**.642
  adult, **P**.640 (Fig.)
  eggs, **P**.640 (Fig.), **P**.642
 prevalence, **P**.647
 protein metabolism, **P**.644
 veterinary importance, **P**.641
Fasciolepis, classification, **P**.641–2
Fascioliasis
 basophils, **I**.68
 clinical manifestations, **P**.650
  acute stage, **P**.650

  biochemical abnormalities, **P**.650
  ectopic infection, **P**.650
  latent phase, **P**.650
 control, **P**.40, **P**.654
 diagnosis, egg morphology, **P**.652–3
 epidemiology, **P**.40, **P**.46 (Tab.)
 geographical distribution, **P**.40, **P**.41 (Fig.)
 immune response, **P**.652
  eosinophils, **I**.70
 pathogenesis/pathology, **P**.651–2
  granuloma formation, **P**.651–2
  immune response, **P**.652
  proinflammatory cytokines, **P**.652
 public health importance, **P**.105 (Tab.)
 transmission, **P**.645
  raw/undercooked food, **P**.647–8
 vaccine trials, **P**.652
Fasciolidae, **P**.583
Fasciolopsis, **P**.583
 public health importance, **P**.44
 structure/life cycle, **P**.583
Fas/Fas ligand mediated apoptosis
 apoptosis, **I**.477
 bacterial immune interference, **I**.655–6
 in cancer, **I**.101
 CD4 cells, **I**.792
  in HIV infection, **I**.792
 CTLs, **I**.422–3, **I**.477
 dendritic cells, **I**.903
  in HIV infection, **I**.792
 NK cells, **I**.81, **I**.101
 signaling complex assembly, **I**.134
 target cell death, **I**.478, **I**.479 (Fig.)
 Vpu protein, **V2**.1327–8
Fas ligand (Fas-L), **I**.288 (Tab.)
 cytotoxic granules, **I**.477
 expression, IL-2 effects, **I**.279–80
 homeostatic function, **I**.480, **I**.480 (Fig.)
 mutations, autoimmune disease, **I**.756
 NK cell cytotoxic granules, **I**.477
 see also Fas/Fas ligand mediated apoptosis
Fast-food, bacterial infection, **B1**.360–1
Fatal familial insomnia (FFI), **V2**.1347,
  V2.1368
Fatigue, babesiosis, **P**.454
Fat malabsorption, giardiasis, **P**.245–6
Fatty acid methyl esters (FAME), **B2**.945
Fatty acids
 Fusobacterium, **B2**.1949
 leptospire growth, **B2**.1870, **B2**.1881
 Plasmodium, **P**.477
 Porphyromonas, **B2**.1924 (Tab.)
 Prevotella, **B2**.1924 (Tab.)
 Pseudomonas, **B2**.1597
 synthesis, **B1**.61
Favus
 history, **M**.5
 tinea favosa, **M**.232, **M**.238
Fc (fragment crystalline), **I**.304
 Ig effector functions, **I**.311–12
Fc receptors, **I**.312–19
 on HSV, **V1**.258, **V1**.258 (Fig.)
 immune evasion, **V1**.312–13
 monoclonal antibody therapy, **I**.354, **I**.357
 neutrophil intracellular signaling, **I**.42

Fc receptors (*Continued*)
  viral receptors, **V1**.211
  see also specific types
Fcα/μR, **I**.317–18
  properties, **I**.313 (Tab.)
  structure, **I**.309 (Fig.), **I**.317
FcαRI (CD89), **I**.317
  neutrophils, **I**.39, **I**.317
  properties, **I**.313 (Tab.)
  structure, **I**.309 (Fig.), **I**.317
FcδR, properties, **I**.313 (Tab.)
FCER1B gene, IgE production, **I**.582
FcεRI, **I**.316
  basophils, **I**.62, **I**.316
  eosinophils, **I**.64, **I**.316
  IgE interaction, **I**.320–1
    antibody change, **I**.321
    receptor change, **I**.320–1
  mast cells, **I**.308, **I**.316
  properties, **I**.313 (Tab.)
  signal transduction, **I**.316
  structure, **I**.309 (Fig.), **I**.316
    ITAM, **I**.316
FcεRII (CD23), **I**.316–17
  IgE interactions, **I**.317
  properties, **I**.313 (Tab.)
  soluble forms, **I**.316–17
  structure, **I**.309 (Fig.), **I**.316–17
  upregulation, airway hypersensitivity, **I**.733–4
FcεRIII, eosinophils, **I**.64
FCG2A gene, dengue virus infection, **I**.588
FcγR
  genes, meningococcal meningitis association, **I**.594
  macrophages, **I**.25
  neutrophils, **I**.39, **I**.43
  prion diseases, **V2**.1384
  structural similarities, **I**.312
  see also specific types
FcγRI (CD64), **I**.314
  cell anchors, **I**.314
  cells, **I**.314
    eosinophils, **I**.64–5
    neutrophils, **I**.39
  cross-linking, **I**.314
  functions, **I**.314
  genes, **I**.314
  IgG interactions, **I**.314
  properties, **I**.313 (Tab.)
  structure, **I**.309 (Fig.), **I**.314
    intracellular domain, **I**.314
    signal transduction, **I**.314
FcγRII (CD32), **I**.314
  eosinophils, **I**.64–5
  properties, **I**.313 (Tab.)
  structure, **I**.309 (Fig.), **I**.314
FcγRIIa
  cells, **I**.314
  meningococcal meningitis, **I**.594
  neutrophils, **I**.39, **I**.314
FcγRIIb
  basophils, **I**.62
  B-cell downregulation, **I**.347
  immunoreceptor tyrosine-based inhibitory motif, **I**.347–8

macrophages, **I**.314
monocytes, **I**.314
FcγRIII (CD16), **I**.315
  eosinophils, **I**.64–5
  HCMV infection, **I**.772
  IgG interactions, **I**.321
    structural changes, **I**.321
  NK cells, **I**.79–80, **I**.627
  properties, **I**.313 (Tab.)
  structure, **I**.309 (Fig.)
FcγRIIIa, **I**.315
FcγRIIIb
  eosinophils, **I**.315
  glycophosphatidylinositol anchor, **I**.315
  neutrophils, **I**.39, **I**.315
FCGR gene, periodontitis association, **I**.595
FcγRIII (CD16), natural killer (NK) cells, **V1**.271–2
FcRn (neonatal receptor), **I**.315–16
  functions, **I**.315
  IgG binding, **I**.315–16, **I**.525
  maternal IgG transfer, **I**.315, **I**.316
  mucosal immune response, **I**.525
  pH dependency, **I**.316
  properties, **I**.313 (Tab.)
  structure, **I**.309 (Fig.), **I**.315
Febrile paroxysms, vivax/ovale (benign tertian) malaria, **P**.482
Febris quintana see Trench fever
Fecal analysis, **P**.150–1, **P**.150 (Tab.)
  amebiasis diagnosis, **P**.150, **P**.220, **P**.268
  Balantidium coli infection, **P**.280
  Chilomastix mesnili infection, **P**.272
  cryptosporidiosis diagnosis, **P**.151
  culture methods, **P**.151
  cyclosporiasis, **P**.415
  diagnosis *see* Diagnosis, parasitic infection
  direct saline wet preparations, **P**.151
  gastrointestinal nematodes, **P**.730
  giardiasis diagnosis, **P**.148, **P**.150, **P**.247–8
  immunoassays, **P**.151
  isosporiasis, **P**.151, **P**.413
  macroscopic examination, **P**.150–1
  microscopic examination, **P**.151
  microsporidiosis diagnosis, **P**.545, **P**.546–7
  molecular diagnostics, **P**.151
    PCR, **P**.151
  proctoscopy, **P**.150 (Tab.)
  Retortamonas intestinalis infection, **P**.273
  sigmoidoscopy, **P**.150 (Tab.), **P**.151
  staining, **P**.151
  string test, **P**.150 (Tab.), **P**.151
  Strongyloides diagnosis, **P**.741
  tapeworm diagnosis, **P**.664
Fecal coliform bacteria test, **B1**.223
Fecal coliforms, **B1**.186 (Tab.)
Fecal excretion, enteroviruses, **V2**.876
Fecal–oral transmission, **B1**.329, **V2**.1403–4
  adenoviruses, **V1**.445
  astroviruses, **V2**.900
  CNS infection, **V2**.1403–4
  Helicobacter pylori infection, **B2**.1578–9
  hepatitis A virus, **V2**.1160–1, **V2**.1172
  hepatitis E virus, **V2**.1160–1, **V2**.1180
  norovirus infection, **V2**.919

poliomyelitis, **V1**.368–9
  rotavirus infection, **V1**.368, **V2**.949–50
Fecal streptococci, airborne concentrations in facilities, **B1**.186 (Tab.)
Fecal streptococci test, **B1**.223–4
Feces
  astroviruses, **V2**.889, **V2**.902
  diarrhoea, **M**.399
    protothecosis, **M**.398–9
  Hepatitis A virus, **V2**.1160–1, **V2**.1169–71
  Hepatitis E virus, **V2**.1160–1
  Prototheca, **M**.398–9
  specimens, **M**.84
Fedchenko A., **P**.10–1
Feedback inhibition, **B1**.75–6
  branching biosynthetic pathways, **B1**.75–6
  concerted, **B1**.75–6
  cumulative, **B1**.75–6
  sequential, **B1**.76
Feet
  chromoblastomycosis, **M**.361–2
  mycetoma *see* Mycetoma
  protothecosis, **M**.397–8
  tinea nigra, **M**.198
  tinea pedis *see* Tinea pedis
Feline astrovirus (FAstV)
  cell culture, **V2**.906
  classification, **V2**.890 (Tab.)
  detection, ELISA, **V2**.899
  genome, **V2**.894 (Tab.)
  human infection, **V2**.903
Feline calicivirus, **V2**.912
Feline coronavirus (FCoV/FIPV), **V1**.392, **V1**.845
  infection, **V1**.841 (Tab.)
  membrane (M) protein, **V1**.837
Feline foamy virus (FFV)
  gene vectors, **V2**.1314
  genome, **V2**.1304–5, **V2**.1307–8
  infection, **V2**.1305
  zoonosis, **V2**.1296
Feline immunodeficiency virus (FIV), **B2**.1209
  emerging infection, **V2**.1651 (Tab.)
  gene therapy vector, **V2**.1592–3
  zoonosis, **V2**.1296
Feline infectious peritonitis, **V1**.845
  'antibody-dependent enhancement,' **V1**.845
  immunopathology, **V1**.279 (Tab.)
Feline infectious peritonitis virus (FIPV), **V1**.824–5
Feline leukemia virus (FeLV)
  cell receptors, **V1**.207 (Tab.)
  oncogenic mechanisms, **V1**.338, **V1**.342 (Tab.)
  receptors, **V1**.246 (Fig.)
  vaccines, **V1**.349
  zoonosis, **V2**.1296
Feline panleukopenia virus (FPV), **I**.871–2
  discovery, **V1**.409
  infection *see* Feline panleukopenia virus (FPV) infection
  morphology/structure, **V1**.412
  pathogenic potential, **V1**.422
Feline panleukopenia virus (FPV) infection
  cell entry, **V1**.416–17

Feline panleukopenia virus (FPV) infection (*Continued*)
  pathogenesis, **V1**.426
Feline spongiform encephalopathy (FSE), **V2**.1363
Female genital tract disease, schistosomiasis japonicum, **P**.631
Female worms, *Onchocerca volvulus,* **P**.782
Femur infection, inflammatory responses, **B1**.689
Fen1, SV40 replication, **V1**.154 (Tab.)
Fenbendazole, toxocariasis therapy, **P**.755
Fentichlor, **B1**.438
Fer-de-lance virus, **V1**.819
'Ferida brava,' **P**.327
'Ferida sêca,' **P**.324, **P**.327
Fermentation, **B1**.54
  Bifidobacterium, **B2**.1025–6
  definition, **B1**.4–5, **B1**.54
  Eubacterium, **B2**.1027, **B2**.1028
  food processing and preservation, **B1**.268 (Tab.)
  historical aspects, **B1**.4–5
Ferrets, *Pneumocystis,* **M**.775–6
Ferridoxin-mediated electron transport, *Dientamoeba fragilis,* **P**.267
Ferritin, **I**.202
Fertility, *Prnd* gene, **V2**.1359–61, **V2**.1361 (Fig.)
Fertilization, *Plasmodium,* **P**.468–71
Fetal infection, **V2**.1444 (Tab.)
  Coxsackie virus, **V2**.1482–3
  diagnostic procedures, **V2**.1444–6, **V2**.1445 (Tab.)
    amniocentesis, **V2**.1445, **V2**.1445 (Tab.)
    biopsy, **V2**.1445 (Tab.)
    chorionic villus sampling, **V2**.1445
    cordocentesis, **V2**.1445 (Tab.)
    direct procedures, **V2**.1445
    interpretation, **V2**.1445
    PCR, **V2**.1444–5
    serology, **V2**.1446 (Tab.)
    ultrasonography, **V2**.1445 (Tab.)
  echoviruses, **V2**.1482–3
  enteroviruses, **V2**.1482–3
  HCMV infection *see* Human cytomegalovirus (HCMV) infection
  hepatitis viruses, **V2**.1474–82
  HIV infection *see* HIV infection
  HPV, **V2**.1444 (Tab.), **V2**.1483–4
  HSV, **V2**.1461–7
  LCMV, **V2**.1483
  mumps, **V1**.749, **V1**.750
  neonatal infection *vs.,* **V2**.1446 (Tab.)
  Parvovirus infection, **V1**.425–6
  rubella *see* Rubella
  syphilis *see* Syphilis, congenital transmission, **V2**.1443–4, **V2**.1444 (Tab.)
    congenital (prenatal), **V2**.1443
    gestational age, **V2**.1444
    maternal antibodies, **V2**.1443–4
    maternal infection frequency, **V2**.1443
    perinatal infection, **V2**.1443
    pregnancy loss, **V2**.1444
    Th2 immune response, **V2**.1443

VZV infection *see* Congenital varicella syndrome (CVS); Varicella-zoster virus infection
  see also Congenital infection; *specific infection; specific viruses*
Fetal liver kinase ligand (FLK2), **I**.85
Fever
  acute phase response, **I**.197–8, **I**.198 (Fig.)
  babesiosis, **P**.454
  human brucellosis, **B2**.1737–8
  see also Pyrogenic exotoxins (PET)
Fever of unknown origin (FUO), cat-scratch disease, **B2**.1892–3
F' formation, conjugation, **B1**.102–3
Fialuridine
  hepatitis B therapy, **V2**.1629
  toxicity, **V2**.1638
Fiber diffraction, helical viruses, **V1**.60
Fibrinogen, **I**.203
  Aspergillus fumigatus binding, **M**.706
  Candida albicans binding, **M**.588
  IL-6 production, **I**.285
Fibrinolytic proteins, acute phase proteins, **I**.203–4
Fibrobacter, **B2**.1930
Fibroblasts
  G-CSF production, **I**.276
  GM-CSF production, **I**.277
  MHC class I antigen presentation, **I**.426–7
  schistosomiasis granulomas, **I**.722–3
Fibronectin
  Staphylococcus aureus adherence, **B1**.687–8
  Treponema pallidum, **B1**.149, **B2**.1840–1
  viral hemorrhagic septicemia virus receptor, **V2**.1108
Fibronectin-binding proteins (Fnb's), **B1**.149
Fibrosarcoma, BCE peptide vaccines, **I**.861 (Tab.)
Fibrosis, African trypanosomiasis, **P**.365
Fibrotic granulomas (type 2), schistosomiasis *see* Schistosomiasis
Fibrous nodules, *Onchocerca,* **I**.685
Field-inversion gel electrophoresis (FIGE), **B2**.894
Fijivirus, **V1**.47–8, **V2**.932
Filamentous fungi
  antifungal susceptibility testing, **M**.157
  susceptibility testing, **M**.157
  see also individual species
Filamentous hemagglutinin (FHA), **B2**.1789, **B2**.1789 (Tab.), **B2**.1792, **B2**.1798, **B2**.1799–800
Filariae, **P**.591
'Filarial dance sign,' **P**.773, **P**.777
Filarial nematodes
  cuticle, **P**.91
  immune response, **P**.91–2
    antigens, **P**.91
    T cells, **P**.91–2, **P**.93 (Fig.)
Filariasis, **P**.591–2, **I**.600–1
  blood transfusions, **P**.27–9
  control
    community participation, **P**.122–3
    stratification of disease, **P**.115
  'endemic normals', **P**.91–2

HLA associations, **I**.600–1
  immune response, **P**.91–2
    T cells, **P**.91–2
  public health importance, **P**.39–40
  see also Lymphatic filariasis
Filariasis Control Movement (FILCO), **P**.123
Filariasis Parents' Association, **P**.123
Filaroidea, **P**.591–2, **P**.782
  Onchocercidae, **P**.591–2
Filifactor alocis, reclassification, **B2**.1946
Filobasidiella, **M**.17–8
  classification, **M**.63, **M**.65 (Tab.)
  Trichosporon, **M**.197
Filobasidiella neoformans, **M**.77
  var. *bacillispora,* **M**.17–8, **M**.639
  var. *neoformans,* **M**.17–8, **M**.639
Filopodia, **P**.178 (Fig.), **P**.179, **P**.201–2
Filoviridae, **V1**.26
  characteristics, **V1**.129 (Tab.), **V1**.177 (Tab.), **V1**.382
  classification, **V1**.27 (Tab.), **V1**.48, **V1**.49 (Tab.)
  characteristics, **V1**.379, **V1**.380 (Tab.)
  phylogeny, **V1**.388
  see also specific viruses
Filoviruses, **V2.1085–101**
  cell culture, **V2**.1091–2
    artificial replication systems, **V2**.1093
    Vero cell line, **V2**.1091
  chemical agent resistance, **V2**.1098
  classification, **V2**.1086
    biohazard, **V2**.1086
    genome analysis, **V2**.1086
  Δ-peptide, **V2**.1091
  genome structure, **V1**.387 (Tab.), **V2**.1088, **V2**.1088 (Fig.)
    gene overlaps, **V2**.1088, **V2**.1092
    intergenic regions, **V2**.1088
    untranslated regions, **V2**.1092
  glycoprotein (GP), **V2**.1089–90, **V2**.1090 (Fig.)
    cell entry, **V2**.1092
    neutralizing antibodies, **V2**.1096
  historical aspects, **V2**.1093
  host range, **V1**.381–2
  immune evasion, **V2**.1096
    IFN antagonist, **V2**.1089
    innate immune response, **V2**.1096
  infection *see* Filovirus infection
  infectivity, **V2**.1086
  isolation/propagation and identification, **V1**.95, **V1**.96 (Tab.)
  large (L) protein, **V2**.1086–8, **V2**.1091
  morphology/structure, **V1**.75–6, **V1**.75 (Fig.), **V1**.128–30, **V2**.1086–8, **V2**.1088 (Fig.)
    matrix proteins, **V1**.75–6
    nucleoproteins, **V1**.75
    protein structures, **V1**.70 (Tab.)
    replication component, **V1**.75
    transport component, **V1**.75
  non structural glycoproteins, **V2**.1091
  nucleoprotein (NP), **V2**.1086–9
  physical agent resistance, **V2**.1098
  polypeptides, **V2**.1089–91
  see also specific types

Filoviruses (*Continued*)
post-translational processing, **V2**.1089, **V2**.1090 (Fig.)
replication, **V2**.1090 (Fig.), **V2**.1091–3
assembly and exit, **V2**.1093
genome replication, **V2**.1092–3
mRNA transcription, **V1**.381
subgenomic RNA synthesis, **V2**.1092
transcription, **V2**.1090 (Fig.), **V2**.1092–3
translation, **V2**.1092–3
virus entry, **V2**.1092
reverse genetics, **V1**.133–4, **V1**.189
RNP complex, **V2**.1086–8
structural proteins, **V2**.1086–8
see also specific types
transmission, **V1**.371 (Tab.)
VP24, **V2**.1091
VP30 (minor nucleoprotein), **V2**.1090–1
VP35 (polymerase cofactor), **V2**.1089
VP40 (matrix protein), **V2**.1089
Filovirus infection, **V2**.1093–8
abortion risk, **V2**.1094
clinical course, **V2**.1094 (Fig.)
convalescence, **V2**.1094
clinical features, **V2**.1094
hemorrhagic fever, **V2**.1094
nonfatal cases, **V2**.1094
diagnosis, **V2**.1096–7, **V2**.1097 (Tab.)
serology, **V2**.1093
differential diagnosis, **V2**.1096
epidemiology, **V2**.1093
immune response, **V2**.1096
humoral, **V2**.1096
IFN activity, **I**.260 (Tab.)
immunosuppression, **V2**.1096
neutralizing antibodies, **V2**.1096
management, **V2**.1097–8
patient isolation, **V2**.1097
supportive therapy, **V2**.1097
mortality, **V2**.1094
outbreaks, **V2**.1085–6, **V2**.1087 (Tab.)
pathology, **V2**.1095
animal models, **V2**.1095
humans, **V2**.1095
pathophysiology, **V2**.1095–6
disseminated intravascular coagulation (DIC), **V2**.1095
extrahepatic targets, **V2**.1095
immunopathology, **V2**.1095–6
visceral organ necrosis, **V2**.1095
transmission, **V2**.1093–4
aerosols, **V2**.1093–4
droplets, **V2**.1093–4
intimate contact, **V2**.1093–4
nosocomial transmission, **V2**.1093–4
vaccine development, **V2**.1097–8
zoonosis, **V2**.1093
see also Hemorrhagic fevers
Filtration, **B1**.453
applications, **B1**.445 (Tab.), **B1**.453
mechanisms of action, **B1**.453
types of filter, **B1**.453
uses, **B1**.453
validation and monitoring, **B1**.454 (Tab.)
viral classification, **V1**.24–5

FimA protein, **B1**.148–9
Fimbriae
Bartonella alsatica, **B2**.1887
Bartonella tribocorum, **B2**.1887
Bordetella, **B2**.1789 (Tab.), **B2**.1799
Enterobacter, **B2**.1342–3
Enterobacteriaceae *see* Enterobacteriaceae
Escherichia, **B2**.1342–3
Klebsiella, **B2**.1342–3
Moraxella, **B2**.1305
M. catarrhalis, **B2**.1307
Proteus, **B2**.1446
Salmonella, **B2**.1399, **B2**.1407
Shigella flexneri, **B2**.1342–3
FimH protein, **B1**.148–9
Finegoldia, **B2**.913–14
classification, **B2**.905 (Tab.)
identification, **B2**.906–7
Finegoldia magna, **B2**.913–14
antibacterial susceptibility/resistance, **B2**.911, **B2**.912
biochemical characteristics, **B2**.908 (Tab.)
classification, **B2**.904–5
definition/characteristics, **B2**.913–14
isolation and maintenance, **B2**.905
normal microbiota, **B2**.910
as normal microbiota, **B1**.296 (Tab.)
pathogenicity and virulence factors, **B2**.910–11
protein L, **B2**.911
Firmicutes, **B2**.1028
First-line responders, smallpox vaccination, **V1**.589, **V1**.590
Fischer's exact test, **I**.574
Fish and fish products, **B1**.279–80
Bacillus infection, **B2**.944
bacterial numbers on fresh produce, **B1**.279
dracunculiasis transmission, **P**.834
erysipeloid, **B2**.971
internal flesh, **B1**.279
microbiology, **B1**.279–80
ocean water temperature, **B1**.279
pathogens, **B1**.279
safety assurance, **B1**.288–9
spoilage, **B1**.279
Fish pathogens
herpesviruses, **V1**.45
microsporidiosis, **P**.541–2, **P**.544
rhabdoviruses, **V2**.1105
Fission yeasts, **M**.73
Fite-Faracou stain, modified, **M**.123 (Tab.)
Fitness of viruses
antiviral chemotherapy resistance, **V2**.1633–4
definition, **V1**.18–9
gains *vs.* losses, **V1**.18–9
quasispecies, **V1**.18–9
Flagella
Aeromonas, **B2**.1527–8
assembly, **B1**.151–2
Bartonella, **B2**.1887
Burkholderia cepacia complex, **B2**.1614
Burkholderia thailandensis, **B2**.1622–3
Chilomastix mesnili, **P**.270–1
composition, **B1**.44, **B1**.151–2
Enterobacteriaceae, **B2**.1339–40, **B2**.1342

function, **B1**.151–2
functions, **B1**.44
Helicobacter, **B2**.1576
Legionella, **B2**.1762 (Tab.)
leptospires, **B2**.1868
protein export system, **B1**.48
protozoa, **P**.179, **P**.179 (Fig.), **P**.180 (Fig.)
structure, **P**.161 (Fig.), **P**.170 (Fig.)
Retortamonas intestinalis, **P**.272–3
Salmonella see Salmonella
Trypanosoma brucei, **P**.353, **P**.355–6
Flagellar pocket, *Trypanosoma brucei*, **P**.355–6
Flagellates, **P**.187–8
blood/tissue, **P**.187–8
classification, **P**.197
cell division, **P**.181
intestinal, **P**.187–8
immune response, **P**.76
species, **P**.76
see also individual species
Flagellins, **B1**.44
Aeromonas, **B2**.1527–8
Burkholderia pseudomallei, **B2**.1614
Burkholderia thailandensis, **B2**.1622–3
Campylobacter, **B2**.1549
dendritic cell activation, **I**.393–4
as pathogen-associated molecular patterns, **I**.896
Salmonella, **B2**.1404
TLR-5 binding, **I**.121
Flame cells *see* Solenocytes (flame cells)
FLASH, death-inducing signaling complex assembly, **I**.134
Flash sterilization, **B1**.447
Flat sour spoilage
Bacillus, **B2**.923–4
food can bulging, **B1**.271, **B1**.283
Flavin adenine mononucleotide (FMN), **B1**.63
Flavins, **B1**.63
Flaviviridae
characteristics, **V1**.139 (Tab.), **V1**.177 (Tab.)
classification, **V1**.27 (Tab.), **V1**.51 (Tab.), **V1**.53–4
see also Flaviviruses; *specific viruses*
Flavivirus
classification, **V1**.53–4, **V2**.993
mRNA structure, **V1**.139
mRNA translation, **V1**.113
multifunctional gene products, **V1**.136–7
protein processing, **V1**.140
see also Flaviviruses
Flaviviruses, **V2**.993–1009
antigens, **V2**.996
classification, **V2**.993
transmission mode, **V2**.993
core (C) protein, **V2**.993, **V2**.995
as antigen, **V2**.996
envelope (E) protein, **V2**.993, **V2**.995, **V2**.996 (Fig.)
as antigen, **V2**.996
gene expression, **V1**.119
genome organization, **V1**.135–6, **V1**.136 (Fig.), **V2**.993–5, **V2**.995 (Fig.)
open reading frame, **V1**.135–6
Hepatitis C virus *vs.*, **V2**.1190, **V2**.1191–2

Flaviviruses (*Continued*)
immune evasion, IFN, **V1**.296
infection *see* Flavivirus infection
isolation/propagation and identification,
V1.95
membrane (M) protein, **V2**.993
morphology/structure, **V1**.138, **V2**.993
virion structure, **V2**.993
mRNA
structure, **V1**.140 (Tab.)
translation, **V1**.113
nonstructural proteins, **V2**.995
see also specific types
NS1 protein, **V2**.996
post-translational protein modification,
V1.225, **V2**.996
proteolytic cleavage, **V1**.121–2
proteins, **V2**.995–6
synthesis, **V1**.115–16
see also specific types
replication, **V2**.996–7
cell receptors, **V1**.138–9, **V2**.996
cell-specific factors, **V1**.136 (Fig.), **V1**.137
cellular entry, **V1**.108–9, **V1**.213
gene expression, **V1**.110
particle assembly/release, **V1**.143–4
see also Flavivirus
Flavivirus infection
arthropod vectors, **V2**.994 (Tab.), **V2**.997–9
mosquito-borne, **V2**.997–9, **V2**.998 (Tab.),
V2.999–1003
tick-borne, **V2**.998 (Tab.), **V2**.1003–4
clinical aspects, **V2**.997, **V2**.997–9
encephalitis (neuromorphic), **V2**.999
febrile illness (pantomorphic), **V2**.999
hemorrhagic fever, **V2**.999
control, **V2**.999
diagnosis, **V2**.999
serology, **V2**.1547
diseases caused by, CNS infection,
V2.1424–6
host cell, effects on, cell membrane
metabolism, **V1**.142
human disease importance, **V1**.135, **V2**.997,
V2.998 (Tab.)
immune response, **V2**.999
IFN activity, **I**.260 (Tab.)
pathogenesis, **V2**.999
cell apoptosis, **V2**.997
host factors, **V2**.999
neural spread, **V1**.244 (Tab.)
pathology, **V2**.997–9
tumors associated, **V1**.331 (Tab.)
vaccines, **V2**.996–7
BCE peptide vaccines, **I**.870–1
Flavobacterium
in foods
fish, **B1**.279
milk, **B1**.233
nosocomial infection, **B1**.401 (Tab.)
waterborne, **B1**.211, **B1**.221
Flavoproteins, **B1**.63
Fleas, *Rickettsia* transmission, **B2**.2037,
B2.2040, **B2**.2041
Fleroxacin, *Haemophilus,* **B2**.1710
Flexal virus, **V2**.1060 (Tab.)

Flexibacter, bioremediation, **B1**.212
FLICE-inhibitory proteins, **I**.135
Flinders Island tick typhus, **B2**.2039 (Tab.),
B2.2040
Flip-flop mechanisms, mutation, **B1**.90–1
Florists, **M**.368
Florphenicol, development, **B1**.482–4
Flow cytometry
antifungal testing, **M**.158
leukocyte adhesion deficiency diagnosis,
I.50–1
neutrophil disorders, **I**.52
Fluconazole, **M**.182–3
adverse effects, **M**.150, **M**.151 (Tab.),
M.152–3, **M**.183–4, **M**.612
AIDS, **M**.644, **M**.651–2
cryptococcosis incidence, **M**.644, **M**.652,
M.653
doses and half-life, **M**.152
drug interactions, **M**.152 (Tab.)
mechanism of action, **M**.70
neutropenia, **M**.152
pharmacokinetics, **M**.150, **M**.150 (Tab.)
prophylaxis
candidiasis, **M**.586, **M**.610–11, **M**.613
cryptococcosis, **M**.653
resistance, **M**.169
Aspergillus, **M**.169
Candida, **M**.169, **M**.170, **M**.174, **M**.585–6,
M.611, **M**.612
Candida albicans, **M**.152, **M**.611–12
Candida glabrata, **M**.169, **M**.174, **M**.585–6
Candida krusei, **M**.586
Condidiobolus, **M**.352
spectrum of activity, **M**.151 (Tab.)
susceptibility testing, **M**.170, **M**.170 (Tab.)
therapy
aspergillosis, **M**.728
Blastoschizomyces capitatus, **M**.626
blepharitis, **M**.297
candidiasis, **M**.257, **M**.610–11, **M**.610 (Fig.),
M.612
coccidioidomycosis, **M**.511
cryptococcosis, **M**.651–2
dermatomycosis, **M**.253
endophthalmitis, **M**.319, **M**.321–4, **M**.326–7
histoplasmosis capsulati, **M**.531
itraconazole *vs.,* **M**.728
keratitis, **M**.311–12, **M**.314
mucocutaneous candidiasis, **M**.189
onychomycosis, **M**.187–8, **M**.187 (Tab.),
M.253
pityriasis versicolor, **M**.185
pityrosporal folliculitis, **M**.185–6
prototheocis, **M**.402
rhino-orbital-cerebral zygomycosis,
M.293–4
sporotrichosis, **M**.379
superficial candidiasis, **M**.189
tinea, **M**.233
tinea barbae, **M**.186, **M**.187 (Tab.)
tinea capitis, **M**.188, **M**.188 (Tab.)
tinea cruris, **M**.186
tinea manuum, **M**.186–7, **M**.187 (Tab.)
tinea pedis, **M**.186–7, **M**.187 (Tab.)
vulvovaginal candidiasis, **M**.189

zygomycosis, **M**.352
Flucoxacillin
pharmacology, **B1**.475
structure, **B1**.474 (Fig.)
'Fluctuation test,' spontaneous mutation,
B1.82–3, **B1**.82 (Fig.)
Flucytosine (5-fluorocytosine)
historical aspects, **M**.147
mechanism of action, **M**.149–50, **M**.176
resistance, **M**.176
Aspergillus, **M**.176
Candida, **M**.176, **M**.585
Candida albicans, **M**.176, **M**.585
Candida glabrata, **M**.176
Condidiobolus, **M**.352
Cryptococcus neoformans, **M**.176
genetic basis, **M**.176
Prototheca, **M**.402
side-effects, **M**.612
susceptibility testing, **M**.170, **M**.170 (Tab.)
therapy
adiaspiromycosis, **M**.821
amphotericin B combination, **M**.149–50,
M.612, **M**.651–2
Blastoschizomyces capitatus, **M**.626
candidiasis, **M**.612
chromoblastomycosis, **M**.364
cryptococcosis, **M**.651–2
keratitis, **M**.308
pythiosis, **M**.425–6
Rhodotorula infection, **M**.627–8
toxicity, **M**.149–50, **M**.364
Flügge, **B1**.371
Fluid mosaic model, **P**.161, **P**.162 (Fig.)
Flukes (digeneans), **P**.573
immunity, **P**.92–5
see also Liver fluke(s); Lung fluke(s);
individual species; specific diseases/
infection
Fluorescein, **B2**.1596
Fluorescein-isothiocyanate (FITC)
Legionella pneumophila, **B2**.1773, **B2**.1774
Pneumocystis, **M**.788
syphilis diagnosis, **B2**.1844–5, **B2**.1847–8
Fluorescence assay, filovirus infection
diagnosis, **V2**.1097 (Tab.)
Fluorescence resonance energy transfer
(FRET)
bacteriology, **B1**.727 (Fig.), **B1**.728
applications, **B1**.728–9
Hepatitis B virus detection, **V2**.1254–5
Hepatitis C virus detection, **V2**.1213–14
Fluorescence, *Veillonella* culture, **B2**.1314
Fluorescent amplified fragment length
polymorphism (FAFLP)
Escherichia, **B2**.1371
Salmonella typing, **B2**.1408–9, **B2**.1411
Fluorescent antibody absorption (FTA-ABS)
test, in syphilis, **B2**.1847–8
cerebrospinal fluid test, **B2**.1848
IgM, **B2**.1848
problems, **B2**.1850–1
Fluorescent antibody test (FAT)
Actinomyces, **B2**.1009
rabies, **V2**.1125

Fluorescent in situ hybridization (FISH), soil bacteria, **B1**.206

Fluorescent microscopy, **B1**.713 (Tab.), **B1**.714

Fluorescent pigments, *Pseudomonas,* **B2**.1596

Fluorescent staining, *Blastocystis hominis,* **P**.566

Fluorescent-treponemal antibody-absorbed (FTA-ABS) test, **B1**.663

Fluorescent treponemal antibody test (FTA), **B1**.746

Fluorocarbon extraction, viral antigens, **V1**.91–2

5-Fluorocytosine *see* Flucytosine (5-fluorocytosine)

Fluoroquinolones
  development, **B1**.492
  plague, **B2**.1466
  Q fever treatment, **B2**.2078
  resistance
    plasmid resistance genes, **B1**.113
    Staphylococcus, **B2**.794 (Tab.), **B2**.804
  spectrum of activity
    Actinobacillus actinomycetemcomitans, **B2**.1664
    Brucella, **B2**.1742
    Campylobacter, **B2**.1548
    Capnocytophaga, **B2**.1677
    Cardiobacterium hominis, **B2**.1672–3
    Escherichia, **B2**.1370
    Legionella, **B2**.1777
    Pasteurella multocida, **B2**.1655
    Tropheryma whippelii, **B2**.1002
    Vibrio, **B2**.1514
  urinary tract infection, **B1**.679
  see also specific types

5-Fluorouracil, mutagen, **V1**.183

FMet-Leu-Phe, intracellular signaling, **I**.222

Foals, *Actinobacillus equuli* infection, **B2**.1665–6

Foamy viruses (FVs), **V1**.6, **V2.1304–21**
  antigens, **V2**.1310–13
    conservation, **V2**.1310 (Fig.)
    see also specific proteins
  Bet protein, **V2**.1312–13
    gene, **V2**.1308
    overexpression, **V2**.1313
  capsid assembly, **V2**.1310
  classification, **V2**.1295
  core antigen (GAG), **V2**.1307, **V2**.1310
    gene, **V2**.1308
    posttranslational modification, **V2**.1310
    structure, **V2**.1310
  ΔTas virus, **V2**.1309, **V2**.1313
  envelope antigens, **V2**.1307, **V2**.1311–12
    budding function, **V2**.1311–12
    gene, **V2**.1308
    leader peptide, **V2**.1311
    posttranslational modification, **V2**.1307
    subviral particle assembly, **V2**.1312
  gene vectors, **V2**.1314–15
    CD34+ cell targeting, **V2**.1315
    Murine leukemia virus *vs.,* **V2**.1314
    resting cells, **V2**.1314–15
  genome, **V2**.1307–10, **V2**.1309 (Fig.)
    env gene, **V2**.1308

gag gene, **V2**.1308
  internal promoter (IP), **V2**.1308
  long terminal repeats, **V2**.1308
  open reading frames, **V2**.1307
  pol gene, **V2**.1308
historical aspects, **V2**.1304
infection *see* Foamy virus infection
isolates, **V2**.1306 (Tab.)
molecular biology, **V2**.1307–13
morphology, **V2**.1305 (Fig.), **V2**.1307–8, **V2**.1308 (Fig.)
natural history, **V2**.1304–7
nonstructural proteins, **V2**.1312–13
  see also specific types
packaging, **V2**.1309–10
polymerase (pol), **V2**.1307
replication, **V2**.1313, **V2**.1313 (Fig.), **V2**.1314 (Fig.)
  full-length cDNA, **V2**.1313
RT antigens (POL), **V2**.1311
structural proteins, **V2**.1309–10
  see also specific types
Tas protein, **V2**.1312
  gene, **V2**.1308
  structure, **V2**.1312
  as transactivators, **V2**.1312

Foamy virus infection, **V2**.1305–6
  cell culture, **V2**.1306–7
  cell interactions, **V2**.1306–7
  diagnosis, **V2**.1315–16
  epidemiology, **V2**.1315
    prevalence, **V2**.1306, **V2**.1315
    transmission *see below*
  human infection, **V2**.1295–6
    human-to-human transmission, **V2**.1296
    serology, **V2**.1295
  species, **V2**.1304
  therapy, **V2**.1316
  transmission, **V2**.1304–5
    close primate contact, **V2**.1306, **V2**.1315

Focal epithelial hyperplasia, HPV associations, **V1**.463 (Tab.), **V1**.465 (Tab.)

Focal hepatitis, human brucellosis, **B2**.1738

Folate metabolism, *Plasmodium,* **P**.477

Folate receptor, filovirus cellular entry, **V2**.1092

Folinic acid, toxoplasmosis, **P**.437

Follicular B cell lymphoma, BCE peptide vaccines, **I**.855 (Tab.)

Follicular dendritic cells (FDCs)
  antigen depot retention, **I**.491, **I**.497
  B cell activation, **I**.326–7
  complement receptor 1, **I**.151
  generation, **I**.493
  prion diseases, **V2**.1377–8, **V2**.1378 (Fig.), **V2**.1379
  see also Dendritic cells

Folliculitis
  AIDS, **M**.14–5
  lipophilic yeasts, **M**.14–5
  Malassezia globosa infection, **M**.213
  tinea capitis, **M**.231–2

Follow-up (incidence) studies, **B1**.314

Fomites, indirect transmission, **V1**.354–5

Fomivirsen, HCMV therapy, **V1**.527, **V2**.1618–19
  AIDS/HIV infection, **V2**.1503

Fonsecaea, **M**.61–3

Fonsecaea compacta
  chromoblastomycosis, **M**.29–30, **M**.357
  histopathology, **M**.89 (Tab.), **M**.128 (Tab.)

Fonsecaea pedrosoi, **M**.22
  ecology, **M**.357–8, **M**.358 (Tab.)
  histopathology, **M**.89 (Tab.), **M**.128 (Tab.)
  infection, **M**.29–30, **M**.30 (Fig.), **M**.356–7, **M**.361–2
    CNS, **M**.743–4
    immune response, **M**.363
    oculomycoses, **M**.278 (Tab.)
    therapy, **M**.364
  morphology, **M**.30 (Fig.), **M**.360, **M**.360 (Fig.), **M**.361 (Fig.)
  pleomorphism, **M**.360, **M**.360 (Fig.), **M**.361 (Fig.)

Fontana-Masson stain, modified, **M**.123 (Tab.), **M**.124

Food(s), **B1.263–92**
  airborne bacteria monitoring, **B1**.189–90
  bacterial infection transmission, **B1**.310, **B1**.361
    cook-chill, **B1**.377
    necrotizing enteritis, **B2**.1118–19
    nosocomial, **B1**.377
    technology changes, **B1**.361–2
    see also individual species
  bacteriocins, **B1**.139
  bacteriology of specific food commodities, **B1**.272–88
  contamination, **B1**.289
  general principles, **B1**.263
  hazard analysis critical control point regulations, **B1**.288–9
  microbial growth influencing factors, **B1**.263–7
    antibacterial properties, **B1**.267
    chilling effect, **B1**.264
    extrinsic factors, **B1**.266–7
    freezing effect, **B1**.264–5
    gaseous atmosphere, **B1**.266
    heating effect, **B1**.265–6
    nutrients, **B1**.267
    other factors, **B1**.267
    pH, **B1**.266–7
    redox potential, **B1**.267
    temperature, **B1**.264–6
    water activity, **B1**.266
  preservation and processing, **B1**.267–72, **B1**.268 (Tab.)
    hurdle technology, **B1**.272
    temperature, **B1**.264
    waterborne bacteria, **B1**.212, **B1**.221
    see also specific methods
  safety assurance, **P**074. **B1**.288–9
  safety regulation, **B1**.289
  see also specific foods

Food and Drug Administration (FDA), vaccine adverse event monitoring, **V2**.1565

Food borne transmission
  astroviruses, **V2**.900–1

Food borne transmission (*Continued*)
  hepatitis A, **V2**.1172
  norovirus infection, **V2**.919–20
  Salmonella Enteritidis bacteriophage type
    4b, **B1**.322
Food chain, biomagnification of pollutants,
  B1.201–2
Food contamination
  Aspergillus, **M**.729
  Sporothrix schenckii, **M**.371
Food handlers, hepatitis A outbreaks, **V2**.1172
Food hygiene
  amebiasis prevention, **P**.214–15
  liver fluke control, **P**.653–4
  lung fluke control, **P**.653–4
  sarcocystosis prevention/control, **P**.449
  Trypanosoma cruzi transmission, **P**.392
Food poisoning, **B1**.310
  case-control studies, **B1**.315–16
  Clostridia, **B1**.203
  cohort studies, **B1**.315
Food Standards Agency, **B1**.330
Foot-and-mouth disease, **V2**.874
  BCE peptide vaccines, **I**.854, **I**.855 (Tab.),
    I.861, **I**.870
  disinfection, **B1**.422–4, **B1**.434
  immune response, **V2**.865
  peptide vaccine design, **I**.870
Foot-and-mouth disease virus (FMDV)
  cell receptors, **V1**.207 (Tab.)
  classification, **V1**.50
  discovery, **V2**.858
  emerging infection, **V2**.1651 (Tab.)
  genome size, **V2**.863–5
  historical aspects, **V1**.24–5
  host cell protein synthesis, **V1**.141
  morphology/structure, **V2**.863
  mutations
    evolution, **V1**.17–8
    phenotypic modifications, **V1**.19
  neutralizing antibodies, **V2**.865
  quasispecies dynamics, **V1**.19
  ribosomal skipping, **V1**.117
  serotypes, **V2**.874
  virus attachment protein (VAP), **V2**.1405–6
  VP proteins, T-helper cell epitope,
    I.862 (Tab.)
'Force of infection , infection models, **I**.948–9
Forestry workers, **M**.368, **M**.369
'Forest-yaws,' **P**.329
Formaldehyde, **B1**.426–7
  action, **B1**.437 (Tab.), **B1**.438, **B1**.439–40
  formaldehyde-releasing agents, **B1**.426–7
  gas, **B1**.429–30
  liquid state, **B1**.426–7
  low temperature steam with formaldehyde,
    B1.429–30, **B1**.447–8, **B1**.454
    applications, **B1**.445 (Tab.)
Formalin
  Histoplasma capsulatum var. *capsulatum*
    decontamination, **M**.520
  virus inactivation, **V1**.91, **V2**.1553
Formic acid, **B1**.422
  fermentation, **B1**.55, **B1**.55 (Fig.)
Formins, **M**.72–3

Formivirsen, **V2**.1618–19
  structure, **V2**.1618 (Fig.)
Formol–ether method, fecal concentration,
  P.151
Formol-gel test, Old World leishmaniasis,
  P.302
Formolized yolk-sac antigen (FYSA), **B2**.1774
Formulary, antibacterial control, **B1**.468
3-Formul-1-butyl pyrophosphate, **I**.440 (Fig.)
N-Formylated peptides, **I**.445
Formyl-methionine-leucine phenylalanine
    (fMLP) receptor, neutrophils, **I**.43, **I**.44
Fort Morgan virus (FMV), **V2**.1010,
    V2.1011 (Tab.)
Fortovase *see* Saquinavir
Forvade *see* Cidofovir
Foscarnet (phosphonoformic acid: PFA),
    V2.1616–17
  HCMV infection, **V1**.526, **V1**.527
    AIDS/HIV infection, **V2**.1503, **V2**.1505
  HHV infection, **V1**.533
  HSV infection, **V1**.512
  Kaposi's sarcoma therapy, **V1**.553, **V2**.1503
  resistance, **V2**.1634–5
  structure, **V2**.1617 (Fig.)
Foscavir *see* Foscarnet (phosphonoformic acid:
    PFA)
Fosfomycin, **B1**.481
4–1BB ligand, **I**.288 (Tab.)
  CD4 T cells, **I**.396
Fourier transformation
  electron microscopy, **V1**.60
  infrared spectroscopy, **V2**.1352,
    V2.1353 (Fig.), **V2**.1354 (Fig.)
Foveavirus, **V1**.27 (Tab.)
Fowl adenovirus A, type species, **V1**.45
Fowl cholera, **B2**.1653–4
Fowl pest *see* Newcastle disease virus (NDV)
Fowlpox virus (FPV)
  cytokine homologue production, **V1**.288
  immune evasion, **V1**.288
  phylogenetic comparison, **V1**.584 (Fig.)
  type species, **V1**.583, **V1**.589
  as vaccine vector, **I**.846, **I**.898
  virion maturation, **V1**.614
Foxes, botulism, **B2**.1074
F plasmid *see* Conjugation, bacterial
F (fusion) protein *see* Measles virus
Fracastora of Verona, **M**.6
Fracastoro, G, **B1**.4
Fractalkine (neurotacin:CX3CL1), **I**.220
Fracture fixation infection
  causative pathogens, **B1**.690–1
  epidemiology, **B1**.684–5, **B1**.686 (Tab.)
  reconstruction, **B1**.697
Fracture infection, inflammatory response,
    B1.689
Frame-shift mutations *see* Point mutations
Frameshift signal
  astrovirus genome, **V2**.894 (Fig.)
  Human astrovirus, **V2**.894 (Fig.)
Framework regions, Igs, **I**.305
France, toxoplasmosis incidence, **P**.436–7
Francisella, **B2**.1752–8
  biochemical properties, **B2**.1753–4
  carbohydrate surface molecules, **B2**.1753–4

  culture, **B2**.1753
  distribution, **B2**.1753
  genomics, **B2**.1756
  growth requirements, **B2**.1753
  history, **B2**.1752
  infection
    immune response in humans and animals,
      B2.1756–7
    immune response in murine model,
      B2.1756–7
    in immunocompromised, **B2**.1753
    serology, **B1**.757, **B2**.1754
    see also Tularemia
  intracellular growth, **B2**.1755
  proteomics, **B2**.1756
Francisella holarctica, **B2**.1752
Francisella nearctica, **B2**.1752
Francisella novicida, **B2**.1753
  distribution, **B2**.1753
  genetics, **B2**.1753
  virulence, **B2**.1753–4
Francisella philomiragia, **B2**.1753
  distribution, **B2**.1753
Francisella tularensis
  bioterrorism, **B1**.189
  biovars, **B2**.1752–3
  capsule, **B2**.1753, **B2**.1754
  classification, **B2**.1752–3, **B2**.2027 (Fig.)
    phylogeny, **B2**.1752, **B2**.1753
    proteomics, **B2**.1756
    species and strains, **B2**.1752–3
  colonial phase variation, **B2**.1754
  distribution, **B2**.1753
  as facultative intracellular bacteria, **B2**.1755
  genetics
    genomics, **B2**.1756
    nucleic acid composition, **B2**.1729 (Tab.)
    variation, **B2**.1755–6
  hosts, **B2**.1753
  infection *see* Tularemia
  intracellular growth, **B2**.1755
  live vaccine strain, **B2**.1755, **B2**.1756–8
  LPS, **B2**.1753–4
  morphology and growth, **B2**.1753
  reservoirs, **B2**.1753
  subspecies *palaearctica,* **B2**.1752
  virulence, **B2**.1753–6
    mutants, **B2**.1755–6
Frankfurters, **B1**.275
Freeze-drying, **B1**.450
  food preservation, **B1**.268–9
Freezing and thawing, **B1**.450
Freezing, food, **B1**.269–70
  effectiveness, **B1**.270
  freeze drying, **B1**.268–9
  fruit, **B1**.283
  integrity of food, **B1**.270
  microbial growth effect, **B1**.264–5
  microbial radiation resistance, **B1**.271
  organoleptic characteristics, **B1**.264
  process, **B1**.270
  refrigeration vs, **B1**.269
  timing, **B1**.270
  vegetables, **B1**.281–2
  see also Chilling food

Frequency distribution of numbers/host, **P**.54

Frequency of vaccination, vaccination models, **I**.962–3

Freshwater, *Aeromonas* habitats, **B2**.1524–5

Freund's complete adjuvant (FCA)
  mechanism of action, **I**.926
  nonhuman use, **I**.927

Freund's incomplete adjuvant (FIA), **I**.927

Friend spleen focus-forming virus (SFFV),
    V1.336

Frontal sinus, respiratory tract, **B1**.606–7

Fructose-6-phosphate, **B1**.57–8
  Bifidobacterium, **B1**.58

Fructose-6-phosphoketolase, **B1**.58

Fructose-6-phosphokinase
    (phosphofructokinase), **B1**.51, **B1**.58,
    B1.59

Fruit bats, Nipah virus, **V1**.817

Fruit cannery workers, **M**.597
  candidiasis, **M**.597

Fruits, **B1**.280, **B1**.282–3
  carbon dioxide in atmosphere, **B1**.283
  emerging bacterial infection, **B1**.360
  handling, **B1**.282
  harvesting, **B1**.282
    losses, **B1**.282
  pH, **B1**.283
  preservation
    canned, **B1**.283
    dried, **B1**.283
    freezing, **B1**.283
    irradiation, **B1**.271
    potassium sorbate treatment, **B1**.283
    sulfite treatment, **B1**.283
  sorting and grading, **B1**.282
  spoilage
    fungal, **B1**.282–3
    molds, **B1**.282–3
    rots, **B1**.282
    yeasts, **B1**.282–3
  storage, **B1**.283
    temperatures, **B1**.283
  water activity, **B1**.283

Frustrated phagocytosis, neutrophils, **I**.40

FTC *see* Emtricitabine

FtsY protein, **B1**.45

FtsZ, **B1**.48

α-Fucosidase, **B2**.1924 (Tab.)

Fülleborn, Friedrich, **P**.9

Fulminant hepatitis, **V2**.1248

Fumagillin
  microsporidiosis chemotherapy, **P**.549
  microsporidiosis keratoconjunctivitis, **P**.549

Fumarase, **B1**.52–3

Fungal pneumonitis, IL-13, **I**.734–5

Fungemia, **M**.86, **M**.87, **B1**.516 (Fig.)
  aspergillosis, **M**.699–700
  Blastoschizomyces capitatus infection, **M**.625
  blood culture, **B1**.512–13
  candidiasis, **M**.13, **M**.586
  causative organisms, **B1**.522
  Coccidioides immitis infection, **M**.513
  definition, **B1**.510, **B1**.511 (Tab.)
  Hansenula anomala infection, **M**.626
  Malassezia furfur infection, **M**.626–7

Malassezia infection, **M**.626–7

Rhodotorula infection, **M**.627

Saccharomyces cerevisiae infection, **M**.628

Trichosporon cutaneum (T. beigelii)
    infection, **M**.629

Trichosporon infection, **M**.629, **M**.630

  uncommon species, **M**.624

Fungi
  antibacterial agents, **B1**.439
    resistance, **B1**.444
  cell culture contamination, **V1**.88
  classification, **P**.195–6
  food
    cereal spoilage, **B1**.284–5
    fruit spoilage, **B1**.282–3
    nuts and seeds, **B1**.286–7
    water activity, **B1**.266
  lichen formation, **B1**.201
  nitrification, **B1**.200
  plant associations, **B1**.197
    biogeochemical transformations, **B1**.199
    carbon:nitrogen (C:N) ratios, **B1**.200
    detection methods, **B1**.205
    growing season and domination, **B1**.198
    nitrogen cycling, **B1**.200

Fungi (kingdom), **M**.43–4, **M**.44, **M**.49–51, **M**.69
  classifications, **M**.49, **M**.51

Fungicides, **B1**.434

Fungistatic agents, **B1**.434

'Fungus balls,' **M**.295–6, **M**.385–6, **M**.394

Funiculo-epididymoorchitis, lymphatic
    filariasis, **P**.773

Furanocoumarin, fish, **B1**.281

Furazolidone
  Blastocystis hominis, **P**.566–7
  giardiasis, **P**.251
  spectrum of activity, **B1**.495

Furfural formation, food, **B1**.267

fur gene, iron-dependent repression, **B1**.165–6

Furovirus, **V1**.27 (Tab.)

Furzeon *see* Enfurvirtide

Fusariosis, **M**.189
  continuous ambulatory peritoneal dialysis -
    associated peritonitis, **M**.754
  diagnosis, **M**.125–7, **M**.751–2
  disseminated, **M**.754
  graft-*versus*-host disease, **M**.754
  histopathology, **M**.125–7, **M**.138 (Fig.),
    M.141 (Fig.)
  mortality rates, **M**.754–5
  mycetoma, **M**.389 (Fig.), **M**.386 (Tab.)
  nails, **M**.754
  nosocomial, **B1**.403
  oculomycoses, **M**.274, **M**.275 (Tab.)
    contact lens contamination, **M**.330–1
    dacryocanaliculitis, **M**.298
    endophthalmitis, **M**.317, **M**.326
    keratitis, **M**.141 (Fig.), **M**.300, **M**.301,
      M.303, **M**.304–5, **M**.307–9, **M**.312, **M**.316,
      M.327
    post surgical, **M**.327
  onychomycosis, **M**.246, **M**.754
  prognosis, **M**.754
  renal, **M**.138 (Fig.)
  risk factors, **M**.754

  therapy, **M**.754
    amphotericin B, **M**.755
    G-CSF, **M**.755
    GM-CSF, **M**.755
    posaconazole, **M**.755
    voriconazole, **M**.153, **M**.755

Fusarium
  antifungal susceptibility, **M**.752 (Tab.)
  cereals, **B1**.284
  echinocandin resistance, **M**.176
  ecology, **M**.753
  environmental source identification, **M**.95
  fruit, **B1**.282
  genus description, **M**.752
  histopathology, **M**.89 (Tab.), **M**.127 (Tab.),
    M.128 (Tab.)
  infection *see* Fusariosis
  morphology, **M**.753, **M**.753 (Fig.)
  mycotoxins, **M**.754
  nuts and seeds, **B1**.286–7
  peanuts, **B1**.286–7

Fusarium dimerum, **M**.753–4
  contact lens contamination, **M**.331
  morphology, **M**.753

Fusarium graminearum, **B1**.284

Fusarium moniliforme, **M**.89 (Tab.)
  histopathology, **M**.138 (Fig.)

Fusarium oxysporum, **M**.249–50, **M**.753–4
  contact lens contamination, **M**.331
  onychomycosis, **M**.246

Fusarium proliferatum, **M**.753–4

Fusarium solani, **M**.89 (Tab.), **M**.249, **M**.753–4,
    M.282 (Fig.)
  amphotericin B resistance, **M**.172
  contact lens contamination, **M**.330–1
  culture, **M**.304 (Fig.)
  histopathology, **M**.138 (Fig.), **M**.141 (Fig.)
  infection
    keratitis, **M**.301–2, **M**.302 (Fig.), **M**.303,
      M.304–5, **M**.316 (Fig.), **M**.327–8
    onychomycosis, **M**.246
    see also Fusariosis

Fusarium venenatum, **M**.753

Fusarium verticillioides, **M**.753–4

Fuselloviridae, **V1**.27 (Tab.), **V1**.43 (Tab.)

Fusidic acid, **B1**.488–9
  mode of action, **B1**.488
  pharmacology, **B1**.489
  resistance, **B1**.488–9
  spectrum of activity, **B1**.488, **B1**.499 (Tab.)
    Actinomyces, **B2**.1011
  structure, **B1**.488, **B1**.488 (Fig.)
  toxicity/adverse effects, **B1**.489

Fusion (F) proteins
  Avian pneumovirus, **V1**.787
  Human metapneumovirus, **V1**.787
  Human respiratory syncytial virus, **V1**.786
  Measles virus *see* Measles virus
  monoclonal antibody therapy, **I**.369
  Mumps virus *see* Mumps virus
  Nipah virus, **V1**.817
  paramyxoviruses *see* Paramyxoviruses
  respiroviruses *see* Respiroviruses
  stabilization, membrane fusion, **V1**.214

Fusion vectors, **B1**.125–6

Fusobacterium, **B2**.1945–56
  antibacterial susceptibility/resistance,
    B2.1949
    antibiotics, **B2**.1949
  antigens, **B2**.1948–9
  cell wall composition, **B2**.1948–9
  classification, **B2**.1913, **B2**.1914, **B2**.1946
  coaggregation, **B2**.1950
  culture, **B2**.1947
    media, **B2**.1949
  definition, **B2**.1945
  differential characteristics, **B2**.1950 (Tab.)
  fatty acids, **B2**.1949
  genetics, **B2**.1947–8
  habitats, **B2**.1946–7
  historical perspective, **B2**.1945–6
  infection
    in animals, **B2**.1945–6
    bacteremia, **B1**.523
    bone and joint infection, **B1**.690–1
    endocarditis, **B1**.533
    gingivitis, **B1**.614
    intracranial abscess, **B1**.585
    oral cavity abscess, **B1**.618
    periodontal abscess, **B1**.614
  intragenic heterogeneity, **B2**.1946
  isolation/identification, **B2**.1949–50
    DNA probes, **B2**.1950
  LPS, **B2**.1948
  metabolism, **B2**.1948
  morphology, **B2**.1947
  normal microbiota, **B1**.296 (Tab.), **B1**.301,
    B2.1950
    mouth, **B1**.609
    nasopharynx, **B1**.609
  outer-membrane, **B2**.1948
  pathogenicity, **B2**.1950–1
  species, **B2**.1946
  virulence factors, **B2**.1950–1
Fusobacterium alocis, **B2**.1946
Fusobacterium canifelium, **B2**.1946
Fusobacterium equinum, **B2**.1946–7
Fusobacterium gonidiaformans
  differential characteristics, **B2**.1950 (Tab.)
  habitats, **B2**.1946
  morphology, **B2**.1947
Fusobacterium mortiferum
  classification, **B2**.1946
  differential characteristics, **B2**.1950 (Tab.)
  habitats, **B2**.1946
  metabolism, **B2**.1948
  morphology, **B2**.1947
Fusobacterium naviforme
  differential characteristics, **B2**.1950 (Tab.)
  habitats, **B2**.1946
  morphology, **B2**.1947
Fusobacterium necrogenes
  differential characteristics, **B2**.1950 (Tab.)
  habitats, **B2**.1946
Fusobacterium necrophorum, **B1**.629
  cell wall and antigens, **B2**.1948
  classification, **B2**.1946
  culture, **B2**.1947
  differential characteristics, **B2**.1950 (Tab.)
  habitats, **B2**.1946–7

infection, **B2**.1951
  Lemierre's syndrome, **B1**.618
leukotoxin, **B2**.1951
metabolism, **B2**.1948
morphology, **B2**.1947
subspecies, **B2**.1946
Fusobacterium nucleatum, **B2**.1945
  cell wall and antigens, **B2**.1948–9
    FomA and porins, **B2**.1948–50
  classification, **B2**.1946
  culture, **B2**.1947
  differentiating characteristics, **B2**.1949 (Tab.),
    B2.1950 (Tab.)
  genetics, **B2**.1947–8
  habitats, **B2**.1946–7
  infection
    intracranial abscess, **B1**.584–5
    stomatitis, **B1**.614
  isolation/identification, **B2**.1949–50
  metabolism, **B2**.1948
  morphology, **B2**.1947, **B2**.1949–50,
    B2.1952 (Fig.)
  normal microbiota role, **B2**.1950
  pathogenicity and virulence factors,
    B2.1950–1
Fusobacterium perfoetens, **B2**.1946
Fusobacterium periodonticum
  classification, **B2**.1946
  habitats, **B2**.1946
  normal microbiota role, **B2**.1950
Fusobacterium plauti-vincenti, **B2**.1945
Fusobacterium polymorphum, **B2**.1945
Fusobacterium prausnitzii, **B2**.1946
Fusobacterium russii
  differential characteristics, **B2**.1950 (Tab.)
  habitats, **B2**.1946–7
Fusobacterium simiae, **B2**.1946–7
Fusobacterium sulci, **B2**.1946
Fusobacterium ulcerans
  classification, **B2**.1946
  differential characteristics, **B2**.1950 (Tab.)
  habitats, **B2**.1946
Fusobacterium varium
  classification, **B2**.1946
  differential characteristics, **B2**.1950 (Tab.)
  habitats, **B2**.1946
  morphology, **B2**.1947
Fuzzy sets, viral species, **V1**.30–1
F value, **B1**.270–1, **B1**.446
Fv antibody fragments, **I**.367, **I**.367 (Fig.),
  I.368 (Fig.)
  monoclonal antibody therapy, 184.78–79
FY gene, **I**.582–3
Fyn tyrosine kinase, **I**.342

G1 glycoprotein
  bunyaviruses *see* Bunyaviruses
  Dugbe virus *see* Dugbe virus
  hantaviruses, **V2**.1031–3
  La Crosse virus, **V2**.1034–5
  nairoviruses, **V2**.1034, **V2**.1038
  phleboviruses, **V2**.1033–4
  Rift Valley fever virus, **V2**.1038
  Uukuniemi virus, **V2**.1034

G1 protein, Crimean–Congo hemorrhagic
  fever virus, **V2**.1034
G2 glycoprotein
  bunyaviruses *see* Bunyaviruses
  Dugbe virus, **V2**.1034
  hantaviruses, **V2**.1031–3
  nairoviruses, **V2**.1034
  phleboviruses, **V2**.1033–4
  Punta Toro virus, **V2**.1038
  Rift Valley fever virus, **V2**.1038–9
  Uukuniemi virus, **V2**.1034
G_2 phase arrest, Vpr (viral protein R),
  V2.1326–7
Gab1 (Grb-2-associated binding protein), BCR
  signaling, **I**.345
gag gene
  foamy viruses, **V2**.1308
  HTLVs, **V2**.1285–7
Gag protein
  cleavage, **V1**.58–9
    retrovirus assembly/maturation, **V1**.78–9
  HIV *see* HIV
  retroviruses, **V1**.78, **V2**.1322–3, **V2**.1591
Galactofuran
  Aspergillus, **M**.712, **M**.713
  Aspergillus fumigatus, **M**.712
Galactomannan, **M**.107
  Aspergillus, **M**.712, **M**.713, **M**.714, **M**.717
    ELISA, **M**.714
  Aspergillus fumigatus, **M**.107, **M**.712, **M**.714
Galactose monomycolate, αβ T cell
  recognition, **I**.443 (Fig.)
Galactose-6-phosphate, inducer in *lac* operon,
  B1.71
Galactose, *Plasmodium* host cell changes,
  P.473
α-Galactosidase
  Porphyromonas identification, **B2**.1924 (Tab.)
  Prevotella identification, **B2**.1924 (Tab.)
β-Galactosidase, **B1**.70
  Porphyromonas identification, **B2**.1924 (Tab.)
  Prevotella identification, **B2**.1924 (Tab.)
  testing for presence, **B1**.223
Galactosyl ceramide, HIV receptor, **V2**.1426–7
Gallbladders
  candidiasis, **M**.600
  giardiasis, **P**.246
Gallen, **M**.5
Galleria mellonella densovirus (*Gm*DNV),
  V1.412, **V1**.413 (Fig.)
Gallibacterium, **B2**.1658
  classification, **B2**.1658–9
  genomospecies 1, **B2**.1658
Gallibacterium anatis, **B2**.1658
  animal infection, **B2**.1654
  characteristics, **B2**.1652 (Tab.)
  classification, **B2**.1650, **B2**.1658–9
Gallicola, **B2**.914
  classification, **B2**.904, **B2**.905 (Tab.)
Gallicola barnesae, **B2**.914
  biochemical characteristics, **B2**.908 (Tab.)
  classification, **B2**.904–5
Galls, plant disease source, **B1**.202
Gallstones, liver flukes, **P**.649
Gametes, *Plasmodium see* Plasmodium
Gametocytes, *Plasmodium*, **P**.468, **P**.473–4

Gamma-aminobutyric acid (GABA), in rabies, **V2**.1409
γδ T-cells, **I**.436–41
    airway hypersensitivity, **I**.737–8
    dendritic epidermal cells, **I**.436–7
        chemokine expression, **I**.437
        development, **I**.436
        epithelial integrity maintenance, **I**.437
        in humans, **I**.437
        Ly49E expression, **I**.437
        NKG2D expression, **I**.436
        progenitors, **I**.436
        Rae expression, **I**.437
        self-antigen recognition, **I**.436
        somatic recombination, **I**.436
        TCR generation, **I**.436
        Th2 response, **I**.437
        tumor protection, **I**.437
    development
        epithelial cells, **I**.527
        IL-7, **I**.527
    infection
        HIV infection, **I**.796–7
        Listeria monocytogenes infection, **I**.526–7
        malaria, **P**.490, **P**.496
        oropharyngeal candidiasis, **M**.263
        viral infection, **V1**.274
        vulvovaginal candidiasis, **M**.265
    intraepithelial lymphocytes, **I**.525–6
    killing mechanism, **I**.472
    knockout mice, babesiosis, **P**.456
    non-epidermal tissues, **I**.438
        bowel cancer, **I**.438
        CD1 proteins, **I**.438
        development, **I**.438
        immunoprotective role, **I**.438
        small intestine, **I**.438
        'stress antigen' recognition, **I**.438
        TCR diversity, **I**.438
    systemic, **I**.438–41
        autoantigen selection, **I**.441
        bacterial infection, **I**.438–41
        biological functions, **I**.440
        derivation, **I**.439
        development, **I**.441
        heat shock protein recognition, **I**.439–40
        increased metabolism, **I**.439
        microbial product recognition, **I**.439, **I**.440
        nonpeptide recognition, **I**.439, **I**.440 (Fig.)
        TCR, **I**.439
    TCR, **I**.436, **I**.439
    see also T-cell receptor (TCR)
γ heavy chain, IgG structure, **I**.307
γ locus, TCR, **I**.450 (Fig.), **I**.451
Gammaherpesvirinae
    characteristics, **V1**.177 (Tab.)
    classification, **V1**.43 (Tab.), **V1**.488–9
    evolution, **V1**.175–6
    see also Gammaherpesviruses
Gammaherpesviruses, **V1**.**559–77**
    genome structure, **V1**.492
    host range, **V1**.489
    immune evasion, **V1**.502–3
        apoptosis interference, **V1**.287, **V1**.324–5
        chemokine disruption, **V1**.288

infection
        immune response, **V1**.285–6
        lymphocyte tropism, **V1**.281
    see also Gammaherpesvirinae
Gamma radiation
    Campylobacter, **B2**.1545
    toxoplasmosis prevention, **P**.439
Gammaretrovirus, **V1**.46, **V2**.1286 (Tab.)
    see also Gammaretroviruses
Gammaretroviruses
    insertional mutagenesis, **V1**.340
    tumors associated, **V1**.331 (Tab.)
    see also Gammaretrovirus
Ganciclovir, **V2**.1613
    HCMV infection, **V1**.526–7, **V2**.1613
        AIDS/HIV infection, **V2**.1502–3, **V2**.1505
        congenital, **V2**.1453
    HHV infection, **V1**.533
    Kaposi's sarcoma therapy, **V1**.553, **V2**.1503
    mechanism of action, **V1**.217–18
    structure, **V2**.1611 (Fig.), **V2**.1613 (Fig.)
Ganglion, HSV latent infection, **V1**.509–10
Gardeners, **M**.368
Gardnerella, **B2**.994–5
    chemotaxonomic characteristics, **B2**.978 (Tab.)
    urinary tract infection, **B1**.678
Gardnerella vaginalis, **B2**.994–5
    antibacterial susceptibility/resistance, metronidazole, **B1**.495
    bacterial vaginosis, **B1**.665–8
    biochemical characteristics, **B2**.993 (Tab.)
    disease associations, **B2**.981 (Tab.)
    habitats, **B2**.978
    normal microbiota, **B1**.296 (Tab.), **B1**.303
Garissa virus infection, **V2**.1047–8
Garki project, malaria epidemiology, **P**.512–13
Garnham, Cyril, *Plasmodium* life cycle, **P**.17
Gas gangrene, **B1**.203, **B2**.1111–16
    associated infection, **B2**.1112, **B2**.1114
    bacteriology, **B2**.1112
    causative agents, **B2**.1112, **B2**.1114
    clinical features, **B2**.1114–15
    diagnosis, **B2**.1115
    experimental studies, **B2**.1113–14
    historical aspects, **B2**.1111
    incidence, **B2**.1111–12
        civilian practice, **B2**.1111–12
        military during war, **B2**.1111
    incubation period, **B2**.1114
    pathogenesis, **B2**.1112–13
        clostridial toxins role, **B2**.1113–14
        tissue anoxia, **B2**.1112–13
    postoperative, **B2**.1111, **B2**.1112–13
    prophylaxis and treatment, **B2**.1115
        antibacterial agents, **B2**.1116
        hyperbaric oxygen, **B2**.1115–16
        surgery, **B2**.1115
        wound debridement, **B2**.1115
    wound tissue anoxia and anaerobic growth, **B2**.1112–13
Gas-liquid chromatography (GLC)
    Fusobacterium, **B2**.1950
    rapidly growing mycobacteria, **B2**.1242
Gas plasmas, sterilization, **B1**.453

Gasteroenteritis, *Aeromonas,* **B2**.1535–6
Gastric acid, giardiasis association, **P**.250
Gastric biopsy, *Helicobacter pylori* infection diagnosis, **B2**.1571 (Tab.)
Gastric cancer
    EBV association, **V1**.571
    Helicobacter pylori infection, **B2**.1580
Gastric mucosa, *Helicobacter pullorum,* **B2**.1564–5
Gastric ulcers
    Helicobacter pylori infection, **B2**.1564, **B2**.1580
    recurrence, **B2**.1574
Gastritis, *Helicobacter pylori* infection, **B1**.365, **B2**.1564
    acute, **B2**.1578, **B2**.1579
    chronic, **B2**.1564–5, **B2**.1578, **B2**.1579
Gastrodiscoides
    classification, **P**.583
    structure/life cycle, **P**.583–4
Gastroenteritis
    astrovirus infection, **V2**.903
    enterovirus infection, **V2**.872
    herbs and spices, **B1**.288
    immunodeficient patients (non-HIV), **V2**.1508–9
    Salmonella Paratyphi B, **B2**.1421
    viral, **B1**.400
    viral isolation/propagation and identification, **V1**.96 (Tab.), **V1**.98
Gastroesophageal reflux disease (GERD), *Helicobacter pylori* infection, **B2**.1580–1
Gastrointestinal bleeding, liver fluke infection, **P**.649
Gastrointestinal nematodes *see* Nematodes, gastrointestinal
Gastrointestinal samples, *Aeromonas* isolation, **B2**.1531–2
Gastrointestinal tract
    decontamination, **B1**.390
    normal defenses, **P**.75
    normal microbiota, **B1**.293–4, **B1**.302–3
        antibiotic-induced changes, **B2**.1119–20
        Bacteroides/Prevotella/Porphyromonas, **B2**.1933
    prototheccosis, **M**.398–9
    surgery, fungal endophthalmitis after, **M**.318
    see also Small intestine
Gastrointestinal tract infection
    adenoviruses, **V1**.444
    aspergillosis, **M**.701, **M**.705
        invasive, **M**.701, **M**.705
    bunyavirus infection, **V2**.1042
    Chagas disease, **P**.386
    epidemiology, **V1**.368–9
    HIV infection *see* HIV infection
    measles, **V1**.723
    nematode infection, **I**.600–1
        HLA association, **I**.600–1
    Pneumocystis carinii infection, **M**.785
    TLR-5, **I**.121
    viral entry, **V1**.237 (Fig.), **V1**.239
        Peyer's patch/M cells, **V1**.240 (Fig.)
    virus shedding, **V1**.249
    Whipple's disease, **B2**.999, **B2**.1001–2, **B2**.1001 (Fig.)

Gastrointestinal tract infection (*Continued*)
  zygomycosis, **M**.20–1
    systemic, **M**.674, **M**.674 (Tab.), **M**.678
    ulceration, **M**.674
  see also specific diseases/infection; specific
    viruses
Gastropods, **B1**.280
Gatifloxacin
  Nocardia, **B2**.1165–6
  spectrum of activity, **B1**.492
GB virus A (GBV-A), emerging infection,
    V2.1650, **V2**.1653 (Tab.)
GB virus B (GBV-B)
  emerging infection, **V2**.1650, **V2**.1653 (Tab.)
  Hepatitis C virus *vs.,* **V2**.1191–2
GB virus-C *see* Hepatitis G virus (HGV)
    infection
Gc globulin, **I**.203
GCP-2 *see* Granulocyte chemoattractant
    protein 2 (GCP-2:CXCL6)
Gelatinase production, *Legionella* species
    identification, **B2**.1762 (Tab.)
Gelatin hydrolysis, **B2**.1351
  Enterobacteriaceae identification,
    B2.1319 (Tab.)
  Enterobacter identification, **B2**.1351
  Klebsiella identification, **B2**.1351
  Proteus identification, **B2**.1351
  Salmonella identification, **B2**.1351, **B2**.1401
  Serratia identification, **B2**.1351
Gemella, **B2**.833–5
  differentiating characteristics, **B2**.906–7
  identification, **B2**.906–7
  normal microbiota, **B1**.296 (Tab.)
Gemella morbillorum
  endocarditis, **B1**.528–9
  as normal microbiota, **B1**.303
Gemifloxacin, spectrum of activity, **B1**.492
Geminiviridae, **V1**.27 (Tab.), **V1**.41 (Tab.)
  see also specific viruses
GenBank
  Aspergillus identification, **M**.688–9
  BLAST program, **B1**.177
Gender effects, hookworm infection, **P**.728
Gene(s)
  ablation by proviral insertion, **V1**.339–40
  acquisition, **B1**.99
  complementation, **V1**.185–6
  disruption during retrovirus insertion,
    V1.339–40
  double-stranded RNA virus genome, **V1**.189
  filovirus overlaps, **V2**.1088, **V2**.1092
  Helicobacter sequence, **B2**.1567–8
  order conservation, **V1**.386–8
  probes, **B1**.225
  tagging, **V1**.338–9
  therapy, cystic fibrosis, **B1**.651
Gene arrays, pathogen-associated microbial
    patterns, **I**.111
Gene cassettes, **B1**.97–8
  mode of action, **B1**.98
  reversibility, **B1**.98
Gene cloning, **B1**.119, **B1**.126–7
  bacterial promoter genes, **B1**.126
  bacteriophage cloning vectors, **B1**.119–20,
    B1.120–1

Brucella, **B2**.1730
complementary DNA, **B1**.126–7
cosmids, **B1**.120–1
discontinuous ('split') genes, **B1**.126–7
Entamoeba histolytica, **P**.206
gene synthesis, **B1**.126
genetically modified plants, **B1**.127
plasmid cloning vectors, **B1**.119–24
  Ara system, **B1**.122–3
  broad host range vectors, **B1**.121
  gene replacement, **B1**.123
  mechanisms, **B1**.126
  PCR amplicon recovery, **B1**.121
  protein expression, **B1**.121–3
  shuttle vectors, **B1**.121
  suicide vectors, **B1**.123–4
  targeted gene modification, **B1**.123
subcloning, **B1**.126
TCR, **I**.449–50
Trypanosoma cruzi, **P**.381–2
vaccine development, **B1**.127
Gene conversion, *Borrelia,* **B2**.1826
Gene expression, **V1**.109–22
  adenoviruses, **V1**.115 (Fig.)
  capping, **V1**.112–13
  control, **V1**.118–19
  coronaviruses, **V1**.119
  flaviviruses, **V1**.110, **V1**.119
  hepadnaviruses, **V1**.111–12
  influenza virus, **V1**.120
  mRNA synthesis, **V1**.105–6, **V1**.112
  Nidovirales order, **V1**.392–3
  polyadenylation, **V1**.112–13
  protein encoding, **V1**.114–8
  transcription control, **V1**.113–8
Gene families, *Borrelia,* **B2**.1823–4
GeneProbe®, *Chlamydia* detection, **B2**.2019
General practitioners, reporting system,
    B1.320, **B1**.321 (Tab.)
General Register Office for England and
    Wales, **B1**.317
Generation times
  macroparasite epidemiology, **P**.52
  microparasite epidemiology, **P**.51
Genera, viral classification, **V1**.26,
    V1.27 (Tab.), **V1**.29, **V1**.35
Gene sequencing
  Candida albicans, **M**.583
  Cryptosporidium parvum, **P**.403–4
Gene switching, variable surface glycoprotein,
    P.362
Gene therapy
  aims, **V2**.1590
  autoimmune diseases, **I**.760
  clinical trials, **V2**.1590–1
  genetic analysis, **V1**.198
  hepatitis B therapy, **V2**.1261
  immune response, **V2**.1590–1
  integration, **V2**.1591
  naked DNA delivery, **V2**.1590–1
  see also specific infection
Gene therapy vectors, **V2**.1595 (Tab.),
    V2.1590–604
  adeno-associated viruses *see* Adeno-
    associated viruses (AAV)

adenoviruses *see* Adenoviruses
Dependovirus, **V1**.428–9
foamy viruses *see* Foamy viruses
HSV *see* Herpes simplex virus(es) (HSVs)
Minute virus of mice, **V1**.426–7
parvoviruses, **V1**.426–7
retroviruses *see* Retroviruses
zoonosis risk, **V2**.1297
Genetically engineered microorganisms, crops
    and insect resistance, **B1**.203–4
Genetically engineered plants, **B1**.127
Genetic analysis, **V1**.182–5
  applications, **V1**.193–9
    drug resistance, **V1**.194
    epitope analysis, **V1**.194
    gene therapy, **V1**.198
    genetic engineered vectors, **V1**.195–8
    immune evasion mechanisms, **V1**.198–9
    molecular epidemiology, **V1**.198
    vaccine development, **V1**.197
    viral attenuation, **V1**.195
    virulence determinant identification,
      V1.194–5
  conditional lethal mutants, **V1**.182–3
  deletion mutants, **V1**.184
  directed mutagenesis, **V1**.183–4, **V1**.184 (Fig.)
    PCR-directed, **V1**.183–4
  linker insertion mutagenesis, **V1**.185
  linker scanning mutagenesis, **V1**.184–5
  mutation rescue, **V1**.185 (Fig.)
  random mutagenesis, **V1**.183
  site-specific mutagenesis, **V1**.183–4
  spontaneous mutants, **V1**.183
'Genetic cassettes'
  coronaviruses, **V1**.835–6
  parvoviruses, **V1**.408
Genetic code, **B1**.13
  discovery, **B1**.13
Genetic engineering, bispecific antibodies,
    I.360
Genetic factors, in population immunity,
    B1.355
Genetic information exchange, *Trypanosoma*
    brucei, **P**.361
Genetic manipulation, **B1**.119–27
  fusion vectors, **B1**.125–6
  gene cloning *see* Gene cloning
  transposition-delivery vectors, **B1**.124–3
Genetic polymorphisms
  CTLA-4 gene *see* CTLA-4 gene
  CYP1A1 gene, **I**.587
  HLA *see* Human leukocyte antigens
    (HLAs); *individual HLA genes*
  IL1 gene cluster, **I**.588
  IL4 gene, **I**.587
  IL8 gene, **I**.587
  IL10 gene, **I**.587–8
  IL12B gene, **I**.582
  MBL gene, **I**.580
  pattern recognition receptors, **I**.124–5
  PRNP gene, **I**.589
  SLC11A1 gene, **I**.579
  TNF gene *see* Tumor necrosis factor-α
    (TNF-α), *TNF* gene
  see also Single nucleotide polymorphisms
    (SNPs)

Genetic recombination, *Plasmodium,* **P.**479
Genetic resistance, tuberculosis, **I.**711
Genetics, **B1.**80–135
  Borrelia taxonomy, **B2.**1821
  chromosomes
    replication, **B1.**81–2
    size, **B1.**81
    structure, **B1.**81
  Fusobacterium, **B2.**1947–8
  gene acquisition, **B1.**98–106
    artificial competence, **B1.**99, **B1.**100
    conjugation *see* Conjugation, bacterial
    natural competence, **B1.**99–100
    protoplast fusion, **B1.**106
    transduction *see* Transduction
    transformation, **B1.**99
  genome analysis, **B1.**81
  historical aspects, **B1.**12–14
  historical perspective, **B1.**81
  mobile elements, **B1.**91–8
    deletions, **B1.**95–6
    duplications, **B1.**95–6
    insertion mechanisms, **B1.**94–5
    insertions, **B1.**95–6
    insertion specificity, **B1.**94–5
    see also specific types
  pulsed-field gel electrophoresis, **B1.**81
  restriction endonucleases, **B1.**81
  of vertebrate viruses, **V1.**174–201
    complementation, **V1.**185–6
      definition, **V1.**185
      gene function, **V1.**185–6
    defective interfering particles *see*
      Defective interfering particles
    interactions, **V1.**187–92
      cross-reactivation, **V1.**189
      host transcript recombination, **V1.**190–1
      marker rescue, **V1.**189
      multiplicity reactivation, **V1.**189
      recombination, **V1.**187–8
      reverse genetics, **V1.**189–90
      reverse transcription, **V1.**188–9
      subunit reassortment, **V1.**191–2
      superinfection exclusion, **V1.**192
      see also specific types
    phenotypic mixing, **V1.**186
    pseudotype formation, **V1.**186
    systems, **V1.**174–5
    variability, **V1.**192–3
      biased hypermutation, **V1.**193
      hypermutation, **V1.**193
      quasi-species, **V1.**192–3
    viral interference, **V1.**186–7
Genetic susceptibility, alveolar echinococcosis,
  P.691
Genetic variability, basic reproductive number
  of infection (R_0), **P.**53–4
Genital fluids, virus shedding, **V1.**249
Genital tract infection, **B1.**657–8, **B1.**658 (Tab.)
  see also Genitourinary tract infection;
    Urinary tract infection; *specific infection*
Genital ulcers
  HIV transmission, **V2.**1500
  Pasteurella bettyae association, **B2.**1657

Genital warts
  HPV-6, **V1.**448–9
  low-risk HPVs, **V1.**448–9
Genitourinary medicine (GUM) clinics,
  B1.320–1, **B1.**321 (Tab.)
Genitourinary tract infection, **M.**600
  animal infection, **M.**602
  blastomycosis, **M.**489
  candidiasis, **M.**599, **M.**600, **M.**603, **M.**609
    see also Vulvovaginal candidiasis (VVC)
  cryptococcosis, **M.**648
    AIDS, **M.**648
  HPV infection *see* Human papillomavirus
    infection
  immune response, **P.**76–7
  mycoplasmas causing *see* Mycoplasma(s)
  Pasteurella aerogenes, **B2.**1656
  Pasteurella bettyae, **B2.**1657
  Pneumocystis carinii infection, **M.**785
  rhinosporidiosis, **M.**459, **M.**460
  spirochaetes
    non-pathogenic, **B2.**1860
    pathogenic *see* Syphilis
  virus entry, **V1.**236–7
  white piedra, **M.**196–7
  women, *Capnocytophaga,* **B2.**1674
  see also Genital tract infection; Urinary tract
    infection; Urinary tract infection (UTIs)
Genitourinary tract, normal microbiota,
  B1.303–4, **B1.**657
  gram-positive anaerobic cocci, **B2.**910
  protective role, **B1.**657
Genome
  scanning
    gene identification, **I.**572
    linkage, **I.**573
  sequencing
    Entamoeba moshkovskii, **P.**219
    epidemiology effects, **P.**50
    Plasmodium, **P.**478
Genome(s), **V1.**176–82
  ambisense coding, **V1.**181, **V1.**181 (Fig.)
  analysis, **B1.**81
    Cryptosporidium, **P.**399, **P.**404
  bacterial pathogenicity, **B1.**177–8
  Borrelia, sequences, **B2.**1823, **B2.**1824 (Fig.)
  Brucella, **B2.**1729–30
    maps, **B2.**1729
  coding potential, **V1.**176–80
    alternate splicing, **V1.**180
    minimum information content, **V1.**180
    nontemplated insertion of nucleotides,
      V1.180
    overlapping reading frames, **V1.**180
    RNA editing, **V1.**180
    small genomes, **V1.**180
  Coxiella burnetii see Coxiella burnetii
  endogenous viruses, **V1.**181–2
  infectious nucleic acid, **V1.**182
  integration and oncogenesis, **V1.**336–40,
    V1.345
  mutation, viral evolution, **V1.**16–7
  persistence and oncogenicity, **V1.**334–5
  Plasmodium, **P.**478–9
  rearrangement, **V1.**16

reengineering, **V1.**56
replication, **V1.**122–5
reverse transcription, **V1.**181–2
segmentation, **V1.**180–1
sequencing
  adeno-associated viruses, **V1.**409–10
  alphaherpesviruses, **V1.**494 (Tab.)
  astroviruses, **V2.**892–3
  betaherpesviruses, **V1.**494 (Tab.)
  herpesviruses, **V1.**494 (Tab.)
  human-specific herpesviruses, **V1.**489
  picornaviruses, **V2.**858
  sapoviruses, **V2.**923
  West Nile virus, **V2.**1002
Genomic groups, *Coxiella burnetii,* **B2.**2074
Genomics
  fungal classification, **M.**49
  vaccine development *see* Subunit vaccines
Genomic species, **B1.**29–30
Genomovars, *Burkholderia cepacia* complex,
  B2.1609, **B2.**1611–12
Genospecies, **B1.**29–30
Genotyping, **V2.**1542
  Bartonella bacilliformis, **B2.**1890
  Chlamydia, **B2.**2018
  Helicobacter, **B2.**1570
  heteroduplex mobility assay, **V2.**1542
  line probe assays, **V2.**1542
  melting curve analysis, **V2.**1542
  PCR, **V2.**1542
  restriction fragment length polymorphisms
    (RFLPs), **V2.**1542
Gentamicin
  gonorrhea treatment, **B1.**662
  joint prostheses, **B1.**392
  PMMA beads delivery in bone and joint
    infection, **B1.**700
  resistance, *Staphylococcus aureus,* **B2.**779–
    80, **B2.**791, **B2.**794 (Tab.), **B2.**804
  spectrum of activity, **B1.**482, **B1.**499 (Tab.)
    Brucella, **B2.**1742
    Citrobacter, **B2.**1476
    Edwardsiella, **B2.**1491–2
    Enterobacter, **B2.**1484–5
    Ewingella, **B2.**1493
    Haemophilus, **B2.**1702 (Tab.)
    Klebsiella, **B2.**1480
    Leclercia, **B2.**1495
    Listeria, **B2.**957–8
    Moellerella, **B2.**1496
    Serratia, **B2.**1488–9
    Yokenella, **B2.**1498
  structure, **B1.**483 (Fig.)
  tularemia treatment, **B2.**1755
Genus subclusters, picornaviruses, **V2.**858–9
Genus, viral classification, **V1.**39
*Geobacillus stearothermophilus (Bacillus
  stearothermophilus),* **B.**922–3
  characteristics, **B2.**935 (Tab.)
  food spoilage, **B2.**923–4
  *see also Bacillus stearothermophilus
    (Geobacillus stearothermophilus)*
Geographical distribution
  African trypanosomiasis, **P.**27 (Fig.),
    P.29–30, **P.**350–1, **P.**367
  alveolar echinococcosis, **P.**677, **P.**702

Geographical distribution (*Continued*)
  Angiostrongylus cantonensis, **P**.804
  ascariasis, **P**.42
  babesiosis, **P**.459
  Bartonella bacilliformis, **B2**.1888
  Bartonella henselae, **B2**.1897
  Borna disease virus, **V2**.1142–3
  Borrelia, **B2**.1819–21
  botulism, **B2**.1066–70
  bovine brucellosis, **B2**.1722
  Brucella abortus, **B2**.1721
  Brucella canis, **B2**.1722
  Brucella melitensis, **B2**.1721
  Brucella suis, **B2**.1720, **B2**.1722
  Carrión's disease, **B2**.1888
  Chromobacterium violaceum, **B2**.1679–80
  cutaneous Old World leishmaniasis,
    P.284 (Fig.)
  cystic echinococcosis, **P**.677, **P**.701
  cysticercosis, **P**.677, **P**.699
  Diphyllobothrium, **P**.658
  Diphyllobothrium latum, **P**.671
  dracunculiasis, **P**.39, **P**.830
  Enterocytozoon bieneusi, **P**.537
  Fasciola gigantica, **P**.647
  Fasciola hepatica, **P**.647
  giardiasis, **P**.37, **P**.249, **P**.250
  glanders, **B2**.1633
  hepatitis B, **V2**.1255
  hepatitis C, **V2**.1209–10
  HTLVs, **V2**.1289, **V2**.1292
  human brucellosis, **B2**.1721
  Hymenolepis nana, **P**.658
  Leishmania aethiopica, **P**.304
  Leishmania donovani, **P**.286 (Tab.), **P**.305
  Leishmania infantum, **P**.286 (Tab.), **P**.305
  Leishmania major, **P**.286 (Tab.), **P**.302
  Leishmania tropica, **P**.286 (Tab.)
  leprosy, **B2**.1203
  liver fluke(s), **P**.646–7
  lung fluke(s), **P**.646–7
  Lyme borreliosis, **B2**.1822
  lymphatic filariasis, **P**.769, **P**.770 (Fig.), **P**.772
  malaria, **P**.34, **P**.35 (Fig.), **P**.464, **P**.465 (Fig.)
    see also under Plasmodium
  melioidosis, **B2**.1628
  microsporidians, **P**.537
  mycetoma, **B2**.1159–60
  onchocerciasis, **P**.785, **P**.792, **P**.792 (Fig.)
  Onchocerciasis Control Programme,
    P.115 (Fig.)
  Paragonimus, **P**.41 (Fig.), **P**.647
  plague, **B2**.1459
  Plasmodium, **P**.473–4, **P**.474–5
    chloroquine resistance, **P**.465 (Fig.),
      P.509–10
    drug resistance, **P**.465 (Fig.), **P**.481 (Fig.)
    see also under Malaria
  Plasmodium falciparum, **P**.473–4
  Plasmodium vivax, **P**.474–5
    chloroquine resistance, **P**.509–10
  polycystic echinococcosis, **P**.677
  rabies, **V2**.1119–20
  Rickettsia, **B2**.2031 (Tab.), **B2**.2037,
    B2.2038 (Fig.)

Schistosoma haematobium, **P**.43, **P**.610
Schistosoma intercalatum, **P**.43, **P**.610
Schistosoma japonicum, **P**.43
Schistosoma mansoni, **P**.43, **P**.610
Schistosoma mekongi, **P**.43
Strongyloides, **P**.42, **P**.739
sulfadoxine–pyrimethamine resistance,
  P.465 (Fig.)
Taenia, **P**.658
tapeworms, **P**.658
trichuriasis, **P**.42
Trypanosoma brucei gambiense, **P**.352
Trypanosoma brucei rhodesiense, **P**.352
Trypanosoma cruzi, **P**.391
tularemia, **B2**.1752, **B2**.1753
visceral leishmaniasis (kala-azar), **P**.285 (Fig.)
Geographic information systems (GIS),
  malaria epidemiology, **P**.512–13
Geographic isolation, rabies control, **V1**.370–1
Geophilic dermatophytes, **M**.45–6, **M**.222–3,
  M.223–5, **M**.227 (Tab.)
Geotrichosis
  histopathology, **M**.128 (Tab.), **M**.134 (Fig.)
  oculomycoses, **M**.280 (Tab.)
Geotrichum, **M**.89 (Tab.)
Geotrichum candidum, histopathology,
  M.128 (Tab.), **M**.134 (Fig.)
Gerbils, *Leishmania major* host, **P**.303
Geriatric and long-stay facilities, nosocomial
  infection, **B1**.394
Germ cells
  SCF effects, **I**.274
  viral infection, **V1**.236
Germinal centers (GCs), **I**.400–1
  B-cell activation, **I**.401
  CD40 ligand (CD40L), **I**.349
  derivation, **I**.401
  formation, **I**.327
  functions, **I**.400
  HIV infection, **I**.797–8
  Ig affinity maturation, **I**.401
  memory B cell generation, **I**.491–2
  plasma cell generation, **I**.491–2
Germiston virus, transcription, **V2**.1035
  nucleotide insertion, **V2**.1035–6
'germ theory of disease', **B1**.4
Germ tube test, **M**.604–5
Gerstmann–Sträussler–Scheinker (GSS)
  disease, **V2**.1347
  dementing form, **V2**.1367
  diagnosis
    amyloid plaques, **V2**.1365
    molecular diagnosis, **V2**.1365
  prion transgenetics, **V2**.1355
  PrP mutations, **V2**.1367
  telencephalic form, **V2**.1367
  transgenic mouse model, **V2**.1355
Gerstmann–Straussler syndrome, *PRNP* gene
  polymorphisms, **I**.589
Gestational age
  congenital varicella syndrome (CVS),
    V2.1455
  fetal infection transmission, **V2**.1444
Getah virus (GETV), **V2**.1011 (Tab.), **V2**.1023
G glycoprotein epitope, respiratory syncytial
  virus, **I**.869

Giant cell pneumonia, measles, **V1**.724
  immunosuppressed, **V2**.1509
Giant cells, granulomatous amebic
  encephalitis, **P**.233
'Giant ulcer,' HIV infection, **I**.799
Giardia
  antigenic variation, **P**.245, **P**.246
  biochemistry, **P**.243–5
  classification, **P**.196–7, **P**.241–2
    groups, **P**.241
    molecular typing, **P**.242
    restriction fragment length polymorphisms,
      P.242
    ribosomal RNA sequencing, **P**.242
  control, **P**.251–2
    ultraviolet treatment, **P**.251
  endocytosis, **P**.164
  energy metabolic pathway, **P**.244
  historical aspects, **P**.13–5, **P**.241
  infection *see* Giardiasis
  isoenzyme studies, **P**.247
  life cycle, **P**.242–3, **P**.242 (Fig.)
    encystation-specific vesicles, **P**.243
  lipids, **P**.245
  molecular detection methods, **P**.250–1
  structure, **P**.242–3, **P**.243 (Fig.)
  toxin, **P**.246–7
  variant surface proteins, **I**.681
  waterborne, **B1**.214, **B1**.218–19
  see also individual species
Giardia agilis, **P**.241
Giardia duodenalis, **P**.187–8
  classification, **P**.191, **P**.241, **P**.242
Giardia lamblia (intestinalis), **P**.241
  attachment to intestine, **P**.242
  biochemistry, **P**.243–5
  classification, **I**.675–6
  classification/terminology, **P**.191, **P**.242
  CRP136 protein, **P**.246–7
  cysts, **P**.242, **P**.243, **P**.244 (Fig.), **P**.245 (Tab.)
  detection, **P**.247
  division, **P**.242
  fusidic acid effects, **B1**.488
  historical aspects, **P**.13–5
  infection *see* Giardiasis
  life cycle, **P**.242–3, **P**.242 (Fig.)
  structure, **P**.242–3, **P**.243 (Fig.)
    cyst wall, **P**.166, **P**.167 (Fig.)
    ventral disc, **P**.171 (Fig.)
  trophozoite, **P**.242, **P**.244 (Fig.), **P**.245 (Tab.)
Giardia muris, **P**.241
  antibacterial susceptibility/resistance, **B1**.434
  immune response, **P**.76
Giardiasis, **P**.241–54
  in AIDS, **P**.76, **P**.247, **P**.251
  asymptomatic, **P**.251
  chemotherapy, **P**.251
    in absence of diagnosis, **P**.251
  chronic, **P**.246
  clinical features, **P**.245–6
    acute, **P**.246
    agammaglobulinemia, **I**.780
  diagnosis, **P**.247–8, **P**.247 (Tab.)
    biopsies, **P**.150
    fecal examination, **P**.148

Giardiasis
  diagnosis (*Continued*)
    fecal samples, **P**.150
    immunoassays, **P**.154, **P**.248
    indirect fluorescent assay, **P**.248
    serological, **P**.247
    string test, **P**.148, **P**.151
  epidemiology, **P**.46 (Tab.), **P**.249–51
    geographical distribution, **P**.37, **P**.249, **P**.250
    outbreaks, **P**.250
    prevalence, **P**.37
    seasonal patterns, **P**.250
  gastric acidity relationship, **P**.250
  historical aspects, **P**.13–5
  immunology, **P**.76, **P**.246
  incubation period, **P**.245
  integrated control, **P**.251–2
  occupations associated, **P**.250
  pathology, **P**.246–7
  prevention, **P**.37, **P**.39
  public health importance, **P**.44, **P**.105 (Tab.)
    travellers/immigrants, **P**.29
  with tapeworm infection, **P**.664
  transmission, **P**.249–50
  vaccination prospects, **P**.252
Gibberella zeae, **B1**.284
Gibbon ape leukemia virus
  cell receptors, **V1**.207 (Tab.)
  receptors, **V1**.246 (Fig.)
Giemsa stain, **M**.88 (Tab.), **B2**.2030
  Bartonella bacilliformis, **B2**.1889
  Chlamydia, **B2**.2017
  mycology, **M**.87
  Pneumocystis, **M**.787–8
Gilchrist, T C, **M**.24
Gill-associated virus (GAV), **V1**.825
  classification, **V1**.392, **V1**.398
Giménez staining procedure, **B2**.2030
Gingival crevice
  Fusobacterium, **B2**.1946, **B2**.1950
  normal microbiota, **B1**.609, **B1**.609 (Tab.)
Gingival sulcus, gram-positive anaerobic cocci, **B2**.910
Gingivitis, **B1**.613–14
  causative organisms, **B1**.614
    spirochaetes, **B2**.1859–60
  clinical features, **B1**.613–14
  historical perspective, **B1**.614
  treatment, **B1**.614
Gingivostomatitis, HSV infection, **V1**.507
Girardi heart cell lines, **B2**.897
Glanders, **B2**.1633–5
  clinical manifestations, **B2**.1633
  control, **B2**.1634
  diagnosis, **B2**.1634
    ELISA, **B2**.1633, **B2**.1634
  epidemiology, **B2**.1633
    geographical distribution, **B2**.1633
    reservoirs, **B2**.1633
    transmission, **B2**.1633
  historical aspects, **B2**.1633
  mortality, **B2**.1634
  outcome/follow-up, **B2**.1634
  pathology/pathogenesis, **B2**.1633–4
    histopathology, **B2**.1634
    host immune response, **B2**.1634
  treatment, **B2**.1634
Glaucoma, rubella, **V2**.973
Glenosporella loboi see Loboa loboi
Gliding filament theory, **P**.170–2, **P**.179–80
Gliotoxin, **M**.707, **M**.709
  Aspergillus fumigatus, **M**.707, **M**.709
Global Alliance for African Human Trypanosomiasis, **P**.110
Global Alliance for Vaccines and Immunization, **V2**.1583
Global Alliance to Eliminate Lymphatic Filariasis, **P**.110
Global Rinderpest Eradication Program (GREP), **V1**.810
Global warming *see* Climate change
Glomerulonephritis
  endocarditis, **B1**.528
  hepatitis C, **V2**.1207
  post-streptococcal, **B1**.244
  prevalence, **I**.748 (Tab.)
Glossina see Tsetse flies *(Glossina)*
Gloves, surgeons', **B1**.388
Glucagon, acute phase response, **I**.208
Glucan(s), **B1**.444
  Aspergillus, **M**.716–17
  endocarditis, **B1**.527
  Paracoccidioides brasiliensis, **M**.542
  Pneumocystis, **M**.765, **M**.783
Glucanase, *Coccidioides immitis*, **M**.504, **M**.506 (Fig.)
Glucantime, **P**.341
  anergic diffuse cutaneous leishmaniasis, **P**.342
Glucocorticoid-responsive elements (GRE), **I**.197
  Hepatitis B virus, **V2**.1230
Glucocorticoids
  acute phase response, **I**.198 (Fig.), **I**.208
  immunodeficiency, **I**.788 (Tab.)
Gluconobacter, **B1**.60
Glucose
  blood:cerebrospinal fluid ratio, **B1**.558–9
  catabolism, **B1**.50–2
    alternative routes, **B1**.58–60
    repression, **B1**.72–3
  dissimilation, *Neisseria*, **B2**.1274–5
  fermentation, **B1**.55
    acid production, **B2**.1319 (Tab.)
    alcohol, **B1**.54
    butanediol formation, **B1**.55
    butanol, **B1**.55–6
    butyrate, **B1**.55–6
    Enterobacteriaceae identification, **B2**.1319 (Tab.)
    formic acid, **B1**.55 (Fig.)
    gas production, **B2**.1319 (Tab.)
    homolactic acid, **B1**.54, **B1**.54 (Fig.)
    Porphyromonas identification, **B2**.1924 (Tab.)
    Prevotella identification, **B2**.1924 (Tab.)
    by *Zymomonas*, **B1**.60
  metabolism
    Plasmodium, **P**.476

Trypanosoma brucei, **P**.359, **P**.359 (Fig.)
  phosphorylation, **B1**.50–1
  pyruvate formation
    hexose diphosphate pathway, **B1**.51, **B1**.51 (Fig.)
    KDPG pathway, **B1**.58
    Pseudomonas, **B1**.59
Glucose-6-dehydrogenase
  deficiency, innate malaria resistance, **P**.485
  Plasmodium, **P**.476
  trypanosomes, **P**.359–60
'glucose effect', **B1**.72–3
Glucose monomycolate, αβ T cell recognition, **I**.443 (Fig.)
Glucose-6-phosphate
  conversion to glyceraldehyde-3-phosphate, **B1**.51
  in hexose monophosphate pathway, **B1**.57–8
Glucose-6-phosphate dehydrogenase (G-6-PD) deficiency, **I**.770, **M**.789
Glucose transporters, larval cestodes, **P**.681–2
β-Glucuronidase (GUS) marker gene, soil bacteria analysis, **B1**.207
β-Glucuronidase, testing for presence, **B1**.223
Glucuronoxylomannan *see Cryptococcus neoformans*
Glutamate
  Fusobacterium metabolism, **B2**.1948
  transport, **B1**.49
Glutamic acid derivatives, Borna disease virus infection, **V2**.1147
Glutamine synthetase, covalent modification, **B1**.76
γ-Glutamyl transferase, leukotriene production, **I**.184–5
Glutaraldehyde (GTA), **B1**.427
  action, **B1**.436, **B1**.437 (Tab.), **B1**.438
    fungi, **B1**.439
    spores, **B1**.439
    viruses, **B1**.440
    ultrasonic waves, **B1**.454
Glutaredoxin, poxviruses, **V1**.598–600
Glutathione
  Entamoeba histolytica, **P**.204–5
  Trypanosoma cruzi, **P**.380
Glutathione *S*-transferases (GSTs)
  Echinococcus granulosus, **P**.682–3
  liver/lung flukes, **P**.652
  parasite immune avoidance mechanisms, **I**.686
  schistosomiasis, **P**.94
    vaccine/vaccination, **P**.620, **P**.633 (Tab.), **P**.634–5
GlyCAM, lymphocyte migration, **I**.508 (Tab.)
Glyceraldehyde-3-phosphate dehydrogenase, schistosomiasis vaccine, **P**.620
Glyceraldehyde-3-phosphate
  conversion to pyruvate, **B1**.54, **B1**.57
  glucose-6-phosphate conversion to, **B1**.51
Glycerol
  facilitated diffusion, **B1**.48–9
  fermentation, Enterobacteriaceae identification, **B2**.1319 (Tab.)
Glycerol, bare skin immunization, **I**.823–4
Glycine metabolism, *Cryptococcus neoformans*, **M**.638
Glycocalix barrier, parasites, **I**.685

Glycocalyx, **P**.168–9, **P**.168 (Fig.), **P**.169 (Fig.)
  functions, **P**.168
Glycocalyx (surface coat), **B1**.432–3
  functions, **B1**.688
  resistance, **B1**.443
Glycogenosis Ib, **I**.765
Glycogen, storage elements, **P**.179
Glycolipids
  CD1a/b/c-reactive αβ T cell binding, **I**.442,
    I.443 (Fig.)
  CD1d-reactive αβ T cell recognition, **I**.441–2,
    I.443 (Fig.)
Glycolysis
  Cryptosporidium parvum, **P**.403
  Trypanosoma brucei, **P**.357, **P**.359
Glycopeptide antibiotics, **B1**.480–1
  mode of action, **B1**.480
  pharmacology, **B1**.481
  resistance to, **B1**.480–1
    enterococci, **B1**.480–1, **B2**.892,
      B2.892 (Tab.)
  spectrum of activity, **B1**.480
  structure, **B1**.480, **B1**.480 (Fig.)
  toxicity, **B1**.481
  see also specific types
Glycophorin-binding protein (GBP),
  Plasmodium, **P**.475–6
Glycophorins, *Plasmodium* cell invasion,
  P.472
Glycophosphatidylinositol (GPI)
  FcγRIIIb, **I**.315
  malaria anti-disease immunity, **P**.493
Glycoprotein(s)
  arteriviruses, **V1**.827
  Avian pneumovirus, **V1**.787–8
  Borna disease virus *see* Borna disease virus
    (BDV)
  coronaviruses, **V1**.76
  Cryptosporidium parvum, **P**.402
  Ebola virus *see* Ebola virus (EBOV)
  Entamoeba histolytica, **P**.202, **P**.205
  Equine arteritis virus, **V1**.827
  filoviruses *see* Filoviruses
  herpesviruses, **V1**.502
  Human respiratory syncytial virus *see*
    Human respiratory syncytial virus
    (HRSV)
  larval cestodes, **P**.682–3
  Marburg virus *see* Marburg virus (MARV)
  Mononegavirales order, **V1**.381
  nonsymmetrical viruses, **V1**.69
  Porcine reproductive and respiratory
    syndrome virus, **V1**.827
  Rabies virus *see* Rabies virus (RABV)
  retroviruses, **V1**.77
  rhabdoviruses *see* Rhabdoviruses
  Vesicular stomatitis virus *see* Vesicular
    stomatitis virus (VSV)
  Zaire ebolavirus, **V2**.1089
Glycoprotein B, HHV-8, **V1**.546
Glycoprotein E, Tick-borne encephalitis virus,
  V1.208, **V1**.209 (Fig.)
Glycoprotein GP$_2$, arteriviruses, **V1**.836 (Tab.),
  V1.839–40
Glycoprotein GP$_3$, arteriviruses, **V1**.836 (Tab.),
  V1.839–40

Glycoprotein GP$_4$
  arteriviruses *see* Arteriviruses
  Equine arteritis virus, **V1**.836 (Tab.)
  Porcine reproductive and respiratory
    syndrome virus *see* Porcine reproductive
    and respiratory syndrome virus
    (PRRSV)
Glycoprotein GP$_5$
  arteriviruses *see* Arteriviruses
  Equine arteritis virus, **V1**.840
Glycoprotein K8.1, HHV-8, **V1**.546
Glycoprotein spikes, attachment proteins
  (viral), **V1**.208
Glycosomes, **P**.177–8
  Trypanosoma brucei, **P**.353, **P**.359
  Trypanosoma cruzi, **P**.377–8, **P**.380
Glycosylation
  cell–virus interactions, **V1**.225
  FcγRIIIa, **I**.315
  Ig structure, **I**.306
  Measles virus hemagglutinin (H) protein,
    V1.717–18
  PrP^C, **V2**.1358 (Fig.)
  viral replication, **V1**.122
Glycosylphosphatidylinositols
  Leishmania, **P**.294–5
  Trypanosoma cruzi, **P**.381
Glyoxisomes, **P**.177–8
Glyoxylate
  bypass, **B1**.53
  cycle, **B1**.53
  production, **B1**.53
Gnathosomiasis
  clinical manifestations/pathology, **P**.820–4
    cutaneous, **P**.820
    eosinophilia, **P**.821
    peripheral leukocytosis, **P**.821
    visceral, **P**.820–1
  diagnosis, **P**.820 (Tab.), **P**.821–4
    immunological methods, **P**.154
Gnathostoma, **P**.592, **P**.818
  infection *see* Gnathosomiasis
  structure/life cycle, **P**.592
  see also individual species
Gnathostoma binucleatum, **P**.818
Gnathostoma doloresi, **P**.818, **P**.823–4
  control, **P**.824
  infection *see* Gnathosomiasis
  life cycle, **P**.823
  morphology, **P**.823
  transmission/epidemiology, **P**.823
Gnathostoma hispidum, **P**.818, **P**.822–3
  control, **P**.823
  infection *see* Gnathosomiasis
  life cycle, **P**.822
  morphology, **P**.822
  transmission/epidemiology, **P**.822
Gnathostoma malaysiae, **P**.818
Gnathostoma nipponicum, **P**.824
  control, **P**.824
  infection *see* Gnathosomiasis
  life cycle, **P**.824
  morphology, **P**.824
  transmission/epidemiology, **P**.824

Gnathostoma spinigerum, **P**.818, **P**.818–22
  classification/morphology, **P**.818–19,
    P.819 (Fig.)
  control, **P**.822
  infection *see* Gnathosomiasis
  life cycle, **P**.819, **P**.821 (Fig.)
  transmission/epidemiology, **P**.819–20
Gnathostomatidae, **P**.592
Gnathostomatoidea, **P**.592
Goat milk, toxoplasmosis, **P**.437
Goats
  Brucella melitensis infection, **B2**.1722
  milk, **B1**.231–2
Goblet cells, **B1**.623 (Fig.)
Golgi-adjunct body, **P**.174, **P**.175 (Fig.)
Golgi apparatus
  apoptosis, **I**.136
  protozoa, **P**.176–7, **P**.177 (Fig.)
  viral transport
    bunyaviruses, **V2**.1039–40
    Hantavirus replication, **V2**.1039–40
    Phlebovirus replication, **V2**.1039–40
Gomori's methenamine silver (GMS) stain,
  M.33, **M**.123 (Tab.), **M**.351–2, **M**.491,
  M.676
  applications, **M**.122, **M**.130, **M**.132
  hematoxylin and eosin stain combination,
    M.123 (Tab.), **M**.124, **M**.351–2, **M**.491
  Histoplasma capsulatum, **M**.533–4
  procedure techniques, **M**.122, **M**.124–5
Gonadotrophin-releasing hormone (GnRH),
  immunocastration vaccines, **I**.875
Gongylonema, **P**.594
Gongylonematidae, **P**.594
Gonococcal arthritis, **B2**.1289
Gonococcal complement fixation test (GFFT),
  Neisseria gonorrhoeae detection, **B1**.751
Gonorrhea, **B1**.658–62
  bacteremia due to, **B1**.522
  behavioural control, **B1**.354
  causative agent, **B1**.658
  clinical features, **B1**.658
    female, **B1**.658, **B2**.1289
    men, **B1**.658, **B2**.1289
    oral, **B1**.658
    oral manifestations, **B1**.658
  complications, **B1**.658
  diagnosis, **B1**.659–61
    confirmatory, **B1**.659–60
    EIAs, **B1**.751
    gonococcal complement fixation test,
      B1.751
    presumptive, **B1**.659
  disseminated gonococcal infection, **B1**.522,
    B1.658
  endocarditis, **B1**.525
  epidemiology and sociology, **I**.954 (Fig.),
    B2.1289, **B2**.1289 (Fig.)
  immune response, blocking antibodies,
    B2.1282
  infection route, **B1**.658
  prevention, **B2**.1292–3
  treatment, **B2**.1277
    alternatives, **B1**.661–2
    antibiotics, **B1**.661
  uncomplicated gonococcal infection, **B1**.658

Gonorrhea (*Continued*)
see also Neisseria gonorrhoeae
Goose parvovirus (GPV), **V1**.410
  infection, **V1**.426
Gordona see Gordonia
Gordonia, **B2**.1137–8, **B2**.1151–3
  antibacterial susceptibility/resistance,
    B2.1145
  classification, **B2**.1137–8
  identification systems and methods,
    B2.1144–5
  lysozyme, **B2**.1144
  microscopic morphology, **B2**.1141–3
  mycolic acids, **B2**.1146
  staining properties, **B2**.1139–40
  see also individual species
Gordonia aichiensis, **B2**.1151
Gordonia bronchialis, **B2**.1151–2
Gordonia erythropolis, **B2**.1152, **B2**.1168
Gordonia rubropertincta, **B2**.1152
Gordonia sputi, **B2**.1152
Gordonia terrae, **B2**.1152–3
'Gordon' method, **B2**.1143–4, **B2**.1161
Gorilla rhadinovirus-1, **V1**.542 (Tab.)
Gougerot–Carteaud (confluent and reticulate
    papillomatosis), **M**.203 (Fig.), **M**.213–14
Gowans, James, **I**.503–4
gp21, HTLVs, **V2**.1285–7
gp22 deficiency, **I**.769
gp41 *see* HIV
gp43 glycoprotein, *Paracoccidioides*
    brasiliensis, **M**.553
gp46, HTLVs, **V2**.1285–7
gp91 deficiency, **I**.769
gp120 *see* HIV
gp160 *see* HIV
g proteins, **V1**.335–6
G proteins, neutrophil intracellular signaling,
    I.42
Gracilibacillus, **B2**.922–3
Graft rejection
  complement pathology, **I**.155–6
  IL-8, **I**.228
  MCP-1 (CCL2), **I**.228
  therapy
    chemokine antagonists, **I**.231–2
    IL-2 blocking, **I**.280
    monoclonal antibody therapy, **I**.357–8
Grafts, intravascular, **B1**.392
Graft-versus-host disease (GvHD)
  fusariosis, **M**.754
  HHV-6 infection, **V1**.530–1
  perforin deficiency, **I**.480
Grahamella, classification, **B2**.2026
Grain storage, airborne bacteria, **B1**.186 (Tab.)
Gramicidin, **B1**.497
Gram-negative bacilli
  airborne concentrations in facilities,
    B1.186 (Tab.)
  endocarditis, **B1**.532
  nosocomial infection, **B1**.377
Gram-negative bacteria
  airborne bacteria, **B1**.186 (Tab.)
    exposure and dispersal, **B1**.189
  antibacterial susceptibility/resistance, **B1**.433,
    B1.436, **B1**.441 (Tab.), **B1**.442

cell wall, **B1**.188
diplococci, **B2**.1270
factors influencing colonization, **B1**.294
food
  eggs, **B1**.278–9
  fish, **B1**.279
  freeze-drying, **B1**.269
  frozen, **B1**.264, **B1**.269–70
  ionizing radiation sensitivity, **B1**.271
  vegetables, frozen, **B1**.281–2
infection
  bacteremia, **B1**.516 (Fig.), **B1**.520, **B1**.522,
    B1.523
  nosocomial infection, **B1**.401 (Tab.)
  pneumonia, **B1**.637
iron scavenging, **B1**.151
see also individual species
Gram-positive anaerobic cocci (GPAC),
    B2.903
antibacterial susceptibility/resistance, **B2**.907,
    B2.911–12
capsules, **B2**.910–11
classification, **B2**.903–5
  changes at genus level, **B2**.904
  currently recognized genera, **B2**.905 (Tab.)
  currently recognized species, **B2**.906 (Tab.)
  new and recent species, **B2**.904–5
  species awaiting description, **B2**.905,
    B2.917
clinical importance, **B2**.910
culture, **B2**.905–6
β-Gal group, **B2**.905, **B2**.908 (Tab.), **B2**.917
genera, **B2**.912–17
  species descriptions, **B2**.912–17
growth requirements, **B2**.905, **B2**.906–7
historical perspective, **B2**.903
identification, **B2**.906–7, **B2**.908 (Tab.)
  16S rRNA probes, **B2**.907
  biochemical characteristics, **B2**.908 (Tab.)
  DNA probes, **B2**.907
  at genus level, **B2**.906–7
  metronidazole sensitivity, **B2**.907
  non-volatile fatty acid groups, **B2**.907
  PCR, **B2**.907
  at species level, **B2**.907
  typing methods, **B2**.911
  volatile fatty acid groups, **B2**.907
infection, **B2**.910
  clinical specimens, **B2**.906–7
  therapy, **B2**.912
isolation and maintenance, **B2**.905–6
normal microbiota, **B2**.907–10
pathogenicity, **B2**.910–11
proteolytic activity, **B2**.910–11
synergistic action, **B2**.910–11
'trisimilis' group, **B2**.905, **B2**.908 (Tab.),
    B2.917
virulence factors, **B2**.910–11
Gram-positive bacteria
  airborne bacteria
    concentrations in facilities, **B1**.186 (Tab.)
    dispersal, **B1**.189
    drying and heat stress, **B1**.188
  antibacterial susceptibility/resistance, **B1**.433,
    B1.441 (Tab.)

  antimicrobial susceptibility/resistance,
    B1.441–2, **B1**.441 (Tab.)
    drug efflux, **B1**.440
    possibly liked to biocide resistance,
      B1.443–4
  catabolite repression, **B1**.73–4
  cell wall, **B1**.188
  cocci
    airborne concentrations in facilities,
      B1.186 (Tab.)
    facultative anaerobes catalase-negative,
      B2.883 (Tab.)
  food
    fish, **B1**.279
    freeze-drying, **B1**.269
    frozen, **B1**.264, **B1**.269–70
    ionizing radiation sensitivity, **B1**.271
    vegetables, frozen, **B1**.281–2
    water activity, **B1**.266
  infection
    bacteremia, **B1**.393, **B1**.516 (Fig.), **B1**.517,
      B1.519–20
    factors influencing colonization, **B1**.294
    nosocomial infection, **B1**.401 (Tab.)
  iron scavenging, **B1**.151
  nonspore-forming, airborne dispersal, **B1**.189
  ribosomes, **B1**.188
  see also individual bacterial genera
Gram stain, **M**.87, **M**.88 (Tab.), **B1**.713–14
  bloodstream infection, **B1**.515–16
  historical aspects, **B1**.6–7
  modified, **M**.123 (Tab.), **M**.124–5
  Veillonella, **B2**.1314–15
'Granular dermatitis,' **M**.412
Granular form, *Blastocystis hominis*, **P**.557,
    P.558, **P**.558 (Fig.)
Granule(s)
  histopathology, **M**.89 (Tab.)
  in vivo formation, **M**.385, **M**.394
Granulicatella, **B2**.862–3
  endocarditis, **B1**.528–9
  metabolism, **B2**.838
  as normal microbiota, **B1**.296 (Tab.)
Granulicatella adiacens, **B1**.529, **B1**.533
Granulocyte chemoattractant protein 2
    (GCP-2:CXCL6), **I**.218 (Tab.)
  ELR motif, **I**.221
Granulocyte-colony stimulating factor
    (G-CSF), **I**.276–7
  in disease
    aspergillosis, **M**.724
    candidiasis, **M**.613
  effects, **I**.276–7
    neutrophils, **I**.36, **I**.43, **I**.274, **I**.276 (Fig.)
  production, **I**.276
    IL-17 effects, **I**.290
  structure, **I**.276
  therapeutic use, **I**.276–7
    fusariosis, **M**.755
    neutropenia, **I**.277
    neutropenia therapy, **I**.47, **I**.50
    Scedosporium infection, **M**.757
    septic shock therapy, **I**.702
    systemic zygomycosis, **M**.678

Granulocyte-macrophage colony-stimulating factor (GM-CSF), **I**.276–7
  in disease
    aspergillosis, **M**.709, **M**.724
    candidiasis, **M**.593
  effects
    basophil chemotaxis, **I**.60
    basophil degranulation, **I**.63
    basophils, **I**.57
    CD8 T cell activation, **I**.427–8
    eosinophil activation, **I**.64
    eosinophil adhesion, **I**.60
    eosinophil chemotaxis, **I**.61
    eosinophils, **I**.57–8
    HIV replication, **V1**.300
    IL-1 stimulation, **I**.277
    IL-2 stimulation, **I**.277
    neutrophil development, **I**.36
    neutrophil priming, **I**.43, **I**.44
    VLA upregulation, **I**.60
  mucosal immune response, **I**.522–3
  production, **I**.277
    eosinophils, **I**.67, **I**.277
    NK cells, **I**.82
  structure, **I**.277
  therapeutic uses, **I**.277
    cryptococcosis, **M**.652–3
    DNA vaccine co-administration, **I**.918, **I**.918 (Tab.)
    fusariosis, **M**.755
    systemic zygomycosis, **M**.678
    vaccine adjuvant, **I**.898
Granulocytes
  as APCs, **I**.112
  Chédiak–Higashi syndrome, **I**.481 (Fig.)
  tuberculosis granulomas, **I**.717
Granulocytopenia, aspergillosis, **M**.698
Granuloma(s)
  CD8 T cells, **I**.709
  definition, **I**.705–6
  in disease, **I**.706 (Tab.)
    Angiostrongylus costaricensis, **P**.810
    aspergillosis, **M**.694
    Brucella infection, **B1**.741, **B2**.1737
    candidiasis, **M**.597
    cryptococcosis, **M**.534
    deep dermatophytic, *Microsporum canis,* **M**.138 (Fig.)
    fascioliasis, **P**.651–2
    histoplasmosis capsulati, **M**.533, **M**.534
      mediastinal, **M**.519
    Listeria monocytogenes infection, **B1**.741
    lymphocytic, cutaneous leishmaniasis, **P**.300
    Mycobacterium terrae infection, **B1**.741
    paracoccidioidomycosis, **M**.553, **M**.554 (Fig.)
    paragonimiasis, **P**.650–1
    schistosomiasis, **P**.604–5, **P**.605 (Fig.), **P**.613–5, **P**.616–17, **P**.629–30
    toxocariasis, **P**.754
    trichinellosis, **P**.762–3
  fibrotic (type 2), **I**.707–8, **I**.708–9
  see also Schistosomiasis

  formation, **I**.705–6
    CD4 T cells, **I**.706–7
    cytokines, **I**.707
    Th1/Th2 cell balance, **I**.706
  functions, **I**.709
  histopathology, **I**.706, **I**.707 (Fig.)
  macrophages, **I**.31, **I**.31 (Fig.)
  necrotic (type 1), **I**.707–8, **I**.708–9
    chemokines, **I**.708
    structure, **I**.708
  see also Tuberculosis
Granuloma inguinale, diagnosis, **B2**.1336
Granulomatosis infantiseptica, **B1**.243
Granulomatosis, lymphomatoid, histoplasmosis capsulati *vs.,* **M**.534
Granulomatous amebic encephalitis (GAE), **P**.226, **P**.229
  chemotherapy, **P**.237
  clinical features, **P**.231
  diagnosis, **P**.235
  epidemiology/control, **P**.236
  in immunosuppressed, **P**.236
  incubation period, **P**.231
  pathology, **P**.233–4, **P**.234 (Fig.)
Granulysin
  CTLs, **I**.477
  cytotoxic granules, **I**.477
  NK cell cytotoxic granules, **I**.82, **I**.99, **I**.477
  target cell death, **I**.478
Granzyme(s), **I**.476–7
  CTLs, **I**.423
  deficiencies, **I**.482
    viral infection, **I**.482
  mechanism of action, **I**.476, **I**.479 (Fig.)
  mice, **I**.477
  NK cell cytotoxic granules, **I**.81
  target cell death, **I**.479 (Fig.)
  tumor rejection, **I**.482 (Tab.)
  viral clearance, **I**.482 (Tab.)
Granzyme A, **I**.476–7
  deficiencies, **I**.482
  target cell death, **I**.478, **I**.479 (Fig.)
Granzyme B
  deficiencies, **I**.482
  target cell death, **I**.478, **I**.479 (Fig.)
Granzyme H, **I**.477
  target cell death, **I**.478
Granzyme K, **I**.476–7
  target cell death, **I**.478
Granzyme M, **I**.476, **I**.477
  apoptosis initiation, **I**.476
  Bid (BH3 domain binding B-cell lymphoma) cleavage, **I**.476
  caspase-dominated DNA cleavage, **I**.476
  caspases cleavage, **I**.476
Graphium eumorphum, **M**.755
Graves' disease
  CTLA-4 gene polymorphisms, **I**.752
  prevalence, **I**.748 (Tab.)
'Gray baby' syndrome, chloramphenicol, **B1**.485
Gray Lung 'virus' disease, **B2**.1964
Grb-2-associated binding protein (Gab1), BCR signaling, **I**.345
Grb2, Ras activation, **I**.346

Green fluorescent protein (GFP), soil bacteria analysis, **B1**.207
Greenhouse worker infection, **M**.222–3
Green sulfur bacteria, **B1**.68
  sulfur oxidation, **B1**.201
Gregg, N McAlister, **V2**.968–9
Gridley's fungus (GF) stain, **M**.123 (Tab.)
  applications, **M**.122, **M**.132
  Histoplasma capsulatum, **M**.533–4
Griesinger, Wilhelm, **P**.9
Griffith, F, **B1**.13
Griscelli's syndrome, **I**.482, **I**.778
Griseofulvin, **M**.184
  drug interactions, **M**.184
  headache, **M**.184
  mechanism of action, **M**.184
  resistance, **M**.177
    dermatophytes, **M**.177
    Trichophyton, **M**.177, **M**.234
  therapy
    dermatomycosis, **M**.253
    dermatophytoses, **M**.184
    dermatophytosis, **M**.11
    mycetoma, **M**.393
    onychomycosis, **M**.187–8, **M**.253
    tinea, **M**.233, **M**.234–5
    tinea barbae, **M**.186, **M**.187 (Tab.)
    tinea capitis, **M**.188, **M**.188 (Tab.)
    tinea cruris, **M**.186
GROα (CXCL1), **I**.218 (Tab.)
  neutrophil production, **I**.47
  structure, **I**.217–19
    ELR motif, **I**.221
  structure–function relationship, **I**.221
GROβ (CXCL2), **I**.218 (Tab.)
GroEL
  Coxiella burnetii, **B2**.2076
  function, **B1**.47–8
GroES, **B1**.47–8
GroESL, *Ehrlichia,* **B2**.2055–6
GROγ (CXCL3), **I**.218 (Tab.)
Groin
  Staphylococcus infection, **B2**.777
  tinea cruris, **M**.228, **M**.231, **M**.234, **M**.239
'Groove sign,' lymphogranuloma venereum, **B2**.2012
Ground beef, microbiology, **B1**.273–4
Ground squirrel hepatitis virus (GSHV)
  discovery, **V2**.1227
  HBx protein, **V2**.1242
Groundwater
  bacteriology of, **B1**.214–15, **B1**.224
  nitrate leaching, **B1**.200
Group A Streptococcus Direct (GASD), **B1**.723 (Tab.)
Group D streptococci, tritrpticin sensitivity, **I**.172
Group-specific globulin, **I**.203
Growth
  bacteria, **B1**.37–42
    balanced and unbalanced, **B1**.38
    culture, **B1**.37–8
      continuous, **B1**.41–2
      liquid culture, **B1**.38
      solid surfaces, **B1**.42

Growth
  bacteria
    culture (*Continued*)
      synchronized, **B1**.38
    curve, **B1**.39–40, **B1**.39 (Fig.)
      batch culture, **B1**.39 (Fig.)
      death phase, **B1**.40
      exponential (logarithmic) phase,
        B1.39–40
      lag phase, **B1**.39
      stationary phase, **B1**.40
    generations, **B1**.38–9
    generation time, **B1**.38
    measurement of cell number, **B1**.38
      colony-forming units, **B1**.38
      pour plate method, **B1**.38
      spread plate method, **B1**.38
    phases, **B1**.39–40
    rate changes, **B1**.40–1
      shift-up and shift-down, **B1**.40–1
    rates, **B1**.38–9
      in chemostats, **B1**.41
  fungal, **M**.70–4
    dimorphism, **M**.21–2, **M**.74–6, **M**.74 (Tab.)
    epiphytic/epilythic, **M**.195
    mold pattern, **M**.70–4, **M**.70 (Fig.), **M**.71,
      M.72 (Fig.)
    mycelium production, **M**.70, **M**.72
    phenotypic switching, **M**.76, **M**.76 (Fig.)
    yeast pattern, **M**.70 (Fig.), **M**.73
    see also individual patterns
Growth factors, **P**.70
  historical aspects/re-evaluation, **I**.10
  keratinocyte production, **I**.820–1
  poxviruses encoding and tumor induction,
    V1.257
  in tumor pathogenesis, **V1**.341
Growth hormone (GH), acute phase response,
  I.208
Growth receptor, interferon-γ receptor *vs.*,
  I.250–1
Growth related oncogene, CNS expression,
  V2.1409
Growth retardation
  ascariasis, **P**.727
  gastrointestinal nematodes, **P**.725
  trichuriasis, **P**.729
Growth temperature, *Borrelia* culture, **B2**.1828
Gruby, D, **M**.6
GuaBA operon, *Shigella* vaccine vectors, **I**.843
Guanarito virus
  animal infection, **V2**.1069–70
  emerging infection, **V2**.1648 (Tab.)
  geographical distribution/carrier and disease,
    V2.1060 (Tab.)
  transmission, **V1**.371 (Tab.)
Guano
  Candida parapsilosis, **M**.586
  Cryptococcus neoformans, **M**.643
Guanosine 5′-diphosphate 3′-diphosphate
  (ppGpp), **B1**.40
  biocide and antibiotic resistance, **B1**.440
Guanylyltransferase, orbiviruses, **V2**.939–40
Guaroa virus, **V2**.1042–3
Guidelines, *Chlamydia trachomatis* infection
  therapy, **B2**.2021

Guillain–Barré syndrome
  BCE peptide vaccines, **I**.855 (Tab.)
  Campylobacter infection, **B2**.1551
  Campylobacter jejuni associated, **B1**.365
  complement pathology, **I**.156
  echovirus infection, **V2**.1424
  hepatitis A vaccine, **V2**.1576
  hepatitis B vaccine, **V2**.1574
  influenza vaccine, **V2**.1577
  Mycoplasma pneumoniae, **B2**.1983
  neuro-AIDS similarity, **V2**.1427–8
  pathogen-induced, **I**.753 (Tab.)
  rabies vaccine, **V2**.1578
  yellow fever vaccine, **V2**.1579–80
Guinea pig(s)
  arenavirus infection, **V2**.1069–70
  listeriosis, **B2**.963
Guinea worm *see* Dracunculiasis; *Dracunculus;
  Dracunculus medinensis*
Guinea Worm Eradication Programme, **P**.110
Gut-associated lymphoid tissue (GALT), **I**.505,
  I.529–32
  HIV infection, **I**.799
  mucosal vaccination, **I**.827
  Peyer's patches *see* Peyer's patches
  structure, **I**.531 (Fig.)
    compartments, **I**.533 (Fig.)
Gymnoascaceae, **M**.486
Gymnophallidae, **P**.582
Gymnophalloidea, **P**.582
Gymnophalloides, **P**.582
  structure/life cycle, **P**.582
Gynecological infection
  Eikenella corrodens, **B2**.1667
  see also Genital tract infection;
    Genitourinary tract infection
Gynecophoric canal, *Schistosoma*, **P**.600–1
Gyrovirus, classification, **V1**.41

H₁ histamine receptor, **I**.64
H1 Influenza virus A *see* Influenza virus A
H1N1 Influenza virus A *see* Influenza virus A
H₂ histamine receptor, **I**.64
H-2 histocompatibility complex, *Babesia
  microti* immunity and, **P**.455–6
H2 Influenza virus A *see* Influenza virus A
H2N2 Influenza virus A *see* Influenza virus A
H₃ histamine receptor, **I**.64
H3 Influenza virus *see* Influenza virus A
H3N2 Influenza virus A *see* Influenza virus A
H3N3 Influenza virus *see* Influenza virus A
H6 protein (topoisomerase), poxviruses,
  V1.169 (Tab.)
Habronemiasis, horses, **M**.412–13
HACEK group, endocarditis, **B1**.532, **B1**.533,
  B1.537, **B1**.540
Haeckel, E H, **B1**.10–1, **P**.189–90
  protozoa definition, **P**.186–7
Haemagogus
  Mayaro virus transmission, **V2**.1023
  yellow fever, **V2**.999
Haemobartonella, classification, **B2**.1964,
  B2.1968
Haemobartonella felis, **B2**.1973–4
Haemonchus, **P**.595

Haemophilus, **B2**.1692–718
  antibacterial susceptibility/resistance,
    B2.1702–4, **B2**.1710
    testing, **B2**.1703–4
  antigens, **B2**.1698–9
  bacteriocins, **B2**.1706
  cell composition, **B2**.1698–9
    capsule, **B2**.1698
    lipo-oligosaccharide, **B2**.1698
    outer-membrane proteins, **B2**.1698–9
    pili, **B2**.1698
  classification, **B2**.1692, **B2**.1699–700
    species, **B2**.1693–4
    see also individual species
  conjugation, **B1**.103
  culture, **B2**.1694–7, **B2**.1709–10
    colonial morphology, **B2**.1696
    growth factors, **B2**.1694–5
    hemolysis, **B2**.1696–7
    physical requirements, **B2**.1695–6
    preservation and storage, **B2**.1702
    V factor, **B2**.1695
    X factor, **B2**.1694–5
  definition, **B2**.1692
  genetics, **B2**.1697–8
    plasmids, **B2**.1697
    population genetics, **B2**.1698
    transduction, **B2**.1697
    transformation, **B2**.1697
    transposons, **B2**.1697
  habitats, **B2**.1694
  historical perspective, **B2**.1692
  infection
    hemolysis, **B2**.1696–7
    intracranial abscess, **B1**.585
    urinary tract infection, **B1**.678
  isolation/identification, **B2**.1700–2, **B2**.1710
    biochemical tests, **B2**.1701–2
    preservation/storage, **B2**.1702
  metabolism, **B2**.1697
  morphology, **B2**.1694, **B2**.1696
  in normal microbiota, **B1**.296 (Tab.), **B1**.301,
    B1.303, **B2**.1706–7
    oral cavity, **B1**.609
  pathogenicity, **B2**.1707–9, **B2**.1710–11
  plasmids, **B2**.1697
  typing methods, **B2**.1704–6, **B2**.1710
    animal strains, **B2**.1706
    biotyping, **B2**.1704–5
    capsule typing, **B2**.1704
    DNA-based methods, **B2**.1705–6
    OMP typing, **B2**.1705
  virulence factors, **B2**.1707–9, **B2**.1710–11
Haemophilus aegyptius, **B2**.1693
  classification, **B2**.1692
    characteristics, **B2**.1693 (Tab.)
  emerging bacterial infection, **B1**.362–3
Haemophilus agni, **B2**.1694
Haemophilus aphrophilus, **B2**.1693–4
  characteristics, **B2**.1693 (Tab.), **B2**.1699–700,
    B2.1699 (Tab.)
  culture, **B2**.1695–6
  infection, endocarditis, **B1**.532
  morphology, **B2**.1696
  in normal microbiota, **B2**.1706, **B2**.1707

Haemophilus aphrophilus, (Continued)
pathogenicity, **B2**.1708

Haemophilus avium, reclassification, **B2**.1650

Haemophilus ducreyi, **B1**.663–5, **B2**.1709–11
antibacterial susceptibility/resistance, **B1**.664–5, **B2**.1710
antibacterial susceptibility testing, **B1**.665
characteristics, **B2**.1693 (Tab.), **B2**.1699–700, **B2**.1699 (Tab.)
culture, **B2**.1695, **B2**.1709–10
colonies, **B1**.664
cytolethal distending toxin, **I**.655
immune evasion, **I**.655
infection *see* Chancroid
isolation/identification, **B2**.1701, **B2**.1710
culture, **B1**.664
microscopy, **B1**.664
molecular detection, **B1**.664
morphology, **B2**.1709
pathogenicity, **B2**.1710–11
typing methods, **B2**.1710

Haemophilus felis, **B2**.1694
characteristics, **B2**.1693 (Tab.)

Haemophilus gallinarum, **B2**.1694

Haemophilus haemoglobinophilus
characteristics, **B2**.1693 (Tab.), **B2**.1699 (Tab.)
morphology, **B2**.1696
pathogenicity, **B2**.1708

Haemophilus haemolyticus
characteristics, **B2**.1693 (Tab.), **B2**.1699–700, **B2**.1699 (Tab.)
culture, **B2**.1696–7
in normal microbiota, **B2**.1706, **B2**.1707

Haemophilus influenzae, **B2**.1693
acapsulate strains, **B1**.573
antibacterial susceptibility/resistance, **B1**.499 (Tab.), **B2**.1702–4
antigens, **B2**.1698–9
capsulate strains, **B1**.573
capsule, **B2**.1698, **B2**.1708
typing, **B2**.1704
cell composition, **B2**.1698–9
fimbriae, **B1**.627
lipo-oligosaccharide, **B1**.627, **B2**.1698
pili, **B2**.1698
characteristics, **B2**.1693 (Tab.), **B2**.1699 (Tab.), **B2**.1700
classification, **B2**.1692
Pittman types, **B1**.757
culture, **B2**.1694–6
preservation and storage, **B2**.1702
genetics, **B2**.1697–8
artificial competence, **B1**.99–100
natural competence, **B1**.99
habitats, **B1**.608–9
hemocin, **B2**.1706
immune evasion
antibody degradation/modification, **I**.662
capsule phase variation, **I**.660–1
complement surface masking, **I**.662–3
LPS variation, **I**.661
outer membrane protein variation, **I**.661
infection
agammaglobulinemia, **I**.780

airway adherence, **B1**.648 (Fig.)
attached to airway mucus, **B1**.623 (Fig.)
bacteremia, **B1**.522, **B1**.573
C3 deficiency, **I**.770–1
chronic bronchitis, **B1**.648
conjunctivitis, **B1**.598, **B1**.599, **B1**.600
in cystic fibrosis, **B1**.650
endocarditis, **B1**.532
epiglottitis, **B1**.613
hyper-IgE syndrome, **I**.49
Ig deficiencies, **I**.781–2
influenza, **V1**.661
keratitis, **B1**.601
keratoconjunctivitis, **B1**.386
Ludwig's angina, **B1**.614–15
neutrophils, **I**.44
otitis media, **B1**.617–18
pneumonia, **B1**.636–7, **B1**.640 (Tab.), **B1**.640–1
sinusitis, **B1**.615, **B1**.615 (Tab.)
vaccines, **I**.424 (Tab.)
BCE peptide vaccines, **I**.855 (Tab.), **I**.861 (Tab.)
development status, **I**.933 (Tab.)
historical aspects, **I**.15
proteasomes, **I**.839
virulence factors promoting, **B1**.627
iron-dependent repression, **B1**.165–6
iron scavenging, **B1**.151
isolation/identification, **B2**.1700–1
biochemical tests, **B2**.1701–2
biotyping, **B2**.1704–5
serology, **B1**.757
typing methods, **B2**.1704–6, **B2**.1705 (Tab.)
laboratory worker immunization, **B1**.767
morphology, **B2**.1694, **B2**.1694 (Fig.), **B2**.1696, **B2**.1696 (Fig.)
in normal microbiota, **B2**.1706–7
outer-membrane proteins, **B2**.1698–9
subtyping, **B2**.1705
pathogenicity, **B2**.1707–8
virulence factors, **B1**.627, **B2**.1707–9
evolution within host, **B1**.173–4

Haemophilus influenzae type b (Hib)
diagnosis, nasopharyngeal swabs, **B1**.560
endotoxin, **B1**.557
infection
bacteremia, **B1**.522, **B1**.573
bone and joint infection, **B1**.690
carriage rates, **B1**.556, **B1**.573
immune response, **B1**.573
meningitis *see Haemophilus influenzae* type b (Hib) meningitis
predisposition factors, **B1**.557
process, **B1**.556
rates, **B1**.572–3
vaccines, **B1**.574
conjugate vaccines, **B1**.574, **I**.935–6
epidemiological evaluation/surveillance, **B1**.323
impact, **B1**.574
MF59 adjuvant, **I**.927
polysaccharide, **B1**.573
resurgence of invasive infection, **B1**.574, **B1**.574 (Fig.)

virulence, **B1**.556
Haemophilus influenzae type b (Hib) meningitis, **B1**.555–6, **B1**.572–4
clinical features, **B1**.573
epidemiology, **B1**.572–3
fatality rate, **B1**.572–3
immunology, **B1**.573
infection route, **B1**.573
management of contacts, **B1**.574
prophylaxis, **B1**.574
treatment, **B1**.573–4
vaccines, **B1**.574

Haemophilus paracuniculus, **B2**.1694
characteristics, **B2**.1693 (Tab.), **B2**.1699 (Tab.)
pathogenicity, **B2**.1708

Haemophilus paragallinarum, **B2**.1694
characteristics, **B2**.1693 (Tab.), **B2**.1699 (Tab.)
culture, **B2**.1695–6
morphology, **B2**.1694, **B2**.1696
pathogenicity, **B2**.1708
reclassification, **B2**.1650
typing methods, **B2**.1706

Haemophilus parahaemolyticus
antibacterial susceptibility/resistance, **B2**.1703
characteristics, **B2**.1693 (Tab.), **B2**.1699 (Tab.), **B2**.1700
culture, **B2**.1696–7
in normal microbiota, **B2**.1706, **B2**.1707

Haemophilus parainfluenzae
antibacterial susceptibility/resistance, **B2**.1703
biotyping, **B2**.1704
characteristics, **B2**.1693 (Tab.), **B2**.1699–700, **B2**.1699 (Tab.)
culture, **B2**.1695
infection
endocarditis, **B1**.532
epiglottitis, **B1**.613
isolation/identification, **B2**.1700, **B2**.1701
biochemical tests, **B2**.1701–2
typing methods, **B2**.1704, **B2**.1705, **B2**.1705 (Tab.)
morphology, **B2**.1694, **B2**.1696
in normal microbiota, **B2**.1706, **B2**.1707
pathogenicity, **B2**.1708

Haemophilus paraphrohaemolyticus
characteristics, **B2**.1693 (Tab.), **B2**.1699 (Tab.), **B2**.1700
culture, **B2**.1695–6
infection, hemolysis, **B2**.1696–7
in normal microbiota, **B2**.1707
pathogenicity, **B2**.1708

Haemophilus paraphrophilus, **B2**.1693–4
antibacterial susceptibility/resistance, **B2**.1703
characteristics, **B2**.1693 (Tab.), **B2**.1699 (Tab.)
culture, **B2**.1695–6
infection, endocarditis, **B1**.532
morphology, **B2**.1696
in normal microbiota, **B2**.1707
pathogenicity, **B2**.1708

Haemophilus parasuis, **B2**.1694
  characteristics, **B2**.1693 (Tab.),
    B2.1699 (Tab.)
  culture, **B2**.1695
  morphology, **B2**.1694, **B2**.1696
  pathogenicity, **B2**.1708
  typing methods, **B2**.1706
Haemophilus pleuropneumoniae, **B2**.1694
  genetics, **B2**.1697
  reclassification, **B2**.1658–9
Haemophilus segnis, **B2**.1693–4
  characteristics, **B2**.1693 (Tab.),
    B2.1699 (Tab.)
  isolation/identification, **B2**.1701
  morphology, **B2**.1696
  in normal microbiota, **B2**.1706, **B2**.1707
  pathogenicity, **B2**.1708
Haemophilus somnus, **B2**.1694
Haemophilus suis, **B2**.1694
Haemosporida, **P**.464
Haemosporidians, classification, **P**.198
Hafnia, **B2**.1493–4
  antibacterial susceptibility/resistance,
    B2.1493
  antigens, **B2**.1493
  classification, **B2**.1493
  culture, **B2**.1493
  definition, **B2**.1493
  habitats, **B2**.1493–4
  identification
    biochemical tests, **B2**.1493
    screening tests, **B2**.1349 (Tab.)
  infection, intestinal, **B2**.1347
  morphology, **B2**.1493
  pathogenicity, **B2**.1493–4
Hafnia alvei, **B2**.1493
  antibacterial susceptibility/resistance,
    B2.1352 (Tab.)
  biochemical tests, **B2**.1319 (Tab.), **B2**.1493
  culture, **B2**.1344
  as normal microbiota, **B1**.296 (Tab.)
  pathogenicity, **B2**.1493–4
Hail, bacteriology of, **B1**.213
Hair
  dermatophytosis, **M**.221, **M**.238
  facial *see* Facial hair
  Pythium, **M**.416–17
  skin immunization, **I**.822, **I**.825
  specimens, **M**.83 (Tab.), **M**.84, **M**.235
Hair perforation test, **M**.237
'Hairpin resolution,' Minute virus of mice
  genome replication, **V1**.419
Hairpin termini, parvovirus replication, **V1**.150
'Hairpin transfer,' parvovirus replication,
  V1.419
Hairy cell leukemia, non-tuberculous
  mycobacteria infection, **B2**.1206
Halazone, **B1**.424
Haliscomenobacter hydrossis, **B1**.212
Halobacterium saccharovorum, **B1**.70
Halocarbons, as terminal electron acceptors,
  B1.67
Halofantrine, malaria therapy, **P**.506
Halogen-releasing agents, **B1**.423 (Tab.)
Halophiles
  food, **B1**.266

metabolism, **B1**.69–70
Hamburgers, contamination, **B1**.361
Hamer, W H, **B1**.336–7, **B1**.342–3
Hamer's model, **B1**.336–7, **B1**.342–3,
  B1.343 (Fig.)
Hamer–Soper model, **B1**.337, **B1**.343
Hamster polyomavirus (HaPyV), **V1**.473
Hand(s)
  decontamination, **B1**.378
  erosio interdigitalis, **M**.597
  mycetoma, **M**.386
  tinea manuum, **M**.232
  tinea nigra, **M**.198
Hand-foot-and-mouth disease (HFMD),
  V2.871–2
Handwashing
  disinfectants, **B1**.378
  healthcare staff, **B1**.377–8
  laboratory-acquired infection prevention,
    B1.766–7
  surgeons, **B1**.388
'Hanging groin,' onchocerciasis, **P**.793
Hanseniaspora, **B1**.283
Hanseniaspora valbyensis, **B1**.282
Hanseniospora, **M**.631, **M**.631 (Tab.)
Hanseniospora guilliermondii, **M**.631,
  M.632 (Tab.)
Hanseniospora uvarum, **M**.631, **M**.632 (Tab.)
Hanseniospora valbyensis, **M**.631, **M**.632 (Tab.)
Hansen's disease *see* Leprosy
Hansenula
  characteristics, **M**.631, **M**.631 (Tab.)
  infection, **M**.625 (Tab.), **M**.626
Hansenula anomala
  characteristics, **M**.631, **M**.631 (Tab.)
  infection, **M**.626
    amphotericin B therapy, **M**.626
    fungemia, **M**.626
Hansenula polymorpha, **M**.626
  characteristics, **M**.631, **M**.631 (Tab.)
Hantaan virus, **V2**.1025, **V2**.1666 (Tab.)
  biosafety level 3 classification, **V2**.1526
  emerging infection, **V2**.1648 (Tab.)
    identification, **V2**.1663–4
  epidemiology, **V2**.1049
  genome structure, **V2**.1031 (Tab.)
  laboratory-acquired infection, **V2**.1517 (Tab.)
  transcription, **V2**.1035
  transmission, **V1**.371 (Tab.)
  vaccines, **I**.933 (Tab.)
Hantavirus, **V2**.1025
  characteristics, **V1**.129 (Tab.)
  classification, **V1**.50, **V2**.1026
    biosafety level 3, **V2**.1526
  genome structure
    consensus sequences, **V2**.1031 (Tab.)
    gene organization, **V2**.1033 (Fig.)
    Golgi transport, **V2**.1039–40
    members, **V2**.1029 (Tab.)
Hantaviruses, **V2**.1666 (Tab.)
  genome structure, **V2**.1031–3
    M (medium) segment, **V2**.1031–3
    S (small) segment, **V2**.1031–3
    geographical distribution, **V2**.1665 (Fig.)
    glycoproteins, **V2**.1031–3

infection *see* Hantavirus infection
prime-and-realign transcription, **V2**.1035–6
rodent hosts, **V2**.1044 (Fig.), **V2**.1049
transmission, **V1**.371–2, **V1**.371 (Tab.)
Hantavirus infection
  clinical manifestations, **V2**.1043–5
  emerging infection, **V2**.1648 (Tab.),
    V2.1663–4
  immune response, **V2**.1041
  serological diagnosis, **V2**.1547
  see also specific diseases/infection
Hantavirus pulmonary syndrome, **V2**.1043–5
  animal models, **V2**.1042
  emerging infection, **V2**.1646–7
  pathogenesis, **V2**.1050
  transmission, **V1**.371 (Tab.)
H antigens
  agglutination tests, **B1**.748
  deficiency, **I**.769
  Enterobacteriaceae, **B2**.1339–40, **B2**.1342
  Escherichia coli, **B2**.1365
  Salmonella see Salmonella
  Salmonella Paratyphi A, **B2**.1404
  Salmonella Typhi, **B1**.744, **B2**.1404–5
  Salmonella Typhimurium, **B2**.1404
Hanzalova virus, **V2**.998 (Tab.)
Haplorchis, **P**.584
Haplosporangium parvum, **M**.26, **M**.811
Haplotype relative risk (HRR),
  immunogenetics, **I**.574
Haptens, **B1**.12
Haptoglobin, **B1**.151, **I**.202–3
  IL-6 effects, **I**.285
Haptoglobin-related protein (hpr),
  trypanosomes, effect on, **P**.352–3
'Hard pad,' **V1**.811–12
Hartmannella, **P**.226
Harvesting, airborne bacteria, **B1**.186 (Tab.)
Hashimoto's thyroiditis, **I**.748 (Tab.)
Haverhill fever, **B2**.1909, **B2**.1910, **B2**.1911
Hawke's group GA7752 *see Edwardsiella
  ictaluri*
Hawkey, McCormick and Simpson medium,
  B2.1436
Hayes, W, **B1**.13
Hazard analysis critical control point
  (HACCP), **B1**.288–9
Hazard groups, microbiological risk
  assessment, **V2**.1520
Hazelnuts, *Clostridium botulinum,* **B1**.287
HBeAg *see* Hepatitis B virus (HBV)
HBsAg *see* Hepatitis B virus (HBV)
HBx protein
  Ground squirrel hepatitis virus, **V2**.1242
  Hepatitis B *see* Hepatitis B virus (HBV)
  Woodchuck Hepatitis B virus, **V2**.1242
HCAP-18
  expression, **I**.174
  genes, **I**.175
  LL37 subunit, **I**.174, **I**.175
    inhibition by bacteria, **I**.175
    LPS binding, **I**.174
    NK cell production by, **I**.175
    T cell production by, **I**.175
  spermatozoa, **I**.175
  structure, **I**.174

HCAP-18 (*Continued*)
  synthesis/storage, **I**.174
HCC-1 (CCL14), **I**.218 (Tab.)
HCC-2 (CCL15), **I**.218 (Tab.)
HCC-4 (CCL16), **I**.218 (Tab.)
HCMV *see* Human cytomegalovirus (HCMV)
hDLG, papillomavirus E6 protein binding,
  V1.460 (Tab.)
Headache, griseofulvin, **M**.184
Head and neck infection, *Eikenella corrodens*,
  B2.1667
Heaf test, **B1**.746
Health and Safety at Work Act (1974),
  V2.1515
Health and Safety Executive (UK), infectious
  material transport, **V2**.1528
Healthcare associated infection *see*
  Nosocomial infection
Healthcare workers
  handwashing, **B1**.766–7
  nosocomial infection spread by, **B1**.377–8
  resident and transient microorganisms on,
    B1.377–8
  varicella vaccines/vaccination, **V2**.1575
  viral infection transmitted by, **B1**.382
  viral infection transmitted to, **B1**.382
Health education
  amebiasis control, **P**.214–15
  cystic echinococcosis control, **P**.701–2
  cysticercosis control, **P**.700–1
  dracunculiasis eradication, **P**.833–4
  liver fluke control, **P**.653–4
  lung fluke control, **P**.653–4
  lymphatic filariasis control, **P**.123
  parasite control, **P**.115
Health Protection Agency (HPA), **B1**.318
Health services, planning/costing, **B1**.323
Health system components, parasite control,
  P.111 (Tab.)
Heart
  aspergillosis, **M**.700, **M**.705
  Pneumocystis carinii infection, **M**.785
Heart disease
  congenitally acquired rubella, **V2**.974
  C-reactive protein, **I**.200, **I**.206
Heart murmur, infective endocarditis,
  B1.534–5
Heart surgery, infection after, **B1**.385
  Nocardia farcinica, **B2**.1162
Heart transplants
  aspergillosis, **M**.704–5
  infection after
    Nocardia asteroides, **B2**.1156
    Nocardia nova, **B2**.1162–3
    Malassezia folliculitis, **M**.213
Heart valves
  histoplasmosis capsulati, **M**.535
  prosthetic, infection, **B1**.392
Heat
  Brucella susceptibility/resistance, **B2**.1733
  dry, **B1**.445 (Tab.), **B1**.446 (Tab.),
    B1.448 (Tab.), **B1**.449, **B1**.454 (Tab.)
  food preservation, **B1**.268 (Tab.), **B1**.270–1
    aseptic packaging, **B1**.271
      heat sterilization in hermetically sealed
        containers, **B1**.270–1

  see also Canned products
  microbial growth effect, **B1**.265–6,
    B1.265 (Fig.)
  pasteurization, **B1**.271
  survivor curve, **B1**.265–6, **B1**.265 (Fig.)
  moist *see* Moist heat
Heating, ventilation, and air-conditioning
  (HVAC), airborne bacteria,
  B1.186 (Tab.)
Heat labile enterotoxin (LT) *see Escherichia
  coli* heat labile enterotoxin (LT)
Heat sensing mechanisms, **B1**.448
Heat shock protein(s) (HSPs), **B1**.74, **B1**.448
  Aspergillus, **M**.106, **M**.107, **M**.694
  Candida, **M**.100, **M**.102–3, **M**.591, **M**.594,
    M.607
  Candida albicans, **M**.101, **M**.102–3
  Candida parapsilosis, **M**.101, **M**.102–3
  Histoplasma capsulatum, **M**.112, **M**.529
  Neisseria, **B2**.1285
  Paracoccidioides brasiliensis, **M**.114, **M**.542
  rapidly growing mycobacteria, **B2**.1244,
    B2.1245 (Fig.)
  systemic γδ T cell recognition, **I**.439–40
  TLRs 4 binding, **I**.926
  viral infection, **V1**.228–9
Heat shock protein-10 (HSP-10), **I**.626
Heat shock protein-60 (HSP-60), **I**.626
Heat shock protein-70 (HSP-70), **I**.626
Heat shock response, **B1**.74
Heat sterilization, **B1**.270–1
Heat stress proteins, *Taenia solium*, **P**.682–3
Heat therapy, sporotrichosis, **M**.379
Heavy chains *see* Immunoglobulin structure
Heavy metal derivatives, **B1**.423 (Tab.), **B1**.428
  action, **B1**.437 (Tab.), **B1**.438
  resistance, **B1**.442
Hedaquinium chloride, **B1**.428
HEF protein *see* Influenza virus C
HeLa cells, contamination of cell lines,
  V1.88–9
Helcococcus kunzii, **B1**.296 (Tab.)
Helical viruses, morphology/structure *see*
  Morphology, viruses
Helicase primase, antiviral target, **V2**.1617–18
Helicases
  arteriviruses, **V1**.834
  DNA virus replication, **V1**.149
  Hepatitis C virus NS3 protein, **V2**.1197
  papillomavirus replication, **V1**.156–7
  poxviruses, **V1**.598–600
Helicobacter, **B2**.**1563–90**
  biochemistry, **B2**.1566 (Tab.), **B2**.1567
  cell walls/antigens, **B2**.1568–9
    Lewis antigen mimicry, **B2**.1569
    lipid A, **B2**.1569
    LPS, **B2**.1568–9
    outer membrane proteins, **B2**.1569
  characteristics, **B2**.1563
  classification, **B2**.1563–4
    phylogenetic analysis, **B2**.1564
  culture, **B2**.1566 (Tab.), **B2**.1567
    microaerobic conditions, **B2**.1567
  genomics, **B2**.1567–8
    general features, **B2**.1568 (Tab.)
    gene sequence, **B2**.1567–8

    plasmids, **B2**.1567–8
    recA gene, **B2**.1567–8
    vacuolating cytotoxin gene, **B2**.1567–8
  habitats, **B2**.1564–6
    gastric/intestinal mucosa, **B2**.1564
  historical perspective, **B2**.1563–4
  infection, **B2**.1564
  metabolism, **B2**.1567
  morphology, **B2**.1567
  as normal microbiota, **B1**.296 (Tab.)
  pathogenicity, **B2**.1576–8
    adhesins, **B2**.1577–8
    CagA pathogenicity island, **B2**.1577
    catalase, **B2**.1576
    flagella, **B2**.1576
    Lewis antigens, **B2**.1577–8
    superoxide dismutase, **B2**.1576
    urease, **B2**.1576
    vasculating cytotoxin, **B2**.1577
  species, **B2**.1564, **B2**.1565 (Tab.), **B2**.1581–4
  typing, **B2**.1569–70
    genotyping, **B2**.1570
    multilocus sequence typing, **B2**.1570
    phenotyping, **B2**.1570
Helicobacter acinonychis, **B2**.1581
Helicobacter aurati, **B2**.1582, **B2**.1583
Helicobacter bilis, **B2**.1582, **B2**.1583
  infection, **B2**.1565–6
Helicobacter bizzozeroni, **B2**.1565 (Tab.),
  B2.1581
  morphology, **B2**.1566–7
Helicobacter canadensis, **B2**.1565 (Tab.),
  B2.1582
  characteristics, **B2**.1566 (Tab.)
  infection, **B2**.1564
Helicobacter canis, **B2**.1565 (Tab.), **B2**.1583
  biochemistry, **B2**.1567
  characteristics, **B2**.1566 (Tab.)
  infection, **B2**.1565–6
Helicobacter cholecystus, **B2**.1583
  infection, **B2**.1565–6
Helicobacter cinaedi, **B2**.1563, **B2**.1565 (Tab.),
  B2.1582–3
  characteristics, **B2**.1566 (Tab.)
  culture, **B2**.1572
  infection, **B2**.1564, **B2**.1565–6
Helicobacter felis, **B2**.1565 (Tab.), **B2**.1581
  biochemistry, **B2**.1567
  infection, **B2**.1564–5
  morphology, **B2**.1566–7
Helicobacter fennelliae, **B2**.1565 (Tab.),
  B2.1582–3
  characteristics, **B2**.1566 (Tab.)
  culture, **B2**.1572
  infection, **B2**.1564
Helicobacter ganmani, **B2**.1565 (Tab.), **B2**.1583
Helicobacter heilmannii, **B2**.1565 (Tab.),
  B2.1581
  classification, **B2**.1564
  infection, **B2**.1564
Helicobacter hepaticus, **B2**.1563,
  B2.1565 (Tab.), **B2**.1583
  characteristics, **B2**.1566 (Tab.)
  genomics, **B2**.1568 (Tab.)
  gene sequence, **B2**.1568

Helicobacter hepaticus, (*Continued*)
infection, **B2**.1565–6
regulatory T cells, **I**.666–7
Helicobacter marmotae, **B2**.1565 (Tab.),
B2.1583
Helicobacter mesocricetorum, **B2**.1583
Helicobacter muricola, **B2**.1565 (Tab.), **B2**.1583
Helicobacter muridarum, **B2**.1583
Helicobacter mustelae, **B2**.1565 (Tab.), **B2**.1581
biochemistry, **B2**.1567
Helicobacter nemestrinae, **B2**.1581
Helicobacter pametensis, **B2**.1565 (Tab.),
B2.1584
Helicobacter pullorum, **B2**.1565 (Tab.),
B2.1584
characteristics, **B2**.1566 (Tab.)
culture, **B2**.1572
gastric mucosa, **B2**.1564–5
infection, **B2**.1564, **B2**.1565–6
Helicobacter pylori, **B2**.1563, **B2**.1565 (Tab.),
B2.1582
antibacterial susceptibility/resistance,
B2.1575–6
metronidazole, **B1**.495
quinolone resistance, **B1**.493 (Tab.)
biochemistry, **B2**.1567
characteristics, **B2**.1566 (Tab.)
culture, **B2**.1570–2, **B2**.1571 (Tab.)
microaerobic conditions, **B2**.1567
selective media, **B2**.1572
specimen transport, **B2**.1571–2
genomics, **B2**.1568 (Tab.)
historical aspects, **B2**.1563–4
immune evasion
B-cell-attracting chemokine
(BCA-1:CXCL13), **I**.230
complement cleavage, **I**.663–4
Fas-mediated apoptosis, **I**.656
IL-10 induction, **I**.654
immunosuppression, **I**.665
LPS variation, **I**.661
MHC class II antigen presentation, **I**.657–8
phagocytic uptake inhibition, **I**.649
regulatory T cells, **I**.666
immunogenetics, **I**.594
infection *see Helicobacter pylori* infection
morphology, **B2**.1566 (Fig.)
as normal microbiota, **B1**.296 (Tab.), **B1**.302
signal transduction, **B1**.167–8
transmission, by endoscopes, **B1**.380
VacA toxin, **I**.657–8
virulence factors, evolution within host,
B1.173–4
Helicobacter pylori infection
clinical consequences, **B2**.1579–81
acute gastritis, **B2**.1578, **B2**.1579
chronic gastritis, **B1**.365, **B2**.1564–5,
B2.1578, **B2**.1579
epidemic hypochlorrhydia, **B2**.1579
extragastric disease, **B2**.1581
gastric malignancy, **B2**.1580
gastric ulceration, **B2**.1580
gastroesophageal reflux disease, **B2**.1580–1
nonulcer dyspepsia, **B2**.1580
peptic ulceration, **B1**.365, **B2**.1580
polymorphonuclear infiltrates, **B2**.1564–5

diagnosis, **B2**.1570–4, **B2**.1571 (Tab.)
culture, **B2**.1570–2, **B2**.1571 (Tab.)
gastric biopsy, **B2**.1571 (Tab.)
histology, **B2**.1571, **B2**.1571 (Tab.)
molecular tests, **B2**.1574
office-based tests, **B2**.1574
rapid urease test, **B2**.1571 (Tab.), **B2**.1572
salivary antibody assays, **B2**.1574
serology, **B2**.1571 (Tab.), **B2**.1573
stool antigen test, **B2**.1571 (Tab.), **B2**.1573
string test, **B2**.1574
urea breath test, **B2**.1571 (Tab.), **B2**.1572–3
urine antibody assays, **B2**.1574
epidemiology, **B2**.1578–9
fecal–oral transmission, **B2**.1578–9
interfamilial spread, **B2**.1578–9
prevalence, **B2**.1578
transmission, **B2**.1578–9
waterborne transmission, **B2**.1579
as zoonosis, **B2**.1578
morphology, **B2**.1567 (Fig.)
mucosal immune response, **I**.522–3
prevention, **B2**.1576
vaccination *see below*
treatment, **B2**.1574–6
first-line therapy, **B2**.1574–5
patient selection, **B2**.1574
second-line therapy, **B2**.1575
vaccines/vaccination, **B2**.1576
cholera enterotoxin adjuvants, **I**.932
development status, **I**.933 (Tab.)
LT adjuvants, **I**.932
Salmonella vectors, **I**.843, **I**.847
Helicobacter rappini, **B2**.1584
Helicobacter rodentium, **B2**.1565 (Tab.),
B2.1584
Helicobacter salomonis, **B2**.1582
morphology, **B2**.1566–7
Helicobacter suncus, **B2**.1565 (Tab.), **B2**.1582
Helicobacter trogontum, **B2**.1583, **B2**.1584
Helicobacter typhlonius, **B2**.1565 (Tab.),
B2.1584
Helicobacter winghamensis, **B2**.1565 (Tab.),
B2.1584
biochemistry, **B2**.1567
characteristics, **B2**.1566 (Tab.)
infection, **B2**.1564
Heller–Vasconcelos procedure, **P**.393
Helmgmosomoides polygrias infection, **I**.70
Helminth(s)
classification, **P.573–99**
enzymes, **P**.88
groups, **P**.574
historical aspects, **P**.5–13
hosts
final (definitive), **P**.573
intermediate, **P**.573
paratenic, **P**.573
identification/morphometric analysis, **P**.574
fixation, **P**.574
histology, **P**.574
mounting, **P**.574
immune evasion, **I**.683–7
antibody blocking, **I**.685–6
antibody class switching, **I**.686

avoidance strategies, **I**.684–5
complement blocking, **I**.685–6
cystatin, **I**.687
cytokine homologues, **I**.687
effector cell inhibition, **I**.686
lymphocyte inhibition, **I**.687
phosphorylcholine secretion, **I**.687
reactive oxygen species defenses, **I**.686
infection *see* Helminth infection
life cycle, **P**.573
nomenclature, **P**.573
see also individual species
Helminth infection, **I**.682–3
animal models, **P**.88–9
chronic infection, **I**.683
concomitant immunity, **I**.683
control, **P**.90
epidemiology, **P**.89
history, **P.5–13**, **P**.4–5
immune response, **P**.90
antibody-dependent cell-mediated
cytotoxicity, **I**.683
antigens, **P**.88
characteristics affecting, **P**.87–9
eosinophils *see* Eosinophil(s)
IL-4, **I**.68, **I**.600
IL-5, **I**.70, **I**.600
IL-9, **I**.282, **I**.600
IL-13, **I**.600
larval stages, **P**.88
Th2 response, **I**.683, **I**.684
T helper cell polarization, **P**.72–3
worm burden, **P**.87–8
longevity, **I**.683
see also specific infection
Helper T cells *see* T-helper cell(s)
Helper viruses, adeno-associated virus
replication, **V1**.160
Helpin *see* Brivudin
Hemadsorption
cell culture, **V2**.1540
Mumps virus, **V1**.747–8
serotyping, **V2**.1542
Hemagglutination inhibition (HI), **V2**.1545
influenza diagnosis, **V1**.675, **V1**.676 (Fig.)
measles diagnosis, **V1**.732
serotyping, **V2**.1542
Hemagglutination tests
glanders diagnosis, **B2**.1634
Helicobacter typing, **B2**.1570
influenza neuraminidase (NA), **V1**.656
Measles virus, **V1**.715
Mumps virus, **V1**.747–8
paramyxoviruses, **V1**.700
rhinovirus infection, **V2**.878
syphilis detection, **B1**.663, **B2**.1848
Hemagglutinin (HA)
conformational change in cell entry,
V1.107–8
Enterococcus, **B2**.897
influenza viruses *see* Influenza viruses
Measles virus *see* Measles virus
processing, **V1**.121
Rubella virus antigens, **V2**.967
structure, **V1**.106, **V1**.107 (Fig.)

Hemagglutinin (HA) (*Continued*)
  virosome vaccines, **I**.838
Hemagglutinin–esterase (HE)
  Bovine coronavirus, **V1**.838–9
  Bovine torovirus, **V1**.838–9
  coronaviruses, **V1**.827, **V1**.836 (Tab.),
    V1.838–9
  Human coronavirus, **V1**.838–9
  Influenza virus C *see* Influenza virus C
  Murine hepatitis virus, **V1**.838–9
  Porcine hemagglutinating encephalomyelitis
    virus, **V1**.838–9
  toroviruses, **V1**.827, **V1**.836 (Tab.), **V1**.838–9
  Turkey coronavirus, **V1**.838–9
Hemagglutinin-neuraminidase (HN)
  Bovine parainfluenza virus 3, **V1**.766
  Human parainfluenzavirus 3, **V1**.766
  Mumps virus *see* Mumps virus
  parainfluenza viruses *see* Parainfluenza
    viruses
  paramyxoviruses *see* Paramyxoviruses
  respiroviruses *see* Respiroviruses
  Sendai virus, **V1**.766
Hemagglutinin noose epitope (HNE), **I**.868–9
Hematocrit centrifugation test, African
  trypanosomiasis diagnosis, **P**.366–7
Hematocrit, Lassa fever, **V2**.1070
Hematogenous route of virus entry to CNS,
  V2.1404–5
Hematopoiesis, **I**.504–5
  acute phase response *see* Acute phase
    response
  APCs, **I**.112, **I**.113 (Fig.)
  dendritic cells, **I**.113, **I**.113 (Fig.)
  Langerhans' cells, **I**.113, **I**.113 (Fig.)
  macrophages, **I**.113 (Fig.)
  monocytes, **I**.113 (Fig.)
  SCF effects, **I**.275 (Tab.)
Hematopoietic stem cells, retrovirus gene
  therapy vectors, **V2**.1592
Hematoxylin and eosin (H&E) stain,
  M.123 (Tab.), **M**.132, **M**.676
  Gomori's methenamine silver stain
    combination, **M**.123 (Tab.), **M**.124,
    M.351–2, **M**.491
  Helicobacter pylori identification, **B2**.1571
  identification, **M**.122, **M**.123 (Tab.), **M**.125
    Basidiobolus, **M**.351–2, **M**.351 (Fig.)
    Blastomyces dermatitidis, **M**.491
    Coccidioides immitis, **M**.513, **M**.516
    Histoplasma capsulatum, **M**.533–4
    limitations, **M**.123 (Tab.)
Hematuria, schistosomiasis, **P**.612–13
Heme oxygenase, acute phase response,
  I.205–6
Heme-scavenging systems, iron sequestering,
  B1.151
Hemianopia, homonymous, **V2**.1417
Hemiascomyetes, **M**.54, **M**.55 (Tab.),
  M.62 (Fig.)
Hemocin, **B2**.1706
Hemocytometer counts, antifungal
  susceptibility testing, **M**.156
Hemodialysis, infection, rapidly growing
  mycobacteria, **B2**.1247, **B2**.1258–9

Hemoglobin
  digestion, *Plasmodium* nutrition, **P**.466,
    P.468, **P**.475
  Neisseria utilizing, **B2**.1284–5
Hemoglobin E persistence, malaria resistance,
  P.478
Hemoglobinopathies
  innate malaria resistance, **P**.485
  pythiosis, **M**.420–2
Hemoglobin S, malaria association, **I**.598
Hemoglobinuria
  babesiosis, **P**.454–5
  falciparum malaria, **P**.482
Hemolysin(s), **I**.654–5
  Burkholderia cepacia complex, **B2**.1615
  Burkholderia thailandensis, **B2**.1624
  Enterococcus, **B2**.894–6
  Escherichia coli protein secretion, **B1**.48
  functions, **B1**.153 (Tab.)
  Proteus, **B2**.1446, **B2**.1447
  Pseudomonas aeruginosa, **B2**.1600, **B2**.1601
β-Hemolysin, *Aeromonas* pathogenicity,
  B2.1535–6
Hemolysis, babesiosis, **P**.456, **P**.459–60
α-Hemolytic species, *Enterococcus*, **B2**.885–6
β-Hemolytic species, *Enterococcus*, **B2**.885–6,
  B2.890–1
Hemolytic–uremic syndrome (HUS), **I**.154,
  B1.273–4
  causative organisms
    Citrobacter freundii, **B1**.250
    Enterobacteriaceae, **B2**.1347
    Escherichia coli, **B1**.241–2, **B1**.249–50,
      B1.255–6, **B2**.1374–5, **B2**.1377
    Shigella dysenteriae serotype 1, **B2**.1387
  emerging bacterial infection, **B1**.360
  outbreaks associated with fast-food, **B1**.361
Hemopexin, **B1**.151, **I**.203
Hemophagocytic syndrome (HPS), **I**.778–9
Hemophilia A, gene therapy, **V2**.1600
Hemophilia, Hepatitis A virus transmission,
  V2.1172–3
Hemopoietic growth factors, **I**.274 (Tab.)
Hemoptysis
  aspergilloma, **M**.696
  histoplasmosis capsulati, **M**.524–5
  paragonimiasis, **P**.649
Hemorrhages *see* Bleeding
Hemorrhagic colitis, case-control study,
  B1.315–16
Hemorrhagic cystitis, BK virus, **V1**.481
Hemorrhagic fevers, **B1**.400
  arenavirus, **V2**.1070
  Argentine, **V2**.1070
  Bolivian, **V2**.1070
  chikungunya, **V2**.1022
  filovirus infection, **V2**.1094
  Venezuelan, **V2**.1070
  see also specific infection
Hemorrhagic fever with renal syndrome
  (HFRS), **V2**.1043
  causative pathogens, **V2**.1045
  emerging infection, **V2**.1663–4
  hypotensive phase, **V2**.1044
  mortality, **V2**.1044
  pathogenesis, **V2**.1050

  treatment, **V2**.1044–5
Hemorrhagic nephritis, BK virus, **V1**.481
Hemorrhagic proctosigmoiditis, *Blastocystis
  hominis* infection, **P**.564
Hemostasis, defect in arenavirus infection,
  V2.1070
Hendersonula toruloidea, **M**.11, **M**.246–7
Hendra virus, **V1**.816
  classification, **V1**.48–9
  C protein, **V1**.816
  emerging infection, **V2**.1648 (Tab.),
    V2.1651 (Tab.)
    species-barrier crossing, **V2**.1657 (Tab.),
      V2.1658
  genome, **V1**.816
  human infection, **V1**.817–18
    clinical features, **V1**.817
    pathogenesis, **V1**.818
  large (L) protein, **V1**.816
  phosphoprotein (P), **V1**.816
    RNA editing, **V1**.816
  transmission, **V1**.817
  type species, **V1**.816
  V protein, **V1**.816
  W protein, **V1**.816
Henipavirus
  characteristics, **V1**.129 (Tab.), **V1**.702 (Tab.)
  classification, **V1**.48–9, **V1**.382, **V1**.700 (Tab.),
    V1.808 (Fig.)
  genome structure/organization,
    V1.387 (Tab.), **V1**.701 (Fig.)
  members, **V1**.382–3
  phylogeny, **V1**.388
  type species *see* Hendra virus
  see also Henipaviruses
Henipaviruses, **V1**.816–18
  attachment (G) protein, **V1**.706
  C protein, **V1**.816
  epidemiology, **V1**.817
  fusion (F) protein, **V1**.705
  genomes, **V1**.816
  infection *see* Henipavirus infection
  large (L) protein, **V1**.816
  phosphoprotein (P), **V1**.816
    RNA editing, **V1**.816
  P protein, **V1**.704
  V protein, **V1**.816
  W protein, **V1**.816
Henipavirus infection
  clinical manifestations, **V1**.817–18
  control, **V1**.818
  laboratory diagnosis, **V1**.818
  pathology, **V1**.817–18
  transmission, **V1**.817
  see also Henipavirus
Hepacivirus
  characteristics, **V1**.177 (Tab.)
  classification, **V1**.53–4, **V2**.993
  mRNA translation, **V1**.113
  protein synthesis, **V1**.115–16
Hepadnaviridae
  characteristics, **V1**.177 (Tab.)
  classification, **V1**.27 (Tab.), **V1**.46–7,
    V1.46 (Tab.)
  definition of, **V2**.1227
  see also Hepadnaviruses; *specific viruses*

Hepadnaviruses, **B1**.435–6
  BCE peptide vaccines, **I**.872
  cell interactions, **V1**.219
    DNA maintenance, **V1**.219
  evolution, **V1**.13
  gene expression, **V1**.111–12
  IFN activity, **I**.260 (Tab.)
  infectivity, **V1**.45–6
  origins, **V1**.12
  reverse transcription, **V1**.181–2
  tumors associated, **V1**.332 (Tab.)
  see also Hepadnaviridae
HEPA filters, biosafety level 3 laboratories,
    V2.1526
Heparan sulfate
  adeno-associated virus binding, **V1**.416–17
  alphavirus E2 glycoprotein, **V2**.1015
  herpesviruses binding, **V1**.106–7
  HSV association, **V1**.502
  Human parainfluenzavirus 3 receptor,
    V1.765–6
  viral receptor, **V1**.209
Heparan sulfate protein glycoprotein (HSPG),
    Plasmodium hepatocyte invasion,
    P.472–3
Hepatic candidiasis, **M**.595, **M**.596 (Fig.),
    M.599–600
Hepatic cirrhosis, schistosomiasis japonicum,
    P.631 (Fig.)
Hepatic fibrosis, schistosomiasis, **P**.612–13,
    P.630 (Fig.)
Hepatic invasive aspergillosis, **M**.701, **M**.705
Hepatic steatosis, hepatitis C, **V2**.1204
Hepatitis
  in AIDS/HIV infection, HCMV infection,
    V2.1505
  antiviral therapy, **V2**.1629–30
    nucleoside analogue prodrugs, **V2**.1629
    nucleotide analogues, **V2**.1629
    resistance, **V2**.1637
  enterically transmitted, **V2**.1160
  enterovirus infection, **V2**.872
  fetal infection, **V2**.1474–82
  fulminant
    hepatitis A, **V2**.1171–2
    hepatitis E, **V2**.1179
  HSV infection
    immunodeficient patients (non-HIV),
      V2.1506
    in pregnancy, **V2**.1463
  mollusks, **B1**.280
  mortality, **P**.29 (Tab.)
  non-A, non-B (NANB), **V2**.1160
  parvovirus infection, **V1**.426
  Q fever, **B2**.2076
  therapy
    IFN-α, **I**.259
    type I INFs, **I**.259
  vaccines
    virosome vaccines, **I**.839
    virus-like particles, **I**.840
Hepatitis viruses
  cytokines, **V1**.303
  isolation/propagation and identification,
    V1.96 (Tab.), **V1**.98
  see also specific viruses

Hepatitis A, **V2**.1169–75, **V2**.1474
  antibodies, **B1**.353 (Fig.)
  cholestatic, **V2**.1172
  clinical features, **V2**.1171–2
  control, **V2**.1474
  control, by hygiene, **B1**.353
  course of infection, **V2**.1064 (Fig.),
    V2.1169–72
    virological/pathological events,
      V2.1064 (Fig.), **V2**.1170
  diagnosis, **V2**.1172
    immunoassays, **V2**.1171
  emerging infection , agricultural practices,
    V2.1660–1
  endemic disease, **B1**.353
  epidemiology, **V1**.369, **V2**.1172–3
    age-relation, **V1**.356–7
    developed countries, **V2**.1173
    fetal infection, **V2**.1475 (Tab.)
    neonatal infection, **V2**.1444 (Tab.),
      V2.1474, **V2**.1475 (Tab.)
    in pregnancy, **V2**.1444 (Tab.),
      V2.1475 (Tab.)
    seasonal outbreaks, **V1**.358
    severity and age relationship, **V2**.1171–2
  fulminant, **V2**.1171–2
  hepatitis B coinfection, **V2**.1248
  histopathology, **V2**.1170
  immune response
    cell-mediated, **V2**.1170–1
    humoral, **V2**.1171
    IL-6, **V1**.303
  mollusks, **B1**.280
  pathogenesis, **V2**.1169–70
  prevalence, **V2**.1173
  prevention, **V2**.1173–5
    human Ig, **V2**.1173–4, **V2**.1567–8,
      V2.1567 (Tab.)
    postexposure, **V2**.1173–4
    vaccines *see below*
  relapsing, **V2**.1172
  vaccines/vaccination, **B1**.353, **V2**.1174–5,
    V2.1552 (Tab.), **V2**.1575–6
    adverse effects, **V2**.1576
    attenuated, **V2**.1174, **V2**.1575–6
    BCE peptide vaccines, **I**.855 (Tab.), **I**.870
    candidate strains, **V2**.1169, **V2**.1174
    development status, **I**.933 (Tab.)
    history, **V1**.8 (Tab.), **V2**.1575–6
    inactivated whole virus, **V2**.1174, **V2**.1576
    recombinant, **V2**.1174–5
    recommendations, **V2**.1576
    USA schedules, **V2**.1560 (Fig.)
    virosomes, **I**.839, **I**.929
  viremia, **V2**.1169–71
Hepatitis A virus (HAV), **V2**.1160, **V2**.1161–
74
  antigenic structure, **V2**.1165–6
    epitopes, **V2**.1166
    monotonicity, **V2**.1166
  antiviral agents, **B1**.434, **B1**.440
  capsid structure, **V2**.1165
  cell cultures, **V2**.1166–7, **V2**.1170
    adaptations and genetic changes for,
      V2.1169

  classification, **V2**.1161, **V2**.1162 (Tab.)
    biosafety level 2, **V2**.1525
    phylogenetic relationships, **V2**.1064 (Fig.),
      V2.1164–5
  cytopathic effect absent, **V2**.1166–7
  detection, **V2**.1160
  epidemiology, Europe, **V1**.250 (Fig.),
    V2.1173
  genetic variation
    cell culture-adapted viruses, **V2**.1169
    between strains, **V2**.1164–5
  genome organization, **V2**.1161–5,
    V2.1163 (Fig.)
    3' non-translated RNA (NTR), **V2**.1163–4
    5' non-translated RNA (NTR), **V2**.1161–3,
      V2.1163 (Fig.)
    internal ribosomal entry site (IRES),
      V2.1163, **V2**.1167
    long open reading frame, **V2**.1161,
      V2.1163
    P1/P2/P3 segments, **V2**.1163
    pyrimidine-rich tract (pY1), **V2**.1161–3
  Hepatitis E virus *vs.*, **V2**.1160–1,
    V2.1161 (Tab.)
  historical aspects, **V2**.1160
  host cell effects, **V2**.869
  'mimotope', **V2**.1166
  molecular detection, **B1**.723 (Tab.)
    quantification, **B1**.722–4
  monoclonal antibodies, **V2**.1165–6
  morphology/structure, **V2**.1161,
    V2.1162 (Fig.)
    absence of envelope, **V2**.1160–1
  mutations
    5'NTR deletion in vaccine strain, **V2**.1174
    for cell culture, **V2**.1169
    neutralization-resistant, **V2**.1166
  non-structural proteins, **V2**.1167–8
    2B and 2C proteins, **V2**.1167, **V2**.1168
    3A and 3B proteins, **V2**.1167, **V2**.1168
    3C^{pro} protein (protease), **V2**.1168
    3D^{pol} (RNA polymerase), **V2**.1168
    functions, **V2**.1167–8
    VP1–2A protein, **V2**.1165, **V2**.1167–8
  polyproteins, **V2**.1163
  see also specific types
  properties, **V2**.1161 (Tab.)
  replication, **V2**.1167
    attachment and penetration, **V2**.1166
    cap-independent translation, **V2**.1163,
      V2.1167
    cell receptor, **V2**.1167
    in cultured cells, **V2**.1166–7
    early events, **V2**.1166
    non-structural protein functions,
      V2.1167–8
    sites, **V2**.1168
  shedding, **V2**.1170, **V2**.1171
  structural (capsid) polypeptides, **V2**.1165
    IA (VP4), **V2**.1165
    IAB (VP0), **V2**.1165
    ID, **V2**.1165, **V2**.1166
    open reading frame encoding, **V2**.1165
    proteolytic cleavage, **V2**.1165
  T-helper cell epitope, **I**.862 (Tab.)
  translation, **V2**.1163

Hepatitis A virus (HAV) (*Continued*)
  transmission, **V1**.239, **V2**.1169–70, **V2**.1172–3
    fecal-oral, **V2**.1160–1, **V2**.1172
    food- and water-borne, **V2**.1172
    parenteral, **V2**.1172–3
  vaccine *see* Hepatitis A
  variants
    GBM strain, **V2**.1169
    genotypes, **V2**.1164
    HM175 strain, **V2**.1169
    simian strains, **V2**.1164, **V2**.1165
  VP1 protein, **I**.870
Hepatitis B, **V2**.1474–8, **V2.1226–68**
  acute, **V2**.1246–8
    alanine aminotransferase (ALT), **V2**.1246, **V2**.1251
    asymptomatic, **V2**.1245–6
    coinfection, **V2**.1248
    diagnosis, **V2**.1246, **V2**.1251
    duration, **V1**.258
    fulminant, **V2**.1248
    HBsAg, **V2**.1246
    occult infection, **V2**.1247–8
    persistence, **V2**.1246–7
    recovery, **V2**.1246–7
    serological markers, **V2**.1247 (Fig.)
    subclinical course, **V2**.1247–8
    viremia, **V2**.1247
  animal models, **V2**.1233
  antiviral therapy, **V2**.1260–1, **V2**.1629–30
    adefovir, **V2**.1629
    cidofovir, **V2**.1616
    fialuridine, **V2**.1629
    lamivudine, **V2**.1629
    penciclovir, **V2**.1614
    ribavirin, **V2**.1629
  carriers
    counseling, **V2**.1256
    serological parameters, **V2**.1252 (Tab.)
  chronic, **V2**.1248–9
    alanine aminotransferase (ALT), **V2**.1248
    clinical features, **V2**.1248–9
    coinfection, **V2**.1249
    diagnosis, **V2**.1251
    disease course, **V2**.1248–9
    HBeAg, **V2**.1248–9
    HBsAg, **V2**.1251
    immunosuppressed patients, **V2**.1249
    neonatal infection, **V2**.1476
    previous infection, **V2**.1248
    serological parameters, **V2**.1247 (Fig.), **V2**.1252 (Tab.)
  cirrhosis, **V2**.1249
    decompensated, **V2**.1248
  clinical course, **V2**.1246–9, **V2**.1246 (Fig.)
  clinical features, **V2**.1245–61
    cirrhosis *see above*
    hepatocellular carcinoma *see below*
  coinfection
    Hepatitis A virus, **V2**.1248
    Hepatitis C virus, **V2**.1248, **V2**.1249
    Hepatitis delta virus, **V2**.1248, **V2**.1249, **V2**.1272
    HIV, **V2**.1248, **V2**.1249

control, **V2**.1256–61, **V2**.1477
  barrier nursing, **V2**.1257
  blood product safety, **V2**.1257–8
  carrier counseling, **V2**.1256
  disinfection, **V2**.1257
  hygiene, **V2**.1256–7
  passive immunization *see below*
  vaccines *see below*
diagnosis, **V2**.1251–5
  acute hepatitis, **V2**.1251
  chronic hepatitis, **V2**.1251
  inapparent infection, **V2**.1251–2
  natural immunity, **V2**.1252–3
  from tissue specimens, **V2**.1253
diagnostic tests, **V2**.1253–5
  anti-HBc test, **V2**.1246, **V2**.1251, **V2**.1253–4, **V2**.1477
  anti-HBs, **V2**.1254
  DNA assay, **V2**.1251–5
  HBeAg, **V2**.1254
  HBsAg, **V2**.1246, **V2**.1251, **V2**.1253, **V2**.1476–7
  IgM anti-HBc, **V2**.1253–4
  serology, **V2**.1546
dynamics, **V2**.1279 (Tab.)
epidemiology, **V1**.283, **V1**.369, **I**.953–4, **I**.954 (Fig.), **V2**.1255–6, **V2**.1272
  age-relation, **V2**.1255
  carriers, **V2**.1629
  geological distribution, **V2**.1255
  incidence, **V2**.1255
  prevalence, **V2**.1255
fetal infection, **V2**.1475 (Tab.)
healthcare staff immunization, **B1**.383
hepatocellular carcinoma, **V2**.1249
  cirrhosis, **V2**.1249
  clinical features, **V2**.1249
  diagnosis, **V2**.1249
historical aspects, **V2**.1226
in HIV infection, **V2**.1248, **V2**.1249, **V2**.1499 (Tab.)
immune response, **V1**.283–4, **V2**.1249–51
  CD4+ T cell responses, **V1**.283
  CD8+ T cell responses, **V2**.1250
  cytokines, **V2**.1250
  detection, **V2**.1252–3
  IFN-γ, **V1**.284
  IL-1, **V1**.296–7
  IL-6, **V1**.303
  innate mechanisms, **V1**.283
  NK cells, **V1**.283
  T-cell response, **V2**.1250
  TNF-α, **V1**.284
immune tolerance, **V2**.1252, **V2**.1252 (Tab.)
immunopathology, **V1**.279 (Tab.), **V1**.303, **V2**.1245
  ICAM-1, **V1**.303
  IFN-γ, **V1**.303
  IL-2, **V1**.303
  immune complexes, **V2**.1250
  TNF-α, **V1**.303
laboratory worker immunization, **B1**.767
neonatal infection, **V2**.1444 (Tab.), **V2**.1475 (Tab.)
  management, **V2**.1477–8

occupational exposure, **B1**.767, **B1**.767 (Tab.)
oncogenicity, **V1**.336, **V1**.338 (Tab.)
passive immunization, **V2**.1259–60
  liver transplants, **V2**.1259
  recommendations, **V2**.1259–60
  see also Hepatitis B immunoglobulin (HBIG)
pathogenesis, **V2**.1249–51
  HBx, **V2**.1249–50
  LHB, **V2**.1249
perinatal infection, **V2**.1476
persistent infection, **V1**.259, **V1**.283, **V1**.373
  diagnosis, **V2**.1251–2
postnatal infection, **V2**.1476
in pregnancy, **V2**.1444 (Tab.), **V2**.1474, **V2**.1475 (Tab.)
  diagnosis, **V2**.1476–7
  management, **V2**.1477
  mother–child transmission, **V2**.1474–6
  transmission rate, **V2**.1476
serological parameters, **V2**.1251 (Tab.)
  HBsAg, **V2**.1252 (Tab.)
transient, **V2**.1247 (Fig.)
transmission, **V1**.369, **V2**.1255–6
  blood/blood products, **V1**.369
  blood/body fluids, **V2**.1255–6
  injury-associated, **V2**.1255–6
  prevention *see* Hepatitis B, control
  sexual contact, **V1**.369, **V2**.1255–6
  vertical, **V1**.369
  yellow fever vaccination (WWII), **V2**.1662
treatment, **V2**.1260–1
  antivirals *see above*
  combination therapy, **V2**.1629–30
  IFN, **V2**.1260
  IFN-α, **V1**.295, **V1**.303, **V2**.1629
  immune modulators, **V2**.1260
  immune therapy, **V2**.1260
vaccines/vaccination, **I**.424 (Tab.), **V2**.1258–9, **V2**.1552 (Tab.), **V2**.1573–4
  adolescents, **V2**.1574
  adults, **V2**.1258
  adverse reactions, **V2**.1258–9, **V2**.1564 (Tab.), **V2**.1574
  BCE peptide vaccines, **I**.855 (Tab.), **I**.861 (Tab.), **I**.872
  children, **V2**.1258, **V2**.1477
  controlled trials, **V1**.365
  CpG adjuvant, **I**.931, **I**.937
  development status, **I**.933 (Tab.)
  DNA vaccines, **I**.825, **V2**.1554
  edible antigens, **I**.828
  escape mutants, **V2**.1259
  GM-CSF adjuvants, **I**.277
  Hepatitis delta virus effects, **V2**.1273
  history, **V1**.8 (Tab.), **V2**.1573
  immune response, **V2**.1574
  inactivated, **V2**.1258
  indications, **V2**.1256, **V2**.1258–9
  infants, **V2**.1574
  ISCOMs adjuvant, **I**.930
  MF59 adjuvant, **I**.927, **I**.929, **I**.937
  MPL/QS-21 adjuvant, **I**.930
  plasma-derived, **V2**.1258
  in pregnancy, **V2**.1562–3

Hepatitis B
vaccines/vaccination (*Continued*)
  pre-/post-testing, **V2**.1259
  recombinant, **I**.15, **V1**.349, **I**.937, **V2**.1258,
    V2.1573
  schedules, **V2**.1560–1, **V2**.1573–4
  skin routes, **I**.822, **I**.823
  USA schedules, **V2**.1559–60, **V2**.1560 (Fig.)
  vaccination programs, **I**.937, **I**.963–4,
    V2.1559 (Tab.)
  virosomes, **I**.839
  WHO recommendations, **V2**.1574
Hepatitis B immunoglobulin (HBIG), **V2**.1566,
    V2.1567 (Tab.)
  neonates, **V2**.1477
  post exposure prophylaxis, **V2**.1567–8
  in pregnancy, **V2**.1481
Hepatitis B surface antigen (HBsAG)
  peptide vaccines, **I**.828
  transgenic plant expression, **I**.828
Hepatitis B virus (HBV), **V2.1226–68**
  antiviral agents, **B1**.434, **B1**.440
  blood product screening, **V2**.1257–8
  cell culture, **V2**.1232–3
  classification, **V2**.1227
  core protein, morphology, **V2**.1228
  detection, nucleic amplification methods,
    V2.1537
  DNA assays, **V2**.1254–5
    NAT technique, **V2**.1254–5
  DNA integration, **V2**.1243–4
  envelope protein, Hepatitis delta virus virion
    structure, **V2**.1233, **V2**.1271
  escape mutants, **V2**.1259
  genome
    DNA structure, **V2**.1230
    integration, **V2**.1244
    organization, **V2**.1231 (Fig.)
    replication, **V1**.123–4, **V1**.124 (Fig.)
  genome structure/function, **V2**.1229–31
    open reading frames, **V2**.1230
    organization, **V2**.1231 (Fig.)
    promoters, **V2**.1230
  genotypes, **V2**.1244–5
    pathogenicity differences, **V2**.1250
    prevalence, **V2**.1244–5
  HBc
    antibodies, **V2**.1250
    antibody test, **V2**.1246, **V2**.1251,
      V2.1253–4
    IgM, **V2**.1253–4
    transgenic mice, **V2**.1250
  HBeAg, **V2**.1241
    chronic infection, **V2**.1248–9
    diagnostic tests, **V2**.1254
    hepatitis B diagnostic tests, **V2**.1254
    loss of production, **V2**.1245
    negative variants, **V2**.1250
  HBe protein, **V2**.1241–2
    conservation, **V2**.1242
    function in life cycle, **V2**.1242
    in serum, **V2**.1242
    synthesis, **V2**.1242
    transgenic mice, **V2**.1250
  HBsAg
    acute hepatitis B, **V2**.1246

chronic hepatitis B, **V2**.1251
chronic infection, **V2**.1251
diagnostic tests, **V2**.1246, **V2**.1251,
  V2.1253
escape mutants, **V2**.1259
particle secretion, **V2**.1226, **V2**.1241
persistence, **V2**.1246
subtypes, **V2**.1244–5
variability mechanism, **V2**.1245
HBs proteins, **V2**.1241
  particle maturation, **V2**.1241
HBx, **V2**.1230, **V2**.1242–3
  deletions, **V2**.1245
  gene, **V2**.1242–3
  immune evasion, **V2**.1242
  oncogenicity, **V2**.1243
  pathogenesis, **V2**.1249–50
  pathogenicity role, **V2**.1249–50
  RNA, **V2**.1234
Hepatitis delta virus interactions, **V2**.1269,
  V2.1271, **V2**.1272
historical aspects, **V2**.1226
hypermutation, **V1**.193
immune evasion, **V1**.325, **V2**.1250–1
immunogenetics, **I**.587
infection, risk categorization, **B1**.762
large HB surface protein (LHBs),
  V2.1227–8
  attachment role, **V2**.1233
  HBV assembly, **V2**.1239–41
  mRNA, **V2**.1235
  pathogenesis, **V2**.1249
  preS domain, **V2**.1233, **V2**.1239–40
  topology, **V2**.1240 (Fig.)
  transgenic mice, **V2**.1249
mannose-binding lectin interaction, **V1**.273
middle HB surface protein (MHBs),
  V2.1227–8
  in attachment, **V2**.1233
  topology, **V2**.1240 (Fig.)
molecular detection, **B1**.723 (Tab.)
  HBsAg, **B1**.383
  hybrid capture assay, **B1**.731
  nucleic acid sequencing, **B1**.732, **B1**.733–4
  quantification, **B1**.722–4
  specimen suitability, **B1**.724
morphology/structure, **V1**.66 (Fig.),
  V2.1227–9, **V2**.1227 (Fig.), **V2**.1228 (Fig.)
  α-structures, **V1**.65
non-structural proteins, **V2**.1241–3
  see also specific types
nosocomial infection, **B1**.382–3
polymerase, **V2**.1229–30
pregenomic RNA, **V2**.1235–6
  encapsidation, **V2**.1235–6
  encapsidation signal ( ), **V2**.1235–6
  genome generation, **V2**.1236–9,
    V2.1237 (Fig.)
protein kinase C, **V2**.1228–9
replication, **V2**.1231–41, **V2**.1232 (Fig.)
  assembly, **V2**.1228, **V2**.1235–9
  attachment, **V2**.1232–3
  envelopment and secretion, **V2**.1239–41
  genome maturation, **V2**.1235–9
  nuclear entry/episomal DNA formation,
    V2.1231, **V2**.1233–4, **V2**.1239

transcription *see below*
translation, **V2**.1234–5
uptake, **V2**.1231
small HB surface protein (SHBs),
  V2.1227–8
  antibodies to, **V2**.1250
  antibody administration, **V2**.1250
  attachment role, **V2**.1233
  HBV assembly, **V2**.1239, **V2**.1241
  topology, **V2**.1240 (Fig.)
  transgenic mice, **V2**.1250
  variability, **V2**.1245
supergenomic RNA, **V2**.1235
surface proteins
  assembly, **V2**.1239
  expression, **V2**.1239
  see also specific types
T-helper cell epitope, **I**.862 (Tab.)
transcription, **V2**.1234–5
  promoters and enhancers, **V2**.1230
transcription factors, **V2**.1235
transgenic mice, **V2**.1250
transmission, **I**.819–20
  blood transfusions, **B1**.380–1
  endoscopes, **B1**.380
  guidelines to minimize during surgery,
    B1.383
type species, **V1**.46–7
vaccine *see* Hepatitis B
variants, **V2**.1244–5
  generation, **V2**.1245
viricides, **B1**.435–6
Hepatitis C, **V2**.1202–8, **V2**.1478–81
  acute, **V2**.1202–3
    asymptomatic individuals, **V2**.1202–3
    biological markers, **V2**.1204 (Fig.)
    liver function tests, **V2**.1202–3
    viremia, **V2**.1203
    virological markers, **V2**.1204 (Fig.)
  animal models, **V2**.1194
  chronic, **V2**.1203
  clinical course, **V2**.1203 (Fig.),
    V2.1204–5
    age-relation, **V2**.1204
    cirrhosis, **V2**.1205
    hepatic steatosis, **V2**.1204
    organ transplants, **V2**.1204
  coinfection
    Hepatitis A virus, **V2**.1248
    Hepatitis B virus, **V2**.1249
    Hepatitis G virus, **V2**.1482
  control, **V2**.1215–17, **V2**.1480
    antiviral treatment, **V2**.1215–16
    genotype effects *see* Hepatitis C virus
      (HCV)
    IFN-α/ribavirin therapy, **V2**.1198, **V2**.1215,
      V2.1215 (Fig.), **V2**.1628
    liver transplantation, **V2**.1216
    vaccines *see below*
  diagnostic tests, **V2**.1210–15
    antigens, **V2**.1210–13
    blood donor screening, **V2**.1213, **V2**.1216
    ELISA *see* Enzyme-linked immunosorbent
      assay (ELISA)
    first generation, **V2**.1211–12

Hepatitis C
  diagnostic tests (*Continued*)
    genome detection, **V2**.1213
    genotyping assays, **V2**.1214–15
    second generation, **V2**.1212
    serology, **V2**.1547
    third generation, **V2**.1212
    viral load measurement, **V2**.1213–14
  dynamics, **V2**.1279 (Tab.)
  emerging infection, **V2**.1647–50,
    V2.1648 (Tab.)
    recognition, **V2**.1653 (Tab.)
  epidemiology, **B1**.382–3, **V2**.1208–10
    geographical distribution, **V2**.1209–10
    molecular epidemiology, **V2**.1210,
      V2.1214–15
    prevalence, **V2**.1189
  extrahepatic manifestations, **V2**.1207–8
    disease association, **V2**.1207
    'essential mixed cryoglobulinemia,'
      V2.1208
    glomerulonephritis, **V2**.1207
    IFN-α/ribavirin therapy, **V2**.1215
    membranoproliferative glomerulonephritis
      (MPGN) type 1, **V2**.1208
    vasculitis, **V2**.1207
  fetal infection, **V2**.1475 (Tab.)
  hepatocellular carcinoma, **V2**.1205
    IFN-α/ribavirin therapy, **V2**.1205
    prevalence, **V2**.1205
  histology, **V2**.1203–4, **V2**.1205 (Fig.)
    liver biopsies, **V2**.1203–4
    lobular hepatitis, **V2**.1203–4
  in HIV infection, **V2**.1504
  host protein synthesis effects, **V1**.120
  immune response
    cell-mediated, **V2**.1206
    genotype effects, **V2**.1201–2
    humoral, **V2**.1206
    IL-6, **V1**.303
    neutralizing antibodies, **V2**.1196,
      V2.1206–7
  immunopathology, **V2**.1207
  Ishak score, **V2**.1204
  Knodell score, **V2**.1204
  liver damage mechanisms, **V2**.1207
  mortality, **V2**.1205 (Fig.)
  mother–infant transmission, **V2**.1209,
    V2.1478–80
    breastfeeding, **V2**.1479–81
    delivery method, **V2**.1480, **V2**.1481
    genotype effects, **V2**.1480
    high risk groups, **V2**.1478–80,
      V2.1479 (Tab.)
    HIV coinfection, **V2**.1478–9
    low risk groups, **V2**.1478, **V2**.1479 (Tab.)
    transmission routes, **V2**.1478
    vertical transmission, **V2**.1478–80
  neonatal infection, **V2**.1444 (Tab.),
    V2.1475 (Tab.)
    diagnosis, **V2**.1480
    management, **V2**.1481
  nosocomial infection, **B1**.382–3
  occupational exposure, **B1**.767, **B1**.767 (Tab.)
  persistence mechanisms, **V2**.1206

  in pregnancy, **V2**.1444 (Tab.),
    V2.1475 (Tab.), **V2**.1478
    diagnosis, **V2**.1480
    management, **V2**.1480–1
    mother–infant transmission *see above*
  prevention, **V2**.1216–17
    blood donor screening, **V2**.1208–9,
      V2.1213, **V2**.1216
    drug abuse, **V2**.1216
    vaccination, **V2**.1216–17
  therapy, IFN-α, **V1**.295, **V1**.303
  transmission, **V2**.1208–9
    blood/blood products, **V2**.1203, **V2**.1208
    intravenous drug users, **V2**.1208
    maternal transmission *see above*
    organ transplants, **V2**.1209
    parenteral transmission, **V2**.1208–9
    sexual behavior, **V2**.1209
  vaccines
    BCE peptide vaccines, **I**.855 (Tab.),
      I.861 (Tab.), **I**.870–1
    development status, **I**.933 (Tab.)
    DNA vaccines, **V2**.1554
    edible antigens, **I**.870–1
    MF59 adjuvant, **I**.929
    subunit vaccine development, **I**.941
Hepatitis C virus (HCV), **V2.1189–225**
  classification, **V1**.53–4
    phylogenetic analysis, **V2**.1192 (Fig.)
  core protein, **V2**.1196
    tests for, **V2**.1211
  detection
    ELISA *see* Enzyme-linked immunosorbent
      assay (ELISA)
    nucleic amplification methods, **V2**.1537
  discovery, **V2**.1189–90
    PCR, **V2**.1190
  E1 protein, **V2**.1196
    neutralizing antibodies, **V2**.1196,
      V2.1206–7
    posttranslational modification, **V2**.1195,
      V2.1196
    in vaccine, **V2**.1217
    variability, **V2**.1201–2
    Yellow fever virus *vs.*, **V2**.1190
  E2 protein, **V2**.1196
    neutralizing antibodies, **V2**.1196,
      V2.1206–7
    posttranslational modification, **V2**.1195,
      V2.1196
    in vaccine, **I**.870–1, **V2**.1217
    variability, **V2**.1201–2
  genetic variability *see below*
  genome, **V2**.1192–3
    open reading frames, **V2**.1194–5
    organization, **V2**.1191 (Fig.)
    replication, **V1**.143, **V2**.1194
    secondary RNA structure, **V2**.1194–5
    untranslated regions, **V2**.1190
  genotypes/genetic variability, **V2**.1199,
    V2.1199–202
    antiviral susceptibility, **V2**.1202
    biological differences, **V2**.1201–2
    evolutionary tree, **V2**.1200 (Fig.)
    geographical distribution, **V2**.1199–201,
      V2.1209–10

    IFN susceptibility, **V2**.1202, **V2**.1215–16
    immune response, **V2**.1201–2
    nomenclature, **V2**.1199–201
    nucleotide sequence variation,
      V2.1199–201
    pathogenicity, **V2**.1202
    recombination, **V2**.1201
  immune evasion, **V2**.1206–7
    NS5A protein, **V2**.1198
  immunogenetics, **I**.587–8
  in vitro culture, **V2**.1193–4
    protein translation, **V2**.1193–4
  molecular detection, **B1**.721, **B1**.723 (Tab.)
    nucleic acid sequencing, **B1**.732, **B1**.733–4
    quantification, **B1**.722–4
    specimen suitability, **B1**.724
    transcription-mediated amplification,
      B1.729–30
  morphology, **V2**.1193, **V2**.1193 (Fig.)
  NS2 protein, **V2**.1197
    post-translational modification, **V2**.1195
  NS3 protein, **V2**.1197
    post-translational modification, **V2**.1195
    tests for, **V2**.1211, **V2**.1212
  NS4A protein, **V2**.1197
    cell-mediated immune response, **V2**.1206
    genotype variability, **V2**.1210–11
    tests for, **V2**.1210–11, **V2**.1212
  NS4B protein, **V2**.1197–8
    cell-mediated immune response, **V2**.1206
    genotype variability, **V2**.1210–11
    tests for, **V2**.1210–11, **V2**.1212
  NS5A protein, **V2**.1198
    gene, **V2**.1198 (Fig.)
    immune evasion, **V2**.1198
    tests for, **V2**.1211, **V2**.1212
  NS5B protein (RdRp), **V2**.1194, **V2**.1198–9
    sequence drift, **V2**.1210
    tests for, **V2**.1211, **V2**.1212
  p7 protein, **V2**.1196
  physicochemical properties, **V2**.1193
    density, **V2**.1193
    resistance to physical agents, **V2**.1193
  prevalence, **B1**.382–3
  proteins, **V2**.1195–9
    nonstructural, **V2**.1195–6
    structural, **V2**.1195–9
    see also specific proteins
  relationship to other viruses, **V2**.1190–2
    flaviviruses, **V2**.1190, **V2**.1191–2
    GB virus B (GBV-B) vs, **V2**.1191–2
    pestiviruses, **V2**.1190–1
    positive-strand RNA viruses, **V2**.1190
    Yellow fever virus *vs.*, **V2**.1190
  replication, **V2**.1193–5
    cell-specific factors, **V1**.136 (Fig.), **V1**.137
    entry/uncoating/release, **V2**.1195
  RNA-dependent RNA polymerase *see above*
  translation, **V2**.1194–5
    initiation, **V2**.1195
    IRES, **V2**.1195
    post-translational modification, **V2**.1195
  transmission
    blood transfusions, **B1**.380–1
    needle contamination, **I**.819–20

Hepatitis C virus (HCV) (*Continued*)
vaccine *see* Hepatitis C
Hepatitis D, **V2**.1271–3, **V2**.1481
clinical manifestations, **V2**.1272
coinfection, **V2**.1271
Hepatitis B virus, **V2**.1248, **V2**.1249,
V2.1272
emerging infection, **V2**.1648 (Tab.)
epidemiology, **V2**.1272–3
hosts, **V2**.1271
incubation period, **V2**.1272
neonatal infection, **V2**.1444 (Tab.),
V2.1475 (Tab.), **V2**.1481
pathogenicity, **V2**.1273
perinatal infection, **V2**.1476
in pregnancy, **V2**.1444 (Tab.),
V2.1475 (Tab.), **V2**.1481
prophylaxis, **V2**.1481
superinfection, **V2**.1271
therapy, **V2**.1273
IFN-α, **V1**.303, **V2**.1273
lamivudine, **V2**.1273
vaccines/vaccination, **V2**.1273
viremia, **V2**.1272
Hepatitis delta virus (HDV), **V2.1269–75**
classification, **V1**.48, **V1**.127–8, **V2**.1269
delta antigen, **V2**.1270
small form, **V2**.1270
detection, **V2**.1272
experimental systems, **V2**.1271
genome, **V2**.1269–70
replication, **V1**.124
sequence isolates, **V2**.1273
helper virus interactions, **V2**.1273
Duck Hepatitis B virus, **V2**.1271
Hepatitis B virus, **V2**.1269, **V2**.1271,
V2.1272
Woodchuck Hepatitis B virus, **V2**.1271
historical aspects, **V2**.1269
phylogenetics, **V2**.1272–3
plant virioids *vs.*, **V2**.1271
protein synthesis, RNA editing, **V1**.116–17
replication, **V2**.1270–1
host RNA polymerase II, **V2**.1270
liver, **V2**.1270
post-transcriptional editing, **V2**.1270
transmission, **V2**.1271–2
liver transplantations, **V2**.1272
virion structure, **V2**.1269–70
Hepatitis B virus envelope protein,
V2.1271
Hepatitis E, **V2**.1480–2
animal models, **V2**.1178–9
cholestatic, **V2**.1179
clinical features, **V2**.1179
course of infection, **V2**.1178–9, **V2**.1179 (Fig.)
diagnosis, **V2**.1179–80
antibody detection, **V2**.1179–80
baculovirus-expressed ORF2 as antigen for
assays, **V2**.1179–80
emerging infection, **V2**.1648 (Tab.)
recognition, **V2**.1653 (Tab.)
epidemiology, **V2**.1180
age-related susceptibility, **V2**.1180
fatalities, **V2**.1179

incubation period, **V2**.1179
neonatal infection, **V2**.1444 (Tab.),
V2.1475 (Tab.), **V2**.1481–2
outbreaks, **V2**.1160, **V2**.1180
perinatal infection, **V2**.1476
in pregnancy, **V2**.1444 (Tab.),
V2.1475 (Tab.), **V2**.1481–2
immune response, **V2**.1179
antibodies, **V2**.1179
protective antibodies, **V2**.1177–8
pathogenesis, **V2**.1178–9
pathology, **V2**.1178–9
prophylaxis, **V2**.1482
transmission, **V2**.1180
fecal-oral, **V2**.1160–1, **V2**.1180
vaccines, **I**.933 (Tab.)
development, **V2**.1180
viremia, **V2**.1178–9
Hepatitis E virus (HEV), **V2**.1175–80,
V2.1178–80
absence of envelope, **V2**.1160–1
animal reservoirs, **V2**.1178
antigenic variants, **V2**.1177–8
caliciviruses *vs.*, **V2**.1175, **V2**.1175 (Tab.)
classification, **V1**.53, **V2**.1175
control, **V2**.1180
discovery and historical aspects, **V2**.1160
endemic, **V2**.1180
genetic variants/clusters of strains, **V2**.1178
genome organization, **V2**.1175–6, **V2**.1175–8,
V2.1176 (Fig.)
open reading frame 2 (ORF2), **V2**.1175–8
open reading frame 3 (ORF3), **V2**.1175–7
open reading frames, **V2**.1175–6
helicase, **V2**.1176–7
Hepatitis A virus *vs.*, **V2**.1160–1,
V2.1161 (Tab.)
morphology and structure, **V2**.1175,
V2.1176 (Fig.)
cryoelectron microscopy, **V2**.1175
properties, **V2**.1161 (Tab.), **V2**.1175 (Tab.)
proteins, **V2**.1176–7
see also specific types
replication, **V2**.1177
RNA polymerase, **V2**.1176–7
rubiviruses *vs.*, **V2**.1175, **V2**.1175 (Tab.)
shedding, **V2**.1179
Hepatitis G virus (HGV) infection,
V2.1444 (Tab.), **V2**.1482
coinfection, **V2**.1482
emerging infection, **V2**.1648 (Tab.)
recognition, **V2**.1650, **V2**.1653 (Tab.)
neonatal infection, **V2**.1475 (Tab.)
perinatal infection, **V2**.1476
in pregnancy, **V2**.1475 (Tab.)
Hepatocellular carcinoma
hepatitis B *see* Hepatitis B
hepatitis C *see* Hepatitis C
Hepatocellular injury, *Ehrlichia chaffeensis*
infection, **B2**.2058–9
Hepatocyte invasion, *Plasmodium*, **P**.472–3
Hepatocytes, HAV replication, **V2**.1169
Hepatolithiasis, clonorchiasis, **P**.649
Hepatomegaly
amebic liver abscess, **P**.208
opisthorchiasis, **P**.649

visceral leishmaniasis (kala-azar), **P**.298
Hepatosplenic candidiasis, **M**.599–600
Hepatosplenomegaly
Chagas disease, **P**.384–5
schistosomiasis, **P**.612–13, **P**.630–1
Hepatotoxicity, azoles, **M**.183–4
Hepatovirus, **V2**.1161
see also Hepatoviruses
Hepatoviruses
cell entry, receptors, **V2**.867 (Tab.)
characteristics, **V2**.861 (Tab.)
classification, **V2**.858, **V2**.859 (Fig.)
properties, **V2**.1162 (Tab.)
size, **V2**.859
see also Hepatovirus
HEPT, **V2**.1621–2
Herbal remedies, nasopharyngeal carcinoma
and, **V1**.572
Herbs, **B1**.287–8
Herceptin, licensing, **I**.355 (Tab.)
Herd immunity, **B1**.341, **B1**.347–53, **I**.957–8,
I.959 (Fig.)
concept, **B1**.341
genetic factors, **B1**.355
historical aspects, **B1**.337
origin of term, **B1**.337
vaccination programs, **B1**.347–53
Hereditary angioedema (HAE), **I**.153–4
Hereditary hemorrhagic telangiectasia,
intracranial abscess complication, **B1**.583
Hermansky–Pudlak disease, **I**.482
Hermetically sealed containers, heat
sterilization, **B1**.265–6, **B1**.270–1, **B1**.275,
B1.283
Heroin addicts, **M**.12–3
Heron Hepatitis B virus (HHBV), **V2**.1227
Herpangina, **V2**.871
Herpes gladiatorum, **V1**.507
Herpes simplex virus(es) (HSVs), **V1**.506–12
adeno-associated virus replication, **V1**.160
antiviral resistance
aciclovir, **V1**.512, **V2**.1501
mechanism, **V1**.512
antiviral susceptibility testing, **V2**.1543
capsid structure, **V2**.1597
cell interactions
host protein synthesis inhibition, **V1**.203
host RNA degradation, **V1**.221
receptors *see below*
transcription factors, **V1**.220
culture, **V1**.511
detection
cytospinning, **V2**.1540–1
ELISA *see* Enzyme-linked immunosorbent
assay (ELISA)
DNA replication, **V1**.218–19
genes
supplemental essential, **V2**.1407–8
temporal control, **V1**.118–19
gene therapy vectors, **V2**.1595 (Tab.),
V2.1597–8
amplicons, **V2**.1598
genome, **V2**.1418–19, **V2**.1420 (Fig.),
V2.1597
packaging, **V1**.67
glycoprotein C, **V1**.510

Herpes simplex virus(es) (HSVs) (*Continued*)
glycoprotein D, **V1**.510
vaccine development, **V2**.1582
host transcript recombination, **V1**.190
immune evasion, **V1**.502, **V1**.510
complement, **V1**.313, **I**.638–9
dendritic cells, **V1**.323, **I**.632
Fc receptor homologues, **V1**.510
IFN effector functions, **V1**.315, **I**.619
Igs, **I**.638
MHC, **V1**.321, **I**.634
infection *see* Herpes simplex virus infection
latency associated transcripts (LATs),
V1.509, **V1**.509 (Fig.), **V2**.1408,
V2.1418–19, **V2**.1420 (Fig.)
life cycle, **V2**.1597–8
membrane-associated glycoproteins, **V1**.502
cell heparan sulfate association, **V1**.502
immune system interaction, **V1**.502
receptors, **V1**.207 (Tab.), **V2**.1405
CNS receptors, **V2**.1406 (Tab.)
complement receptors, **V1**.257–8
Fc receptors, **V1**.258, **V1**.258 (Fig.)
glycoprotein C, **V1**.207
replication, **V2**.1418–19
in CNS, **V2**.1418–19, **V2**.1419 (Fig.)
virulence, genes of cellular origin, **V1**.257–8
see also Herpes simplex virus 1 (HSV-
1); Herpes simplex virus type 2 (HSV-2)
Herpes simplex virus infection, **V1**.506–12
antiviral therapy, **V1**.507, **V1**.511–12
cidofovir, **V2**.1616
clinical features, **V1**.506–8
children, **V2**.1420
CNS features *see below*
cold sores, **V1**.507, **V1**.507 (Fig.)
encephalitis *see below*
eye, **V1**.507
genital, **V1**.506–7
keratitis, **V1**.507
mucocutanous ulceration, **V2**.1500
neonates, **V2**.1419–20
oral, **V1**.506–7, **V1**.507 (Fig.), **V2**.1419
skin infection, **V1**.507
CNS infection, **V1**.507, **V2**.1418–21,
V2.1419–20
acute, **V2**.1407–8
T-cell response, **V1**.304
complications, **V2**.1420
control/therapy, **V1**.511–12, **V2**.1421
antivirals *see above*
vaccines *see below*
diagnosis, **V1**.511
bronchoalveolar lavage, **V2**.1506
cytopathology, **V2**.1534 (Tab.)
ELISA *see* Enzyme-linked immunosorbent
assay (ELISA)
HSV-1 *vs* HSV-2, **V1**.511
encephalitis, **V1**.245, **V1**.507, **V1**.511,
V2.1419–20
clinical features, **V2**.1419–20
diagnosis, **V1**.511, **V2**.1421
immunocompetent patients, **V2**.1421
pathology, **V2**.1420 (Fig.)
treatment, **V2**.1421

entry/migration route, **V2**.1405, **V2**.1418,
V2.1419–20
epidemiology, **V1**.508
bone marrow transplants, **V2**.1506
fetal infection, **V2**.1461–7
HIV infection *see below*
neonatal infection *see below*
in pregnancy *see below*
genital infection
classification, **V2**.1462–3, **V2**.1463 (Tab.)
clinical features, **V1**.507
nonprimary first episode, **V2**.1463
primary infection, **V2**.1462–3
recurrent, **V2**.1463
in HIV infection, **V2**.1498, **V2**.1500–1
in children, **V2**.1504–5
exposure prevention, **V2**.1500–1
treatment, **V2**.1501
host cell relationship, **V2**.1420
nonhomologous end joining (NHEJ)
pathway, **V1**.169–70
immune response, **V1**.284–5, **V1**.510
adaptive immune response, **V1**.284–5
antibodies, **V1**.510, **V2**.1421
CD4+ T cells, **V1**.284–5
CD8+ T cells, **V1**.285
cell-mediated immune response, **V1**.284–5
complement, **V1**.284
defensin actions, **I**.168
dendritic cells, **V1**.284
IL-18, **I**.290–2
INFs, **V1**.271, **V1**.284–5
innate immune response, **V1**.284
NK cells, **I**.94–6, **V1**.284, **V1**.510
T cells, **V1**.510
immunocompromised patients, **V1**.508
non-HIV, **V2**.1506
immunopathology, **V1**.279 (Tab.)
infection route, **V1**.506–7
keratitis, *Acanthamoeba* keratitis *vs*, **P**.236
latent infection, **V1**.260, **V1**.261, **V1**.506–7,
V1.509–10, **V2**.1408, **V2**.1418–19,
V2.1420–1, **V2**.1598
aciclovir, **V2**.1638
famciclovir, **V2**.1638
nerve growth factor, **V2**.1418
reactivation, **V1**.261, **V2**.1598
neonatal infection, **V1**.507–8, **V2**.1419,
V2.1444 (Tab.), **V2**.1464–5
clinical manifestations, **V2**.1465
diagnosis, **V2**.1465–6
immune response, **V2**.1465
incidence, **V2**.1464
management, **V2**.1467
mortality, **V2**.1465
pathogenesis, **V2**.1464–5
transmission, **V2**.1464–5
pathology and pathogenesis, **V1**.508–10,
V2.1420 (Fig.)
persistent infection, **V1**.373, **V1**.509
in pregnancy, **V1**.508, **V2**.1444 (Tab.),
V2.1461–4, **V2**.1463
cesarean section delivery, **V2**.1466
diagnosis, **V2**.1465–6
disseminated infection, **V2**.1463
epidemiology, **V2**.1461–2

hepatitis, **V2**.1463
management, **V2**.1466–7
transmission risk factors, **V2**.1464
reactivation, **V1**.507, **V1**.509–10, **V2**.1418,
V2.1421
recurrent, **V2**.1421
immune response, **V1**.510
transmission, **V1**.508, **V2**.1418, **V2**.1419–20
vaccines/vaccination
development, **V1**.511, **I**.933 (Tab.),
V2.1552 (Tab.), **V2**.1582
DNA vaccines, **V2**.1554
intranasal route, **I**.831–2
MF59 adjuvant, **I**.929
MPL/QS-21 adjuvant, **I**.930
skin application, **I**.823
Herpes simplex virus type 1 (HSV-1)
antibody effects, **V1**.278
biosafety level 2 classification, **V2**.1525
cell interactions, host RNA degradation,
V1.221
characteristics, **V1**.489 (Tab.)
classification, **V1**.44
DNA replication
origin of replication, **V1**.500
proteins, **V1**.500
entry into cells, **V2**.1418
gene delivery system, cytokines, **V1**.305
genome replication, **V1**.148 (Tab.),
V1.163–8, **V1**.164 (Fig.), **V1**.167 (Fig.)
alkaline nuclease, **V1**.165 (Tab.)
dUTPase, **V1**.165 (Tab.)
elongation, **V1**.166–7
ICP8 (UL29), **V1**.165–6, **V1**.165 (Tab.)
initiation, **V1**.166
lagging-strand replication, **V1**.166–7
leading-strand replication, **V1**.166–7
nonessential viral gene products, **V1**.166
origin recognition proteins, **V1**.149 (Tab.)
origins of replication, **V1**.164
OriL, **V1**.164
OriS, **V1**.164, **V1**.166
ribonucleotide reductase, **V1**.165 (Tab.)
thymidine kinase, **V1**.165 (Tab.)
UL5/UL8/UL52, **V1**.165, **V1**.165 (Tab.)
UL9, **V1**.149 (Tab.), **V1**.165–6
UL30/UL40, **V1**.165, **V1**.165 (Tab.)
UL42, **V1**.165 (Tab.)
uracil N glycosylase, **V1**.165 (Tab.)
viral proteins, **V1**.149 (Tab.), **V1**.164–6,
V1.165 (Tab.)
see also specific proteins
genome sequences, **V1**.494 (Tab.)
genome structure, **V1**.148 (Tab.), **V1**.163–4,
V1.164 (Fig.), **V1**.492, **V1**.493,
V1.493 (Fig.), **V1**.509, **V2**.1418–19,
V2.1420 (Fig.)
gene arrangement, **V1**.495 (Fig.)
inverted sequence repeats, **V1**.163–4
latency-associated transcripts (LATs),
V1.495
nested arrangement, **V1**.495
U$_L$, **V1**.163–4
U$_S$, **V1**.163–4
hypermutation, **V1**.193
immune evasion, **V1**.287

Herpes simplex virus type 1 (HSV-1)
  (*Continued*)
  infection *see* Herpes simplex virus type 1
      (HSV-1)
  isolation/propagation, **V1**.98
  latency associated transcripts (LATs),
      V1.509, **V1**.509 (Fig.), **V2**.1418–19,
      V2.1420 (Fig.)
  morphology/structure, **V1**.490 (Fig.)
  nucleotide metabolism
    deoxyuridine triphosphatase (dUTPase),
        V1.500
    ribonucleotide reductase, **V1**.499
    thymidine kinase, **V1**.499, **V1**.511–12
    uracil-DNA glycosylase, **V1**.500
  proteins, **V1**.496 (Tab.)
    see also specific types
  replication, **V1**.491 (Fig.), **V2**.1418
    in CNS, **V2**.1418, **V2**.1419 (Fig.)
    host cell, effects on, **V1**.491
Herpes simplex virus type 1 (HSV-1) infection,
    V1.506–7
  clinical features, **V1**.506–7
  cytokine response, **V1**.301–2
  diagnosis, **V1**.511
  epidemiology, **V1**.508
  in HIV infection, **V2**.1499 (Tab.)
  immunopathology, **V1**.280
  medical importance, **V1**.162
  neonatal infection, prognosis, **V2**.1465
  in pregnancy
    diagnosis, **V2**.1465–6
    incidence, **V2**.1461–2
  transmission, sexual activity, **V2**.1500
  vaccine development, **I**.898, **V2**.1582
Herpes simplex virus type 2 (HSV-2)
  biosafety level 2 classification, **V2**.1525
  characteristics, **V1**.489 (Tab.)
  classification, **V1**.44
  genome sequences, **V1**.494 (Tab.)
  genome structure, **V1**.492, **V1**.493 (Fig.)
  infection *see* Herpes simplex virus type 2
      (HSV-2) infection
  medical importance, **V1**.162
  recombination, HHV-1, **V1**.187
Herpes simplex virus type 2 (HSV-2) infection,
    V2.1418–21
  antibodies, **V1**.508–9
  brivusin therapy, **V2**.1614
  clinical features, **V1**.506–7
  CNS, **V2**.1420–1
  diagnosis, **V1**.511
  epidemiology, **V1**.508
  in HIV infection, **V2**.1499 (Tab.)
  neonatal infection
    diagnosis, **V2**.1466
    prognosis, **V2**.1465
  in pregnancy
    abortion, **V2**.1463
    diagnosis, **V2**.1465–6
    incidence, **V2**.1461–2
  transmission, sexual activity, **V2**.1500
  vaccine development, **V2**.1582
Herpes (Trichophyton) tonsurans, **M**.220
Herpesviridae, **V1**.488–9
  characteristics, **V1**.177 (Tab.)

classification, **V1**.26, **V1**.27 (Tab.),
    V1.43 (Tab.), **V1**.44–5
  fish viruses, **V1**.45
  phenotypic analysis, **V1**.44–5
  species differences, **V1**.44
  see also Herpesviruses; *specific viruses*
Herpesvirus ateles
  characteristics, **V1**.542 (Tab.)
  genome sequences, **V1**.494 (Tab.)
Herpesvirus B, **V1**.371 (Tab.)
Herpesvirus, classification, **V1**.53
Herpesviruses, **V1.488–505**
  adeno-associated virus replication, **V1**.160
  cell entry mechanisms, **V1**.213
  cell interactions, DNA maintenance, **V1**.219
  cell receptors, **V1**.106–7, **V1**.207 (Tab.)
    CNS, **V2**.1406 (Tab.)
  classification, **V1**.488–9
    amino acid sequences, **V1**.497–8
    historical aspects, **V1**.26
  DNA packaging, **V1**.501
  DNA replication, **V1**.217, **V1**.500
    DNA polymerase, **V1**.500
    origin of replication, **V1**.500
    proteins, **V1**.500
  evolution, **V1**.498
    non-mammalian, **V1**.498
    phylogenetic tree, **V1**.498 (Fig.)
  gene function, **V1**.498–503
    control, **V1**.498–9
    determination, **V1**.498
    IE genes, **V1**.498–9
    transcriptional regulators, **V1**.499
  genetic content, **V1**.493–8
    arrangement/expression, **V1**.493
    protein-coding genes, **V1**.493
    splicing, **V1**.493
  genome replication, **V1**.162–8
    polymerases, **V1**.147–8
    replication compartments/centers,
        V1.170–1
  genome structure, **V1**.488, **V1**.492–3,
      V1.492 (Fig.), **V1**.494 (Tab.)
    heterogeneity, **V1**.493
    HHVs, **V1**.492–3
  heparin sulfate binding, **V1**.106–7
  human-specific, **V1**.489, **V1**.489 (Tab.)
    genome sequences, **V1**.489
    historical aspects, **V1**.489
  ICP0 protein, **V1**.498–9
  ICP4 protein, **V1**.498–9
  ICP22 protein, **V1**.498–9
  ICP27 protein, **V1**.498–9
  IE genes, **V1**.498–9
    function, **V2**.1597–8
  immune evasion
    chemokines, **V1**.288, **I**.622
    complement, **V1**.230, **V1**.287, **V1**.313
    cytokine receptors, **V1**.318
    cytokines, **V1**.316–17, **I**.621, **I**.623
    death-receptor inhibitors, **I**.626–7
    Fc receptors, **V1**.312–13
    IFN-receptor analogue production, **V1**.230
    latency, **V1**.311
    MHC, **V1**.287, **I**.637

infection *see* Herpesvirus infection
isolation/propagation and identification,
    V1.96 (Tab.), **V1**.98
medical importance, **V1**.162
mixed cell culture, **V1**.88
morphology/structure, **V1**.490, **V1**.490 (Fig.)
  electron cryomicroscopy, **V1**.490
  lipid envelope, **V1**.490
  nuclear transit, **V1**.216
nucleotide metabolism, **V1**.499–500
  deoxyuridine triphosphatase (dUTPase),
      V1.500
  dihydrofolate reductase, **V1**.500
  ribonucleotide reductase, **V1**.499
  thymidine kinase, **V1**.499
  thymidylate synthase, **V1**.500
  uracil-DNA glycosylase, **V1**.500
origins, **V1**.175–6
recombination, adenoviruses, **V1**.187
replication, **V1**.490–1, **V1**.491 (Fig.)
  cell entry, **V1**.490–1
  gene functions, **V1**.491
  host cell, effects on, **V1**.491
  mRNA synthesis, **V1**.110
  nuclear transfer, **V1**.490–1
  packaging, **V1**.491
  transcription, **V1**.491
  virion maturation, **V1**.491
species range, **V1**.488
virion structure, **V1**.501–2
  capsid, **V1**.501
  degree of complexity, **V1**.501
  envelope, **V1**.502
  membrane-associated glycoproteins,
      V1.502
  scaffold proteins, **V1**.501
  tegument, **V1**.502
VP16 protein, **V1**.498, **V2**.1597–8
see also Herpesviridae; *specific viruses*
Herpesvirus infection
  adeno-associated virus coinfection,
      V2.1598–9
  animal models, **V2**.1609, **V2**.1609 (Tab.)
  antiviral therapy
    cidofovir, **V2**.1616
    combination, **V2**.1618
    immunomodulators, **V2**.1618
    latent infection, **V2**.1638
    penciclovir, **V2**.1614
    resistance, **V2**.1634–5, **V2**.1635 (Tab.)
  caspase deficiency, **I**.776
  diagnosis, serology, **V2**.1547
  hemophagocytic syndrome, **I**.778
  in HIV infection, **V2**.1498, **V2**.1499–503,
      V2.1499 (Tab.)
    in children, **V2**.1504–5
    disease progression, **V2**.1499–500
    phenotypic mixing, **V2**.1500
  host cell DNA metabolism, **V1**.217
  immune response, **V1**.284–6
    cytokines, **V1**.301–3
    IL-1, **V1**.296–7
    macrophage avoidance, **I**.30
    NK cells, **I**.94–5, **V1**.272

Herpesvirus infection (*Continued*)
immunodeficient patients (non-HIV),
V2.1506–8
infection, IFN activity, **I**.260 (Tab.)
infection process, **V1**.241 (Tab.)
latent infection, **V1**.260, **V1**.284, **V1**.345,
V2.1499
neural spread, **V1**.244 (Tab.)
oncogenicity, **V1**.332 (Tab.), **V1**.342 (Tab.)
pathogenesis, **V1**.502–3
persistent, **V1**.373
transmission, **V1**.371 (Tab.), **V1**.488
vaccines, **V1**.349
Herpesvirus saimiri (HVS), **V1**.543
characteristics, **V1**.542 (Tab.)
genome sequences, **V1**.494 (Tab.)
IL-17 homologue, **V1**.317–18
immune evasion
apoptosis interference, **V1**.287
complement, **V1**.287, **V1**.313
cytokine homologues, **V1**.317–18, **I**.620
oncogenic mechanisms, **V1**.342 (Tab.)
vFLIP, **V1**.287
Herpesvirus sylvilagus, characteristics,
V1.542 (Tab.)
Herpes zoster *see* Varicella-zoster virus (VZV)
Herpetic stromal keratitis, pathogen induced,
I.753 (Tab.)
Herpetic whitlows, nosocomial infection,
B1.400
Herpid *see* Idoxuridine
Herpotrichiellaceae, **M**.61–3, **M**.359
HERV-K18.1, superantigens, **I**.564
Heteroduplex mobility assay, **V2**.1542
Heterogenous nuclear ribonucleoprotein
(hnRNP) complex proteins, **V1**.137
Heterolactic acid fermentation pathway, **B1**.58
Heterophile-negative infectious
mononucleosis, **V1**.521
Heterophyes, **P**.584
Heterophyidae, **P**.584
Heterothallic fungi, *Histoplasma capsulatum*
var. *capsulatum,* **M**.520
Heterotrophic plate count test for water,
B1.221–2, **B1**.222 (Tab.)
Heterotrophs, in water, **B1**.221–2,
B1.222 (Tab.)
Hexacanth, **P**.576
Hexachlorophane, action, **B1**.437 (Tab.)
Hexokinase, **B1**.50–1
Hexose diphosphate (HDP) pathway, **B1**.50–2,
B1.51 (Fig.)
Entamoeba histolytica, **P**.204
glucose-6-phosphate conversion to
glyceraldehyde-3-phosphate, **B1**.51
glucose phosphorylation, **B1**.50–1
glyceraldehyde-3-phosphate conversion to
pyruvate, **B1**.51–2
intermediates, **B1**.57, **B1**.57 (Fig.)
pentoses conversion to, **B1**.57
pyruvate dehydrogenase complex, **B1**.52
Hexose monophosphate (HMP) pathway,
B1.57–8
Plasmodium, **P**.476
Hexoses, oxidative pathway, **B1**.59–60
Hexylresorcinol, **B1**.430
Hickman catheters, infection, **B1**.391

Hierarchical system, viral classification, **V1**.26,
V1.38–9
High-density lipoproteins (HDLs)
acute phase response, **I**.207
serum amyloid A association, **I**.204–5
High-dose antigen, mucosal tolerance
induction, **I**.542
High efficiency particulate air (HEPA) filters,
B1.763, **B1**.765 (Tab.), **M**.729
filters, **B1**.453
High endothelial venules (HEVs), lymphocyte
extravasation, **I**.503
High frequency of recombination (Hf6–110),
B1.102–3
High-grade squamous intraepithelial lesions
(HGSIL), HPV infection, **V1**.465–6
Highlands J virus (HLV), **V2**.1010,
V2.1011 (Tab.)
Highly active antiretroviral therapy
(HAART), **I**.800–1
cryptococcosis incidence, **M**.644, **M**.651,
M.652, **M**.653
cryptosporidiosis effects, **P**.407, **P**.410
development, **V2**.1606
HCMV infection in AIDS/HIV infection,
V2.1502
HIV therapy, **I**.800–1, **V2**.1336
latency, **V2**.1638–9
in pregnancy, **V2**.1473
immune reconstitution, **I**.799
introduction of, **I**.791
Kaposi's sarcoma therapy, **V1**.553
memory CD4+ T cell effects, **I**.800–1
microsporidiosis, **P**.550
PCP, **M**.764, **M**.783–4
thymus effects, **I**.798
High performance liquid chromatography
(HPLC), **B2**.1242–3
IFN-α purification, **I**.238–41, **I**.240 (Fig.),
I.241 (Fig.), **I**.242 (Fig.)
High-risk human papillomaviruses
(HR-HPVs)
cervical cancer, **V1**.448–9
cervical cancer link, **V1**.459
E6 proteins, **V1**.455–6, **V1**.459
E7 proteins, **V1**.455–6, **V1**.459, **V1**.461
High temperature short time (HTST)
pasteurization, **B1**.232, **B1**.236,
B1.236 (Fig.)
Hilar lymph nodes, histoplasmosis capsulati,
M.534–5
Hinge region, **I**.306
b12 anti-HIV-gp120 monoclonal antibody,
I.319
IgD, **I**.309
IgE structure, **I**.320
Hip joint infection, inflammatory responses,
B1.689
Hippocampus development, Borna disease
virus infection, **V2**.1147–8
Hippocrates, **M**.5
Hippurate hydrolysis, *Legionella,*
B2.1762 (Tab.)
Hirame rhabdovirus, classification, **V1**.385–6
Histamine
basophils, **I**.62, **I**.63–4

effects, **I**.66–7
airway hypersensitivity pathology, **I**.731–2
cytokine production, **I**.66
monocytes, **I**.67
Th2 cell stimulation, **I**.66–7
poisoning, **B1**.252
receptors, **I**.64
signaling, **I**.66–7
release
complement, **I**.62
parasitic infection, **I**.68–9
scombroid poisoning, **B1**.280
Histamine carboxylase, **I**.64
Histamine-releasing factors, **I**.62
Histidine permease system, *Salmonella*
Typhimurium, **B1**.49
Histomonas meleagridis, Dientamoeba fragilis
vs., **P**.266
Histone acetylation, somatic recombination,
I.328–9
Histones, *Trypanosoma brucei,* **P**.361
Histopathological diagnosis, **M**.121–2
defining features, **M**.125
histomorphology, **M**.89 (Tab.), **M**.90–1
identification, **M**.125–30
immunofluorescence, **M**.34, **M**.130–2
immunohistochemistry, **M**.130–2,
M.130 (Tab.)
infection
adiaspiromycosis, **M**.815
aspergillosis, **M**.710–11, **M**.710 (Fig.),
M.711 (Fig.), **M**.717
Blastomyces dermatitidis, **M**.89 (Tab.),
M.491, **M**.492 (Fig.)
candidiasis, **M**.89 (Tab.), **M**.594–5
Coccidioides immitis, **M**.89 (Tab.),
M.510–11, **M**.516
co-infection, **M**.121–2, **M**.142 (Fig.)
Conidiobolus, **M**.351–2
dermatophytes, **M**.89 (Tab.), **M**.128 (Tab.),
M.238
Histoplasma capsulatum var. *capsulatum*
see Histoplasma capsulatum var.
capsulatum
Paracoccidioides brasiliensis, **M**.89 (Tab.),
M.543 (Fig.), **M**.553, **M**.554 (Fig.),
M.555 (Fig.)
penicilliosis marneffei, **M**.567–8
rhinosporidiosis, **M**.462, **M**.463 (Fig.),
M.464 (Fig.), **M**.470
inflammatory response, **M**.127, **M**.130
microscopic evaluation, **M**.121–2
morphology, **M**.125, **M**.126 (Tab.),
M.127 (Tab.)
mycology, **M**.87
stains/staining, **M**.33, **M**.87, **M**.88 (Tab.),
M.122–5
applications, **M**.122, **M**.123 (Tab.)
hosts inflammatory response
determination, **M**.122
limitations, **M**.123 (Tab.), **M**.124
Mucin stains, **M**.123 (Tab.), **M**.124
pigmented fungi, **M**.124
tissue components *vs.,* **M**.122
terminology, **M**.131 (Tab.), **M**.132
see also Specimens, mycology

Histopathology
  Carrión's disease, **B2**.1890–1
  cat-scratch disease diagnosis, **B2**.1898
  opisthorchiasis, **P**.651, **P**.651 (Fig.)
  rabies, **V2**.1122, **V2**.1122 (Fig.)
Histoplasma capsulatum, **M**.519–22
  dimorphism, **M**.22–3, **M**.22 (Fig.), **M**.74
  echinocandin resistance, **M**.154
  Emmonsia, **M**.810 (Tab.), **M**.811, **M**.817, **M**.820
  geographical distribution, **M**.519
  growth, **M**.73
  heat shock proteins, **M**.112
  histopathology, **M**.89 (Tab.)
  history, **M**.22 (Fig.), **M**.23, **M**.519–22
  in HIV infection, **I**.795
  identification
    Gomori's methenamine silver stain, **M**.533–4
    Gridley's fungus stain, **M**.533–4
    hematoxylin and eosin stain, **M**.533–4
    nucleic acid probes, **M**.91
    PCR, **M**.112
    serology, **M**.92
  infection *see* Histoplasmosis
  macrophage dysfunction, **I**.795
  meiotic stage, **M**.24, **M**.811–12, **M**.819–20
  natural history, **M**.519–22
  TNF-α suppression, **I**.652
  varieties, **M**.519
Histoplasma capsulatum var. *capsulatum,* **M**.519, **M**.520
  classification, **M**.520
  Coccidioides immitis vs., **M**.531, **M**.532, **M**.534
  decontamination procedures for, **M**.520
  detection
    complement fixation test, **M**.532
    culture, **M**.532
    exoantigen test, **M**.111
    histopathology, **M**.87 (Fig.), **M**.126 (Tab.), **M**.128 (Tab.), **M**.133 (Fig.), **M**.533–5, **M**.534 (Fig.)
    microscopy, **M**.565, **M**.565 (Fig.), **M**.569
    stains, **M**.122, **M**.124, **M**.125
  Emmonsia, **M**.810 (Tab.)
  geophilism, **M**.520
  historical aspects, **M**.4, **M**.519–22
  infection *see* Histoplasmosis
  macrophage, **M**.525, **M**.526 (Fig.)
  morphology, **M**.126 (Tab.), **M**.526 (Fig.), **M**.527 (Fig.), **M**.535 (Fig.)
    cleistothecia and ascospores, **M**.520
    conversion from mycelial to yeast forms, **M**.521, **M**.525
    dimorphism, **M**.22–3
    saprophytic form, **M**.520
  natural history, **M**.519–22
  NK cell binding, **M**.525–6, **M**.527 (Fig.)
  phagocytosis, **M**.525, **M**.526–7
    by endothelial cells, **M**.526–7, **M**.528 (Fig.)
    neutralization of phagolysosome pH, **M**.525
  relationship with var. *duboisii,* **M**.520–1
  virulence, **M**.525

Histoplasma capsulatum var. *duboisii,* **M**.22–3, **M**.22 (Fig.), **M**.24, **M**.519, **M**.521–2
  geographical distribution, **M**.521
  geophilic nature, **M**.521
  histopathology, **M**.126 (Tab.), **M**.128 (Tab.), **M**.133 (Fig.)
  historical aspects, **M**.521–2
    discovery, **M**.521
  infection *see Histoplasma capsulatum* var. *duboisii,* infection
  isolation and identification, **M**.521
  morphology, **M**.126 (Tab.)
  natural history, **M**.520–2
  relationship with var. *capsulatum,* **M**.520–1
Histoplasma capsulatum var. *duboisii,* infection, **M**.535–7
  aardvarks, **M**.521–2
  AIDS, **M**.535–7
  birds, **M**.535–6
  diagnosis, **M**.537
    histopathology, **M**.537
    radiography, **M**.536
  disseminated, **M**.521, **M**.537, **M**.536 (Fig.)
  host range, **M**.521–2
  incubation period, **M**.522
  oculomycoses, **M**.288, **M**.295
  osteocytic lesions, **M**.536
  serology, **M**.110–11, **M**.112
  subcutaneous abscesses, **M**.536 (Fig.)
  therapy, **M**.537
  see also Histoplasmosis
Histoplasma capsulatum var. *farciminosum,* **M**.22–4, **M**.519
  historical aspects, **M**.522
  infection, **M**.24
    diagnosis, **M**.537
    histopathology, **M**.537
    horses, **M**.522, **M**.536
    ocular, **M**.537
    therapy, **M**.537
    see also Histoplasmosis
  macro-/microconidia, **M**.522
  natural history, **M**.522
Histoplasmin, **M**.93 (Tab.), **M**.111, **M**.532–3
  delayed type hypersensitivity to, **M**.529
  Histoplasma capsulatum var. *capsulatum* detection, **M**.532
  skin test, **M**.111, **M**.532–3
Histoplasmoma, **M**.524–5, **M**.533
Histoplasmosis, **M**.519–40, **M.531–7**
  African, **M**.24
  AIDS (*see* AIDS, concomitant infection)
  animal infection
    birds, **M**.520
    equine cases, **M**.519
  causative agents (*see Histoplasma capsulatum; Histoplasma capsulatum* var. *duboisii*)
  clinical features
    adrenal gland enlargement, **M**.523–4, **M**.524 (Fig.)
    broncholithiasis, **M**.524–5
    cerebritis, **M**.523–4
    granulomas, **M**.533, **M**.534
    heart valves, **M**.535
    hilar lymph nodes, **M**.584–5

  clinical forms, **M**.523–5
  diagnosis, **M**.125–7, **M**.531–7
    culture, **M**.532
    direct examination, **M**.531
    PCR, **M**.94
    samples, **M**.531
    serology (*see below*)
    time course for tests, **M**.533 (Fig.)
  differential diagnosis, **M**.531, **M**.534
  disseminated, **M**.523–4, **M**.524 (Fig.)
    abscesses, **M**.536 (Fig.)
    bone marrow, **M**.532 (Fig.)
    mechanism, **M**.526–7
    therapy, **M**.530–1
  epidemiology, **M**.11, **M**.12, **M**.23, **M**.24
  epizootic lymphangitis, **M**.24
  histopathology, **M**.128 (Tab.), **M**.133 (Fig.), **M**.533–7, **M**.534 (Fig.)
    extrapulmonary, **M**.535
    pulmonary, **M**.533–4
  history, **M**.23–4
  host range, **M**.520
  immune response, **M**.522–31, **M**.525–9
    acquired immunity, **M**.527–8, **M**.529
    antibody-dependent cellular cytotoxicity, **M**.525–6, **M**.529
    CD4 cells, **M**.527–8
    CD8 cells, **M**.527–8
    cell-mediated immune response, **M**.527, **M**.528–9
    delayed-type hypersensitivity, **M**.527, **M**.529
    innate immunity, **M**.525–7
  mediastinal fibrosis, **M**.524, **M**.524 (Fig.)
    therapy, **M**.531
  mediastinal granulomas, **M**.519
    therapy, **M**.520
  oculomycoses, **M**.275 (Tab.), **M**.288, **M**.318, **M**.325
    endophthalmitis, **M**.317
    keratitis, **M**.305
  outbreaks, **M**.520
  pericarditis, **M**.523, **M**.534–5
    therapy, **M**.530
  pulmonary infection, **M**.523, **M**.523 (Fig.)
    calcification, **M**.534
    caseous necrosis, **M**.533–4
    cavitary, **M**.533–4
    chronic, **M**.523, **M**.523 (Fig.)
    granulomas, **M**.533, **M**.534
    recurrent hemoptysis, **M**.524–5
    therapy, **M**.529–30
  resistance to reinfection, **M**.527
  rheumatological syndromes, **M**.523
    therapy, **M**.530
  serology/serological diagnosis, **M**.92, **M**.93 (Tab.), **M**.110–11, **M**.110–12, **M**.111–12, **M**.532–3
    antibody assays, **M**.111–12
    antigen detection, **M**.112
    EIAs, **M**.532
  specimen site selection, **M**.83 (Tab.)
  therapy, **M**.529–31, **M**.530 (Tab.)
    amphotericin B, **M**.529–30, **M**.530 (Tab.), **M**.531
    fluconazole, **M**.531

Histoplasmosis (*Continued*)
  vaccine development, **M**.529
    heat shock proteins, **M**.529
    ribosomes, **M**.527
'Histoplasmosis duboisis,' **M**.521
History
  of bacteriology, **B1**.3
    19th century, **B1**.8 (Tab.)
    20th century, **B1**.9 (Tab.), **B1**.10
    classification/discovery, **B1**.8 (Tab.),
      B1.9 (Tab.), **B1**.11, **B1**.13
      Actinomyces, **B2**.1005–6
      Arcobacter, **B2**.1553–4
      Campylobacter, **B2**.1541–2
      Citrobacter, **B2**.1474–5
      Clostridium, **B2**.1089–90
      Edwardsiella, **B2**.1491
      Enterobacter, **B2**.1474–5
      Escherichia, **B2**.1360
      Klebsiella, **B2**.1477
      Lactobacillus, **B2**.863
      Legionella, **B2**.1761–4
      Listeria, **B2**.953–4
      Serratia, **B2**.1487
      Shigella, **B2**.1386
      Staphylococcus, **B2**.771–2
      Streptococcus, **B2**.833–5
    communicable disease, **B1**.4
    culture, **B1**.6, **B1**.9–11
    definitions, **B1**.10–1
    fermentation and putrefaction, **B1**.4–5
    filters, **B1**.8–9
    genetics, **B1**.12–4
    immunity, **B1**.7–8
    macromolecules, **B1**.12
    nonmedical applications, **B1**.9–10
    pathogenic bacteria, **B1**.5–9
    staining, **B1**.6–7
    theory of infectious disease transmission,
      B1.336–8
    see also individual species; specific diseases/
      infection
  of fungi, **M**.4–6
    medical mycology, **M**.30–3
  of immunology, **I**.5–18
    computer technology, **I**.9
    empirical view, **I**.11–2
    infection *vs.* hereditary disease, **I**.9
    innate response reassessment, **I**.9
    molecular biology, **I**.9–11
    'new age' of infection/immunity, **I**.7–9
    postmodern perspective, **I**.16–7
    primoinfection, **I**.9
    'return' of infectious diseases, **I**.6–7
    selective theory, **I**.9
    unification mechanisms, **I**.12–4
  of parasitology, **P**.3–23
    helminth infection, **P**.4–5, **P**.5–13
    phases, **P**.5
    protozoal infection, **P**.4–5, **P**.13–8
    protozoology, **P**.189–90
    see also individual species
  virus research, **V1**.3–10
    antiviral therapy, **V1**.9 (Tab.)
    classification of viruses, **V1**.7–8

  discovery of viruses, **V1**.3
  host range and pathogenicity, **V1**.4
  immune response, **V1**.4
  immunization, **V1**.8 (Tab.)
  propagation, **V1**.3–4, **V1**.4–5
  quantification of viruses, **V1**.4
  virus properties, **V1**.5–7
HIV, **I**.789, **V2**.1322–45
  antiretroviral resistance, **V2**.1333–6
    mechanisms, **V2**.1336–8
    nonnucleoside reverse transcriptase
      inhibitors, **V2**.1336
    point mutations, **V2**.1337 (Fig.)
  antiviral susceptibility testing, **V2**.1543
  basic reproduction number, **B1**.340 (Tab.)
  budding, **V2**.1324
  CA protein, **V1**.78–9, **V1**.78 (Fig.),
    V2.1323–4
  capsid, **V1**.78–9, **V1**.78 (Fig.)
  CCR5 binding, **I**.227–8
  cell culture, **V2**.1539
  cell interactions, host RNA processing/
    transport, **V1**.221
  cell receptors, **V1**.207, **V1**.207 (Tab.),
    V1.246–7, **V1**.246 (Fig.), **V1**.247 (Fig.),
    V2.1426–7
    antibody-mediated enhancement, **V1**.211
    CD4, **V1**.207, **V1**.209, **V1**.246–7,
      V1.246 (Fig.), **V1**.247 (Fig.), **I**.389,
      V2.1323
    coreceptors *see below*
    galactosyl ceramide, **V1**.209, **V2**.1426–7
    gp120, **V1**.246–7
  cellular entry, **V1**.106, **V1**.211–12, **V2**.1323
    fusin, **V1**.212
    GAG polyprotein cleavage, **V1**.58–9
    inhibition by antibody, **V1**.277
    plasma membrane fusion, **V1**.108
  characteristics, **V1**.135
  chemokines, **I**.227–8
  coreceptors, **V1**.247, **V1**.247 (Fig.), **V2**.1323
    CCR5, **V1**.247, **V1**.247 (Fig.), **V1**.253,
      V2.1323
    CXCR4, **V1**.106, **I**.227–8, **V1**.247, **V1**.253,
      I.584–5, **V2**.1323
  defensin actions, **I**.168
  description, **B1**.435–6
  diversity, clinical impact, **V2**.1331–2
  Env glycoproteins, **V2**.1323–4
  fusion protein, **V1**.214
  Gag polyprotein, **V1**.78–9, **V2**.1323–4
  gene expression, **V2**.1407
  genetically-engineered cell culture, **V1**.88
  genetic variation, **V2**.1330
    enzyme infidelity, **V2**.1330
    mutation rate, **V2**.1330, **V2**.1336–7
    recombination, **V2**.1330
  genome, **I**.789, **V2**.1322–4
  gp41, **V1**.77, **V2**.1323–4
    peptide vaccines, **I**.871
  gp120, **I**.62, **V1**.77, **V1**.207
    peptide vaccines, **I**.871
    synthesis, **V2**.1323–4
    toxicity to CNS, **V2**.1428
  gp160, **V1**.77, **I**.862 (Tab.)
  historical aspects, **V2**.1322

  host susceptibility, **V1**.265, **V1**.265 (Tab.)
  immune evasion, **V1**.282
    CD8 interference *in vivo*, **I**.636–7
    chemokines, **V1**.319, **I**.621–2
    complement, **V1**.287, **V1**.313, **I**.639
    factor H, **I**.639
    IFN effector functions, **V1**.315, **I**.619
    MHC, **V1**.322, **I**.472, **I**.636, **I**.796,
      V2.1327–8
    mutation, **V1**.286
    NK cell interference, **I**.629–30
  inactivation
    biocide sensitivity, **B1**.434
    UV radiation, **B1**.451
  infection of CD4- astroglial cells, **V2**.1426–7
  killer cell Ig receptor, **I**.793
  long terminal repeats (LTR), neurovirulence
    and tropism, **V2**.1406–7
  macrophage mannose receptor, **I**.795
  macrophage-tropic, **V1**.247 (Fig.), **V1**.253,
    V1.253 (Tab.), **V1**.273
  mannose-binding lectin interaction, **V1**.273
  MA protein, **V1**.78–9, **V2**.1323–4
  molecular detection, **B1**.721, **B1**.723 (Tab.)
    microarrays, **B1**.736
    nucleic acid sequence-based amplification,
      B1.729–30
    nucleic acid sequencing, **B1**.732, **B1**.733–4
    nucleic amplification methods, **V2**.1537
    quantification, **B1**.722–4
    specimen suitability, **B1**.724
  morphology/structure, **V1**.70 (Tab.)
  Nef protein, **I**.789, **V2**.1329
    CD4 downregulation, **V2**.1329
    integrin signal transduction, **V2**.1326
    lymphocyte activation, **I**.789
    MHC class I downregulation, **I**.789, **I**.793
    pathogenicity effects, **V2**.1329
    regulatory functions, **V2**.1326
    T-cell activation, **V2**.1329
    N-terminal myristolaytion, **V1**.122
    virion incorporation, **V2**.1329
  nucleocapsid (NC), **V1**.77–9, **V1**.78 (Fig.),
    V2.1323–4
  p6^Gag protein, **V2**.1323–4
  pol gene, **V2**.1336–7
  Pol polyprotein, **V1**.78
  regulator proteins, **V2**.1326
    see also specific proteins
  replication, **V2**.1322–4, **V2**.1335 (Fig.)
    cell entry *see above*
    cell specificity, **V2**.1323
    cellular factors, **V2**.1324–6
    cyclophilin A (CypA), **V2**.1324–5
    dynamics, **V2**.1329–30
    GM-CSF, **V1**.300
    IFN effects, **V1**.300–1
    IL-1, **V1**.300
    M-CSF, **V1**.300
    preintegration complex (PIC), **V2**.1323
    Th1/Th2 balance, **V1**.300–1
    TNF-α, **V1**.300
  reverse transcriptase complex (RTC),
    V2.1323
  Rev protein, **V2**.1326

HIV (*Continued*)
rev-response element, **V1**.221
Tat protein, **I**.789, **V2**.1326
vaccine development, **I**.941
T-cell-tropism, **V1**.247 (Fig.), **V1**.253, **V1**.253 (Tab.)
transmission
blood transfusions, **B1**.380–1
to healthcare staff, **B1**.382
needle contamination, **I**.819–20
ubiquitin proteasome system (UPS), **V2**.1323
viral budding, **V2**.1325
Vif (virus infectivity factor) phosphoprotein, **V2**.1328
apolipoprotein B mRNA editing enzyme (APOBEC3G), **V2**.1325–6, **V2**.1328
infectivity regulation, **V2**.1328
regulatory functions, **V2**.1326
virion assembly, **V2**.1328
Vpr (viral protein R), **V2**.1323, **V2**.1326–7
G$_2$ phase arrest, **V2**.1326–7
host cell interaction, **V2**.1325
nuclear targeting, **V2**.1326–7
nucleoplasmic shuttling, **V2**.1327
regulatory functions, **V2**.1326
structure, **V2**.1327
see also HIV-1; HIV-2
HIV-1
antigenic variation, **V1**.262
antiviral resistance, detection, **V1**.194
circulating recombinant forms (CRFs), **V2**.1330–1
classification, **V2**.1322–3
CNS receptors, **V2**.1406 (Tab.)
ELISA, HIV-2 *vs.,* **V2**.1331
emerging infection, **V2**.1648 (Tab.)
species-barrier crossing, **V2**.1657 (Tab.)
gene therapy vector, **V2**.1592–3
genetics, HIV-2 *vs.,* **V2**.1331
gp120, neutralizing antibodies, **V2**.1332–3
infection, perinatal transmission, **V2**.1471
mutations, **V1**.17–8
antiretroviral inhibitor resistance, **V1**.19
recombination, **V1**.188–9
'species-jumping,' **V2**.1657
subtypes, **V2**.1330–1
geographical distribution, **V2**.1331, **V2**.1331 (Fig.)
Main (M), **V2**.1330–1
Non-M-Non-O (N), **V2**.1330–1
Outlier (O), **V2**.1330–1
vaccine development effects, **V2**.1332–3
variability, **V2**.1332–3
variant form evolution, **V1**.15
Vpr protein, **V2**.1327
Vpu protein, **V2**.1327–8
CD4 degradation, **V2**.1327–8
Fas-mediated apoptosis, **V2**.1327–8
ion channel interaction, **V2**.1326
MHC class I interference, **V2**.1327–8
regulatory functions, **V2**.1326
structure, **V2**.1328
HIV-2
classification, **V2**.1322–3
CNS receptors, **V2**.1406 (Tab.)

ELISA, HIV-1 *vs.,* **V2**.1331
emerging infection, **V2**.1648 (Tab.)
species-barrier crossing, **V2**.1657 (Tab.)
gene therapy vector, **V2**.1592–3
genetics, HIV-1 *vs.,* **V2**.1331
perinatal transmission, **V2**.1471
'species-jumping,' **V2**.1657
Vpx protein, **V2**.1327
HIV-exposed but persistently HIV-sero-negative subjects (HEPS), **V2**.1333
vaccine development, **V2**.1333
HIV infection, **V1**.298–301, **I**.788 (Tab.), **I**.789–801
antiretroviral therapy, **V2**.1333–6, **V2**.1334 (Tab.), **V2**.1335 (Fig.), **V2**.1619–21
Combined Antiretroviral Therapy (CART), **V2**.1330, **V2**.1333–4, **V2**.1336
HAART *see* Highly active antiretroviral therapy (HAART)
multiple resistance, **V2**.1636
in pregnancy, **V2**.1473
protease inhibitors, **V2**.1336
resistance, **V2**.1636
reverse transcriptase inhibitors, **V2**.1334–6
see also specific drugs
autoimmunity in, **V2**.1428
B cells, **I**.795–6
activation, **I**.795
B-cell lymphoma generation, **I**.795–6
memory cell loss, **I**.795
mucosa, **I**.799–800
CD4+ T-cells, **V1**.242, **V1**.281, **V1**.299, **I**.790 (Fig.), **I**.791–3
activation-induced cell death, **I**.792
apoptosis, **I**.791–2
cytopathicity, **I**.791
cytotoxicity, **I**.791
dysfunction, **I**.791
impaired production, **I**.792–3
infection, **V1**.299
migration patterns, **I**.792
mucosa, **I**.799–800
opportunistic infection *vs.,* **I**.800 (Fig.)
CD8+ T-cells, **V1**.281, **I**.793–4
cell markers, **I**.793
impaired maturation, **I**.793
MHC binding, **I**.793
mucosa, **I**.799–800
reduced homing, **I**.793
cells
basophils, **I**.55, **I**.70–1
B cells *see above*
dendritic cells, **I**.794
eosinophils, **I**.55, **I**.71
intraepithelial lymphocytes, **I**.799–800
lamina propria lymphocytes, **I**.799
macrophages, **I**.794–5
monocytes *see* Monocyte(s)
neutrophils, **I**.796
NK cells, **I**.96, **I**.796, **I**.799–800
T cells
assessment, **V2**.1544–5
CD4+ T-cells *see above*
CD8+ T-cells *see above*
γδ T cells, **I**.796–7

Th1/Th2 ratio, **V1**.298
in children, **V2**.1472–3
clinical course, **I**.789–91
acute phase, **V1**.299
cell-associated viremia, **V1**.242
chronic asymptomatic phase, **I**.790
clinical latency, **V1**.299
cutaneous manifestations, **I**.790
HIV-exposed but persistently HIV-sero-negative subjects (HEPS), **V2**.1333
incubation period, **V2**.1656
morbidity, **P**.26 (Fig.)
p24 antigen-capture assay, **I**.790
PCR, **I**.790
persistent, **V1**.373
primary infection, **I**.789–90
'rapid progressors,' **I**.790
seroconversion rates, cohort study, **B1**.314
seronegativity, **I**.790
'slow progressors,' **I**.790
viremia, **V2**.1329–30
of CNS, **V2**.1426–8
autoimmunity, **V2**.1428
CD4- astroglial cells, **V2**.1426–7
clinical features, **V2**.1427–8
cytokines produced, **V2**.1428
encephalopathy, **V2**.1427 (Fig.)
immune response, **V2**.1413
mechanisms of CNS disturbances, **V2**.1428
neurovirulence, **V2**.1407
pathology, **V2**.1408, **V2**.1427 (Fig.), **V2**.1428
route, **V2**.1426–7
toxic HIV products, **V2**.1428
coinfection, **V2**.1498–504, **V2**.1499 (Tab.)
CD4+ T cell numbers *vs.,* **I**.800 (Fig.)
in children, **V2**.1504–6
HAART, **V2**.1498
see also HIV infection, concommitant infection; *specific infection*
control, **V2**.1473
behavioral changes, **V2**.1659
measles vaccination, **V1**.736
vaccine development *see below*
cytokines, **V1**.299–301, **I**.791, **I**.797
IFN-α, **V1**.295, **V1**.299, **V1**.302 (Fig.)
IFN-β, **V1**.299, **I**.797
IFN-γ, **V1**.299, **I**.793, **I**.797
IL-1, **V1**.296–7, **V1**.299
IL-2, **I**.797
IL-4, **V1**.298, **V1**.301, **I**.793, **I**.797
IL-5, **I**.793
IL-6, **V1**.297, **V1**.299
IL-7, **I**.797
IL-8, **V1**.299
IL-10, **I**.797
IL-12, **V1**.298, **I**.797
IL-15, **I**.797
IL-16, **I**.793, **I**.797
replication down-regulation, **V1**.300–1
replication up-regulation, **V1**.299–300
TNF-α, **V1**.299
transforming growth factor-β (TGF-β), **V1**.298–9, **V1**.301

HIV infection (*Continued*)

diagnosis

diversity effects, **V2**.1331–2

ELISA *see* Enzyme-linked immunosorbent assay (ELISA)

dynamics, **V2**.1279 (Tab.)

emerging infection, **V2**.1648 (Tab.)

entry/invasion of host, **V1**.237, **V2**.1426–7

epidemiology, **V1**.370

case-finding, **B1**.347

modeling approaches, **B1**.337–8

models, **V1**.370

prevalence, **V2**.1656 (Fig.)

transmission *see below*

fetal infection, **V2**.1444 (Tab.), **V2**.1471–2, **V2**.1471–4

diagnosis, **V2**.1472

gastrointestinal mucosa, **I**.799–800

immune activation, **I**.799

mucosal immunodeficiency, **I**.799–800

'giant ulcer,' **I**.799

health services, planning/costing, **B1**.323

historical aspects, **I**.789

immune reconstitution, **I**.800–1

immune response, **V1**.281

assessment, **V2**.1544

CD4 T cell infection, **V1**.281, **V2**.1498

CD8+ T cell responses, **V1**.281

complement activation, **V2**.1413

cytokines *see above*

inflammatory response, **V1**.299

secretory IgA, **I**.799–800

viral production *vs.,* **V2**.1330

immunodeficiency in, **V1**.341

immunogenetics, **I**.584–6

HLA polymorphisms, **I**.586

latency, HAART (HAART), **V2**.1638–9

lymphadenopathy, **I**.797

lymph nodes, **I**.797–8

germinal centers, **I**.797–8

lymphadenopathy, **I**.797

reservoir, **I**.797–8

mortality, **P**.26 (Fig.), **P**.29 (Tab.)

Mx proteins, **V1**.301

neonatal infection, **V2**.1444 (Tab.), **V2**.1471–2

asymptomatic, **V2**.1471–2

diagnosis, **V2**.1472–3, **V2**.1546–7

management, **V2**.1473–4

2'-5' oligo adenylate synthetase, **V1**.301

oncogenic mechanisms, **V1**.342 (Tab.)

oxidative burst, **I**.796

pandemic, impact on tuberculosis, **B2**.1199

pathogenicity, **V1**.298–9

diversity effects, **V2**.1332

phagocytosis, **I**.795, **I**.796

in pregnancy, **V2**.1444 (Tab.)

antiretroviral therapy, **V2**.1473

delivery, **V2**.1473

diagnosis, **V2**.1472

effects of, **V2**.1471

infant transmission, **V2**.1471

management, **V2**.1473

perinatal transmission, **V2**.1471

transmission routes, **V2**.1471

prevalence studies, **B1**.313–14, **B1**.314 (Fig.)

protection

CCR2b gene deletions, **I**.585

CCR5 gene deletions, **I**.585

CCR5 polymorphisms, **V1**.265, **I**.585

SDF1 gene point mutations, **I**.586

protein kinase R (PKR) activation, **V1**.301

replication, **V1**.298–9

RNaseL, **V1**.301

routine serological surveillance, **B1**.321–2

TCR signaling, **I**.793

therapy

antiretroviral therapy *see above*

azole antifungals in, **M**.152

chemokine blocking, **I**.231

IL-2, **I**.280

thymus, **I**.792–3, **I**.798–9

dysplasia, **I**.798

immune reconstitution, **I**.799

precocious involution, **I**.798

target cells, **I**.798–9

thymitis, **I**.798

transmission, **V1**.370

diversity effects, **V2**.1332

epidemiological modeling, **V1**.365

occupational exposure, **B1**.767, **B1**.767 (Tab.)

gloves protection, **B1**.765

needle stick injury and risk, **B1**.767, **B1**.767 (Tab.)

sexual, **V1**.237, **V1**.239

sexual contact, **V1**.370

vaccine development, **V1**.349, **I**.839, **I**.933 (Tab.), **V2**.1332–3

attenuated viral vectors, **I**.846, **I**.898

BCE peptide vaccines *see* Peptide vaccines

BCG vector, **I**.845

development status, **I**.933 (Tab.)

DNA vaccines, **I**.920–1, **V2**.1333, **V2**.1554

escape mutants, **V2**.1332

historical aspects/re-evaluation, **I**.16

HIV-exposed but persistently HIV-sero-negative subjects (HEPS), **V2**.1333

intranasal route, **I**.832

Listeria vector, **I**.845

live attenuated viral carriers, **V2**.1333

live vaccines, **I**.903

attenuated viral vectors, **I**.846, **I**.898

BCG vectors, **I**.845

delivery route, **I**.904

Vibrio cholerae vectors, **I**.843–4

MF59 adjuvant, **I**.929

MPL/QS-21 adjuvant, **I**.930

neutralizing antibodies, **V2**.1332

'prime-boost immunization,' **I**.846

subtype range, **V2**.1332

subunit vaccine development, **I**.938, **I**.941

Tat protein, **I**.941

trials, **V2**.1333

Vibrio cholerae vectors, **I**.843–4

virosomes, **I**.839

virus-like particles, **I**.841

see also AIDS

HIV infection, concomitant infection

Balantidium coli infection, **P**.279–80

cryptosporidiosis, **P**.45, **P**.409

cyclosporiasis, **P**.45, **P**.414, **P**.415–16

Entamoeba gingivalis infection, **P**.221

enteric infection, **V2**.1504

gastrointestinal nematode infection, **P**.730

Hepatitis C virus, **V2**.1478–9

Hepatitis G virus, **V2**.1482

HTLV, **I**.803

malaria, **P**.494–5, **P**.513

microsporidiosis, **P**.45, **P**.537, **P**.539

ocular, **P**.540–1

oropharyngeal candidiasis, **M**.256, **M**.262–3

parasitic infection association, **P**.97

see also individual infection

Pneumocystis carinii, **I**.795

Strongyloides, **P**.739–40

toxoplasmosis, **I**.677

tuberculosis, **I**.592–3

HLA *see* Human leukocyte antigens (HLAs)

HLA-A

EBV infection association, **I**.588

HIV infection association, **I**.586

HLA-A9, tuberculosis association, **I**.592

HLA-A11, leprosy association, **I**.590–1

HLA-A26, leishmaniasis association, **I**.597

HLA-A30, Chagas disease association, **I**.597

HLA-B

EBV infection association, **I**.588

HIV infection association, **I**.586

HPV infection association, **I**.588

HLA-B5, malaria association, **I**.598

HLA-B14, tuberculosis association, **I**.592

HLA-B27

ankylosing spondylitis association, **I**.577, **I**.594–5, **I**.752, **I**.752 (Tab.)

reactive arthritis association, **I**.752, **I**.752 (Tab.)

HLA-B40, schistosomiasis association, **I**.601

HLA-B53, malaria association, **I**.598–9

HLA-C, HIV infection association, **I**.586

HLA-DB, hepatitis C association, **I**.587–8

HLA-DM, antigen processing/presentation, **I**.383

HLA-DPA1, nematode infection association, **I**.600–1

HLA-DPB1 association, tuberculosis, **I**.592

HLA-DP, schistosomiasis association, **I**.601

HLA-DQ

diabetes mellitus type I association, **I**.752, **I**.758

nematode infection association, **I**.600–1

schistosomiasis association, **I**.601

HLA-DQA1

Helicobacter pylori infection association, **I**.594

hepatitis Bs association, **I**.587

tuberculosis association, **I**.592

HLA-DQB1

diabetes mellitus type I association, **I**.577

Helicobacter pylori infection association, **I**.594

hepatitis B association, **I**.587

hepatitis C association, **I**.587–8

malaria association, **I**.598

tuberculosis association, **I**.592

HLA-DQB1 (Continued)
  variant Creutzfeldt–Jakob disease
    association, **I**.589
HLA-DQw1, leprosy association, **I**.590–1
HLA-DR
  autoimmune disease association, **I**.751
  diabetes mellitus type I association, **I**.752,
    I.752 (Tab.)
  multiple sclerosis association, **I**.751–2,
    I.752 (Tab.)
  reactive arthritis association, **I**.752 (Tab.)
  rheumatoid arthritis association, **I**.751,
    I.752 (Tab.)
  schistosomiasis association, **I**.601
  SLE association, **I**.758
HLA-DR2
  hepatitis B association, **I**.587
  leprosy association, **I**.590–1
  subdivisions, **I**.576–7
  tuberculosis association, **I**.592
HLA-DR3
  diabetes mellitus type I association, **I**.577
  hepatitis C association, **I**.588
  leprosy association, **I**.590–1
  tuberculosis association, **I**.592
HLA-DR4
  diabetes mellitus type I association, **I**.577
  hepatitis C association, **I**.588
HLA-DR5, hepatitis C association, **I**.587–8
HLA-DR6, hepatitis B association, **I**.587
HLA-DR7
  hepatitis B association, **I**.587
  hepatitis C association, **I**.588
HLA-DRB1
  Chagas disease association, **I**.597
  hepatitis B association, **I**.587
  hepatitis C association, **I**.587–8
  leprosy association, **I**.591
  malaria association, **I**.598–9
HLA-DRB5, malaria association, **I**.598
HLA-E, CD8+ T-cells interactions, **I**.443–5,
  I.444 (Fig.)
HMPC *see* Cidofovir
Hodgkin's disease
  EBV infection, **V1**.566 (Tab.), **V1**.571
  immunodeficiency, **I**.788 (Tab.)
Holoenzyme, **B1**.74
Homobasidiomycetes, **M**.63
Homolactic acid fermentation, **B1**.54,
  B1.54 (Fig.)
Homologous serum jaundice, **V2**.1160
Homology-guided recombination, TCR
  rearrangements, **I**.452–3
Homosexuals, amebic infection, **P**.213
Homothetogenic fission, **P**.181, **P**.183 (Fig.)
Honey, infant botulism, **B2**.1069–70
'Honeymoon period,' vaccination, **B1**.346,
  B1.346 (Fig.), **I**.960
Hooke, R, **M**.6, **M**.20
Hookworm(s), **P**.589
  egg morphology, **P**.716 (Fig.), **P**.717
  epidemiology, **P**.46 (Tab.)
  historical aspects, **P**.8–9
  life cycle, **P**.717
  mortality, **P**.28 (Tab.), **P**.29 (Tab.), **P**.42
  transmission, **P**.89

see also Ancylostoma duodenale; Necator
  americanus
Hookworm infection
  clinical manifestations, **P**.727–8
    cognitive performance, **P**.728
    gender effects, **P**.728
    iron-deficiency anemia, **P**.725, **P**.727–8,
      P.727 (Fig.)
    worker productivity, **P**.728
  control, **P**.130
  diagnosis, **P**.149–50
    culture, **P**.151
    immunological methods, **P**.154
  epidemiology/population biology
    age-related prevalence, **P**.722, **P**.722 (Fig.)
    infection predisposition, **P**.724
    intensity, **P**.723–4, **P**.723 (Fig.)
    number of worms per host, **P**.724,
      P.724 (Fig.)
  immune response, **P**.90, **P**.729–30
  public health importance, **P**.105 (Tab.)
Hop protein family, *Helicobacter,* **B2**.1569
Hordevirus, **V1**.27 (Tab.)
Horizontal transmission, plasmid genes, **B1**.110
Hormones
  changes, acute phase response *see* Acute
    phase response
  cytokines *vs.,* **I**.273, **I**.274 (Fig.)
Horses
  Actinobacillus infection, **B2**.1665–6
  bites *see* Bites
  botulism, **B2**.1074
  habronemiasis, **M**.412–13
  histoplasmosis, **M**.519, **M**.522, **M**.536
  pythiosis, **M**.412–13
  rhinosporidiosis, **M**.456–7, **M**.472
Hortaea, **M**.199
Hortaea (Phaeoannellomyces) werneckii,
  M.195, **M**.199, **M**.199 (Fig.)
  ecology, **M**.199
  genetic analysis, **M**.199
  histopathology, **M**.89 (Tab.)
  phylogeny, **M**.199
Horticulture, **M**.368, **M**.376
Hospital-acquired infection *see* Nosocomial
  infection
Hospital Episode Statistics, **B1**.321
Hospitals, **B1**.433
  bacterial evolution, **B1**.30
  cleaners, **M**.706
  data collection, **B1**.321
  handwashing, **B1**.766–7
  infection *see* Nosocomial infection
  worker infection, **M**.238–9, **M**.706
Host–bacteria interactions
  colonization, factors affecting, **B1**.294
  disease or transient/prolonged colonization,
    B1.294
  factors affecting, **B1**.294–5
  response to infection, **B1**.310
Host cell penetration, microsporidiosis, **P**.531
Host factors, affecting CNS infection
  development, **V2**.1406–7
Host genetic factors
  epidemiology effects, **P**.55, **P**.56–7
  gastrointestinal nematode infection, **P**.725

schistosomiasis predisposition, **P**.55
Host initiation factor cleavage, **V1**.115–16
Host molecule incorporation, immune evasion,
  I.684
Host population stratification, microparasite
  epidemiology, **P**.51
Host range
  historical aspects, **V1**.4
  Mononegavirales order, **V1**.381–2
  parvoviruses, **V1**.422–3
  respirovirus fusion (F) protein, **V1**.766–8
  restriction
    influenza viruses, **V1**.652–3, **V1**.653–5,
      V1.666–7
    papillomavirus infection, **V1**.451
Host RNA polymerase II, Hepatitis delta virus
  replication, **V2**.1270
Hosts
  definitive *see* Definitive hosts
  intermediate *see* Intermediate hosts
  see individual species
Host-specific tropism, bacterial adherence,
  B1.147–8
Host tissues, bacterial infiltration, **B1**.152–3
Host transcript recombination, **V1**.190–1
Hot-water heaters/systems, airborne bacteria,
  B1.186 (Tab.)
HPr protein, **B1**.50
hTERT, papillomavirus E6 protein effects,
  V1.460 (Tab.)
HTLV *see* Human T-cell leukemia viruses
  (HTLV)
HTLV-1 *see* Human T-cell leukemia virus 1
  (HTLV-1)
HTLV-2 *see* Human T-cell leukemia virus 2
  (HTLV-2)
HTLV-associated arthropathy (HAA),
  V2.1290–1
HTLV-associated myelopathy(HAM)/tropical
  spastic paraparesis (TSP), **I**.802,
  V2.1289, **V2**.1290, **V2**.1429–30
  antivirals, **V2**.1290
  CD8+ T cells, **V2**.1290
  chemokines, **V2**.1429–30
  clinical features, **V2**.1429
  corticosteroid therapy, **V2**.1290
  cytokines, **V2**.1429–30
  experimental model, **V2**.1430
  IFN-α therapy, **V2**.1292
  pathogenesis/pathology, **V2**.1429–30
  prevalence and host factors affecting,
    V2.1406–7
HTLV-associated uveitis (HU), **V2**.1290
HtrA2/Omni, mitochondria apoptosis, **I**.132
HtrA gene, **I**.842
HtrA stress-induced protein, **B2**.1736
Hülle cells, **M**.666–7
Human adenovirus
  origin recognition proteins, **V1**.149 (Tab.)
  viral proteins, **V1**.149 (Tab.)
Human adenovirus 2, **V1**.68 (Fig.)
Human adenovirus C, **V1**.45
Human anaplasmosis *see Anaplasma*
  phagocytophilum (Ehrlichia
  phagocytophilia), infection (human
  anaplasmosis)

Human anti-mouse antibody response
(HAMA), I.362
Human astrovirus (HAstV)
cell culture, V2.889, V2.906
classification, V2.890 (Tab.)
electron microscopy, V2.890–1
genome, V2.894 (Tab.)
frameshift signal, V2.894 (Fig.)
sequencing, V2.892–3, V2.899
prevalence, V2.901–2
replication, V2.894–5
seroconversion, V2.901–2
serotypes, V2.899
virion-associated proteins, V2.891–2
Human astrovirus 1, V1.53
Human behavior
epidemiology effects, P.54–7
schistosomiasis predisposition, P.54–5,
P.56 (Fig.)
Human chorionic gonadotrophin (hCG),
I.875
Human coronavirus (HCoV), V1.824–5
genome structure, V1.828 (Fig.)
hemagglutinin-esterase (HE), V1.838–9
infection see Human coronavorus (HCoV)
infection
nsp15, V1.834
replicase (RNA polymerase), V1.833 (Fig.)
Human coronavirus 229E, V1.207 (Tab.)
Human coronavirus OC43, V1.207 (Tab.)
Human coronavorus (HCoV) infection,
V1.841–3, V1.841 (Tab.)
diagnosis, V1.842
immune response, V1.841–2
incubation period, V1.841–2
lower respiratory tract, V1.841–2
seasonality, V1.841–2
Human cytomegalovirus (HCMV), V1.520–7
adeno-associated virus replication, V1.160
characteristics, V1.489 (Tab.)
CNS receptors, V2.1406 (Tab.)
detection
cytospinning, V2.1540–1
nucleic amplification methods, V2.1537
genome sequences, V1.494 (Tab.)
genome structure, V1.493, V1.493 (Fig.)
immediate/early promoter, DNA vaccines,
I.910
immune evasion
antibody, V1.287
antigen processinf/presentation,
V1.229–30, I.633
apoptosis mitochondrial pathways,
V1.324–5
chemokine receptors, V1.319–20, I.622
chemokines, I.621–2
complement, V1.287, V1.313, I.639
cytokines, V1.318
dendritic cells, V1.323, I.632
leukocyte Ig-like receptors, I.630
MHC, V1.287, V1.322, I.634, I.637
MHC expression, I.472
mitochondrial apoptosis inhibitors, I.627
NK cells, V1.322–3, I.628, I.629
receptor homologues, V1.318, I.620–1

infection see Human cytomegalovirus
(HCMV) infection
isolation/propagation and isolation, V1.98
shell vial culture, V1.87
molecular detection, B1.723 (Tab.)
hybrid capture assay, B1.731
nucleic acid sequence-based amplification,
B1.729–30
organ transplants, aspergillosis risk factors,
M.701
origin of replication, V1.500
phosphoprotein 65 (pp65), V1.524–5
phosphoprotein 150 (pp150), V1.524–5
superantigens, I.563–4
Human cytomegalovirus (HCMV) infection
acute infection, V1.521 (Tab.)
in AIDS/HIV infection see AIDS,
concomitant infection
antiviral therapy, V1.526–7, V2.1618–19
fomivirsen therapy, V2.1618–19
ganciclovir, V2.1613
maribavir (1263W94) therapy, V2.1619
resistance, V2.1636
valganciclovir, V2.1619
chronic infection, V1.521 (Tab.)
clinical course, NK cells, I.94–5, I.97–9
binding interference, I.97–9
deficiencies, I.772
LY49 receptors, I.97
clinical manifestations, V1.521–2,
V1.521 (Tab.), V2.1502
atherosclerosis association, V1.521
cytomegalic inclusion disease (CID),
V1.521
heterophile-negative infectious
mononucleosis, V1.521
multi-organ disease, V1.520–1
congenital disease, V2.1447, V2.1448–9
asymptomatic infection, V2.1449
clinical manifestations, V2.1448–9,
V2.1449 (Tab.)
consecutive pregnancies, V2.1448
diagnosis, V2.1449
future measures, V2.1453
mental deficiencies, V2.1448–9
public health impact, V2.1453–4
sequelae, V2.1449 (Tab.)
control, V1.526–7
antiviral therapy see above
Ig prophylaxis (CMV IVIG) see below
vaccines see below
diagnosis, V1.525–6, V2.1507
cytopathology, V2.1534 (Tab.)
DNA detection, V1.526
early infection detection, V1.525, V1.526
PCR, V1.526
recent vs. past infection, V1.526
serology, V2.1547
epidemiology, V1.520–3
body fluid transmission, V1.522
fetal infection, V1.523
immune deficits, V1.522–3
intravenous drug users, V2.1502
neonates, V1.521
perinatal infection, V2.1450
postnatal infection, V2.1450

FcγRIII (CD16), I.772
fetal infection, V1.523, V2.1444 (Tab.),
V2.1446–54
abortion, V2.1447
diagnosis, V2.1451
immune response, V2.1448
leukocytes, V2.1448
pathogenesis, V2.1448
primary maternal infection, V2.1447
recurrent maternal infection, V2.1447–8
transovarian transmission, V2.1448
twin pregnancies, V2.1448
Ig prophylaxis (CMV IVIG), V2.1567 (Tab.)
organ transplants, V2.1566–7
prophylaxis in pregnancy, V2.1452
immune response, V1.524–5
antibody responses, V1.524, V1.525
cell-mediated, V1.524
chemokines, I.228
IFN-α, V1.295
IFN-γ, V1.524–5
IL-1, V1.296–7
immunodeficient patients (non-HIV),
V2.1507
immunogenetics, I.588–9
latent infection, V1.260, V1.520–1, V2.1446
macrophage infection, V1.273
medical importance, V1.162, V2.1582
mortality, V1.521
neonatal infection, V2.1444 (Tab.),
V2.1450
breastfeeding, V2.1450, V2.1452
diagnosis, V2.1451–2
management, V2.1452–3
perinatal transmission, V2.1450
nosocomial, B1.400
pathogenesis, V1.523–4
host cell damage, V1.523–4
host inflammation, V1.523–4
nonlytic mechanisms, V1.523–4
viral load vs., V1.523–4
in pregnancy, V2.1446–50
diagnosis, V2.1450–1, V2.1547
epidemiology, V2.1446–7
immune response, V2.1447–8
management, V2.1452
primary infection, V2.1447
recurrent infection, V2.1447–8
T cell deficiency, V1.274
transmission, V1.524 (Tab.)
blood products, V2.1507
breastfeeding, V2.1452
sexual transmission, V2.1502
vertical transmission, V2.1446–7
transplants, V2.1507
in transplants, V1.521–2, V1.522–3
cell-mediated immune response, V1.524–5
immunosuppressive drugs, V1.521–2
mortality, V1.521–2
pneumonia, V1.521–2
steroid use, V1.521–2
vaccines/vaccination, V1.527, I.933 (Tab.)
congenital infection prevention, V2.1453
development, V2.1582
live attenuated, V2.1582

Human cytomegalovirus (HCMV) infection
vaccines/vaccination (*Continued*)
    MF59 adjuvant, **I**.929
    subunit, **V2**.1582
Human endogenous retroviruses (HERV),
    V1.176
    superantigens, **I**.556 (Tab.), **I**.563–6
Human foamy virus (HFV) *see* Prototypic
    foamy virus (PFV)
Human Genome Project, **I**.10
Human granulocytic ehrlichiosis (HGE) *see*
    Anaplasma phagocytophilum (Ehrlichia
    phagocytophilia), infection (human
    anaplasmosis)
Human growth hormone therapy, iatrogenic
    Creutzfeldt–Jakob disease (iCJD),
    V2.1366–7
Human herpesviruses
    in AIDS/HIV infection, **V2**.1500
    CD4 expression, **V2**.1500
    promiscuous transactivators, **V2**.1500
Human herpesvirus 1 (HHV-1) *see* Herpes
    simplex virus type 1 (HSV-1)
Human herpesvirus 2 (HHV-2) *see* Herpes
    simplex virus type 2 (HSV-2)
Human herpesvirus 3 (HHV-3) *see*
    Varicella-zoster virus (VZV)
Human herpesvirus 4 (HHV-4) *see*
    Epstein–Barr virus (EBV)
Human herpesvirus 5 (HHV-5) *see* Human
    cytomegalovirus (HCMV)
Human herpesvirus 6 (HHV-6), **V1**.527–33
    cell culture, **V1**.530, **V2**.1539
    characteristics, **V1**.489 (Tab.)
    CNS receptors, **V2**.1406 (Tab.)
    genome sequences, **V1**.494 (Tab.)
    genome structure, **V1**.492, **V1**.493,
        V1.493 (Fig.)
    immune evasion, **V1**.530–1
        chemokine receptors, **V1**.319–20, **I**.622
        chemokines, **V1**.319, **I**.621–2
        IL-6, **V1**.301–2
    isolation/propagation and identification,
        V1.98
        initial isolation, **V1**.527
    medical importance, **V1**.162
    multiple sclerosis, **V2**.1418
    peripheral blood mononuclear cells, **V2**.1418
Human herpesvirus 6 (HHV-6) infection
    in AIDS/HIV infection *see* AIDS,
        concomitant infection
    clinical manifestations, **V1**.527–9
        multiple sclerosis associations, **V1**.527–8
        neurotropism, **V1**.527–8
        seizures, **V1**.527–8
    control, **V1**.533
    diagnosis, **V1**.532–3
        immunoassays, **V1**.532–3
        PCR, **V1**.532–3
        serology, **V1**.533
    emerging infection, **V2**.1648 (Tab.)
    epidemiology, **V1**.529–30
        seroprevalence, **V1**.529
        transmission, **V1**.530
    exanthem subitum (roseola), **V1**.527–8
    immune response, **V1**.531–2
        cell-mediated, **V1**.532

chemokines, **I**.228
humoral, **V1**.532
IL-1β, **V1**.301–2
passively-acquired immunity, **V1**.531–2
TNF-β, **V1**.301–2
immunocompromised hosts, **V1**.528–9
latent infection, **V1**.528–9
pathogenesis, **V1**.530–1
    chemokine receptor coding, **V1**.530–1
    CNS dysfunction, **V1**.531
    graft-versus-host disease, **V1**.530–1
    lymphokine induction, **V1**.530–1
    viral load, **V1**.530–1
reactivation, HHV-7 infection, **V1**.531
rubella *vs.,* **V2**.970
TNF-α induction, **V1**.296
in transplants, **V1**.528–9, **V1**.529–30
Human herpesvirus 7 (HHV-7), **V1**.527–33
    CD4 receptors, **V1**.209
    cell culture, **V2**.1539
    characteristics, **V1**.489 (Tab.)
    discovery, **V1**.489
    genome sequences, **V1**.494 (Tab.)
    genome structure, **V1**.493, **V1**.493 (Fig.)
    infection *see* Human herpesvirus 7 (HHV-7)
        infection
    isolation/propagation and identification,
        V1.98
        initial isolation, **V1**.527
    medical importance, **V1**.162
    peripheral blood mononuclear cells, **V2**.1418
Human herpesvirus 7 (HHV-7) infection
    in AIDS/HIV infection *see* AIDS,
        concomitant infection
    clinical manifestations, **V1**.527–9
    control, **V1**.533
    diagnosis, **V1**.532–3
        immunoassays, **V1**.532–3
        PCR, **V1**.532–3
        serology, **V1**.533
    emerging infection, **V2**.1648 (Tab.)
    epidemiology, **V1**.529–30
        seroprevalence, **V1**.529
        transmission, **V1**.530
    immune response, **V1**.531–2
        cell-mediated, **V1**.532
        humoral, **V1**.532
    pathogenesis, **V1**.530–1
        HHV-6 reactivation, **V1**.531
    rubella *vs.,* **V2**.970
    in transplants, **V1**.529–31
Human herpesvirus 8 (HHV-8: Kaposi's
    sarcoma-associated herpesvirus
    (KSHV)), **V1**.345, **V1.541–58**
    CC chemokine analogues, **V1**.550
    cell culture, **V1**.544–5
    characteristics, **V1**.489 (Tab.), **V1**.542 (Tab.)
    classification, **V1**.541–3
        related primate rhadinoviruses, **V1**.541–3
    discovery, **V1**.489, **V1**.541
    gene expression regulation, **V1**.499
    genome sequences, **V1**.494 (Tab.)
    genome structure, **V1**.492, **V1**.493, **V1**.543–4,
        V1.544 (Fig.)
        nucleotide sequence, **V1**.543–4

    open reading frames, **V1**.543–4
    glycoproteins, **V1**.546
        glycoprotein B, **V1**.546
        glycoprotein K8.1, **V1**.546
    immune evasion, **V1**.548–50
        apoptosis, **V1**.287, **V1**.323, **V1**.324–5
        chemokine homologues, **V1**.288, **V1**.319,
            I.621–2
        chemokine receptor homologues,
            V1.319–20, **I**.622
        cytokine homologues, **V1**.288, **V1**.317–18,
            I.620
        IFN regulatory factors, **V1**.548,
            V1.549 (Tab.)
        IFN signal transduction, **V1**.315, **I**.619
        MHC interference, **V1**.322, **I**.635–6
        NK cell interference, **I**.630
    infection *see* Human herpesvirus 8 infection;
        Kaposi's sarcoma
    inflammatory cytokine coding, **V1**.548–50
        chemokines, **V1**.550
        viral IL-6, **V1**.548–50, **V1**.549 (Tab.)
        viral IL-8 receptor, **V1**.549 (Tab.), **V1**.550
    isolation/propagation and identification,
        V1.98
    K8/K-BZIP, **V1**.545–6
        ORF50 regulation, **V1**.545–6
    K12 (Kaposin), **V1**.548, **V1**.549 (Tab.)
    k-cyclin (cyclin D homologue), **V1**.546,
        V1.548, **V1**.549 (Tab.), **V1**.555
        retinoblastoma phosphorylation, **V1**.548
        S cycle entry, **V1**.548
    latent nuclear antigen (LANA-1), **V1**.546–7,
        V1.549 (Tab.), **V1**.555
        p53 inhibition, **V1**.546–7
        S-phase entry effects, **V1**.546–7
    molecular biology, **V1**.543–50
    morphology/structure, **V1**.543
    nucleotide metabolism, **V1**.500
    ORF45-protein, **V1**.545
    peripheral blood mononuclear cells, **V2**.1418
    replication and transcription activator
        (ORF50/K-RTA), **V1**.545
    vFLIPs, **V1**.287, **V1**.323, **V1**.546, **V1**.548,
        V1.549 (Tab.)
    viral macrophage inhibitory proteins,
        V1.549 (Tab.), **V1**.550
    virus-coded proteins, **V1**.544–8, **V1**.549 (Tab.)
        latent proteins, **V1**.546–8
        lytic regulatory proteins, **V1**.545–6
        viral capsid proteins, **V1**.546
        virion proteins, **V1**.546
        see also individual proteins
Human herpesvirus 8 (HHV-8) infection,
    V1.550
    in AIDS/HIV infection *see* AIDS,
        concomitant infection
    B-cell lymphoma generation, in HIV
        infection, **I**.795–6
    clinical manifestations, **V1**.551–4
        multifocal Castleman's disease, **V1**.550,
            V1.554
        primary effusion lymphoma, **V1**.550,
            V1.553–4
        primary infection, **V1**.551–2
    emerging infection, **V2**.1648 (Tab.)
        medical practices, **V2**.1660

Human herpesvirus 8 (HHV-8) infection
emerging infection (*Continued*)
recognition, **V2**.1653 (Tab.)
epidemiology, **V1**.551
geographical effects, **V1**.551
transmission routes, **V1**.551–2
immune response
chemokines, **I**.228
NK cells, **I**.96
immunosuppressed patients, **V1**.550
latent infection, **V1**.544–5
medical importance, **V1**.162
pathogenesis, **V1**.554–5
'cytokine model,' **V1**.554–5
k-cyclin (cyclin D homologue), **V1**.555
latent nuclear antigen (LANA-1), **V1**.555
oncogenes, **V1**.554
S cycle entry, **V1**.555
transmembrane proteins, **V1**.555
temporal gene expression, **V1**.547 (Fig.)
see also Kaposi's sarcoma
Human histamine-releasing factor (HRF), **I**.62
Humanization, monoclonal antibodies, **I**.333,
I.365, **I**.366 (Fig.)
Human lactoperoxidase, **I**.521
Human leukocyte antigens (HLAs)
chromoblastomycosis, **M**.359
class I, **I**.405–6
gene structure, **I**.576 (Fig.)
immunogenetics, **I**.576–7
KIR interactions, **I**.88
class II
expression deficiencies, **I**.776
gene structure, **I**.576 (Fig.)
immunogenetics, **I**.576–7
class III, immunogenetics, **I**.577–8
disease associations
Ascaris lumbricoides infection, **I**.600–1
Chagas disease, **I**.597
Crohn's disease, **I**.577
filarial nematode infection, **I**.600–1
gastrointestinal nematode infection,
I.600–1
inflammatory bowel disease, **I**.577
leishmaniasis, **I**.597
leprosy *see* Leprosy
malaria, **I**.379–80, **P**.485–6, **I**.598
Onchocerca volvulus infection, **I**.600–1
paracoccidioidomycosis, **M**.545
periodontal disease, **I**.577
reactive arthritis, **I**.577
rheumatoid arthritis, **I**.577
schistosomiasis, **I**.601
toxoplasmosis association, **I**.597
trypanosomiasis association, **I**.597
tuberculosis, **I**.591–2
ethnicity differences, **I**.405–6
genetic map, **I**.406 (Fig.)
immunogenetics, **I**.576–7
case–control studies, **I**.577
linkage disequilibrium mapping, **I**.577
polymorphisms, **I**.576
EBV infection, **I**.588
hepatitis B, **I**.587
hepatitis C, **I**.587–8

HIV infection, **I**.586
peptide-binding specificities, **I**.576–7
see also individual HLA genes
see also specific genes
Human metapneumovirus (hMPV),
V1.783–806
animal models, **V1**.790
emerging infection, **V2**.1648 (Tab.)
recognition, **V2**.1653 (Tab.)
epidemiology, **V1**.798
fusion (F) protein, **V1**.787
genome structure, **V1**.785 (Fig.)
isolation/propagation and identification,
V1.99
matrix (M) protein, **V1**.788–9
morphology, **V1**.787, **V1**.788 (Fig.)
Human papillomaviruses (HPVs)
cell interactions, **V1**.220
epithelial tropism, **V1**.454–5
immune evasion, **V1**.325
infection *see* Human papillomavirus
infection
replication
DNA polymerase α primase, **V1**.457
DNA polymerase δ, **V1**.457
E1 expression, **V1**.457
E2 expression, **V1**.457
proliferating nuclear cell antigen (PCNA),
V1.457
regulation, **V1**.457
replication protein A, **V1**.457
replication protein C (RPC), **V1**.457
topoisomerases, **V1**.457
structural proteins, **I**.872
structure, **I**.872
see also Papillomaviruses; *specific viruses*
Human papillomaviruses, molecular detection
hybrid capture assay, **B1**.731
nucleic acid sequencing, **B1**.732, **B1**.733–4
Human papillomavirus infection,
V1.463 (Tab.), **V2**.1483–4
aerodigestive tract, **V1**.463 (Tab.), **V1**.464,
V1.465 (Fig.), **V1**.465 (Tab.)
in AIDS/HIV infection, **V1**.338,
V2.1499 (Tab.), **V2**.1503–4
cidofovir therapy, **V2**.1616
clinical aspects, **V1**.462–4
diagnosis, **V1**.467, **V2**.1484
cytopathology, **V2**.1533–4, **V2**.1534 (Tab.)
serology, **V1**.467
emerging infection, **V2**.1647, **V2**.1648 (Tab.)
recognition, **V2**.1653 (Tab.)
epidemiology, **V1**.373–4
epidermodysplasia verruciformis *see*
Epidermodysplasia verruciformis
EVER gene mutations, **I**.772
fetal infection, **V2**.1444 (Tab.), **V2**.1483–4
genital tract infection, **V1**.463 (Tab.),
V1.464–7
anogenital cancers, **V1**.463 (Tab.),
V1.465–7
cervical intraepithelial neoplasia (CIN),
V1.465–6
condyloma acuminata, **V1**.463 (Tab.),
V1.464–5, **V1**.466 (Fig.)

high-grade squamous intraepithelial
lesions (HGSIL), **V1**.465–6
oncogenesis mechanisms, **V1**.467
squamous intraepithelial lesions,
V1.463 (Tab.), **V1**.464–5, **V1**.465–7,
V1.466 (Fig.)
immune response, **V1**.467–8
neutralizing antibodies, **V1**.468
persistent infection, **V1**.468
subunit vaccines, **V1**.468
T helper cells type 1, **V1**.467–8
immunodeficiency diseases/disorders, **I**.772
immunogenetics, **I**.588
juvenile laryngeal papillomatosis *see*
Juvenile laryngeal papillomatosis (JLP)
koilocytic dysplasia, **V1**.465 (Tab.)
laryngeal papillomas, **V1**.449 (Fig.),
V1.463 (Tab.)
latent infection, **V1**.453
leukoplakias, **V1**.463 (Tab.), **V1**.465 (Tab.)
management, **V2**.1484
neonatal infection, **V2**.1444 (Tab.), **V2**.1484
nongenital skin warts, **V1**.462–3,
V1.462 (Fig.), **V1**.463 (Tab.)
classification, **V1**.462–3
immunosuppression, **V1**.462–3
specific type association, **V1**.462–3
non-melanoma skin cancer, **V1**.464
oncogenesis, **V1**.336, **V1**.342 (Tab.),
I.865 (Tab.)
cervical cancer, **V2**.1647
epidemiological evidence, **V1**.373–4
laryngeal cancer, **V1**.463 (Tab.)
mechanisms, **V1**.338 (Tab.)
nasal cancer, **V1**.463 (Tab.)
oral cancer, **V1**.463 (Tab.)
oral epithelial dysplasia, **V1**.465 (Tab.)
in pregnancy, **V2**.1444 (Tab.), **V2**.1483–4
respiratory infection, **V2**.1647
transmission, **V1**.467
type association, **V1**.463 (Tab.)
vaccines/vaccination, **V2**.1552 (Tab.),
V2.1581–2
BCE peptide vaccines, **I**.855 (Tab.), **I**.872
development, **I**.933 (Tab.), **V2**.1581–2
DNA vaccines, **V2**.1554
MF59 adjuvant, **I**.929
MPL/QS-21 adjuvant, **I**.930
subunit vaccines, **V1**.468
virus-like particles, **I**.840–1
Human papillomavirus-6 (HPV-6) infection
aerodigestive tract papillomas, **V1**.464
Buschke–Lowenstein tumors, **V1**.465
genital warts, **V1**.448–9
juvenile laryngeal papillomatosis (JLP),
V2.1483
recurrent respiratory papillomatosis (RRP),
V1.464
Human papillomavirus-11 (HPV-11) infection
aerodigestive tract papillomas, **V1**.464
Buschke–Lowenstein tumors, **V1**.465
genital warts, **V1**.448–9
juvenile laryngeal papillomatosis (JLP),
V2.1483
recurrent respiratory papillomatosis (RRP),
V1.464

Human papillomavirus-11 (HPV-11) infection
(*Continued*)
  vaccine development, **V2**.1581–2
Human papillomavirus-16 (HPV-16)
  genome organization, **V1**.451 (Fig.),
    V1.452 (Fig.)
  structure/morphology, **V1**.450 (Fig.)
  T-helper cell epitope, **I**.862 (Tab.)
  transcription map, **V1**.452 (Fig.)
  URR structure, **V1**.457 (Fig.)
  vertical transmission, **V1**.467
Human papillomavirus-16 (HPV-16) infection
  in AIDS/HIV infection, **V2**.1503
  Buschke–Lowenstein tumors, **V1**.465
  cervical cancer, **V1**.448–9
  early gene expression, **V1**.454
  recurrent respiratory papillomatosis (RRP),
    V1.464
  tonsillar carcinomas, **V1**.464
  vaccine development, **I**.902, **V2**.1581–2
Human papillomavirus-18 (HPV-18) infection
  in AIDS/HIV infection, **V2**.1503
  cervical cancer, **V1**.448–9
  early gene expression, **V1**.454
  recurrent respiratory papillomatosis (RRP),
    V1.464
  vaccine development, **V2**.1581–2
Human papillomavirus-31 (HPV-31) infection,
    V1.454
Human papillomavirus-33 (HPV-33) infection,
    V1.464
Human parainfluenza virus infection, **V1**.774–7
  vaccine development, **V1**.776
  see also specific diseases/infection
Human parainfluenza virus 1, **V1**.763
  classification, **V1**.382–3
  infection *see* Croup
    (laryngotracheobronchitis)
  vaccine development, **V1**.775–6
  V protein, **V1**.704
Human parainfluenzavirus 2, **V1**.744
  classification, **V1**.382–3
  croup *see* Croup (laryngotracheobronchitis)
  immune evasion, **V1**.315
Human parainfluenzavirus 3, **V1**.763
  cell receptors, **V1**.765–6
  classification, **V1**.382–3
  C proteins, **V1**.771
  hemagglutinin-neuraminidase (HN)
    active site, **V1**.765 (Fig.)
    functions, **V1**.766
  infection *see* Croup
    (laryngotracheobronchitis)
  vaccine development, **V1**.775–6
Human parainfluenza virus 4, **V1**.382–3
Human parainfluenza virus 4a, **V1**.744
Human parainfluenza virus 4b, **V1**.744
Human parechovirus, **V1**.50–2
Human parvovirus B19 *see* Parvovirus B19
    virus
Human respiratory syncytial virus (HRSV),
    V1.783–806
  animal models, **V1**.790
  antibody effects, **V1**.278
  attenuation measurement, **V1**.195
  cell penetration, **V1**.789

classification, **V1**.385, **V1**.784–5
cytopathic effects, **V1**.94 (Fig.)
fusion (F) protein, **V1**.786
  TLR-4 binding, **I**.121
genome structure, **V1**.381, **V1**.785 (Fig.),
    V1.789
glycoprotein (G), **V1**.786, **V1**.796–7,
    V1.797 (Fig.)
  cell attachment, **V1**.786
  CXC3 chemokine receptor binding,
    V1.786, **V1**.789
  polymorphisms, **V1**.789
history, **V1**.783–4
hypermutation, **V1**.193
immune evasion, **V1**.787
  chemokine homologue production,
    I.622
  chemokine homologues, **V1**.319
  IFN antagonism, **V1**.787
infection *see* Human respiratory syncytial
    virus (HRSV) infection
isolation/propagation and identification,
    V1.96 (Tab.), **V1**.99
  mixed cell culture, **V1**.88
  shell vial culture, **V1**.87
large (L) protein, **V1**.787
  transcription initiation, **V1**.789
M2–1 protein, **V1**.708
M2 (matrix) protein, **V1**.787
molecular epidemiology, **V1**.198
morphology/structure, **V1**.785–6,
    V1.786 (Fig.)
  protein structures, **V1**.70 (Tab.)
M (matrix) protein, **V1**.787
multinucleated syncytia formation, **V1**.213
NS proteins, **V1**.708, **V1**.787
nucleocapsid (N) protein, **V1**.787
phosphoprotein (P), **V1**.787
SH protein, **V1**.786–7
strains, **V1**.783–4, **V1**.789
transcription, **V1**.702–3
viral assembly, **V1**.774
Human respiratory syncytial virus (HRSV)
    infection, **V1**.241 (Tab.), **V1**.790–8
  children, **B1**.400
  clinical manifestations, **V1**.790–3
  diagnosis, **V1**.791–2
    cytopathology, **V2**.1534 (Tab.)
    serology, **V1**.791–2
  differential diagnosis, **V1**.791–2
  epidemiology, **V1**.365–6, **V1**.797–8
    adults, **V1**.791, **V1**.797–8
    age-relation, **V1**.356–7, **V1**.790–1,
      V1.797–8
    children, **V1**.783–4, **V1**.797–8
    immunodeficiency, **V1**.783–4
    nosocomial pneumonia, **V1**.798
    seasonality, **V1**.366, **V1**.783–4,
      V1.784 (Fig.)
  history, **V1**.783–4
  in HIV infection, **V2**.1499 (Tab.)
    in children, **V2**.1505–6
  immune response, **V1**.790–1, **V1**.793–6
    adaptive immune response, **V1**.794–6
    cell-mediated immune response,
      V1.795–6

chemokines, **V1**.793–4
collectins, **V1**.793–4
cytokines, **V1**.793–4
eosinophils, **I**.71
humoral response, **V1**.794–5
IL-6, **V1**.297
IL-7, **V1**.297–8
IL-13, **I**.734–5
innate immunity, **V1**.793–4
mucosal immune response, **I**.522–3
SP-A, **V1**.793–4
SP-D, **V1**.793–4
TNF-α induction, **V1**.296
immunodeficiency, **V1**.783–4
immunogenetics, **I**.587
immunopathology, **V1**.796–7
  glycoprotein (G), **V1**.796–7,
    V1.797 (Fig.)
  Th1/Th2 balance, **V1**.796
management, **V1**.792
  intravenous Igs, **V1**.792, **V2**.1567,
    V2.1567 (Tab.)
  peptide fusion inhibitors, **V1**.792
  ribavirin therapy, **V2**.1628
  supportive care, **V1**.792
nosocomial, **B1**.372, **B1**.374, **B1**.390, **B1**.400
periodicity, **B1**.633 (Fig.)
self-limiting, **V1**.792
vaccines, **V1**.792–3
  attenuated vaccines, **V1**.793
  BCE peptide vaccines, **I**.855 (Tab.),
    I.861 (Tab.), **I**.869
  development status, **I**.933 (Tab.)
  G glycoprotein epitope, **I**.869
  monophosphoryl lipid adjuvant, **I**.929
  reverse genetics, **V1**.793
  subunit vaccines, **V1**.793
  trial failure, **V1**.792–3, **V1**.796
Human rhinovirus (HRV)
  cellular entry, **V1**.139
  protein processing, **V1**.140
Human T-cell leukemia viruses (HTLV),
    I.801–2
  cell culture systems, **V1**.88
  genome, **I**.801
  infection *see* Human T-cell leukemia viruses
    (HTLV), infection
  Rex, **I**.802
  Strongyloides coinfection, **P**.739–41
  Tax, **I**.801–2
Human T-cell leukemia viruses (HTLV),
    infection, **I**.788 (Tab.), **I**.801–3
  diseases/infection, **I**.801, **I**.802–3
    cryptococcal meningitis, **I**.802–3
    Pneumocystis carinii infection, **I**.802–3
    Strongyloides infection, **I**.803
  epidemiology, **I**.801
    transmission, **I**.801
    world distribution, **I**.801
  GM-CSF production effects, **I**.277
  HIV co-infection, **I**.803
  IL-2 receptor, **I**.802
  immunosuppression, **I**.802–3, **I**.804 (Fig.),
    I.805 (Fig.)
  natural course, **I**.802
    gene transcription effects, **I**.801–2

Human T-cell leukemia viruses (HTLV)
(*Continued*)
  TNF gene polymorphisms, **I**.586
  see also Adult T-cell leukemia/lymphoma
    (ATL)
Human T-cell leukemia virus 1 (HTLV-1),
    V2.1285–94, **V2**.1428–30
  detection, PCR, **V2**.1542
  genetic diversity, **V2**.1289
  genome organization, **V2**.1285–8,
    V2.1287 (Fig.)
    env gene, **V2**.1285–7
    gag gene, **V2**.1285–7
    open reading frames, **V2**.1287–8
    pol gene, **V2**.1285–7
    pro gene, **V2**.1285–7
    transcriptional control sequences,
      V2.1285–7
  gp21, **V2**.1285–7
  gp46, **V2**.1285–7
  historical aspects, **V2**.1285
  infection *see* Human T-cell leukemia virus 1
    (HTLV-1) infection
  morphology, **V2**.1285
  p12^I protein, **V2**.1287–8
  p13^{II} protein, **V2**.1287–8
  p15 protein (NC), **V2**.1285–7
  p19 protein (MA), **V2**.1285–7
  p24 protein (CA), **V2**.1285–7
  replication, **V2**.1288–9
    cell receptor, **V2**.1288
    cellular infection, **V2**.1288–9
  reverse transcriptase, **V2**.1285–7
  Rex protein, **I**.802, **V2**.1287
    homology, **V2**.1289
  structural proteins, **V2**.1285–7
    see also specific types
  subtypes, **V2**.1289
  Tax protein, **I**.801–2, **V2**.1287
    homology, **V2**.1289
  transformation by, **V1**.336
Human T-cell leukemia virus 1 (HTLV-1)
    infection, **V2**.1289–92
  adult T-cell leukemia *see* Adult T-cell
    leukemia/lymphoma (ATL)
  arthropathy, **V2**.1290–1
  CD4+ T cell infection, **V1**.282, **V2**.1288
  emerging infection, **V2**.1648 (Tab.)
  epidemiology, **V2**.1292–3
    geographical distribution, **V2**.1289,
      V2.1292
  host cell interactions, **V2**.1288
  HTLV-associated myelopathy/tropical
    spastic paraparesis *see* HTLV-associated
    myelopathy(HAM)/tropical spastic
    paraparesis (TSP)
  immune response
    IL-1, **V1**.296–7
    IL-6, **V1**.297
  immunosuppressive effects, **V2**.1291
  infective dermatitis, **V2**.1290–1
  inflammatory diseases, **V2**.1290–1
  laboratory diagnosis, **V2**.1293–4
    antigen detection, **V2**.1294
    blood films, **V2**.1290 (Fig.)
    nucleic acid detection, **V2**.1294

  reverse transcriptase assays, **V2**.1294
  serology, **V2**.1293–4
  virus isolation, **V2**.1294
  myelopathy *see* HTLV-associated
    myelopathy(HAM)/tropical spastic
    paraparesis (TSP)
  oncogenesis, **V1**.342 (Tab.)
    multi-step process, **V1**.345
  Sjögren's syndrome, **V2**.1290–91
  transmission, **V2**.1292–3, **V2**.1429
    cell-to-cell contact, **V2**.1288
    injecting drug use, **V2**.1293
    microtubule reorientation, **V2**.1288
    saliva, **V2**.1292–3
    sexual transmission, **V2**.1292
    vertical transmission, **V2**.1292
  treatment, **V2**.1291–2
  tropical paraparesis *see* HTLV-associated
    myelopathy(HAM)/tropical spastic
    paraparesis (TSP)
  uveitis, **V2**.1290
Human T-cell leukemia virus 2 (HTLV-2),
    V2.1285–94
  genetic diversity, **V2**.1289
  genome organization, **V2**.1285–8,
    V2.1287 (Fig.)
    env gene, **V2**.1285–7
    gag gene, **V2**.1285–7
    open reading frames, **V2**.1287–8
    pol gene, **V2**.1285–7
    pro gene, **V2**.1285–7
    transcriptional control sequences,
      V2.1285–7
  gp21, **V2**.1285–7
  gp46, **V2**.1285–7
  historical aspects, **V2**.1285
  infection *see* Human T-cell leukemia virus 2
    (HTLV-2) infection
  morphology, **V2**.1285
  p12^I protein, **V2**.1287–8
  p13^{II} protein, **V2**.1287–8
  p15 protein (NC), **V2**.1285–7
  p19 protein (MA), **V2**.1285–7
  p24 protein (CA), **V2**.1285–7
  replication, **V2**.1288–9
    cell receptor, **V2**.1288
    cellular infection, **V2**.1288–9
  reverse transcriptase, **V2**.1285–7
  Rex protein, **I**.802, **V2**.1287
    homology, **V2**.1289
  structural proteins, **V2**.1285–7
    see also specific types
  subtypes, **V2**.1289
  Tax protein, **I**.801–2, **V2**.1287
    homology, **V2**.1289
Human T-cell leukemia virus 2 (HTLV-2)
    infection, **V2**.1289–92, **V2**.1291
  CD4+ T cell tropism, **V2**.1288
  CD8+ T cell tropism, **V2**.1288
  emerging infection, **V2**.1648 (Tab.)
  epidemiology, **V2**.1292–3
    geographical distribution, **V2**.1289,
      V2.1292
  host cell interactions, **V2**.1288
  immunosuppressive effects, **V2**.1291
  inflammatory diseases, **V2**.1290–1

  laboratory diagnosis, **V2**.1293–4
    antigen detection, **V2**.1294
    blood films, **V2**.1290 (Fig.)
    nucleic acid detection, **V2**.1294
    reverse transcriptase assays, **V2**.1294
    serology, **V2**.1293–4
    virus isolation, **V2**.1294
  transmission, **V2**.1292–3
    cell-to-cell contact, **V2**.1288
    injecting drug use, **V2**.1293
    microtubule reorientation, **V2**.1288
    saliva, **V2**.1292–3
    sexual transmission, **V2**.1292
    vertical transmission, **V2**.1292
  treatment, **V2**.1291–2
Human tetanus immunoglobulin (HTIG),
    B2.1066
Human T-lymphotrophic virus type 1
    (HTLV-1) *see* Human T-cell leukemia
    virus 1 (HTLV-1)
Human T-lymphotrophic virus type 2
    (HTLV-2) *see* Human T-cell leukemia
    virus 2 (HTLV-2)
Human torovirus (HToV)
  infection, **V1**.841 (Tab.)
  tissue culture, **V1**.846
Humerus infection, inflammatory responses,
    B1.689
Humidifiers (portable), airborne bacteria,
    B1.186 (Tab.)
Humira, licensing, **I**.355 (Tab.)
Humoral immune response, H **P**.69–70,
    V1.270, **B1**.741–6
  antibody course, **B1**.741 (Fig.), **B1**.742–3
    IgG, **B1**.742, **B1**.743
    IgM, **B1**.742–3
  antibody 'titers' definition, **B1**.742
  bacterial infection, **I**.647
    human brucellosis, **B1**.744–5, **B2**.1737
    immune interference *see* Immune evasion,
      bacteria
    syphilis, **B1**.745–6
  cellular immune response *vs.*, **I**.489–90,
    I.490 (Fig.), **I**.490 (Tab.)
    protective immunity, **I**.489
  in CNS, **V2**.1411–13
  discovery, **B1**.7
  DNA vaccine modulation, **I**.917
  fungal infection
    allergic bronchopulmonary aspergillosis,
      M.708
    aspergilloma, **M**.708–9
    candidiasis *see* Candidiasis
    cryptococcosis, **M**.645
    invasive aspergillosis, **M**.709
    oropharyngeal candidiasis, **M**.260, **M**.263
    vulvovaginal candidiasis, **M**.260, **M**.266
  ILs, **P**.70–2
  kinetics, **I**.492, **I**.492 (Fig.)
  mucosal vaccination, **I**.828
  parasitic infection, **P**.68, **P**.69–70
    amebiasis, **P**.208–9
    Chagas disease, **P**.385
    cryptosporidiosis, **P**.406–7
    echinococcosis, **P**.689
    hookworms, **P**.729–30

Humoral immune response
  parasitic infection (*Continued*)
    leishmaniasis, **P**.300
    Naegleria fowleri infection, **P**.232
    onchocerciasis, **P**.795
    trichomoniasis, **P**.258–9
    trypanosomiasis, **P**.80–1
  primary, **I**.303
  secondary infection, **I**.492–3
  seroepidemiology, **B1**.743–4
    antibody functions, **B1**.743
    antigen persistence, **B1**.743
    antigens *vs.* immunogens, **B1**.743
    antigen variety, **B1**.743
  suppression, in LCMV infection, **V2**.1075
  viral infection
    acute bronchiolitis pathogenesis, **V1**.776
    adenovirus infection, **V1**.445
    alphavirus infection, **V2**.1018
    arenaviruses, **V2**.1072
    arterivirus infection, **V1**.840
    bunyavirus infection, **V2**.1041
    coronaviruses, **V1**.840
    EBV infection, **V1**.568–9, **V1**.569 (Fig.),
      V1.570
    filovirus infection, **V2**.1096
    hepatitis A, **V2**.1171
    hepatitis C, **V2**.1206
    hepatitis E, **V2**.1179
    HHV-6 infection, **V1**.532
    HHV infection, **V1**.532
    influenza, **V1**.663–4
    measles, **V1**.726–7
    mumps, **V1**.751
    subacute sclerosing panencephalitis
      (SSPE), **V1**.731
    viral immune interference *see* Immune
      evasion, viruses
  see also Antibodies; Immunoglobulin(s)
Hurdle technology, food preservation, **B1**.272
Hv1 gene, **I**.587
Hv2 gene, **I**.587
Hyaline hyphomycetes, **M**.274, **M**.275 (Tab.)
Hyalohyphomycosis
  AIDS, **M**.750–1
  categories, **M**.749, **M**.750 (Tab.)
  cutaneous, **M**.138 (Fig.)
  deep-seated phaeohyphomycosis *vs.*, **M**.740
  definition, **M**.749
  diagnosis, **M**.751–2
    culture, **M**.751
    histology, **M**.751
    microscopy, **M**.751
    molecular, **M**.752
  etiological agents, **M**.749, **M**.750 (Tab.)
    see also individual species
  histopathology, **M**.128 (Tab.), **M**.138 (Fig.),
    M.139 (Fig.)
  patients at risk, **M**.750–1
  phaeohyphomycosis *vs.*, **M**.740
  prevention, **M**.752
  specimen site selection, **M**.83 (Tab.)
Hyalomma, Crimean–Congo hemorrhagic
  fever virus transmission, **V2**.1049–50
Hyaloplasm, **P**.169

Hyaluronidase
  Balantidium coli, **P**.278–9
  Clostridium perfringens, **B2**.1113
  functions, **B1**.153 (Tab.)
Hybrid Capture®, **B1**.723 (Tab.), **B1**.731,
  B1.731 (Fig.)
Hybridization, **M**.34
Hybridization assays
  aerobic actinomycetes, **B2**.1147
  Brucella, **B2**.1729
  Burkholderia, **B2**.1609
  Burkholderia mallei, **B2**.1632
  Buttiauxella, **B2**.1338
  Citrobacter, **B2**.1338
  Enterobacter agglomerans complex, **B2**.1337
  Enterobacter cloacae, **B2**.1338
  Enterobacteriaceae, **B2**.1318, **B2**.1338–9
  Enterococcus, **B2**.884–5, **B2**.887, **B2**.890
  Proteus vulgaris, **B2**.1338
  Rahnella aquatilis, **B2**.1338
  Trichomonas vaginalis diagnosis, **P**.261
  Yersinia classification, **B2**.1338
Hydatid cysts, **P**.579
  Echinococcus, **P**.679
  Echinococcus granulosus, **P**.680–1,
    P.681 (Fig.)
  Echinococcus multilocularis, **P**.680,
    P.682 (Fig.)
  historical aspects, **P**.12–3
  see also Echinococcosis
Hydatosis *see* Echinococcosis
Hydrocele, lymphatic filariasis, **P**.773–4,
  P.774 (Fig.)
Hydrocephalus
  congenital toxoplasmosis, **P**.430, **P**.430 (Fig.)
  neurocysticercosis, **P**.687–8, **P**.687 (Fig.),
    P.692–3
Hydrochloric acid, **B1**.422
Hydrogenosomes, **P**.172 (Fig.), **P**.174, **P**.177–8
  Blastocystis hominis, **P**.557, **P**.561
  Trichomonas vaginalis, **P**.256, **P**.256 (Fig.)
Hydrogen peroxide, **B1**.428–9
  action, **B1**.437 (Tab.)
    on spores, **B1**.428–9, **B1**.439
  generation by trypanosomes, **P**.360
  stress response, **B1**.65
Hydrogen sulfide production, **B1**.201
  Brucella, **B2**.1731
  Enterobacteriaceae identification,
    B2.1319 (Tab.)
Hydrolases, *Candida albicans* virulence factor,
  M.259
Hydronephrosis, schistosomiasis, **P**.612–13,
  P.613 (Fig.)
Hydrophobins, **M**.71, **M**.78
Hydrops fetalis
  fetal Parvovirus B19 virus infection, **V2**.1468
  nonimmune *see* Nonimmune hydrops fetalis
Hydrostatic pressure, sterilization, **B1**.450,
  B1.454
5,6-Hydroxydihydrothymine, **B1**.451,
  B1.452 (Fig.)
5-Hydroxyeicosatetraenoic acid (5-HETE),
  neutrophils, **I**.186
12-Hydroxy-5,8,10-heptadecatraenoic acid
  (HHT), **I**.189

5-Hydroxyperoxide eicosatetraeonate
  (5HPTE), **I**.181
  biosynthesis, **I**.182 (Fig.)
  structure, **I**.182 (Fig.)
1-Hydroxyphenazine, **B1**.650
Hydroxypyridones, **M**.233
8-Hydroxyquinoline, **B1**.428
3β-Hydroxysteroid hydrogenase, poxvirus
  immune evasion, **V1**.622
Hygiene
  alveolar echinococcosis control, **P**.702
  bacterial disease control by, **B1**.353–4
  cystic echinococcosis control, **P**.701–2
  giardiasis prevention, **P**.251–2
  hepatitis B control, **V2**.1256–7
  viral infection prevention, oncogenic viruses,
    V1.348
Hygiene hypothesis, **P**.96–7, **I**.738–9
  endotoxin effects, **I**.738–9
  IL-10, **I**.739
  mycobacteria, **I**.739
Hymenolepididae, **P**.578, **P**.677
Hymenolepis, **P**.576, **P**.677
  autoinfection, **P**.576
  classification, **P**.578
  reproductive system, **P**.661
  structure/life cycle, **P**.578
  see also individual species
Hymenolepis diminuta, **P**.670–1
  control, **P**.671
  infection *see Hymenolepis diminuta* infection
  life cycle, **P**.670–1
  morphology/structure, **P**.670
Hymenolepis diminuta infection, **I**.70
  clinical manifestations, **P**.671
    food supply, **P**.663
  diagnosis, **P**.671
  immune response, **P**.663
    concomitant immunity, **P**.663
  location in host, **P**.662–3
  pathogenesis/pathology, **P**.671
  transmission/epidemiology, **P**.671
Hymenolepis nana, **P**.669–70
  control, **P**.670
    chemotherapy, **P**.670
    prophylaxis, **P**.670
  geographical distribution, **P**.658
  infection
    clinical manifestations, **P**.670
    diagnosis, **P**.670
    immunity, **P**.670
    location in host, **P**.662, **P**.670
    pathogenesis/pathology, **P**.670
  life cycle, **P**.669–70, **P**.670 (Fig.)
    intermediate hosts, **P**.669–70
  morphology/structure, **P**.659, **P**.669
  public health importance, **P**.44
  transmission/epidemiology, **P**.670
    prevalence, **P**.658
    as zoonosis, **P**.669
Hymenomycetes, **M**.63, **M**.65 (Tab.)
Hyperactive malarial splenomegaly (tropical
  splenomegaly syndrome), **P**.484,
  P.501 (Tab.)
  in pregnancy, **P**.484

Hyperammonaemic encephalopathy, **B2**.1447
Hyperbaric oxygen therapy, **M**.678, **B1**.701
Hyperemia, acute phase response, **B1**.739
Hypereosinophilic syndrome, toxocariasis,
  P.754
Hypergammaglobulinemia
  cystic echinococcosis, **P**.694–6
  malaria, **P**.501 (Tab.)
Hyper IgD syndrome, **I**.309
Hyper-IgE syndrome (Job's syndrome),
  I.48 (Tab.), **I**.49, **I**.770
  fungal infection, **I**.770
  Haemophilus influenzae infection, **I**.49
  immunogenetics, **I**.575–6
  Staphylococcus aureus infection, **I**.49, **I**.770
Hyper-IgM syndrome, **I**.384, **I**.778, **I**.781
  AID gene mutations, **I**.781
  CD40 deficiency, **I**.778
  molecular basis, **I**.332
  X-linked, **I**.778
Hyperimmune gammaglobulin, mumps
  prevention, **V1**.752
Hyperimmune sera, **V1**.92–3
Hyperinfection
  Capillaria philippiensis, **P**.745
  Strongyloides, **P**.740–1
Hyperkeratosis, onchocerciasis, **P**.794
Hypermutation
  biased *see* Biased hypermutation
  Hepatitis B virus, **V1**.193
  HSV type-1 (HSV-1), **V1**.193
  Human respiratory syncytial virus, **V1**.193
  retroviruses, **V1**.193
  variability, **V1**.193
  Vesicular stomatitis virus, **V1**.193
Hyperparasitaemia, *Plasmodium*
  gametocytogenesis, **P**.468
Hyperpyrexia, human brucellosis, **B2**.1737–8
Hypersensitivity measurement, **B1**.746–7
  evoked IFN-γ assays, **B1**.747
Hypersensitivity pneumonitis, **B2**.1137–8,
  B2.1170
Hypersensitivity reactions
  Anisakis, **P**.815–16
  ascariasis, **P**.726
  delayed *see* Delayed-type hypersensitivity
    (DTH)
  measles vaccination, **V1**.736
  schistosomiasis, **P**.615–16
  toxocariasis, **P**.754
Hypersensitivity type I, **I**.308
Hypersensitivity type IV *see* Delayed-type
  hypersensitivity (DTH)
Hypertriglyceridemia, acute phase response,
  I.207
Hypervariability, JC virus, **V1**.475–6
Hypervariable regions
  αβ TCRs, **I**.460–1
  Ig heavy chains, **I**.305
  Ig light chains, **I**.305
  see also Complementarity-determining
    regions (CDRs)
Hyphae
  angiotropism, **M**.717
  Aspergillus, **M**.689–90, **M**.717
  Candida albicans as pathogen, **M**.258–9

Coccidioides immitis, **M**.503, **M**.504
  growth, **M**.70, **M**.70 (Fig.), **M**.71, **M**.72 (Fig.)
  histopathology, **M**.87, **M**.88 (Fig.),
    M.89 (Tab.), **M**.125, **M**.127 (Tab.),
    M.128 (Tab.)
  spore-bearing, **M**.76–7
  vegetative, **M**.76–7
  zygomycete, **M**.659, **M**.676, **M**.676 (Fig.)
Hyphal wall protein-1 (HWP-1), **M**.259
Hyphomyces destruens, **M**.412–13
Hyphomycetes, classification, **M**.49, **M**.51
'Hyphomycosis,' **M**.412
Hypnozoites
  malaria relapses, **P**.471
  Plasmodium, **P**.471
  Plasmodium ovale, **P**.471
  Plasmodium vivax, **P**.471
Hypochlorites, **B1**.424
  action, **B1**.437 (Tab.)
Hypochlorous acid, **B1**.425
Hypocomplementemic urticarial vasculitis
  (HUVS), **I**.155
Hypoderaeum, **P**.582–3
Hypogammaglobulinemia
  cryptosporidiosis, **P**.407
  malaria, **P**.488
  X-linked proliferative syndrome, **I**.779
Hypoglycemia
  cerebral malaria in children, **P**.483
  falciparum malaria, **P**.481–2
  malaria in pregnancy, **P**.484
Hypoiodous acid, **B1**.425
Hypokalaemia, amphotericin B causing,
  M.148–9
Hypotension, septic shock, **I**.700
Hypoviridae
  classification, **V1**.27 (Tab.), **V1**.47 (Tab.),
    V1.48
  see also specific viruses
Hypoxanthine–guanine phosphoribosyl
  transferase (HGPRT), monoclonal
  antibodies generation, **I**.333
Hypr virus, **V2**.998 (Tab.)

I3L gene, **V1**.611
I-309 (CCL1), **I**.218 (Tab.)
Iatrogenic Creutzfeldt–Jakob disease (iCJD),
  V2.1365–7
  human growth hormone therapy etiology,
    V2.1366–7
  molecular genetic studies, **V2**.1367
  prevalence, **V2**.1366
  surgical transmission, **V2**.1365–6
  transmission, **V2**.1366 (Tab.)
  see also Creutzfeldt–Jakob disease (CJD)
IBD5 gene, **I**.581
ICAM-1 *see* Intracellular adhesion molecule 1
  (ICAM-1: CD45)
ICAM1 gene, **I**.582–3
  malaria, **I**.599–600
Ice, bacteriology of, **B1**.213
Ice cream, **B1**.250–1
  microbiological quality of, **B1**.251
Ichthyophthirius multifiliis, structure,
  P.171 (Fig.), **P**.174 (Fig.)
ICP0 protein, herpesviruses, **V1**.498–9

ICP4 protein, herpesviruses, **V1**.498–9
ICP8 (UL29), HSV-1 replication, **V1**.165–6,
  V1.165 (Tab.)
ICP22 protein, herpesviruses, **V1**.498–9
ICP27 protein, herpesviruses, **V1**.498–9
Ictalurid herpesvirus 1, **V1**.45
Ictalurivirus
  classification, **V1**.45
  genome sequences, **V1**.494 (Tab.)
'Icythism,' **B2**.1038
Idaeovirus, **V1**.27 (Tab.)
IDDMK1.2, superantigens, **I**.564
Identical by descent (IBD), linkage, **I**.573
Identification
  bacteria, **B1**.19–22, **B1**.28, **B1**.29
    chemical composition, **B1**.22 (Tab.), **B1**.24,
      B1.32–3
    classification *vs.*, **B1**.20
    enzyme tests, **B1**.22 (Tab.), **B1**.24
    fingerprinting, **B1**.22 (Tab.), **B1**.25
    keys, **B1**.20
    mathematical, **B1**.20, **B1**.21 (Tab.)
    numerical, **B1**.20, **B1**.21 (Tab.)
    serology, **B1**.22 (Tab.), **B1**.24
    see also individual species
  fungi
    history, **M**.33–4
    immunodiagnosis, **M**.34–5
      antibodies, **M**.34–5
      circulating antigens, **M**.35
      see also individual assays
  viruses, **V1**.34–5, **V1**.90–3
    diagnostic properties, **V1**.34
    reagent preparation for, **V1**.90–3
      antigens, **V1**.90–2
      controls, **V1**.91
      high-titre antisera, **V1**.92–3
      monoclonal antibodies, **V1**.93
    reference types, **V1**.34
    specimens, **V1**.93–100
      from cell cultures, **V1**.93–4
      from chick embryo cultures, **V1**.94
      collection and transport, **V1**.93
      infection diagnosis, **V2**.1533
      isolation procedures, **V1**.93–5
      from laboratory animal, **V1**.94–5
      specific viruses, **V1**.95–100
      specimen collection, **V1**.93
      specimen types, **V1**.93
  see also Classification
Idiopathic CD4 lymphocytopenia, **I**.779
Idoxuridine, **V2**.1615
Idurin *see* Idoxuridine
IE genes, herpesviruses, **V1**.498–9
IFNGR1 gene
  defects, **I**.575
  familial eosinophilia association, **I**.581
  intracellular bacterial infection, **I**.589
  malaria association, **I**.599
  mutations, **I**.571–2
  schistosomiasis association, **I**.601
IFNGR2 gene
  intracellular bacterial infection, **I**.589
  mutations, **I**.571–2

Igα (CD79a)
  autosomal recessive agammaglobulinemia,
    I.780
  BCR, **I**.339
  pre-BCR, **I**.340–1
Igβ (CD79b)
  BCR, **I**.339
  pre-BCR, **I**.340–1
Igh gene
  allelic exclusion, **I**.324
  gene rearrangement, **I**.323
Igl gene rearrangement, **I**.323, **I**.324
'Ig-like fold,' Ig structure, **I**.305
Ikaros
  B cell development, **I**.324
  NK cell development, **I**.85
IKKγ deficiency, **I**.772
IL1A gene, **I**.578
IL1B gene, **I**.578
  Helicobacter pylori infection, **I**.594
IL1 gene cluster
  hepatitis C, **I**.588
  immunogenetics, **I**.578–9, **I**.578 (Fig.)
  meningococcal meningitis association, **I**.594
  periodontitis association, **I**.595
  tuberculosis association, **I**.591–2
  variable number tandem repeats, **I**.578
IL1R1 gene, **I**.578–9
IL1R2 gene, **I**.578–9
IL1RN gene, **I**.578
IL1RNVNTR gene, **I**.594
IL2 gene, **I**.584
  periodontitis association, **I**.595
IL3 gene, **I**.580
IL3RA gene, **I**.582
IL4 gene, **I**.580, **I**.584
  periodontitis association, **I**.595
  respiratory syncytial virus infection, **I**.587
IL5 gene, **I**.580
IL8 gene, respiratory syncytial virus infection,
    I.587
IL9 gene, **I**.580
IL10 gene, **I**.582–3
  EBV infection, **I**.588
  periodontitis association, **I**.595
  polymorphisms, hepatitis C, **I**.587–8
IL12B gene
  intracellular bacterial infection, **I**.589
  mycobacterial infection association, **I**.582
  polymorphisms, **I**.582
  salmonellosis association, **I**.593
IL13 gene, **I**.580
'Ilaga,' **P**.324
ILC *see* Cutaneous T-cell attracting chemokine
    (CTACK:CCL27)
Ileum, normal microbiota, **B1**.302
Ilhéus virus, **V2**.998 (Tab.), **V2**.1003
Ilizarov method, **B1**.698
Imidazoles, **M**.183 (Tab.), **M**.233
  Aspergillus otomycosis, **M**.700–1
  superficial candidiasis, **M**.189
  vulvovaginal candidiasis, **M**.189
  see also individual drugs
Imidazoquinoline, **I**.121–2

Imipenem
  melioidosis treatment, **B2**.1631,
    B2.1631 (Tab.)
  spectrum of activity, **B1**.478–80,
    B1.499 (Tab.)
  Cardiobacterium hominis, **B2**.1672–3
  Enterobacter, **B2**.1484–5
  Haemophilus, **B2**.1702 (Tab.)
  Klebsiella, **B2**.1480
  Listeria, **B2**.957–8
  Nocardia, **B2**.1165–6
  structure, **B1**.479 (Fig.)
Imipenem-cilastatin, intracranial abscess,
    B1.588
Imiquimod
  adenovirus infection therapy, **V2**.1631
  papillomavirus therapy, **V2**.1631
  structure, **V2**.1618 (Fig.)
Immune complex disease
  antibody-mediated immunopathology,
    V1.287
  Parvovirus B19 virus infection, **V1**.430–1
Immune complexes
  amebiasis, **P**.209
  Borna disease virus infection, **V2**.1150
  clearance
    C1 complement protein, **I**.155
    C4 complement protein, **I**.155
    complement *see* Complement
    erythrocytes, **I**.147
  deposition, SLE, **I**.757
  FcγRIII binding, **I**.315
  hepatitis B, **V2**.1250
  infectious, smoldering infection, **V1**.262
  neutrophil abnormalities, **I**.49
Immune evasion
  bacteria, **B1**.153–4, **I.645–74**
    antigenic variation, **I**.660–1
      capsules, **I**.660–1
      lipooligosaccharide, **I**.661
      LPS, **I**.661
      point mutations, **I**.660
      proteins, **I**.661
    antigen presentation, **I**.657–60
      MHC class I, **I**.659–60
      MHC class II, **I**.657–9
    apoptosis modulation, **I**.654
      caspase interference, **I**.655
      DNA damage, **I**.655
      Fas-mediated apoptosis, **I**.655–6
      pore-forming toxins, **I**.654–5
      type III secretion system, **I**.655
    bacterial pathogenicity, **B1**.153–5
    cellular immunity, **I**.664–8
      immunosuppression, **I**.665
      regulatory T cells, **I**.666–8
      superantigens, **I**.668
      T cells, **I**.664–5
      Th1/Th2 balance, **I**.665–6
    complement, **I**.662–4, **I**.663 (Fig.)
      cleavage, **I**.663–4
      inhibitory protein binding, **I**.664
      membrane attack complex inhibition,
        I.664
      shedding, **I**.663

  surface masking, **I**.662–3
  cytokine modulation, **I**.651–4
    IL-10 induction, **I**.652–4
    IL-12, **I**.652
    TNF-α, **I**.652
    transforming growth factor-β, **I**.652–4
  dendritic cell maturation, **I**.656, **I**.667–8
  humoral response, **I**.660–2, **I**.660 (Fig.)
    antibody-binding proteins, **I**.661–2
    antibody degradation/modification, **I**.662
  phagocytosis, **I**.647–51, **I**.648 (Fig.)
    chemotaxis inhibition, **I**.648
    escape to cytoplasm, **I**.650
    lysosomal killing resistance, **I**.651
    lysosome fusion inhibition, **I**.650
    nonlysosomal organelles, **I**.650–1
    uptake inhibition, **I**.649
  see also individual species
parasites, **I**.420–1, **I.675–91**
  cysticercosis, **P**.691
  echinococcosis, **P**.691
  Entamoeba histolytica, **P**.209
  glutathione peroxidases, **I**.686
  Leishmania major, **P**.77–8
  malaria *see* Malaria
  Plasmodium, **P**.62
  Schistosoma, **P**.92–3, **P**.93–4, **P**.94–5
  Toxoplasma gondii, **P**.77, **P**.85–6
  toxoplasmosis, **P**.78–9
  transmission dynamics, **P**.62
  Trypanosoma, **P**.62
  Trypanosoma cruzi, **P**.77, **P**.86, **P**.87,
    P.385–6
  see also individual species
protozoa infection, **I**.679–82
  antigen variation, **I**.680–1
  intracellular refuges, **I**.681–2
  see also individual species
viruses, **I.617–44**, **V1**.229–30, **V1**.286–8, **I**.420,
    V1.311–29
  adaptive immune response, **V1**.311–12,
    I.630–9
  see also specific mechanisms
  antibodies, **V1**.287, **V1**.313 (Fig.)
  antigen presentation, **V1**.320–3,
    V1.321 (Fig.)
    dendritic cells, **V1**.323
    MHC class I, **V1**.321–2
    MHC class II, **V1**.322
    MHC interference, **V1**.287, **V2**.1206–7
  apoptosis, **V1**.287, **V1**.323–5, **V1**.324 (Fig.),
    V1.603 (Fig.), **I**.625 (Fig.), **I**.626–7
    caspase inhibitors, **V1**.324, **I**.625 (Fig.),
      I.627
    death-receptor inhibitors, **I**.625 (Fig.),
      I.626–7
    mitochondrial apoptosis inhibitors,
      I.625 (Fig.), **I**.627
    signal blocking, **V1**.323
  CD8 interference *in vivo*, **I**.636–7
  CD8 T cell epitope variation, **I**.636
  cell signaling molecules, **I**.618–23
    see also specific molecules
  chemokines, **V1**.288, **V1**.319–20, **V1**.619,
    I.621–3, **V1**.622
    binding proteins, **V1**.320, **I**.622–3

Immune evasion
  viruses
    chemokines (*Continued*)
      homologues, **V1**.319, **I**.620 (Fig.), **I**.621–2
      receptor homologues, **V1**.319–20, **I**.620 (Fig.), **I**.622
    complement, **V1**.230, **V1**.287, **V1**.311–12, **V1**.313, **V1**.313 (Fig.), **V1**.619–20
    inhibitory factor recruitment, **V1**.313
    regulatory protein analogues, **V1**.313
    Cowpox virus *see* Cowpox virus
    cytokines, **V1**.288, **V1**.298 (Tab.), **V1**.315–9, **V1**.316 (Fig.), **I**.619–21, **I**.639
      binding proteins, **V1**.318–19, **I**.621
      expression/activation interference, **V1**.316, **I**.623
      homologues, **V1**.317–18, **V1**.317 (Fig.), **I**.620, **I**.620 (Fig.)
      receptor homologues, **V1**.317 (Fig.), **V1**.318, **I**.620–1, **I**.620 (Fig.)
      signal transduction, **V1**.316–17
    dendritic cells, **I**.630–2, **I**.632 (Fig.)
    genetic analysis, **V1**.198–9
    humoral immunity, **V1**.312–13, **I**.638–9, **I**.638 (Fig.)
      antibodies, **I**.638
      Fc receptors, **V1**.312–13
      genetic variability, **V1**.312
    inflammation inhibitors, **V1**.286
    INFs, **V1**.199, **V1**.228, **V1**.230, **V1**.286–7, **V1**.296, **V1**.311–12, **V1**.313–5, **V1**.314 (Fig.), **I**.618–19, **I**.618 (Fig.), **V1**.619, **V1**.620
      antagonism, **V1**.787
      effector functions, **V1**.315, **I**.619
      receptors/binding proteins, **V1**.314–15, **I**.619
      signal transduction, **V1**.315, **I**.619
    innate cellular immunity, **I**.627–30
      see also specific mechanisms
    innate immune response, **V1**.311–12
    MHC class I antigen presentation, **I**.420, **I**.632–6
      antigen processing, **I**.633, **I**.633 (Fig.), **I**.635 (Fig.)
      expression modulation, **I**.637
      MHC degradation, **I**.634, **I**.636 (Fig.)
      MHC synthesis, **I**.634, **I**.635 (Fig.)
      molecule removal, **I**.635–6, **I**.636 (Fig.)
      peptide-loading complex, **I**.633–4, **I**.635 (Fig.)
      TAP transport, **I**.633
    mutation rates, **I**.420
    NK cell interference, **V1**.287, **V1**.311–12, **V1**.321 (Fig.), **V1**.322–3, **I**.628–30, **I**.629 (Fig.)
      infected cell recognition, **I**.628–30
      leukocyte Ig-like receptors, **I**.630
      MHC class I homologues, **V1**.322–3
    superantigens, **I**.637–8
    see also specific viruses
Immune modulators, hepatitis B treatment, **V2**.1260
Immune-privileged sites, cysticercosis, **P**.691
Immune reconstitution inflammatory syndrome, **I**.800–1

Immune response, **P**.67, **P**.68–73, **P**.69 (Fig.), **B1**.175–7, **V1.270–91**
  acquired *see* Adaptive immune response
  activated macrophage, **P**.68–9
  acute infection, **V1**.258
  adaptive *see* Adaptive immune response
  adiaspiromycosis diagnosis, **M**.816–17
  analysis, **V2**.1544–7
  anatomical barriers, **B1**.175–6
  antigen processing/presentation, **P**.68
  antiviral chemotherapy, **V2**.1606
  bacterial antagonism, **B1**.176
  cellular *see* Cell-mediated immune response
  common pattern recognition, **B1**.176–7
  CTLs, **P**.68
  cytokine network *see* Cytokine(s)
  dermatophytes, **M**.232–3
  development, **B1**.339
  emerging viral infection, **V2**.1655
  entomophthoromycosis (entomophthoramycosis), **M**.347, **M**.350
  evasion *see below*
  evasion of *see* Immune evasion
  gene therapy, **V2**.1590–1
  granulomatous response, **B1**.741–7
    causative organisms, **B1**.741
    latent infection, **B1**.741
  herpesviruses interaction, **V1**.257–8, **V1**.258 (Fig.)
  historical aspects, **V1**.4, **B1**.7–8
  humoral *see* Humoral immune response; *specific components*
  humoral response, **P**.69–70
  inactivated (killed) vaccines, **V2**.1556
  against infection *vs.* against disease, **B1**.339
  innate *see* Innate immune response
  innate immunity, **B1**.175
  iron-binding, **B1**.151
  keratitis, **M**.314–15
  Mumps virus vaccination, **V1**.751
  natural immunity, **B1**.339
  neutralizing antibodies, **V2**.1115–16
  NK cells, **P**.68
  nutritional restriction, **B1**.176
  parasite recognition, **P**.68
  PCP in AIDS, **M**.792, **M**.793–4, **M**.794–6
  population, genetic factors, **B1**.355
  privileged site infection, **B1**.747–8
  role, **P**.67
  viral infection, **B1**.435–6, **V1**.618–19
  see also Acute phase response; Immunoserology; *individual infection; individual species; specific diseases/ infection; specific viruses/infection*
'Immune surveillance hypothesis,' **I**.421
Immune system reconstitution
  HAART, **I**.799
  HIV infection, **I**.799, **I**.800–1
Immune therapy, hepatitis B treatment, **V2**.1260
Immune tolerance *see* Tolerance
Immunity
  concomitant (premunition) *see* Concomitant immunity (premunition)

development
  basic reproductive number of infection effects, **P**.53–4, **P**.54 (Fig.)
  malaria, **P**.53–4, **P**.54 (Fig.)
helminths, **P**.87–96
  antigens, **P**.88
  characteristics affecting, **P**.87–9
  cytokines released, **P**.88
  filarial nematodes, **P**.91–2
  flukes, **P**.94
  intestinal, **P**.89–91
  larval tapeworms, **P**.95–6
  nematodes, **P**.89–91
  tapeworms, **P**.95–6
partial
  epidemiology, **I**.955
  infection models, **I**.956
protective *see* Protective immunity
protozoa, **P**.75–6
  amebae, **P**.75
  ciliates, **P**.76
  coccidians, **P**.76
  depression by HIV, **P**.74–5
  flagellates, **P**.76
  intestinal, **P**.75
  macrophage-inhabiting protozoa, **P**.77
  tissue-inhabiting protozoa, **P**.85–7
  in urinogenital tract, **P**.76–7
temporary, epidemiology, **I**.955
transmission dynamics effects *see* Transmission dynamics
Immunization
  active *see* Vaccination; Vaccine(s)
  passive *see* Passive immunization
Immunization Action Coalition, **V2**.1583
Immunization Practices Advisory Committee (ACIP), measles vaccination recommendations, **V1**.735–6
Immunoassays, **P**.153–4
  African trypanosomiasis, **P**.367
  alveolar echinococcosis, **P**.694
  amebiasis, **P**.154
  Anisakis infection, **P**.817–18
  antibody detection, **P**.153–4
  antigen detection, **P**.154
  Bartonella henselae, **B2**.1897
  bunyavirus infection diagnosis, **V2**.1050
  Canine distemper virus diagnosis, **V1**.812
  cryptosporidiosis, **P**.154
  cystic echinococcosis, **P**.694–6
  dracunculiasis, **P**.832
  Equine arteritis virus infection, **V1**.846–7
  fecal samples, **P**.151
  giardiasis, **P**.154
  gnathosomiasis, **P**.154
  Hepatitis A virus, **V2**.1171
  Hepatitis delta virus, **V2**.1272
  hepatitis E, **V2**.1179
  HHV, **V1**.532–3
  hookworm infection, **P**.154
  lymphatic filariasis, **P**.776–7
  malaria, **P**.154, **P**.488, **P**.503–4, **P**.504 (Fig.)
  melioidosis diagnosis, **B2**.1630
  microsporidiosis, **P**.154, **P**.536, **P**.546
  monoclonal antibodies, **I**.333

Immunoassays (*Continued*)

neurocysticercosis, **P**.693–4

Newcastle disease virus diagnosis, **V1**.816

onchocerciasis, **P**.791

Parvovirus B19 virus infection diagnosis, **V1**.430

Peste-des-petits-ruminants virus diagnosis, **V1**.811

pharyngitis diagnosis, **B1**.611

rinderpest diagnosis, **V1**.810

sapovirus detection, **V2**.924–5, **V2**.925–6

schistosomiasis, **P**.606

severe acute respiratory syndrome (SARS), **V1**.842–3

toxocariasis, **P**.154

toxoplasmosis, **P**.154

trichinellosis, **P**.154, **P**.765, **P**.766 (Fig.)

trichomoniasis, **P**.258–9

vaccine response, **V2**.1558

see also Immunoserology; *individual techniques; specific assays*

Immunoblotting

Anisakis diagnosis, **P**.817

Aspergillus, **M**.712–13

Borrelia detection, **B2**.1829

Pythium insidiosum, **M**.424 (Fig.)

syphilis test, **B2**.1849–50

see also Western blotting

Immunochemotherapy, anergic diffuse cutaneous leishmaniasis, **P**.342

Immunochromatographic strip tests, syphilis detection, **B2**.1850

Immunocompetency, cryptosporidiosis, **P**.409

Immunocompromised patients

microbiological risk assessment, **V2**.1519

oncogenicity in, **V1**.346–7

virus infection, **V2.1498–512**

adenovirus infection, **V1**.444

diagnosis, **V2**.1498

HHV-6 infection, **V1**.528–9

HSV infection, **V1**.508

Minute virus of mice infection, **V1**.426

non-HIV infection, **V2**.1506–10

Parvovirus infection, **V1**.426

varicella (chickenpox), **V1**.513

see also specific infection; specific viruses

see also HIV infection; Immunodeficiency diseases/disorders; Immunosuppressed patients

Immunoconjugates

adverse effects, **I**.359

antigen choice, **I**.358–9

immunogenicity of, **I**.359

Immunocytochemistry, progressive multifocal leucoencephalopathy (PML), **V2**.1418

Immunodeficiency diseases/disorders, **I**.766 (Tab.), **I.765–85**

acquired, **I.787–815**

causes, **I**.787–9, **I**.788 (Tab.)

adaptive immunity, **I**.773–82

AIDS *see* AIDS; HIV infection

antibody, respiratory tract infection, **B1**.626

B cell diseases/infection, **I**.766 (Tab.), **I**.779–82, **I**.780 (Fig.)

autosomal recessive agammaglobulinemia, **I**.780

IgG isotype deficiencies, **I**.781–2

with bone abnormalities, **I**.766 (Tab.), **I**.777

complement deficiencies, **B1**.564

congenital asplenia, **I**.771

emerging bacterial infection, **B1**.362

genomic instability, **I**.766 (Tab.), **I**.776–7

Bloom syndrome, **I**.777

centromeric instability and facial anomalies, **I**.777

DNA ligase 4 deficiency, **I**.776

Nigmegan breakage syndrome, **I**.777

granulocyte production deficiencies, **I**.765–7

hospital-acquired bacteremia, **B1**.393

HPV infection, **I**.772

innate/adaptive immunity, **I**.766 (Tab.), **I**.772–3

innate immunity, **I**.765–72

intravenous Ig, **V2**.1566

measles vaccination, **V1**.736

mycobacterial infection susceptibility, **I**.772–3

NEMO/IKKγ deficiency, **I**.772

neutrophil function disorders, **I**.766 (Tab.), **I**.767–70, **I**.768 (Fig.)

actin dysfunction, **I**.769

chronic granulomatous disease *see* Chronic granulomatous disease (CGD)

glucose-6-phosphate dehydrogenase deficiency, **I**.770

lymphocyte adhesion deficiency *see* Leukocyte adhesion deficiency (LAD)

Papillon-Lefévre syndrome, **I**.770

RAC-2 deficiency, **I**.769

specific granule deficiency, **I**.769

NK cell disorders, **I**.772

Parvovirus B19 virus infection, **V1**.431–2

perforin-dependent cytolysis deficiencies, **I**.778–9

plasma protein disorders, **I**.766 (Tab.), **I**.770–1

pneumonia, **B1**.644–5

Pseudomonas infection, **B2**.1593

rapidly growing mycobacteria, **B2**.1249, **B2**.1259

Salmonella antibacterial susceptibility/ resistance, **B2**.1414

smallpox, **V1**.586–7

T cell diseases/infection, **I**.766 (Tab.), **I**.773–6

caspase 8 deficiency, **I**.776

CD3 deficiency, **I**.775

chronic mucocutaneous candidiasis, **I**.779

diGeorge syndrome, **I**.774–5

HLA class II expression deficiencies, **I**.776

idiopathic CD4 lymphocytopenia, **I**.779

IL-2 receptor α chain deficiency, **I**.775–6

nude phenotype, **I**.775

purine nucleoside phosphorylase deficiency, **I**.775

severe combined immunodeficiency *see* Severe combined immunodeficiency (SCID)

TAP deficiencies, **I**.776

thymic defects, **I**.774–5

ZAP-70 deficiency, **I**.775

tuberculosis, **I**.713

undescribed deficiencies, **I**.771–2

see also Immunocompromised patients; Immunosuppressed patients; *specific diseases/infection*

Immunodiagnostic tests

candidiasis diagnosis, **M**.591, **M**.606

identification of fungi *see* Identification, fungi; *individual assays*

Immunodiffusion (ID) assays, **B1**.718

Coccidioides immitis, **M**.514–15

Histoplasma capsulatum var. *capsulatum* detection, **M**.532

pythiosis, **M**.421–2

Pythium insidiosum, **M**.423–4

Immunodominance, **I**.404

Immunodominant antigens, *Plasmodium*, **P**.486, **P**.488

Immunoelectroosmophoresis (IEOP), **B1**.749

Immunofluorescence (IF) assays

African trypanosomiasis, **P**.367

amebiasis, **P**.211–12

arenaviruses, **V2**.1068–9, **V2**.1076

Avian infectious bronchitis virus infection, **V1**.844

bacteria, **B1**.718, **B1**.719

blastomycosis, **M**.491, **M**.492, **M**.496

Chlamydia, **B2**.2017–18

in diagnosis, **V2**.1535

direct *see* Direct immunofluorescence

HSV infection, in pregnancy, **V2**.1465

indirect *see* Indirect immunofluorescence

Legionella, **B2**.1773

limitations, **V2**.1535

melioidosis, **B2**.1630

microsporidiosis, **P**.536, **P**.546

mycology, **M**.33, **M**.34, **M**.130–2

Pneumocystis, **M**.788

Porcine transmissible gastroenteritis virus infection, **V1**.844–5

rabies diagnosis, **V2**.1125

VZV detection, **V1**.516

Immunofluorescent antibody tests (IFATs), **B1**.749

cryptosporidiosis, **P**.408–9

Legionella detection, **B1**.752

malaria diagnosis, **P**.488, **P**.503 (Fig.)

Rickettsia detection, **B1**.752–3

Strongyloides diagnosis, **P**.741–2

see also Indirect fluorescent antibody test (IFAT)

Immunogenetics, **I.571–614**

association, **I**.574–5

Bonferroni correction method, **I**.574

case–control studies, **I**.574

Fischer's exact test, **I**.574

haplotype relative risk, **I**.574

linkage disequilibrium methods, **I**.574

linkage *vs.*, **I**.574

single nucleotide polymorphisms, **I**.575

transmission disequilibrium test, **I**.574

bacterial infection, **I**.589–95

Helicobacter pylori infection, **I**.594

intracellular bacteria, **I**.589–90

leprosy *see* Leprosy

Neisseria meningitidis, **I**.594

see also Meningococcal disease (meningitis)

Immunogenetics
  bacterial infection (*Continued*)
    periodontitis, **I**.595
    Salmonella infection, **I**.593–4
      see also Salmonellosis
    tuberculosis, **I**.591–3
      see also Tuberculosis
  clinical phenotype definition, **I**.572
    qualitative traits, **I**.572
    quantitative traits, **I**.572
  commonly investigated genes, **I**.576–84,
      I.585 (Fig.)
    chromosome 5 gene cluster, **I**.580–2,
        I.581 (Fig.)
    chromosome 17, **I**.582, **I**.583 (Fig.),
        I.584 (Fig.)
    complement genes, **I**.579–80
    HLA, **I**.576–7
    HLA class III, **I**.577–8
    IgE-influencing genes, **I**.580–2
    ILA1 gene cluster, **I**.578–9, **I**.578 (Fig.)
    mannose-binding lectin, **I**.579–80
  fungal infection, **I**.595–6
  gene identification, **I**.572
    candidate gene testing, **I**.572
    genome scanning, **I**.572
  genetic control testing, **I**.572
    co-infection, **I**.572
    familial clustering of disease, **I**.572
    nutritional status, **I**.572
    racial differences, **I**.572
    segregation analysis, **I**.572
    twin studies, **I**.572
  helminth infection, **I**.600–1
    filarial nematodes, **I**.600–1
    gastrointestinal nematodes, **I**.600–1
    schistosomiasis, **I**.601
      see also Schistosomiasis
  linkage, **I**.572–4
    animal models, **I**.572–3
    identical by descent, **I**.573
    knockout mice, **I**.572–3
    LOD score, **I**.573
    microsatellite markers, **I**.573
    model-dependent analysis, **I**.573
    model-free analysis, **I**.573
    necessary *vs.* susceptibility loci, **I**.573–4
    nonparametric linkage, **I**.573
    nonparametric methods, **I**.573
    polymorphism information content, **I**.573
    transgenic mice, **I**.572–3
    variance component methods, **I**.573
  protozoal infection, **I**.596–600
    leishmaniasis, **I**.596–7
      see also Leishmaniasis
    malaria, **I**.597–600
      see also Malaria
  single gene control, **I**.575–6
    adaptive immune response defects, **I**.575
    innate immune response defects, **I**.575
  viral infection, **I**.584–9
    hepatitis B, **I**.587
    hepatitis C, **I**.587–8
    HIV infection, **I**.584–6
    respiratory syncytial virus, **I**.587

    *see also individual genes; specific diseases/
        infection*
Immunogenicity
  immunoconjugates, **I**.359
  monoclonal antibody therapy, **I**.362, **I**.365–6
Immunoglobulin(s)
  affinity maturation, germinal centers, **I**.401
  C1 complement protein binding, **I**.142–3
  classes, **I**.307–11
    see also individual classes
  class switching *see* Class switching
  deficiencies
    infection, **I**.781–2
    respiratory tract infection, **B1**.626
  diversity generation, **I**.328
    class switch recombination *see* Class
        switching
    somatic recombination *see* Somatic
        recombination, Igs
    V(D)J recombination, **I**.328
  effector functions, **I**.311–12
    complement fixation, **I**.312
    Fc region, **I**.311–12
    neutralization, **I**.312
  genes, **I**.328–32
    J genes, **I**.328
    regulated rearrangement, **I**.322–3
    V genes, **I**.328
  as host defence mechanism in lung, **B1**.624
  membrane, **I**.310
  metabolism, **I**.310, **I**.311 (Tab.)
  oropharyngeal candidiasis, **M**.260
  prophylaxis *see* Passive immunization
  receptors, **I**.312–19
    polymeric receptor *see* PIgR (polymeric
        immunoglobulin receptor)
    see also under Fc receptors
  somatic hypermutation *see* Somatic
      hypermutation, Igs
  structure *see* Immunoglobulin structure
  synthesis, **I**.321–8
    BcR heavy chains, **I**.332
    clonal selection theory, **I**.321–2
    defects, **I**.575–6
      see also specific diseases/infection
    IL-6, **I**.285
    in measles, **I**.806
    see also B cell development
  see also Antibodies
Immunoglobulin A (IgA), **P**.69–70, **V1**.276–7,
    I.307–8
  bacterial infection, **I**.647
    blocking by meningococci, **B1**.564
    immune evasion, **I**.662
  candidiasis, **M**.260–1
    vulvovaginal, **M**.260, **M**.266
  class switching, **I**.331
    mucosal immune response, **I**.535–6
    see also Class switching
  common mucosal immune system, **I**.534
  deficiencies, **I**.781
    drug-induced, **I**.781
    immunogenetics, **I**.575–6
  detection in serum, **V2**.1546–7
  functions, **I**.537 (Fig.)

IgA1 protease, **B1**.556
monomeric forms, **I**.308 (Fig.)
nasal-associated lymphoid tissue, **I**.533–4
oral immunization, **I**.539–40
parasitic infection
  intestinal nematode infection, **P**.90
  trichomoniasis, **P**.258–9
  trichuriasis, **P**.90
polymeric forms, **I**.308 (Fig.)
  mucosal immune response, **I**.524–5
receptors
  Fcα/μR interactions, **I**.317–18
  pIgR binding, **I**.318–19
  transport, **I**.537–8
  see also individual receptors
secondary humoral immune response, **I**.308
secretory *see* Secretory immunoglobulin A
    (sIgA)
structure
  α heavy chain, **I**.307
  glycosylation, **I**.306
subtypes *see specific subtypes*
synthesis
  CD4+ T cells, **I**.536
  cytokine control, **I**.536–7, **I**.537 (Fig.)
  IL-5, **I**.536
  IL-6, **I**.536–7
Th1 responses, **I**.540 (Fig.)
viral infection
  Hepatitis A virus targeting to liver,
      V2.1167
  measles, **V1**.726–7
  mumps, **V1**.756
    nephropathy, **V1**.748–9
  picornaviruses, **V1**.282
  rhinoviruses, **V2**.874
  rotavirus infection, **V2**.952–3
  rubella, **V2**.972
  viral cell entry inhibition, **V1**.278
Immunoglobulin A1 (IgA1), **I**.307–8
  effector functions, **I**.311 (Tab.)
  metabolism, **I**.311 (Tab.)
  molecular properties, **I**.307 (Tab.)
Immunoglobulin A2 (IgA2), **I**.307–8
  effector functions, **I**.311 (Tab.)
  metabolism, **I**.311 (Tab.)
  molecular properties, **I**.307 (Tab.)
Immunoglobulin D (IgD), **I**.309
  effector functions, **I**.311 (Tab.)
  metabolism, **I**.311 (Tab.)
  molecular properties, **I**.307 (Tab.)
  receptors, **I**.318
    see also specific receptors
  structure, **I**.306 (Fig.)
    glycosylation, **I**.306
    hinge region, **I**.309
  subacute sclerosing panencephalitis, **V1**.731
Immunoglobulin E (IgE), **P**.69–70, **I**.308
  class switching, **I**.327, **I**.331
  in diseases/infection
    airway hypersensitivity, **I**.732–3, **I**.733–4
    in allergic reactions, **I**.308
    hypersensitivity type I, **I**.308
    in parasitic infection, **I**.308

Immunoglobulin E (IgE) (*Continued*)
  effector functions, **I**.311 (Tab.)
    basophil activation, **I**.62
  elevated levels, liver/lung fluke infection,
    P.653
  immunogenetics, **I**.580–2
  metabolism, **I**.310, **I**.311 (Tab.)
  molecular properties, **I**.307 (Tab.)
  parasitic infection
    alveolar echinococcosis, **P**.689
    ascariasis, **P**.729
    cystic echinococcosis, **P**.689
    gastrointestinal nematodes, **P**.90, **P**.725
    onchocerciasis, **P**.794–5, **P**.795, **P**.796
    schistosomiasis, **P**.94, **P**.631–2
    Strongyloides infection, **P**.741
    toxocariasis, **P**.754
  receptors, **I**.316–17
    FcεRI interaction *see* FcεRI
    FcεRII (CD23) interactions, **I**.317
    interaction, **I**.320–1
    see also specific receptors
  structure, **I**.306 (Fig.)
    deviations, **I**.310 (Fig.)
    hinge region, **I**.320
Immunoglobulin G (IgG), **P**.69–70, **V1**.276–7,
  I.307
  avidity differences, **B1**.742
  complement fixation, **I**.312
  deficiencies, **I**.781–2
  function in airways, **B1**.624
  levels during infection, **B1**.742, **B1**.743
  metabolism, **I**.310
  mucosal immune response, **I**.524–5
  parasitic infection
    African trypanosomiasis, **P**.365
    hookworms, **P**.729–30
    onchocerciasis, **P**.795
  receptors, **I**.312–5
    FcγRI (CD64) interactions, **I**.314
    FcγRIII (CD16) interactions *see* FcγRIII
    (CD16)
    FcRn (neonatal receptor) binding, **I**.315–
    16, **I**.525
    interaction, **I**.321
    see also under Fc receptors; specific
    receptors
  structure
    γ heavy chain, **I**.307
    glycosylation, **I**.306
  subacute sclerosing panencephalitis, **V1**.731
  subclasses, **P**.69–70, **I**.307
    deficiencies, **I**.781–2
    see also individual types
  viral infection, **I**.618
    alphaviruses, **V2**.1018
    hepatitis A, **V2**.1171
    HHV-6, **V1**.532
    mumps, **V1**.755, **V1**.756
    Parvovirus B19 virus infection, in
    pregnancy, **V2**.1469
    rubella, **V2**.972
  vulvovaginal candidiasis, **M**.266
Immunoglobulin G1 (IgG1)
  bacterial toxin neutralization, **I**.647

complement fixation, **I**.142, **I**.307
  deficiency, **I**.781–2
  effector functions, **I**.311 (Tab.)
  intestinal nematode infection, **P**.90
  measles, **V1**.726–7
  metabolism, **I**.311 (Tab.)
  molecular properties, **I**.307 (Tab.)
  rubella, **V2**.972
  structure, **I**.306 (Fig.), **I**.319–20
    deviations, **I**.310 (Fig.)
    disulfide bridges, **I**.306
Immunoglobulin G2 (IgG2)
  Blastocystis hominis infection, **P**.563–4
  class switching, **I**.327
  deficiency, **I**.781–2
  effector functions, **I**.311 (Tab.)
    complement fixation, **I**.142
    opsonization, **I**.647
  metabolism, **I**.311 (Tab.)
  molecular properties, **I**.307 (Tab.)
  schistosomiasis, **P**.94
  structure, **I**.306 (Fig.)
    disulfide bridges, **I**.306
Immunoglobulin G3 (IgG3)
  class switching, **I**.327
  effector functions, **I**.311 (Tab.)
    complement fixation, **I**.142, **I**.307
  measles, **V1**.726–7
  metabolism, **I**.310, **I**.311 (Tab.)
  molecular properties, **I**.307 (Tab.)
  rubella, **V2**.972
  structure, **I**.306 (Fig.)
    disulfide bridges, **I**.306
Immunoglobulin G4 (IgG4)
  deficiency, **I**.781–2
  effector functions, **I**.311 (Tab.)
    complement fixation, **I**.142
  filariasis, **P**.91
  metabolism, **I**.311 (Tab.)
  molecular properties, **I**.307 (Tab.)
  onchocerciasis, **P**.795
  schistosomiasis, **P**.94
  structure, **I**.306 (Fig.)
    disulfide bridges, **I**.306
Immunoglobulin M (IgM), **I**.307
  capture assays, hepatitis A, **V2**.1172
  detection in serum, **V2**.1546
  effector functions, **I**.311 (Tab.)
    C1 complement protein binding, **I**.142
    C1q interaction, **I**.312
    complement fixation, **I**.307, **I**.312
    opsonization, **I**.307
    viral infection, **I**.618
  initial infection, **V1**.276–7
  levels during infection, **B1**.742–3
  metabolism, **I**.311 (Tab.)
  molecular properties, **I**.307 (Tab.)
  monomeric forms, **I**.308 (Fig.)
  parasitic infection
    African trypanosomiasis, **P**.365
    Chagas disease, **P**.385, **P**.389
    hyperactive malarial splenomegaly
      (tropical splenomegaly syndrome), **P**.484
    onchocerciasis, **P**.795
    schistosomiasis, **P**.94

polymeric forms, **I**.308 (Fig.)
  mucosal immune response, **I**.524–5
  primary humoral immune response, **I**.303,
    I.307
  receptors, **I**.317–18
    Fcα/μR interactions, **I**.317–18
    pIgR binding, **I**.318–19
    see also individual receptors
  secretory, **I**.309–10
  structure
    J chain, **I**.307
    μ heavy chain, **I**.307
  syphilis
    EIA test, **B2**.1849, **B2**.1850 (Tab.)
    fluorescent antibody absorption test,
      B2.1848
    immunoblotting, **B2**.1849–50
  T helper cells, **P**.69–70
  viral infection
    alphavirus infection, **V2**.1018
    HCMV infection, **V1**.525, **V1**.526
    hepatitis A, **V2**.1171, **V2**.1172
    HHV-6 infection, **V1**.532
    infectious mononucleosis (IM), **V1**.568–9
    measles, **V1**.726–7
    mumps, **V1**.751, **V1**.755, **V1**.756
    Parvovirus B19 virus infection, in
      pregnancy, **V2**.1469
    rubella, **V2**.972
Immunoglobulin structure, **I**.303, **I**.303–6,
  I.304 (Fig.), **I**.319–21
  in BCR, **I**.339
  disulfide bonds, **I**.306
  enzyme digestion, **I**.304
  F(ab)'₂, **I**.304
  Fab (fragment antibody binding), **I**.304
  Fc (fragment crystalline), **I**.304
  glycosylation, **I**.306
  heavy chains, **I**.303–4, **I**.304 (Fig.)
    constant domain interactions, **I**.319
    constant region, **I**.305
    framework regions, **I**.305
    hypervariable regions, **I**.305
    pre-BCR, **I**.340–1
    surface expression in B cell development,
      I.323
    variable region, **I**.305
  hinge region, **I**.306
  J chain, **I**.309–10
  light chains, **I**.303–4, **I**.304 (Fig.)
    constant region, **I**.304
    framework regions, **I**.305
    hypervariable regions, **I**.305
    kappa, **I**.309, **I**.323
    lambda, **I**.309, **I**.323
    rearrangement in B-cell development,
      I.324
    surface expression in B cell development,
      I.304
    variable region, **I**.304
  primary structure, **I**.304–5
  quaternary structure, **I**.305–6
    constant domain interactions, **I**.305
    intermolecular forces, **I**.305–6
    variable domain interactions, **I**.305

Immunoglobulin structure (*Continued*)
  secondary structure, **I**.305
    β pleated sheets, **I**.305
    disulfide bonds, **I**.305
    'Ig-like fold,' **I**.305
  tertiary structure, **I**.305
Immunoglobulin superfamily, viral receptors, **V1**.209
Immunohistochemical (IHC) techniques, syphilis diagnosis, **B2**.1844–5
Immunohistochemistry, **M**.130–2, **M**.130 (Tab.)
  chemokine patient studies, **I**.229
  filovirus infection diagnosis, **V2**.1096–7, **V2**.1097 (Tab.)
  Pythium insidiosum, **M**.424–5
Immunologically-priviliged sites, **V1**.261
  peripheral tolerance, **I**.749
Immunological memory *see* Memory
Immunological synapse *see* T-cell receptor (TCR)
Immunological tolerance *see* Tolerance
Immunomagnetic bead separation, *Giardia* detection, **P**.250–1
Immunomodulatory agents
  candidiasis therapy, **M**.597, **M**.611
  in meningococcal disease, **B1**.567
Immunopathology
  malaria, **P**.500, **P**.501 (Tab.)
  of viral infection, **V1**.278–80, **V1**.292, **V1**.312
    antibody-mediated, **V1**.279, **V1**.279 (Tab.)
      antibody-dependent enhancement (ADE), **V1**.287
      immune complex disease, **V1**.287
    filovirus infection, **V2**.1095–6
    hepatitis C, **V2**.1207
    rabies, **V2**.1125
    T-cell-mediated, **V1**.279–80, **V1**.279 (Tab.)
      delayed-type hypersensitivity, **V1**.280
    Th1/Th2 balance, **V1**.292–3
Immunoperoxidase assays (IPA), virus inactivation, **V1**.91
Immunoprecipitation assays, **B1**.749
  double diffusion, **B1**.749
Immunoprophylaxis, parasite control, **P**.112–15
Immunoradiometric assay (IRMA), *Bacillus anthracis* endospore detection, **B2**.930
Immunoreceptor tyrosine-based activation motifs (ITAMs)
  BCR, **I**.341
  CD3, **I**.460
  FcεRI, **I**.316
  FcγRII (CD32), **I**.314
  NK cell receptors, **I**.90
  ZAP-70 binding, **I**.775
Immunoreceptor tyrosine-based inhibitory motifs (ITIMs)
  FcγRII (CD32), **I**.314
  FcγRIIB, **I**.347–8
  NK cells, **I**.87–8
Immunoserology, **B1.738–59**
  advantages, **B1**.738
  antibody detection, **B1**.748–50
    applications, **B1**.750–4
      see also individual infection
    direct visualization, **B1**.748–9
    indirect visualization, **B1**.749–50

histoplasmosis, **M**.532–3
molecular assays *vs.,* **B1**.738, **B1**.755–6
near-patient testing, **B1**.753–4
  controls, **B1**.754
  inappropriate use, **B1**.754
  safety, **B1**.754
organism characterization, **B1**.754–6
  applications, **B1**.756–8
    see also individual species
  non cultural diagnosis, **B1**.738, **B1**.754
saliva testing, **B1**.753
see also Immune response; Immunoassays; Serology/serological diagnosis; *specific assays/techniques*
Immunosorbent agglutination assay (ISAGA), toxoplasmosis diagnosis, **P**.434–5
Immunostimulating particles (ISCOMs), **I**.930–1
  intranasal vaccine delivery, **I**.864
  mechanism of action, **I**.930
Immunostimulation, CpG motifs, **I**.911–12, **I**.916
Immunostimulatory sequence (ISS), CpG motifs, **I**.911
Immunosuppressed patients, **M**.12
  African trypanosomiasis, **P**.365–6
  amebiasis, **P**.209
  aspergillosis *see* Aspergillosis
  autoimmune disease therapy, **I**.760
  bacterial immune interference, **I**.665
  Blastocystis hominis infection, **P**.563
  candidiasis, **M**.13, **M**.580, **M**.585, **M**.589
  Carrión's disease, **B2**.1888–9
  Chagas disease, **P**.86
  chromoblastomycosis, **M**.359
  chronic hepatitis B, **V2**.1249
  coccidioidomycosis, **M**.508–10, **M**.516
  CpG motifs, **I**.912
  cryptococcosis *see* Cryptococcosis
  cryptosporidiosis, **P**.399, **P**.409–10
  diagnostic accuracy, **M**.82, **M**.86
  EBV-associated lymphomas after, **V1**.570–1
  Echinococcus granulosus, **P**.96
  granulomatous amebic encephalitis, **P**.236
  HCMV infection in transplants, **V1**.521–2
  histoplasmosis, **M**.23
  HTLV infection, **I**.802–3, **I**.804 (Fig.), **I**.805 (Fig.)
  HTLV transmission, **V2**.1291
  IL-17 therapy, **I**.290
  inactivated (killed) vaccines, **V2**.1563
  leishmaniasis, **P**.339
  malaria, **P**.491, **P**.501 (Tab.)
  measles, mumps and rubella (MMR) vaccine, **V2**.1563
  nongenital skin warts, **V1**.462–3
  paracoccidioidomycosis, **M**.550
  PCP *see* Pneumocystis pneumonia (PCP)
  penicilliosis marneffei, **M**.562
  progressive multifocal leucoencephalopathy (PML), **V1**.477
  protot'hecosis, **M**.398–9, **M**.401
  pyrogenic exotoxins, **I**.561–2
  rabies, **V2**.1124–5
  reduced phagocytosis in, **B1**.626
  serology, **M**.92

sporotrichosis, **M**.375
subunit vaccines, **V2**.1563
superantigens, **I**.561–2
Taenia solium cysticercus, **P**.685–6
Trichomonas vaginalis infection, **P**.258
trichomoniasis, **P**.258
trichosporonosis, **M**.109, **M**.629
varicella vaccines/vaccination, **V2**.1575
viruses causing, **V1**.341, **V1**.342 (Tab.)
  filovirus infection, **V2**.1096
  HHV-8 infection, **V1**.550
  LCMV, **V2**.1074–5
  measles *see* Measles
zygomycosis, **M**.21
  systemic, **M**.672–3
see also Immunocompromised patients; Immunodeficiency; Transplants; *specific infection*
Immunosuppressive therapy
  immunodeficiency, **I**.788 (Tab.)
  withdrawal, cryptococcosis therapy, **M**.652
Immunotherapy
  candidiasis *see* Candidiasis
  cryptococcosis, **M**.652–3
  LCMV infection, **V2**.1077
  leishmaniasis, **P**.342–3
  mucocutaneous/mucosal leishmaniasis, **P**.342
  tumor virus infection, **V1**.350
Immunotoxins, **I**.358–9
  antibody fragments, **I**.369
Impingement samplers, airborne bacteria monitoring, **B1**.190
'Imported malaria,' **P**.514–15
Importins, Hepatitis B virus nuclear entry, **V2**.1234
Inactivated live vaccine, Rabies virus, **V2**.1126
Inactivated poliomyelitis vaccine (Salk: IPV), **V2**.879–80, **V2**.1552 (Tab.), **V2**.1560 (Fig.)
  adverse effects, **V2**.1564 (Tab.)
    see also Vaccine-related poliomyelitis
  in developing countries, **V2**.1573
  development, **V2**.1571–2
  historical aspects, **V2**.1572
  in pregnancy, **V2**.1562–3
  schedule, **V2**.1572
Inactivation factor (IF), **B1**.446
Inactivation procedures, viruses, **V1**.91
Inapparent infection, poliomyelitis, **V2**.870
Incidence
  cumulative, **B1**.310
  infection models, **I**.948–9
    rates, **I**.949–50
  number of susceptibles *vs.,* **I**.949, **I**.949 (Fig.)
  prevalence *vs.,* **I**.948, **I**.948 (Fig.)
  rates, **B1**.310
  see also Epidemiology
Incidence rate (density), **V1**.359–60
Incidence studies, **B1**.313–14, **B1**.314 (Fig.)
Inclusion conjunctivitis, **B2**.2012, **B2**.2013–14, **B2**.2013 (Fig.)
Incompatibility groups *see* Plasmid(s)
Incoscint, licensing, **I**.355 (Tab.)
Incubation periods, **B1**.310, **B1**.338, **B1**.338 (Fig.)
  amebiasis, **P**.207

Incubation periods (*Continued*)
  astrovirus infection, **V2**.903–4
  Chagas disease, **P**.385
  definition, **V1**.356
  giardiasis, **P**.245
  granulomatous amebic encephalitis (GAE),
    P.231
  Human coronavirus infection, **V1**.841–2
  malaria, **P**.511
    vivax/ovale (benign tertian) malaria, **P**.482
  mumps, **V1**.748
  prion diseases, **V2**.1356
  rabies, **V2**.1117–18
  rubella, **V2**.969
  sapovirus infection, **V2**.924
India ink, **M**.88 (Tab.), **B2**.934–7, **B2**.947
Indian tick typhus, **B2**.2039 (Tab.)
India, parasitic disease importance, **P**.27 (Fig.)
Indinavir, **V2**.1623–4
  resistance, **V2**.1336
    point mutations, **V2**.1337 (Fig.)
  structure, **V2**.1624 (Fig.)
Indirect fluorescent antibody test (IFAT)
  Anaplasma phagocytophilum infection,
    B2.2063–4
  babesiosis, **P**.456, **P**.457
  Bartonella, **B2**.1897
  Bartonella bacilliformis, **B2**.1890
  Borrelia detection, **B2**.1829
  Chagas disease, **P**.389
  Ehrlichia chaffeensis human infection,
    B2.2063–4
  Legionella pneumophila, **B2**.1761–4, **B2**.1774
  malaria, **P**.503
    blood transfusions, **P**.506
  microsporidiosis, **P**.546
  mumps diagnosis, **V1**.754, **V1**.755–6
  Old World leishmaniasis, **P**.302
  Pneumocystis, **M**.793–4
  see also Immunofluorescent antibody tests
    (IFATs)
Indirect hemagglutination assay (IHA)
  amebiasis, **P**.154, **P**.208
  Chagas disease, **P**.389
  cystic echinococcosis, **P**.694–6
  malaria, **P**.503
  melioidosis, **B2**.1630
Indirect immunofluorescence assay (IFA),
    V2.1535, **V2**.1545
  amebiasis, **P**.154
  cystic echinococcosis, **P**.694–6
  filovirus infection diagnosis, **V2**.1091–2,
    V2.1096–7, **V2**.1097 (Tab.)
  giardiasis, **P**.248
  intestinal protozoa, **P**.154
  measles diagnosis, **V1**.732
  melioidosis diagnosis, **B2**.1630
  Q fever diagnosis, **B2**.2077
Indium labeled white scan, osteomyelitis,
    B1.694
Individuals, populations *vs.*, **I**.948
Indoles
  Enterobacteriaceae identification,
    B2.1319 (Tab.)
  Porphyromonas identification, **B2**.1924 (Tab.)
  Prevotella identification, **B2**.1924 (Tab.)

Providencia, **B2**.1451
Indolicidin, **I**.172
Indoor feeding (endophagy), mosquito
    (*Anopheles*), **P**.470
Inducer exclusion, **B1**.50
Inducers (inducible promoters), **B1**.71
  recombinant gene expression, **B1**.122
Inducible co-stimulatory molecule (ICOS),
    I.395, **I**.399
  APC interactions, **I**.392 (Fig.)
Inducible nitric oxide synthase (iNOS), **P**.73
  acute phase response, **I**.205–6
  IL-17 effects, **I**.290
  leishmaniasis, **I**.596
  macrophages, **I**.26
  malaria association, **I**.599
  polymorphisms, malaria susceptibility,
    P.485–6
  regulation, **P**.73
  septic shock, **I**.700
  TLR stimulus, **I**.697
  see also Nitric oxide (NO)
Industrial facilities, endotoxin exposure, **B1**.189
Industrialized nations, rubella epidemiology,
    V2.970
Indwelling medical devices, **B1**.390–2
  cerebrospinal fluid shunts, **B1**.392
  infection associated, **B1**.390–2
  intravascular cannulae, **B1**.391–2
  intravascular devices
    emerging bacterial infection, **B1**.361
    endocarditis associated, **B1**.524–5, **B1**.525–6
  intravascular grafts, **B1**.392
  see also specific types
Inermicapsifer, **P**.577
Inermicapsifer madagascariensis, **P**.674
Infantile genetic agranulosis, **I**.47
Infants
  bacterial colonization, **B1**.293
  diarrhea
    Escherichia coli, enteroaggregative,
      B2.1378–9
    Escherichia coli, enteropathogenic,
      B2.1373–4
    Escherichia coli, enterotoxigenic, **B2**.1375
  enteritis, *Escherichia coli*, enteropathogenic,
    B2.1372–4
  influenza, **V1**.661
  meningitis, **B1**.557
    Haemophilus influenzae type b (Hib),
      B1.573
  susceptibility to viral infection, **V1**.263
  vaccines/vaccination, **V2**.1559
    hepatitis B vaccines/vaccination, **V2**.1574
  see also Children; Neonatal infection
Infected dusts, indirect transmission, **V1**.355
Infection(s)
  bacterial
    antigenic variation, **I**.661
    barriers, **B1**.294
    cell wall, phagocytosis effects, **I**.645–6
    chronic diseases due to, **B1**.365
    course in populations, **B1**.339–41
    CXCR1, **I**.227
    CXCR2, **I**.227
    definition, **B1**.294

DNA
  septic shock, **I**.696
  TLR-8 binding, **I**.122
  TLR binding, **I**.696
  encapsulated
    polysaccharide vaccines, **I**.935
    Wiskott–Aldrich syndrome, **I**.777–8
  epidemiology, **I**.953
    see also Epidemiology of infection
  IFN-γ deficiency, **I**.288
  immune interference *see* Immune evasion
  induced apoptosis *see* Apoptosis
  intracellular *see* Intracellular pathogens
  neutrophil abnormalities, **I**.50
  NK cells, **I**.79, **I**.99–100
  recurrent, lectin pathway deficiencies,
    I.152–3
  secondary, trichuriasis, **P**.728
  spreading factors, **B1**.152, **B1**.153 (Tab.)
  stages, **B1**.338–9, **B2**.1953 (Fig.)
  systemic γδ T cells, **I**.438–41
  toxins, induced apoptosis, **I**.136–7
  transmission principles, **B1**.338–9
  as vaccine vectors *see* Vaccines, live;
    individual species
disease *vs.*, **I**.948
fungal
  hyper-IgE syndrome, **I**.770
  joint prostheses, **B1**.392
  neutrophil abnormalities, **I**.50
  nosocomial, **B1**.374, **B1**.403
  therapy, **M**.182, **M**.182–5
mathematical models, **I**.948–50
  basic reproduction number (R_0), **I**.955–6
    epidemic threshold value, **I**.956
    secondary cases, **I**.955
  chemotherapy effects, **I**.950
  dynamic equilibria, **I**.956–7
    endemic infection, **I**.956–7
    susceptible removal, **I**.957, **I**.958 (Fig.)
  effective reproduction number *(R)*,
    B1.340, **I**.956
    potential transmission, **I**.956
    vaccination campaign effects, **B1**.346
  host population effects, **I**.956
    damped oscillations, **I**.956
    host arrival, **I**.956
    partial immunity effects, **I**.956
  incidence *vs.* prevalence, **I**.948, **I**.948 (Fig.)
  individual *vs.* populations, **I**.948
  infection *vs.* disease, **I**.948
  political complications, **I**.950
  simple dynamic models, **I**.949–50
    epidemic shape, **I**.950, **I**.950 (Fig.)
    flow diagram, **I**.950 (Fig.)
    incidence rates, **I**.949–50
    recovery rates, **I**.949–50
  statistical complications, **I**.950
  susceptibility, **I**.948–9
  transmission dynamics, **I**.948–9
    'force of infection,' **I**.948–9
    incidence, **I**.948–9
    incidence *vs.* number of susceptibles,
      I.949, **I**.949 (Fig.)
    random transmission, **I**.948–9

Infection(s)
mathematical models (*Continued*)
  see also Epidemiology of infection;
    Vaccination, mathematical models
parasitic
  chronic disease, I.675, I.680
  cytokines, I.679–80
  IgE, I.308
  IL-3 effects, I.275–6
  immune evasion *see* Immune evasion
  immunity, CD8 T cells, I.420–1
  importance of, P.46 (Tab.), P.24–49
    age-relation, P.25
    demography, P.25
    disability adjusted life year (DALY),
      P.25, P.25 (Fig.), P.27 (Fig.), P.28 (Tab.)
    geographical areas, P.25, P.27 (Fig.)
    helminth parasites, P.39–44
    mortality, P.24, P.28 (Tab.), P.29 (Tab.)
    new diseases/infection, P.44–5
    non-helminth parasites, P.29–39
      intestinal protozoa, P.37–9
    population movement, P.25–9
      air travel, P.29
      blood transfusions, P.27–9
      conflict-related, P.25–6
      control costs, P.26–7
      economic immigrants, P.26–7
      intestinal parasites, P.26–7
    prevalence, P.24–5
    socioeconomic groups, P.25
    World Bank studies, P.24–5
    see also specific diseases/infection
  intracellular *see* Intracellular pathogens
  neutrophil abnormalities, I.50
  NK cells, I.79, I.100
  pathogen-associated molecular patterns,
    I.679–80
  pattern recognition receptors, I.679–80
  protozoa, I.675–9
  TLRs, I.679–80
  transforming growth factor-β, I.297
  see also individual species; individual types
viral
  acute *see* Acute infection
  basophils *see* Basophils
  CD8 T cells, I.419–20
  cellular susceptibility, V1.247–8,
    V1.265 (Tab.)
  chronic, epidemiology, V1.373–4
  eosinophils *see* Eosinophil(s)
  epidemiology *see* Epidemiology of
    infection, viral infection
  gastroenteritis, B1.400
  granzyme deficiencies, I.482
  IFN-γ deficiency, I.288
  immune interference *see* Immune evasion,
    viruses
  incubation period, V1.356
  infectious dose, V1.355–6
  initial biosynthesis, V1.216 (Tab.)
  of *Leishmania*, P.335
  meningoencephalitis, HLA class II
    expression deficiency, I.776
  MHC effects, I.472
  neonatal, B1.395

neutrophil abnormalities, I.49
new *see* Emerging infection
NK cells, I.79, I.94–9
nosocomial, B1.374, B1.395, B1.400
otitis media, B1.617
pathogenicity, V1.356
persistent *see* Persistent viral infection
productive *see* Cell–virus interactions
secondary attack rate (SAR), V1.356
therapy
  IFN-α, I.258–9
  type I IFN, I.258–9
  TNF-α, I.286
transmission
  blood transfusions, B1.380–1
  tissue donation, B1.381
virulence, V1.356
see also individual viruses
see also individual infection; specific
  organisms
Infection Control Committee, B1.406
Infection Control Doctor (ICD), B1.406
Infection Control Link Nurse (ICLN),
  B1.407–8
Infection Control Nurse (ICN), B1.406
Infection Control Team (ICT), B1.404, B1.406
Infection mode, transmission of infection(s),
  I.951 (Tab.)
Infection rates, influenza, V1.669
Infection resistance, cross-sectional surveys,
  P.56–7
Infectious bronchitis virus (IBV)
  envelope (E) protein, V1.831–2, V1.837
  genome
    sequencing, V1.397–8
    structure, V1.828 (Fig.)
  infection, V1.841 (Tab.)
  replicase (RNA polymerase), V1.833 (Fig.)
  type species, V1.392, V1.824–5
Infectious bursal disease virus, V1.48
Infectious Diseases Society of America
  (IDSA), pneumonia treatment
  guidelines, B1.638, B1.639 (Tab.)
Infectious dose, definition, V1.355–6
Infectious hematopoietic necrosis virus
  classification, V1.385–6
  genome structure, V2.1112 (Fig.)
Infectious immune complexes, smoldering
  infection, V1.262
Infectious jaundice, V2.1160
Infectious mononucleosis (IM), V1.567–9
  clinical features, V1.568
  complications, V1.568
  diagnostic tests, V1.568–9
  epidemiology, V1.567–8
    observational studies, V1.364
  immune response, V1.568–9, V1.569 (Fig.)
  immunodeficient patients (non-HIV),
    V2.1507–8
  pathogenesis, V1.568
  spread, V1.567–8
  see also Epstein–Barr virus (EBV) infection
Infectious salmon anemia virus, V1.50
Infective biting rate, onchocerciasis, P.785–6
Infective density of vector, onchocerciasis,
  P.785–6

Infective dermatitis, HTLV type 1 (HTLV-1)
  infection, V2.1290, V2.1291
Infective endocarditis *see* Endocarditis,
  infective
Infective spondylitis, causative pathogens,
  B1.690
Infectivity, period, B1.338, B1.338 (Fig.)
INFGR1 gene, I.582
INFGR2 gene, I.582
Infiltration, bacterial pathogenicity, B1.152–3
Inflammatory bowel disease (IBD)
  animal models, I.753
  Chlamydia pneumoniae infection, B2.2017
  Escherichia coli, diffusely adherent link,
    B1.148–9
  HLA association, I.577
  prostaglandin E$_2$, I.188
Inflammatory chemokines *see* Chemokine(s)
Inflammatory cytokines *see* Proinflammatory
  cytokines
Inflammatory diseases, HTLV type 1 (HTLV-
  1) infection, V2.1290–1
Inflammatory lesions, African trypanosomiasis,
  P.365
Inflammatory neuropathies, neuro-AIDS,
  V2.1428
Inflammatory responses
  bacterial infection, I.645
  Borna disease virus infection, V2.1148
  C5a complement protein, I.154
  chemokine disease models, I.228–9
  chemokine receptors, I.227
  chronic, host-pathogen interactions, I.109–11
  cytokines *see* Proinflammatory cytokines
  defensins, I.520–1
  dermatophytosis, M.232–3
  fungal infection diagnosis, M.127, M.130
  histopathology, M.127, M.130
  historical aspects/re-evaluation, I.5–6, I.11
  HIV infection, V1.299
  IFN-γ effects, I.288
  inhibitors, V1.286
    Lassa virus, V2.1072
  lymphocyte migration, I.512
  Molluscum contagiosum virus infection,
    V1.619
  onchocerciasis, P.781
  opisthorchiasis, P.651
  prostacyclins, I.189
  prostaglandin E$_2$, I.188
  rhinovirus infection, V2.873
  therapy
    chemokine antagonists, I.231
    RANTES antagonists, I.231
  toxoplasmosis, P.434
  trichinellosis, P.762–3
  Trichophyton infection, M.232
  see also specific diseases/infection
Infliximab, mechanism of action, I.357
Influenza
  adults, V1.660–1
  antiviral therapy, V1.679–80
    amantadine, V2.1625–6
  basic reproduction number, B1.340 (Tab.)
  clinical manifestations, V1.660–5

Influenza (*Continued*)
complications, **V1**.661
in elderly patients, **V1**.661
lower respiratory tract infection, **V1**.661
pneumonia, **V1**.367
pregnancy, **V1**.661
primary influenza pneumonia, **V1**.661
secondary bacterial infection, **V1**.661
upper respiratory tract infection, **V1**.661
control, **V1**.677–80
chemotherapy *see above*
neuraminidase inhibitors, **V1**.680
vaccine *see below*
diagnosis, **V1**.674–7
embryonated egg isolation, **V1**.674
molecular methods, **V1**.676–7
point-of-care tests, **V1**.675
serology, **V1**.675, **V2**.1546–7
tissue culture isolation, **V1**.674–5
ecology, **V1**.671–4
bird reservoirs, **V1**.641 (Fig.), **V1**.672
emerging infection, **V2**.1648 (Tab.)
mutation, **V2**.1653
reassortment, **V2**.1654
epidemics, **V1**.635 (Tab.)
pandemics *vs.,* **V1**.668–9
epidemiology, **V1**.367, **V1**.667–74
age-relation, **V1**.367
antigenic drift, **V1**.367, **V1**.668–9
antigenic shift, **V1**.367, **V1**.669–71
in HIV infection, **V2**.1499 (Tab.)
infection rates, **V1**.669
monitoring/surveillance, **V1**.360–1,
V1.361 (Fig.)
seasonality, **V1**.367, **V1**.668
subtype effects, **V1**.367
transmission, **V1**.667–8
immune response, **V1**.662–5
adaptive, **V1**.663
humoral, **V1**.663–4
IL-1, **V1**.296–7
IL-18, **I**.290–2
innate, **V1**.662–3
intrasubtypic, **V1**.663–4
NK cells, **I**.96
persistence, **V1**.663–4
T-cell responses, **V1**.664–5
Th1/Th2 ratio, **V1**.298
TNF-α induction, **V1**.296
immunogenetics, **I**.588–9
immunopathology, **V1**.280
infants/children, **V1**.661
laboratory worker immunization, **B1**.767
morbidity, **V1**.668–9
mortality, **V1**.669
complications, **V1**.669
'excess mortality,' **V1**.669, **V1**.671 (Tab.)
influenza A *vs.* influenza B, **V1**.669
prediction, **V1**.669
nosocomial, **B1**.400
pandemics, **V1**.367, **V1**.634–5
epidemics *vs.,* **V1**.668–9
pathogenesis, **V1**.661–2
columnar epithelial cells, **V1**.661–2

vaccines/vaccination, **V1**.677–9,
V2.1552 (Tab.), **V2**.1576–7
adverse effects, **V2**.1577
at-risk groups, **V1**.677, **V2**.1561, **V2**.1577
attenuated bacterial vectors, **I**.902
attenuated viral vectors, **I**.846
BCE peptide vaccines, **I**.855 (Tab.),
I.869–70
development status, **I**.933 (Tab.)
DNA vaccines, **V2**.1554
effectiveness, **V1**.679, **V2**.1576–7
epidemiological modeling, **V1**.365
formulations, **V1**.678–9, **V1**.678 (Tab.)
GM-CSF adjuvants, **I**.277
history, **V1**.8 (Tab.)
immune response, **V1**.679
inactivated, **V2**.1576–7
intranasal route, **I**.831–2
ISCOMs adjuvant, **I**.930–1
live, attenuated, **V2**.1555 (Tab.), **V2**.1577
MF59 adjuvant, **I**.927–9
in pregnancy, **V2**.1562–3
programs, **V1**.367, **V2**.1559 (Tab.)
proteasomes, **I**.839
skin application, **I**.823, **I**.825
USA schedules, **V2**.1559–60,
V2.1560 (Fig.), **V2**.1577
virosomes, **I**.838–9, **I**.929
virus-like particles, **I**.840
Influenza viruses, **V1.634–98**
animal infection, **V1**.652
antigenic drift, **V1**.668–9
epidemics, **V1**.668
morbidity effects, **V1**.668–9
antigens, **V1**.665–7
see also specific antigens
apoptosis, **V1**.662
cell entry, **V1**.58–9, **V1**.106, **V1**.107 (Fig.),
V1.241 (Tab.)
endocytosis, **V1**.107–8
inhibition by antibody, **V1**.277
neuraminidase, **V1**.212
receptor binding/membrane fusion, **V1**.213
cell interactions
host RNA processing/transport, **V1**.221
host RNA synthesis, **V1**.221
classification, **V1**.636–7
dendritic cell importance, **V1**.273
E1B, **V1**.221
E4, **V1**.221
gene expression, **V1**.120
genetic engineering, **V1**.195–7
genome, **V1**.639–60
coding strategies, **V1**.644 (Fig.)
potential maximization, **V1**.133
segment structure, **V1**.642 (Fig.)
subunit reassortment, **V1**.192
hemagglutinin (HA), **V1**.71, **V1**.647–53
acylation, **V1**.652
antibody-binding sites, **V1**.664
as antigen, **V1**.664, **V1**.665
antigenic variation, **V1**.653, **V1**.670 (Fig.)
assembly, **V1**.650–1
as attachment protein, **V1**.207
attenuated viral vaccine, **I**.898

cleavage, **V1**.651
conformational change in cell entry,
V1.107–8, **V1**.214–15, **V1**.214 (Fig.),
V1.649–50, **V1**.650 (Fig.)
evolutionary rates, **V1**.669 (Tab.)
folding, **V1**.650–1
functions, **V1**.766
glycosylation, **V1**.225
intracellular transport, **V1**.650–1
membrane fusion, **V1**.213–14,
V1.214 (Fig.), **V1**.649–50, **V1**.649 (Fig.)
monomeric structure, **V1**.648 (Fig.)
oligosaccharide side chains, **V1**.651
peptide vaccines, **I**.869–70
pH effects, **V1**.649–50
post-translational modifications, **V1**.224–5
receptor binding, **V1**.642, **V1**.652–3
receptor specificity, **V1**.652
structure, **V1**.106, **V1**.107 (Fig.), **V1**.208,
V1.208 (Fig.), **V1**.639, **V1**.639 (Fig.),
V1.648–9, **V1**.650 (Fig.)
translation/processing, **V1**.646
virosome adjuvants, **I**.929
historical aspects, **V1**.634–6
egg inoculation, **V1**.636
seroarcheology, **V1**.635
vaccine development, **V1**.636
virus isolation, **V1**.635–6
host range restriction, **V1**.652–3, **V1**.666–7
identification, **V1**.96 (Tab.), **V1**.98–9
immune evasion
genetic variability, **V1**.312
IFN interference, **V1**.230
infection *see* Influenza
isolation/propagation, **V1**.96 (Tab.), **V1**.98–9
M1 protein, **V1**.656–7
as antigen, **V1**.666
cold-adapted strains, **V1**.657
membrane interactions, **V1**.646
nuclear export function, **V1**.656–7
viral budding, **V1**.639, **V1**.656
'zinc-finger' motif, **V1**.657
M2 protein, **V1**.657
as antigen, **V1**.666
cell attachment, **V1**.642
functions, **V1**.657
ion channel activity, **V1**.645 (Fig.), **V1**.657
morphology/structure, **V1**.71
mixed cell culture, **V1**.88
morphology/structure, **V1**.637–9,
V1.637 (Fig.), **V1**.638 (Fig.),
V1.639 (Fig.), **V1**.640 (Fig.)
hemagglutinin, **V1**.71
internal structure, **V1**.641 (Fig.)
M2 protein, **V1**.71
M proteins, **V1**.69–70, **V1**.637–8
neuraminidase, **V1**.71
nucleocapsids, **V1**.71
pleomorphism, **V1**.637–8
M proteins, **V1**.69–70, **V1**.637–8
MX protein, **V1**.662
NB protein, **V1**.656
neuraminidase (NA), **V1**.654–6
as antigen, **V1**.665–6
assembly, **V1**.656
folding, **V1**.656

Influenza viruses
  neuraminidase (NA) (*Continued*)
    hemagglutinin activity, **V1**.656
    host range restriction, **V1**.655, **V1**.666–7
    intracellular transport, **V1**.656
    reverse genetics, **V1**.654
    sialidase activity, **V1**.655–6
    structure, **V1**.639, **V1**.639 (Fig.),
      V1.655 (Fig.), **V2**.1626–7
    three-dimensional structure, **V1**.655
    viral entry/release, **V1**.655–6
  NS1 protein, **V1**.221
  NS2 (NEP) protein, **V1**.659
    as antigen, **V1**.666
    nuclear transport, **V1**.646
  nuclear transit, **V1**.216
  nucleoprotein (NP), **V1**.653–4
    as antigen, **V1**.665
    host range restriction, **V1**.653–4, **V1**.666–7
    matrix (M) protein binding, **V1**.216
    maturation, **V1**.653–4
    morphology, **V1**.654 (Fig.)
  PA protein, **V1**.647
    structure, **V1**.639
    transcription/translation, **V1**.642
  PB1 protein, **V1**.646–7
    structure, **V1**.639
    transcription/translation, **V1**.642
  PB2 protein, **V1**.647
    host range restriction, **V1**.647
    structure, **V1**.639
    transcription/translation, **V1**.642
  polymerase proteins, **V1**.646–7
    as antigens, **V1**.665
    structure, **V1**.647 (Fig.)
    see also specific types
  polypeptides, **V1**.646–59
    see also specific proteins
  replication, **V1**.642–6, **V1**.645 (Fig.)
    attachment/uncoating, **V1**.642,
      V1.645 (Fig.)
    budding, **V1**.646
    nucleus, **V1**.131
    transcription, **V1**.642–6
    translation, **V1**.642–6
    viral morphogenesis, **V1**.646
  reverse genetics, **V1**.659–60, **V1**.660 (Fig.)
  ribonucleoprotein complex
    morphology, **V1**.654 (Fig.)
    structure, **V1**.639
  as vaccine vector, **I**.846
  virulence, HA cleavage, **V1**.651
Influenza virus A
  amantidine resistance, **V2**.1636
  antigenic shift, **V1**.669–71
    pandemics, **V1**.669–71
  apoptosis induction, **V1**.662
  cell entry, **V1**.642
    cell receptors, **V1**.207 (Tab.)
  characteristics, **V1**.129 (Tab.)
  chemotherapy, **V1**.679–80
  classification, **V1**.50
  epidemiology, **V1**.667
  evolution, host species effects, **V1**.18
  fusion protein, **V1**.214

genome, **V1**.639–40, **V1**.643 (Tab.)
  coding strategies, **V1**.644 (Fig.)
  conserved sequences, **V1**.640–1
  RNA segments, **V1**.636–7
  segment reassortment, **V1**.16
H1N1 subtype, **V1**.667
  epidemics, **V1**.634–5
  pandemics, **V1**.671
  virulence, **V1**.660–1
H1 subtype, **V1**.652
  pandemic, **V1**.671
H2N2 subtypes
  epidemics, **V1**.634–5
  mortality, **V1**.669
  pandemics, **V1**.671
  virulence, **V1**.660–1
H2 subtype
  pandemic, **V1**.671
  receptor specificity, **V1**.653
H3N2 subtype, **V1**.667
  mortality, **V1**.669
  virulence, **V1**.660–1
H3N3 subtype, epidemics, **V1**.634–5
H3 subtype
  pandemic, **V1**.671
  receptor specificity, **V1**.653
hemagglutinin (HA), **V1**.636–7,
  V1.643 (Tab.)
  antigenic drift, **V1**.668
  receptor specificity, **V1**.652
  structure, **V1**.639
  translation/processing, **V1**.646
historical aspects, **V1**.636 (Fig.)
infection
  croup (laryngotracheobronchitis), **V1**.774
  influenza *see* Influenza
M1 protein, **V1**.643 (Tab.)
  coding strategies, **V1**.644 (Fig.)
M2 protein, **V1**.643 (Tab.)
  coding strategies, **V1**.644 (Fig.)
  translation/processing, **V1**.646
M gene, **V1**.641–2
morphology/structure, **V1**.72 (Fig.), **V1**.637–
  8, **V1**.637 (Fig.), **V1**.638 (Fig.)
  protein structures, **V1**.70 (Tab.)
neuraminidase (NA), **V1**.636–7,
  V1.643 (Tab.)
  antibody escape mutants, **V1**.666
  antigenic drift, **V1**.668
  antigenic sites, **V1**.665–6
  structure, **V1**.639
  translation/processing, **V1**.646
nonstructural proteins, **V1**.646
  see also specific types
NP protein, **V1**.643 (Tab.)
  antigenic variation, **V1**.665
NS1 protein, **V1**.643 (Tab.), **V1**.658
  as antigen, **V1**.666
  apoptosis induction, **V1**.658
  coding strategies, **V1**.644 (Fig.)
  functional domains, **V1**.658
  genetics, **V1**.641
  IFN inhibition, **V1**.658
  post-transcriptional modification, **V1**.658

NS2 protein
  coding strategies, **V1**.644 (Fig.)
  genetics, **V1**.641
  NS gene, **V1**.641
  pandemics, virulence, **V1**.671
  PA protein, **V1**.643 (Tab.)
  PB1-F2 polypeptide, **V1**.646–7, **V1**.665
    apoptosis, **V1**.662
  PB1 protein, **V1**.643 (Tab.)
  PB2 protein, **V1**.643 (Tab.)
  phylogenetic studies, **V1**.672
  recombination, **V1**.16
    virulence effects, **V1**.15–6
  reverse genetics, **V1**.659–60, **V1**.660 (Fig.)
    live attenuated vaccine, **V1**.660
  structural proteins, **V1**.646
    see also specific types
  subtypes, **V1**.637
    see also specific types
Influenza virus B
  apoptosis induction, **V1**.662
  BM2 protein, **V1**.657–8
  cell entry, **V1**.642
  cell receptors, **V1**.207 (Tab.)
  characteristics, **V1**.129 (Tab.)
  chemotherapy, **V1**.679–80
  classification, **V1**.50
  epidemiology, **V1**.667
  genome, **V1**.639–40
    coding strategies, **V1**.644 (Fig.)
    conserved sequences, **V1**.640–1
    RNA segments, **V1**.636–7
  hemagglutinin (HA), **V1**.636–7
    antigenic drift, **V1**.668
    structure, **V1**.639
  historical aspects
    isolation, **V1**.635–6
    prevalence, **V1**.636 (Fig.)
  infection *see* Influenza
  M1 protein
    coding strategies, **V1**.644 (Fig.)
    phosphorylation, **V1**.657
  M gene, **V1**.641–2
  morphology/structure, **V1**.72, **V1**.73 (Fig.),
    V1.637–8
    protein structures, **V1**.70 (Tab.)
  NA gene, **V1**.641, **V1**.642
  NB protein, **V1**.642, **V1**.656
    translation/processing, **V1**.646
  neuraminidase (NA), **V1**.636–7, **V1**.642
    antigenic drift, **V1**.668
    coding strategies, **V1**.644 (Fig.)
    structure, **V1**.639
  nonstructural proteins, **V1**.646
    see also specific types
  structural proteins, **V1**.646
    see also specific types
Influenza virus C
  cell entry, **V1**.642
    esterase, **V1**.212
    receptors, **V1**.207 (Tab.)
  characteristics, **V1**.129 (Tab.)
  classification, **V1**.50
  CM2 protein, **V1**.658
    coding strategies, **V1**.644 (Fig.)

Influenza virus C (*Continued*)
  genome, **V1**.639–40
    coding strategies, **V1**.644 (Fig.)
    RNA segments, **V1**.636–7
  hemagglutinin–esterase (HEF) fusion
      protein, **V1**.636–7, **V1**.659
    translation/processing, **V1**.646, **V1**.659
  historical aspects, isolation, **V1**.635–6
  infection see Influenza
  M1 protein, **V1**.644 (Fig.)
  M gene, **V1**.641–2
    splicing, **V1**.641–2
  morphology/structure, **V1**.72, **V1**.637–8,
      V1.640 (Fig.)
    protein structures, **V1**.70 (Tab.)
  nonstructural proteins, **V1**.646
  P42 protein, **V1**.644 (Fig.)
  structural proteins, **V1**.646
Infundibulum, respiratory tract, **B1**.606–7
Infusion fluid contamination, **B1**.384
Inhalation, airborne bacteria, **B1**.188
Inhibition enzyme immunoassay, *Aspergillus,*
    M.714–15
Inhibitors of apoptosis (IAPs), **I**.135, **I**.624
Inhibitory receptors, NK cells *see* Natural
    killer (NK) cells
Injecting drug use, HTLV transmission,
    V2.1293
Injections, gas gangrene after, **B2**.1089,
    B2.1111, **B2**.1113
Injury, acute phase response induction, **I**.194
Inkoo virus, **V2**.1042–3
Innate immune response, **I**.111–12, **B1**.175–7,
    V1.270–4
  acute phase proteins, **I**.199–202
  adaptive immunity *vs.,* **I**.377 (Tab.)
  anatomical barriers, **B1**.175–6
  bacterial infection, **I**.645–6, **I**.646 (Fig.)
    alternative complement pathway, **I**.645
    cellular activation, **I**.651–2
      see also Pattern recognition
    inflammatory response, **I**.645
  cellular immunity, **I**.112–13
    viral immune interference, **I**.627–30
      see also specific mechanisms
    see also individual cell types
  commensal bacterial antagonism, **B1**.176
  common pattern recognition, **B1**.176–7
  complement, **I**.141
    see also Complement
  cytokines, **I**.403
    see also Cytokine(s)
  diseases/infection
    bacterial infection *see above*
    immunodeficiency diseases/disorders,
      I.765–72
    immunogenetics, **I**.575
    viral infection *see below*
  fungal infection
    candidiasis *see* Candidiasis
    vulvovaginal candidiasis, **M**.266
  history, **I**.111–12
  immune evasion, **I**.311–12
  immunodeficiency diseases/disorders,
    I.766 (Tab.), **I**.772–3
  mechanical removal, **B1**.176

mucosa *see* Mucosal immune response
nutritional restriction, **B1**.176
parasitic infection
  toxoplasmosis, **P**.78–9
  trichomoniasis, **P**.258
pattern recognition receptors, **I**.645
prion diseases *see* Prion diseases
reassessment, **I**.9
self recognition, **I**.112
time scales, **V1**.271 (Fig.)
viral infection, **I**.617
  filovirus immune evasion, **V2**.1096
  hepatitis B, **V1**.283
  HSV infection, **V1**.284
  Human respiratory syncytial virus
      infection, **V1**.793–4
  influenza, **V1**.662–3
  measles, **V1**.727
  norovirus infection, **V2**.920–1
*see also specific diseases/infection; specific
    organisms*
Innate resistance, malaria, **P**.485–6
Inoculation site, rabies, **V2**.1120, **V2**.1120 (Fig.)
Inoculation, spread of infection, **B1**.380–4
  accidental, **B1**.382
Inositol 1,4,5-triphosphate (IP$_3$), BCR
    signaling, **I**.344–5
Inoviridae, **V1**.27 (Tab.), **V1**.41 (Tab.)
  see also specific viruses
Insect cell lines, **V1**.87
  orbivirus replication, **V2**.940
Insecticide(s)
  African trypanosomiasis vector control,
      P.369
  bioremediation, **B1**.201
  Chagas disease control, **P**.394–5
  environmental effects, **P**.126
  malaria control, **P**.517
    impregnated bednets, **P**.517
  Old World leishmaniasis control, **P**.308
  resistance
    Onchocerciasis Control Programme,
        P.787–8
    triatomine bugs, **P**.394–5
  temephos, water treatment, **P**.833–4
Insects
  bacterial pathogens, **B1**.203–4
  mycoplasma pathogenicity, **B2**.1964,
      B2.1965–6
  spiroplasmas association, **B2**.1965
  vectors *see* Arthropod vectors; Vector(s)
Insertional mutagenesis, retrovirus integration
    into host genome, **V2**.1593–4
Insertion-like elements, mycoplasma, **B2**.1982
Insertion mechanisms, mobile elements,
    B1.94–5
Insertion sequences (IS), **B1**.80, **B1**.91–4
  classification, **B1**.93–4
  DNA viruses *vs.,* **V1**.12
  historical perspective, **B1**.91
  mobile elements, **B1**.95–6
  size, **B1**.91
  structure, **B1**.91
    inverted repeat sequence, **B1**.91
  typing, *Salmonella,* **B2**.1409, **B2**.1410
  ubiquity, **B1**.96–7

In situ bioremediation (ISB), **B1**.202
in situ DNA hybridization, **V2**.1536
  Aspergillus, **M**.94
  Candida detection, **M**.94
  chemokine patient studies, **I**.229
  progressive multifocal leucoencephalopathy
      (PML), **V2**.1418
Institutions
  gram-negative bacillary pneumonia, **B1**.637
  hepatitis A outbreaks, **V2**.1172, **V2**.1173
  Mycoplasma pneumoniae pneumonia, **B1**.633
Institut Pasteur, **M**.32–3, **V1**.90
Instruments
  nosocomial infection from, **B1**.379–80
  sterilization, **B1**.388
Insulin injection, gas gangrene after, **B2**.1111
Insulin-like growth factor-I, **I**.208
Insulin-like growth factor-II, **I**.63
Integrase, retrovirus replication, **V1**.58
Integrative conjugative elements (ICE), **B1**.99
Integrin(s)
  actions/effects
    lymphocyte migration, **I**.508 (Tab.)
    macrophage development, **I**.21
    NK cell regulation, **I**.85
  analogues, *Candida albicans* virulence
      factors, **M**.259
  basophils, **I**.59 (Tab.)
  Ebola virus receptors, **V2**.1092
  eosinophils, **I**.59 (Tab.)
  inside-out signaling, **I**.24 (Tab.)
  intracellular bacteria, **I**.649
  leukocyte adhesion deficiency, **I**.47–8,
      I.767–9
  microbial recognition, **I**.24 (Tab.)
  neutrophil interactions, **I**.38
  signal transduction, **V2**.1326
  structure, **I**.507
  see also specific types
Integrin α$_4$β$_1$ (VLA-4), **I**.507–9, **I**.508 (Tab.)
  cytokine upregulation, **I**.60
Integrin α$_4$β$_7$
  expression, **I**.507
  lymphocyte migration, **I**.506, **I**.507–9,
      I.508 (Tab.)
  memory T cells, **I**.227
  mucosal addressin-cell adhesion molecule-1
      binding, **I**.227
Integrin α$_4$β$_7$, prion disease, **V2**.1374
Integrin α6β4, papillomavirus binding, **V1**.451
Integrin α$_L$β$_2$ (LFA-1: CD11a) *see* Leukocyte
    function antigen-1 (LFA-1: CD11a)
Integrons, **B1**.97–8
  transposon, **B1**.97–8
Intercalcating agents, mutagens, **V1**.183
Interchromosomal recombination, **B1**.88 (Fig.)
Interdigital candidiasis, **M**.189
Interfamilial spread, *Helicobacter pylori*
    infection, **B2**.1578–9
Interference microscopy, soil bacteria analysis,
    B1.207
Interferon(s), **P**.70, **V1**.226–8, **V1**.271,
    V1.293–6, **V1**.294 (Fig.)
  actions, **V1**.227–8, **V1**.227 (Fig.),
      V1.294 (Fig.)
    adenosine-deaminase ADAR1, **V1**.295

Interferon(s)
actions (*Continued*)
ISG20, **V1**.295
LCMV lysis, **V2**.1073
MHC, **V1**.294
Mx proteins, **V1**.271, **V1**.294–5
NK cells, **V1**.272, **V1**.292–3
2'-5' oligo adenylate synthetase, **V1**.228, **V1**.271, **V1**.294–5, **V1**.313–14
protein kinase R (PKR), **V1**.271, **V1**.286–7, **V1**.294–5, **V1**.313–14
specificity, **V1**.228
tumor virus infection prevention, **V1**.349
antiviral effects, **I**.483, **V1**.618–19
adenoviruses, **V1**.445, **V2**.1596–7
bunyaviruses, **V2**.1041–2
filoviruses, **V2**.1089
HHV-6, **V1**.532
HHV-8, **V1**.548, **V1**.549 (Tab.)
HIV, **V1**.300–1
HSV, **V1**.284
Influenza virus A, **V1**.658
respirovirus, **V1**.773–4
Variola virus, **V1**.620
viral immune interference *see* Immune evasion, viruses
CNS expression, **V2**.1409–10
crosstalk with other cytokines, **V1**.296
discovery, **V1**.8–9
historical aspects/re-evaluation, **I**.10
IFN-specific response elements (IRES), **V1**.227
immune evasion *see* Immune evasion
induction, **V1**.226–7, **V1**.293
pattern recognition, **I**.123
production
CD8 T cells, **I**.421–2
dendritic cells, **I**.123
keratinocytes, **I**.820–1
signal transduction, **V1**.227, **V1**.293–4, **I**.618–19
Janus-activated kinase (JAK) kinases, **V1**.294, **V1**.315
signal transducers and activators of transcription (STAT), **V1**.294, **V1**.315
therapeutic uses, **V1**.295
hepatitis B, **V2**.1260
rhinovirus infection, **V2**.879
type I, **V1**.293, **I**.237–71
actions/effects, **I**.237
antiviral activity, **I**.260 (Tab.)
diversity of, **I**.255–6
macrophage deactivation, **I**.27
NK cell development, **I**.86, **I**.96
classes, **I**.237, **I**.247, **I**.247 (Tab.)
historical research, **I**.237
induction, **I**.237
measles, **V1**.727
nomenclature, **I**.240–1, **I**.241–2
purification, **I**.237–8
HPLC, **I**.237–8
therapeutic uses, **I**.237, **I**.258–61, **I**.259 (Tab.)
adverse effects, **I**.261
autoantibodies due to, **I**.261
cancers, **I**.258

clinical trials, **I**.258–9, **I**.261
hepatitis, **I**.259
rhinovirus infection, **I**.259
signaling effects, **I**.259–61
viral infection, **I**.258–9
see also specific types
type II, **V1**.293
classes, **I**.247, **I**.247 (Tab.)
see also individual types
Interferon-α (IFN-α), **P**.70, **V1**.226, **I**.237, **V1**.293, **V1**.294 (Fig.)
activity/effects, **I**.28 (Tab.), **I**.245–6
acute phase protein expression, **I**.197
antiproliferative, **I**.245, **I**.245 (Tab.)
antiviral, **I**.245, **I**.245 (Tab.), **I**.260 (Tab.)
IL-12 downregulation, **V1**.296
IL-15 induction, **V1**.296
MHC activation, **V1**.271
NK cell effects, **V1**.271
NK cell stimulation, **I**.245, **I**.245 (Tab.), **I**.246 (Tab.)
other INFs *vs.*, **I**.255–6
cytopathic inhibition assay, **I**.238
genes, **V1**.271, **V1**.293
induction/secretion, **V1**.226–7
nomenclature, **I**.240–1, **I**.241–2
production, **I**.28 (Tab.)
CpG stimulation, **I**.911, **I**.931
in vitro production, **I**.238, **I**.238 (Fig.)
purification, **I**.238–43, **I**.239 (Fig.), **I**.243 (Tab.)
HPLC, **I**.238–41, **I**.240 (Fig.), **I**.241 (Fig.), **I**.242 (Fig.)
receptor, gene *see IFNGR1* gene; IFNGR2 gene
recombinant, **I**.244–5, **I**.245 (Tab.)
species of, **I**.241–2
structure
amino acid sequences, **I**.240–3
carbohydrate content, **I**.243
functional unit, **I**.246–7, **I**.246 (Fig.)
therapeutic uses, **I**.258–61, **V1**.295
adult T-cell leukemia, **V2**.1291–2
cancers, **I**.258
hepatitis, **I**.259
hepatitis B, **V1**.295, **V1**.303
hepatitis C, **V1**.295, **V1**.303, **V2**.1198, **V2**.1215, **V2**.1215 (Fig.)
hepatitis D, **V1**.303, **V2**.1273
HTLV-associated myelopathy(HAM)/ tropical spastic paraparesis (TSP), **V2**.1292
papillomaviruses, **V1**.295
rhinoviruses, **V1**.295
viral infection, **I**.258–9
viral infection
adenoviruses, **V1**.295
HCMV, **V1**.295
HIV, **V1**.299, **V1**.300, **V1**.301, **V1**.302 (Fig.)
influenza, **V1**.662–3
Interferon-β (IFN-β), **P**.70, **V1**.226, **I**.237, **V1**.293, **V1**.294 (Fig.)
activity/effects, **I**.28 (Tab.)
MHC activation, **V1**.271
neutrophil priming, **I**.43, **I**.44
NK cell effects, **V1**.271

other INFs *vs.*, **I**.255–6
amino acid sequences, **I**.242–3
genes, **V1**.271, **V1**.293
induction/secretion, **V1**.226–7
nomenclature, **I**.241–2
production, **I**.28 (Tab.)
in vitro production, **I**.243, **I**.243 (Fig.)
purification, **I**.243–5, **I**.243 (Tab.)
recombinant, **I**.247
species of, **I**.241–2
therapeutic uses
in HIV infection, **V1**.299, **I**.797
multiple sclerosis therapy, **I**.259
Interferon-γ (IFN-γ), **P**.70, **V1**.226, **I**.237, **I**.287–8, **V1**.293, **V1**.294 (Fig.)
activity/effects, **I**.28 (Tab.), **P**.72–3, **I**.288
acute phase protein expression, **I**.197
APC stimulation, **I**.288
CD8 T cell activation, **I**.427–8
chemokines, **I**.224
class switching, **I**.327
direct antiviral effect, **V1**.295
IL-2 synergy, **I**.279–80
IL-4 antagonist, **I**.288
IL-17 synergy, **I**.290
inflammation, **I**.288
intercellular adhesion factor expression, **I**.820–1
keratinocytes, **I**.820–1
macrophage activation, **I**.27, **I**.288
MHC class I expression, **I**.288
MHC class II expression, **I**.820–1
mucosal immune response, **I**.524
neutrophil priming, **I**.43
nitric oxide generation, **I**.288
nitric oxide synthase regulation, **P**.73
prostaglandin production, **I**.187
T helper cell polarization, **P**.73, **I**.288, **I**.398–9
CNS expression, **V2**.1409
deficiency/defects
bacterial infection, **I**.288
intracellular bacterial infection, **I**.589–90
viral infection, **I**.288
in diseases/infection
African trypanosomiasis, **P**.80
AIDS-dementia complex (ADC), **V1**.304
aspergillosis, **M**.708, **M**.709
Burkholderia thailandensis infection, **B2**.1625
candidiasis, **M**.259–60, **M**.593
Chagas disease, **P**.86
Coccidioides immitis, **M**.510
cryptococcosis, **M**.645
cryptosporidiosis, **P**.407
EBV, **V1**.302–3
HCMV, **V1**.524–5
hepatitis B, **V1**.284, **V1**.303
histoplasmosis capsulati, **M**.527–8
in HIV infection, **V1**.299, **V1**.300, **I**.793, **I**.797
HSV, **V1**.284–5, **V1**.301–2
HTLV-1-associated myelopathy/tropical spastic paraparesis (HAM/TSP), **V2**.1429–30
human brucellosis, **B2**.1737

Interferon-γ (IFN-γ)
in diseases/infection (*Continued*)
influenza, **V1**.664–5
intestinal nematode infection, **P**.90
intracellular bacterial infection, **I**.589
isosporiasis, **P**.412–13
larval cestode disease, **P**.690
leishmaniasis, **P**.77–8, **I**.679
malaria, **I**.599
malaria immunity, **P**.490–1
measles, **V1**.726, **I**.805–6, **V2**.1433
onchocerciasis, **P**.795–6
PCP, **M**.795
Plasmodium, **P**.83
poxviruses, **V1**.620
pythiosis, **M**.427
salmonellosis, **I**.593
schistosomiasis, **P**.616, **I**.719
pathology, **P**.94–5
toxoplasmosis, **P**.79, **P**.432–3
tuberculosis, **I**.711
tumor rejection, **I**.478
viral clearance, **I**.478
Yersinia infection, **I**.138
genes, **V1**.271, **V1**.293
granuloma formation, **I**.708
schistosomiasis, **I**.720
tuberculosis, **I**.715
immunogenetics, **I**.582–3
induction/synthesis, **V1**.226–7
IL-1, **V1**.296–7
IL-18, **V1**.620–1
by T cells, **V2**.1170–1
overproduction, **I**.288
production, **I**.28 (Tab.), **I**.287–8
CD4 T cells, **I**.395
CpG stimulation, **I**.911
CTL production, **I**.478
DNA vaccines, **I**.896
IL-12 effects, **I**.288
macrophages, **I**.28
NK cells, **I**.81–2, **I**.99, **I**.287–8, **I**.478
prostaglandin E$_2$ effects, **I**.188
superantigen stimulation, **I**.561
T cells, **I**.287–8
Th1 cells, **I**.224, **I**.287–8, **I**.397
proteasomes, **I**.411
purification, **I**.243 (Tab.)
structure, **I**.287
therapeutic uses
cryptococcosis, **M**.652–3
cryptosporidiosis, **P**.406–7, **P**.410
systemic zygomycosis, **M**.678
as vaccine adjuvant, **I**.898
DNA vaccine co-administration, **I**.896,
I.918, **I**.918 (Tab.)
Interferon-γ receptor (IFN-γR), **I**.248–52,
V1.620
chromosomal location, **I**.248–9
erythropoietin receptor *vs.,* **I**.250
functional complex, **I**.249
gene *see IFNGR1* gene; *IFNGR2* gene
growth receptor *vs.,* **I**.250–1
ligand binding, **I**.249, **I**.252 (Fig.)
mutations, **I**.772

nomenclature, **I**.248 (Tab.)
signal transduction, **I**.248–50, **I**.250 (Fig.)
Jak-STAT, **I**.249
soluble analogues, myxoma virus, **I**.687
structure, **I**.248, **I**.250 (Fig.)
accessory chain, **I**.251–2
chain interaction, **I**.249–50, **I**.251 (Fig.)
IFN-γR1 chain, **I**.249
IFN-γR2 chain, **I**.249
Th1 *vs.* Th2 cells, **I**.251–2
Interferon-inducible protein 10 (IP-
10:CXCL10), **I**.47, **I**.218 (Tab.)
CNS expression, **V2**.1409
DNA vaccine co-administration, **I**.912–13,
I.918 (Tab.)
granuloma formation, **I**.708
Lassa virus, suppression of, **V2**.1072
structure, **I**.221
function relationship, **I**.221
T cell chemotaxis, **I**.224
Interferon-κ (IFN-κ), **I**.237, **V1**.293,
V1.294 (Fig.)
genes, **V1**.293
Interferon-λ (IFN-λ), **V1**.293, **V1**.294 (Fig.)
Interferon receptors, **I**.247
analogue production, poxviruses, **V1**.230
gene polymorphisms, malaria susceptibility,
P.485–6
genes *see specific genes*
nomenclature, **I**.247, **I**.248 (Tab.)
signal transduction, **I**.247
type I, **I**.252–6
binding diversity, **I**.255–6
cDNA clones, **I**.253
chromosomal location, **I**.252–3
cloning, **I**.247
competition binding studies, **I**.247
expression in hamster cells, **I**.254
IFN-αR1 chain, **I**.254–5
IFN-αR2c chain, **I**.255
nomenclature, **I**.248 (Tab.)
signal transduction, **I**.256–8, **I**.258 (Fig.)
structure, **I**.253, **I**.258 (Fig.)
YAC clones, **I**.253
type II *see* Interferon-γ receptor (IFN-γR)
Interferon-regulatory factor-3 (IRF-3), **I**.122–3
papillomavirus E6 protein effects,
V1.460 (Tab.)
Interferon-specific response elements (IRES),
V1.227
Interferon-τ (IFN-τ), **I**.237
Interferon-ω (IFN-ω), **V1**.226, **I**.237, **V1**.293,
V1.294 (Fig.)
activity, **I**.255–6
genes, **V1**.271
Intergenic regions
filoviruses, **V2**.1088
pneumoviruses, **V1**.701
Intergenic suppression, base pair substitutions,
B1.86–7
Interhuman transmission, *Chilomastix mesnili,*
P.270
Interleukin(s), **P**.70–2, **P**.71 (Tab.)
aspergillosis, **M**.724
candidiasis, **M**.592–3
cell-mediated immune response, **P**.70–2

coccidioidomycosis, **M**.510
historical aspects/re-evaluation, **I**.10
humoral immune response, **P**.70–2
keratinocyte production, **I**.820–1
PCP, **M**.795
pro-inflammatory, **P**.70–2
trichinellosis, **P**.764–5
see also individual types
Interleukin-1 (IL-1), **P**.70–2, **P**.71 (Tab.),
I.284–5, **V1**.296–7
actions/effects, **I**.284–5, **I**.293 (Fig.)
acute phase proteins, **I**.284–5
acute phase response, **I**.194–5, **I**.195–6,
I.195 (Fig.), **I**.197
antigen presentation, **I**.384
basophils, **I**.58, **I**.63
defensin induction, **I**.168, **I**.520–1
dendritic cell activation, **I**.378, **I**.393–4
E-selectin expression, **I**.506–7
IFN-γ synthesis, **V1**.296–7
IL-6 production, **I**.284–5
IL-13 suppression, **I**.294–7
mucosal immune response, **I**.522–3, **I**.525
neutrophil priming, **I**.43, **I**.44
prostaglandin production, **I**.187
septic shock, **I**.697
gene cluster, **I**.578 (Fig.)
see also IL1 gene cluster
IL-1α, **I**.283–4
eosinophil production, **I**.67
IL-1β *vs.,* **I**.285 (Tab.)
IL-17 synergy, **I**.290
infection
adenovirus infection, **V1**.296–7
AIDS-dementia complex (ADC), **V1**.304,
V2.1428
EBV infection, **V1**.296–7
HCMV infection, **V1**.296–7
hepatitis B, **V1**.296–7
herpesvirus infection, **V1**.296–7
HIV infection, **V1**.296–7, **V1**.299–300
HSV type 1 (HSV-1) infection, **V1**.301–2
HTLV-1 infection, **V1**.296–7
influenzavirus infection, **V1**.296–7
malaria, **P**.490–1, **P**.495–6
measles, **V1**.727
neurocysticercosis, **P**.690
schistosomiasis, **P**.616
toxoplasmosis, **P**.78–9
knockout animal models, **I**.195–6
measles receptor antagonist, **V1**.727
production, **I**.284
IL-17 effects, **I**.290
intradermal DNA vaccine delivery,
I.912–13
keratinocytes, **I**.820–1
Langerhans' cells, **I**.821
macrophages, **I**.284
monocytes, **I**.284
neutrophils, **I**.36, **I**.46, **I**.47
prostaglandin E$_2$ effects, **I**.188
receptor
genes, **I**.578–9
TLRs *vs.,* **I**.116

Interleukin-1 (IL-1) (*Continued*)
  therapeutic applications
    DNA vaccine co-administration,
      I.918 (Tab.)
    intranasal vaccine adjuvant, **I**.832
Interleukin-1β (IL-1β), **I**.283–4
  apoptosis, **V1**.621
  HHV-6 infection, **V1**.301–2
  IL-1α *vs.*, **I**.285 (Tab.)
  poxvirus immune evasion, **V1**.621
  soluble binding protein
    Cowpox virus, **V1**.585–6
    Vaccinia virus, **V1**.318, **V1**.585–6, **V1**.621
  Toll-like receptors effects, **V1**.621
Interleukin-1β converting enzyme (ICE) *see*
    Caspase-1
Interleukin-1 receptor antagonist (IL-1Ra),
    I.204, **I**.292
  effects, **I**.292, **I**.293 (Fig.)
  genetics, **I**.292
  production, **I**.292
    IL-10 effects, **I**.292–3
  septic shock therapy, **I**.702
Interleukin-1 receptor-associated kinase
    (IRAK), **I**.122
Interleukin-2 (IL-2), **P**.70–2, **P**.71 (Tab.),
    I.279–80
  actions/effects, **P**.72–3, **I**.279–80
    CD8 T cell activation, **I**.427–8
    CTLA-4 expression, **I**.279–80
    eosinophil chemotaxis, **I**.61
    Fas ligand expression, **I**.279–80
    HIV protection, **I**.797
    measles, **I**.804–5, **I**.805–6
    neutrophil priming, **I**.43
    NK cell regulation, **I**.85–6
    NK cells, **I**.279–80
    T cells, **I**.224
    Th1/Th2 differentiation, **I**.279–80
    T helper cell expansion, **I**.279–80
  blocking, allograft rejection prevention, **I**.280
  CNS expression in viral infection, **V2**.1409
  gene *see IL2* gene
  IFN-γ synergy, **I**.279–80
  IL-12 synergy, **I**.279–80
  infection
    Borna disease virus infection, **V2**.1149–50
    candidiasis, **M**.259–60
    Chagas disease, **P**.385
    cryptococcosis, **M**.645, **M**.652–3
    EBV infection, **V1**.302–3
    hepatitis B immunopathology, **V1**.303
    HSV type 1 (HSV-1) infection, **V1**.301–2
    HTLV-1-associated myelopathy/tropical
      spastic paraparesis (HAM/TSP),
      V2.1429–30
    measles, **V1**.726
    neurocysticercosis, **P**.690
    schistosomiasis, **P**.614
  inhibition, IL-10, **I**.293–4
  knockout mice, **I**.280
  local gene expression, **V1**.305
  Measles virus receptor secretion, **V1**.726
  monoclonal antibody therapy, **I**.357
  production, **I**.279
    prostaglandin E$_2$ effects, **I**.188

regulatory T cells, **I**.751
    superantigen stimulation, **I**.561
    T cells, **I**.279
  receptor, **I**.279, **I**.279 (Fig.)
    α chain deficiency, **I**.775–6
    γc chain, **I**.575
    HTLV infection, **I**.802
    X-linked SCID, **I**.575
  structure, **I**.279
  therapeutic uses, **I**.280
    as adjuvant, **I**.878–9, **I**.918, **I**.918 (Tab.)
    cancer, **I**.280
    HIV, **I**.280
Interleukin-2 (IL-2)/interferon-γ (IFN-γ)
    pathway, diseases/infection, **I**.772–3,
    I.773 (Fig.)
Interleukin-3 (IL-3), **P**.70–2, **P**.71 (Tab.),
    I.275–6
  actions/effects, **I**.275
    basophils, **I**.55, **I**.56–60, **I**.63, **I**.66
    eosinophils, **I**.55, **I**.57–8, **I**.60, **I**.61, **I**.64,
      I.275
    erythroid cells, **I**.275
    on macrophages, **I**.275
    mast cells, **I**.275
    megakaryocytes, **I**.275
    neutrophils, **I**.36, **I**.275
    parasitic infection, **I**.275–6
    VLA upregulation, **I**.60
  IL3 gene, **I**.580
  IL-11 synergy, **I**.279
  local release, **I**.275
  production, **I**.275
    eosinophils, **I**.67, **I**.275
    mast cells, **I**.275
    neutrophils, **I**.46
    T cells, **I**.275
  receptor, *IL3RA* gene, **I**.582
  SCF interaction, **I**.275
  structure, **I**.275
Interleukin-4 (IL-4), **P**.70–2, **P**.71 (Tab.),
    I.280–1, **V1**.298
  actions/effects, **P**.72–3, **V1**.298
    basophils, **I**.58, **I**.66
    B cells, **I**.280, **I**.348–9
    CD4 T cell production, **I**.395
    CD8 T cell activation, **I**.427–8
    class switching, **I**.327, **I**.331
    eosinophils, **I**.60
    eotaxin release, **I**.61
    Ig class switching, **I**.280
    IL-8 down regulation, **I**.280
    macrophage activation, **I**.27
    mast cell proliferation, **I**.275
    nitric oxide synthase regulation, **P**.73
    proinflammatory cytokine downregulation,
      I.280
    prostaglandin production, **I**.187
    septic shock therapy, **I**.702
    T cells, **I**.224, **I**.280, **I**.281 (Fig.)
    Th2 cells, **I**.66, **I**.280, **I**.281 (Fig.), **I**.399
    T helper cell polarization, **P**.73
    VCAM-1 expression, **I**.60, **I**.280
  in diseases/infection
    airway hypersensitivity, **I**.732–3, **I**.735

airway remodeling, **I**.732
    diabetes development, **I**.280–1
    EBV infection, **V1**.302–3
    experimental allergic encephalitis
      development, **I**.280–1
    filarial nematode infection, **P**.91, **P**.92
    Giardia infection, **P**.76
    granuloma formation, **I**.708
    helminth infection, **I**.68, **I**.600
    histoplasmosis capsulati, **M**.528
    HIV infection, **V1**.298, **V1**.301, **I**.793, **I**.797
    influenza, **V1**.664–5
    intestinal amebae, **P**.75
    leishmaniasis, **P**.74, **P**.77–8, **I**.280, **I**.679
    malaria immunity, **P**.491
    measles, **V1**.298
    in measles, **I**.805–6
    onchocerciasis, **P**.795
    Schistosoma infection, **I**.68
    schistosomiasis, **P**.94, **P**.613, **P**.614–15
    Sindbis virus infection, **V1**.298
  gene *see IL4* gene
  IFN-γ antagonist, **I**.288
  IL-11 synergy, **I**.279
  oral tolerance, **I**.544
  production, **I**.280
    basophils, **I**.280
    eosinophils, **I**.280
    macrophages, **I**.28
    mast cells, **I**.280
    MF59 adjuvant, **I**.927
    NK cells, **I**.280
    prostaglandin E$_2$ effects, **I**.188
    T cells, **I**.28 (Tab.), **I**.280
    Th2 cells, **I**.224, **I**.280, **I**.397
  receptors, **I**.279 (Fig.)
    asthma, **I**.581–2
    γc chain, **I**.575
  SCF interaction, **I**.275
  structure, **I**.280
  therapeutic uses, **I**.28 (Tab.), **I**.280–1
    DNA vaccine co-administration, **I**.918,
      I.918 (Tab.)
Interleukin-5 (IL-5), **P**.70–2, **P**.71 (Tab.),
    I.277–9
  actions/effects, **P**.72–3, **I**.277, **I**.278
    basophils, **I**.55, **I**.57, **I**.58–60, **I**.63, **I**.278
    B-cell activation, **I**.348–9
    CD4 T cell production, **I**.395
    eosinophils, **I**.57–8, **I**.61, **I**.64, **I**.278,
      I.278 (Fig.)
    IgA synthesis, **I**.536
  in diseases/infection
    airway hypersensitivity, **I**.736
    airway remodeling, **I**.732
    asthma, **I**.735, **I**.736
    EBV infection, **V1**.302–3
    Echinococcus infection, **P**.96
    in eosinophilia, **I**.278, **I**.278 (Fig.)
    helminth infection, **I**.70, **I**.600
    HIV infection, **I**.793
    influenza, **V1**.664–5
    neurocysticercosis, **P**.690
  eosinophilia, **P**.69
  gene, *IL5* gene, **I**.580

Interleukin-5 (IL-5) (*Continued*)
    knockout mice, helminth infection, **I**.70
    local gene expression, **V1**.305
    nitric oxide synthase regulation, **P**.73
    production, **I**.277
        CD4+ T cells, **I**.57
        CD8+ T cells, **I**.57
        eosinophils, **I**.67
        mast cells, **I**.277
        MF59 adjuvant, **I**.927
        NK cells, **I**.57
        T cells, **I**.277
        Th2 cells, **I**.224, **I**.280
    structure, **I**.277
    therapeutic uses, DNA vaccine co-
        administration, **I**.918 (Tab.)
Interleukin-6 (IL-6), **P**.70–2, **P**.71 (Tab.),
        I.285–6, **V1**.297
    actions/effects, **I**.285
        α1-antichymotrypsin production, **I**.285
        acute phase response, **I**.195–6, **I**.195 (Fig.),
            I.285
        basophils, **I**.57
        C-reactive protein production, **I**.285
        dendritic cell activation, **I**.393–4
        fibrinogen production, **I**.285
        haptoglobulin production, **I**.285
        IgA synthesis, **I**.536–7
        Ig production, **I**.285
        mucosal immune response, **I**.522–3
        serum amyloid A production, **I**.285
    Burkholderia LPS effects, **B2**.1617
    in diseases/infection
        in AIDS/HIV infection, **V1**.297, **V1**.299,
            V1.304
        CNS infection, **V1**.303–4, **V2**.1409
        Dengue fever, **V1**.297
        DNA virus infection, **V1**.297
        EBV infection, **V1**.302–3
        hepatitis viruses, **V1**.303
        HSV type 1 (HSV-1) infection, **V1**.301–2
        HTLV-1 infection, **V1**.297
        Human respiratory syncytial virus
            infection, **V1**.297
        influenza, **V1**.662–3
        malaria, **P**.490, **P**.495–6
        neurocysticercosis, **P**.690
        RNA virus infection, **V1**.297
        schistosomiasis, **P**.614–15
        SIV infection, **V1**.297
        toxoplasmosis, **P**.79
    IL-11 synergy, **I**.279
    knockout animal models, **I**.195–6
    local gene expression, **V1**.305
    production, **I**.285
        CpG stimulation, **I**.911–12, **I**.931
        IL-1 effects, **I**.284–5
        IL-17 effects, **I**.290
        neutrophils, **I**.46, **I**.47
        prostaglandin E$_2$ effects, **I**.188
        Th2 cells, **I**.280
    receptor, **I**.285
    structure, **I**.285

therapeutic uses
    DNA vaccine co-administration, **I**.896,
        I.912–13, **I**.918, **I**.918 (Tab.)
    intranasal vaccine adjuvant, **I**.832
    TNF-α, **V1**.296
    viral homologue, **I**.620
        HHV-8 analogue coding, **V1**.301–2,
            V1.317–18, **V1**.548–50, **V1**.549 (Tab.)
Interleukin-7 (IL-7), **P**.71 (Tab.), **I**.281–2,
        V1.297–8
    actions/effects, **I**.281
        B cell development, **I**.281, **I**.323, **I**.341
        CD4 T cell long-term persistence, **I**.392
        γδ T-cell development, **I**.527
        NK cell actions, **I**.281
        T cell development, **I**.281
    in diseases/infection, in HIV infection, **I**.797
    Human respiratory syncytial virus infection,
        V1.297–8
    production, **I**.281
    receptors, **I**.279 (Fig.)
        γc chain, **I**.575
    structure, **I**.281
    therapeutic uses, DNA vaccine co-
        administration, **I**.912–13, **I**.918 (Tab.)
Interleukin-8 (IL-8), **P**.70–2, **P**.71 (Tab.),
        I.218 (Tab.), **V1**.297–8
    actions/effects
        basophil chemotaxis, **I**.60
        eosinophil chemotaxis, **I**.60, **I**.61
        graft rejection, **I**.228
        IL-13 suppression, **I**.294–7
        mucosal immune response, **I**.522–3, **I**.525
        neutrophils, **I**.37, **I**.43
    activity measurement, two-well chambers,
        I.223
    Burkholderia LPS effects, **B2**.1617
    candidiasis resistance, **M**.259–60
    cloning, **I**.220
    CNS expression, **V2**.1409
    gene, *IL8* gene, **I**.587
    HIV infection, **V1**.299
    Human respiratory syncytial virus infection,
        V1.793–4
    intracellular signaling, **I**.222
    production
        IL-4 effects, **I**.280
        IL-17 effects, **I**.290
        neutrophils, **I**.47
    receptor deficiencies, **I**.229–30
    receptor, HHV-8 coding, **V1**.549 (Tab.),
        V1.550
    structure, **I**.217–19, **I**.220
        dimerization, **I**.220 (Fig.)
        mutagenesis studies, **I**.221
    suppression of, Lassa virus, **V2**.1072
    synthetic antagonists, **I**.231–2
    therapeutic uses, DNA vaccine
        co-administration, **I**.918, **I**.918 (Tab.)
Interleukin-9 (IL-9), **P**.70–2, **P**.71 (Tab.),
        I.281–2
    actions/effects, **I**.282
        T cell differentiation, **I**.282, **I**.282 (Fig.)
    in diseases/infection, **I**.283 (Fig.)
        airway remodeling, **I**.732
        allergic asthma, **I**.735

        helminth infection, **I**.282, **I**.600
        Trichuris muris infection, **I**.282
    IL9 gene, **I**.580
    production, **I**.281–2
    receptors, **I**.279 (Fig.)
        γc chain, **I**.575
    structure, **I**.281
Interleukin-10 (IL-10), **P**.70–2, **P**.71 (Tab.),
        I.291, **I**.293–4, **V1**.297–8
    actions/effects, **I**.28 (Tab.), **P**.72–3, **I**.291,
        I.293–4
        dendritic cell maturation, **I**.750
        IL-12 inhibition, **I**.288–9
        macrophage deactivation, **I**.27
        mucosal immune response, **I**.525
        oral tolerance, **I**.544
        prostaglandin production, **I**.187
        T cells, **I**.224
        Th2 cell differentiation, **I**.399
    cells producing, **P**.72–3
    in diseases/infection
        airway hypersensitivity, **I**.737, **I**.739–40
        chronic parasitic infection, **I**.680, **I**.683
        EBV infection, **V1**.302–3
        filarial nematode infection, **P**.92
        in HIV infection, **I**.797
        HSV type 1 (HSV-1) infection, **V1**.301–2
        intestinal amebae infection, **P**.75
        intestinal nematode infection, **P**.90
        leishmaniasis, **P**.74, **P**.77–8, **I**.679
        lymphatic filariasis, **P**.775–6
        malaria, **P**.83, **P**.491
        onchocerciasis, **P**.796
        schistosomiasis, **P**.615, **P**.616
            pathology, **P**.94–5
        schistosomiasis granulomas, **I**.720
        septic shock therapy, **I**.702
        toxoplasmosis, **P**.79
    gene *see IL10* gene
    homologue secretion, EBV, **I**.687
    hygiene hypothesis, **I**.739
    immunogenetics, **I**.582–3
    nitric oxide synthase regulation, **P**.73
    production, **I**.28 (Tab.), **I**.292
        bacterial immune interference, **I**.652–4
        B cells, **I**.292
        CD4 T cells, **I**.395
        CpG stimulation, **I**.911
        neutrophils, **I**.46
        NK cells, **I**.82, **I**.292
        regulatory T cells, **I**.751
        T cells, **I**.292
        Th2 cells, **I**.280
    related cytokines, **I**.294
        effects, **I**.294
        production, **I**.294
        structure, **I**.294
    structure, **I**.292
    therapeutic uses, DNA vaccine co-
        administration, **I**.912–13, **I**.918 (Tab.)
    viral homologue, **I**.620
Interleukin-11 (IL-11), **P**.71 (Tab.), **I**.278–9
    actions/effects, **I**.279
    in diseases/infection, **I**.279
    production, **I**.279, **I**.279 (Tab.)

Interleukin-11 (IL-11) (*Continued*)
 SCF synergy, **I**.279
 structure, **I**.278–9
 synergy, **I**.279
Interleukin-12 (IL-12), **P**.70–2, **P**.71 (Tab.),
  I.288–9, **V1**.298
 actions/effects, **I**.28 (Tab.), **I**.288–9
  acute phase response, **I**.195 (Fig.)
  antigen presentation, **I**.384
  antiviral properties, **V1**.318–19
  CD4+ T cell effect, **V1**.298
  CD4 T-cells/dendritic cell interactions,
   I.394
  CD8 T cell activation, **I**.427–8
  downregulation, IFN-α (IFN-α), **V1**.296
  eosinophils, **I**.57
  IL-2 synergy, **I**.279–80
  IL-10 inhibition, **I**.288–9
  IL-13 suppression, **I**.294–7
  IL-18 synergy, **I**.290
  macrophage activation, **I**.27
  NK cell development, **I**.86, **I**.96, **I**.288
  T cell, **I**.288
  T cells, **I**.224
  Th1 cells, **I**.29, **I**.288, **I**.398–9
  T helper cell polarization, **P**.73
 in diseases/infection
  airway hypersensitivity *see* Airway
   hypersensitivity/hyperreactivity
  bacterial immune interference, **I**.652
  Chagas disease, **P**.86
  histoplasmosis capsulati, **M**.528
  HIV infection, **V1**.298
  HIV protection, **I**.797
  influenza, **V1**.663
  intestinal nematode infection, **P**.90
  leishmaniasis, **P**.77–8
  malaria, **P**.83
  measles, **V1**.727–9
  schistosomiasis, **P**.614–15
  toxoplasmosis, **P**.78–9
  tuberculosis granulomas, **I**.715
 gene *see IL12B* gene
 mutations, **I**.772–3
 production, **I**.28 (Tab.), **I**.288–9
  CpG effects, **I**.911, **I**.931
  dendritic cells, **I**.288–9
  ISCOMs adjuvant requirements, **I**.930
  Langerhans' cells, **I**.821
  macrophages, **I**.28
  superantigen stimulation, **I**.561
 receptors
  deficiency, **I**.589
  mutations, **I**.772
 structure, **I**.288
 superantigen stimulation, **B1**.157
 suppression, heat labile enterotoxin, **I**.652
 therapeutic uses
  cryptococcosis therapy, **M**.652–3
  DNA vaccine co-administration, **I**.896,
   I.912–13, **I**.918, **I**.918 (Tab.)
  schistosomiasis granuloma therapy, **I**.723
  TCE peptide vaccines, **I**.879
  vaccine adjuvant, **I**.832, **I**.898

Interleukin-13 (IL-13), **P**.70–2, **P**.71 (Tab.),
  I.297
 actions/effects, **I**.28 (Tab.), **P**.72–3, **I**.294–7
  basophils, **I**.58, **I**.66
  eosinophils, **I**.60
  eotaxin release, **I**.60–1
  macrophage activation, **I**.27
  prostaglandin production, **I**.187
 in diseases/infection, **I**.294–7
  airway hypersensitivity *see* Airway
   hypersensitivity/hyperreactivity
  airway remodeling, **I**.732
  chronic obstructive pulmonary disease,
   I.734–5
  fungal pneumonitis, **I**.734–5
  helminth infection, **I**.600
  intestinal nematode infection, **P**.90
  leishmaniasis, **P**.77–8
  onchocerciasis, **P**.795
  respiratory syncytial virus infection,
   I.734–5
  schistosomiasis, **P**.614–15
  schistosomiasis granulomas, **I**.720, **I**.722
 genetics, **I**.295 (Fig.)
 IL13 gene, **I**.580
 production, **I**.28 (Tab.), **I**.294
  macrophages, **I**.28
  mast cells, **I**.294
  NK cells, **I**.82
  Th2 cells, **I**.280, **I**.294
 receptor, asthma, **I**.581–2
 structure, **I**.294
 therapeutic uses, septic shock therapy, **I**.702
Interleukin-14 (IL-14), **P**.71 (Tab.)
Interleukin-15 (IL-15), **P**.70–2, **P**.71 (Tab.),
  I.282–4
 actions/effects, **I**.282, **I**.284 (Fig.)
  eosinophils, **I**.58
  macrophage activation, **I**.27
  NK cells, **I**.85–6, **I**.100, **I**.282, **I**.284 (Fig.)
 in diseases/infection, **I**.282
  in HIV infection, **I**.797
 increased expression, **I**.282
 induction, **V1**.296
 production, **I**.282
 receptors, **I**.279 (Fig.)
  γc chain, **I**.575
 structure, **I**.282
 therapeutic uses, **I**.282–3
  DNA vaccine co-administration, **I**.912–13,
   I.918, **I**.918 (Tab.)
Interleukin-16 (IL-16), **P**.70–2, **P**.71 (Tab.),
  I.289–90
 actions/effects, **I**.289
  antigen-induced cell death, **I**.289
  T cells, **I**.289
 in HIV infection, **I**.793, **I**.797
 measles, **V1**.727
 production, **I**.289
  CD8 T cells, **I**.289
  intraepithelial αβ T cells, **I**.441
 structure, **I**.289
Interleukin-17 (IL-17), **P**.70–2, **P**.71 (Tab.),
  I.289–90
 actions/effects, **I**.290

Herpesvirus saimiri (HVS) homologue,
  V1.317–18
 IL-1 synergy, **I**.290
 IL-17B, **I**.290
 IL-17C, **I**.290
 IL-17F, **I**.290
 production, **I**.290
 structure, **I**.289–90
 therapeutic uses, **I**.290
 TNF-α synergy, **I**.290
 viral homologue, **I**.620
Interleukin-18 (IL-18), **P**.70–2, **P**.71 (Tab.),
  I.290–1
 actions/effects, **I**.28 (Tab.), **I**.290–1,
  I.291 (Fig.)
  antigen presentation, **I**.384
  basophil histamine release, **I**.62
  IFN-γ induction, **V1**.620–1
  macrophages, **I**.27
  NK cells, **I**.86, **I**.290
  Salmonella typhimurium infection, **I**.290–2
  Sendai virus infection, **I**.290–2
  Th1 cells, **I**.290, **I**.398–9
  vaccinia virus infection, **I**.290–2
  viral binding protein, **I**.621
  Yersinia enterocolitica infection, **I**.290–2
 antiviral properties, **V1**.318–19
 binding protein
  Molluscum contagiosum virus, **V1**.318–19,
   V1.621
  poxviruses, **V1**.314–15, **V1**.318–19,
   V1.620–1
 in diseases/infection, **I**.290–2
  diabetes mellitus type I, **I**.290–2
  experimental autoimmune
   encephalomyelitis, **I**.290–2
  leishmaniasis, **P**.77–8
  malaria, **P**.83
  toxoplasmosis, **P**.78–9
 IL-12 synergy, **I**.290
 production, **I**.28 (Tab.), **I**.290, **I**.291 (Fig.)
  CpG stimulation, **I**.911
  dendritic cells, **I**.290
  macrophages, **I**.28, **I**.290
 receptor, **I**.290
 structure, **I**.290
 therapeutic uses, DNA vaccine co-
  administration, **I**.918, **I**.918 (Tab.)
Interleukin-19 (IL-19), **I**.294
 production, **I**.294
 receptor, **I**.279 (Fig.)
 structure, **I**.294
Interleukin-20 (IL-20), **I**.294
 effects, **I**.294
 production, **I**.294
 structure, **I**.294
Interleukin-21 (IL-21), **I**.283–4
 actions/effects, NK cells, **I**.86, **I**.283–4
Interleukin-22 (IL-22), **I**.294
 acute phase protein expression, **I**.197
 effects, **I**.294
 production, **I**.294
 structure, **I**.294
Interleukin-23 (IL-23), **I**.292
Interleukin-24 (IL-24), **I**.294
 effects, **I**.294

Interleukin-24 (IL-24) (*Continued*)
  production, **I**.294
  structure, **I**.294
Interleukin-25 (IL-25), **I**.292
Interleukin-26 (IL-26), **I**.294
  effects, **I**.294
  production, **I**.294
    T cells, **I**.294
  structure, **I**.294
Interleukin-27 (IL-27), **I**.284
  Th1 cell differentiation, **I**.398–9
Intermediate hosts
  Angiostrongylus cantonensis, **P**.803
  Clonorchis, **P**.646
  Diphyllobothrium latum, **P**.671–2
  Echinococcus granulosus, **P**.684, **P**.701
  Echinococcus multilocularis, **P**.701, **P**.702
  Echinococcus vogeli, **P**.684–5
  epidemiology (viral infection), **V1**.353–4
  Fasciola gigantica, **P**.646
  Fasciola hepatica, **P**.646
  Hymenolepis nana, **P**.669–70
  Opisthorchis, **P**.646
  Paragonimus, **P**.646
  Schistosoma, **P**.602, **P**.603 (Tab.)
  Schistosoma haematobium, **P**.603 (Tab.),
    P.611 (Tab.), **P**.612, **P**.612 (Fig.)
  Schistosoma japonicum, **P**.603 (Tab.), **P**.628,
    P.628 (Fig.)
  Schistosoma malayensis, **P**.603 (Tab.), **P**.628
  Schistosoma mansoni, **P**.603 (Tab.),
    P.611 (Tab.), **P**.612, **P**.613 (Fig.)
  Schistosoma mekongi, **P**.603 (Tab.), **P**.628
  Taenia saginata saginata, **P**.665
  Taenia solium, **P**.668, **P**.684
  tapeworms, **P**.662
  Wuchereria bancrofti, **P**.771
Intermittent presumptive treatment (IPT),
  malaria, **P**.493–4
Intermolecular spreading, **I**.756
Internal promoter (IP), foamy viruses, **V2**.1308
Internal ribosome entry sites (IRES)
  Hepatitis A virus, **V2**.1163, **V2**.1167
  Hepatitis C virus, **V2**.1195
  picornaviruses, **V1**.188
  poliovirus neurovirulence, **V2**.1407
  protein synthesis, **V1**.222–3
  single-stranded positive-sense RNA virus
    replication, **V1**.58
Internal transcribed spacer (ITS) regions
  Aspergillus identification, **M**.688–9
  Toxocara, **P**.751
International Air Transport Association
  (IATA), **V2**.1528–9
International Antigenic Typing Scheme
  (IATS), **B2**.1602
International Civil Aviation Organization
  (ICAO), **V2**.1528–9
International Code of Botanical
  Nomenclature, **M**.44
*International Code of Virus Classification and
  Nomenclature*, **V1**.29, **V1**.40, **V1**.176–80
  type species definition, **V1**.32
International Commission for Disease, animal
  reservoir control, **P**.118

International Commission for the Certification
  of, dracunculiasis control, **P**.123–4
International Committee for Systematic
  Bacteriology (ICSB), **B1**.15, **B1**.16, **B1**.18
  Enterobacteriaceae nomenclature/
    classification, **B2**.1335–6
  nomenclature changes, **B1**.32
International Committee on the Taxonomy of
  Viruses (ICTV), **V1**.26–9, **V1**.378
  anellovirus classification, **V2**.1277
  database, **V1**.35
  establishment, **V1**.38–9
  negative-strand RNA viruses classification,
    V1.127–8
  Nidovirales order establishment, **V1**.390–2
  orthoretrovirus nomenclature, **V2**.1322–3
  poxvirus nomenclature, **V1**.595–6
  subcommittees, **V1**.26–9, **V1**.39
  website details, **V1**.39
International Development Targets, **P**.103–6
*International Journal of Systemic and
  Evolutionary Microbiology* (IJSEM),
  B1.18
  nomenclature changes, **B1**.32
International Journal of Systemic Bacteriology
  (IJSB), **B1**.18
  nomenclature changes, **B1**.32
International Society of Human and Animal
  Mycology (ISHAM), **M**.3, **M**.9, **M**.30–1
International Task Force for Disease
  Eradication
  control *vs.* eradication, **P**.108–9
  cysticercosis as erradicable disease, **P**.120
International Union Against Tuberculosis and
  Lung Disease (IUTLD), **B2**.1200
International Union of Microbiological
  Societies (IUMS), **B1**.18, **V1**.38–9
International Water Decade, **P**.123–4
Internet, nomenclature changes, **B1**.32
Interrupted mating experiments, conjugation,
  B1.102–3, **B1**.102 (Fig.)
Intertrigo, candidal, **M**.189, **M**.595, **M**.609
Interventional phase, emerging viral infection,
  V2.1667
Intervention studies, **B1**.313
Interviews, epidemiological, **B1**.311
Intestinal amebiasis *see* Amebiasis
Intestinal bacteria, Enterobacteriaceae
  infection, **B2**.1347
Intestinal coccida *see* Coccidia
Intestinal tapeworms *see* Cestodes (intestinal
  tapeworms)
Intestine *see* Gastrointestinal tract
Intimate contact, filovirus transmission,
  V2.1093–4
Intraabdominal infection, *Pasteurella
  multocida* causing, **B2**.1654–5
Intracellular adhesion molecule(s) (ICAMs)
  antigen presentation, **I**.383, **I**.384
  granuloma formation, **I**.708
  see also individual types
Intracellular adhesion molecule 1 (ICAM-1:
  CD45)
  actions/effects
    B cell activation, **I**.326
    CTL killing, **I**.474
    lymphocyte migration, **I**.508 (Tab.)

  macrophage development, **I**.21
  mucosal immune response, **I**.524
  CD4 T cells/APC interactions, **I**.392 (Fig.)
  CNS expression, **V2**.1410
  deficiency, **I**.774
  expression
    IFN-γ, **I**.820–1
    keratinocytes, **I**.820–1
    TLR stimulus, **I**.697
  gene *see ICAM1* gene
  hepatitis B immunopathology, **V1**.303
  immunogenetics, **I**.582–3
  induction, by lymphotoxin, **I**.286–7
  inhibition, by IL-10, **I**.292–3
  lymphocyte trafficking into CNS, **V2**.1410–11
  malaria, **I**.599
  neutrophil interactions, **I**.38
  polio receptor, **V2**.866
  polymorphisms, malaria susceptibility,
    P.485–6
  rhinovirus cellular receptor, **V1**.208–9,
    V1.210 (Fig.)
  structure, **V1**.246 (Fig.)
  upregulation in malaria, **P**.496–7
Intracellular adhesion molecule 2 (ICAM-2)
  lymphocyte migration, **I**.508 (Tab.)
  neutrophil interactions, **I**.38
Intracellular adhesion molecule-3 (ICAM-3),
  I.396
Intracellular bacteria
  iron scavenging, **B1**.151
  see also individual species
Intracellular bridges, smoldering infection,
  V1.261
Intracellular enveloped virus (IEV),
  poxviruses, **V1**.596–7, **V1**.613 (Fig.)
Intracellular mature virus (IMV)
  poxviruses *see* Poxviruses
  Vaccinia virus, **V1**.586
Intracellular pathogens
  entry into cells, **I**.649–50
    actin cytoskeleton, **I**.649–50
    adressins, **I**.649
    complement, **I**.649
    integrins, **I**.649
  escape to cytoplasm, **I**.650
  IFN-γ, **I**.589
    defects, **I**.589–90
  IL-12 receptor deficiency, **I**.589
  IL-18, **I**.290–2
  immune response, **I**.403
    avoidance, **I**.403
  immunogenetics, **I**.589–90
  infected cell identification, **I**.403
    see also Major histocompatibility complex
      (MHC) class I
  intracellular refuges, **I**.681–2
  protective immunity, **I**.489
  see also individual species
Intracellular signaling
  C5a, **I**.222
  chemokines, **I**.222–3
  fMet-Leu-Phe, **I**.222
  IL-8, **I**.222
  prostaglandin, **I**.188–9

Intracellular signaling (*Continued*)
SDF-1, **I.**222
Intracerebral calcification, congenital
toxoplasmosis, **P.**430 (Fig.)
Intrachromosomal recombination,
B1.88 (Fig.)
Intracranial abscess (brain abscess),
B1.581–9
anatomical site, **B1.**582 (Fig.), **B1.**582 (Tab.)
bacteriology, **B1.**584–6, **B1.**584 (Tab.)
causative organisms
Gordania terrae, **B2.**1152–3
Nocardia asteroides, **B2.**1157–8
clinical presentation, **B1.**586, **B1.**586 (Tab.)
contiguous spread, **B1.**582–3
development stages, **B1.**584
diagnostic methods, **B1.**586–7, **B1.**587 (Fig.)
epidemiology, **B1.**581–2
hematogenous spread, **B1.**583, **B1.**584 (Tab.)
pathogenesis and pathophysiology, **B1.**583–4
predisposing conditions, **B1.**582–3,
B1.582 (Tab.), **B1.**584 (Tab.),
B1.589 (Tab.)
treatment, **B1.**587–9
antibiotics, **B1.**587–9, **B1.**589 (Tab.)
surgery, **B1.**589
see also Subdural empyema
Intracranial pressure, cryptococcosis, **M.**652
Intradermal hypersensitivity test, human
brucellosis, **B2.**1741
Intraepithelial αβ T cells *see* αβ T-cells
Intraepithelial lymphocytes (IELs), **I.**522,
I.525–9
αβ T cells *see* αβ T-cells
CD7 expression, **I.**525–6
c-kit effects, **I.**527–8
CTLs, **I.**525–6
cytokine production, **I.**527
definition, **I.**525–6
distribution, **I.**526 (Fig.)
epithelial cell interactions, **I.**527–9,
I.528 (Fig.)
γδ T cells, **I.**525–6
see also γδ T-cells
gastrointestinal candidiasis, **M.**262
HIV infection, **I.**799–800
Listeria monocytogenes infection, **I.**526–7
mucosal barrier, **I.**527
origin/function, **I.**525–7
SCF effects, **I.**527–8
Intra-erythrocytic development, *Plasmodium*,
P.467–8
Intramolecular spreading, **I.**756
Intramuscular injections, viral infection by,
V1.238 (Fig.), **V1.**239
Intranasal vaccine delivery *see* Vaccination,
nasal administration
Intrapartum transmission
hepatitis B, **V2.**1474
hepatitis C, **V2.**1478
HIV, **V2.**1471
Intrathecal antibodies, virus infection, **V2.**1413
Intrathymic selection, αβ TCRs, **I.**456
Intrauterine contraceptive devices
Actinomyces, **B1.**669
bacterial vaginosis, **B1.**665

Intrauterine transmission, **V2.**1444 (Tab.)
hepatitis B, **V2.**1474–6
Parvovirus B19 virus infection, **V2.**1470
see also Fetal infection; Neonatal infection
Intravascular cannulae
colonization, **B1.**391
organisms, **B1.**391
nosocomial infection, **B1.**391–2
Intravascular grafts, infection, **B1.**392
Intravenous drug use
endocarditis, **B1.**526, **B1.**527
fungal endophthalmitis, **M.**318
HCMV infection, **V2.**1502
Hepatitis A virus transmission, **V2.**1172–3
hepatitis C transmission, **V2.**1208
pneumonia in HIV infection, **B1.**645
spinal epidural abscess, **B1.**592
tetanus association, **B2.**1065
Intravenous immunoglobulin (IVIG)
enterovirus control, **V2.**878
hepatitis A prevention, **V2.**1173–4
Human respiratory syncytial virus infection,
V1.792
see also Passive immunization
Intravitreal injection
amphotericin B, **M.**319
corticosteroids, **M.**320
dexamethasone, **M.**320
endophthalmitis, **M.**320
Intubation, pneumonia after, **B1.**389–90
Invariant chain Ii
antigen processing/presentation, **I.**382–3
mouse mammary tumor virus superantigen
vs., **I.**563
Invariant surface glycoprotein (ISG),
trypanosomes, **P.**355
Invasins, **B1.**152
Invasion, bacterial, **B1.**152–3
Invasive aspergillosis *see* Aspergillosis
Inverted repeat (IR) sequence, insertion
sequences, **B1.**91
Inverted terminal repeats (ITR)
adeno-associated viruses, **V1.**159–60,
V2.1599
Dependovirus, **V1.**409–10
HSV-1 genome, **V1.**163–4
Investigative phase, emerging viral infection,
V2.1665
Invirase *see* Saquinavir
in vitro culture *see* Cell culture, viruses;
Culture
in vitro fertilization, *Chlamydia trachomatis*
infection, **B2.**2012
in vitro replication, Mumps virus, **V1.**747,
V1.747 (Fig.)
in vivo expression technology (IVET),
genomics and bacterial pathogenicity,
B1.177, **B1.**178
Iodamoeba bütschlii, **P.**187, **P.**200, **P.**218,
P.223–4
cysts, **P.**223–4, **P.**224 (Fig.)
identification from other species, **P.**223–4
infection
immune response, **P.**218–19
treatment withholding, **P.**220
life cycle, **P.**219

trophozoites, **P.**223–4
Iodamoeba, classification, **P.**197, **P.**218
Iodides
pythiosis, **M.**425
sporotrichosis, **M.**28
Iodine, **B1.**425
action, **B1.**437 (Tab.)
autoimmune thyroid disease, **I.**756
giardiasis prevention, **P.**251–2
Iododeoxyuridine, structure, **V2.**1611 (Fig.)
Iodophors, hand disinfection, **B1.**378
Iodoquinol (di-iodohydroxyquinoline)
Blastocystis hominis, **P.**566–7
Dientamoeba fragilis infection, **P.**269
Ion-exchange resins, in *Clostridium difficile*
infection, **B2.**1123
Ion gradient-linked transport systems, **B1.**49
Ionizing radiation sterilization, **B1.**450–1,
B1.454 (Tab.)
DNA repair, **B1.**271, **B1.**451
food, **B1.**268 (Tab.), **B1.**271–2, **B1.**289,
B1.451
meat, **B1.**274
poultry, **B1.**271–2, **B1.**278
mechanisms of action, **B1.**450–1
microbial sensitivity, **B1.**450
public's perception, **B1.**271–2, **B1.**289
resistance, **B1.**450
thermoradiation, **B1.**454
uses, **B1.**445 (Tab.), **B1.**451
validation and monitoring, **B1.**454 (Tab.)
see also Radiation
Ion metabolism, *Plasmodium see* Plasmodium
Ion transport, across cell membrane, **P.**161–2
myo-Inositol fermentation, Enterobacteriaceae
identification, **B2.**1319 (Tab.)
IP10 *see* Interferon-inducible protein 10
(IP-10:CXCL10)
Ippy virus, geographical distribution/carrier
and disease, **V2.**1060 (Tab.)
IRF1 gene, **I.**580
IRF-3, Measles virus nucleocapsid (N) protein
interaction, **V1.**716
Iridoviridae
characteristics, **V1.**177 (Tab.)
classification, **V1.**27 (Tab.), **V1.**43 (Tab.),
V1.44
major capsid protein, **V1.**44
see also specific viruses
Irkut virus, **V2.**1104
Iron
acute phase response, **I.**208
Bordetella growth, **B2.**1793
diphtheria toxin expression, **B2.**981
Neisseria acquisition proteins, **B2.**1284–5
Plasmodium, **P.**478
scavenging systems, **B1.**151
terminal electron acceptor, **B1.**67
Iron-deficiency anemia
gastrointestinal nematodes, **P.**725
hookworm infection, **P.**725, **P.**727–8,
P.727 (Fig.)
trichuriasis, **P.**719–20, **P.**728–9
Iron-dependent repression, bacterial sensory
pathway, **B1.**165–6

Iron receptors, *Cryptococcus neoformans,* **M**.641–2

Iron regulated proteins, *Yersinia enterocolitica,* **B2**.1469

Iron-superoxide dismutase, trypanosomes, **P**.360

Irradiation *see* Ionizing radiation sterilization

Irrigation workers, giardiasis, **P**.250

Irritable bowel syndrome (IBS), *Blastocystis hominis* infection, **P**.563–4

ISA-51, TCE peptide vaccines, **I**.878–9

Isavirus
  characteristics, **V1**.129 (Tab.)
  classification, **V1**.50

Ischemia–reperfusion injury, **I**.155–6, **I**.155 (Tab.)
  C5 blocking antibody therapy, **I**.158

ISG20, interferon actions, **V1**.295

Ishak score, hepatitis C, **V2**.1204

Isla Vista virus, **V2**.1666 (Tab.)

Isocahedral viruses, morphology/structure *see* Morphology, viruses

Isocitrate dehydrogenase, **B1**.52, **B1**.53–4

Isocitrate lyase, **B1**.53–4

Isoenzyme characterization
  amebiasis diagnosis, **P**.220
  Bifidobacterium classification, **B2**.1026
  Blastocystis hominis, **P**.561
  Leishmania braziliensis, **P**.326
  Leishmania panamensis, **P**.329
  protozoa classification, **P**.192
  Trypanosoma brucei classification, **P**.352
  Trypanosoma cruzi, **P**.382–3, **P**.382 (Fig.)
  see also Zymodemes

Isoerythritol, *Brucella* culture, **B2**.1734

Isoforms, Borna disease virus nucleoprotein (N), **V2**.1140

Isolated environments, parasite control, **P**.110

Isolation of patients, control of bacterial infection, **B1**.328–9

Isoniazid (INH), **B1**.436–8, **B1**.481
  biocide-antibiotic linked resistance, **B1**.443
  Mycobacterium, **B2**.1217–18, **B2**.1222–3
    M. tuberculosis, **B2**.1197, **B2**.1200, **B2**.1217–18

Isopentyl pyrophosphate, systemic γδ T cell binding, **I**.439, **I**.440 (Fig.)

Isoprenoid quinones, Actinomycetes, aerobic, **B2**.1145

Isopropanol, **B1**.427
  action, **B1**.438

Isopropyl alcohol exposure, glove protection efficiency, **B1**.765–6

Isoprotanes, **I**.189–90

Isoquinoline derivatives, **B1**.428

Isospora belli, **P**.188
  classification, **P**.410–11
    Toxoplasma vs., **P**.411
  historical aspects, **P**.18, **P**.410–11
  infection *see* Isosporiasis
  life cycle, **P**.411–12
    cysts, **P**.411–12
    excystation, **P**.411
    sporozoites, **P**.411
  molecular biology, **P**.412

morphology, **P**.412 (Fig.)
  eggs, **P**.413 (Fig.)

Isospora, oocysts, **P**.167 (Fig.)

Isosporiasis, **P**.410–14
  chemotherapy, **P**.414
  clinical aspects, **P**.412
    in AIDS, **P**.97, **P**.412
    extra-intestinal manifestations, **P**.412
    self-limiting diarrhea, **P**.412
  diagnosis, **P**.413, **P**.413 (Fig.)
    fecal examination, **P**.413
    fecal samples, **P**.151
    PCR, **P**.413
  epidemiology, **P**.413–14
    AIDS, **P**.413–14
    cryptosporidiosis *vs.,* **P**.414
  immunology, **P**.76, **P**.412–13
    CD4 T cells, **P**.412–13
    IFN-γ production, **P**.412–13
    immunity to reinfection, **P**.412–13
    T helper cells, type 1, **P**.412–13
  infection recurrence, **P**.411–12
  pathology, **P**.413
    villous atrophy, **P**.413

Isothiazolones, **B1**.423 (Tab.), **B1**.427
  action, **B1**.437 (Tab.)

Isotope scanning, bone and joint infection diagnosis, **B1**.694

Israeli spotted fever, clinical manifestations, **B2**.2039 (Tab.)

Issatchenkia orientalis, **M**.582

I-TAC *see* CXCL11

ITAM *see* Immunoreceptor tyrosine-based activation motifs (ITAMs)

Itching, onchocerciasis, **P**.793

ITIM *see* Immunoreceptor tyrosine-based inhibitory motifs (ITIMs)

Itraconazole, **M**.182–3
  adverse effects, **M**.151 (Tab.), **M**.152, **M**.183–4
  aspergillosis, **M**.719, **M**.722–3, **M**.727–9
    amphotericin B *vs.,* **M**.728
    children, **M**.729
    fluconazole *vs.,* **M**.729
    lung transplants, **M**.703, **M**.704
    neonates, **M**.726
    safety, **M**.728–9
  Blastoschizomyces capitatus infection, **M**.626
  blepharitis, **M**.297
  candidiasis, **M**.257, **M**.611, **M**.612–13
    superficial, **M**.189
  chromoblastomycosis, **M**.364
  coccidioidomycosis, **M**.511
  cryptococcosis, **M**.651
  dermatomycosis, **M**.252, **M**.253
  doses and half-life, **M**.152
  drug interactions, **M**.152 (Tab.)
  endophthalmitis, **M**.319
  histoplasmosis capsulati, **M**.530, **M**.530 (Tab.), **M**.531, **M**.531 (Tab.)
  keratitis, **M**.311
  lobomycosis, **M**.434–5
  mechanism of action, **M**.70
  microsporidiosis, **P**.550
  keratoconjunctivitis, **P**.549

mucocutaneous candidiasis, **M**.189

nondermatophyte mold infection, **M**.189

onychomycosis, **M**.187–8, **M**.187 (Tab.), **M**.252, **M**.253

oral, **M**.728

paracoccidioidomycosis, **M**.552

penicilliosis marneffei, **M**.569

phaeohyphomycosis, **M**.745

pharmacokinetics, **M**.150, **M**.150 (Tab.), **M**.151–2

piedra, **M**.186

pityriasis versicolor, **M**.185, **M**.211

pityrosporal folliculitis, **M**.185–6

protothecosis, **M**.402

resistance, **M**.174
  Condidiobolus, **M**.352

rhino-orbital-cerebral zygomycosis, **M**.293–4

Scedosporium, **M**.757

spectrum of activity, **M**.151 (Tab.)

sporotrichosis, **M**.379

susceptibility testing, **M**.170, **M**.170 (Tab.)

tinea, **M**.233, **M**.234, **M**.235

tinea barbae, **M**.186, **M**.187 (Tab.)

tinea capitis, **M**.188, **M**.188 (Tab.)

tinea cruris, **M**.186

tinea manuum, **M**.186–7, **M**.187 (Tab.)

vulvovaginal candidiasis, **M**.189

white piedra, **M**.197

zygomycosis, **M**.352

iuc gene, *Shigella* vaccine vectors, **I**.843

Ivanovsky, Dmitri, **V1**.24

Ivasin, *Yersinia,* **B2**.1468

Ivermectin
  adverse reactions, **P**.789
  anti-nematode activity, **P**.789
  Ascaris lumbricoides, **P**.789
  development of, **P**.128
  discovery, **P**.10
  echinococcosis treatment, **P**.698–9
  onchocerciasis therapy, **P**.787, **P**.788–9, **P**.789–90
    community trials, **P**.789
    cost/economics, **P**.789
    morbidity control, **P**.790
    see also Community-directed treatment with ivermectin (CDTI)
  Strongyloides control, **P**.742
  Strongyloides stercoralis, **P**.789
  Wuchereria bancrofti, **P**.789

Ixodes
  Anaplasma phagocytophilum transmission, **B2**.2062–3
  Central European encephalitis transmission, **V2**.1003
  increase of exposure, **B1**.362
  life cycle, **B2**.1822
  Russian spring-summer encephalitis transmission, **V2**.1003

Ixodes dammini
  Babesia life cycle, **P**.452–3, **P**.458
  life cycle, **P**.458

Ixodes pacificus, **B1**.362

Ixodes persulcatus, **B2**.2050–1

Ixodes ricinus, **B1**.362
  Babesia divergens life cycle, **P**.458–9

Ixodes scapularis, **B1**.362

J2 protein (thymidine kinase), **V1**.169 (Tab.)
J3R gene, **V1**.609
Jaagsiekte sheep retrovirus (JSRV), **V1**.336
JAM proteins, lymphocyte migration,
  I.508 (Tab.)
Janeway lesions, infective endocarditis,
  B1.534–5, **B1**.534 (Fig.)
Janus-activated kinase (JAK) kinases,
  interferon signal transduction, **V1**.294,
  V1.315
Japan
  food-borne botulism, **B2**.1067–9
  schistosomiasis control programs, **P**.628
Japanese encephalitis (JE), **V2**.1001,
  V2.1424–5
  emerging infection, **V2**.1648 (Tab.)
    ecological changes, **V2**.1663
  epidemiology, **V1**.373, **V2**.997
  pathogenesis, **V2**.1424–5
  pathology, **V2**.1424–5
  transmission, **V1**.372 (Tab.)
  vaccines/vaccination, **V2**.1425,
    V2.1552 (Tab.), **V2**.1577–8
    adverse effects, **V2**.1577–8
    BCE peptide vaccines, **I**.855 (Tab.)
    development, **V2**.1555
    history, **V1**.8 (Tab.)
    inactivated, **V2**.1577–8
    live, attenuated, **V2**.1578
    recommendations, **V2**.1578
    schedules, **V2**.1577–8
Japanese encephalitis (JE) virus, **V2**.998 (Tab.)
  ELISA, **V2**.1425
  geographical distribution, **V2**.1424
  infection *see* Japanese encephalitis (JE)
  infection route, **V2**.1404, **V2**.1424
  release from nerve terminals, **V2**.1405
  transmission, **V2**.1424
Japanese Journal of Medical Mycology, **M**.31
Japanese spotted fever, **B2**.2039 (Tab.),
  B2.2040
Jarisch–Herxheimer reaction, early syphilis,
  B2.1857
Jaundice, **V2**.1160
  babesiosis, **P**.454–5
  obstructive, liver fluke infection, **P**.649
J (joining) chain
  genes, **I**.328
  IgM structure, **I**.307
  Ig structure, **I**.309–10
  pIgR interactions, **I**.318–19
JC virus (JCV), **V1**.474–80, **V2**.1416
  cell entry, **V1**.474
  c-Jun transcription factor, **V1**.476–7
  evolution, **V1**.475–6
  genome, **V1**.475 (Fig.)
    transcription factor binding, **V1**.475 (Fig.),
    V1.476–7
  immunohistochemistry, **V1**.480 (Fig.)
  infection *see* JC virus (JCV) infection
  neurotropic features, **V1**.477
  NF-1 transcription factor, **V1**.476–7
  NFκB proteins, **V1**.476–7
  nucleotide sequence analysis, **V1**.474–5
  regulatory region, **V1**.475–6, **V1**.475 (Fig.)
    hypervariability, **V1**.475–6

TATA box, **V1**.475–6
  Sp-1 transcription factor, **V1**.476–7
  species infected, **V1**.473
  T antigen, **V1**.473–4, **V1**.476
  Tst-1 transcription factor, **V1**.476–7
JC virus (JCV) infection
  cancer associations, **V1**.478–80
    animal models, **V1**.478–9
    human, **V1**.479–80
    nonhuman primates, **V1**.479
    non-neural, **V1**.480
    transgenic animals, **V1**.479
  in HIV infection, **V2**.1499 (Tab.), **V2**.1504
  host cytokine effects, **V1**.477
  host growth factor effects, **V1**.477
  immunodeficient patients (non-HIV),
    V2.1509–10
  infection route, **V2**.1416
  progressive multifocal leukoencephalopathy
    see Progressive multifocal
    leucoencephalopathy (PML)
Jejunum, normal microbiota, **B1**.302
J elements, TCR, **I**.450, **I**.451
Jena virus, **V2**.926
Jenner, Edward, **V1**.4, **I**.487, **V1**.579–80,
  V1.580 (Fig.), **I**.895, **V2**.1578
Jeryl Lynn strain, Mumps virus vaccination,
  V1.753
JHM virus (murine coronavirus)
  encephalomyelitis, **V2**.1411–12
  immune response, antibodies, **V2**.1413
jMPV, SH glycoproteins, **V1**.787–8
JNK pathway, Vav activation by, **I**.345–6
Job's syndrome *see* Hyper-IgE syndrome
  (Job's syndrome)
Johne's disease (paratuberculosis), **B2**.1182
Joining chain *see* J (joining) chain
Joint(s)
  penicilliosis marneffei, **M**.567
  specimens, **M**.83 (Tab.), **M**.84
  sporotrichosis, **M**.374–5, **M**.377
Joint infection *see* Bone/joint infection
Joint prostheses, infection, **B1**.392
  reduction, **B1**.375, **B1**.375 (Fig.)
Jonesia denitrificans, **B2**.958
Jordans tartrate, Enterobacteriaceae
  identification, **B2**.1319 (Tab.)
Journal de Mycologie Médicale, **M**.31
Journal of Medical and Veterinary Mycology
  (JMVM), **M**.31, **M**.32
Junctional adhesion molecule 1 (JAM1),
  V2.933
Junctional diversity, TCR, **I**.454
Junction resolution, **V1**.419, **V1**.420
Junin virus, **V2**.1059
  animal infection, **V2**.1069–70
  arenavirus cross-reactivity, **V2**.1069
  classification, **V2**.1060–1
  emerging infection, **V2**.1648 (Tab.)
  genome, **V2**.1066
  geographical distribution/carrier and disease,
    V2.1060 (Tab.)
  infection
    antiviral agents, **V2**.1078
    chronic, **V2**.1071
    clinical features, **V2**.1071

histopathology, **V2**.1071
  immune response, **V2**.1073
  immunotherapy, **V2**.1077–8
  pathogenesis, **V2**.1071
  isolation from tissue specimens,
    V2.1076 (Tab.)
  laboratory-acquired infection, **V2**.1517 (Tab.)
  RNA detection, **V2**.1075–6
  S RNA segment, **V2**.1064 (Fig.)
  transmission, **V1**.371–2, **V1**.371 (Tab.)
  vaccine (Candid:1), **V2**.1076
JUN, papillomavirus E7 protein effects,
  V1.461 (Tab.)
Juquitiba virus, **V2**.1666 (Tab.)
Juvenile laryngeal papillomatosis (JLP),
  V2.1483, **V2**.1484

K3L gene, **V1**.620, **V1**.624
K12 (Kaposin), **V1**.548, **V1**.549 (Tab.)
Kala-azar *see* Leishmaniasis, Old World,
  visceral (kala-azar)
Kaletra *see* Lopinavir
Kanamycin
  Brucella, **B2**.1742
  Enterobacter, **B2**.1484–5
  Ewingella, **B2**.1493
  gonorrhea treatment, **B1**.662
  Leclercia, **B2**.1495
  structure, **B1**.483 (Fig.)
  Yokenella, **B2**.1498
K-antigens, **B1**.154
  Enterobacteriaceae, **B2**.1339–40, **B2**.1343
  Escherichia coli, **B2**.1364–5
Kaposi's sarcoma, **V1**.550, **V1**.552–3
  epidemiology, **V1**.551, **V1**.552
  historical aspects, **V1**.541
  Mycoplasma penetrans association, **B2**.1985
  NK cells, **I**.96
  pathology, **V1**.552–3
    histology, **V1**.552–3
  signs/symptoms, **V1**.552, **V1**.553 (Fig.)
  therapy, **V1**.553, **V2**.1503
    counseling, **V2**.1503
    foscarnet (phosphonoformic acid; PFA),
      V2.1503
  variants, **V1**.552
  see also Human herpesvirus 8 (HHV-8)
    infection
Kaposi's sarcoma-associated herpesvirus
  (KSHV) *see* Human herpesvirus 8
  (HHV-8: Kaposi's sarcoma-associated
  herpesvirus (KSHV))
Kappa light chains, **I**.309, **I**.323
Karshi virus, **V2**.998 (Tab.)
Kartagener's syndrome, **B1**.626
Karyokinesis, **P**.228
Karyopherins, Hepatitis B virus nuclear entry,
  V2.1234
Karyoplasm, protozoa, **P**.173
Karyotyping
  Blastocystis hominis, **P**.562
  Candida, **M**.583–4
  protozoa classification, **P**.193
Kasokero virus infection, **V2**.1047
Katayama fever, **P**.629–30
  historical aspects, **P**.11

Katayama fever (*Continued*)
  see also Schistosomiasis
Kato–Katz smears
  gastrointestinal nematodes, **P**.730
    infection intensity, **P**.723
  schistosomiasis, **P**.149–50, **P**.606
Kauffmann–White nomenclature, *Salmonella*,
    B1.757, **B2**.1402, **B2**.1403 (Tab.)
Kawasaki's disease
  superantigens, **I**.562
  Yersinia pseudotuberculosis infection, **I**.563
K/BxN mouse model, rheumatoid arthritis,
    I.759
k-cyclin (cyclin D homologue), HHV-8,
    V1.546, **V1**.548, **V1**.549 (Tab.), **V1**.555
KDPG, **B1**.58
KDPG aldolase, **B1**.58
KDPG hexose cycle, **B1**.59
KDPG pathway (Entner–Doudoroff pathway),
    B1.58–9, **B1**.59 (Fig.), **B2**.1274–5
  Acetobacter, **B1**.60
  enteric bacteria, **B1**.58–9
  nonmethanogenic archaea, **B1**.70
  other aerobic bacteria, **B1**.60
Kedougou virus (KEDV), **V2**.998 (Tab.)
'Keep-up, catch-up, follow-up' schedule,
    measles vaccine schedule, **V1**.735–6
Kennel cough, **B2**.1810
Keratin intermediate filament, papillomavirus
    E4 protein association, **V1**.458
Keratinocytes
  cytokines produced, **I**.820–1
    chemokines, **I**.820–1
    colony-stimulating factors, **I**.820–1
    growth factors, **I**.820–1
    ILs, **I**.820–1
    INFs, **I**.820–1
    TNF, **I**.820–1
  defensins, **I**.168
  IFN-γ actions, **I**.820–1
  immune surveillance, **I**.820–1
  intercellular adhesion molecule 1 expression,
    I.820–1
  MHC class II expression, **I**.820–1
  papillomavirus infection, **V1**.451–3
Keratitis, **M**.300–16, **B1**.601–2
  causal agents/infection
    Absidia corymbifera, **M**.301–2
    Acremonium, **M**.303, **M**.328
    Acremonium kiliense, **M**.328
    aspergillosis, **M**.300, **M**.301, **M**.302, **M**.306,
      M.307–9, **M**.316
    Aspergillus flavus, **M**.302 (Fig.), **M**.312,
      M.313 (Fig.), **M**.327–8
    Aspergillus fumigatus, **M**.303, **M**.305,
      M.327–8
    Beauveria bassiana, **M**.328
    Bipolaris, **M**.301–2
    Blastomyces dermatitidis, **M**.305
    candidiasis *see* Candidiasis
    cryptococcosis, **M**.648
    Curvularia, **M**.301–2, **M**.307–9, **M**.313,
      M.313 (Fig.), **M**.327–8
    Exophiala dermatitidis, **M**.328
    Exserohilum, **M**.301–2

Fusarium, **M**.300–1, **M**.303, **M**.307–9,
    M.312, **M**.316, **M**.327, **M**.754
Fusarium solani, **M**.301–2, **M**.302 (Fig.),
    M.303, **M**.304–5, **M**.316 (Fig.), **M**.327–8
histoplasmosis, **M**.305
Lasiodiplopodia theobromae, **M**.301–2,
    M.309, **M**.313, **M**.316
Mycobacterium chelonae, **B2**.1252
Nocardia asteroides, **B2**.1158–9
Paecilomyces, **M**.282–3, **M**.303, **M**.316
Paecilomyces lilacinus, **M**.316
Pythium insidiosum, **M**.301–2, **M**.305,
    M.316
Rhodotorula, **M**.328
Scedosporium apiospermum, **M**.301–2,
    M.313–14, **M**.327–8
sporotrichosis, **M**.305
trauma association, **M**.301
  clinical manifestations, **B1**.601
  diagnosis, **M**.301, **B1**.601–2
    PCR, **M**.306
    scrapings and culture, **M**.302–3,
      M.303 (Fig.), **M**.304, **M**.304 (Fig.)
  histopathology, **M**.303, **M**.304–5, **M**.305 (Fig.)
  immune response, **M**.314–15
  incidence, **M**.300
  infecting agents, **B1**.601
  post surgical, **M**.327
  predisposing factors, **B1**.601
  risk factors, **M**.301
    contact lens association, **M**.330–1
  sclerosing, onchocerciasis, **P**.793–5
  therapy, **M**.306
    amphotericin B therapy, **M**.307–8, **M**.312
    azoles, **M**.308–9
    chlorhexidine, **M**.307
    clotrimazole, **M**.309
    corticosteroids, **M**.315
    econazole, **M**.309
    fluconazole, **M**.311–12, **M**.314
    flucytosine, **M**.308
    itraconazole, **M**.311
    ketoconazole, **M**.310, **M**.312
    miconazole, **M**.309, **M**.313
    natamycin, **M**.308, **M**.312
    polyenes, **M**.307–8
    polyhexamethylene biguanides, **M**.306–7
    pyrimidines, **M**.308
    selection of antifungal therapy, **M**.312
    silver sulfadiazine, **M**.307
    surgical, **M**.315
  treatment, **B1**.602
  types, **M**.300
Keratoconjunctivitis
  causative organisms, **B1**.386
  microsporidiosis, **P**.540–1
Keratosis palmoplantarus with
    periodontopathia, **I**.482
Kerecid *see* Idoxuridine
KETc antigens, peptide vaccine design, **I**.874–5
Keterah virus infection, **V2**.1048
Ketoconazole, **M**.151 (Tab.), **M**.183 (Tab.)
  AIDS, **M**.611
  absorption, **M**.611
  doses and half-life, **M**.152
  drug interactions, **M**.152 (Tab.)

mechanism of action, **M**.70
pharmacokinetics, **M**.150, **M**.150 (Tab.),
    M.151–2
resistance, *Condidiobolus*, **M**.352
side-effects, **M**.151 (Tab.), **M**.152–3,
    M.183–4, **M**.234, **M**.551, **M**.611
spectrum of activity, **M**.151 (Tab.)
therapy
  adiaspiromycosis, **M**.821
  atopic dermatitis, **M**.213
  blepharitis, **M**.297
  candidiasis, **M**.257, **M**.609–10
  coccidioidomycosis, **M**.511
  endophthalmitis, **M**.319, **M**.320, **M**.326–7
  keratitis, **M**.310, **M**.312
  mucocutaneous candidiasis, **M**.189
  mycetoma, **M**.393
  onychomycosis/dermatomycosis therapy,
    M.253
  paracoccidioidomycosis, **M**.551
  penicilliosis marneffei, **M**.571
  piedra, **M**.186
  pityriasis versicolor, **M**.185, **M**.211
  pityrosporal folliculitis, **M**.185–6
  prototheccosis, **M**.402
  seborrheic dermatitis, **M**.185, **M**.212
  tinea, **M**.233–4
  tinea barbae, **M**.186
  tinea capitis, **M**.188–9
  tinea nigra, **M**.186
  white piedra, **M**.197
  zygomycosis, **M**.352
2-Keto-3-deoxyoctonate (KDO), **B1**.160
  Enterobacteriaceae LPS, **B2**.1340
2-Keto-3-deoxy-6-phosphogluconate (KDPG),
    B1.58–9, **B1**.59 (Fig.)
α-Ketoglutarate, **B1**.53
  trypanosomes, **P**.357
9-Ketoisomerase, **I**.186–7
11-Ketoisomerase, **I**.186–7
Ketol–enol tautomerism, **V1**.57, **V1**.58 (Fig.)
Ketolides, *Mycoplasma*, **B2**.1992
9-Ketoreductase, **I**.186–7
  prostaglandin production, **I**.187
Keyhole limpet hemocyanin, as carrier protein,
    I.862–3, **I**.869
Khabarovsk virus, **V2**.1666 (Tab.)
Khujand virus (KHUV), **V2**.1104
KID50, *Proteus*, **B2**.1447
Kidney
  amphotericin B, **M**.611–12
  candidiasis, **M**.595, **M**.600
  as immunologically privileged site, **V1**.261
  transplants *see* Renal transplants
Kidney disease *see* Renal diseases/infection
Kidney stones, **B2**.1446
Kilham rat virus (KRV)
  discovery, **V1**.409
  oncotropism, **V1**.423
Killed vaccines *see* Vaccine(s)
Killer cell immunoglobulin receptor (KIR),
    I.80, **I**.87, **I**.88–9, **I**.96 (Tab.),
    V1.272
killing mechanism, **I**.472

Killer cell immunoglobulin receptor (KIR)
(*Continued*)
  NK cell activation, **I**.88 (Fig.), **I**.90, **I**.92, **I**.94,
    I.628
    polymorphisms, **I**.96 (Tab.)
  NK cell development, **I**.85
  upregulation, HIV infection, **I**.793
'Killer yeast' phenomenon, **B2**.1145
Kinetics, enzyme reactions, **B1**.45
Kinetodesmal fibrils, **P**.170–2
Kinetoplastea, **P**.350
Kinetoplastida, **I**.675–6
Kinetoplasts, **P**.174, **P**.174 (Fig.)
  Leishmania, **P**.296
  Trypanosoma brucei, **P**.353
  Trypanosoma cruzi, **P**.377–8
  Trypanosoma vivax, **P**.174 (Fig.)
Kinetosome (basal body), **P**.179–80
  structure, **P**.161 (Fig.)
King A medium, **B2**.1596
King B medium, **B2**.1596
Kingella
  antibacterial susceptibility/resistance,
    B2.1671
  classification, **B2**.1668–9
  clinical significance, **B2**.1669–70
  culture and identification, **B2**.1670–1
  habitats, **B2**.1649–50
  normal microbiota, **B1**.296 (Tab.)
  taxonomy, **B2**.1668–9
Kingella denitrificans
  antibacterial susceptibility/resistance,
    B2.1671
  characteristics, **B2**.1668 (Tab.), **B2**.1670–1
  classification, **B2**.1668–9
  clinical significance, **B2**.1670
  culture, **B2**.1670–1
Kingella indologenes
  antibacterial susceptibility/resistance,
    B2.1671
  classification, **B2**.1271, **B2**.1668–9
Kingella kingae
  antibacterial susceptibility/resistance,
    B2.1671
  characteristics, **B2**.1668 (Tab.), **B2**.1670–1
  classification, **B2**.1668–9
  clinical significance, **B2**.1669–70
  culture, **B2**.1670–1
  identification, **B2**.1671
  infection, **B2**.1669–70
    bone and joints, **B1**.690
    endocarditis, **B1**.532
  taxonomy, **B2**.1668–9
Kingella oralis, **B2**.1668 (Tab.)
Kinyoun acid-fast stain, **B2**.1140
Kinyoun acid-fast stain, mycobacteria,
    M.123 (Tab.)
Kirby–Bauer test, **B1**.498
KIR gene defects, **I**.576
Kit ligand (KL) *see* Stem cell factor (SCF:
    c-kit)
Klebsiella, **B2**.1476–83
  antibacterial susceptibility/resistance, **B1**.433,
    B2.1480
    quinolone resistance, **B1**.493 (Tab.)

antigens, **B2**.1480–1
  virulence effects, **B2**.1340
biochemistry, **B2**.1479–80
  lactose fermentation, **B1**.115
  nitrogen fixation, **B1**.201
capsules, **B2**.1343
characteristics, **B2**.1476
classification, **B2**.1477
  to *Raoultella* genus, **B2**.1336
culture, **B2**.1477–9
  morphology, **B2**.1345
definition, **B2**.1476
fimbriae, **B2**.1342–3
infection
  bacteremia, **B1**.520–1
  intestinal, **B2**.1347
  nosocomial *see below*
isolation/identification
  gelatin liquefaction, **B2**.1351
  historical perspective, **B2**.1351
  screening tests, **B2**.1349 (Tab.)
  typing methods, **B2**.1481
morphology, **B2**.1477–8
non-motility, **B2**.1342
as normal microbiota, **B1**.296 (Tab.)
nosocomial infection, **B1**.372, **B1**.397,
    B1.398 (Tab.)
  food-borne, **B1**.377
  spread by contact with staff, **B1**.378
pathogenicity, **B2**.1482–3
plasmids, **B1**.115
temperature susceptibility/resistance,
    B2.1345–6
waterborne, **B1**.212–13, **B1**.220–1, **B1**.222–3
  testing, **B1**.223
Klebsiella aerogenes see Klebsiella pneumoniae
Klebsiella ascorbata, **B2**.1319 (Tab.)
Klebsiella cryocrescens, **B2**.1319 (Tab.)
Klebsiella edwardsii see Klebsiella pneumoniae
Klebsiella georgiana, **B2**.1319 (Tab.)
Klebsiella granulomatis
  antibacterial susceptibility/resistance,
    B2.1480
  characteristics, **B2**.1330 (Tab.)
  classification, **B2**.1336
    changes in, **B2**.1336
  pathogenicity, **B2**.1482–3
Klebsiella (Calymmatobacterium)
    granulomatis, **B1**.665
  classification, **B1**.665
Klebsiella mobilis see Enterobacter aerogenes
Klebsiella ornithinolytica, **B2**.1477
  biochemical tests, **B2**.1319 (Tab.)
Klebsiella oxytoca, **B2**.1477
  antibacterial susceptibility/resistance,
    B2.1480
  antigens, **B2**.1481
  biochemical tests, **B2**.1319 (Tab.), **B2**.1479
  characteristics, **B2**.1479 (Tab.)
  classification, **B2**.1477
  infection
    extraintestinal, **B2**.1346–7
    nosocomial, **B1**.398 (Tab.)
  pullunase secretion system, **B1**.48
  waterborne, **B1**.220

Klebsiella ozaenae, **B2**.1477
  antigens, **B2**.1480–1
  biochemical tests, **B2**.1319 (Tab.),
    B2.1479–80
  classification, **B2**.1477
Klebsiella planticola, **B2**.1477
  biochemical tests, **B2**.1319 (Tab.), **B2**.1479
  classification, **B2**.1477
Klebsiella pneumoniae, **B2**.1477
  antibacterial susceptibility/resistance,
    B1.499 (Tab.), **B2**.1480
    β-lactamase resistance, **B1**.472–3
    intrinsic, **B2**.1352 (Tab.)
  antigens, **B2**.1480–1
    K-antigens, **B1**.154
  characteristics, **B2**.1479 (Tab.)
  classification, **B2**.1477
  complement surface masking, **I**.662–3
  culture morphology, **B2**.1345 (Tab.)
  infection, **B2**.1346
    epiglottitis, **B1**.613
    extraintestinal, **B2**.1346–7
    immune system avoidance, **B1**.154
    intracranial abscess, **B1**.585
    nosocomial infection, **B1**.398 (Tab.)
    pneumonia, **B1**.637
  isolation/identification
    biochemical tests, **B2**.1319 (Tab.), **B2**.1479
    problem strains, **B2**.1348–50
  pathogenicity, **B2**.1482
  subspecies *ozaenae see Klebsiella ozaenae*
  subspecies *rhinoscleromatis see Klebsiella
    rhinoscleromatis*
  tritrpticin sensitivity, **I**.172
  virulence factors, **B1**.154
  waterborne, **B1**.211–12, **B1**.220
Klebsiella rhinoscleromatis, **B1**.629, **B2**.1477
  antibacterial susceptibility/resistance,
    B2.1480
  antigens, **B2**.1481
  biochemical tests, **B2**.1319 (Tab.),
    B2.1479–80
  classification, **B2**.1477
  infection, rhinoscleroma, **B1**.616
Klebsiella terrigena, **B2**.1477
  biochemical tests, **B2**.1319 (Tab.)
  classification, **B2**.1477
Klebsiella trevisanii, **B2**.1477
Klebsiella variicloa, **B2**.1477
Kloeckera apiculata, fruit, **B1**.282
Kluyvera, **B2**.1494–5
  antibacterial susceptibility/resistance,
    B2.1494
  biochemical tests, **B2**.1494
  classification, **B2**.1494
  culture, **B2**.1494
  definition, **B2**.1494
  habitats, **B2**.1494–5
  pathogenicity, **B2**.1494–5
  species 3, **B2**.1494
Kluyvera ascorbata, **B2**.1494
  antibacterial susceptibility/resistance,
    B2.1494
  classification, **B2**.1494
  pathogenicity, **B2**.1494–5
Kluyvera cochleae, classification, **B2**.1336

Kluyvera cryocrescens, **B2**.1494
  antibacterial susceptibility/resistance,
      B2.1494
    intrinsic, **B2**.1352 (Tab.)
  pathogenicity, **B2**.1494–5
Kluyvera georgiana, **B2**.1494
Kluyveromyces marxianus, **M**.582
Kluyveromyces marxianus, fruit, **B1**.283
'Knobs'
  Plasmodium, **P**.473, **P**.473 (Fig.), **P**.475
  Plasmodium falciparum, **P**.473, **P**.473 (Fig.)
  Plasmodium malariae, **P**.473, **P**.473 (Fig.),
      P.475
Knockout animal models
  β-only T-cells, **I**.445
  historical aspects/re-evaluation, **I**.7–8
  IL-1, **I**.195–6
  IL-6, **I**.195–6
  IL-10, **I**.653
  linkage, **I**.572–3
  salmonellosis, **I**.593–4
Knodell score, hepatitis C, **V2**.1204
Kobuvirus, **V1**.50–2
Koch phenomenon, delayed-type
    hypersensitivity, **I**.709–10
Koch, Robert, **V1**.3, **P**.4, **B1**.6, **B1**.7
Koch's postulates, **B1**.7, **V1**.364
Kocuria, as normal microbiota, **B1**.296 (Tab.),
    B1.304
Köhler, Georges, **I**.7, **I**.10
Koilocytic dysplasia, HPV association,
    V1.465 (Tab.)
Kokobera virus (KOKV), **V2**.998 (Tab.)
Koplik's spots, **V1**.722–3
  measles, **I**.803–4
Korean hemorrhagic fever virus
  emerging infection, **V2**.1663–4
  transmission, **V1**.371 (Tab.)
Kostmann's syndrome, **I**.765
Kotonkan virus, morphology, **V2**.1105
Koutango virus, **V2**.998 (Tab.)
Kovacs oxidase, **B2**.1319 (Tab.)
Kozak sequence, **V1**.114
Krebs cycle, *Schistosoma,* **P**.605–6
Krotoski, Wojciech, *Plasmodium* life cycle,
    P.17
Kunjin virus (KUNV), **V2**.998 (Tab.)
  immune evasion, **V1**.296
  particle assembly/release, **V1**.143–4
Kunjin virus, immune evasion, **V1**.296
Kupffer cells
  cutaneous leishmaniasis, **P**.300
  Mycobacterium leprae, **B2**.1204
  Plasmodium hepatocyte invasion, **P**.472–3
  viral infection, **V1**.241
Ku proteins
  deficiency, **I**.330
  somatic recombination, **I**.330
Kuru, **V1**.7, **V2**.1347
  bovine spongiform encephalopathy *vs.,*
      V2.1363
  incidence, **V2**.1347
  transmission, **V2**.1366 (Tab.)
Kussmaul breathing, malaria in children, **P**.484
Kwashiorkor, malaria, **P**.493
Kwon-Chung, K J, **M**.16–8

Kyasanur forest disease, **V2**.1004
  public health importance, **V2**.997
Kyasanur forest disease virus, **V2**.998 (Tab.)
Kytococcus sedentarius, as normal microbiota,
    B1.296 (Tab.)

L1A1 gene, **M**.102
L1 gene sequence, papillomaviruses,
    V1.449–50
L1 protein, papillomaviruses, **V1**.450, **V1**.462
L2 protein, papillomaviruses, **V1**.450, **V1**.462
Laboratories, **V2**.1523–8
  access, **V2**.1520–3
  biosafety level 1, **V2**.1524–5
    facilities, **V2**.1525
    practices, **V2**.1523 (Tab.)
    requirements, **V2**.1524 (Tab.)
  biosafety level 2, **V2**.1525–6
    agent classification, **V2**.1525
    design, **V2**.1525–6, **V2**.1525 (Fig.)
    practices, **V2**.1523 (Tab.)
    requirements, **V2**.1524 (Tab.)
  biosafety level 3, **V2**.1526
    agent classification, **V2**.1526
    design, **V2**.1526, **V2**.1527 (Fig.),
        V2.1528 (Fig.)
    HEPA filters, **V2**.1526
    practices, **V2**.1523 (Tab.), **V2**.1526
    requirements, **V2**.1524 (Tab.)
  biosafety level 4, **V2**.1526–8
    agent classification, **V2**.1526
    cabinet-line, **V2**.1527, **V2**.1528 (Fig.)
    design, **V2**.1526–7, **V2**.1528 (Fig.)
    filoviruses, **V2**.1086
    practices, **V2**.1523 (Tab.), **V2**.1527–8
    requirements, **V2**.1524 (Tab.)
    'suit laboratory,' **V2**.1527, **V2**.1529 (Fig.)
  data reporting systems, **B1**.319–20,
      B1.321 (Tab.)
  see also Laboratory safety
Laboratory-acquired infection, **V2**.1516–17,
    V2.1517 (Tab.)
  aerosol transmission, **V2**.1516
  analytic phase/preanalytic phase testing,
      B1.760
  brucellosis, **B2**.1721, **B2**.1733–4
  contaminated surfaces, **B1**.761
  definition, **B1**.760
  epidemiology of, **B1**.760–1
  first account, **B1**.760
  human factors, **B1**.761
  laboratory department statistics, **B1**.761
  needlestick injury *see* Needlestick injury
  prevention and control, **B1**.764–5
    immunization, **B1**.767
    see also Laboratory safety
  transmission routes, **B1**.761
Laboratory animals
  housing, **V1**.90
  virus isolation from, **V1**.94–5
  virus propagation, **V1**.90, **V1**.94–5
Laboratory diagnosis *see* Diagnosis
Laboratory Response Network (LRN), **B1**.768

Laboratory safety, **B1.760–8**, **M**.92, **V2.1515–31**
  aerosols
    generation, **B1**.765
    protection from, **B1**.764–5
  agent categorization, **V2**.1521 (Tab.),
      V2.1523 (Tab.)
  biological safety cabinets, **B1**.764–5,
      B1.765 (Tab.)
  biological safety officer, **V2**.1520–3
  bioterrorism, **B1**.767–8
  centrifuges, **V2**.1520–3
  classification systems, **B1**.762–4
    environments, **B1**.762–3
    organisms, **B1**.762
    practices/behaviors, **B1**.763–4
    risk clarification, **B1**.760–1
    see also below
  clothing, **B1**.765–6
    biosafety level 3, **B1**.763–4
    gloves, **B1**.765–6
    masks, **B1**.764
    respiratory protective devices, **B1**.764–5
  code of safety practices, **V2**.1516, **V2**.1520–3
  components, **V2**.1518
  containment levels, **V2**.1520
  development, **V2**.1518
  emerging viral infection, **V2**.1518
  handwashing, **B1**.766–7
  level 1 (BL1), **B1**.763
  level 2 (BL2), **B1**.763
  level 3 (BL3), **B1**.763–4
  level 4 (BL4; maximum), **B1**.763, **B1**.764
  microbiological risk assessment, **V2**.1516,
      V2.1518–20
    hazard groups, **V2**.1520
    immunocompromised individuals, **V2**.1519
    legislation, **V2**.1519
    medical surveillance policy, **V2**.1519–20
    occupational infection, **V2**.1518
    relative risk, **V2**.1519
    risk quantification, **V2**.1519
  personal protective equipment, **V2**.1518,
      V2.1520–3
  practices, **B1**.763
  quality assurance materials, **B1**.761
  quality management, **B1**.761–2
    laboratory safety officer, **B1**.762
    risk assessment, **B1**.761–2
  'sharps,' **V2**.1520–3
  waste, **V2**.1528
  see also Laboratories
Laboratory workers
  botulism, **B2**.1076
  clothing *see* Laboratory safety
  handwashing, **B1**.766–7
  immunization, **B1**.767
LA-Candida Antigen Detection System, **M**.100
Lac operon, **B1**.80–1
Lacrimal canaliculitis, candidiasis, **M**.601
Lacrimal duct, respiratory tract, **B1**.606–7
La Crosse virus
  cell attachment/entry, **V2**.1034
    G1 glycoprotein, **V2**.1034–5
  epidemiology, **V2**.1048–9
  morphology/structure, **V2**.1026–8

La Crosse virus (*Continued*)
  passive viremia, **V1**.241 (Fig.)
  transcription termination, **V2**.1037
  transmission, **V2**.1048–9
  viremia determining localization/virulence,
    V1.245, **V1**.245 (Tab.)
β-Lactam antibiotics, **B1**.471–3
  mode of action, **B1**.471, **B1**.472 (Fig.)
    Gram-positive *vs.* Gram-negative, **B1**.471
    penicillin-binding proteins, **B1**.471
  pharmacology, time-dependency, **B1**.470
  resistance, **B1**.471–3
    Acinetobacter, **B1**.472–3
    Aeromonas, **B1**.472–3
    β-lactamases *see* β-Lactamases
    Brucella, **B2**.1742
    Burkholderia cepacia complex, **B2**.1610–11
    Enterococcus, **B2**.891–2, **B2**.892 (Tab.)
    porin mutations, **B1**.473
    Staphylococcus, **B2**.793–802, **B2**.794 (Tab.)
    Stenotrophomonas maltophilia, **B2**.1637
    'tolerance,' **B1**.471
  spectrum of activity
    Actinomyces, **B2**.1011
    Aeromonas, **B2**.1534
    Campylobacter, **B2**.1548
    Edwardsiella, **B2**.1491–2
    Enterobacter, **B2**.1484–5
    Gram-positive *vs.* Gram-negative, **B1**.471
    Klebsiella, **B2**.1480
    Legionella, **B2**.1777
    Staphylococcus, **B2**.793–802
  structure, **B1**.471, **B1**.471 (Fig.)
  toxicity/adverse effects, **B1**.473
  see also specific types
β-Lactamase inhibitors, **B1**.478
  structure, **B1**.479 (Fig.)
β-Lactamases, **B1**.471–3
  Bacteroides/Prevotella/Porphyromonas,
    B2.1930, **B2**.1935
  Capnocytophaga, **B2**.1677
  classification, **B1**.472
  Eikenella corrodens, **B2**.1668
  Enterococcus, **B2**.892
  Legionella, **B2**.1762 (Tab.)
  Moraxella (Branhamella) catarrhalis,
    B2.1307–8
  Neisseria meningitidis, **B1**.566
  Pasteurella multocida, **B2**.1655
  plasmid resistance genes, **B1**.111–12,
    B1.112–13
  Neisseria, **B2**.1277, **B2**.1291–2
  Proteus, **B2**.1441–4
  SHV-1 enzymes, **B1**.472–3
  TEM-1 enzymes, **B1**.472–3
  TEM-2 enzymes, **B1**.472–3
  Yersinia enterocolitica, **B2**.1465–6
Lactate dehydrogenase, contraceptive
    vaccines, **I**.875
Lactate dehydrogenase-elevating virus (LDV),
    V1.825
  classification, **V1**.53
  GP$_2$ glycoprotein, **V1**.839
  infection, **V1**.841 (Tab.)
  infectious immune complexes, **V1**.262

macrophage infection, **V1**.273
  major surface glycoprotein (MSG), **V1**.838
  membrane (M) protein, **V1**.837
  subgenomic RNA, **V1**.831–2
Lactenin, food, **B1**.267
Lactic acid, **B1**.422
  as aerial disinfectant, **B1**.430
  formation from pyruvate, **B1**.54, **B1**.54 (Fig.)
  meat, **B1**.272
Lactic acid bacteria, **B1**.54
  vegetables, frozen, **B1**.281–2
  see also individual species
Lactic acid dehydrogenase, **B1**.54
Lactobacillaceae, **B2**.833
  cereals, **B1**.284–5
Lactobacillus, **B2**.863–7
  antibacterial susceptibility/resistance,
    intrinsic anti-glycopeptide activity,
    B1.480
  antigens, **B2**.865–6
  applications
    in cheesemaking, **B1**.252
    as probiotic, **B1**.666–8
  attenuated vaccine vectors, **I**.830–1
  cell wall, **B2**.865–6
  classification, **B2**.866
  culture, **B2**.865
  genus definition, **B2**.863
  habitats, **B1**.657, **B2**.863–4
    meat and meat products, **B1**.273
  historical perspective, **B2**.863
  immune evasion
    antibody degradation/modification, **I**.662
    regulatory T cells, **I**.666
  infection, endocarditis, **B1**.532–3
  metabolism, **B2**.865
    nutritional requirements, **B2**.865
  morphology, **B2**.864–5
  in normal microbiota, **B1**.296 (Tab.), **B1**.301,
    B1.303, **B2**.867
    oral cavity, **B1**.609
  pathogenicity, **B2**.866–7
  physical/chemical agents susceptibility/
    resistance, **B2**.866
    pasteurization, **B1**.232–3
  species, **B2**.864 (Fig.)
  see also individual species
Lactobacillus acidophilus, **B2**.863
  freeze-dried food, **B1**.269
  habitats, **B1**.657, **B2**.863–4
  S layer, **B1**.155
Lactobacillus brevis
  catabolite repression, **B1**.50
  cell wall, **B2**.865–6
  habitats, **B2**.863–4
Lactobacillus buchneri
  cell wall, **B2**.865–6
  histamine poisoning, **B1**.252
Lactobacillus bulgaricus
  morphology, **B2**.864–5
  as yogurt starter, **B1**.249
Lactobacillus casei, **B2**.863
  antigens, **B2**.866, **B2**.866 (Tab.)
  cell wall, **B2**.865–6
  dendritic cell infection, **I**.656

habitats, **B2**.863–4
  immune evasion, **I**.656
  morphology, **B2**.864–5
Lactobacillus cellobiosus
  cell wall, **B2**.865–6
  habitats, **B2**.863–4
Lactobacillus coleohominis, **B2**.863–4
Lactobacillus crispatus, **B1**.657, **B2**.863–4
Lactobacillus delbrueckii, **B2**.863
Lactobacillus fermentum
  antigens, **B2**.866 (Tab.)
  cell wall, **B2**.865–6
  habitats, **B1**.657, **B2**.863–4
Lactobacillus gasseri, **B2**.863–4
Lactobacillus helveticus, **B2**.866 (Tab.)
Lactobacillus hordniae, **B2**.864–5
Lactobacillus jensenii, **B1**.657, **B2**.863–4
Lactobacillus lactis
  antigens, **B2**.866 (Tab.)
  catabolite repression, **B1**.50
  morphology, **B2**.864–5
Lactobacillus leichmannii, **B2**.864–5
Lactobacillus mucosae, **B2**.863–4
Lactobacillus odontolyticus, **B2**.863
Lactobacillus paracasei, **B2**.863–4
Lactobacillus paracasei, immune evasion,
    I.666–7
Lactobacillus plantarum, **B2**.863
  antigens, **B2**.866 (Tab.)
  cell wall, **B2**.865–6
  morphology, **B2**.864–5
Lactobacillus reuteri, **B2**.863–4
Lactobacillus reuteri, immune evasion
  dendritic cell suppression, **I**.656
  TNF-α suppression, **I**.652
Lactobacillus rhamnosus, **B2**.863–4
Lactobacillus ruminis, **B2**.863–4
Lactobacillus salivarius, **B2**.863–4
Lactobacillus vaginalis, **B2**.863–4
Lactobacillus viridescens
  canned cured meats, **B1**.275
  cell wall, **B2**.865–6
Lactobacillus xylosus, **B2**.864–5
Lactococcus, **B2**.833–5
  antigens, **B2**.842
  classification, **B2**.889
  as normal microbiota, **B1**.296 (Tab.)
  phenotypic characteristics, **B2**.888 (Tab.),
    B2.889
Lactococcus lactis
  cheesemaking, **B1**.252
  nisin production, **B2**.1046–7
Lactoferrin, **B1**.430, **I**.521
  in airway secretion, **B1**.623
  innate immune response, **B1**.176
  meningococcal requirement, **B1**.563
  receptors, *Neisseria gonorrhoeae*, **B2**.1285
Lactoperoxidase (LP), **B1**.430
  food, **B1**.268 (Tab.)
  host resistance to bacterial infection, **B1**.176
Lactose fermentation
  Enterobacteriaceae, **B2**.1335
  Enterobacteriaceae identification,
    B2.1319 (Tab.)
  Klebsiella, **B1**.115

Lactose fermentation (*Continued*)
  plasmids, **B1**.115
  Porphyromonas identification, **B2**.1924 (Tab.)
  Prevotella identification, **B2**.1924 (Tab.)
  Yersinia enterocolitica, **B1**.115
Lactose operon
  Escherichia coli, **B1**.70–1, **B1**.71 (Fig.)
  repressor, **B1**.70–1
  Staphylococcus aureus, **B1**.71
Lactose permease, **B1**.70–1
LacY, *E. coli*. lactose transporter, **B1**.49
Lady Windermere's syndrome, **B2**.1207–8
Lagenidium, **M**.414–16, **M**.420
Lagging-strand DNA replication
  DNA virus replication, **V1**.149–50,
    V1.150 (Fig.)
  HSV-1 replication, **V1**.166–7
  SV40 replication, **V1**.153–4
Lagochilascaris, **P**.590
Lagos bat virus, **V2**.1103–4
Lagovirus, **V2**.912
  phylogenetic analysis, **V2**.917 (Fig.)
Laguna Negra virus, **V2**.1666 (Tab.)
Lake Victoria marburgvirus, **V1**.381
Lake waters, **B1**.214, **B1**.221
Lamb(s)
  Bordetella parapertussis, **B2**.1810
  Escherichia coli, O157:H7 reservoirs,
    B1.274
  λ5 gene mutations, **I**.780
  pre-BCR, **I**.340–1
Lambda light chains, **I**.309, **I**.323
  see also Somatic recombination, Igs
Lambda phage, renaming, **V1**.40
Lambl V., **P**.14–5
LamB porin, **B1**.43
λ1 protein *see* Reoviruses
λ2 protein *see* Reoviruses
λ3 protein *see* Reoviruses
Lamina propria, microsporidiosis, **P**.538
Lamina proproa lymphocytes, HIV infection,
  I.799
Laminar air flow (LAF) units, **B1**.453
  aspergillosis prevention, **M**.730
Lamivudine, **V2**.1620
  hepatitis B therapy, **V2**.1260–1, **V2**.1629
    resistance, **V2**.1261
  hepatitis D therapy, **V2**.1273
  HIV infection, **V2**.1334
    resistance, **V2**.1337 (Fig.)
  HTLV-associated myelopathy(HAM)/
    tropical spastic paraparesis (TSP),
    V2.1290
  resistance, **V2**.1637
  structure, **V2**.1620 (Fig.)
Lancefield, R, **B1**.12
Landfills, airborne bacteria, **B1**.186 (Tab.)
Landsteiner, Karl, **B1**.12, **I**.748
Land use patterns, emergence/resurgence of
  infection, **B1**.362
Langat virus, **V2**.998 (Tab.)
Langerhans' cells, **I**.393–4, **I**.820
  antigen presentation, **I**.821
  common mucosal immune system, **I**.534–5
  cutaneous leishmaniasis, **P**.300

cytokine production, **I**.821
development, **I**.22
DNA vaccines, **I**.912–13, **I**.916
  bare skin routes, **I**.825
hematopoiesis, **I**.113, **I**.113 (Fig.)
immune surveillance, **I**.820–1
MHC expression, **I**.821
nasal-associated lymphoid tissue, **I**.533
Langerhans, Paul, **I**.8
Langeron, M, **M**.10, **M**.32–3
Lantibiotics, **B1**.136–7, **B1**.137–8
Laos, schistosomiasis control programs,
  P.636–7
La-Piedad Michoacean-Mexico virus,
  V1.818–19
Lapudrine–dapsone (Lapdap®), **P**.506
LARC *see* CCL20
Large intestine, normal microbiota, **B1**.302–3
Large (L) protein
  Avian pneumovirus, **V1**.788
  bunyaviruses *see* Bunyaviruses
  filoviruses, **V2**.1086–8, **V2**.1091
  Hendra virus, **V1**.816
  henipaviruses, **V1**.816
  Human respiratory syncytial virus *see* Human
    respiratory syncytial virus (HRSV)
  Marburg virus, **V2**.1091
  Measles virus, **V1**.713–15, **V1**.716 (Fig.),
    V1.717
  Mumps virus, **V1**.745, **V1**.746 (Tab.)
  Nipah virus, **V1**.816
  respiroviruses *see* Respiroviruses
  rhabdoviruses *see* Rhabdoviruses
  Zaire ebolavirus, **V2**.1091
  see also RNA-dependent RNA polymerase
Large T antigen, SV40 *see* Simian virus 40
  (SV40)
Larva currens, *Strongyloides*, **P**.740
Larvae, *Toxocara*, **P**.751 (Fig.)
Larval cestodes, **P**.677–712
  general biology, **P**.681–3
    aerobic/anaeorbic pathways, **P**.681
    calcareous corpuscles, **P**.681–2
    excretory systems, **P**.681–2
    glucose transporters, **P**.681–2
    glycoproteins, **P**.682–3
    nutrition, **P**.681–2
  infection *see* Cysticercosis; Echinococcosis
  life cycle, **P**.684–5
  location in host, **P**.685–6
  morphology/structure, **P**.678–81
  see also Cestodes (intestinal tapeworms);
    individual species
Larva migrans, **P**.587–8
Laryngeal cancer, HPV associations,
  V1.463 (Tab.)
Laryngeal papillomas, HPV associations,
  V1.449 (Fig.), **V1**.463 (Tab.)
Laryngitis, causative organisms, **B1**.629
Laryngotracheal infection, **B1**.629
Laryngotracheobronchitis *see* Croup
  (laryngotracheobronchitis)
Larynx, normal microbiota, **B1**.302
Lasiodiplodia theobromae, **B1**.286–7

Lasiodiplopodia theobromae infection,
  M.278 (Tab.), **M**.284, **M**.285 (Fig.)
  endophthalmitis, **M**.323
  keratitis, **M**.301–2, **M**.309, **M**.313, **M**.316
  scleritis, **M**.316
Lassa fever, **V2**.1070
  antiviral treatment, **V2**.1078
  clinical features, **V2**.1070
  immune response, **V2**.1073
  pathogenesis, **V2**.1072
  in pregnancy, **V2**.1070
  transmission, **V1**.371 (Tab.)
Lassa virus, **V2**.1060
  animal infection
    clinical features, **V2**.1070
    histopathology, **V2**.1071
    pathogenesis, **V2**.1071
  arenavirus cross-reactivity, **V2**.1069
  biosafety level 4 classification, **V2**.1526
  chronic infection, **V2**.1071
  cytokine suppression, **V2**.1072
  detection, **V2**.1069
  emerging infection, **V2**.1648 (Tab.)
  geographical distribution/carrier and disease,
    V2.1060 (Tab.)
  immune evasion, **V2**.1072
  immunotherapy, **V2**.1077
  inflammation suppression, **V2**.1072
  isolation from tissue specimens,
    V2.1076 (Tab.)
  laboratory-acquired infection, **V2**.1517 (Tab.)
  transmission, **V2**.1070, **V2**.1071
  vaccine, **V2**.1076–7
    recombinant, **V2**.1076–7
Last memory differentiation model, **I**.495,
  I.496 (Fig.)
Latamoxef
  development, **B1**.480
  structure, **B1**.479 (Fig.)
Latency-associated transcripts (LATs),
  V2.1408
  HSV, **V1**.509, **V1**.509 (Fig.), **V2**.1408,
    V2.1418–19, **V2**.1420 (Fig.)
  HSV-1, **V1**.495
Latent nuclear antigen (LANA-1) *see* Human
    herpesvirus 8 (HHV-8: Kaposi's
    sarcoma-associated herpesvirus
    (KSHV))
Latent period of infection, **P**.61 (Tab.), **B1**.338,
  B1.338 (Fig.)
Latent viral infection, **V1**.259, **V1**.259 (Fig.),
  V1.260–1, **V1**.345, **V2**.1408
  antiviral chemotherapy, **V2**.1638–9
  cell types, **V1**.260
  HCMV infection, **V1**.520–1
  initial immune response, **V1**.261
  neurons, **V1**.260–1
  non-dividing cells, **V1**.260–1
  nonproductive infection, **V1**.204, **V1**.206
  reactivation, **V1**.261
  see also specific viruses
Late-onset epilepsy, neurocysticercosis,
  P.686–7
Late transcription factors, poxviruses,
  V1.599 (Tab.)

Latex agglutination test (LAT), **V2**.1545

American visceral leishmaniasis, **P**.335–6

Angiostrongylus costaricensis diagnosis, **P**.810

Burkholderia pseudomallei, **B2**.1619

cystic echinococcosis diagnosis, **P**.694–6

malaria diagnosis, **P**.503

melioidosis, **B2**.1630

rubella, **V2**.978

syphilis detection, **B2**.1849

VZV infection, in pregnancy, **V2**.1456–7

Latino virus

chronic infection, **V2**.1071

geographical distribution/carrier and disease, **V2**.1060 (Tab.)

Laurolinium acetate, **B1**.428

Laveran C., **P**.17

LBP, microbial recognition, **I**.24 (Tab.)

LC16m8 strain, Vaccinia virus, **V1**.591

Lck, TCR signaling, **I**.395

LD78β (CCL3L1), **I**.218 (Tab.)

LDL receptor-related protein, α2-macroglobulin, **I**.202

'Leader-primed transcription' model, *Nidovirales* order, **V1**.399–401

Leading-strand DNA replication

DNA viruses, **V1**.149–50, **V1**.150 (Fig.)

HSV-1, **V1**.166–7

SV40, **V1**.153–4

Lead, resistance to, **B1**.114

Leafhopper spiroplasma, **B2**.1985–6

Leafspots, plant disease source, **B1**.202

'Leaky phenotype,' **I**.774

Leber's disease, gene therapy, **V2**.1600

Lechiguanas virus, **V2**.1666 (Tab.)

Lecithinases

Burkholderia thailandensis, **B2**.1624

Clostridium perfringens, **B2**.1099, **B2**.1113–14

functions, **B1**.153 (Tab.)

Lecithodendriidae, **P**.585

Leclercia, **B2**.1495

antibacterial susceptibility/resistance, **B2**.1495

biochemical tests, **B2**.1495

classification, **B2**.1495

culture, **B2**.1495

definition, **B2**.1495

habitats, **B2**.1495

pathogenicity, **B2**.1495

Leclercia adecarboxylata

biochemical tests, **B2**.1319 (Tab.)

pigment production, **B2**.1345

Lectins

food, **B1**.267

Helicobacter typing, **B2**.1570

Lecythophora hoffmannii infection, **M**.283–4

Lecythophora mutabilis infection, **M**.278 (Tab.), **M**.283–4

Lederberg, J, **B1**.13

'Leeches,' **M**.412

van Leeuwenhoek, A, **M**.6, **M**.20

Legionella, **B2**.1761–85

as airborne bacteria, **B1**.188–9

concentrations in facilities, **B1**.186 (Tab.)

antibacterial susceptibility/resistance, **B2**.1776–7

antibiotics, **B2**.1776–7

antigens, **B2**.1770–1

somatic O antigens, **B2**.1770–1

cell wall composition, **B2**.1770

chemical/physical agent susceptibility/resistance, **B2**.1777

classification, **B2**.1771, **B2**.1772 (Fig.)

species, **B2**.1762 (Tab.), **B2**.1774–5, **B2**.1775 (Fig.)

taxonomy, **B2**.1771, **B2**.1772 (Fig.)

culture, **B2**.1768, **B2**.1771–3

colonies, **B2**.1768, **B2**.1768 (Fig.), **B2**.1769 (Fig.)

growth requirements, **B2**.1768, **B2**.1769

definition, **B2**.1761

flagella, **B2**.1771

genetics, **B2**.1769–70

DNA homology, **B2**.1769–70

plasmids, **B2**.1770

habitats, **B2**.1766–7

immune evasion, **I**.651

infection *see* Legionellosis

isolation/identification, **B2**.1771–6

antibody detection, **B1**.752

culture, **B2**.1771–3

EIAs, **B1**.752, **B1**.758, **B2**.1773

epidemiological typing, **B2**.1775–6

immunofluorescent antibody tests, **B1**.752

immunoserology, **B1**.758, **B2**.1548, **B2**.1774

molecular methods, **B2**.1773–4

ribotyping, **B2**.1775

species identification, **B2**.1774–5

stains/staining, **B2**.1773

urinary antigen, **B2**.1773

LPS, **B2**.1770–1

metabolism, **B2**.1769

morphology, **B2**.1767–8

pathogenicity, **B2**.1777–9

PHB granules, **B2**.1767, **B2**.1767 (Fig.)

physical/chemical agent susceptibility/resistance, **B2**.1777

viable but nonculturable state, **B2**.1769

virulence factors, **B2**.1777–9

waterborne, **B1**.211, **B1**.220

analysis, **B1**.221

Legionella adelaidensis, **B2**.1762 (Tab.)

Legionella anisa, **B2**.1762 (Tab.)

identification, **B2**.1775 (Fig.)

infection, **B2**.1765

Legionella beliardensis, **B2**.1762 (Tab.)

Legionella birminghamensis, **B2**.1762 (Tab.)

Legionella bozemanii, **B2**.1762 (Tab.)

classification, **B2**.1771

Legionella brunensis, **B2**.1762 (Tab.)

Legionella busanensis, **B2**.1762 (Tab.)

Legionella cherrii, **B2**.1762 (Tab.)

Legionella cincinnatiensis, **B2**.1762 (Tab.)

Legionella drozanskii, **B2**.1762 (Tab.)

Legionella dumoffii, **B2**.1762 (Tab.)

classification, **B2**.1771

epidemiological typing, **B2**.1775–6

Legionella erythra, **B2**.1762 (Tab.)

identification, **B2**.1774–5, **B2**.1775 (Fig.)

somatic 'O' antigens, **B2**.1770

Legionella fairfieldensis, **B2**.1762 (Tab.)

Legionella fallonii, **B2**.1762 (Tab.)

Legionella feeleii, **B2**.1762 (Tab.)

infection, **B2**.1765

Legionella geestiana, **B2**.1762 (Tab.)

classification, **B2**.1771

identification, **B2**.1775

Legionella genomospecies 1, **B2**.1762 (Tab.)

Legionella gormanii, **B2**.1762 (Tab.)

classification, **B2**.1771

Legionella gratiana, **B2**.1762 (Tab.)

Legionella gresilensis, **B2**.1762 (Tab.)

genetics, **B2**.1769–70

Legionella hackeliae, **B2**.1762 (Tab.)

Legionella israelensis, **B2**.1762 (Tab.)

Legionella jamestownensis, **B2**.1762 (Tab.)

Legionella jordanis, **B2**.1762 (Tab.)

Legionella lansingensis, **B2**.1762 (Tab.)

Legionella londiniensis, **B2**.1762 (Tab.)

Legionella longbeachae, **B2**.1762 (Tab.)

pathogenicity, **B2**.1766

Legionella lytica, **B2**.1762 (Tab.)

Legionella maceachernii, **B2**.1762 (Tab.)

classification, **B2**.1771

Legionella micdadei, **B1**.635, **B2**.1762 (Tab.)

classification, **B2**.1771

culture, **B2**.1768

infection, **B2**.1765

Legionella moravica, **B2**.1762 (Tab.)

Legionella nautarum, **B2**.1762 (Tab.)

Legionella oakridgensis, **B2**.1762 (Tab.)

identification, **B2**.1774

metabolism, **B2**.1769

Legionella parisiensis, **B2**.1762 (Tab.)

Legionella pneumophila, **B2**.1762 (Tab.)

as airborne bacteria, **B1**.188

concentrations in facilities, **B1**.186 (Tab.)

dispersal, **B1**.188

sampling, **B1**.190–1

antibacterial susceptibility/resistance, **B1**.433

antigens, **B2**.1770–1

somatic 'O' antigens, **B2**.1770

type IV pili, **B2**.1779

cell wall composition, **B2**.1770–1

classification, **B2**.1771, **B2**.2027, **B2**.2027 (Fig.)

taxonomy, **B2**.1771

culture, **B1**.635

colonies, **B2**.1768, **B2**.1768 (Fig.)

discovery, **B1**.634

genetics, **B2**.1769–70

DOT/ICM gene, **B2**.1779

MIP gene, **B2**.1778–9

growth phase, **B2**.1778

habitats and sources, **B2**.1767

identification, **B2**.1771–6, **B2**.1775 (Fig.)

antibody level estimation, **B2**.1774

epidemiological typing, **B2**.1775–6

molecular methods, **B2**.1773–4

organism or components demonstration, **B2**.1773

serogroup I antigenuria test, **B1**.635

urinary antigen EIAs, **B2**.1773

Legionella pneumophila, (*Continued*)
  immune evasion
    lysosomal killing resistance, **I.**651
    nonlysosomal organelles, **I.**650
  infection *see* Legionellosis; Legionnaires'
    disease
  metabolism, **B2.**1769
  morphology, **B2.**1767–8, **B2.**1767 (Fig.),
    B2.1768 (Fig.)
  pathogenicity, **B2.**1766, **B2.**1777–9
  physical/chemical agent susceptibility/
    resistance, **B2.**1777
  virulence factors, **B1.**627–8, **B2.**1777–9
    genetic determinants, **B2.**1778–9
Legionella quarteirensis, **B2.**1762 (Tab.)
Legionella quinlivanii, **B2.**1762 (Tab.)
Legionella rowbothamii, **B2.**1762 (Tab.)
Legionella rubrilucens, **B2.**1762 (Tab.)
  identification, **B2.**1774–5
  somatic 'O' antigens, **B2.**1770
Legionella sainthelensi, **B2.**1762 (Tab.)
  somatic 'O' antigens, **B2.**1770
Legionella santicrusis, **B2.**1762 (Tab.)
  somatic 'O' antigens, **B2.**1770
Legionella shakespeari, **B2.**1762 (Tab.)
Legionella spiritensis, **B2.**1762 (Tab.)
Legionella steigerwaltii, **B2.**1762 (Tab.)
Legionella taurinensis, **B2.**1762 (Tab.)
  identification, **B2.**1774–5
Legionella tusconensis, **B2.**1762 (Tab.)
Legionella wadsworthii, **B2.**1762 (Tab.)
Legionella waltersii, **B2.**1762 (Tab.)
Legionella worsleiensis, **B2.**1762 (Tab.)
Legionellosis
  animal models, **I.**593–4
  causative agents, **B2.**1766
  entry into cells, complement, **I.**649
  epidemiology, **B2.**1764
  intracellular replication, **B2.**1778
  macrophages, **I.**30
  neutrophils, **I.**44
  NK cell actions, **I.**99
  nosocomial, **B1.**390, **B2.**1766
  serological diagnosis, **B1.**635
  vaccines, **I.**933 (Tab.)
Legionnaires' disease, **B1.**634–6
  antibacterial susceptibility/resistance,
    B1.635–6
  clinical features, **B1.**634, **B2.**1764–5
  control of source, **B1.**329
  diagnosis, **B1.**635, **B2.**1771–6
  epidemiology, **B2.**1765–6
    emerging bacterial infection, **B1.**362
    outbreaks, **B1.**635
  history, **B2.**1761–4
  mode of spread, **B1.**188–9, **B1.**375–6
  nosocomially-acquired, **B1.**375–6, **B1.**640-1,
    B2.1766
    factors associated, **B1.**375
  pathogenesis/transmission, **B1.**634–5
  prevention, **B1.**636
  treatment, **B1.**635–6
  see also Legionella pneumophila
Legislation
  microbiological risk assessment, **V2.**1519

milk products, **B1.**233–4, **B1.**236
Legs, chromoblastomycosis, **M.**361–2
Legumes
  microbiology, **B1.**286, **B1.**287
  Rhizobium relationship, **B1.**197
Leifsonia, **B2.**992–4
  chemotaxonomic characteristics,
    B2.978 (Tab.)
  habitats, **B2.**978
Leifsonia acquatica, **B2.**992–4
  biochemical characteristics, **B2.**993 (Tab.)
Leiper R.T., **P.**10–1
Leishman-Donovan bodies, **P.**313
Leishmania, **P.**188, **I.**678–9, **P.283–312**
  AIDS, **P.**97
  amastigotes, **P.**285–6
    development, **P.**292–4, **P.**293 (Fig.)
    flagellar pocket, **P.**287
    glycosome, **P.**287–8
    identification, **P.**301
    kinetoplast, **P.**287–8, **P.**296
    as obligate intracellular parasites, **P.**294
    structure, **P.**286–8
    ultrastructure, **P.**288 (Fig.)
  classification, **P.**190–2, **P.**197, **P.**283–5, **P.**313,
    P.318, **I.**675–6
    anomalies/changes, **P.**191
    DNA technology, **P.**193
    species, **P.**318, **P.**318–34
    subgenera, **P.**318–34
    techniques used in, **P.**284–5
  culture, **P.**301
  detection, **P.**301
  DNA, **P.**287, **P.**296
    analysis, **P.**284–5
    maxicircles, **P.**296
  ectoenzymes and ATPase, **P.**295–6
  genetics, **P.**296
  historical aspects, **P.**13, **P.**16
  hosts, **P.**283–4
  hybrids, **P.**332–5
  immune evasion
    antigenic complexity, **I.**680
    intracellular refuges, **I.**678–9, **I.**681
    variant surface glycoproteins, **I.**680
  immunogenetics, **I.**589
  infection *see* Leishmaniasis
  isoenzyme analysis, **P.**284
  kinetoplast DNA, **P.**287, **P.**296
  life cycle, **P.**285–94, **P.**287 (Fig.), **I.**678
    in macrophage, **P.**77, **P.**283–4
    mammalian host, **P.**292–4
    promastigote development, **P.**289–92,
      P.290 (Fig.)
    sandflies, **P.**288–92
  New World (neotropical), **P.**334–5
    distribution/diseases caused by,
      P.319 (Tab.)
    genetic exchange, **P.**334
    genetics, **P.**334–5
    species, **P.**318
    see also Leishmaniasis, New World
  Old World, **P.283–312**
    genetics, **P.**296
    life cycle, **P.**285–94

  molecular biology, **P.**296
  species included, **P.**283
  surface membrane biochemistry, **P.**295–6
  surface membrane structure, **P.**291,
    P.294–5
  transmission, **P.**283–4, **P.**288–9, **P.**294
  see also Leishmaniasis, Old World
  paramastigotes, **P.**289
  pellicle, **P.**162, **P.**163 (Tab.)
  promastigotes, **P.**285–6
    development, **P.**289–92, **P.**290 (Fig.),
      P.291 (Fig.)
    ectoenzymes, **P.**295–6
    flagellum, **P.**288, **P.**288 (Fig.)
    forms/types, **P.**289
    haptomonad form, **P.**289, **P.**291–2,
      P.291 (Fig.)
    lipophosphoglycan, **P.**291–2, **P.**294–5
    metacyclic, **P.**288–9, **P.**291–2, **P.**291 (Fig.)
    nectomonads, **P.**289, **P.**291, **P.**291 (Fig.)
    procyclic form, **P.**289, **P.**291 (Fig.)
    structure, **P.**288
    ultrastructure, **P.**288, **P.**288 (Fig.)
  surface membrane, **P.**291, **P.**294–5
    biochemistry, **P.**295–6
    gp63, **P.**294–5
    lipophosphoglycan, **P.**291–2, **P.**294–5
  Viannia (subgenus), **P.**318
    species, **P.**326–32
  viral infection and virus-like particles in,
    P.335
  virulence factors, **I.**678
  zymodemes, **P.**284
    cladogram, **P.**286 (Fig.)
  see also Leishmaniasis; *individual species*
Leishmania aethiopica, **P.**283
  cladogram, **P.**286 (Fig.)
  geographical distribution/hosts, **P.**286 (Tab.),
    P.304
  infection, **P.**286 (Tab.)
    cutaneous, **P.**297
    diffuse cutaneous leishmaniasis, **P.**298
    epidemiology, **P.**304
    see also Leishmaniasis, Old World
  transmission, prevention, **P.**308
  vectors, **P.**304
Leishmania amazonensis, **P.**324
  amastigotes, **P.**325 (Fig.)
  disease caused by, **P.**316 (Fig.), **P.**324,
    P.336 (Fig.), **P.**337 (Fig.)
    see also Leishmaniasis, New World
  distribution, **P.**324
  mammalian hosts, **P.**324
  sandfly hosts, **P.**324
Leishmania arabica, **P.**286 (Fig.)
Leishmania aristidesi, **P.**324–5
  disease caused by, **P.**325
    see also Leishmaniasis, New World
  distribution, **P.**324
  mammalian hosts, **P.**324
  sandfly hosts, **P.**324–5
Leishmania braziliensis, **P.**318, **P.**326, **P.**326–7,
    P.327
  classification
    DNA technology, **P.**193
    isoenzyme analysis, **P.**326

Leishmania braziliensis, (Continued)
  disease caused by, **P**.327
    see also Leishmaniasis, New World
  distribution, **P**.326
  mammalian hosts, **P**.326, **P**.326–7
  metastatic lesions, **P**.314, **P**.315 (Fig.)
  sandfly hosts, **P**.327
Leishmania braziliensis/L. guyanensis hybrid,
  P.333
Leishmania braziliensis/L. panamensis hybrid,
  P.332
Leishmania braziliensis/L. peruviana hybrid,
  P.333
Leishmania chagasi, **P**.188, **P**.305
  disease caused by, **P**.336 (Fig.)
    see also Leishmaniasis, New World
  Leishmania infantum relationship, **P**.285
    see also Leishmaniasis, Old World
Leishmania colombiensis, **P**.331
  disease caused by, **P**.331
    see also Leishmaniasis, New World
  distribution/hosts, **P**.331
Leishmania deanei, **P**.333–4
  disease caused by, **P**.334
    see also Leishmaniasis, New World
  distribution/hosts, **P**.333–4
Leishmania donovani, **P**.283, **P**.318
  cladogram, **P**.286 (Fig.)
  classification, **P**.191
  geographical distribution, **P**.286 (Tab.),
    P.305
  hosts, **P**.286 (Tab.)
  immune response, **P**.77–8
  infection, **P**.286 (Tab.)
    biopsies, **P**.153
    blood culture, **P**.152–3
    C-reactive protein, **I**.199–200
    cutaneous, **P**.297
    epidemics, **P**.305
    epidemiology, **P**.304–5
    insusceptibility, **P**.305
    post kala-azar leishmaniasis, **P**.298
    visceral leishmaniasis (kala-azar), **P**.298
    see also Leishmaniasis, Old World
  integrated control, **P**.308
  structure
    amastigote, **P**.165 (Fig.)
    pellicle, **P**.165 (Fig.)
  transmission, prevention, **P**.308
  vectors, **P**.305
    see also Leishmaniasis, New World
Leishmania enriettii, **P**.322–3
  disease caused by, **P**.323
    see also Leishmaniasis, New World
  distribution, **P**.322
  mammalian hosts, **P**.322
  sandfly hosts, **P**.322
Leishmania equatorensis, **P**.331–2
    see also Leishmaniasis, New World
Leishmania forattinii, **P**.325–6
  disease caused by, **P**.326
    see also Leishmaniasis, New World
  distribution/hosts, **P**.325–6

Leishmania garnhami, **P**.325
  disease caused by, **P**.325
    see also Leishmaniasis, New World
  distribution/hosts, **P**.325
Leishmania gerbilli, **P**.286 (Fig.)
Leishmania guyanensis, **P**.328–9
  disease caused by, **P**.317 (Fig.), **P**.329,
    P.337 (Fig.)
    metastatic lesions, **P**.329
    see also Leishmaniasis, New World
  distribution, **P**.328
  Leishmania panamensis vs., **P**.329
  mammalian hosts, **P**.328
  sandfly hosts, **P**.328–9
Leishmania guyanensis complex, **P**.329
    see also Leishmaniasis, New World
Leishmania herreri, **P**.334
    see also Leishmaniasis, New World
Leishmania hertigi, **P**.333
  absence of infection in humans, **P**.333
  distribution/hosts, **P**.333
Leishmania infantum, **P**.188, **P**.283, **P**.285
  cladogram, **P**.286 (Fig.)
  geographical distribution, **P**.286 (Tab.),
    P.305
  infection, **P**.286 (Tab.)
    cutaneous, **P**.297
    epidemiology, **P**.305–6
    HIV coinfection, **P**.298–9
    subclinical, **P**.297
    visceral leishmaniasis (kala-azar), **P**.298
    see also Leishmaniasis, Old World
  Leishmania chagasi relationship, **P**.285
  Old/New World distribution, **P**.305
  reservoir hosts, **P**.118, **P**.286 (Tab.), **P**.305–6
  vectors, **P**.305–6
  zymodemes, **P**.284, **P**.286 (Fig.)
Leishmania infantum chagasi, **P**.318–22
  disease caused by, **P**.322
    kala-azar, **P**.322
    see also Leishmaniasis, New World
  distribution, **P**.318–20
  mammalian hosts, **P**.118, **P**.320–1
  sandfly hosts, **P**.321–2
Leishmania killicki, **P**.304
  cladogram, **P**.286 (Fig.)
    see also Leishmaniasis, Old World
Leishmania lainsoni, **P**.329–30
  disease caused by, **P**.330
    see also Leishmaniasis, New World
  distribution/hosts, **P**.329–30
Leishmania lindenbergi, **P**.332
  disease caused by, **P**.332
    see also Leishmaniasis, New World
  distribution/hosts, **P**.332
Leishmania major, **P**.283
  cladogram, **P**.286 (Fig.)
  geographical distribution, **P**.286 (Tab.),
    P.302
  identification, **P**.301
  immune evasion, **P**.77–8
  immune response, **P**.77–8, **P**.299–300
    mouse model, **P**.77–8
  infection, **P**.286 (Tab.)
    cutaneous, **P**.297

  epidemiology, **P**.302–4
    outbreaks, **P**.303
    transmission, **P**.303
    see also Leishmaniasis, Old World
  life cycle, in sandflies, **P**.292
  reservoir hosts, **P**.118, **P**.286 (Tab.), **P**.303
  vectors, **P**.286 (Tab.), **P**.303
Leishmania mexicana, **P**.323
  classification, DNA technology, **P**.193
  disease caused by, **P**.323
    see also Leishmaniasis, New World
  distribution, **P**.323
  mammalian hosts, **P**.323
  sandfly hosts, **P**.323
Leishmania naiffi, **P**.330–1
  disease caused by, **P**.331
    see also Leishmaniasis, New World
  distribution/hosts, **P**.330–1
Leishmania panamensis, **P**.329
  disease caused by, **P**.329
    see also Leishmaniasis, New World
  distribution/hosts, **P**.329
  isoenzyme characterization, **P**.329
  Leishmania guyanensis vs., **P**.329
Leishmania peruviana, **P**.328
  disease caused by, **P**.328
    see also Leishmaniasis, New World
  distribution/hosts, **P**.328
Leishmania pifanoi, **P**.323–4
  disease caused by, **P**.323–4
    see also Leishmaniasis, New World
  distribution, **P**.323
  mammalian hosts, **P**.323
  sandfly hosts, **P**.323
Leishmania shawi, **P**.330
  disease caused by, **P**.330, **P**.331 (Fig.)
    see also Leishmaniasis, New World
  distribution/hosts, **P**.330
Leishmaniasis, **P**.188
  cell infection
    CD4 T cells, **I**.390
    macrophages, **I**.30
  control
    animal reservoir hosts, **P**.118–19
    chemotherapy/chemoprophylaxis,
      P.144 (Tab.)
    diagnosis, **P**.143 (Tab.)
    stratification of disease, **P**.115, **P**.134 (Tab.)
    vector/reservoir control, **P**.145 (Tab.)
  cutaneous, **P**.33, **P**.188
    control, **P**.33, **P**.107 (Tab.)
    skin biopsies, **P**.153
  epidemics, **P**.142 (Tab.)
    urbanization, **P**.117
  epidemiology, **P**.33, **P**.46 (Tab.)
  experimental infection
    cytokines, **P**.74, **P**.77–8
    T cell subsets, **P**.74, **P**.77–8
    immune response, **P**.77–8, **I**.596
      IFN-γ, **I**.679
      IL-4, **I**.280, **I**.679
      IL-10, **I**.679
    immune response, **P**.77–8, **I**.679
    inducible nitric oxide synthase, **I**.596
    killing mechanisms, **P**.77–8

Leishmaniasis
  immune response (*Continued*)
    NK cell actions, **I**.100
    T helper cell subsets, **P**.72–3, **P**.77–8
    TNF-α, **I**.596
    transforming growth factor-β, **I**.679
  immunogenetics, **I**.596–7
    animal models, **I**.596
    HLA-A26, **I**.597
    HLA associations, **I**.597
    human studies, **I**.596–7
    LTA gene, **I**.596
    Nramp1 gene, **I**.596
    Scl-1 gene, **I**.596
    SLC11A1 (NRAMP1) gene, **I**.597
    SLC11A1 gene polymorphisms, **I**.579
    TNF gene, **I**.596, **I**.597
  'lupoid', **P**.298
  mortality, **P**.28 (Tab.), **P**.29 (Tab.)
  pathogenesis, **I**.596, **I**.678–9
  public health importance, **P**.33, **P**.105 (Tab.)
  transmission, **I**.596
  vaccine development/vaccination, **P**.78,
    P.307
    BCG vector, **I**.845
    CpG adjuvant, **I**.931
    development status, **I**.933 (Tab.)
  visceral, **P**.188
    conflict-related effects, **P**.107 (Tab.)
    diagnosis, **P**.129–30
  see also Leishmaniasis, New World;
    Leishmaniasis, Old World
Leishmaniasis, New World, **P**.188, **P.313–49**
  AIDS, **P**.339, **P**.341
  American visceral (AVL), **P**.315
    clinical features, **P**.335–6, **P**.336 (Fig.)
    diagnosis, **P**.335–6
    differential diagnosis, **P**.335
    genetic susceptibility, **P**.334–5
    prevention/control, **P**.339–40
    species causing, **P**.324
    treatment, **P**.341
  anergic diffuse cutaneous (ADCL), **P**.314–
    15, **P**.316 (Fig.), **P**.324 (Fig.)
    clinical features, **P**.338–9
    differential diagnosis, **P**.338
    immunochemotherapy, **P**.342
    response to drugs, **P**.342
    severity, **P**.338
    signs indicating treatment need, **P**.342
    species causing, **P**.323–4, **P**.338
    treatment, **P**.342
  clinical features, **P**.335–9
  cutaneous, **P**.313–14, **P**.314 (Fig.)
    borderline disseminated, **P**.338–9
    clinical features, **P**.331 (Fig.), **P**.336–7
    control, **P**.33, **P**.119, **P**.340
    diagnosis, **P**.336–7
    differential diagnosis, **P**.336
    hazards of treatment, **P**.341
    immunotherapy, **P**.342–3
    incidence, **P**.313–14
    localized, **P**.338–9
    prevention, **P**.340
    simple lesions, **P**.336

species causing, **P**.325, **P**.327, **P**.328, **P**.329,
    P.330, **P**.331, **P**.332
  treatment, **P**.33, **P**.341
historical aspects, **P**.16, **P**.313
immune response in, **P**.314–15
immunocompromised, **P**.339
mucocutaneous/mucosal, **P**.314 (Fig.)
  clinical features, **P**.337–8
  complications, **P**.338
  differential diagnosis, **P**.338
  immunotherapy, **P**.342–3
  incidence, **P**.337
  metastases, **P**.337
  nose, **P**.337–8
  pathology, **P**.338
  prevention/control, **P**.340
  species causing, **P**.327
  treatment, **P**.338, **P**.341–2
neotropical cutaneous leishmaniasis (NCL),
    P.313
prevention/control, **P**.339–41
reservoirs
  domestic animals, **P**.316–17
  humans, **P**.317
  peridomestic hosts, **P**.317
  sylvatic hosts, **P**.315–16
transmission, **P**.316–17
treatment, **P**.341–2
  effectiveness/responses, **P**.315, **P**.341
  immunotherapy, **P**.342–3
vaccine development, **P**.342–3
vectors, **P**.313, **P**.315–16, **P**.317–18
  control, **P**.339–40
  ecology, **P**.340
Leishmaniasis, Old World, **P**.188, **P.283–312**
  chemotherapy, **P**.306–7
    allopurinol, **P**.307
    amphotericin B, **P**.307
    aromatic diamidines, **P**.306–7
    liposome preparations, **P**.307
    miltefosine, **P**.307
    monomycin/paromomycin and
      aminosidine, **P**.307
    pentavalent antimonials, **P**.306
  clinical features, **P**.296–8
  cutaneous, **P**.283
    clinical features, **P**.296–8
    diagnosis, **P**.301
    geographical distribution, **P**.284 (Fig.)
    immune response, **P**.299
    location of *Leishmania,* **P**.285
    pathology, **P**.300
    species causing, **P**.297
    treatment, **P**.306
    urban, **P**.304
    vaccination, **P**.307
    'wet' and 'dry' lesions, **P**.297
  diagnosis, **P**.300–2
    clinical, **P**.301
    immunological, **P**.302
    molecular biology, **P**.301–2
    parasitological, **P**.301–2
    travel history, **P**.300–1
  differential diagnosis, **P**.301

diffuse cutaneous (DCL), **P**.298, **P**.314–15
  clinical features, **P**.298
diversity, **P**.296–7, **P**.297 (Fig.)
epidemiology, **P**.302–6
experimental, immune response, **P**.300
historical aspects, **P**.16
HIV coinfection, **P**.298–9, **P**.301
immunology, **P**.299–300
  antibodies, **P**.300
  cell-mediated, **P**.299–300
  cutaneous disease, **P**.299
  host genetic variability, **P**.299
  T helper cell subsets, **P**.300
integrated control, **P**.307–8
mucosal, 'espundia' comparison, **P**.338
pathology, **P**.300
  group I anergic, **P**.300
post kala-azar (PKDL), **P**.298
  clinical features, **P**.298
recidivans, **P**.298, **P**.300
spectrum, **P**.297, **P**.297 (Fig.)
subclinical infection, **P**.297
transmission, **P**.302
vaccination, **P**.307
visceral (kala-azar), **P**.33, **P**.188, **P**.283, **P**.322
  clinical diagnosis, **P**.301
  clinical features, **P**.298
  economic costs, **P**.33
  epidemics, **P**.305
  geographical distribution, **P**.285 (Fig.)
  immune response, **P**.299
  location of *Leishmania,* **P**.285
  pathology, **P**.300
  prevalence, **P**.302
  treatment, **P**.306
  use of term, **P**.322
Leishmaniasis recidivans, **P**.298
  diagnosis, **P**.301
Leishmania tropica, **P**.283
  cladogram, **P**.286 (Fig.)
  classification, **P**.191
  geographical distribution, **P**.286 (Tab.)
  hosts, **P**.286 (Tab.)
  identification, **P**.301
  infection, **P**.286 (Tab.)
    cutaneous, **P**.297, **P**.304
    epidemiology, **P**.304
    visceral, **P**.304
  see also Leishmaniasis, Old World
  transmission, prevention, **P**.308
Leishmania utingensis, **P**.332
  disease caused by, **P**.332
  see also Leishmaniasis, New World
  distribution/hosts, **P**.332
Leishmania venezuelensis, **P**.325
  disease caused by, **P**.325
  see also Leishmaniasis, New World
  distribution/hosts, **P**.325
Leishmaniavirus, **P**.335
Leishmanin test, **P**.302, **P**.336–7
Leishmanioma, **P**.297
Lemierre's disease (necrobacillosis), **B1**.629,
    B2.1951
Lemierre's syndrome, **B1**.618–19

Leminorella, **B2**.1495–6
  antibacterial susceptibility/resistance,
    B2.1496
  biochemical tests, **B2**.1495–6
  classification, **B2**.1495
  culture, **B2**.1495–6
  definition, **B2**.1495
  habitats, **B2**.1496
  as normal microbiota, **B1**.296 (Tab.)
  pathogenicity, **B2**.1496
Leminorella grimontii, **B2**.1495
  biochemical tests, **B2**.1319 (Tab.), **B2**.1495–6
  classification, **B2**.1495
  culture, **B2**.1495–6
  habitats, **B2**.1496
  pathogenicity, **B2**.1496
Leminorella richardii
  biochemical tests, **B2**.1319 (Tab.)
  classification, **B2**.1495
  culture, **B2**.1495–6
Lemonnierin, **B2**.1597
Lenampicillin, **B1**.475
Lenercept, mechanism of action, **I**.357
Lentiviridae
  CNS receptors, **V2**.1406 (Tab.)
  see also specific viruses
Lentivirus
  classification, **V1**.46, **V2**.1286 (Tab.)
  human disease, **V2**.1285
  see also Lentiviruses
Lentiviruses
  characteristics, **V2**.1284
  gene therapy vectors, **V2**.1592–3,
    V2.1595 (Tab.)
  persistent infection, **V1**.260–1, **V1**.260 (Fig.)
  replication, cell specificity, **V2**.1323
  translation, splicing mechanisms, **V1**.114–15
  tumors associated, **V1**.331 (Tab.)
  Vpr protein, conservation, **V2**.1327
  see also Lentivirus
Leopard skin *see* Depigmentation
Lepidoptera (butterflies and moths), **B1**.203–4
Leporipoxvirus, **V1**.588
  classification, **V1**.579 (Tab.), **V1**.582, **V1**.594
  phylogenetics, **V1**.583
  taxonomy, **V1**.595 (Tab.)
Lepromin, **B2**.1185
Lepromin reaction, **B2**.1221
  early and late reactions, **B2**.1221
Leprosy, **B1**.188, **I**.590, **B2**.1182, **B2**.1203–5
  animals, **B2**.1182, **B2**.1204
  borderline, **B2**.1204–5
  causative organism *see Mycobacterium
    leprae*
  clinical features, **B2**.1204
    erythema nodosum leprosum reaction,
      B2.1205
  diagnosis, **B2**.1205
    skin, **B2**.1205, **B2**.1221
  epidemiology, **B2**.1203–4
    case numbers, **B2**.1203
    environmental factors, **B1**.188, **B2**.1203
    genetic factors, **B2**.1203
    geographical distribution, **B2**.1203
    WHO estimates of prevalence, **B2**.1203

family studies, **I**.590
history, **B2**.1203–4
HLA association, **I**.590
  HLA-A11, **I**.590–1
  HLA-DQw1, **I**.590–1
  HLA-DR2, **I**.590–1
  HLA-DR3, **I**.590–1
  HLA-DRB1, **I**.591
  linkage studies, **I**.590
  SLC11A1 (NRAMP1) gene, **I**.591
  TAP2, **I**.591
  VDR codon, **I**.591
immunogenetics, **I**.590–1
  HLA polymorphisms, **I**.590
lepromatous, **B2**.1204, **B2**.1205
prophylaxis, **B2**.1220–1
  chemoprophylaxis, **B2**.1221
reversal reaction, **B2**.1205
Ridley-Jopling classification, **B2**.1204
susceptibility, **I**.590
treatment, **B2**.1219–20
  'cured' patients, **B2**.1203
  dapsone resistance, **B2**.1203, **B2**.1220
  multidrug therapy, **B2**.1203, **B2**.1220
  WHO regimens, **B2**.1220 (Tab.)
tuberculoid, **B2**.1204
twin studies, **I**.590
Leptin, acute phase response, **I**.208–9
Leptonema, **B2**.1865–6
  definitions, **B2**.1865–6
  growth, **B2**.1870
    measurements, **B2**.1870
  morphology, **B2**.1867–8
Leptonema illini, **B2**.1878 (Tab.)
Leptosphaeria, identification, **M**.89 (Tab.),
    M.390
Leptosphaeria senegalensis, **M**.27, **M**.28 (Fig.),
    M.89 (Tab.), **M**.387, **M**.390, **M**.390 (Tab.),
    M.392 (Tab.)
  histopathology, **M**.128 (Tab.)
Leptosphaeria tompkinsii, **M**.27, **M**.89 (Tab.),
    M.390
Leptospira, **B2**.**1865–84**
  antibacterial susceptibility/resistance,
    B2.1881
  antigens, **B2**.1875–6
  classification, **B2**.1876–7
  definitions, **B2**.1865–6
  detection
    complement fixation tests, **B1**.753
    in environment, **B2**.1879
  flagella, **B2**.1867–8, **B2**.1867 (Fig.)
  glycolipoprotein, **B2**.1876
  growth requirements, **B2**.1869–73
  habitats, **B2**.1867
  historical perspective, **B2**.1866–7
  LPS, **B2**.1875
  microscopic appearance, **B2**.1867 (Fig.),
    B2.1868–9
  molecular biology, **B2**.1873–5
    CIRCE element, **B2**.1874–5
    genetic analysis drawbacks, **B2**.1875
    insertion sequence elements, **B2**.1874
    plasmids, **B2**.1875
    RNA genes, **B2**.1874

system development, **B2**.1875
morphology, **B2**.1867–9
non-pathogenic species, **B2**.1866, **B2**.1876,
  B2.1877 (Fig.)
pathogenic species, **B2**.1866, **B2**.1876,
  B2.1877 (Fig.)
  virulence factors, **B2**.1881
species, **B2**.1866
transmission modes, waterborne, **B1**.212
vaccines, **I**.933 (Tab.)
virulence factors, **B2**.1880–1
Leptospira alexanderi, **B2**.1878 (Tab.)
Leptospira biflexa, **B2**.1865, **B2**.1866
  genome, **B2**.1874, **B2**.1875
  growth, **B2**.1871, **B2**.1881
  metabolism, **B2**.1873
  serovars/serogroups, **B2**.1878 (Tab.)
Leptospira borgpetersenii, **B2**.1871, **B2**.1874
  LPS, **B2**.1875
  serovars/serogroups, **B2**.1878 (Tab.)
Leptospiraceae, **B2**.1865–6, **B2**.1876
Leptospira inadai, **B2**.1878 (Tab.)
Leptospira interrogans, **I**.119, **B2**.1865
  genome, **B2**.1874
  growth requirements, **B2**.1871, **B2**.1875 (Fig.)
    selective media, **B2**.1872–3
  LPS, **B2**.1875
  mastitis, **B1**.230
  serovars/serogroups, **B2**.1878 (Tab.)
Leptospira kirschneri, **B2**.1878 (Tab.)
Leptospiral granules, **B2**.1868, **B2**.1868 (Fig.)
Leptospira meyeri, **B2**.1873
Leptospira noguchii, **B2**.1878 (Tab.)
Leptospira pomona, **B2**.1867
Leptospira santarosai, **B2**.1871, **B2**.1878 (Tab.)
Leptospira weilii, **B2**.1878 (Tab.)
Leptospires, **B2**.1865
  antibacterial susceptibility/resistance,
    B2.1880
  antigens, **B2**.1875–6, **B2**.1877 (Fig.)
    LipL. surface proteins, **B2**.1875–6, **B2**.1881
    LPS, **B2**.1876
  biochemistry
    fatty acids, **B2**.1870, **B2**.1881
    glycolipoproteins, **B2**.1876, **B2**.1881
  classification, **B2**.1876–7
    genetic and species, **B2**.1876–7
    non-pathogenic species, **B2**.1866, **B2**.1876,
      B2.1881, **B2**.1877 (Fig.)
    pathogenic species *see below*
    phenotypic typing methods, **B2**.1877
    phylogenetic relationships, **B2**.1876,
      B2.1877 (Fig.)
    serotyping *see below*
  culture, **B2**.1869–73
    autoagglutination, **B2**.1871
    growth requirements *see below*
    indicator media, **B2**.1872–3
    liquid media, **B2**.1871
    low-protein media, **B2**.1873
    media, **B2**.1872–3
    oleic acid–albumin media, **B2**.1872
    protein-free media, **B2**.1873
    semisolid media, **B2**.1871–3
    serum media, **B2**.1872

Leptospires
culture (*Continued*)
solid media, **B2**.1872, **B2**.1873
flagella, **B2**.1867–8, **B2**.1867 (Fig.)
antigen typing, **B2**.1877
growth, **B2**.1871–2
cell division, **B2**.1869–70
growth requirements, **B2**.1869–73
atmospheric conditions, **B2**.1870–1
carbon sources, **B2**.1871
nitrogen sources, **B2**.1871
osmolarity, **B2**.1870
oxidation–reduction potential, **B2**.1870
pH, **B2**.1870
purine/pyrimidines, **B2**.1871
temperature, **B2**.1870
habitats, **B2**.1867
as normal microbiota, **B2**.1880
history, **B2**.1866–7
infection *see* Leptospirosis
isolation/identification, **B2**.1877–80
environmental specimens, **B2**.1879
microscopic agglutination test, **B2**.1879–80
PCR, **B2**.1879, **B2**.1880
restriction endonuclease analysis, **B2**.1880
serotyping *see below*
specimen types, **B2**.1879
typing of isolates, **B2**.1877, **B2**.1879–80
metabolism, **B2**.1873
microscopy, **B2**.1867
appearance, **B2**.1867 (Fig.), **B2**.1868–9
monoclonal antibodies to, **B2**.1877
morphology and visualization, **B2**.1867–9
methods of observation, **B2**.1867, **B2**.1868–9
motility, **B2**.1869
OmpL1, **B2**.1875–6, **B2**.1881
pathogenic species, **B2**.1866, **B2**.1876, **B2**.1877 (Fig.), **B2**.1880–1
virulence factors, **B2**.1881
replicons, **B2**.1874
serotyping, **B2**.1867, **B2**.1877
serogroups, **B2**.1877, **B2**.1878 (Tab.)
serovars, **B2**.1877, **B2**.1878 (Tab.)
structure
cell wall, **B2**.1867–8
flagella *see above*
lipid content, **B2**.1867–8
spheroplasts, **B2**.1868, **B2**.1868 (Fig.)
virulence factors, **B2**.1875–6, **B2**.1880–1
Leptospirosis, **B2**.1866, **B2**.1881
diagnosis, **B1**.524
economic losses, **B2**.1866
emerging bacterial infection, climate changes, **B1**.362
historical aspects, **B2**.1866–7
natural/acquired resistance, **B2**.1881
pathology and pathogenesis, **B2**.1881
Leptotrichia, **B2**.1945, **B2**.1951–3
antibacterial susceptibility/resistance, **B2**.1953
cell wall composition, **B2**.1953
classification, **B2**.1914, **B2**.1915, **B2**.1952
culture, **B2**.1952–3
definition, **B2**.1951

differentiating characteristics, **B2**.1949 (Tab.)
habitats, **B2**.1952
historical perspective, **B2**.1945–6, **B2**.1951–2
isolation/identification, **B2**.1953
metabolism, **B2**.1952–3
morphology, **B2**.1952
pathogenicity, **B2**.1953
Leptotrichia buccalis, **B1**.296 (Tab.), **B2**.1945, **B2**.1951–2
antibacterial susceptibility/resistance, **B2**.1953
classification, **B2**.1952
differentiating characteristics, **B2**.1949 (Tab.)
isolation/identification, **B2**.1953
morphology, **B2**.1952, **B2**.1953 (Fig.)
pathogenicity, **B2**.1953
Lesions
lobomycosis, **M**.431, **M**.431 (Fig.), **M**.432 (Fig.), **M**.433 (Fig.)
melioidosis, **B2**.1629
onchocerciasis, **P**.793
Letrazuril, cryptosporidiosis, **P**.410
Lettuce necrotic yellows virus (LNYV)
genome structure, **V2**.1112 (Fig.)
type species, **V1**.385–6, **V2**.1105
Leucine-rich proteins
macrophage pathogen recognition, **I**.23
microbial recognition, **I**.24 (Tab.)
Leuckart, Rudolf, **P**.9
Balantidium coli, **P**.275
Leuconostoc
intrinsic anti-glycopeptide activity, **B1**.480
as normal microbiota, **B1**.296 (Tab.)
Leucoplakia, candidiasis, **M**.598
Leufactin, **I**.769
Leukemia inhibitory factor (LIF)
IL-17 effects, **I**.290
neutrophil abnormalities, **I**.49
Leukemia, VZV vaccination, **V1**.516
Leukocyte(s) *see* Lymphocyte(s)
Leukocyte adhesion deficiency (LAD), **I**.47–8, **I**.48 (Tab.), **I**.767–9, **I**.768 (Fig.)
diagnosis, **I**.50–1, **I**.50 (Tab.)
flow cytometry, **I**.50–1
integrins, **I**.767–9
signs/symptoms, **I**.47–8
therapy, **I**.50
bone marrow transplants, **I**.50
type I, **I**.47–8, **I**.767–9
type II, **I**.48, **I**.769
Leukocyte-endogenous mediator (LEM), **B1**.176
Leukocyte function antigen-1 (LFA-1: CD11a)
B cell activation, **I**.326
CD4 T cells/APC interactions, **I**.392 (Fig.), **I**.396
eosinophils, **I**.60
ligands, **I**.512–13
lymphocyte migration, **I**.507, **I**.508 (Tab.)
TCR–superantigen binding, **I**.560
Leukocyte function antigen-3 (LFA-3)
DNA vaccine co-administration, **I**.919 (Tab.)
mucosal immune response, **I**.524
Leukocyte receptor cluster (LRC), **I**.88, **I**.89, **I**.94, **I**.95 (Fig.)

Leukopenia
Anaplasma phagocytophilum infection, **B2**.2060
Colorado tick fever virus infection, **V2**.942–3
Ehrlichia chaffeensis infection, **B2**.2057–9
measles, **I**.803
Leukoplakias
HPV association, **V1**.463 (Tab.), **V1**.465 (Tab.)
oral hairy, **V1**.572–3
oral hairy, HIV infection, **B2**.1151
Leukoscan, licensing, **I**.355 (Tab.)
Leukotriene(s) (LTs), **I**.184–5
actions, **I**.185
airway hypersensitivity, P032., **I**.731–2
biosynthesis, **I**.182 (Fig.)
drug development, **I**.185
excretion, **I**.184–5
γ-glutamyl transferase, **I**.184–5
history of, **I**.184
neutrophil recruitment, **I**.37
receptors, **I**.185
see also specific types
Leukotriene A$_4$, **I**.184
Leukotriene A$_4$ hydrolase, **I**.184
Leukotriene B$_4$ (LTB$_4$), **B1**.625
actions/effects, **I**.185
basophil chemotaxis, **I**.60
blood vessel contraction, **I**.185
eosinophil chemotaxis, **I**.61
neutrophil priming, **I**.44
biosynthesis, **I**.182 (Fig.)
production, **I**.181, **I**.185
neutrophils, **I**.46, **I**.184, **I**.185
receptors, **I**.185–6
structure, **I**.182 (Fig.)
Leukotriene C$_4$ (LTC$_4$)
blood vessel contraction, **I**.185
production, **I**.181, **I**.182 (Fig.)
basophils, **I**.64
mast cells, **I**.184
structure, **I**.182 (Fig.)
Leukotriene D$_4$
blood vessel cotraction, **I**.185
production, **I**.181, **I**.182 (Fig.), **I**.184
structure, **I**.182 (Fig.)
Leukotriene E$_4$
production, **I**.181, **I**.182 (Fig.), **I**.184
structure, **I**.182 (Fig.)
Levamisole, **P**.807–8
Levinea amalonatica see Citrobacter amalonaticus
Levinea malonatica see Citrobacter diversus
Leviviridae, **V1**.27 (Tab.), **V1**.51 (Tab.)
see also specific viruses
Levofloxacin
formulations, **B1**.493
Haemophilus, **B2**.1702 (Tab.)
spectrum of activity, **B1**.492
Lewis antigens, *Helicobacter,* **B2**.1569, **B2**.1577–8
Lewis rats, Borna disease virus infection, **V2**.1145–6
LexA, repair of UV-induced DNA damage, **B1**.451–2

Lice, **B2**.2027–30
  Rickettsia transmission, **B2**.2037, **B2**.2041
Lichens, formation, **B1**.201
Lidocaine, **P**.393
Life expectancy (humans), **P**.24
Life expectancy (parasite)
  malaria epidemiology, **P**.511
  onchocerciasis, **P**.792–3
  Schistosoma mansoni, **P**.60 (Tab.)
  Trichuris trichiuria, **P**.60 (Tab.)
  Wuchereria bancrofti, **P**.60 (Tab.)
Ligase chain reaction (LCR), **B1**.731,
  B1.732 (Fig.), **V2**.1537–8
  Chlamydia diagnosis, **B2**.2006–7, **B2**.2019
Light chains
  Ig structure *see* Immunoglobulin structure
  pre-BCR, **I**.340–1
LightCycler®, **B1**.723 (Tab.), **B1**.725, **B1**.728,
  B1.729
Light-harvesting (LH) complexes, **B1**.67
Lignin-degrading enzymes, **B1**.199–200
'Limax amebae', **P**.226
Limestone Canyon virus, **V2**.1666 (Tab.)
Limosoides sigmoidontis infection, **I**.70
Limulus amebocyte lysate assays, **B1**.191
Limulus lysate test, **B1**.559
Lincomycin
  Actinomyces, **B2**.1011
  structure, **B1**.488 (Fig.)
Lincosamides, **B1**.487–8
  mode of action, **B1**.487–8
  pharmacology, **B1**.488
  resistance, **B1**.488
    Staphylococcus, **B2**.794 (Tab.), **B2**.803
  spectrum of activity, **B1**.487
  structure, **B1**.487, **B1**.488 (Fig.)
  toxicity/adverse effects, **B1**.488
Line probe assays, **V2**.1542
Linezolid, **B1**.489
  spectrum of activity, **B1**.499 (Tab.)
  structure, **B1**.490 (Fig.)
Linkage analysis
  epidemiology, **P**.50
  Plasmodium chloroquine resistance, **P**.479
Linkage disequilibrium methods, **I**.574
  HLA class III, **I**.578
Linkage studies, leprosy association, **I**.590
Linker insertion mutagenesis, **V1**.185
Linker scanning mutagenesis, **V1**.184–5
Linnaeus, C, **P**.6, **B1**.11, **P**.189–90
Lipases
  Burkholderia cepacia complex, **B2**.1615
  Burkholderia thailandensis, **B2**.1624
  Enterobacteriaceae identification,
    B2.1319 (Tab.)
  Porphyromonas identification, **B2**.1924 (Tab.)
  Prevotella identification, **B2**.1924 (Tab.)
  Pseudomonas aeruginosa, **B2**.1601
Lipid(s)
  analysis, **B1**.24
  bacterial, **B1**.42
  Borrelia metabolism, **B2**.1827–8
  Brucella, **B2**.1724–5
  Burkholderia cepacia complex, **B2**.1613
  Burkholderia thailandensis, **B2**.1621

Malassezia growth requirements, **M**.205–6
Mononegavirales order, **V1**.381
  synthesis, **B1**.61
  see also specific types
Lipid A
  Enterobacteriaceae LPS, **B2**.1340–1
  Helicobacter, **B2**.1569
Lipid-associated amphotericin B *see*
  Amphotericin B
Lipid(s), *Blastocystis hominis*, **P**.561
Lipid envelope, herpesviruses, **V1**.490
Lipid inflammatory mediators, neutrophils *see*
  Neutrophil(s)
Lipid membranes, nonsymmetrical viruses,
  V1.69
Lipid metabolism
  acute phase response, **I**.207
  Entamoeba histolytica, **P**.204
  Plasmodium see Plasmodium
  tapeworms, **P**.662
  Trypanosoma brucei, **P**.360–1
Lipid preparations, for polyene antifungal
  agent transport, **M**.149, **M**.149 (Tab.)
  see also individual antifungal agents
Lipid rafts
  BCR signaling, **I**.342
  influenza hemagglutinin assembly, **V1**.651
  Measles virus hemagglutinin (H) protein,
    V1.720–1
  nonsymmetrical viruses, **V1**.69
  paramyxoviruses, **V1**.72
  retroviruses, **V1**.77
Lipid transferases, microbial recognition,
  I.24 (Tab.)
Lipoarabinomannan (LAM), **I**.652–3, **B2**.1184
Lipo-oligosaccharide (LOS), **B1**.157–8
  antigenic variation, **I**.661
  Bordetella, **B2**.1789 (Tab.), **B2**.1796
  Haemophilus, **B2**.1698
  Haemophilus influenzae, **B2**.1698
  Neisseria, **B2**.1288
  structure and function, **B1**.158
Lipophilic yeasts, **M**.14–5
Lipophosphoglycan, **P**.291–2, **P**.294–5
Lipopolysaccharide (LPS), **B1**.43, **I**.110
  acute phase response induction, **I**.196–7
  airborne bacteria
    concentrations in facilities, **B1**.186 (Tab.)
    drying and heat stress, **B1**.188
  antigenic variation, **I**.661
  biosynthesis, genetic loci involved, **B1**.160
  classical complement pathway activation,
    I.142
  defensin induction, **I**.520–1
  definition, **B1**.147
  dendritic cell activation, **I**.393–4
  discovery, **B1**.12, **I**.110
  E-selectin expression, **I**.506–7
  host resistance and common pattern
    recognition, **B1**.176–7
  LL37 binding, **I**.174
  as pathogen-associated molecular patterns,
    I.896
  regions, **B1**.158
  release in gram-negative infection, **B1**.159
  in septic shock, **B1**.159, **I**.696

species
  Aeromonas, **B2**.1527, **B2**.1535
  Bacteroides/Porphyromonas, **B2**.1936–7
  Bordetella, **B2**.1789 (Tab.), **B2**.1796
  Brucella, **B2**.1724–6, **B2**.1726 (Fig.),
    B2.1736, **B2**.1737
  Burkholderia cepacia complex,
    B2.1613–14, **B2**.1617
  Burkholderia mallei, **B2**.1632–3
  Burkholderia thailandensis, **B2**.1621–2
  Chlamydia, **B2**.2008–9, **B2**.2019
  Coxiella burnetii, **B2**.2073, **B2**.2075
  Enterobacteriaceae *see* Enterobacteriaceae
  Escherichia coli see Escherichia coli
  Francisella tularensis, **B2**.1753–4
  Fusobacterium, **B2**.1948
  Helicobacter, **B2**.1568–9
  Legionella, **B2**.1770–1
  Leptospira, **B2**.1875
  Moraxella (Branhamella) catarrhalis,
    B2.1307
  Neisseria meningitidis, **B1**.158, **B1**.564
  Porphyromonas gingivalis, **B2**.1936–7
  Proteus, **B2**.1444
  Pseudomonas, **B1**.158–9
  Salmonella see Salmonella
  Shigella, **B1**.158, **B2**.1390
  Veillonella, **B2**.1314
  Vibrio, **B2**.1511
  Yersinia, **B2**.1461
  structure, **B1**.158, **B1**.159 (Fig.)
  TLRs, **I**.696
    TLRs 4 binding, **I**.926
  as virulence factor, **B1**.157–60
Lipopolysaccharide-binding protein (LBP),
  I.114 (Tab.), **I**.115–16, **I**.200
  discovery, **I**.110
  epithelial cells, **I**.115–16
  septic shock, **I**.696
  single nucleotide polymorphisms, **I**.124
Lipoprotein envelope, Rubella virus,
  V2.959–60
Lipoproteins
  in bacterial cell walls, **B1**.43
  Brucella, **B2**.1724
Liposome formulations of drugs, Old World
  leishmaniasis, **P**.307
Liposomes
  DNA vaccine delivery, **I**.917
  intranasal vaccine delivery, **I**.831
  skin immunization, **I**.822
Lipoteichoic acid (LTA), **I**.22, **B1**.43
  group D streptococci, **B2**.887
  septic shock, **I**.696
  TLR recognition, **I**.696
Lipothrixviridae, **V1**.27 (Tab.), **V1**.43 (Tab.)
  see also specific viruses
Lipoxins, **I**.186
Lipoxygenases, **I**.184
  arachidonic acid production, **I**.181–4
  neutrophil production, **I**.46
  structure, **I**.184
5-Lipoxygenases, **I**.184
  eosinophils, **I**.57, **I**.184
  lipoxin production, **I**.186

15-Lipoxygenases, **I**.186
Liquid sterilization systems, **B1**.453–4
LIR receptors, NK cell receptors, **I**.90
Listeria, **B2**.953–65
  antibacterial susceptibility/resistance,
    B2.957–8
  antigens, **B2**.956–7, **B2**.957 (Tab.)
  biochemical properties, **B2**.955, **B2**.959–61
  cell wall structure, **B2**.956–7
  characteristics, **B2**.955, **B2**.959–61,
    B2.960 (Tab.)
  classification, **B2**.953, **B2**.958
  definition, **B2**.953
  genetics, **B2**.955–6
    plasmids, **B2**.956
    transposons, **B2**.956
  habitats, **B2**.954–5
    in milk, **B1**.231–2
  infection *see* Listeriosis
  isolation/identification, **B2**.958–63
    genus, **B2**.959–61
    nucleic acid-based methods, **B2**.962
    selective techniques, **B2**.959
    serotyping, **B2**.961
    species differentiation, **B2**.961
    typing methods, **B2**.961–2
  metabolism, **B2**.955
  morphology, **B2**.955
  in normal microbiota, **B2**.962
  pathogenicity, **B2**.953–4, **B2**.962
  virulence factors, **B2**.962
    internalins, **B1**.152
Listeria grayi, **B2**.953
  antigens, **B2**.957 (Tab.)
  characteristics, **B2**.960 (Tab.)
  classification, **B2**.958
  identification, **B2**.961
  pathogenicity, **B2**.954, **B2**.962–3
Listeria innocua, **B2**.953
  antibacterial susceptibility/resistance, **B2**.958
  antigens, **B2**.957 (Tab.)
  classification, **B2**.958, **B2**.960 (Tab.)
  genetics, **B2**.956
  isolation/identification, **B2**.959
  pathogenicity, **B2**.954, **B2**.964–5
Listeria ivanovii, **B2**.953
  antigens, **B2**.957, **B2**.957 (Tab.)
  characteristics, **B2**.955, **B2**.960 (Tab.)
  classification, **B2**.958
  isolation/identification, **B2**.959, **B2**.961
  pathogenicity, **B2**.954, **B2**.962–5
Listeria monocytogenes, **B2**.953
  antibacterial susceptibility/resistance, **B2**.958
  antigens, **B2**.956–7, **B2**.957 (Tab.)
  bacteriocin use in food industry, **B1**.139
  biochemical properties, **B2**.955
  cell wall structure, **B2**.956–7
  characteristics, **B2**.955, **B2**.960 (Tab.)
  classification, **B2**.958
  in foods, **B2**.954
    butter, **B1**.250
    cheese, **B1**.254–5
    hazard analysis, **B1**.288
    ice cream, **B1**.251
    meat and meat products, **B1**.273–4

    milk, **B1**.230–1, **B1**.231–2, **B1**.235,
      B1.242–3
    poultry, **B1**.276
    storage temperature, **B1**.264
    vegetables, **B1**.282
    yogurt, **B1**.249
  genetics, **B2**.955–6
  growth
    animal
      models, **B2**.962–3
      mammalin cell invasion mechanisms,
        B2.964–5, **B2**.964 (Fig.)
      tissue culture, **B2**.963–5
  habitats, **B2**.954–5
  immune evasion
    IL-10 induction, **I**.652, **I**.653, **I**.654
    MHC class I antigen presentation,
      I.659–60
    MHC class II antigen presentation, **I**.658–9
    pore-forming toxins, **I**.655
  infection *see* Listeriosis
  isolation/identification, **B2**.958–63
    typing methods, **B2**.961–2
  metabolism, **B2**.955
  in normal microbiota, **B1**.296 (Tab.),
    B2.962
  pathogenicity, **B2**.953–4, **B2**.962,
    B2.964 (Fig.), **B2**.965 (Fig.)
  as vaccine vector, **I**.845, **I**.899, **I**.902
    BCG vectors, **I**.844–5
    immune system targeting, **I**.902
  virulence factors
    ActA, **B1**.152–3, **B1**.154 (Fig.)
    listeriolysin O, **B1**.152, **B1**.154 (Fig.)
Listeria pneumophilia, immune evasion
  IL-10 induction, **I**.652
  LPS variation, **I**.661
  outer membrane protein variation, **I**.661
Listeria seeligeri, **B2**.953
  antigens, **B2**.957 (Tab.)
  characteristics, **B2**.955, **B2**.960 (Tab.)
  classification, **B2**.958
  isolation/identification, **B2**.959
  pathogenicity, **B2**.954, **B2**.962–5
Listeria welshimeri, **B2**.953
  antibacterial susceptibility/resistance,
    B2.958
  antigens, **B2**.957 (Tab.)
  classification, **B2**.958, **B2**.960 (Tab.)
  isolation/identification, **B2**.959
  pathogenicity, **B2**.954, **B2**.962–3
Listeriosis, **B2**.953–4, **B2**.962–5
  animals, **B2**.953–4
    experimental models, **B2**.962–3
  bacteremia, **B1**.520
  bone and joint infection, **B1**.690–1
  dendritic cell infection, **I**.656
  endocarditis, **B1**.532–3
  endophthalmitis, **B1**.603
  entry into cells, **I**.649
    bacterial proteins, **I**.649
    complement, **I**.649
    escape to cytoplasm, **I**.650
  food-borne
    cheese, **B1**.254–5
    ice cream, **B1**.251

    milk, **B1**.242–3
    vegetables, **B1**.282
  genital tract infection, **B1**.669
  granulomatous response, **B1**.741
  immune response, **I**.376–7
    αβ T cells, **I**.445
    CD8 T cell responses, **I**.420
    γδ T-cells, **I**.526–7
    IL-18, **I**.290–2
    intraepithelial lymphocytes, **I**.526–7
    macrophages, **I**.27
    mucosal immune response, **I**.522–3
    NK cell actions, **I**.99
  infiltration of host tissues, **B1**.152–3,
    B1.154 (Fig.)
  intracranial abscess, **B1**.585–6
  mastitis, **B1**.230
  meningitis, **B1**.555
  pathogenesis, **B2**.964–5
  reactive arthritis, **I**.594–5
  TLR-5, **I**.121
  vaccines
    attenuated vectors, **I**.902
    BCG vector, **I**.844–5
    development status, **I**.933 (Tab.)
    Salmonella vaccine vector, **I**.901
Lister, J, **B1**.6, **B1**.370–1
Listonella anguillarum, **B2**.1507
Lithotrophy, **B1**.67
Live-attenuated vaccines *see* Vaccines, live
Live attenuated viral carriers, HIV vaccine
    development, **V2**.1333
Liver
  abscesses, melioidosis, **B2**.1627,
    B2.1627 (Fig.)
  aspergillosis, **M**.701, **M**.705
  babesiosis, **P**.456
  candidiasis, **M**.595, **M**.596 (Fig.), **M**.599–600
  hepatitis A, **V2**.1171–2
  Hepatitis delta virus replication, **V2**.1270
  PCP, **M**.785
Liver biopsy
  hepatitis C, **V2**.1203–4
  Hepatitis delta virus, **V2**.1272
Liver enzymes, hepatitis A, **V2**.1171
Liver fluke(s), **P.640–57**
  classification, **P**.641–2
  control, **P**.653–4
    anthelmintic treatment, **P**.653–4
    food safety programs, **P**.653–4
    health education, **P**.653–4
    sanitation improvement, **P**.653–4
  general biology, **P**.643–4
    movement, **P**.643–4
    nutrition, **P**.645
    physiological adjustments, **P**.643–4
  historical aspects, **P**.11–2
  infection *see below*
  life cycles, **P**.644–5
    definitive hosts, **P**.645–6
    developmental stages, **P**.646
  morphology/structure, **P**.642–3
    adults, **P**.642
    oral/ventral suckers, **P**.642
    reproductive system, **P**.642

Liver fluke(s)
  morphology/structure (*Continued*)
    solenocytes (flame cells), **P**.642
  prevalence, **P**.640
  transmission/epidemiology, **P**.645, **P**.646–8
    distribution in communities, **P**.648
    geographic distribution, **P**.646–7
    location in host, **P**.648
    raw/undercooked food, **P**.647
    social factors, **P**.647–8
    see also individual species
Liver fluke infection
  clinical aspects, **P**.648–53
    clinical manifestations, **P**.649–50
    pathogenesis/pathology, **P**.651–2
  diagnosis, **P**.652–3
  immune response, **P**.652
    enzyme antigens, **P**.652
Liver function tests, acute hepatitis C,
  V2.1202–3
Liver-stage antigen 3 (LSA-3) *see* Malaria
Liver stones, liver flukes, **P**.649
Liver transplantation
  alveolar echinococcosis treatment, **P**.699
  aspergillosis, **M**.701
  hepatitis B passive immunization, **V2**.1259
  hepatitis C control, **V2**.1216
  Hepatitis delta virus transmission, **V2**.1272
  Nocardia asteroides infection, **B2**.1157
Live vaccines *see* Vaccines, live
LL37 subunit *see* HCAP-18
'Llaga,' **P**.328
Loa loa
  historical aspects, **P**.10
  infection *see* Loiasis
Loboa loboi, **M**.430
  classification, **M**.430, **M**.434
  histology, **M**.126 (Tab.), **M**.128 (Tab.),
    M.133 (Fig.)
    stains, **M**.122
  infection *see* Lobomycosis
  morphology, **M**.126 (Tab.)
  spread, **M**.432
Lobomycosis (Lobo's disease), **M**.430,
  M.432 (Fig.)
  clinical features, **M**.431–2
  commonly affected areas, **M**.431
  diagnosis, **M**.125–7, **M**.433–4
  dolphins, **M**.430, **M**.431, **M**.432, **M**.433
  ethnic background, **M**.430–1
  etiologic agent *see* Loboa loboi
  evolution, **M**.432
  farmers/farm workers, **M**.431
  gender predilection, **M**.430
  geographical distribution, **M**.430,
    M.431 (Tab.)
  histopathology, **M**.121–2, **M**.128 (Tab.),
    M.133 (Fig.), **M**.433, **M**.433 (Fig.),
    M.434 (Fig.)
  history, **M**.430
  immune response, **M**.434
  lesions, **M**.431, **M**.431 (Fig.), **M**.432 (Fig.),
    M.433 (Fig.)
  lymph nodes, **M**.432, **M**.434
  occupational exposure and inoculation,
    M.431

onset, **M**.432
prognosis, **M**.432
skin smear, **M**.433, **M**.433 (Fig.)
spread, **M**.432
therapy, **M**.434–5
  clofazimine, **M**.434
  itraconazole, **M**.434–5
  miconazole, **M**.434–5
ulceration, **M**.431
Unna band, **M**.433–4
Lobopodia, **P**.178 (Fig.), **P**.179, **P**.201–2, **P**.227
Lobo's disease *see* Lobomycosis (Lobo's
  disease)
Lobsters, **B1**.279–80
Lobular hepatitis, hepatitis C, **V2**.1203–4
Local control programs, **P**.109
Local hyperemia, acute phase response, **B1**.739
Local irritation/itching, *Enterobius
  vermicularis,* **P**.731
Localized cutaneous leishmaniasis, **P**.338–9
Localized infection, monitoring/surveillance,
  V1.361
Localized juvenile periodontitis (LJP)
  Actinobacillus actinomycetemcomitans
    infection, **B2**.1662, **B2**.1663
  Capnocytophaga infection, **B2**.1674
Lockean view, **B1**.13
Locomotion
  Balantidium coli, **P**.276
  Clonorchis sinensis, **P**.644
  liver flukes, **P**.643–4
  protozoa, **P**.169–72, **P**.170 (Fig.), **P**.178 (Fig.),
    P.179–80
    flagella and cilia, **P**.179–80, **P**.179 (Fig.),
      P.180 (Fig.)
      'A' and 'B' tubules, **P**.179–80
      kinetosome (basal body), **P**.179–80
      microtubules, **P**.179–80
    gliding filament theory, **P**.169–72, **P**.179–80
    pseudopodia, **P**.179
    lobopodia and filopodia, **P**.178 (Fig.)
LOD score, linkage, **I**.573
Loiasis, **I**.600
  diagnosis, **P**.143 (Tab.)
  historical aspects, **P**.10
London School of Tropical Medicine,
  foundation, **P**.9–10
Longitudinal (incidence) studies, **B1**.314
Long terminal repeats (LTRs), **V1**.337 (Fig.)
  foamy viruses, **V2**.1308
  retroviruses, **V1**.188, **V1**.337 (Fig.)
  in transformation, **V1**.335–6
Loopingout/excision model, TCR
  rearrangements, **I**.453–4
Looss A., **P**.8–9
Lopinavir (ritonavir), **V2**.1623, **V2**.1624
  HIV resistance, **V2**.1337 (Fig.)
  resistance, **V2**.1623
  structure, **V2**.1624 (Fig.), **V2**.1625 (Fig.)
Loracarbef
  development, **B1**.480
  structure, **B1**.479 (Fig.)
Louping ill, **V2**.1004
Louping ill virus, **V2**.998 (Tab.)
Low-density lipoprotein(s) (LDLs), **I**.207

Low density lipoprotein (LDL) receptor
  Hepatitis C virus receptor/co-receptor,
    V2.1195
  rhinovirus cell receptors, **V1**.209
Low-density lipoprotein receptor domain A,
  I.476 (Fig.)
Low-density lipoprotein receptor-related
  (LPR) proteins, *Plasmodium* hepatocyte
  invasion, **P**.472–3
Lower respiratory tract infection *see*
  Respiratory tract infection
Low-risk human papillomaviruses (LR-HPVs)
  E6 protein, **V1**.455–6, **V1**.459
  E7 protein, **V1**.455–6, **V1**.459, **V1**.461
  genital warts, **V1**.448–9
Low temperature steam with formaldehyde
  (LTSF), **B1**.429–30, **B1**.445 (Tab.),
  B1.447–8, **B1**.454
L (large) segment, bunyavirus genome,
  V2.1028–31, **V2**.1039
L-selectin (CD62L), **I**.505–6
  DNA vaccine co-administration, P048.,
    I.919 (Tab.)
  expression in HIV infection, **I**.792
  lymphocyte migration, **I**.506, **I**.508 (Tab.)
  molecular interactions, **I**.506
  peripheral lymph node addressins
    interactions, **I**.506
  sialy-Lewis^x structure interactions, **I**.506
LTA gene, **I**.577–8
  leishmaniasis, **I**.596
  periodontitis association, **I**.595
Ludwig's angina, **B1**.614–15
Lumbar–peritoneal shunts
  cryptococcosis therapy, **M**.652
  CSF withdrawal, **M**.652
  intracranial pressure reduction, **M**.652
Lumbar puncture, **B1**.557–8
  contraindications and hazards, **B1**.557–8
Lumpy skin disease virus, **V1**.584 (Fig.)
Lung cancer, TCE peptide vaccines,
  I.865 (Tab.)
Lung fluke(s), **P**.592, **P.640–57**
  classification, **P**.641–2
  control, **P**.653–4
    anthelmintic treatment, **P**.653–4
    food safety programs, **P**.653–4
    health education, **P**.653–4
    sanitation improvement, **P**.653–4
  general biology, **P**.643–4
  historical aspects, **P**.11–2
  infection *see below*
  life cycles, **P**.644–5
    definitive hosts, **P**.645–6
    developmental stages, **P**.646
  morphology/structure, **P**.642–3
    adults, **P**.642
    oral/ventral suckers, **P**.642
    reproductive system, **P**.642
    solenocytes (flame cells), **P**.642
  prevalence, **P**.640
  transmission/epidemiology, **P**.646–8
    distribution in communities, **P**.648
    geographic distribution, **P**.646–7
    location in host, **P**.648
    raw/undercooked food, **P**.647

Lung fluke(s)
transmission/epidemiology (*Continued*)
social factors, **P**.647–8
see also individual species
Lung fluke infection
clinical aspects, **P**.648–53
clinical manifestations, **P**.650
pathogenesis/pathology, **P**.650–1
diagnosis, **P**.652–3
immune response, **P**.652
enzyme antigens, **P**.652
Lung function tests, PCP diagnosis, **M**.788
Lung(s)
abscesses
amebic liver abscess, **P**.208
causative agents, **B1**.644
diagnosis and treatment, **B1**.644
multiple, **B1**.644
pneumonia complication, **B1**.643–4
aspergillosis, **M**.699 (Fig.)
invasive, **M**.698–9, **M**.719–26
biopsy, PCP, **M**.787
blastomycosis, **M**.489, **M**.490–2, **M**.497
candidiasis, **M**.600
chromoblastomycosis, **M**.361–2
cryptococcosis, **M**.646–7, **M**.649–50,
M.650 (Fig.)
histoplasmosis capsulati *see* Histoplasmosis
capsulati
inflammation, **B1**.625
intracranial abscess complication, **B1**.583
normal microbiota, **B1**.302
sporotrichosis, **M**.367, **M**.375
transplantation
in cystic fibrosis, **B1**.651
Nocardia asteroides infection, **B2**.1157
zygomycosis, **M**.20–1
systemic, **M**.674, **M**.674 (Tab.), **M**.678
Lung transplants, aspergillosis *see* Aspergillosis
Lutenizing hormone-releasing hormone
(LHRH), **I**.875
Luteoviridae, **V1**.27 (Tab.), **V1**.51 (Tab.)
see also specific viruses
Lutzomyia, **P**.283–4
see also individual species
Lutzomyia cruciata, **P**.317
Lutzomyia cruzi, **P**.321–2
Lutzomyia evansi, **P**.321
Lutzomyia longipalpis, **P**.317, **P**.321
Lutzomyia ylephilator, **P**.317
Lwoff, A., **V1**.6
Ly49 genes
dendritic epidermal γδ T cells, **I**.437
NK cells, **I**.89
Ly49 receptors, **I**.88 (Fig.), **I**.90, **I**.92, **I**.94
NK cells, **I**.87, **I**.88 (Fig.), **I**.89, **I**.92, **I**.94
development, **I**.92
Lyme borreliosis, **B2**.1818
clinical features, **B2**.1821
bacteremia, **B2**.1828–9
cutaneous manifestations, **B2**.1828
meningitis in, **B1**.575
epidemiology, **B2**.1822–3
animal reservoirs, **B2**.1822–3
climate effects, **B2**.1823

geographic range, **B2**.1822
Ixodes life cycle, **B2**.1822
history, **B2**.1818–19
identification, **B2**.1828–32
PCR-based methods, **B2**.1829
samples, **B2**.1828
serology, **B1**.753, **B2**.1829–30
reactive arthritis, **I**.594–5, **I**.752–3
pathogen induced, **I**.753 (Tab.)
strain-specific pathology, **B2**.1821
transmission, **B1**.362
vaccine
BCG vector, **I**.845, **I**.901–2
development status, **I**.933 (Tab.)
outer surface protein, **I**.938
recombinant DNA vaccines, **I**.938
Lymnaea, **P**.646
Lymphadenitis
cat-scratch disease, **B2**.1891
rhinosporidial, **M**.465, **M**.470
streptococcal, **B1**.244
toxoplasmosis, **P**.431
Lymphadenopathy
African trypanosomiasis, **P**.364, **P**.365
chronic bilateral cervical, **B2**.1249
erysipeloid, **B2**.971
in HIV infection, **I**.797
infectious mononucleosis (IM), **V1**.568
regional, cat-scratch disease, **B2**.1891–2
toxoplasmosis, **P**.431
Lymphangitis
epizootic
histoplasmosis farciminosi, **M**.24
horses, **M**.522
erysipeloid, **B2**.971
Lymphatic filariasis, **I**.683, **P.769–80**
clinical manifestations, **P**.39, **P**.773–5
acute dermatotolymphangitis, **P**.773
acute infection, **P**.773
adenolymphangitis, **P**.773
chronic infection, **P**.773–4
chyluria, **P**.774
elephantiasis, **P**.774, **P**.774 (Fig.)
funiculo-epididymoorchitis, **P**.773
hydrocele, **P**.773–4, **P**.774 (Fig.)
lymphedema, **P**.774, **P**.774 (Fig.)
subclinical (asymptomatic), **P**.773
tropical pulmonary eosinophilia, **P**.774–5
uninfected, exposed individuals, **P**.775
control, **P**.122–3, **P**.777–8
chemotherapy/chemoprophylaxis,
P.144 (Tab.)
community-directed programs, **P**.122
control programs, **P**.777–8
diagnosis, **P**.143 (Tab.)
DNA diagnosis, **P**.130
Filariasis Control Movement, **P**.123
Filariasis Parents' Association, **P**.123
Global Alliance to Eliminate Lymphatic
Filariasis, **P**.110
health education, **P**.123
organizations, **P**.123
stratification of disease, **P**.139 (Tab.)
vector elimination, **P**.109, **P**.122–3

vector/reservoir control, **P**.39–40,
P.145 (Tab.), **P**.778
diagnosis, **P**.776–7
'filarial dance sign,' **P**.773, **P**.777
immunoserology, **P**.776–7
PCR-based methods, **P**.777
peripheral blood microfilariae, **P**.776
ultrasound, **P**.773, **P**.777
urine examination, **P**.152
epidemiology, **P**.39, **P**.46 (Tab.), **P**.769,
P.772–3
age dynamics, **P**.772–3
gender, **P**.772
geographical distribution, **P**.769,
P.770 (Fig.), **P**.772
historical aspects, **P**.9–10, **P**.769–71
immune response, **P**.91–2, **I**.683, **P**.775–6
antibody responses, **P**.776
basophils, **I**.68
eosinophils, **I**.68–70
IL-10, **P**.775–6
immunoregulation, **P**.776
T cell subsets, **P**.93 (Fig.), **P**.775–6
transforming growth factor-β, **P**.775–6
immunogenetics, **I**.600
mortality, **P**.28 (Tab.)
pathogenesis/pathology, **P**.775
histamine release, **I**.68–9
worm death, **P**.775
public health importance, **P**.39–40,
P.105 (Tab.)
treatment, **P**.39–40, **P**.777
ivermectin, **P**.789
vaccine development, **I**.933 (Tab.)
subunit vaccines, **I**.941
*see also Brugia malayi; Brugia timori;
Wuchereria bancrofti; individual species*
Lymphedema
Kaposi's sarcoma, **V1**.552
lymphatic filariasis, **P**.774, **P**.774 (Fig.)
Lymph node biopsy, African trypanosomiasis
diagnosis, **P**.367
Lymph node enlargement, onchocerciasis,
P.793, **P**.795
Lymph nodes
CD4 T cells, **I**.389
HIV infection *see* HIV infection
lobomycosis, **M**.432, **M**.434
mycetoma, **M**.388
PCP, **M**.785
prototheosis, **M**.407–8
pythiosis, **M**.418–19
rhinosporidiosis, **M**.464–5, **M**.465 (Fig.)
structure, **I**.505
Lymphoblastoid cell line (LCL), EBV
immortalization, **V1**.559, **V1**.565–6
Lymphocryptovirus, **V1**.494 (Tab.)
Lymphocystivirus, **V1**.44
Lymphocyte(s)
activation
Nef, **I**.789
platelet-activating factor, **I**.191
acute phase response, **I**.206
adhesion to brain capillaries, **V2**.1411,
V2.1411 (Fig.)
in cerebrospinal fluid, **B1**.558, **B1**.558 (Tab.)

Lymphocyte(s) (*Continued*)
  culture, historical aspects/re-evaluation, **I**.10
  defensin expression, **I**.168
  HCMV infection, **V2**.1448
  Ig-like receptors, viral immune interference,
    I.630
  inhibition
    helminths, **I**.687
    phosphorylcholine, **I**.687
  measles, **I**.805–6
  migration/homing, **I**.503–7, **V2**.1410–11,
    I.503–17
    adhesion molecules, **I**.508 (Tab.)
      CD24 (heat stable antigen), **I**.506–7
      cutaneous lymphocyte-associated
        antigen, **I**.507, **I**.508 (Tab.)
      E-selectin, **I**.506–7, **I**.508 (Tab.)
      leukocyte function antigen-1, **I**.507,
        I.508 (Tab.)
      L-selectin, **I**.506, **I**.508 (Tab.)
      P-selectin, **I**.506–7, **I**.508 (Tab.)
      P-selectin glycoprotein ligand-1, **I**.506–7,
        I.508 (Tab.)
    chemokines, **I**.226–7, **I**.509–12
      CXCR5, **I**.226
    firm adhesion, **I**.507–9
    inflammatory tissue, **I**.512
    integrins
      integrin $\alpha_4\beta_1$ (VLA-4), **I**.507, **I**.508 (Tab.)
      integrin $\alpha_4\beta_7$, **I**.506, **I**.507, **I**.508 (Tab.)
    multistep process, **I**.505, **I**.513 (Fig.)
    Peyer's patches, **I**.511
    routes, **I**.504 (Fig.)
    secondary lymphoid tissue, **I**.511
      antigen-activated lymphocytes, **I**.511
      B cells, **I**.512
      extravasation, **I**.503
      naive lymphocytes, **I**.511
      Th1/Th2 cells, **I**.511–12
    T cells, **I**.226
    tethering/rolling, **I**.505–7
      adhesion molecules, **I**.505
      selectins, **I**.505–6
    see also Diapedesis
    in *Mycoplasma pneumoniae* pneumonia,
      B1.634
    neutrophil interactions, **I**.45 (Fig.)
    passage into CNS in viral infection, **V2**.1410–
      11
    prion diseases *see* Prion diseases
    trafficking to vascular endothelium,
      V2.1410–11, **V2**.1411 (Fig.)
    in urine, **B1**.673
    see also B cell(s); T cell(s)
Lymphocyte-mediated cytotoxicity, **I.471–85**
  anti-tumor defense, **I**.483
  antiviral defence, **I**.483
    infected cell apoptosis, **I**.483
  autoimmunity, **I**.472
  cell self-protection, **I**.477–8
    adhesion ring, **I**.477–8
    perforin half-life, **I**.477–8
    serpins, **I**.477–8
  cell types, **I**.471–2
  cytotoxic granules, **I**.472, **I**.473 (Fig.), **I**.474–7
    Fas ligand, **I**.477

  see also Fas ligand (Fas-L)
    granulysin, **I**.477
    granzymes *see* Granzyme(s)
    killing mechanisms, **I**.479 (Fig.)
    perforin *see* Perforin
    serglycine, **I**.475
    structure, **I**.472–3
  diseases/infection, **I**.481–2
    see also specific diseases/infection
  genetic defects, **I**.480–1
    APC death, **I**.481
    fratricide, **I**.481
    see also specific defects
  killing mechanisms, **I**.474
    adhesion ring, **I**.474 (Fig.)
    apoptosis, **I**.471–2
    surface receptor specificity, **I**.471–2
  target self-death, **I**.478
  see also Cytotoxic T cell(s) (CTLs); Natural
    killer (NK) cells
Lymphocytic choriomeningitis
  acute, **V2**.1072
  animal infection, **V2**.1069–70
    histopathology, **V2**.1068 (Fig.), **V2**.1071
    immune response, **V2**.1072
  chronic infection, **V2**.1071
  clinical features, **V2**.1070
  CNS pathology, **V2**.1073–4
  congenital disease, **V2**.1444 (Tab.), **V2**.1483
  diagnosis, **V2**.1075
  immune response, **V2**.1072–3
    cell-mediated immunity, **V2**.1072
    cytotoxic T cells, **V2**.1072–4
    humoral, **V2**.1412
    immune complexes, **V2**.1073
    NK cells, **I**.96
    T cells, **V2**.1072–3
  immunopathology, **V2**.1073–5
  neonates, **V2**.1411–12
  pathogenesis, animals, **V2**.1071
  plasma viremia, **V1**.242 (Fig.)
  treatment, **V2**.1077
    IFN, **V2**.1073
  vaccine, **V2**.1077
  wasting disease, **V2**.1072
  see also Lymphocytic choriomeningitis virus
    (LCMV) infection
Lymphocytic choriomeningitis virus (LCMV),
    V2.1059
  arenavirus cross-reactivities, **V2**.1069
  cell entry, **V2**.1064–5
  defective interfering (DI) particles, **V2**.1062
  gene expression, **V2**.1065–6
  genome, non-coding regions, **V2**.1066
  glycoprotein (GP), **V2**.1077
  host cell receptors, **V2**.1064–5
  infection *see* Lymphocytic choriomeningitis;
    Lymphocytic choriomeningitis virus
    (LCMV) infection
  LCMV Armstrong, **V2**.1064, **V2**.1074–5
  LCMV Docile, **V2**.1074–5
  LCMV-WE virus, **V2**.1064, **V2**.1074–5
  lysis, **V2**.1073–4
  monoclonal antibodies, **V2**.1069

  nucleic acid localization, **V2**.1075–6,
    V2.1075 (Fig.)
  nucleoprotein (NP), **V2**.1077
  polypeptides, **V2**.1067–8
  reassortant viruses, **V2**.1064
  replication
    host enzymes role, **V2**.1066–7
    host-virus interactions, **V2**.1066
  virulence, **V2**.1064–5
  virus assembly, **V2**.1067 (Fig.)
Lymphocytic choriomeningitis virus (LCMV)
    infection
  CNS, **V1**.304
  diagnosis, isolation from tissue specimens,
    V2.1076 (Tab.)
  epidemiology, **V2**.1060 (Tab.)
  immune response, NK cells, **I**.96–7
  immunopathology, **V1**.279 (Tab.)
    T cells, **V1**.279–80
  immunosuppression, **V2**.1074–5
    cell-mediated immunity, **V2**.1075
    humoral immunity, **V2**.1075
  infectious immune complexes, **V1**.262
  murine model, **V2**.1072
  persistent infection, **V1**.259, **V1**.260 (Fig.),
    V2.1072
    immune complexes, **V2**.1073
    immunosuppression in, **V2**.1074
    immunotherapy, **V2**.1077
  transmission, **V1**.371 (Tab.), **V2**.1070–1
  vaccine, **I**.902, **V2**.1077
  see also Lymphocytic choriomeningitis
Lymphocytic encephalitis, Porcine
    reproductive and respiratory syndrome
    virus infection, **V1**.847
Lymphocytosis, in infectious mononucleosis
    (IM), **V1**.568
Lymphogranuloma venereum (LGV) *see*
    Chlamydia trachomatis infection
Lymphoid cell growth factors, **I**.274 (Tab.),
    I.279–84
Lymphoid interstitial pneumonitis (LIP),
    V2.1505
Lymphoid stem cells (LSCs), **I**.323
Lymphoid tissue, structure/organization,
    I.504–5
Lymphoid tumors, TCR recombination, **I**.454
Lymphokine-activated killer (LAK) cells, **I**.286
Lymphokines *see* Cytokine(s); *individual types*
Lymphoma cells, EBV, **V1**.248–9
Lymphomas
  AIDS-related, **I**.795–6
  BCE peptide vaccines, **I**.861 (Tab.)
  EBV infection in immunosuppressed, **V1**.570
  large-cell, **V1**.570
  pathogenesis, **V1**.341
  T cell in EBV infection, **V1**.571
  see also Hodgkin's disease
Lymphomatoid granulomatosis, histoplasmosis
    capsulati *vs.*, **M**.533
Lymphopenia, measles, **I**.804, **I**.805
Lymphoproliferative assays, rubella, **V2**.981
Lymphoproliferative syndrome, X-linked,
    V1.568
Lymphotactin (XCL1:XCL2)
  dendritic epidermal $\gamma\delta$ T cell, **I**.437

Lymphotactin (XCL1:XCL2) (*Continued*)
  structure, **I**.220
Lymphotoxin *see* Tumor necrosis factor-β
    (TNF-β: lymphotoxin)
Lymphotrophic parvovirus (LPV), species
    infected, **V1**.473
Lymphotropism, prion diseases, **V2**.1380
Lyn tyrosine kinase
  BCR signaling, **I**.342
  structure, **I**.343 (Fig.)
Lysine decarboxylase, Enterobacteriaceae
    identification, **B2**.1319 (Tab.)
Lysine, *Fusobacterium* metabolism, **B2**.1948
Lysins, **B1**.42–3
Lysis centrifugation, of blood cultures, **M**.86
Lysis centrifugation system (ISOLATOR),
    B1.515 (Tab.), **B1**.516
Lysogenic conversion, *Salmonella* O antigen,
    B2.1402–4
Lysosomal cationic proteins *see* Defensins
Lysosomal storage diseases, **I**.31
Lysosomes
  primary, **P**.177
  protozoa, **P**.177
  secondary, **P**.177
Lysostaphin, **B1**.436
Lysozyme, **B1**.294, **B1**.430, **B1**.436,
    B1.437 (Tab.)
  in airway secretion, **B1**.623
  Brucella resistance, **B2**.1723–4
  food, **B1**.267, **B1**.268 (Tab.)
  innate immune response, **B1**.175–6
  innate mucosal immune response, **I**.521
Lyssavirus
  characteristics, **V1**.129 (Tab.)
  classification, **V1**.385, **V2**.1103–4
  genome structure, **V1**.387 (Tab.)
  members, **V1**.385–6
Lyssaviruses
  genome
    pseudogenes, **V2**.1112
    structure, **V2**.1112 (Fig.)
  infection, immune response, **V2**.1115–16
  morphology, **V2**.1106 (Fig.)
Lytic viruses, high titer persistent infection,
    V1.258–9, **V1**.259–60

M1 protein *see* Influenza viruses
M2–1 protein, paramyxoviruses, **V1**.708–9
M2–2 protein, paramyxoviruses, **V1**.708–9
M2 genes, paramyxoviruses, **V1**.700
M2 protein
  influenza virus, **V1**.71
  Influenza virus A *see* Influenza virus A
M2 (matrix) protein, Human respiratory
    syncytial virus, **V1**.787
M2 pyruvate kinase binding, papillomavirus
    E7 protein effects, **V1**.461 (Tab.)
M13 cloning vectors, site-directed mutation,
    B1.89
M27-A2 methodology, **M**.608
Mabthera, licensing, **I**.355 (Tab.)
MacCallum-Goodpasture stain, **M**.123 (Tab.),
    M.124–5
Machupo virus, **V2**.1059
  arenavirus cross-reactivity, **V2**.1069

classification, **V2**.1060–1
geographical distribution/carrier,
    V2.1060 (Tab.)
infection, **V2**.1060 (Tab.)
  animal infection, **V2**.1069–70
  chronic, **V2**.1071
  emerging infection, **V2**.1648 (Tab.)
  immune response, **V2**.1073
  pathogenesis, **V2**.1071
  isolation from tissue specimens,
    V2.1076 (Tab.)
  transmission, **V1**.371–2, **V1**.371 (Tab.),
    V2.1071
Maciel virus, **V2**.1666 (Tab.)
Macracanthorhynchus, **P**.597
  structure, **P**.596 (Fig.)
Macrobroth dilution methods, antifungal
    susceptibility testing, **M**.156, **M**.157
Macrococcus, **B2**.772
Macroglobulin (α_2) *see* α_2-Macroglobulin
Macroglobulinemia, African trypanosomiasis,
    P.365
Macrolides, **B1**.486–7
  cat-scratch disease treatment, **B2**.1898–9
  mode of action, **B1**.487
  pharmacology, **B1**.487
  pharyngitis treatment, **B1**.611
  resistance, **B1**.487
    Bacteroides/Prevotella/Porphyromonas,
      B2.1931
    plasmid-mediated enzymes, **B1**.487
    Staphylococcus, **B2**.794 (Tab.), **B2**.803
  spectrum of activity, **B1**.486–7
    Actinomyces, **B2**.1011
    Borrelia, **B2**.1830
    Brucella, **B2**.1742
    Campylobacter, **B2**.1548
    Lactobacillus, **B2**.866
    Legionella, **B2**.1777
    Mycobacterium avium complex, **B2**.1209,
      B2.1222
    Mycoplasma, **B2**.1992
    Pasteurella multocida, **B2**.1655
  structure, **B1**.486, **B1**.486 (Fig.)
  toxicity/adverse effects, **B1**.487
  see also specific types
Macronucleus, *Balantidium coli*, **P**.276–7,
    P.277 (Fig.), **P**.278 (Fig.)
Macroparasites, **P**.67
  epidemiology *see* Epidemiology of infection,
    parasitic infection
Macrophage(s), **V1**.272–3, **I.21–34**
  activation, **I**.27, **P**.68–9
    adjuvants, **I**.926
    gene expression, **I**.27
    IFN-γ, **I**.27, **I**.288
    IL-3, **I**.275
    IL-4, **I**.27
    IL-12, **I**.27
    IL-13, **I**.27, **I**.294–7
    IL-15, **I**.27
    IL-18, **I**.27
    immune activation, **I**.27
    innate, **I**.27
    M-CSF, **I**.277

antigen presentation, **I**.29–30, **I**.112, **I**.378,
    P.489–90
  CD4 T cells, **I**.394
antimicrobial mechanisms, **I**.25–7, **B1**.624–5
  antibody-dependent cellular cytotoxicity
      (ADCC), **V1**.273
  apoptosis, **I**.27
  cellular activation, **I**.27
  inducible nitric oxide synthase, **I**.26
  ingestion *see below*
  myeloperoxidase, **I**.26
  NADPH oxidase, **I**.26
  pH, **I**.25
  physical barriers, **I**.25
  reactive oxygen intermediates, **I**.26
  superoxide ions, **I**.26
  transferrin receptors, **I**.25
apoptosis
  caspase-1, **I**.137–8
  NF-κB, **I**.138
  Salmonella, **I**.137–8
  SipB, **I**.137
  Yersinia, **I**.138
  YopJ/P, **I**.138
CpG binding/signal transduction, **I**.911
cytokines produced, **I**.27–8, **I**.28 (Tab.),
    V1.272–3, **I**.378, **B1**.624
  G-CSF production, **I**.276
  GM-CSF production, **I**.277
  IFN-γ, **I**.28
  IL-1, **I**.284
  IL-4, **I**.28
  IL-12, **I**.28
  IL-13, **I**.28
  IL-18, **I**.28, **I**.290
  platelet-activating factor production, **I**.191
deactivation, **I**.27
in diseases/infection, **I**.31
  Alzheimer's disease, **I**.31
  amebiasis, **P**.209
  atherosclerosis, **I**.31
  Brucella survival, **B2**.1736
  Burkholderia intracellular infection,
    B2.1615–16
  Chagas disease, **P**.86
  cutaneous/mucocutaneous candidiasis,
    M.261–2
  deficiencies, **I**.31
  granulomas, **I**.31, **I**.31 (Fig.)
  histoplasmosis capsulati, **M**.525,
    M.526 (Fig.), **M**.528–9
  HIV infection, **I**.794–5
  human brucellosis, **B2**.1737
  Leishmania killing, **P**.77
  Listeria monocytogenes infection, **I**.27
  localized inflammation, **I**.31
  lysosomal storage diseases, **I**.31
  malaria, **P**.489–90
  mycobacterial infection, **I**.27
  parasitic infection, **P**.68
  prion diseases, **V2**.1383
  rheumatoid arthritis, **I**.31
  schistosomiasis granulomas, **I**.722–3
  trichomoniasis, **P**.258
  tuberculosis granulomas, **I**.712–13

Macrophage(s)
in diseases/infection (*Continued*)
viral infection, **V1**.273
functions, **B1**.624
homeostasis, **I**.27, **I**.30–1
cell clearance, **I**.31
substrate catalysis, **I**.31
intracellular pathogens, **I**.30, **B1**.625
Francisella tularensis growth, **B2**.1755
Mycobacterium tuberculosis, **I**.30
protozoa inhabiting, **P**.77–80
Leishmania, **P**.283–4
see also individual species
microbial ingestion, **I**.24–5, **I**.26 (Fig.)
coiling phagocytosis, **I**.25
endocytosis, **I**.25, **I**.26 (Fig.)
macropinocytosis, **I**.25, **I**.26 (Fig.)
phagocytosis *see below*
phagosome, **I**.25
transmembrane activation signals, **I**.24
morphology, **I**.22
origins/development, **I**.21–2, **I**.22 (Fig.),
I.113 (Fig.)
cytokines, **I**.21–2
heterogeneity, **I**.22, **I**.23 (Fig.)
integrins, **I**.21
surface markers, **I**.21
oxidative burst, HIV infection, **I**.794–5
pathogen avoidance, **I**.30
pathogen recognition, **I**.22–4
pathogen-associated microbial patterns,
I.22
pattern recognition receptors, **I**.22–3,
I.24 (Tab.)
see also individual types
Peyer's patches, **I**.532, **I**.538
phagocytosis, **I**.24–5, **I**.26 (Fig.), **V1**.273
complement receptors, **I**.25
FcγR, **I**.25
Leishmania, **P**.292–4
pulmonary, **B1**.624
receptors, **I**.22–4
Fcα/μR, **I**.317–18
FcγRI (CD64), **I**.314
FcγRIIa, **I**.314
FcγRIIb, **I**.314
ruffled membranes, **M**.528–9
secreted compounds, **I**.27–9, **P**.68–9
chemokines, **I**.27–9
complement, **I**.27
cytokines *see above*
defensins, **I**.168
5-lipoxygenase, **I**.184
prostacyclins, **I**.189
prostaglandins, **I**.187
thromboxanes, **I**.189
surface markers, NKG2D receptor, **I**.90
therapeutic uses, DNA vaccine priming,
I.916
types
alveolar, **B1**.624–5
dendritic, **B1**.624
interstitial, **B1**.624
intravascular, **B1**.624
mucosa, HIV infection, **I**.799–800

see also Monocyte(s)
Macrophage chemotactic protein (MCP),
V2.1409
Macrophage-colony stimulating factor
(M-CSF), **I**.277
actions/effects, **I**.277
neutrophil development, **I**.36
cryptococcosis therapy, **M**.652–3
HIV replication, **V1**.300
structure, **I**.277
tissue expression, **I**.277
Macrophage inflammatory protein(s) (MIPs)
CNS expression, **V2**.1409
HHV-8 analogues, **V1**.549 (Tab.), **V1**.550
HTLV-1-associated myelopathy/tropical
spastic paraparesis (HAM/TSP),
V2.1429–30
Human respiratory syncytial virus infection,
V1.793–4
Macrophage inflammatory protein 1α (MIP-
1α), **I**.218 (Tab.)
basophils, **I**.64
chemotaxis, **I**.58
histamine release, **I**.62
CD8+ T cells, **I**.793
DNA vaccine co-administration, **I**.912–13,
I.918 (Tab.)
immunogenetics, **I**.582
structure, **I**.217–19, **I**.220
dimerization, **I**.220 (Fig.)
Macrophage inflammatory protein 1β (MIP-1β:
CCL4), **I**.218 (Tab.), **I**.582
structure, **I**.217–19
T cell chemotaxis, **I**.224
Macrophage mannose receptor (MMR), **I**.795
Macrophage migration inhibitory factor (MIF),
I.204, **P**.209
anemia in malaria, **P**.499
histoplasmosis capsulati, **M**.529, **M**.530 (Fig.)
septic shock, **I**.697
Macrophomia phaseolina, **B1**.286–7
Macropinocytosis
DNA vaccine uptake, **I**.913
macrophages, **I**.25, **I**.26 (Fig.)
Macroscopic examination, fecal samples,
P.150–1
MAdCAM-1, lymphocyte migration,
I.508 (Tab.)
'Mad cow disease' *see* Bovine spongiform
encephalopathy (BSE)
Madura foot, **B2**.1159–60
see also Mycetoma
Madurella, **M**.390–1, **M**.392 (Tab.)
Madurella grisea
histopathology, **M**.128 (Tab.)
identification, **M**.89 (Tab.), **M**.390 (Fig.),
M.390 (Tab.), **M**.391, **M**.392 (Tab.)
mycetoma, **M**.388 (Fig.)
Madurella mycetomatis, **M**.27, **M**.28 (Fig.)
geographical distribution, **M**.387
histopathology, **M**.89 (Tab.), **M**.128 (Tab.)
identification, **M**.89 (Tab.), **M**.390–1,
M.390 (Tab.), **M**.392 (Tab.)
ketoconazole therapy, **M**.393
melanin, **M**.387
Maedi-visna virus, **V1**.273
Maggots, bone and joint infection, **B1**.701

MagNA Pure LC, **B1**.725
Magnesium ions, alternative complement
pathway activation, **I**.145
Magnetic resonance imaging (MRI), **I**.360
alveolar echinococcosis, **P**.694
Angiostrongylus cantonensis infection, **P**.806
bone and joint infection, **B1**.694–5,
B1.695 (Fig.)
CNS infection
intracranial abscess diagnosis, **B1**.586–7,
B1.587 (Fig.)
spinal epidural abscess, **B1**.594
subdural empyema, **B1**.591–2, **B1**.592 (Fig.)
cryptococcal meningoencephalitis, **M**.649
in diagnosis, **P**.153
echinococcosis, **P**.694
fascioliasis, **P**.650
fetal HCMV infection, **V2**.1451
neurocysticercosis, **P**.692
VZV infection, **V2**.1457
Main (M) subtype, HIV-1, **V2**.1330–1
Majocchi's dermatophytic granuloma, **M**.186,
M.232
Major basic protein (MBP), **I**.65
Major capsid protein, iridovirus classification,
V1.44
Major facilitator superfamily (MFS), **B1**.440
Major histocompatibility complex (MHC)
activation
IFN-α (IFN-α), **V1**.271
IFN-β (IFN-β), **V1**.271
CD8+ T cell binding, HIV infection, **I**.793
class I *see below*
class II *see below*
class III *see LTA* gene; Tumor necrosis
factor-α (TNF-α), *TNF* gene
CNS expression, **V2**.1409–10, **V2**.1415
genes, autoimmune disease, **I**.751–2
historical aspects/re-evaluation, **I**.12
IFN effects, **V1**.294
immune evasion, **V1**.287
Myxoma virus, **V1**.619
poxviruses, **V1**.619
Trypanosoma, **I**.681–2
viral infection, **I**.472, **I**.640
lack of, NK cell killing mechanism, **I**.472
nonclassic, intraepithelial αβ T cell
recognition, **I**.441
peptide–TCR interactions *see* T-cell receptor
(TCR), MHC–peptide interactions
viral infection, **I**.472
see also Human leukocyte antigens (HLAs)
Major histocompatibility complex (MHC)
class I, **P**.68, **P**.82, **V1**.248, **V2**.1410,
I.403–18
antigen presentation, **I**.29, **V1**.275
bacterial infection, **I**.646–7, **I**.659–60
CD8 T cells, **I**.877
DNA vaccine priming, **I**.914
endothelial cells, **I**.426–7
epithelial cells, **I**.426–7
fibroblasts, **I**.426–7
Ib molecule, **I**.29
Listeria vaccine vector, **I**.845
live vaccines, **I**.902

Major histocompatibility complex (MHC)
class I (*Continued*)
  antigen processing, **V1**.275, **I**.405–15,
    I.409 (Fig.), **I**.425 (Fig.), **I**.426–7
    MHC class II *vs.,* **I**.380
    viral antigens, **I**.419–20
  assembly/surface expression, **I**.408–9
    β2-microglobulin, **I**.405, **I**.408–9, **I**.428–9
    IFN-γ effects, **I**.288
    Langerhans' cells, **I**.821
    Nef downregulation, **I**.789
  cell expression, **I**.29
  in exosomes, **I**.415
  immune evasion, **V1**.321–2
    bacterial infection, **I**.659–60
    viruses, **I**.420
    see also Immune evasion, viruses
  induction, lymphotoxin, **I**.286–7
  ISCOMs adjuvant, **I**.930
  Ly49 receptor binding, **I**.89
  Nef down regulation, **I**.793
  NK cells, **I**.88, **I**.88 (Fig.)
  peptide binding, **I**.406–8, **I**.428–9
    binding motifs, **I**.407 (Tab.)
    binding rules, **I**.406–7
    endosomal targeting, **I**.415
    exogenous, **I**.407–8
    experimental determination, **I**.406–7
    generation, **I**.409–10
      see also Antigen processing; Ubiquitin–
      proteasome pathway
    proteasome role, **I**.412
    T cell binding, **I**.429
  Salmonella vaccine vector, **I**.899–901
  smoldering infection, **V1**.261–2
  structure, **I**.405–6, **I**.405 (Fig.)
    α3 domain, **I**.405
    β2-microglobulin, **I**.405
  SV40 binding, **V1**.473–4
  virosome vaccines, **I**.838
Major histocompatibility complex (MHC) class
  II, **P**.68, **I**.379–81, **V2**.1410
  antigen presentation, **I**.29, **V1**.274–5, **I**.555,
    I.375–87
    bacterial infection, **I**.646–7, **I**.657–9
    BCG vaccine vector, **I**.844
    CD4 T cells *see* CD4+ T-cell(s)
    heat labile enterotoxin interference, **I**.659
  antigen processing, **V1**.274–5, **I**.382–3
    MHC class I *vs.,* **I**.380
  bare lymphocyte syndrome, **I**.575
  CD4 T cells/APC interactions, **I**.392 (Fig.)
  cell expression, **I**.29
  CNS expression, **V2**.1410
  eosinophils, **I**.67
  expression
    adjuvant effects, **I**.926
    CpG adjuvant effects, **I**.931
    IFN-γ actions, **I**.820–1
    IL-10 effects, **I**.292–3
    keratinocytes, **I**.820–1
    Langerhans' cells, **I**.821
  genetics, **I**.379
  immune evasion, **V1**.322
    bacterial infection, **I**.657–9

  peptide binding, **I**.380
    affinity, **I**.380–1
    sequence motifs, **I**.381
    T cell binding, **I**.380, **I**.381
  polymorphism, **I**.379–80
  pyrogenic exotoxin binding, **I**.558–9
  structure, **I**.29, **I**.380, **I**.405 (Fig.)
  superantigen binding, **B1**.157, **I**.463, **I**.558–9
    TCR interactions, **I**.559–60
  virosome vaccines, **I**.838
Major outer membrane protein (MOMP),
  Chlamydia, **B2**.2007, **B2**.2008–9
  serovars, **B2**.2018
Major surface glycoproteins (MSGs)
  arteriviruses *see* Arteriviruses
  Equine arteritis virus, **V1**.838
  Lactate dehydrogenase-elevating virus,
    V1.838
  Pneumocystis, **M**.774, **M**.775, **M**.792
  Porcine reproductive and respiratory
    syndrome virus, **V1**.838
Major surface proteins, *Toxoplasma gondii*
  antigens, **P**.428
Malabsorption
  giardiasis, **P**.245–6
  Mycobacterium avium complex infection,
    B2.1209
  Strongyloides, **P**.740
Malaria, **P**.464–528
  'airport ,' **P**.29, **P**.511, **P**.514–15
  anemia, **P**.498–9, **P**.501 (Tab.)
    dyserythropoiesis, **P**.499
    erythrophagocytosis, **P**.499
    macrophage inhibitory factor, **P**.499
    mechanisms, **P**.495
  'baggage,' **P**.511, **P**.514–15
  Burkitt lymphoma (BL) and, **V1**.570
    risk, **V1**.349
  causative organisms, **P**.188–9, **P**.464
    see also under Plasmodium
  cerebral, **P**.481–2
    in children, **P**.482–3
    coma, **P**.498
    hypoglycemia, **P**.483
    lymphotoxin, **P**.495
    neurological damage, **P**.498
    nitric oxide role, **P**.83–4
    opisthotonos, **P**.483, **P**.483 (Fig.)
    pathology/pathophysiology, **P**.498,
      P.499 (Fig.)
    retinal hemorrhages, **P**.481, **P**.481 (Fig.)
    T helper cells, type 1, **P**.498
    tumor necrosis factor-α, **P**.498
  chemoprophylaxis, **P**.510
    community level, **P**.510
    in pregnancy, **P**.510
    principles, **P**.510
  chemotherapy, **P**.506–10
    amodiaquine, **P**.506
    atovaquone–proguanil, **P**.506
    chloroquine, **P**.506
    combination therapy, **P**.506–8
    costs of, **P**.34
    failure definitions, **P**.511 (Tab.)
    halofantrine, **P**.506

    intermittent presumptive treatment,
      P.493–4
    lapudrine–dapsone, **P**.506
    mefloquine, **P**.506
    pryronaridine, **P**.506
    qinghaosu, **P**.128
    quinine, **P**.506
    sulfadoxine–pyrimethamine, **P**.506
    tafenoquine, **P**.506
    treatment protocols, **P**.507 (Tab.),
      P.508 (Tab.), **P**.509 (Tab.), **P**.510 (Tab.)
  in children, **P**.482–4
    adults *vs.,* **P**.483 (Tab.)
    anemia, **P**.482–3
    economic costs, **P**.36
    Kussmaul breathing, **P**.484
    metabolic acidosis, **P**.482–4
    retinal hemorrhages, **P**.482
    splenomegaly, **P**.482
  circumsporozoite protein, **I**.676, **I**.681
    peptide vaccine design, **I**.873, **I**.874
    T-helper cell epitope, **I**.862 (Tab.)
  clinical aspects, **P**.480–4, **I**.676
    anemia *see above*
    autoimmunity, **P**.501 (Tab.)
    Burkitt's lymphoma, **P**.501 (Tab.)
    clinical manifestations, **P**.480–2
    hyperactive malarial splenomegaly *see*
      Hyperactive malarial splenomegaly
      (tropical splenomegaly syndrome)
    hypergammaglobulinemia, **P**.501 (Tab.)
    hypogammaglobulinemia, **P**.488
    immunosuppression, **P**.501 (Tab.)
    kwashiorkor, **P**.493
    malnutrition, **P**.493
    nephrotic syndrome, **P**.501 (Tab.)
    riboflavin (vitamin B2) deficiency, **P**.493
    thrombocytopenia, **P**.501 (Tab.)
    tropical splenomegaly syndrome *see*
      Hyperactive malarial splenomegaly
      (tropical splenomegaly syndrome)
    vitamin A deficiency, **P**.493
    zinc deficiency, **P**.493
  control, **P**.36–7, **P**.38 (Tab.), **P**.517–19,
    P.518 (Fig.)
    African Initiative on Malaria, **P**.518
    chemotherapy/chemoprophylaxis,
      P.144 (Tab.)
    community participation, **P**.124, **P**.517
    conflict-related effects, **P**.107 (Tab.)
    costs, **P**.36–7
    DDT, **P**.517
    diagnosis, **P**.129, **P**.143 (Tab.)
    efficacy, **P**.36
    historical aspects, **P**.517
    insecticide-impregnated bednets, **P**.517
    insecticides, **P**.517
    Medicines for Malaria Venture, **P**.110,
      P.518
    Multilateral Initiative on Malaria, **P**.110,
      P.518
    primary health care, **P**.517–18
    Roll Back Malaria *see* Roll Back Malaria
    stratification of disease, **P**.115, **P**.131 (Tab.)
    Vector Control Research Centre, **P**.124

Malaria
  control (*Continued*)
    vector/reservoir control, **P**.109, **P**.125–6, **P**.145 (Tab.)
  diagnosis, **P**.500–6
    blood films, **P**.152, **P**.501 (Fig.)
    clinical diagnosis, **P**.500–1
    DNA hybridization, **P**.504
    drug-resistance, **P**.150, **P**.154
    epidemiology, **P**.500, **P**.505–6
    immunoassays, **P**.154, **P**.488, **P**.503–4, **P**.504 (Fig.)
      see also individual assays
    immunofluorescence antibody test, **P**.488, **P**.503 (Fig.)
    indirect hemagglutination assay, **P**.503
    latex agglutination assays, **P**.503
    method applicability, **P**.505
    method appraisal, **P**.505
    molecular biology, **P**.504–5, **P**.505 (Fig.)
    parasitemia, **P**.500–1
    parasitological methods, **P**.501–3, **P**.501 (Fig.)
    PCR see Polymerase chain reaction (PCR)
    quantitative buffy coat see Quantitative buffy coat (QBC), malaria diagnosis
    radioimmunoassay see Radioimmunoassays (RIAs)
    returning travelers, **P**.149
    RNA hybridization, **P**.504
    transfusion malaria, **P**.27–9, **P**.505–6
  differential diagnosis, **P**.500, **P**.502 (Tab.)
    babesiosis, **P**.454
  drug resistance, **P**.509–10
    babesiosis vs, **P**.458
    mechanisms, **P**.509
    monitoring, **P**.509
    see also Plasmodium, drug resistance
  epidemics, **P**.34, **P**.142 (Tab.)
  epidemiology, **P**.46 (Tab.), **P**.511–15
    agricultural development projects, **P**.34, **P**.512–13
    anthropogenic change effects, **P**.34, **P**.36, **P**.145 (Tab.)
    climate change effects, **P**.103–6, **P**.512–13
    clinico-epidemiological approach, **P**.513
    conceptual diagrams, **P**.513, **P**.515 (Fig.)
    conflict, **P**.34, **P**.513–14
    deforestation, **P**.34, **P**.512–13
    Duffy blood group determinants polymorphisms, **P**.512
    ecological classification, **P**.513
    environmental effects, **P**.512–13
    epidemic malaria, **P**.34, **P**.513–14
    Garki project, **P**.512–13
    geographical distribution, **P**.34, **P**.35 (Fig.), **P**.464, **P**.465 (Fig.)
    geographic information systems, **P**.512–13
    HIV infection, **P**.513
    host effects, **P**.512
    imported malaria, **P**.514–15
    incubation periods, **P**.511
    migration, **P**.513–14
    non-endemic transmission, **P**.511, **P**.514–15
    nutrition effects, **P**.512
    parasite effects, **P**.511

    parasite life span, **P**.511
    Plasmodium falciparum: P. vivax ratios, **P**.145 (Tab.)
    pre-patency period, **P**.511
    prevalence in UK, **P**.515 (Fig.)
    prevalence vs. age, **P**.58 (Fig.)
    reinfection, **P**.471 (Fig.)
    stable populations, **P**.36
    stable vs. unstable, **P**.512 (Tab.), **P**.513
    stratification, **P**.513
    vector effects, **P**.512
    world prevalence, **P**.33–4, **P**.464
  falciparum (malignant tertian), **P**.464, **P**.480–2
    anemia, **P**.481
    blood film diagnosis, **P**.152
    cerebral see Above, cerebral
    complications, **P**.482 (Tab.)
    hemoglobinuria, **P**.482
    hypoglycemia, **P**.481–2
    immune response, **P**.81, **P**.82–5, **I**.938–9
      neutrophils, **I**.39–40, **I**.43, **I**.44
    management, **P**.507 (Tab.), **P**.509 (Tab.)
    natural history effects, **P**.148–9
    parasitemia levels, **P**.473–4
    pulmonary edema, **P**.482
    renal dysfunction, **P**.481
    retinal hemorrhages, **P**.480–1
  gametocytogenesis induction, **P**.468
  historical aspects, **P**.16–7
  HLA associations, **I**.379–80, **I**.598
    HLA-B5, **I**.598
    HLA-B53, **I**.598–9
    HLA-DQB1, **I**.598
    HLA-DRB1, **I**.598–9
    HLA-DRB5, **I**.598
  hyperendemic, **V1**.570
  immune response, **P**.74, **P**.81–5, **P**.485–95, **P**.489 (Fig.)
    acquired immunity, **P**.486
    AIDS interactions, **P**.494–5
    antibodies, **P**.488–9
    antibody-dependent cellular cytotoxicity, **P**.490
    antibody-dependent cellular inhibition, **P**.489
    anti-disease immunity, **P**.486, **P**.492–3
    antigens involved, **P**.82–3, **P**.486, **P**.488, **P**.487 (Tab.)
    CD8 T cell responses, **I**.420
    chemoprophylaxis effects, **P**.493–4
    C-reactive protein, **P**.490
    CTLs, **P**.82, **P**.490
    cytokines, **P**.490–1
      see also individual cytokines
    development, **P**.53–4, **P**.54 (Fig.), **P**.514 (Fig.)
    epidemiological evidence, **P**.488
    gametocyte stage, **P**.83
    IFN-γ, **P**.490–1, **I**.599
    IL-1, **P**.490–1
    IL-4, **P**.491
    IL-6, **P**.490
    IL-10, **P**.491
    immunodepression, **P**.97
    innate resistance, **P**.485–6

    liver-stage antigens, **P**.82, **P**.83, **P**.84–5
    lymphotoxin, **P**.491
    macrophages, **P**.489–90
    maternal immunity transfer, **P**.486
    merozoite stage, **P**.82–3
    NK cell actions, **I**.100
    nutritional status, **P**.493
    opsonization, **P**.489
    protective immunity, **I**.676
    reactive oxygen intermediates, **P**.490–1
    soluble mediators, **P**.490–1
    sporozoite antigens, **P**.82, **P**.84
    sterile immunity, **P**.486
    T cells, **P**.82, **P**.490
    γδ T cells, **P**.490, **P**.496
    T helper cells, **P**.83
    T helper cells, type 1, **P**.490–1
    T helper cells, type 2, **P**.491
    transmission-blocking immunity, **P**.488
    tumor necrosis factor-α, **P**.490–1
  immunogenetics, **I**.597–600
    animal models, **I**.598
    CD31 gene, **I**.600
    CD36, **I**.599–600
    CD36 gene, **I**.599–600
    Duffy blood group, **I**.599
    hemoglobin S association, **I**.598
    ICAM1 gene, **I**.599–600
    IFNGR1 gene, **I**.599
    TNF gene, **I**.598–9
  'imported,' **P**.514–15
  inducible nitric oxide synthase, **I**.599
  intensity vs. age, **P**.58 (Fig.)
    behavioral changes, **P**.57
  malariae (quartan), **P**.464, **P**.475
    clinical manifestations, **P**.482
    immune response, **I**.938–9
    nephrotic syndrome, **P**.482
    treatment, **P**.510 (Tab.)
  morbidity, **P**.26 (Fig.)
    costs of, **P**.34, **P**.36
  mortality, **P**.26 (Fig.), **P**.28 (Tab.), **P**.29 (Tab.), **P**.34
    costs of, **P**.34, **P**.36
  parasite aggregation, **P**.55–6
  parasitemia waves, **P**.471
  past infection effects, **P**.54, **P**.54 (Fig.)
  pathology/pathophysiology, **P**.495–500
    anemia, **P**.498–9
    cytoadherence receptor upregulation, **P**.496–7
    cytokine production induction, **P**.496
    direct effects, **P**.495
    IL-1, **P**.495–6
    IL-6, **P**.495–6
    immunopathology, **P**.500, **P**.501 (Tab.)
    indirect effects, **P**.495–7
    malarial paroxysm, **P**.497–8
    oxygen-derived free radicals, **P**.497
    species specific, **P**.497–500
    T helper cells, type 1, **P**.496
    tumor necrosis factor-α, **P**.495–6, **P**.496 (Fig.), **P**.497–8
  in pregnancy
    chemoprophylaxis, **P**.510

Malaria
  in pregnancy (*Continued*)
    clinical aspects, **P**.484
    hyperactive malarial splenomegaly, **P**.484
    hypoglycemia, **P**.484
    pathology/pathophysiology, **P**.499–500
    pulmonary edema, **P**.484, **P**.484 (Fig.)
    treatment, **P**.506
    vertical transmission, **P**.484
  premunition, **P**.493
  public health importance, **P**.25, **P**.33–7,
    P.105 (Tab.)
  recrudescences, **P**.471, **P**.471 (Fig.), **P**.475
    long-term survival, **P**.471
    relapses *vs.*, **P**.471
  'refeeding,' **P**.493
  relapses, **P**.471, **P**.471 (Fig.)
    hypnozoites, **P**.471
    recrudescences *vs.*, **P**.471
  ring-infected erythrocyte surface antigen,
    P.488–9, **I**.873, **I**.874
  susceptibility, **P**.485–6
  'taxi-rank,' **P**.511, **P**.514–15
  thrombospondin-related anonymous protein,
    I.873
  transmission, **B1**.354–5
    theories, **B1**.336–7
  vaccines/vaccination, **P**.84–5, **B1**.355,
    P.515–17, **I**.901–2
    antigens, **P**.486
    attenuated viral vectors, **I**.846
    BCE peptide vaccines, **I**.855 (Tab.), **I**.873,
      I.874
    BCG vectors, **I**.901–2
    blood stage targets, **P**.84–5, **P**.515–16
    'cocktail' vaccines, **P**.84, **P**.516–17
    development, **P**.84–5, **I**.938–9
    development status, **I**.933 (Tab.)
    DNA vaccines, **I**.920–1
    liver stage targets, **P**.84
    MPL/QS-21 adjuvant, **I**.930
    peptide *see* Peptide vaccines
    'prime-boost immunization,' **I**.846
    recombinant antigens, **P**.516–17
    Salmonella vectors, **I**.842–3
    sexual stage target, **P**.85
    Spf66, **P**.85, **P**.516–17
    sporozoite target, **P**.84, **P**.516–17
    subunit vaccine development, **I**.938,
      I.940–1
    synthetic antigens, **P**.516–17
    targets, **P**.84–5, **P**.515–17, **P**.516 (Fig.)
    transmission-blocking, **P**.515–16
    virosome vaccines, **I**.839
  vector control, **B1**.354–5
  vectors *see* Anopheles
  vivax/ovale (benign tertian), **P**.464, **P**.474–5
    blood films, **P**.152
    clinical manifestations, **P**.482
    febrile paroxysms, **P**.482
    immune response, **I**.938–9
    incubation period, **P**.482
    malarial paroxysm, **P**.497
    splenic rupture, **P**.482
    thrombocytopenia, **P**.482
    treatment, **P**.510 (Tab.)

  see also Plasmodium
Malariae malaria *see* Malaria
Malarial paroxysm, **P**.497–8
Malarone® (Atovaquone®-proguanil),
  P.506
Malassezia, **M**.202–3
  characteristics, **M**.203–9, **M**.631–2,
    M.632 (Tab.)
  classification, **M**.63, **M**.65 (Tab.)
  cultures, **M**.204, **M**.205 (Fig.)
    maintenance in collections, **M**.208–9
  definition, **M**.202
  ecology, **M**.209
  growth requirements, **M**.204
    lipids, **M**.205–6
  history, **M**.14–5, **M**.202
  identification, **M**.203, **M**.203 (Fig.),
    M.204 (Fig.), **M**.205 (Fig.)
    amplified fragment length polymorphisms,
      M.215–16
    molecular methods, **M**.214–16
    new species, **M**.206–7
    pulsed field gel electrophoresis, **M**.215
    random amplified polymorphic DNA,
      M.215
    restriction fragment length polymorphism,
      M.215
    ribosomal DNA sequencing, **M**.215
    ribosomal RNA sequencing, **M**.215
    in vitro, **M**.203
    in vivo, **M**.204, **M**.216
  infection *see Malassezia* infection
  phylogeny, **M**.202–3
  taxonomy, **M**.202–3, **M**.208–9
  typing, **M**.215
Malassezia dermatis
  atopic dermatitis, **M**.213
  culture, **M**.206–7
  identification, **M**.206–7
Malassezia furfur
  culture, **M**.204–5, **M**.205 (Fig.)
    collections, **M**.208–9
  ecology, **M**.209
  history, **M**.14–5, **M**.15 (Fig.)
  identification, **M**.204–5, **M**.205 (Fig.)
    histopathology, **M**.89 (Tab.), **M**.128 (Tab.),
      M.138 (Fig.)
    molecular methods, **M**.215
  infection, **M**.626
    amphotericin B therapy, **M**.627
    atopic dermatitis, **M**.213
    catheter colonization, **M**.626–7
    fungemia, **M**.626–7
    onychomycosis, **M**.214
    pityriasis versicolor, **M**.210, **M**.211
    seborrheic dermatitis, **M**.212
  morphology, dimorphism, **M**.74
  taxonomy, **M**.202–3
  var. *orbiculare*, **M**.14–5
  var. *ovale*, **M**.14–5
Malassezia globosa
  ecology, **M**.209
  identification, **M**.205 (Fig.), **M**.207,
    M.207 (Fig.), **M**.216
  culture, **M**.205 (Fig.), **M**.207
  molecular methods, **M**.215

  infection
    atopic dermatitis, **M**.213
    folliculitis, **M**.213
    pityriasis versicolor, **M**.210, **M**.210 (Fig.),
      M.211 (Fig.)
    seborrheic dermatitis, **M**.212
  taxonomy, **M**.202–3
Malassezia infection, **M**.185, **M**.203, **M**.209–14,
  M.625 (Tab.), **M**.626
  blepharitis, **M**.296–7
  catheters, **M**.626–7
  conjunctivitis, **M**.299
  folliculitis, **M**.213
    heart transplants, **M**.213
  fungemia, **M**.626–7
  immune response, **M**.211, **M**.212
  neonatal pustulosis, **M**.214
  oculomycoses, **M**.280 (Tab.), **M**.286–7
  therapy, **M**.183 (Tab.)
    azoles, **M**.182–3
    selenium sulfide, **M**.185
    tolnaftate, **M**.185
  see also specific infection
Malassezia obtusa
  culture, **M**.205 (Fig.), **M**.207
  ecology, **M**.209
  identification, **M**.205 (Fig.), **M**.207
  taxonomy, **M**.202–3
Malassezia pachydermatis, **M**.14–5, **M**.626,
  M.627, **M**.631–2
  culture, **M**.205–6
    collections, **M**.208–9
  ecology, **M**.209
  identification, **M**.205–6, **M**.206 (Fig.)
    molecular methods, **M**.215, **M**.216
  infection
    amphotericin B therapy, **M**.627
    otitis externa, **M**.247–8
    otitis in dogs, **M**.214
  taxonomy, **M**.202–3
Malassezia restricta
  culture, **M**.205 (Fig.), **M**.208
  ecology, **M**.209
  identification, **M**.205 (Fig.), **M**.207, **M**.216
  infection
    atopic dermatitis, **M**.213
    seborrheic dermatitis, **M**.212
  taxonomy, **M**.202–3
Malassezia slooffiae
  culture, **M**.205 (Fig.), **M**.206, **M**.208
    collections, **M**.208–9
  identification, **M**.205 (Fig.), **M**.206, **M**.208,
    M.208 (Fig.)
    molecular methods, **M**.215
  infection
    pityriasis versicolor, **M**.210
    seborrheic dermatitis, **M**.212
  taxonomy, **M**.202–3
Malassezia sympodialis, **M**.14–5, **M**.202, **M**.626,
  M.627
  culture, **M**.205 (Fig.), **M**.206
    collections, **M**.208–9
  ecology, **M**.209

Malassezia sympodialis, (Continued)
  identification, **M**.205 (Fig.), **M**.206, **M**.206 (Fig.), **M**.207 (Fig.)
    molecular methods, **M**.215
  infection
    AIDS, **M**.627
    atopic dermatitis, **M**.213
    neonatal pustulosis, **M**.214
    otitis, **M**.214
    pityriasis versicolor, **M**.210
    seborrheic dermatitis, **M**.212
  taxonomy, **M**.202–3
Malassezia tropica, **M**.211
Malassez, L, **M**.14–5
Malate, production, **B1**.53
Malate synthase, **B1**.53–4
MALDI-TOF mass spectrometry, **B1**.25
Males, rubella vaccination programs, **V2**.982
Male worms, *Onchocerca volvulus,* **P**.782
Malignant catarrhal fever virus, **V2**.1651 (Tab.)
Malignant external otitis, **B1**.618
Malignant melanoma
  metastases *see* Metastatic malignant melanoma
  TCE peptide vaccines, **I**.865 (Tab.), **I**.877
  therapy, IFN-α, **I**.258
Malignant tertian malaria *see* Malaria; Malaria, falciparum (malignant tertian)
Malinowski medium, **B2**.1436
Malleobactin, *Burkholderia thailandensis,* **B2**.1624
Malmstein, Petr Henrik, **P**.275
Malnutrition
  enterovirus infection, **V2**.870
  malaria, **P**.493
  measles, **I**.804
  neutrophil abnormalities, **I**.49
Malonate utilization, Enterobacteriaceae identification, **B2**.1319 (Tab.)
Malpighi, M, **M**.6, **M**.20
Maltese cross, *Babesia,* **P**.456–7
Malt extract agar, **M**.662
Maltose fermentation, Enterobacteriaceae identification, **B2**.1319 (Tab.)
Mamastrovirus, **V1**.53
Mammalian cells, orbivirus replication, **V2**.940
Mammals, aquatic, morbillivirus infection, **V1**.812–15
Mammastrovirus
  classification, **V2**.890 (Tab.)
  sequence phylogeny, **V2**.900 (Fig.)
Mammomonogamus, **P**.595
Manganese, terminal electron acceptor, **B1**.67
Mannans, **M**.93 (Tab.)
  Candida, **M**.587, **M**.590–1, **M**.607
  Candida albicans, **M**.99
  Candida glabrata, **M**.99
  Candida krusei, **M**.99
  Candida parapsilosis, **M**.99
  Candida tropicalis, **M**.99
Mannheimia, **B2**.1653, **B2**.1658, **B2**.1658 (Tab.)
  classification, **B2**.1650, **B2**.1653
  habitats, **B2**.1649–50
  species, **B2**.1658, **B2**.1658 (Tab.)
  taxonomy, **B2**.1650–3

Mannheimia glucosida, **B2**.1658 (Tab.)
  classification, **B2**.1653
Mannheimia granulomatis, **B2**.1658 (Tab.)
  classification, **B2**.1653
Mannheimia haemolytica, **B2**.1658 (Tab.)
  classification, **B2**.1653
  infection, **I**.173
    in animals, **B2**.1654
  virulence factors, **B2**.1653–4
    fibrogen-binding proteins, **B2**.1654
    leukotoxin, **B2**.1654
Mannheimia ruminalis, **B2**.1658 (Tab.)
  classification, **B2**.1653
Mannheimia varigena, **B2**.1658 (Tab.)
  classification, **B2**.1653
D-Mannitol
  Aspergillus, **M**.713
  fermentation, Enterobacteriaceae identification, **B2**.1319 (Tab.)
Mannitol cycle, *Cryptosporidium parvum,* **P**.403
Mannose-binding lectin (MBL), **I**.143 (Tab.), **V1**.273
  acute phase response, **I**.200
  classical complement pathway, **V1**.273
  deficiency, **I**.152
  gene *see MBL* gene
  immunogenetics, **I**.579–80
  lectin pathway activation, **I**.144 (Fig.), **I**.145–6, **I**.145 (Fig.)
  microbial recognition, **I**.24 (Tab.)
  polymorphisms, **I**.580
  septic shock, **I**.697–8
  structure, **I**.201 (Fig.)
Mannose binding protein-associated serine protease (MASP), **I**.143 (Tab.), **I**.200
  lectin pathway activation, **I**.144 (Fig.), **I**.145–6, **I**.145 (Fig.)
  septic shock, **I**.697–8
D-Mannose fermentation, Enterobacteriaceae identification, **B2**.1319 (Tab.)
Mannose monomycolate, **I**.443 (Fig.)
Mannose-resistance and eluting hemagglutinins (MREHA), **B2**.1399
Mansonella, **P**.591
  structure/life cycle, **P**.591
Manson, Patrick, **P**.4, **P**.9–11
  loiasis, **P**.10
Mantel-Haenszel method, **B1**.316
M antigen, *Brucella melitensis* LPS, **B2**.1725, **B2**.1726 (Fig.)
Mantoux test, **B1**.746
Manubrium, microsporidians, **P**.529–31
Manufacturing practices
  airborne bacteria, **B1**.186 (Tab.)
  bioremediation, **B1**.201–2
MAP kinases, yeasts, **M**.73
  virulence, **M**.79–80
Maporal virus, **V2**.1666 (Tab.)
MA protein *see* HIV
Marantic endocarditis, **B1**.526–7
Marburg virus (MARV), **I**.6–7, **V1**.744
  animal models, **V2**.1095
  cell culture, **V2**.1091–2
    artificial replication systems, **V2**.1093
  cellular receptor, **V2**.1092

  classification, **V1**.48, **V1**.382–3, **V2**.1086
    biosafety level 4, **V2**.1526
  epidemiology, **V2**.1093
  genome structure, **V1**.387 (Tab.), **V2**.1088, **V2**.1088 (Fig.)
    gene overlap, **V2**.1088
  glycoprotein (GP), **V2**.1089–90
    transcription, **V2**.1093
  historical aspects, **V2**.1085
  infection
    emerging infection, **V2**.1648 (Tab.)
    laboratory-acquired infection, **V2**.1517 (Tab.)
    outbreaks, **V2**.1085–6, **V2**.1087 (Tab.)
    risk categorization, **B1**.762
    transmission, **V1**.371 (Tab.)
  infectivity, particle size, **V2**.1086
  large (L) protein, **V2**.1091
  morphology/structure, **V1**.75 (Fig.), **V2**.1088 (Fig.)
    nucleocapsids, **V1**.71
  nucleoprotein (NP), **V2**.1086–8
  VP24, **V2**.1091
  VP30 (minor nucleoprotein), **V2**.1090–1
  VP35 (polymerase cofactor), **V2**.1089
  VP40 (matrix protein), **V2**.1089
Mardivirus, **V1**.494 (Tab.)
Marek's disease virus type 1, **V1**.494 (Tab.)
Marek's disease virus type 2, **V1**.494 (Tab.)
Maribavir (1263W94)
  HCMV therapy, **V2**.1619
  structure, **V2**.1619 (Fig.)
Marinibacillus, **B2**.922–3
Marker rescue, **V1**.189
Marker rescue mapping, **V1**.615–16
Marmoset lymphocryptovirus, **V1**.494 (Tab.)
Marshallagia, **P**.595
Mason–Pfizer monkey virus
  cell interactions, **V1**.221
  envelope antigens, **V2**.1311
MASP *see* Mannose binding protein-associated serine protease (MASP)
Mass action model and assumption, **B1**.337, **B1**.342
Mass culture, *Coxiella burnetii,* **B2**.2074
Mass screening programs, cystic echinococcosis, **P**.688
Mass treatment strategies, parasite control, **P**.128
Mastadenovirus, **V1**.45
Mastadenoviruses, **V1**.439
Mast cell(s)
  airway hypersensitivity, **I**.731–2, **I**.735
  cytokines produced, **I**.735
    GM-CSF, **I**.277
    IL-3, **I**.275
    IL-4, **I**.280
    IL-5, **I**.277
    IL-13, **I**.294
  leukotriene B$_4$, **I**.185
  prostacyclin, **I**.189
  prostaglandin, **I**.187
  differentiation, IL-9 effects, **I**.282
  FcεRI, **I**.308, **I**.316
  leukotriene C$_4$ synthase, **I**.184
  5-lipoxygenase, **I**.184

Mast cell(s) (*Continued*)
  proliferation
    IL-3 effects, **I**.275
    IL-4 effects, **I**.275
    IL-10 effects, **I**.293–4
    SCF, **I**.275
  septic shock, **I**.699–700
  Th1/Th2 differentiation, **I**.399
Mast cell growth factor (c-kit ligand) *see* Stem
    cell factor (SCF: *c-kit*)
Mastitis, **B1**.230, **B1**.239, **B1**.244–5
  Arcobacter, **B2**.1557
  bovine, **M**.399–400, **M**.407
    protothecal, **M**.399–400, **M**.407
  Campylobacter, **B2**.1550
  candidiasis, **M**.602
  Mycobacterium smegmatis, **B2**.1261
Mastocytosis, IL-15, **I**.282
Mastoiditis, **B1**.617–18
  acute, pathogenesis, **B1**.617
  rapidly growing mycobacteria, **B2**.1253,
    B2.1255
  subdural empyema, **B1**.590, **B1**.591 (Tab.)
Mastomys, arenaviruses associated,
    V2.1060 (Tab.), **V2**.1061
Matakieff, E, **M**.14–5, **M**.15 (Fig.)
Maternal antibodies, fetal infection
    transmission, **V2**.1443–4
Maternal immunity transfer, malaria, **P**.486
Maternal rubella *see* Rubella
Maternal transmission routes, definition,
    I.951 (Tab.)
Mathematical Identification, **B1**.20,
    B1.21 (Tab.)
Mathematical models
  definition, **I**.947
  infection *see* Infection(s), mathematical
    models
  vaccination *see* Vaccination, mathematical
    models
Mathevotaenia, **P**.577
Mating studies, *Emmonsia*, **M**.819–20
Matrilysin *see* Matrix metalloproteinase-7
    (MMP-7)
Matrix-assisted laser desorption ionization-
    time-of-flight (MALDI-TOF) mass
    spectrometry, **B1**.25
Matrix metalloproteinase(s) (MMPs)
  Burkholderia, **B2**.1615
  EDTA-sensitive, in *Proteus*, **B2**.1440
  HTLV-1-associated myelopathy/tropical
    spastic paraparesis (HAM/TSP),
    V2.1429–30
  tuberculosis granulomas, **I**.717
Matrix metalloproteinase-7 (MMP-7)
  α-defensin biosynthesis, **I**.170
  defensin induction, **I**.520–1
Matrix (M) proteins
  Avian pneumovirus, **V1**.788–9
  Borna disease virus *see* Borna disease virus
    (BDV)
  coronaviruses, **V1**.76
  Ebola virus, **V1**.69–70
  filoviruses, **V1**.75–6
  Human metapneumovirus, **V1**.788–9
  Human respiratory syncytial virus, **V1**.787
  influenza virus, **V1**.69–70

Mumps virus, **V1**.746, **V1**.746 (Tab.)
  orthomyxoviruses, **V1**.71
  paramyxoviruses, **V1**.703, **V1**.705
  Rabies virus, **V2**.1114
  rhabdoviruses *see* Rhabdoviruses
  Vesicular stomatitis virus *see* Vesicular
    stomatitis virus (VSV)
  VSV, **V1**.69–70
Matzinger, Polly, **I**.13
Maurer's clefts, **P**.468, **P**.469 (Fig.)
  Plasmodium classification, **P**.464
Maximum Likelihood (ML), **M**.47–8
Maximum Parsimony (MP), **M**.48
Mayaro virus (MAYV), **V2**.1011 (Tab.),
    V2.1023
  emerging infection, **V2**.1662
Mayer's mucicarmine stain, **M**.123 (Tab.),
    M.124
Mayonnaise, bloody diarrhea outbreak, **B1**.279
MBL2 gene, **I**.600–1
MBL-associated serine proteases (MASPs) *see*
    Mannose binding protein-associated
    serine protease (MASP)
MBL gene
  polymorphisms, **I**.580
  tuberculosis association, **I**.591–2, **I**.592–3
MC66, poxvirus apoptosis inhibition, **V1**.624
MC159R, poxvirus apoptosis inhibition,
    V1.624–5
M cells *see* Microfold (M) cells
MCM7, papillomavirus E6 protein effects,
    V1.460 (Tab.)
MDC *see* CCL22
MDC (CCL22), **I**.218 (Tab.)
Meaban virus, **V2**.1004
Measles, **I**.788 (Tab.), **I**.803–6
  acute, **V1**.722–3
    pathogenesis, **V1**.725–9
  animal models, **V2**.1433
  atypical, **V1**.723–4
  basic reproduction number, **B1**.340 (Tab.)
  chronic disease association, **V1**.725
  clinical course, **V1**.723 (Fig.), **I**.803–4,
    I.804 (Fig.)
    lymphopenia, **I**.805
  clinical features, **V1**.722–3, **V1**.722–5
    acute infection, **V2**.1431
    gastrointestinal symptoms, **V1**.723
    Koplik's spots, **V1**.722–3, **I**.803–4
    lymphopenia, **I**.804
    postinfectious encephalitis (PIE) *see below*
    tuberculosis reactivation, **I**.804
  CNS infection, **V2**.1404–5, **V2**.1431–3
    encephalitis, **V2**.1431
    infection routes, **V2**.1432
    pathogenesis, **V2**.1431
    postinfectious encephalitis (PIE) *see below*
    triggers, **V2**.1433
    virus-host interactions, **V2**.1432–3
  complications, **V1**.724–5, **I**.804, **V2**.1431–2
    CNS infection *see above*
    giant cell pneumonia, **V1**.724
    subacute sclerosing panencephalitis
      (SSPE) *see* Subacute sclerosing
      panencephalitis (SSPE)

control
  of outbreaks, **B1**.347
  vaccines *see below*
diagnosis, **V1**.732–4
  cell culture, **V1**.733
  cytopathology, **V2**.1534 (Tab.)
  microscopy, **V1**.732
  RT-PCR, **V1**.733
  serology, **V1**.732–3, **V2**.1547
  symptoms, **V1**.732
  viral RNA isolation/detection, **V1**.733–4
elimination campaign, **B1**.346
emerging infection, **V2**.1648 (Tab.)
epidemics
  Hamer's theory, **B1**.336–7, **B1**.342–3,
    B1.343 (Fig.)
  historical aspects, **B1**.336–7
  mathematical modeling, **B1**.342
epidemiology, **V1**.731–2, **I**.954 (Fig.)
  dynamics, **V2**.1661–2
  outbreaks, **V1**.712
  transmission, **V1**.722–3, **V1**.731
  vaccinated populations, **V1**.731
  vaccination effects, **V1**.712, **V1**.714 (Fig.),
    V1.731–2
  worldwide mortality, **V1**.732
epidemiology, mathematical modelling,
    B1.351–2
eradicable disease, **V2**.1569–70
historical aspects, **V1**.712
in HIV infection, **V2**.1499 (Tab.)
immune response, **V1**.726–9
  activation, **V1**.726–7, **V1**.726 (Fig.)
  cell-mediated, **V2**.1414
  cellular, **V1**.726
  cytokines
    IFN-γ, **I**.805–6
    IL-2, **I**.804–5, **I**.805–6
    IL-4, **I**.805–6
  delayed-type hypersensitivity, **I**.804
  humoral, **V1**.726–7
  IL-4, **V1**.298
  innate, **V1**.727
  nonspecific, **V1**.727
immunodeficient patients (non-HIV),
    V2.1509
immunogenetics, **I**.588
immunopathology, **V1**.279 (Tab.)
induced immunosuppression, **V1**.727–9,
    I.804–6
  APCs, **V1**.727–9, **V1**.728 (Tab.)
  B cells, **V1**.728 (Tab.)
  cytokines, **I**.806
  delayed-type hypersensitivity, **V1**.727–9
  dendritic cells, **I**.805
  hemagglutinin, **I**.805
  Ig production, **I**.806
  IL-12 depletion, **V1**.727–9
  lymphocytes, **I**.805–6
  monocytes, **I**.804–5
  opportunistic infection, **V1**.727–9
  T cells, **V1**.727–9, **V1**.728 (Tab.),
    V1.729 (Fig.)
  Th1 responses, **I**.805
laboratory worker immunization, **B1**.767

Measles (*Continued*)
  malnutrition, **I**.804
  mortality, **V2**.1431
    reduction by vaccination, **V1**.735–6
  neurological complications, **V1**.723,
    V1.724–5
    CSF pleocytosis, **V1**.723
    see also specific diseases/infection
  nitric oxide, **I**.804–5
  pathogenesis, **V1**.725–31, **V2**.1431
    animal models, **V1**.725
  persistent infection, **V1**.721, **V2**.1408,
    V2.1431, **V2**.1434 (Fig.)
    pathogenesis, **V1**.729–31
    tissue culture, **V1**.721
    see also specific diseases/infection
  postinfectious encephalitis (PIE), **V1**.724
    reduction by vaccination, **V1**.735–6
    treatment, **V1**.734
  prevention, **V1**.734–6
    vaccine *see below*
  serological surveillance, **B1**.351, **B1**.352 (Fig.)
  susceptibility, of infants, **V1**.263
  susceptibility/resistance, **B1**.351
  transmission, **V1**.722–3
    age-specific, **B1**.352, **B1**.352 (Fig.)
    modelling, **B1**.351–2
  treatment, **V1**.734
    at-risk groups, **V1**.734
  vaccination schedules, **V2**.1560–1, **V2**.1569
    'keep-up, catch-up, follow-up' schedule,
      V1.735–6
    two-dose schedule, **V1**.734, **V1**.735–6
    USA schedules, **V2**.1559–60
  vaccines/vaccination, **B1**.348, **I**.424 (Tab.),
    V2.1431, **V2**.1569–70
    adverse effects, **V1**.723–4, **V1**.734–6,
      V2.1564 (Tab.)
    age recommendations, **V1**.722
    campaign effect, **B1**.352–3
    contraindications, **V1**.736
    developing countries, **V1**.734
    development status, **I**.933 (Tab.)
    effect on transmission, **B1**.352–3
    efficacy, **V1**.712, **V1**.735–6
    hemagglutinin noose epitope peptides,
      I.868–9
    hemagglutinin peptides, **I**.868
    historical aspects, **V1**.8 (Tab.), **V2**.1569
    immunocompromised patients, **V2**.1509
    live attenuated, **V1**.734–5, **V2**.1555 (Tab.)
    mortality reduction, **V2**.1569
    postinfectious encephalitis (PIE), **V1**.735–6
    programs, **V2**.1559 (Tab.)
    schedules *see above*
    strains, **V1**.734–5, **V2**.1569
    strategy (England/Wales), **B1**.351–3
    uptake, **B1**.351
    wild-type strains *vs.,* **V1**.722
    see also Measles, mumps and rubella
      (MMR) vaccine
Measles inclusion body encephalitis (MIBE),
    V1.724–5, **V2**.1431
  biased hypermutation, **V1**.193
  immunodeficient patients (non-HIV),
    V2.1509

pathogenesis, **V1**.729–30
subacute sclerosing panencephalitis *vs.,*
    V1.724–5
Measles, mumps and rubella (MMR) vaccine,
    B1.324, **I**.424 (Tab.), **V1**.752–3,
    V2.1555 (Tab.), **V2**.1568–71
  adverse effects, **B1**.325–6, **V2**.1564 (Tab.)
  contraindications, **V2**.1562–3
    immunosuppressed, **V2**.1563
  introduction and usage, **B1**.351
  Mumps virus vaccination, **V1**.752–3
  possible adverse effects, **V2**.984
  in pregnancy, **V2**.1562–3
  USA schedules, **V2**.1559–60, **V2**.1560 (Fig.)
  vaccination program models, **I**.963
Measles virus, **I**.803, **V1.712–43**
  biased hypermutation, **V1**.193
  cell entry, **V1**.701–2, **V1**.719 (Fig.)
    cell receptors, **V1**.207 (Tab.)
  classification, **V1**.382–3, **V1**.712–13
    biosafety level 2, **V2**.1525
  CNS receptors, **V2**.1406 (Tab.), **V2**.1432
  C proteins, **V1**.705, **V1**.715–16, **V1**.717
  envelope proteins, **V1**.717–18
  F_1/F_2 protein, **V1**.716 (Fig.)
  fusion (F) protein, **I**.862 (Tab.), **I**.868
    cell entry, **V1**.713–15
    function, **V1**.717
    peptide vaccine design, **I**.868
    structure, **V1**.718
    synthesis, **V1**.718
    T-helper cell epitope, **I**.862 (Tab.)
  genetic characterization, **V1**.722
  genome structure, **V1**.713 (Fig.), **V1**.715–8,
    V1.785 (Fig.)
    'rule of six,' **V1**.715
  genotypes, **V1**.721–2
  hemagglutinin (H) protein, **V1**.715,
    V1.716 (Fig.), **I**.805, **I**.868
    antibodies to, **V1**.726–7
    CD46 binding, **V1**.718–20, **V1**.719 (Fig.),
      V1.719 (Tab.)
    CD150 binding, **V1**.718–20, **V1**.719 (Fig.),
      V1.719 (Tab.)
    cell entry, **V1**.713–15, **V1**.718–20
    function, **V1**.717
    glycosylation, **V1**.717–18
    lipid raft recruitment, **V1**.720–1
    structure, **V1**.717–18
    Toll-like receptor 2 interaction, **V1**.718–20,
      V1.719 (Tab.)
  immune evasion, **V1**.705
    dendritic cells, **I**.631–2
    ICAM- 1 expression, **V2**.1410
    IFN signal transduction, **V1**.315
  isolation/propagation and identification,
    V1.96 (Tab.), **V1**.99
  large (L) protein, **V1**.713–15, **V1**.716 (Fig.),
    V1.717
  matrix (M) protein, **V1**.703
  membrane (M) proteins, **V1**.713–15, **V1**.718
  morphology/structure, **V1**.74 (Fig.), **V1**.713–
    22, **V1**.713 (Fig.), **V1**.714 (Fig.)
    proteins *see individual proteins*

nucleocapsid (N) protein, **V1**.71, **V1**.713–15,
    V1.716 (Fig.)
  antibodies to, **V1**.726–7
  detection in CNS, **V1**.729–30
  gene structure, **V1**.715
  IRF-3 interaction, **V1**.716
  phosphoprotein (P) binding, **V1**.716,
    V1.720–1
  strain variability, **V1**.721–2
phosphoprotein (P), **V1**.713–15, **V1**.716 (Fig.)
  detection in CNS, **V1**.729–30
  nucleocapsid (N) protein binding, **V1**.716,
    V1.720–1
  phosphorylation, **V1**.717
proteins, **V1**.716–8, **V1**.716 (Fig.)
  nonstructural proteins, **V1**.715–16,
    V1.716–17
  see also individual proteins
receptors, **I**.803
replication, **V1**.713 (Fig.), **V1**.718–21
  assembly, **V1**.720–1
  budding, **V1**.720–1
  multiple genome packaging, **V1**.713–15
  receptor interactions, **V1**.718–20
R protein, **V1**.715–16
signaling lymphocyte attachment molecule
    (SLAM), **V1**.701–2
thermolability, **V1**.713–15
transcription, **V1**.715
  initiation, **V1**.720–1
vaccine *see* Measles
V protein, **V1**.715–16, **V1**.717
Meat and bone meal (MBM), bovine
    spongiform encephalopathy
    transmission, **V2**.1348, **V2**.1362
Meat/meat products, **B1.272–6**
  composition, **B1**.272
  cooked, **B1**.275
  cured, **B1**.274–5
  dried, **B1**.276
  edible offal, **B1**.273
  fecal contamination at production, **B1**.273,
    B1.274
  fermented and acidulated sausages, **B1**.275–6
  intestinal *Sarcocystis,* **P**.448, **P**.449
  packaging, **B1**.273, **B1**.274–5
    oxygen-impermeable films, **B1**.273
  perishable, **B1**.274–5
  preservation
    canned, **B1**.275
    ionizing radiation, **B1**.271–2, **B1**.274
    pH, **B1**.272
    refrigerated holding, **B1**.273
    salted, **B1**.274–5
    smoking, **B1**.274–5
  production, **B1**.273–4
  redox potential, **B1**.273
  safety assurance, **B1**.288–9
    government reforms, **B1**.289
  sarcocystosis prevention, **P**.449
  slaughter process, **B1**.273–4
  texture, **B1**.272
  toxoplasmosis after consumption, **P**.436–7
  uncured, **B1**.275
  see also Poultry

Mebendazole
alveolar echinococcosis, **P.**699
Angiostrongylus costaricensis infection, **P.**810
Blastocystis hominis infection, **P.**566–7
Capillaria philippiensis infection, **P.**747
cystic echinococcosis, **P.**698–9
Enterobius vermicularis infection, **P.**732
toxocariasis, **P.**755
trichinellosis, **P.**765–6
MEC (CCL28), **I.**218 (Tab.)
CCR10 binding, **I.**227
mecA gene (methicillin resistance), **B1.**111
Mechanical transmission, **V1.**355
norovirus infection, **V2.**919
Mecillinam
pharmacology, **B1.**475
spectrum of activity, **B1.**475
structure, **B1.**474 (Fig.)
Médecins Sans Frontières, **P.**103–6
Media, specimen transport, **V2.**1533
Mediastinal fibrosis, histoplasmosis, **M.**524,
M.524 (Fig.), **M.**531
Mediastinal granuloma, histoplasmosis, **M.**530
Mediastinal lymphadenopathy, histoplasmosis,
M.523
Mediastinitis, histoplasmosis, **M.**524,
M.524 (Fig.)
Medical mycology, **M.**3–4
education, **M.**32–3
historical developments, **M.**30–3
literature, **M.**31–2
milestones, **M.**4–6
research, **M.**32–3
Medical records, in epidemiology, **B1.**311
Medical surveillance policy, microbiological
risk assessment, **V2.**1519–20
Medicines Control Authority (MCA), **B1.**324
Medicines for Malaria Venture (MMV), **P.**110,
P.518
Mediterranean spotted fever, **B2.**2039–40,
B2.2039 (Tab.)
clinical manifestations, **B2.**2039–40,
B2.2039 (Tab.)
discovery, **B2.**2027–30
transmission and vectors, **B2.**2037–8
treatment, **B2.**2043
Mefloquine, **P.**341
malaria therapy, **P.**506
Megacins, **B1.**136–7, **B1.**139
Megacolon
Chagas disease, **P.**386, **P.**388 (Fig.)
toxic, **B2.**1121–2
treatment, **P.**393, **P.**393 (Fig.)
Megaesophagus
Chagas disease, **P.**387 (Fig.)
treatment, **P.**393
Megakaryocytes, IL-3 effects, **I.**275
Megasphaera, **B2.**1312
biochemical detection, **B2.**1312, **B2.**1314–15
differential characteristics, **B2.**1313 (Tab.)
habitats, **B2.**1313
historical perspective, **B2.**1312
possible infection, **B2.**1314
Megasphaera cerevisiae, **B2.**1313
Megasphaera elsdenii, **B1.**296 (Tab.), **B2.**1313
culture, **B2.**1314

Megasphaera micronuciformis, **B2.**1313
Meglumine antimoniate, Old World
leishmaniasis, **P.**306
Melanin
Cryptococcus neoformans, **M.**642
Madurella mycetomatis, **M.**387
muriform bodies, **M.**362–3, **M.**364
phaeoid fungi, **M.**742
Wangiella dermatitidis, **M.**746
Melanin stains, **M.**123 (Tab.)
Melanoides, fluke intermediate host, **P.**646
Melanoma *see* Malignant melanoma
Melarsoprol, African trypanosomiasis, **P.**371
Melibiose fermentation, Enterobacteriaceae
identification, **B2.**1319 (Tab.)
Melioidosis, **B2.**1626–32
clinical manifestations, **B2.**1626–8,
B2.1627 (Fig.)
acute suppurative parotitis, **B2.**1628,
B2.1628 (Fig.)
latent infection, **B2.**1626
lesions, **B2.**1629
liver abscesses, **B2.**1627, **B2.**1627 (Fig.)
localized, **B2.**1627–8
mild infection, **B2.**1626
necrotizing pneumonitis, **B1.**644
septicemic meloidosis, **B2.**1626–7
septic foci, **B2.**1627
subclinical infection, **B2.**1626
tuberculosis *vs.,* **B2.**1627–8
control, **B2.**1631
vaccine development, **B2.**1631
diagnosis, **B2.**1630
culture, **B2.**1630
ELISA, **B2.**1621, **B2.**1630
immunoassays, **B2.**1630
indirect immunofluorescence, **B2.**1630
microscopy, **B2.**1630
epidemiology, **B2.**1628–9
animal hosts, **B2.**1628–9
geographical distribution, **B2.**1628
reservoirs, **B2.**1628
surface water, **B2.**1628
transmission, **B2.**1628–9
as zoonosis, **B2.**1628
immune response, anti-LPS antibodies,
B2.1622
mortality, **B2.**1626–7, **B2.**1632
as opportunistic disease, **B2.**1629
pathology/pathogenesis, **B2.**1629–30
bacteremia, **B2.**1629
in diabetes mellitus, **B2.**1629
histopathology, **B2.**1629
immune response, **B2.**1629–30
treatment, **B2.**1631
acute phase, **B2.**1631
antibacterial s, **B2.**1631, **B2.**1631 (Tab.)
outcome/follow-up, **B2.**1632
relapse prevention, **B2.**1631
supportive, **B2.**1631
Melons, **B1.**283
Melting curve analysis, genotyping, **V2.**1542
Membrane-active agents, **B1.**436–8
Membrane-associated glycoproteins,
herpesviruses, **V1.**502

Membrane attack complex (MAC), **B1.**158–9
bacterial immune interference, **I.**664
deficiency, **I.**770–1
formation, **I.**146
mechanism of action, **I.**146
pathological effects, **I.**154
see also C7 complement protein; C8
complement protein; C9 complement
protein; Complement membrane attack
pathway
Membrane attack complex/perforin (MACPF)
domain, **I.**475, **I.**476 (Fig.)
Membrane attack pathway *see* Complement
membrane attack pathway
Membrane cofactor protein (MCP:CD46),
I.150 (Tab.), **I.**151, **V2.**1413
deficiency, **I.**154
measles, **V1.**725–6, **I.**804–5
measles virus binding, **I.**803
Measles virus hemagglutinin (H) protein
binding, **V1.**718–20, **V1.**719 (Fig.),
V1.719 (Tab.)
structure, **V1.**718–20
Membrane filters, **B1.**453
Membrane-fusion protein (MFP), **B1.**440
Membrane permeabilization, defensins, **I.**168–9
Membrane potential destruction, bacteriocins,
B1.137–8
Membrane (M) proteins
arteriviruses *see* Arteriviruses
Canine enteric coronavirus, **V1.**837
coronaviruses *see* Coronaviruses
Equine arteritis virus, **V1.**840
Feline coronavirus, **V1.**837
flaviviruses, **V2.**993
Lactate dehydrogenase-elevating virus,
V1.837
Measles virus, **V1.**713–15, **V1.**718
Murine hepatitis virus *see* Murine hepatitis
virus (MHV)
toroviruses, **V1.**827, **V1.**836 (Tab.)
Membranes, leakage, **B1.**436–8
Membranoproliferative glomuleronephritis
(MPGN), **V2.**1208
complement pathology, **I.**155 (Tab.)
factor H deficiency, **I.**154
Memory, **I.**487–501
cellular *see* Memory T cells
cellular differentiation, **I.**490–5
duration, **I.**497–8, **I.**497 (Tab.)
generation, **I.**503
humoral *see* Memory B cells
maintenance, **I.**495–8
antigen-dependent, **I.**496, **I.**497 (Tab.)
antigen depots, **I.**496–7
antigen-independent, **I.**496, **I.**497–8,
I.497 (Tab.)
microbial persistence, **I.**496–7
see also Protective immunity; Vaccination
Memory B cells, **I.**490–3
affinity maturation, **I.**491
development, **I.**492 (Fig.)
CD4 T cells, **I.**493
class switching, **I.**327–8
generation, **I.**493
germinal centers, **I.**491–2

Memory B cells (*Continued*)
  HIV infection, **I**.795
  kinetics, **I**.492 (Fig.)
    secondary infection, **I**.492–3
  memory T cells *vs.,* **I**.490, **I**.494 (Tab.)
  naïve B cells *vs.,* **I**.491 (Tab.)
  persistence, antigen absence, **I**.497–8
  Peyer's patches, **I**.538
  plasma cells *vs.,* **I**.491 (Tab.)
Memory lymphocytes, **I**.225
Memory T cells, **I**.493–5
  CD4+ T cell, HAART effects, **I**.800–1
  cell surface markers, **I**.495–6, **I**.495 (Tab.)
  'central' type, **I**.495, **I**.496 (Fig.)
  chemokine receptors
    CCR4, **I**.227
    CCR5, **I**.225
    CCR7, **I**.225
    CCR9, **I**.227
    CCR10, **I**.227
  clonal burst size *vs.,* **I**.494 (Fig.)
  CTLs, **I**.471
  cutaneous lymphocyte-associated antigen
      expression, **I**.227
  CXCR3, **I**.225
  decreasing potential hypothesis, **I**.495,
      I.496 (Fig.)
  'effector' type, **I**.495, **I**.496 (Fig.)
  influenza HA effects, **V1**.665
  integrin $\alpha_4\beta_7$ expression, **I**.227
  last memory differentiation model, **I**.495,
      I.496 (Fig.)
  memory B cells *vs.,* **I**.490, **I**.494 (Tab.)
  nonlymphoid tissue homing, **I**.227
  persistence, antigen absence, **I**.497–8
  Peyer's patches, **I**.538
Menangle virus, **V1**.818–19
Menaquinones, **B2**.1915
  Actinomycetes, aerobic, **B2**.1145
Mendoza's vaccine, **M**.426
Mengo virus, **V2**.862, **V2**.863
Meningeal arachnoiditis, **P**.686–7
Meningitis, **B1**.555–80
  anthrax, **B2**.931
  aseptic (viral) *see* Aseptic meningitis (viral)
  causative agents, **B1**.555
    Absidia corymbifera, **M**.661
    aspergillosis, **M**.697, **M**.705
    Blastoschizomyces capitatus, **M**.625–6
    candidiasis, **M**.600, **M**.612
    coccidioidomycosis, **M**.508, **M**.511,
        M.515–16
    cryptococcal, **M**.18, **M**.92, **M**.110
    Enterobacter sakazaki, **B1**.247
    Escherichia coli, **B1**.574–5
    gram-positive anaerobic cocci, **B2**.910
    Haemophilus, **B2**.1708
    Haemophilus influenzae type b (Hib) *see*
        Haemophilus influenzae type b (Hib)
        meningitis
    histoplasmosis capsulati, **M**.523–4, **M**.535
    listeriosis, **B1**.243
    Lyme borreliosis, **B1**.575
    Mycobacterium tuberculosis see below
    Neisseria meningitidis see below

    Pseudallescheria boydii, **M**.19
    Sporothrix schenckii, **M**.377–8
    Staphylococcus aureus, **B1**.574
    streptococcus, **B1**.244–5
    streptococcus group B, **B1**.574
    Streptococcus pneumoniae, pneumococcal
        meningitis
    syphilitic, **B1**.575
  clinical features, **B1**.557
  diagnosis, **B1**.557–60
    biochemical analysis, **B1**.558–9
    cerebrospinal fluid, **B1**.557–9
    culture, **B1**.559
    immunoassays, **B1**.559
    lumbar puncture, **B1**.557–8
    microscopy, **B1**.559
    nasopharyngeal swabs, **B1**.560
    PCR, **B1**.559
    peripheral blood, **B1**.559–60
    serology, **B1**.560
  fungal, **B1**.555
    clinical features, **B1**.557
  immunoserology, **B1**.757–8
  intracranial abscess complication, **B1**.583,
      B1.585–6
  meningococcal *see* Meningococcal disease
  miscellaneous types, **B1**.575
  mortality, **P**.29 (Tab.), **B1**.555
  neonatal, **B1**.574–5
    causative organisms, **B1**.574
    rates, **B1**.574
  pathophysiology, **B1**.555–7
    acquisition, **B1**.556
    exposure, **B1**.556
    meningeal invasion, **B1**.556–7
    mucosal invasion, **B1**.556
    respiratory viral infection role, **B1**.556
  pneumococcal *see* Pneumococcal meningitis
  predisposing factors, **B1**.557
  subdural empyema, **B1**.590, **B1**.591,
      B1.591 (Tab.)
  therapy, **M**.531
  tuberculous, **B1**.558–9, **B1**.575, **B2**.1202
    incidence, **B1**.575
    symptoms and diagnosis, **B1**.575
    treatment, **B1**.575
'Meningitis belt', **B1**.562, **B1**.562 (Fig.)
Meningococcal disease (meningitis), **B1**.555,
    B1.560–9
  age-specific incidence, **B1**.563 (Fig.), **B1**.565,
      B2.1289
    immunity relationship, **B1**.339,
        B1.339 (Fig.)
  carriage, **B1**.563–4
    affecting factors, **B1**.563–4
    age-specific incidence, **B1**.563
  clinical features, **B1**.565–6
    pneumonia, **B1**.637
    septicemia, **B1**.565–6
    skin lesions/rash, **B1**.565–6
  complement deficiency, **I**.153, **I**.594
  epidemiology, **B1**.561–3, **B1**.569 (Fig.),
      B2.1289
    'meningitis belt,' **B1**.562, **B1**.562 (Fig.)
    seasonal variations, **B1**.562
    temperate climates, **B1**.562–3, **B1**.563 (Fig.)

FcγRIIA deficiency, **I**.594
  historical perspective, **B1**.560–1
  immunity, **B1**.564–5, **B1**.564 (Fig.)
    age-dependence, **B1**.565
    blocking IgA antibodies, **B1**.564
    host factors, **B1**.564–5
    Ig A, **B1**.564
    Neisseria lactamica, **B1**.564
  immunogenetics, **I**.594
    angiotensin-converting enzyme gene, **I**.594
    FcγR genes, **I**.594
    IL1 gene cluster, **I**.594
  management, **B1**.561, **B1**.566–7
    antibiotics, **B1**.566–7, **B1**.566 (Fig.),
        B2.1291
    novel therapies, **B1**.567
    secondary cases and clusters, **B1**.567
    steroids and immunomodulators, **B1**.567
  mortality, **B1**.565–7
  nosocomial infection, **B1**.374
  notifications, **B1**.322–3, **B1**.561 (Fig.)
    in UK, **B1**.560–1, **B1**.565 (Fig.)
  prevention, **B2**.1292
    chemoprophylaxis, **B1**.567
    vaccine *see below*
  properidin deficiency, **I**.152
  secondary cases/clusters, **B1**.567
  vaccine, **B1**.567–9
    serogroup B, **B1**.568–9
    serogroups A+C, **B1**.568, **B1**.568 (Tab.)
    UK national program, **B1**.322–3
Meningococcemia, antibiotics for, **B2**.1291
Meningococci group B vaccines, **I**.939
Meningoencephalitis
  amebic, **B1**.575
  anthrax, **B2**.931
  Colorado tick fever virus infection, **V2**.942–3
  cryptococcosis, **M**.18, **M**.637–8, **M**.643,
      M.645–6, **M**.646 (Tab.), **M**.647 (Tab.),
      M.648–51
    AIDS, **M**.645–6, **M**.646 (Tab.),
        M.647 (Tab.), **M**.649, **M**.651
    computed tomography, **M**.649
    Cryptococcus neoformans var. *gattii,* **M**.646
    Cryptococcus neoformans var. *grubii,*
        M.646
    Cryptococcus neoformans var. *neoformans,*
        M.646
    diagnosis, **M**.648–9
    prognosis, **M**.653
    therapy, **M**.650–3
  mumps, **V2**.1430
  rubella, **V2**.974
  viruses causing, frequencies, **V2**.1416 (Tab.)
  West Nile virus, **V2**.1002
Men who have sex with men (MSM), syphilis,
    B2.1841
Mercaptides, **B1**.438
Mercury, **B1**.428
  action, **B1**.437 (Tab.), **B1**.438
  ammoniated, **M**.197
  resistance, **B1**.114, **B1**.442
    Pseudomonas, **B1**.114
    Staphylococcus, **B2**.794 (Tab.), **B2**.804–5
Merkel cells, **I**.820

Merogony
  Cryptosporidium parvum, **P**.400
  microsporidians, **P**.531, **P**.535
  see also Schizogony
Meronts
  Encephalitozoon, **P**.534
  Enterocytozoon, **P**.531–2, **P**.534
  Enterocytozoon bieneusi, **P**.531–2,
    P.532 (Fig.), **P**.534 (Fig.)
  Pleistophora, **P**.535
  Trachipleistophora, **P**.534
  Vittaforma, **P**.535
  Vittaforma corneae, **P**.540 (Fig.)
Meropenem, **B1**.478–80
  Cardiobacterium hominis, **B2**.1672–3
  Haemophilus, **B2**.1702 (Tab.)
  Klebsiella, **B2**.1480
  melioidosis treatment, **B2**.1631
  structure, **B1**.479 (Fig.)
Merozoites
  Cryptosporidium parvum, **P**.400
  formation, **P**.184 (Fig.)
  Plasmodium see Plasmodium
  Sarcocystis, **P**.443–5, **P**.446 (Fig.)
Merozoite surface proteins (MSP)
  Plasmodium, **I**.676
  see also Malaria
Mesh pili, *Burkholderia,* **B2**.1614
Mesocestoides, **P**.578, **P**.674
Mesocestoides corti infection, **I**.70
Mesocestoididae, **P**.578–9
Mesomycetozoea, **M**.69
Mesophiles
  Aeromonas strains, **B2**.1529
  temperature range for growth, **B1**.264
Mesoplasma
  characteristics, **B2**.1958 (Tab.)
  classification, **B2**.1967
  metabolism, **B2**.1969
Mesosomes, **B2**.1594
Messenger RNA (mRNA), **B1**.42
Metabisulfites, **B1**.429
Metabolic acidosis, malaria in children,
    P.482–4
Metabolism (bacterial), **B1.37–79**
  aerobic respiration, **B1**.63–5
  anaerobic respiration *see* Anaerobic
    respiration
  Archaebacteria, **B1**.68–70
  biosynthetic reactions, **B1**.60–3
    amino acids, **B1**.60
    fatty acids and lipids, **B1**.61
    nitrogen fixation, **B1**.63
    one-carbon compounds incorporation,
      B1.61–3
    purine/pyrimidines, **B1**.60–1
    small molecules, **B1**.60–1
    TCA cycle intermediates, **B1**.61
  carbohydrate catabolism in genus
    Pseudomonas, **B1**.59–60
  catabolic and anabolic pathways, **B1**.45
  catabolic pathways, **B1**.50–60
    acetate as carbon source, **B1**.53–4
    alternative routes of carbohydrate
      catabolism, **B1**.58–60

ethanol fermentation, **B1**.56
glucose fermentations, **B1**.54–6
hexose diphosphate pathway, **B1**.50–2,
  B1.51 (Fig.)
pentoses fermentation, **B1**.57–8
propionic acid fermentations, **B1**.56
tricarboxylic acid cycle, **B1**.52–3
DNA synthesis, **B1**.46–8
positive control, **B1**.71–2
regulatory mechanisms
  biosynthetic operons, **B1**.70–2
  catabolic operons, **B1**.70
  cell division regulation, **B1**.48
  covalent modification, **B1**.76
  DNA synthesis, **B1**.46–8
  enzyme action alterations, **B1**.75–6
  enzyme activity, **B1**.75–6
  global control networks, **B1**.72–5
    cyclic AMP role, **B1**.73
    σ factors, **B1**.74–5
    two-component signal transduction,
      B1.75
  negative control, **B1**.45–6
  physiological processes regulation, **B1**.70–2
  protein folding, **B1**.47–8
  protein secretion, **B1**.48
  protein synthesis, **B1**.46–8
  RNA synthesis, **B1**.46–8
soil bacteria, quantification, **B1**.205–8
structure and organization of the bacterial
  cell, **B1**.42–6
Metacercaria, **P**.580
Metacestodes, *Echinococcus vogeli,* **P**.680–1
Metachromatic granules, **B2**.981 (Fig.)
Metacyclic forms, *Trypanosoma brucei,*
  P.357–8
Metacyclogenesis, **P**.381
Metagonimus, **P**.584
Metalloenzymes, *Burkholderia thailandensis,*
  B2.1624
Metallothionein, acute phase response, **I**.206
Metapneumovirus, **V1.783–806**
  animal models, **V1**.790
  characteristics, **V1**.129 (Tab.), **V1**.701 (Tab.)
  classification, **V1**.48–9, **V1**.382,
    V1.700 (Tab.)
  genome structure/organization,
    V1.387 (Tab.), **V1**.701 (Fig.),
    V1.785 (Fig.), **V1**.789
  members, **V1**.385
  proteins, **V1**.787–9
  type species *see* Avian pneumovirus (APV)
  virus assembly, **V1**.790
  virus replication, **V1**.789–90
  in vitro culture, **V1**.790
Metarhizium, oculomycoses, **M**.275 (Tab.)
Metastatic malignant melanoma
  Simian virus 40, **V1**.483
  TCE peptide vaccines, **I**.865 (Tab.)
Metastrongyloidea, **P**.592
  Angiostrongylidae, **P**.592
Metaviridae
  classification, **V1**.27 (Tab.), **V1**.46 (Tab.),
    V1.47
  infectivity, **V1**.45–6
  see also specific viruses

Metazoa, **P**.159–60, **P**.186, **P**.189–90
Metchnikoff, E, **B1**.7
Methane
  bacterial carbon source, **B1**.62
  methanol formation, **B1**.62, **B1**.63
  methanol reduction, **B1**.68–9
  production *see* Methanogenesis
Methane mono-oxygenase (MMO), **B1**.62
Methanobacterium, **B1**.69
Methanobacterium thermoautotrophicum,
  B1.44
Methanobrevibacter ruminantium, **B1**.44
Methanogenesis, **B1**.68–9
  energetics, **B1**.69
  first step, **B1**.68
Methanogens
  carbon dioxide fixation, **B1**.199
  metabolism, **B1**.63, **B1**.68, **B1**.69
Methanol
  adverse reactions, **B1**.325–6
  sodium hypochlorite, **B1**.432
Methanosarcina, **B1**.69
Methanosarcinaceae, **B1**.44
Methanotrophs, **B1**.62
Methenamine silver stain, **M**.88 (Tab.)
  Coccidioides immitis, **M**.516
  mycology, **M**.87
Methicillin-gentamycin resistant
    Staphylococcus aureus (MGRSA),
    B1.442, **B2**.779–80, **B2**.791,
    B2.794 (Tab.), **B2**.804
Methicillin-resistant *Staphylococcus aureus*
    (MRSA), **B1**.442, **B2**.793–802
  bone and joint infection
    clinical manifestations, **B1**.685 (Tab.)
    device-related, **B1**.690
    epidemiology, **B1**.685
  epidemiological surveillance, **B1**.323
  evolution, **B1**.30
  identification, **B2**.807–8
    EIA detection, **B1**.756
  infection
    bacteremia, **B1**.517–18
    bone and joints *see above*
    endocarditis, **B1**.526, **B1**.539–40
    intracranial abscess, **B1**.585, **B1**.588–9
    nosocomial *see below*
  molecular detection, **B1**.723 (Tab.)
    cycling probe technology, **B1**.731–2
  nasal carriage eradication, **B2**.814
  nosocomial infection
    bacteremia, **B1**.393–4
    pneumonia, **B1**.389
  prevention/control, **B1**.396
  transposons, **B1**.111
  vaccine development, **B2**.815–16
Methicillin-resistant *Staphylococcus*
    epidermidis (MRSE), **B2**.801
Methicillin, structure, **B1**.474 (Fig.)
Methisazone, **V2**.1631
  structure, **V2**.1631 (Fig.)
Methisazone, historical aspects, **V1**.9 (Tab.)
Methotrexate, immunodeficiency, **I**.788 (Tab.)
2-C-Methyladenosine, hepatitis C therapy,
  V2.1216
Methyl bromide, **B1**.430

Methylene blue, **M**.88 (Tab.)

Methylenomycin production, *Streptomyces coelicolor*, **B1**.113–14

7-Methylguanylate, mRNA, **V1**.112

N-Methylisothiazol-3-one (MIT), **B1**.427

Methylmalonyl-CoA-pyruvate transcarboxylase, **B1**.56

Methyl mercaptan, **B2**.1936

Methylobacterium, **B1**.603

Methyl red, Enterobacteriaceae identification, **B2**.1319 (Tab.)

4-Methylumbelliferyl-β-D-glucuronidase (MUG), **B1**.223, **B1**.225

Metrifonate, **P**.622

Metrocytes, *Sarcocystis*, **P**.443–5

Metronidazole
  adverse effects, **P**.251
  amebiasis, **P**.213
  bacterial vaginosis treatment, **B1**.666–8
  Balantidium coli infection, **P**.281
  Blastocystis hominis infection, **P**.566–7
  CNS infection
    intracranial abscess, **B1**.588–9, **B1**.589 (Tab.)
    subdural empyema, **B1**.591 (Tab.)
  Dientamoeba fragilis infection, **P**.269
  Entamoeba gingivalis infection, **P**.220
  gas gangrene, **B2**.1115–16
  giardiasis, **P**.251
  gingivitis treatment, **B1**.614
  periodontal abscess, **B1**.614
  pharmacology, **B1**.495
  resistance, **B1**.495
    Bacteroides, **B2**.1931, **B2**.1935
    Helicobacter pylori, **B2**.1575
  Retortamonas intestinalis infection, **P**.273
  spectrum of activity, **B1**.495, **B1**.499 (Tab.)
    Actinobacillus actinomycetemcomitans, **B2**.1664
    Actinomyces, **B2**.1011
    Clostridium, **B2**.1064–5
    Clostridium difficile, **B2**.1123
    gram-positive anaerobic cocci, **B2**.907, **B2**.911, **B2**.912
    Helicobacter pylori, **B2**.1574–5
    Treponema pallidum, **B2**.1839–40
  structure, **B1**.495 (Fig.)
  in tetanus, **B2**.1066
  trichomoniasis, **P**.262

Mezlocillin
  Pasteurella multocida, **B2**.1655
  structure, **B1**.474 (Fig.)

MF59 adjuvant, **I**.927–9, **V2**.1557
  age-relation, **I**.927, **I**.929
  chemokine receptor 2, **I**.927
  composition, **I**.927
  depot effect, **I**.927
  IL-4 induction, **I**.927
  IL-5 induction, **I**.927
  licensing, **I**.927
  repeated immunizations, **I**.929
  safety, **I**.929
  Th2 response, **I**.927
  vaccines
    Haemophilus influenzae type b, **I**.927
    HCMV, **I**.929

Hepatitis B virus, **I**.927, **I**.929, **I**.937

Hepatitis C virus, **I**.929

HIV-1, **I**.929

HPV, **I**.929

HSV, **I**.929

influenza virus, **I**.929

Neisseria meningitidis group C, **I**.927

versatility, **I**.927

M'Fadyean stain, *Bacillus anthracis*, **B2**.934–7, **B2**.947

M gene
  Influenza virus A, **V1**.641–2
  Influenza virus B, **V1**.641–2

Micafungin, **M**.154
  characteristics, **M**.155 (Tab.)
  Paecilomyces infection, **M**.758

Mice
  Actinobacillus muris infection, **B2**.1665–6
  athymic (nude), histoplasmosis, **M**.528
  BALB/c, babesiosis, **P**.455
  congenitally athymic, amebic liver abscesses, **P**.210
  epidemic studies, **B1**.337
  listeriosis in, **B2**.963
  SCID *see* Severe combined immunodeficient (SCID) mice

Mice Minute virus (MMV) *see* Minute virus of mice (MMV)

Michaelis constant (K_m), **B1**.45

Michaelis–Menten kinetics, **B1**.45

Micheli, P A, **M**.6

Miconazole, **M**.147, **M**.183 (Tab.)
  Condidiobolus resistance, **M**.352
  mechanism of action, **M**.70
  therapy
    candidiasis, **M**.609–10
    endophthalmitis, **M**.319, **M**.320, **M**.326–7
    keratitis, **M**.309, **M**.313
    lobomycosis, **M**.434–5
    mycetoma, **M**.393
    Scedosporium, **M**.757
    tinea nigra, **M**.186
    vulvovaginal candidiasis, **M**.189

Microaerobic conditions, *Helicobacter pylori* culture, **B2**.1567

Microaerophiles
  bacteria, meat and meat products, **B1**.273
  Plasmodium, **P**.478

Microagglutination, tularemia diagnosis, **B2**.1754

Microarrays, **B1**.736
  in viral infection diagnosis, **V2**.1538

Microbacterium, **B2**.992
  biochemical characteristics, **B2**.993 (Tab.)
  chemotaxonomic characteristics, **B2**.978 (Tab.)
  disease associations, **B2**.981 (Tab.)
  habitats, **B2**.978

Microbial surface components recognizing adhesive matrix molecules (MSCRAMM), **B1**.149, **B1**.527

Microbiological risk assessment (MRA) *see* Laboratory safety

Microbiology, **B1**.3
  pure and applied, **B1**.3
  see also individual species; individual subjects

Microbiota, normal, **B1**.296 (Tab.)
  blood/cerebrospinal fluid/body fluids, **B1**.305
  body tissues, **B1**.305
  colonization prevalence estimation, **B1**.295
  disruption effects, **B1**.293–4, **B1**.305
  factors affecting, **B1**.294
    environmental/nutritional, **B1**.294
    host factors, **B1**.294
    microbial factors, **B1**.294
  function, **B1**.293–4, **B1**.305
  gastrointestinal tract *see* Gastrointestinal tract
  general considerations, **B1**.293–5
  genitourinary tract *see* Genitourinary tract, normal microbiota
  respiratory tract, **B1**.295–302, **B1**.302, **B1**.609, **B1**.628
  skin *see* Skin
  species, **B1**.296 (Tab.)
    see also individual species
  transient and prolonged colonization, **B1**.294–5

Microbodies, **P**.177–8

Microcins, **B1**.136–8

Microcirculation, septic shock, **I**.700, **I**.701

Micrococcaceae, **B1**.284–5

Micrococcus, **B2**.771–2
  airborne bacteria, **B1**.189
  habitats, **B1**.211
  normal microbiota, **B1**.296 (Tab.)
  pasteurization, **B1**.232–3
  waterborne, **B1**.221

Micrococcus foetidus, **B2**.903

Micrococcus luteus, **B1**.304

Microconidia, **M**.78–9

Microcystis aeruginosa, rhinosporidiosis *vs.*, **M**.439–40

Microfilaments, cytoskeleton, **I**.37–8

Microfilariae, **P**.91, **P**.591
  historical aspects, **P**.9–10
  see also Onchocerca volvulus

Microfold (M) cells, **I**.532
  Peyer's patches *see* Peyer's patches
  prion diseases, **V2**.1374, **V2**.1375 (Fig.)
  stratified epithelium, **I**.827
  viral entry, **V1**.240 (Fig.)

Microgamont, **P**.171 (Fig.)

Microhemagglutination assays, *Treponema pallidum*, **B2**.1848

Micromonas, **B2**.914
  classification, **B2**.905 (Tab.)
  definition/characteristics, **B2**.914
  identification, **B2**.906–7

Micromonas micros, **B2**.914
  antibacterial susceptibility/resistance, **B2**.911
  biochemical characteristics, **B2**.908 (Tab.)
  classification, **B2**.904–5
  clinical importance, **B2**.910
  identification, **B2**.907
  isolation and maintenance, **B2**.905, **B2**.906
  as normal microbiota, **B1**.296 (Tab.), **B2**.910
  pathogenicity and virulence factors, **B2**.910–11

Micromonospora, **B2**.1143

Micronemes (toxonemes), **P**.178, **P**.423
  Babesia, **P**.452
Micronucleus, *Balantidium coli,* **P**.276–7,
    P.278 (Fig.)
Micronutrients, acute phase response, **I**.207–8
Microophthalmia, congenital toxoplasmosis,
    P.430 (Fig.)
Microparasites, **P**.67
  epidemiology *see* Epidemiology of infection,
      parasitic infection
Microparticles, as adjuvants, **I**.928 (Tab.)
Microphthalmia, rubella, **V2**.973
Microsatellites
  Cryptosporidium parvum, **P**.404
  Leishmania analysis, **P**.284–5
  linkage, **I**.573
  polymorphism, **I**.580
Microscilla, bioremediation, **B1**.212
Microscopic agglutination test (MAT),
    leptospires, **B2**.1879–80
Microscopy, **B1**.713–14, **B1**.713 (Tab.)
  applications, **B1**.712–13, **B1**.713 (Tab.)
    Bartonella classification, **B2**.1887
    Chlamydia infection diagnosis, **B2**.2017
    gonorrhea diagnosis, **B1**.659
    melioidosis diagnosis, **B2**.1630
    soil bacteria analysis, **B1**.207
  bacterial morphology *see* Morphology,
      bacteria
  darkfield microscopy *see* Dark-field
      microscopy
  development, **B1**.3
  electron *see* Electron microscopy
  fecal samples, **P**.151
  fluorescent, **B1**.713 (Tab.), **B1**.714
  history, **M**.6, **M**.33
  infection diagnosis, **M**.121–2
  interference, **B1**.207
  measles diagnosis, **V1**.732
  phase contrast microscopy *see* Phase-contrast
      microscopy
MicroSeq®, **B1**.733
Microsphaeropsis, oculomycoses, **M**.278 (Tab.)
Microsphaeropsis olivacea
  endophthalmitis, **M**.323
  infection, endophthalmitis, **M**.323
Microspora, structure, **P**.166–8, **P**.168 (Fig.)
Microsporidians, **P**.189
  classification, **P**.198, **P**.529, **P**.534–5, **P**.537,
      P.538, **P**.539–42
  geographical distribution, **P**.537
  historical aspects, **P**.18, **P**.535–6, **P**.539–40
  infection *see* Microsporidiosis
  morphology, **P**.538 (Fig.), **P**.542 (Fig.)
  physical/chemical agent susceptibility, **P**.550
    autoclaving, **P**.550
    cytochalasin D, **P**.550
    demecolcine, **P**.550
    disinfectants, **P**.550
    itraconazole, **P**.550
    nifedipine, **P**.550
    pH, **P**.550
    ultraviolet radiation, **P**.550
  public health importance, **P**.44
  structure/life cycle, **P**.529–33
    binary fission, **P**.531–2, **P**.532–4

chromosomal separation, **P**.533
manubrium, **P**.529–31
merogony, **P**.531, **P**.535
meronts, **P**.531–2, **P**.532 (Fig.), **P**.534,
    P.534 (Fig.), **P**.535, **P**.540 (Fig.)
multilayered interlaced network, **P**.529–31
multiple (sequential) fission, **P**.532–3
nucleus, **P**.529–31
plasmotomy, **P**.531–2
polaroplast, **P**.529–31
polar tube, **P**.529–31, **P**.531 (Fig.)
proliferation, **P**.531
sporegonic stage, **P**.535
spores, **P**.529, **P**.530 (Fig.), **P**.531 (Fig.),
    P.532–3, **P**.532 (Fig.), **P**.533 (Fig.)
sporoblasts, **P**.532–3
sporogonial plasmodium, **P**.533 (Fig.)
sporogonic stage, **P**.532 (Fig.), **P**.534
sporogony, **P**.531, **P**.535
sporonts, **P**.532–3, **P**.532 (Fig.)
sporophorous vesicles, **P**.532–3,
    P.533 (Fig.), **P**.534, **P**.535, **P**.542
sporoplasm, **P**.531, **P**.531 (Fig.),
    P.532 (Fig.)
  in vitro culture, **P**.541, **P**.546, **P**.548
    albendazole effects, **P**.548
  see also individual species
Microsporidiosis, **P.529–55**
  AIDS/HIV infection *see* AIDS, concomitant
      infection; HIV infection, concomittant
      infection
  animal models, **P**.540
  avian infection, **P**.544
  chemotherapy, **P**.548–50
    albendazole, **P**.548, **P**.549–50
    fumagillin, **P**.549
    octreotide, **P**.548
    thalidomide, **P**.549
  cryptosporidiosis co-infection, **P**.546–7
  diagnosis, **P**.545–8
    Calcifluor staining, **P**.546, **P**.547 (Fig.)
    chromotrope 2R, **P**.546
    culture, **P**.547, **P**.548
    direct immunofluorescence, **P**.151
    Entero-test, **P**.546
    fecal samples, **P**.545, **P**.546–7
    immunoassays, **P**.154, **P**.536, **P**.546
    see also individual assays
    molecular biology, **P**.547
    small-intestine biopsy, **P**.545–6, **P**.545 (Fig.)
    Uvitex 2B staining, **P**.546
  disseminated infection, **P**.542–3
    treatment, **P**.549–50
  enteric infection, **P**.537–9, **P**.538
    acalculous cholecystitis, **P**.539
    in Africa, **P**.538
    cholangitis, **P**.539
    cholecystitis, **P**.539
    crypt hyperplasia, **P**.537
    diarrhea, **P**.537
    elderly, **P**.539
    HIV infection, **P**.537, **P**.539
    lamina propria, **P**.538
    organ transplant patients, **P**.539
    travelers' diarrhea, **P**.539

treatment, **P**.548, **P**.549
epidemiology, **P**.543–5
fish infection, **P**.541–2, **P**.544
historical aspects/re-evaluation, **I**.8–9,
    P.535–6
immune response, **P**.87
immune status effects, **P**.536–43
  organ transplants, **P**.537
immune system reconstitution, **P**.550
ocular, **P**.539–41
  corneal stromal infection, **P**.539–40, **P**.543
  HIV infection, **P**.540–1
  keratoconjunctivitis, **P**.540–1
  treatment, **P**.549
progression, **P**.543
public health importance, **P**.45
serological surveys, **P**.536
serology, **P**.536
transmission, **P**.543–4
  host cell penetration, **P**.531
as zoonoses, **P**.543, **P**.544–5
Microsporidium
  classification, **P**.190–1, **P**.198, **P**.535
  historical aspects, **P**.535–6
  see also Microsporidians; Microsporidiosis
Microsporum, **M**.61, **M**.220, **M**.221 (Tab.),
    M.222, **M**.222 (Tab.), **M**.223 (Tab.),
    M.224 (Tab.)
  classification, **M**.45–6, **M**.61, **M**.229
  histopathology, **M**.128 (Tab.)
  infection
    blepharitis, **M**.297
    therapy, **M**.233
  morphology, **M**.222, **M**.222 (Tab.),
      M.224 (Tab.)
Microsporum audouinii, **M**.224 (Tab.),
    M.227 (Tab.)
  classification, **M**.229–30
  epidemiology, **M**.227–8
  geographical distribution, **M**.228–9,
      M.229 (Tab.)
  history, **M**.220
  infection, **M**.231–2
Microsporum canis, **M**.224 (Tab.), **M**.227 (Tab.)
  classification, **M**.229–30
  epidemiology, **M**.225, **M**.227, **M**.228
  geographical distribution, **M**.228–9,
      M.229 (Tab.)
  history, **M**.9–10
  identification, **M**.236, **M**.237
    histopathology, **M**.138 (Fig.)
  infection, **M**.231–2
    deep dermatophytic granuloma,
        M.138 (Fig.)
    oculomycoses, **M**.275 (Tab.)
    therapy, **M**.188, **M**.233
  teleomorph, **M**.10–1
  transmission, **M**.223, **M**.239
  var. *canis,* **M**.224 (Tab.)
  var. *distortum,* **M**.224 (Tab.)
    geographical distribution, **M**.229 (Tab.)
  var. *equinum,* **M**.229 (Tab.)
Microsporum cookei, **M**.224 (Tab.),
    M.227 (Tab.)
  geographical distribution, **M**.229 (Tab.)
Microsporum equinum, **M**.237

Microsporum ferrugineum, **M**.224 (Tab.),
  M.227 (Tab.)
  geographical distribution, **M**.229 (Tab.)
  history, **M**.9–10
  infection, **M**.231–2
Microsporum fulvum, **M**.224 (Tab.)
  geographical distribution, **M**.229 (Tab.)
Microsporum gallinae, **M**.224 (Tab.), **M**.227,
  M.227 (Tab.)
  geographical distribution, **M**.229 (Tab.)
  history, **M**.9–10
Microsporum gypseum, **M**.223, **M**.224 (Tab.),
  M.225
  ecology, **M**.223, **M**.225
  epidemiology, **M**.225
  geographical distribution, **M**.229 (Tab.)
  infection, **M**.231–2
  teleomorph, **M**.10–1
  transmission, **M**.222–3, **M**.225, **M**.227
Microsporum nanum, **M**.223, **M**.224 (Tab.),
  M.225, **M**.227, **M**.227 (Tab.)
  geographical distribution, **M**.229 (Tab.)
Microsporum persicolor, **M**.224 (Tab.), **M**.225,
  M.227 (Tab.)
  geographical distribution, **M**.229 (Tab.)
  history, **M**.9–10
Microsporum praecox, **M**.224 (Tab.),
  M.227 (Tab.)
  geographical distribution, **M**.229 (Tab.)
Microsporum racemosum, **M**.224 (Tab.),
  M.227 (Tab.)
  geographical distribution, **M**.229 (Tab.)
Microsporum simii, **M**.225
Microsporum vanbreuseghemii, **M**.224 (Tab.),
  M.227 (Tab.)
  geographical distribution, **M**.229 (Tab.)
Microthrix parvicella, bioremediation, **B1**.212
Microtubule organizing centres (MTOCs),
  P.169–70
Microtubules, **P**.170–2
  cytoskeleton, **I**.37–8
  in flagella/cilia, **P**.179–80
  protozoa, **P**.162, **P**.169–72, **P**.170–2
  reorientation, HTLV transmission, **V2**.1288
  subpellicular, **P**.162, **P**.163 (Tab.),
    P.165 (Fig.), **P**.170–2
Microviridae, **V1**.27 (Tab.), **V1**.41 (Tab.)
  see also specific viruses
Microwaves, food processing and preservation,
  B1.268 (Tab.)
MIC titrations, antibacterial susceptibility
  testing, **B1**.498
Middleburg virus (MIDV), **V2**.1010,
  V2.1011 (Tab.)
Middle ear, anatomy, **B1**.606
MIF tests, *Chlamydia* detection, **B2**.2019
Mig (CXCL9), **I**.218 (Tab.)
Migration
  epidemics, **P**.117, **P**.127
  malaria epidemiology, **P**.513–14
Migration inhibitory factor (MIF)
  historical aspects/re-evaluation, **I**.10
  homologue secretion, **I**.687
Miksuokella multiacidus, **B1**.296 (Tab.)
Miliary blastomycosis, **M**.489
Miliary tuberculosis, **I**.711

Milk, **B1**.229–45
  associated infection/outbreaks, **B1**.234–45
    microbiological investigation, **B1**.236–7
  cows' milk, **B1**.229–31
  ewes' milk, **B1**.231–2
  goats' milk, **B1**.231–2
  heat treatment, **B1**.232–3, **B1**.236 (Fig.)
    pasteurization, **B1**.232–3
    sterilized, **B1**.233
    thermized, **B1**.233
    ultra-heat treated, **B1**.233
  legislation, **B1**.230, **B1**.236
    quality control tests, **B1**.233–4
    unpasterized milk restrictions, **B1**.234
  powdered, **B1**.245–8
  see also individual bacterial species
Milk powder, **B1**.245–8
'Milky-spore disease,' **B1**.203–4
Millennium Development Goals, **P**.103–6
Miller's vaccine, **M**.426
Milochevitch, S, **M**.10
Milstein, Cesar, **I**.7, **I**.10
Miltefosine, **P**.307
'Mimotope', **V2**.1166
Mimotopes, BCE peptide vaccines, **I**.854,
  I.861 (Tab.)
Mimp 1 (CARD10), **I**.347
MinC, **B1**.48
MinE, **B1**.48
Mineral salts, as adjuvants, **I**.928 (Tab.)
Miners infection, **M**.228
  sporotrichosis, **M**.368–9
  tinea pedis, **M**.228
Mini-exon genes, **P**.381
'Minimal cell' concept, **B2**.1975
Minimum bactericidal concentration (MBC),
  B1.497–8
Minimum information content, genomes,
  V1.180
Minimum inhibitory concentration (MIC),
  M.168–9, **B1**.497–8
Mink, botulism, **B2**.1074
Mink enteritis virus (MEV), **I**.855 (Tab.),
  I.871–2
Minocycline
  Nocardia, **B2**.1165–6
  resistance, **B1**.485
  structure, **B1**.485 (Fig.)
  Vibrio, **B2**.1514
'Minor' illness, poliomyelitis, **V2**.870
Minute virus of mice (MMV)
  allotropic specificity, **V1**.422
  capsids, **V1**.420–1
  DNA strand polarization, **V1**.42
  gene products, **V1**.157–8
  gene therapy vector, **V1**.426–7
  gene transcription, **V1**.414 (Fig.)
  genome replication, **V1**.148 (Tab.),
    V1.157–9, **V1**.158 (Fig.)
    elongation, **V1**.158–9
    'hairpin resolution,' **V1**.419
    initiation, **V1**.158
    junction resolution, **V1**.420
    NS1 protein, **V1**.149 (Tab.), **V1**.158,
      V1.418–19
    origin recognition proteins, **V1**.149 (Tab.)

  origins of replication, **V1**.157
  parvovirus initiation factor (PIF), **V1**.158
  proliferating cellular nuclear antigen
    (PCNA), **V1**.158–9
  replicative form (RF) intermediates,
    V1.158
  'rolling hairpin,' **V1**.158, **V1**.418–20,
    V1.419 (Fig.)
  viral proteins, **V1**.149 (Tab.)
genome structure, **V1**.148 (Tab.), **V1**.414,
  V1.414 (Fig.)
infection *see* Minute virus of mice (MMV)
  infection
morphology/structure, **V1**.412
pathogenic potential, **V1**.422
sialoglycoprotein binding, **V1**.422–3
tissue specificity, **V1**.422–3
type species, **V1**.409
Minute virus of mice (MMV) infection
  acid environment exposure, **V1**.417
  cell entry, **V1**.416–17
  initial transcription, **V1**.418
  pathogenesis
    immunocompromised hosts, **V1**.426
    mature hosts, **V1**.426
  sialoglycoprotein binding, **V1**.416–17
MIP-3α *see* CCL20
MIP-3β *see* Epstein–Barr virus-induced
  receptor ligand chemokine
  (ELC:CCL19)
Mip protein, Q fever pathogenesis, **B2**.2077
Miracidia, **P**.580
  Schistosoma, **P**.602
Mis-sense mutations *see* Point mutations
Mites, *Rickettsia* transmission, **B2**.2037
Mitochondria
  apoptosis *see* Apoptosis
  division, **P**.174
  DNA
    Aspergillus, **M**.715
    Candida, **M**.103, **M**.608
    Hortaea (Phaeoannellomyces) werneckii,
      M.199
    Sporothrix schenckii, **M**.371–2, **M**.378,
      M.378 (Fig.)
    Entamoeba histolytica, **P**.202
    Plasmodium, **P**.466
    protozoa, **P**.173–4, **P**.174 (Fig.)
  respiratory chain, **B1**.63–4
Mitochondria-permeability transition (MPT),
  I.133
Mitogen-activated protein (MAP) kinases
  apoptosis functions, **I**.626
  CpG binding/signal transduction, **I**.911
  neutrophil intracellular signaling, **I**.42, **I**.43
  Vav activation by, **I**.345–6
Mitogenic factor, *Streptococcus pyogenes see*
  Streptococcus pyogenes
Mitogillin, **M**.694
  Aspergillus restrictus, **M**.694
Mitosporic fungi, classification, **M**.49, **M**.51
Mitsuda reaction (lepromin reaction), **B2**.1221
Mitten crabs, *Paragonimus* intermediate host,
  P.646
Mixed acid fermentation, **B1**.55
Mixed cell culture, **V2**.1541

MLS antibacterials, *Enterococcus* resistance, **B2**.892 (Tab.)

MMR vaccine *see* Measles, mumps and rubella (MMR) vaccine

Møarboxylase test, *Aeromonas* identification, **B2**.1532

Mobala virus, **V2**.1060 (Tab.)

mob genes, **B1**.110

Mobile elements, deletions, **B1**.95–6

Mobiluncus
  bacterial vaginosis, **B1**.665, **B1**.666
  normal microbiota, **B1**.296 (Tab.), **B1**.303

Mobiluncus curtisii, **B1**.666

Mobiluncus mulieris, **B1**.666

Model-dependent analysis, linkage, **I**.573

Model-free analysis, linkage, **I**.573

Modified agglutination test (MAT), toxoplasmosis, **P**.435

Modified atmosphere packaging, **B1**.281, **B1**.282

Modified vaccinia virus Ankara (MVA), as vaccine vector, **I**.846–7, **I**.897 (Tab.), **I**.898–9
  malaria, **P**.84
  peptide vaccines, **I**.879

Moellerella, **B2**.1496
  antibacterial susceptibility/resistance, **B2**.1496
  biochemical tests, **B2**.1496
  culture, **B2**.1496
  definition, **B2**.1496
  habitats, **B2**.1496
  non-motility, **B2**.1342
  pathogenicity, **B2**.1496

Moellerella morganii, **B2**.1319 (Tab.)

Moellerella wisconsensis, **B2**.1496
  biochemical tests, **B2**.1319 (Tab.), **B2**.1496
  culture, **B2**.1496
  habitats, **B2**.1496
  as normal microbiota, **B1**.296 (Tab.)
  pathogenicity, **B2**.1496

Mogibacterium, **B2**.1028

Mogibacterium timidum
  differential characteristics, **B2**.1029 (Tab.)
  pathogenicity, **B2**.1029–30

Moist heat, **B1**.445–9, **B1**.454 (Tab.)
  mechanisms of action, **B1**.448–9
  resistance to, **B1**.449
  terminology, **B1**.445–6
  time-temperature relationships, **B1**.448 (Tab.)
  types of process, **B1**.446–8
  uses, **B1**.445 (Tab.)
  validation and monitoring, **B1**.454 (Tab.)

Mokola virus, **V2**.1106 (Fig.)

Mold fungi, pigmented
  infection *see* Phaeohyphomycosis
  see Phaeoid (dematiaceous) fungi

Molds
  antibacterial agents, **B1**.433–4
  cereal spoilage, **B1**.284
  fruit spoilage, **B1**.282, **B1**.283
  herbs and spices, **B1**.287

Molecular assays, **B1**.721–2, **B1**.723 (Tab.)
  benefits, **B1**.721–2

identification, **B1**.22 (Tab.), **B1**.25–6, **B1**.32–3
  Aeromonas, **B2**.1532
  Enterobacteriaceae, **B2**.1351
  inhibitors presence, **B1**.724
  performance, **B1**.722–4
  precision and accuracy measurements, **B1**.722
  quantitative standardization, **B1**.722–4
  specimen suitability, **B1**.724
  see also specific techniques

Molecular beacon probes, **B1**.727 (Fig.), **B1**.728
  applications, **B1**.728–9

Molecular biology
  amebiasis diagnosis, **P**.220
  Babesia, **P**.453
  Giardia diagnosis, **P**.250–1
  intestinal amebae, **P**.219
  Isospora belli, **P**.412
  malaria diagnosis, **P**.504–5, **P**.505 (Fig.)
  microsporidiosis diagnosis, **P**.547
  Old World *Leishmania*, **P**.296, **P**.301–2
  onchocerciasis diagnosis, **P**.791–2
  opportunistic amebae, **P**.229–31
  parasite epidemiology *see* Epidemiology of infection, parasitic infection
  Toxoplasma gondii, **P**.428–9
  Trichomonas vaginalis, **P**.256–7
  see also individual species

Molecular chaperones, *Entamoeba histolytica*, **P**.202

'Molecular clock' hypothesis, **M**.47–8

Molecular epidemiology, **B1**.735–6

Molecular markers, fungi classification, **M**.47

Molecular mimicry
  autoimmune disease, **I**.753–4
  Coxsackie virus infection, **V1**.283
  experimental allergic encephalitis, **I**.753
  historical aspects/re-evaluation, **I**.12–3
  onchocerciasis visual damage, **P**.795
  therapy-resistant Lyme arthritis, **I**.753–4, **I**.754 (Fig.)

Molecular taxonomy
  dermatophytes, **M**.229–31
  Giardia classification, **P**.242
  Taenia solium, **P**.683

Molecular testing, of fungi, **M**.92–5
  nucleic acid detection, **M**.94–5
    epidemiological typing, **M**.95
    PCR, **M**.94
    in situ hybridization, **M**.94
  see also individual species; specific assays

Mollicutes (class) *see* Mycoplasma(s)

Molluscipoxvirus
  classification, **V1**.579 (Tab.), **V1**.582, **V1**.594
  phylogenetics, **V1**.583
  taxonomy, **V1**.595 (Tab.)

Molluscum contagiosum virus (MCV), **V1**.587–8, **V1**.594
  genome structure, **V1**.587–8
  HIV infection, **V1**.587–8
  host range, **V1**.603 (Fig.)
  immune evasion
    apoptosis interference, **V1**.323, **V1**.325, **V1**.603 (Fig.)

chemokine homologues, **V1**.319, **I**.621–2
  chemokine receptor analogues, **V1**.622
  cytokine binding proteins, **I**.621
  genes, **V1**.603 (Fig.)
  IL-18 binding protein, **V1**.318–19, **V1**.621
  NK cells, **V1**.322–3, **I**.628
  infection *see* Molluscum contagiosum virus infection
  phylogenetic comparison, **V1**.584 (Fig.)
  type species, **V1**.583
  vFLIPs, **V1**.323

Molluscum contagiosum virus infection
  cytopathology, **V2**.1534 (Tab.)
  in HIV infection, **V1**.587–8, **V2**.1499 (Tab.)
  inflammation, **V1**.619

Molluskicides, schistosomiasis control programs, **P**.127, **P**.635–6

Mollusks, **B1**.280
  harvesting, **B1**.280
  hepatitis A outbreaks, **B1**.280
  primary septicemia, **B1**.280
  purification, **B1**.280
  seafood-associated illness, **B1**.280
  toxins, **B1**.280
  Vibrio, **B1**.280
  viruses, **B1**.280
  wound infection, **B1**.280

Molokai virus, **V2**.1103–4

Moloney murine leukemia virus (MoMLV)
  gene therapy vector, **V2**.1590–1, **V2**.1593–4
  immune response, **V1**.281
  vertical transmission, **V1**.281

Monascus bisporus, **B1**.283

Monensin, **B1**.497

Moniezia, **P**.577

Monilia, **M**.580

Moniliformida, **P**.597

Moniliformidae, **P**.597

Moniliformis, **P**.597

Monitoring procedures, hazard analysis critical control point system, **B1**.288

Monkeypox, **V1**.587
  emerging infection, **V2**.1648 (Tab.), **V2**.1651 (Tab.)
    behavioral factors, **V2**.1659–60
  laboratory worker immunization, **B1**.767
  mortality, **V1**.587
  outbreaks, **V1**.587

Monkeypox virus, **V1**.594
  classification, **V1**.583
  phylogenetics, **V1**.585
  transmission, **V1**.371 (Tab.)

Monkeys
  Hepatitis A virus genotypes, **V2**.1164
  hepatitis E models, **V2**.1178–9

le Monnier, G., **M**.8–9

Monobactams, **B1**.480
  structure, **B1**.471 (Fig.), **B1**.479 (Fig.)
  Vibrio, **B2**.1514
  see also specific types

Monoclonal antibodies, **I**.332–3, **B1**.754–5
  African trypanosomiasis diagnosis, **P**.367
  Bacillus anthracis, **B2**.937
  characterization, **I**.353–4
  Entamoeba histolytica, **P**.211

Monoclonal antibodies (*Continued*)
 generation, **I.**332–3
 historical aspects, **I.**7
 humanization, **I.**333
 phage display, **I.**333
 preparation, **V1.**93
 production quantities, **I.**353–4
 PrP^Sc, **V2.**1365
 sequential BCE identification, **I.**854
 Trichomonas vaginalis, **P.**261
 Tropheryma whippelii, **B2.**1002
Monoclonal antibodies, therapy, **I.**332–3, **I.353–74**
 antibody fragments, 184.76–83
  effector functions, **I.**369–71
  fusion proteins, **I.**369
  Fv-based constructs, **I.**367–8
  immunotoxins, **I.**369
  radioimmunoconjugates, **I.**369
  recombinant bispecific antibodies, **I.**369–70, **I.**370 (Fig.)
  see also specific fragments
 artificial effector functions, **I.**358–62
  see also ADEPT (Antibody Directed Enzyme Pro-drug Therapy); Immunotoxins; Radioimmunoconjugates
 bispecific antibodies, **I.**360–2, **I.**361 (Fig.)
  cell activation, **I.**361
  chemical methods, **I.**360
  genetic engineering, **I.**360
  tumor immunology, **I.**361
  virally infected cells, **I.**361
 blocking by, **I.**357–8
 chimerisation, **I.**365, **I.**366 (Fig.)
 complement recruitment, **I.**354
 deimmunization, **I.**365–6
 drawbacks, **I.**362
  antigen loss, **I.**362
  antigen properties, **I.**362
  immunogenicity, **I.**362, **I.**365–6
  pharmacokinetics, **I.**358, **I.**362
  serum sickness development, **I.**362
 Fc-mediated killing, **I.**354, **I.**357
 genetic engineering, **I.**362–71
  see also individual techniques
 graft rejection therapy, **I.**357–8
 history, **I.**353
 humanization, **I.**365, **I.**366 (Fig.)
 immunoassays, **I.**333
 licensing, **I.**354, **I.**355 (Tab.)
 polyclonal antibodies *vs.*, **I.**353–4
 signaling by, **I.**358
 specific diseases/infection
  candidiasis, **M.**267
  Crohn's disease therapy, **I.**357
  rheumatoid arthritis, **I.**357
  rhinovirus infection therapy, **V2.**879
  septic shock treatment, **B1.**393
 target killing, **I.**354–62
 tolerance induction, **I.**366
 veneering, **I.**365–6
Monoclonal antibody-resistant (MAR) mutants, **V1.**252
 detection, **V1.**194

Monocyte(s)
 actions/effects
  acute phase response, **I.**207
  as APCs, **I.**112, **I.**376
 CD4 expression, **I.**794
 chemotaxis
  defensins, **I.**169
  HIV infection, **I.**794–5
 cytokines produced
  G-CSF production, **I.**276
  IL-1, **I.**284
  IL-19, **I.**294
  IL-20, **I.**294
  IL-24, **I.**294
  leukotriene B$_4$ production, **I.**185
  platelet-activating factor production, **I.**191
  prostaglandin production, **I.**187
  thromboxane production, **I.**189
 defensin expression, **I.**168
 in diseases/infection
  HIV infection, **V1.**242, **I.**794–5
  measles, **I.**803, **I.**804–5
 hematopoiesis, **I.**113 (Fig.)
 histamine effects, **I.**67
 IL-13 effects, **I.**294–7
 receptors
  CC chemokines, **I.**223–4
  FcγRI (CD64), **I.**314
  FcγRIIa, **I.**314
  FcγRIIb, **I.**314
 TNF-α effects, **I.**286
 viruses replicating in, **V1.**243 (Tab.)
 see also Macrophage(s)
Monocyte chemoattractant protein 1 (MCP-1: CCL2), **I.**218 (Tab.)
 actions/effects
  basophil chemotaxis, **I.**58
  basophil histamine release, **I.**62
  eosinophil rolling, **I.**60
  graft rejection, **I.**228
  mucosal immune response, **I.**522–3
  T cell chemotaxis, **I.**224
 airway hypersensitivity, **I.**734
 antagonists, inflammatory disease therapy, **I.**231
 gene deletion effects, **I.**228
 macrophage production, **I.**28–9
 structure, **I.**221
  amino terminal region, **I.**221
Monocyte chemoattractant protein 2 (MCP-2: CCL8), **I.**218 (Tab.)
 actions/effects
  basophil cytokine production, **I.**66
  eosinophil chemotaxis, **I.**61
 basophil histamine release, **I.**62
 intradermal DNA vaccine delivery, **I.**912–13
 structure, amino terminal region, **I.**221
Monocyte chemoattractant protein 3 (MCP-3: CCL7), **I.**218 (Tab.)
 actions/effects
  basophil chemotaxis, **I.**58
  basophil cytokine production, **I.**66
  basophil histamine release, **I.**62
 structure, **I.**220
  amino terminal region, **I.**221

Monocyte chemoattractant protein 4 (MCP-4: CCL13), **I.**218 (Tab.)
 basophil cytokine production, **I.**66
 structure, **I.**221
Monocyte chemotactic protein-1/CC chemokine ligand-2 (MCP-1/CCL2), aspergillosis, **M.**707–8
Monocyte-derived chemokine (MDC), **I.**734
Monod, O, **M.**19
Monoethyl phosphate, systemic $\gamma\delta$ T cell binding, **I.**440 (Fig.)
Monohydroeicosatetraenoic acids, **I.**186
Monolayers, **V1.**86–7
Monomorphic forms, *Trypanosoma brucei*, **P.**356–7
Monomycin, **P.**307
Mononaghela virus, **V2.**1666 (Tab.)
Mononegavirales order, **V1.**26, **V1.378–89**
 antibody-mediated neutralization, **V1.**381
 characteristics, **V1.**129 (Tab.), **V1.**379 (Tab.)
 classification, **V1.**42, **V1.**48–9, **V1.**127–8, **V1.**390–2, **V1.**808 (Fig.)
  morphology/biochemistry, **V1.**379
 establishment, **V1.**378–9
 gene order conservation, **V1.**386–8
 general properties, **V1.**380–2, **V1.**380 (Tab.)
  electron microscopy, **V1.**380–1
 genome replication, **V1.**381
 genome structure, **V1.**381, **V1.**387 (Tab.)
 glycoproteins, **V1.**381
 health importance, **V1.**381–2
 host ranges, **V1.**381–2
 lipids, **V1.**381
 members, **V1.**48
 morphology, **V1.**380–1
 mRNA transcription, **V1.**381
 nucleocapsid proteins, **V1.**381
 phospholipids, **V1.**381
 phylogenetics, **V1.**384 (Fig.), **V1.**388
 proteins, **V1.**381
  conservation, **V1.**384 (Fig.), **V1.**388
 RNA structure, **V1.**381
 taxonomy, **V1.**378–9
 see also specific viruses
Mononuclear phagocytes (MPs)
 histoplasmosis capsulati, **M.**534
 M-CSF effects, **I.**277
 neutrophil interactions, **I.**45 (Fig.)
Monophosphoryl lipid (MPL) adjuvant, **I.**926, **I.**929–30
 aluminum salt combination, **I.**929–30
 composition, **I.**929
 cytokine production, **I.**929
 hepatitis B vaccine, **I.**937
 QS-21 combination, **I.**930
 Th1 cell responses, **I.**929
 vaccines used, **I.**929–30
Monospot test, **V1.**568–9
Monte-Carlo simulation models, **B1.**331–2, **V1.**364–5
Montenegro (leishmanin) skin test, **P.**302, **P.**336–7
Monthly biting rate (MBR), onchocerciasis, **P.**785–6
Mopeia virus
 genome, **V2.**1066

Mopeia virus (*Continued*)
  geographical distribution/carrier and disease,
    V2.1060 (Tab.)
Moraxella, **B2**.1305
  antibacterial susceptibility testing, **B2**.1306
  characteristics, **B2**.1303 (Tab.), **B2**.1305
  classification, **B2**.1271, **B2**.1302
  clinical significance, **B2**.1306
  colony characteristics, **B2**.1305
  fimbriae, **B2**.1305
  in fish, **B1**.279
  infection
    conjunctivitis, **B1**.599
    keratitis, **B1**.601
  in meat and meat products, **B1**.273
  microbiology, **B2**.1305
  natural competence, **B1**.99
  in poultry, **B1**.277–8
  species, **B2**.1305
    animal-associated, **B2**.1306
    minor, **B2**.1306
  taxonomic delineation, **B2**.1302
  waterborne, **B1**.221
  see also individual species
Moraxella atlantae, **B2**.1306
Moraxella bovis, **B2**.1306
Moraxella canis, **B2**.1306
Moraxella caprae, **B2**.1306
Moraxella (Branhamella) catarrhalis, **B2**.1271,
    B2.1306–8
  antibacterial susceptibility/resistance,
    B2.1307–8
    β-lactamase, **B2**.1307–8
  characteristics, **B2**.1303 (Tab.), **B2**.1306–7
  classification, **B2**.1271, **B2**.1307
  colony characteristics, **B2**.1306–7
  epidemiology, **B2**.1307
  fimbriae, **B2**.1307
  hemagglutination, **B2**.1307
  infection
    chronic bronchitis, **B1**.648
    clinical significance, **B2**.1307
    conjunctivitis, **B1**.599
    nasopharynx colonization, **B1**.295–300,
      B2.1307
    otitis media, **B1**.617–18
    sinusitis, **B1**.615, **B1**.615 (Tab.)
    therapeutic options, **B2**.1307–8
    vaccines, **I**.933 (Tab.)
  LPS, **B2**.1307
  microbiology, **B2**.1306–7
  morphology, **B2**.1306
  normal microbiota, **B1**.296 (Tab.)
  outer membrane proteins, **B2**.1307
  pathogenic factors, **B2**.1307
  pili, **B2**.1307
  virulence, **B2**.1307
Moraxella caviae, **B2**.1306
Moraxellaceae, **B2**.1301–2
Moraxella cuniculi, **B2**.1306
Moraxella equi, **B2**.1306
Moraxella kingae, **B2**.1668–9
Moraxella lacunata, **B2**.1305–6
Moraxella lincolnii, **B2**.1306
Moraxella nonliquefaciens, **B2**.1305

Moraxella osloensis, **B2**.1306
Moraxella ovis, **B2**.1306
Morbidity
  ascariasis, **P**.725, **P**.726 (Tab.)
  gastrointestinal nematodes, **P**.725
  reporting system
    GPs, **B1**.320
    laboratory, **B1**.319
  trichuriasis, **P**.725
Morbidity and Mortality Weekly Report,
    V2.1583
Morbillivirus
  characteristics, **V1**.129 (Tab.), **V1**.702 (Tab.)
  classification, **V1**.48–9, **V1**.382, **V1**.700 (Tab.),
    V1.808 (Fig.)
  members, **V1**.382–3
  phylogenetic tree, **V1**.808 (Fig.)
  see also Morbilliviruses
Morbilliviruses
  animal infection, **V1.807–22**
    aquatic mammals, **V1**.812–15
    impact of, **V1**.807
    see also individual infection
  attachment (H) protein, **V1**.706–7
    conservation, **V1**.706–7
  cell attachment/penetration, **V1**.701–2
  genome structure/organization,
    V1.387 (Tab.), **V1**.701 (Fig.)
    conservation, **V1**.784–5, **V1**.785 (Fig.)
    intergenic regions, **V1**.701
  immune evasion, **V1**.704
    IFN signaling inhibition, **V1**.704
  P protein, **V1**.704
  see also Measles virus; *Morbillivirus*
Moredun Bordetella medium, **B2**.1791
Morganella, **B2**.1447–50
  biochemical characteristics, **B2**.1448–9
  characteristics, **B2**.1435
  definition, **B2**.1447–8
  general properties, **B2**.1448–50
  infection
    intestinal, **B2**.1347
    nosocomial infection, **B1**.398 (Tab.)
  motility, **B2**.1448
  nomenclature and classification, **B2**.1447–8
    culture and hemolytic strains, **B2**.1448
    screening tests, **B2**.1349 (Tab.)
    type species, **B2**.1448
Morganella morganii, **B1**.296 (Tab.),
    B2.1448–50
  antibacterial susceptibility/resistance,
    B2.1449–50
    intrinsic, **B2**.1352 (Tab.)
  biochemical tests, **B2**.1442 (Tab.), **B2**.1448–9
  in feces, **B2**.1449
  infection, **B2**.1449–50
    keratitis, **B1**.601
  subspecies, **B2**.1448
    subsp *morganii*, **B2**.1448–9
    subsp *sibonii*, **B2**.1448–9
  typing, **B2**.1449
    biogroups, **B2**.1448–50
    biotyping, **B2**.1441
Morpholines, **M**.233

Morphological alteration and disintegration
    test (MADT), hepatitis B control,
    V2.1257
Morphology
  bacteria
    microscopy, **B1**.22–3, **B1**.23 (Fig.)
    see also individual species
  fungi, **M**.69, **M**.125
    fungal classification, **M**.45, **M**.46 (Tab.),
      M.49, **M**.51
    see also individual species
  viruses, **V1.57–85**
    helical viruses, **V1**.58, **V1**.59–60,
      V1.59 (Fig.)
      electron microscopy, **V1**.59–60,
        V1.59 (Fig.), **V1**.60 (Fig.)
      fiber diffraction, **V1**.60
      nucleic acids, **V1**.59
      nucleocapsids, **V1**.59
      symmetry, **V1**.6
    historical aspects, **V1**.6
    isocahedral viruses, **V1**.58, **V1**.60–9,
      V1.64 (Fig.), **V1**.66 (Fig.)
      capsid assembly, **V1**.65–7
      connectorless capsids, **V1**.63
      conserved architecture, **V1**.67–9,
        V1.68 (Fig.)
      electron microscopy, **V1**.62
      flexibility, **V1**.63
      methodology, **V1**.62
      as protective container, **V1**.61–2
      protein folds, **V1**.63–5
      'quasi-equivalence,' **V1**.62–3
      structure–function relationship, **V1**.62
      triangulation rule, **V1**.62–3
      X-ray crystallography, **V1**.62
    nonsymmetrical viruses, **V1**.69–79
      glycoproteins, **V1**.69
      lipid membranes, **V1**.69
      lipid rafts, **V1**.69
      negative-strand RNA viruses, **V1**.69–79
      protein structures, **V1**.70 (Tab.)
      receptor binding, **V1**.69
    receptor-binding proteins, **V1**.58, **V1**.67–9
    transport components, **V1**.58
      formation *vs.* decapsidation, **V1**.58
    see also specific viruses
Mortality
  data, **B1**.319
  gastrointestinal nematodes, **P**.725
Mortierella, **M**.664
Mortierellales, **M**.660–1
  classification, **M**.54 (Tab.)
Mortierella polycephala, **M**.660–1, **M**.664
Mortierella wolfii, **M**.660–1, **M**.664, **M**.664 (Fig.)
Mortuary, airborne bacteria, **B1**.186 (Tab.)
'Morula cells of Mott,' African
    trypanosomiasis, **P**.365
Mosquitoes
  alphavirus transmission, **V2**.1018
  Bacillus pathogenic strains, **B2**.929
  flavivirus infection, **V2**.997–9, **V2**.998 (Tab.),
    V2.999–1003
  flavivirus transmission, **V2**.1424
  see also individual species
Mossman virus, **V1**.699, **V1**.819

Mosso das Pedras virus (MDPV),
V2.1011 (Tab.)

Moss, sphagnum, **M**.368, **M**.369, **M**.371

Most probable number (MPN) estimates,
B1.204

Motility, bacterial
Enterobacteriaceae identification,
B2.1319 (Tab.)
pathogenicity, **B1**.151–2
'runs' and tumbling', **B1**.44
swarming, **B1**.152
see also Fimbriae; Flagella

Motor axonal neuropathy, *Campylobacter*
infection, **B2**.1551

Mouse cytomegalovirus (MCMV) *see* Murine
cytomegalovirus (MCMV)

Mouse hepatitis virus *see* Murine hepatitis
virus (MHV)

Mouse mammary tumor virus (MMTV)
immune evasion, superantigen, **V1**.286
immune response, **V1**.281
infection course, **I**.563
insertional mutagenesis, **V1**.340
oncogenic mechanisms, **V1**.342 (Tab.)
superantigens, **V1**.341, **I**.556 (Tab.), **I**.563,
I.637–8
invariant chain Ii *vs.*, **I**.563
sequence conservation, **I**.563

Mouth *see* Oral cavity

Moxidectin, **P**.790

Moxifloxacin
Nocardia, **B2**.1165–6
spectrum of activity, **B1**.492, **B1**.499 (Tab.)

MPIF-2 *see* Eotaxin-2 (CCL24)

M proteins
adhesion, **B1**.149
historical aspects, **B1**.12
Streptococcus pyogenes, **I**.556 (Tab.), **I**.565

MR1-reactive αβ T cells, **I**.443, **I**.444 (Fig.)

mRNA
capping, poxviruses *see* Poxviruses
7-Methylguanylate, **V1**.112
positive strand RNA viruses *see* RNA
viruses, positive-strand
splicing, Borna disease virus, **V2**.1139–40
transcription, **V1**.112
adenoviruses, **V1**.110
DNA viruses, **V1**.110
gene expression, **V1**.105–6
herpesviruses, **V1**.110
Mononegavirales order, **V1**.381
papovaviruses, **V1**.110
Pneumovirus, **V1**.790
translation, **V1**.113

MS2 bacteriophage (*Leviviridae*), **B1**.140

M (medium) segment, bunyavirus genome,
V2.1028–31, **V2**.1038–9

MTT (tetrazolium salt), **M**.453
antifungal testing, **M**.157

Mucambo virus (MUCV), **V2**.1011 (Tab.)

Mucate fermentation, Enterobacteriaceae
identification, **B2**.1319 (Tab.)

Mucin stains, **M**.123 (Tab.), **M**.124

Muckle–Wells syndrome, caspase-recruitment
domain single nucleotide
polymorphisms, **I**.125

Mucociliary clearance, **B1**.623
defects, **B1**.626
Pseudomonas pigments effect, **B1**.650

Mucocutaneous, candidiasis *see* Candidiasis,
cutaneous/mucocutaneous

Mucocutaneous leishmaniasis *see*
Leishmaniasis, New World

Mucocutaneous syndromes, enterovirus
infection, **V2**.871–2

Mucocutanous ulceration, HSV infection,
V2.1500

Mucopolysaccharides
Ascaris lumbricoides eggs, **P**.715
tapeworms, **P**.662

Mucor, **M**.660, **M**.660 (Tab.), **M**.665
histopathology, **M**.89 (Tab.)
history, **M**.6, **M**.9, **M**.20–1
infection
oculomycoses, **M**.287
rhino-orbital-cerebral zygomycosis,
M.290–1, **M**.292 (Fig.)
morphology, **M**.665, **M**.665 (Fig.)
thermotolerance, **M**.665, **M**.665 (Tab.)

Mucoraceae, **M**.660 (Tab.)

Mucorales, **M**.20–1, **M**.347, **M**.660,
M.660 (Tab.)
classification, **M**.53, **M**.54 (Tab.)
culture, **M**.676–7
infection, **M**.672–3, **M**.674 (Tab.)
experimental, **M**.677

Mucor amphibiorum, **M**.665–6, **M**.665 (Tab.)

Mucor circinelloides, **M**.9, **M**.665, **M**.665 (Tab.),
M.666

Mucor corymbifera, **M**.20

Mucor hiemalis, **M**.665 (Tab.), **M**.666

Mucor indicus, **M**.665 (Tab.), **M**.666

Mucormycosis *see* Zygomycosis

Mucor racemosus, **M**.20, **M**.665, **M**.665 (Tab.),
M.666–7

Mucor ramosissimus, **M**.660, **M**.665,
M.665 (Tab.), **M**.667
histopathology, **M**.128 (Tab.)

Mucor rhizopodiformis, **M**.20

Mucor, vegetables, **B1**.282

Mucosa-associated lymphoid tissue (MALT),
P.75, **I**.505, **I**.529–30
mucosal vaccination, **I**.827–8
structure, **I**.529–30
see also Common mucosal immune system
(CMIS); *individual tissues*

Mucosa-associated lymphoid tissue (MALT)
lymphomas, *Helicobacter pylori*
infection, **B2**.1580

Mucosal addressin-cell adhesion molecule-1
(MadCAM-1), **I**.227

Mucosal immune response
cytokines, **I**.535–7
GM-CSF, **I**.522–3
IFN-γ, **I**.524
IL-1, **I**.522–3, **I**.525
IL-6, **I**.522–3
IL-8, **I**.522–3, **I**.525
IL-10, **I**.525
dendritic cells, **I**.538
in diseases/infection, **I**.522–3
Vibrio cholerae infection, **I**.528–9
IgA class switching, **I**.535–6

induction, **I**.537–41
antigen presentation, **I**.524
APCs, **I**.538
site structure, **I**.531 (Fig.)
innate, **I**.519–22, **I**.520 (Fig.)
cathelin-associated peptides, **I**.521
defensins, **I**.520–1
see also Defensins
eosinophil peroxidase, **I**.521
human lactoperoxidase, **I**.521
lactoferrin, **I**.521
lysozyme, **I**.521
myeloperoxidase, **I**.521
NK cells, **I**.519
phospholipase A$_2$, **I**.521
secretory leukocyte protease inhibitor,
I.521
as innate/acquired bridge, **I**.522–5,
I.523 (Fig.)
antigen presentation, **I**.524
chemokines, **I**.522–4
see also individual chemokines
cytokines, **I**.522–4
see also individual cytokines
IgG, **I**.524–5
physical barrier, **I**.519, **I**.522
polymeric IgA, **I**.524–5
polymeric IgM, **I**.524–5
intercellular adhesion molecule 1, **I**.524
intraepithelial lymphocytes *see*
Intraepithelial lymphocytes (IELs)
lymphocyte function-associated antigen-3,
I.524
monocyte chemoattractant protein 1, **I**.522–3
receptors
FcRn (neonatal receptor), **I**.525
pIgR (polymeric Ig receptor), **I**.525
TLRs, **I**.523–4
SCF, **I**.522–3
systemic organization, **I**.529–35
effector tissues, **I**.534–5
inductive sites, **I**.530–4
see also individual systems
T cells, **I**.535–7
IgA synthesis control, **I**.536–7
TNF-α, **I**.522–3, **I**.525
tolerance induction, **I**.541–6
high-dose antigen, **I**.542
mechanisms, **I**.542 (Fig.)
microfold (M) cells, **I**.532
T cell anergy, **I**.542–3
T cell mediation, **I**.542–3
see also Oral tolerance
vaccination *see* Vaccination, mucosal routes
see also Common mucosal immune system
(CMIS); Secretory immunoglobulin A
(sIgA); *individual infection*

Mucosal leishmaniasis *see* Leishmaniasis, New
World

Mucous membranes
bacterial infection barrier, **B1**.176
specimens, **M**.83 (Tab.), **M**.86 (Tab.)
virus entry, **V1**.236
virus shedding, **V1**.249

Mucus
goblet cells secreting, **B1**.623 (Fig.)

Mucus (*Continued*)
　mucosal immune response, **I**.522
　respiratory tract, **B1**.607–8, **B1**.623
Mueller–Hinton agar, **B2**.1793–4
　Campylobacter, **B2**.1548
Muleshoe virus, **V2**.1666 (Tab.)
Muller's ratchet, fitness, **V1**.18–9
Multiceps, **P**.579
Multi-colony stimulating factor *see* Interleukin-
　3 (IL-3)
Multidrug and toxic compound extrusion
　(MATE), efflux pumps and antibiotic
　resistance, **B1**.440
Multidrug efflux pumps, **B1**.443
Multidrug resistance (MDR), **B1**.566, **B1**.571
　Plasmodium, **P**.506
　tuberculosis, **B1**.399
Multifocal Castleman's disease, **V1**.550,
　V1.554, **V2**.1503
Multilateral Initiative on Malaria (MIM),
　P.110, **P**.518
Multilayered interlaced network,
　microsporidians, **P**.529–31
Multilocus enzyme electrophoresis (MLEE)
　Burkholderia cepacia, **B2**.1615
　Enterococcus, **B2**.894
　Escherichia, **B2**.1371
　Legionella, **B2**.1771
　rapidly growing mycobacteria, **B2**.1244–6
　Salmonella, **B2**.1407
　Salmonella Agona, **B2**.1416–17
　Salmonella Choleraesuis, **B2**.1417
　Salmonella Dublin, **B2**.1418
　Salmonella Paratyphi A, **B2**.1420–1
　Salmonella Paratyphi B, **B2**.1421
　Salmonella Typhimurium, **B2**.1407
Multilocus enzyme studies
　Haemophilus, **B2**.1698, **B2**.1704
　Listeria, **B2**.962
　Malassezia., **M**.216
　Vibrio, **B2**.1516
Multilocus restriction typing, *Burkholderia
　cepacia*, **B2**.1615
Multilocus sequence typing (MLST), **M**.47,
　M.47 (Tab.), **B1**.736
　Burkholderia thailandensis typing, **B2**.1623–4
　Escherichia, **B2**.1371
　Helicobacter, **B2**.1570
　Helicobacter typing, **B2**.1570
　Salmonella, **B2**.1407
Multinucleated giant cells, *Burkholderia
　thailandensis* infection, **B2**.1625
Multinucleated syncytia formation, cell–virus
　interactions, **V1**.213
Multiple (sequential) fission, microsporidians,
　P.532–3
Multiple myeloma, immunodeficiency,
　I.788 (Tab.)
Multiple organ dysfunction syndrome
　(MODS), **B1**.511 (Tab.)
　HCMV infection, **V1**.520–1
Multiple organ failure (MOF)
　complement activation, **I**.698–9
　definition, **I**.695
　see also Septic shock

Multiple sclerosis (MS)
　animal model *see* Experimental allergic
　　encephalitis (EAE)
　axonal loss, **I**.757
　complement pathology, **I**.155 (Tab.), **I**.156
　demyelination mechanisms, **I**.757
　HHV-6, **V1**.527–8, **V2**.1418
　HLA-DR association, **I**.751–2, **I**.752 (Tab.)
　IFN-β therapy, **I**.259
　IL-15, **I**.282
　measles association, **V1**.725
　pathogen induced, **I**.753 (Tab.)
　prevalence, **I**.748 (Tab.)
　seborrheic dermatitis, **M**.211–12
　Th1/Th2 balance, **I**.755–6
Multiplex PCR, HTLV, **V2**.1294
Multiplex polymerase chain reaction, syphilis
　detection, **B2**.1852–3
Multiplicity of infection (MOI), cell–virus
　interactions, **V1**.203
Multiplicity reactivation, **V1**.189
Multivacuolar forms, *Blastocystis hominis*,
　P.557, **P**.560, **P**.560 (Fig.), **P**.561 (Fig.)
μ1 protein *see* Reoviruses
μ2 protein, reoviruses *see* Reoviruses
μ heavy chain
　autosomal recessive agammaglobulinemia,
　　I.780
　IgM structure, **I**.307
Mumps
　aseptic meningitis, **V1**.750
　clinical features, **V1**.748, **V1**.749–50
　　arthritis, **V1**.750
　　CNS *see below*
　　deafness, **V1**.750
　　electrocardiographic abnormalities, **V1**.750
　　endolymphatic labyrinthitis, **V1**.750
　　epididymitis, **V1**.749
　　fetal infection, **V1**.749, **V1**.750
　　heart effects, **V1**.748
　　IgA nephropathy, **V1**.748–9
　　meningitis *see below*
　　oophoritis, **V1**.748, **V1**.749
　　orchitis, **V1**.748, **V1**.749
　　pancreatitis, **V1**.750
　　parotid gland infection, **V1**.748, **V1**.749
　　renal dysfunction, **V1**.748–50
　　testicular atrophy, **V1**.748, **V1**.749
　　thyroiditis, **V1**.750
　CNS manifestations, **V1**.749–50, **V2**.1430–1
　　cerebrospinal fluid pleocytosis, **V1**.748,
　　　V1.749–50, **V1**.756
　　clinical features, **V2**.1430, **V2**.1430–1
　　diagnosis, **V2**.1430–1
　　incidence, **V2**.1430
　　meningoencephalitis, **V2**.1430
　　pathogenesis/pathology, **V2**.1430
　　postinfectious encephalomyelitis, **V1**.748,
　　　V1.749–50
　diagnosis, **V1**.755–6
　　antigen, **V1**.755–6
　　recent/current infection, **V1**.755–6
　　RNA, **V1**.755–6
　　samples, **V1**.755–6
　　serology, **V1**.755
　　virus, **V1**.755–6

differential diagnosis, **V1**.754
epidemiology, **V1**.751–2
　ages affected, **V1**.751–2
　fetal infection, **V1**.749, **V1**.750
　incubation period, **V1**.748
　outbreaks, **V1**.753
　seasonal variation, **V1**.751–2, **V1**.751 (Fig.)
　transmission, **V1**.748, **V2**.1404
eradicable disease, **V2**.1570
immune response, **V1**.751
　cell-mediated immunity, **V1**.751
　humoral immunity, **V1**.751
　IgA, **V1**.756
　IgG, **V1**.755, **V1**.756
　IgM, **V1**.751, **V1**.755, **V1**.756
　neutralizing antibodies, **V1**.751
　secretory IgA, **V1**.748, **V1**.751
laboratory investigations, **V1**.754–6
　immunity determination, **V1**.754
laboratory worker immunization, **B1**.767
meningitis, **V1**.748
　diagnosis, **V1**.756
pathogenesis, **V1**.748–9
　viral detection, **V1**.748
prevention, **V1**.752–4
　hyperimmune gammaglobulin, **V1**.752
　vaccination *see below*
treatment, **V1**.752
vaccines/vaccination, **B1**.348, **I**.424 (Tab.),
　V1.752–4
　adverse effects, **V2**.1564 (Tab.), **V2**.1570
　at-risk age cohort, **V1**.753
　complications, **V1**.753
　contraindications, **V1**.753
　historical aspects, **V1**.8 (Tab.), **V2**.1570
　immune response, **V1**.751
　incidence since introduction, **V1**.753
　Jeryl Lynn strain, **V1**.753
　killed vaccines, **V1**.752
　live-attenuated vaccines, **V1**.752–3,
　　V2.1555 (Tab.)
　Rubini strain, **V1**.754
　schedules, **V2**.1560–1
　strains, **V1**.753–4, **V2**.1570
　Urabe Am 9 strain, **V1**.753–4
　USA schedules, **V2**.1559–60
　see also Measles, mumps and rubella
　　(MMR) vaccine
Mumps virus, **V1**.744–62
biological properties, **V1**.747–8
　hemadsorption, **V1**.747–8
　hemagglutination, **V1**.747–8
　in vitro replication, **V1**.747, **V1**.747 (Fig.)
classification, **V1**.382–3, **V1**.744
fusion (F) protein, **V1**.746, **V1**.746 (Tab.)
　cell penetration, **V1**.747
genome structure, **V1**.745–7, **V1**.746 (Fig.),
　V1.785 (Fig.)
　noncoding regions, **V1**.746–7
　organization, **V1**.745
hemagglutinin-neuraminidase (HN) protein,
　V1.745–6, **V1**.746 (Tab.)
　cell penetration, **V1**.747
historical aspects, **V1**.744
immune evasion, **V1**.315

Mumps virus (*Continued*)

infection *see* Mumps

isolation/propagation and identification, **V1**.99

large protein (L), **V1**.745, **V1**.746 (Tab.)

matrix (M) protein, **V1**.746, **V1**.746 (Tab.)

morphology, **V1**.744, **V1**.745 (Fig.)

neurotropism, **V2**.1430

nucleocapsid associated protein (NP), **V1**.745, **V1**.746 (Tab.)

phosphoprotein (P), **V1**.745, **V1**.746 (Tab.)

small hydrophobic (SH) protein, **V1**.708, **V1**.746, **V1**.746 (Tab.)

diversity, **V1**.746

stability, **V1**.745

strain variation, **V1**.746–7

mutation rates, **V1**.747

vaccine *see* Mumps

Mupirocin, **B1**.490

structure, **B1**.490 (Fig.)

topical application, **B1**.490

Mural endocarditis, **B1**.526–7

Muramic acid, **B1**.42–3

Murein polypeptides, **B1**.24

Muridae, arenaviruses associated, **V2**.1061

Muriform bodies, **M**.89 (Tab.), **M**.356, **M**.357 (Fig.), **M**.362–3, **M**.364

melanin, **M**.362–3, **M**.364

Murine astrovirus (MAstV), **V2**.890 (Tab.)

Murine cytomegalovirus (MCMV)

genome sequences, **V1**.494 (Tab.)

immune evasion

CD8 interference *in vivo,* **I**.637

chemokine receptor, **I**.622

chemokines, **V1**.319, **I**.621–2

dendritic cell maturation, **V1**.323

MHC, **V1**.322, **I**.634–5, **I**.635–7

NK cells, **V1**.322–3, **I**.628, **I**.630

infection, immune response, **V1**.285

NK cells, **I**.96, **I**.97, **V1**.272, **V1**.285

deficiencies, **I**.97

Murine gammaherpesvirus 68 (MHV-68)

characteristics, **V1**.542 (Tab.)

genome sequences, **V1**.494 (Tab.)

immune evasion

CD8 interference *in vivo,* **I**.637

chemokine binding proteins, **I**.622–3

chemokine receptor homologues, **I**.622

MHC degradation, **I**.634

infection, **V1**.285–6

Murine hepatitis virus (MHV)

accessory proteins, **V1**.835–6

cell receptor, **V1**.207 (Tab.), **V1**.246 (Fig.), **V1**.838

classification, **V1**.392

double membrane vesicles, **V1**.835

envelope (E) protein, **V1**.831–2, **V1**.837

genome

expression strategies, **V1**.829 (Fig.)

non-translated region, **V1**.827

packaging, **V1**.827

structure, **V1**.828 (Fig.)

hemagglutinin-esterase (HE), **V1**.838–9

immune evasion

apoptosis mitochondrial pathways, **V1**.324–5

complement, **V1**.287

MHC class I interference, **V1**.322

infection, **V1**.841 (Tab.)

membrane (M) protein

antibody responses, **V1**.840

budding, **V1**.837

nucleocapsid (N) protein, **V1**.832

protein processing, **V1**.141

recombination, **V1**.15

replicase (RNA polymerase), **V1**.833 (Fig.)

intracellular localization, **V1**.835

RNA-dependent RNA polymerase activity, **V1**.833–4

replication, cell-specific factors, **V1**.136 (Fig.)

Murine leukemia virus (MuLV)

capsid, **V1**.78–9

envelope antigens, **V2**.1311

erythroleukemia, **V1**.339–40

gene vectors, foamy viruses *vs.,* **V2**.1314

oncogenic mechanisms, **V1**.342 (Tab.)

receptors, **V1**.246 (Fig.)

virulence and neoplasm types, **V1**.253–4

Murine Minute virus *see* Minute virus of mice (MMV)

Murine neonates, enterovirus infection, **V2**.877

Murine polyomavirus (MPV), immune evasion, **V1**.315, **I**.619

Murine rotavirus, enterotoxin NSP4, **I**.829

Murine typhus *see* Typhus, murine

Muromegalovirus, **V1**.494 (Tab.)

Murray Valley encephalitis, **V2**.1003, **V2**.1424, **V2**.1426

transmission, **V1**.372 (Tab.)

Murray Valley encephalitis virus (MVEV), **V2**.998 (Tab.), **V2**.1424, **V2**.1426

Mus, arenaviruses associated, **V2**.1060 (Tab.), **V2**.1061

Muscle biopsy, **P**.153, **P**.153 (Tab.)

trichinellosis diagnosis, **P**.153, **P**.765

Muscovy duck parvovirus (MDPV), **V1**.410

Musculoskeletal infection *see* Bone/joint infection

Musculoskeletal pains, onchocerciasis, **P**.794

Musculoskeletal symptoms, infective endocarditis, **B1**.535

Mussels, **B1**.280

Mutagens/mutagenesis, **B1**.82, **B1**.83

alkylating agents, **B1**.84–5, **V1**.183

attenuation of viruses, **V1**.251–2, **V1**.254–5

5-Azacytidine, **V1**.183

base analogues, **V1**.183

5-Bromodeoxyuridine, **V1**.183

deaminating agents, **V1**.183

directed

picornaviruses, **V1**.183–4

poxviruses, **V1**.183–4

5-Fluorouracil, **V1**.183

insertional

modes/methods, **V1**.339 (Fig.)

retroviral, **V1**.338–40

intercalating agents, **V1**.183

nitrous acid, **B1**.84–5

proflavine, **B1**.85–6

site-specific mutagenesis, genetic analysis, **V1**.183–4

Mutants/mutations, **B1**.82–91

attenuation, **V1**.251–2, **V1**.254–5

conditional lethal, **V1**.334

definition, **B1**.82

emerging viral infection, **V2**.1652–4

flip-flop mechanisms, **B1**.90–1

genetically engineered, **V1**.252

HIV genetic variation, **V2**.1330, **V2**.1336–7

induction, **B1**.82

macrolesions, **B1**.87

microlesions, **B1**.84–6

base substitution suppression, **B1**.86–7

see also Point mutations

mutagenesis, **B1**.83–4

detection, **B1**.83–4

measurement, **B1**.83

replica plating, **B1**.84

mutator (*mut*) genes, **B1**.89

parvoviruses, **V1**.407

replication errors, **B1**.87, **B1**.88 (Fig.)

site-directed, **B1**.89–90

M13 cloning vectors, **B1**.89

PCR, **B1**.89–90, **B1**.90 (Fig.)

spontaneous, **B1**.82–3, **B1**.89, **V1**.183

'fluctuation test,' **B1**.82–3, **B1**.82 (Fig.)

temperature-sensitive, **V1**.251–2

ultraviolet light, **B1**.87–9

viral evolution, **V1**.19

Mutator (*mut*) genes, **B1**.89

MVA strain, Vaccinia virus, **V1**.591

Mx gene/locus, **V1**.265

MxGTPase, microbial recognition, **I**.24 (Tab.)

Mx proteins

HIV infection, **V1**.301

IFN actions, **V1**.294–5

INFs, **V1**.271

Myalgic encephalomyelitis (postviral fatigue syndrome), **V2**.871

Myasthenia gravis (MG)

BCE peptide vaccines, **I**.855 (Tab.)

complement pathology, **I**.155 (Tab.)

NK cells, **I**.103

pathogen induced, **I**.753 (Tab.)

Mycelium, **M**.70, **M**.72

Aspergillus, **M**.690

Mycetoma, **M**.385–6, **M**.388, **M**.388 (Fig.), **M**.394

actinomycotic, **M**.140 (Fig.)

causative agents, **M**.27, **M**.28 (Fig.), **M**.386, **M**.386 (Tab.), **M**.390–1

aspergillosis, **M**.386 (Tab.)

eumycotic black grain, **M**.139 (Fig.)

eumycotic white grain, **M**.139 (Fig.)

Exophiala jeanselmei, **M**.386 (Tab.), **M**.390, **M**.390 (Tab.)

Fusarium, **M**.386 (Tab.), **M**.389 (Fig.)

see also individual species

clinical features, **M**.388, **M**.388 (Fig.)

abscesses, **M**.385

bone, **M**.389

foot, **M**.386, **M**.388, **M**.388 (Fig.), **M**.394

hands, **M**.386

Mycetoma
　clinical features (*Continued*)
　　pseudomycetoma, **M**.138 (Fig.), **M**.386,
　　　M.392, **M**.394
　diagnosis, **M**.388–92
　　culture, **M**.389–90
　　microscopy, **M**.389
　　serology, **M**.391–2
　epidemiology, **M**.387–8
　epidemiology, agriculture/agricultural
　　workers, **M**.388
　etiologic agents
　　Actinomadura, **B2**.1150, **B2**.1159–60
　　Nocardia brasiliensis, **B2**.1159–60
　　Streptomyces somaliensis, **B2**.1169
　geographical distribution, **M**.387–8,
　　B2.1159–60
　histopathology, **M**.127, **M**.128 (Tab.),
　　M.139 (Fig.), **M**.392, **M**.392 (Tab.)
　　stains, **M**.124–5
　history, **M**.27, **M**.386
　immune response, **M**.387
　metastasis, **M**.388
　nomenclature, **M**.385–6
　pathogenesis, **M**.386, **M**.386–7
　specimens, **M**.83 (Tab.), **M**.389
　therapy, **M**.393
　　amphotericin B, **M**.393
　　griseofulvin, **M**.393
　　surgery, **M**.393
　treatment, **B2**.1159–60
Mycobacteria
　antibacterial susceptibility/resistance, **B1**.427,
　　B1.433, **B1**.436, **B1**.441, **B1**.441 (Tab.)
　　quinolones, **B1**.492
　blood cultures, **B1**.524
　infection
　　bacteremia, **B1**.524
　　nosocomial infection, **B1**.399–400
Mycobacteria (slow-growing)
　antigens, **B2**.1185–6
　　tuberculins, **B2**.1185
　cell-wall structure and components,
　　B2.1183–5
　　lipids, **B2**.1183–4
　　lipoarabinomannan, **B2**.1184
　　mycolic acids, **B2**.1184
　　mycosides, **B2**.1184–5
　　trehaloses, **B2**.1184
　characteristics, **B2**.1181–6
　chemical/physical agent susceptibility/
　　resistance, **B2**.1216–17
　classification, **B2**.1181–2
　culture, **B2**.1190, **B2**.1191–2
　　growth conditions, **B2**.1192
　　liquid media, **B2**.1191–2
　　solid media, **B2**.1191
　definition, **B2**.1181–2
　genetics, **B2**.1186–9
　habitats, **B2**.1182
　identification, **B2**.1189–97, **B2**.1192–5
　　acid-fast smear microscopy, **B2**.1190
　　biochemical tests, **B2**.1192
　　direct amplification tests, **B2**.1194
　　DNA sequencing, **B2**.1193–4
　　genotype, **B2**.1193–4

　　mycolic acid analysis, **B2**.1192
　　PCR, **B2**.1193
　　phenotypic tests, **B2**.1192
　　restriction enzyme analysis, **B2**.1193
　metabolism, **B2**.1182–3
　　carbon sources, **B2**.1182
　　iron acquisition, **B2**.1182–3
　　nitrogen sources, **B2**.1182
　　pathways, **B2**.1183
　morphology, **B2**.1181
　mycolic acids, **B2**.1192
　nutritional requirements, **B2**.1182–3
　specimen collection, **B2**.1190
　see also individual species
Mycobacteria, Kinyoun acid-fast stain,
　　M.123 (Tab.)
Mycobacteria non-tuberculous (NTM),
　　B2.1205–7
　classification, **B2**.1182
　colonization *vs.* infection, **B2**.1206
　infection, **B2**.1205–7, **B2**.1206 (Tab.)
　　AIDS patients *see* AIDS, concomitant
　　　infection
　　colonization *vs.*, **B2**.1206
　　extrapulmonary, **B2**.1222–3
　　immunocompetent hosts, **B2**.1206
　　pseudoinfection, **B2**.1216
　　pulmonary, **B2**.1206–7, **B2**.1222
　　　treatment, **B2**.1222
　　species frequently involved, **B2**.1206 (Tab.),
　　　B2.1207–13
　　species rarely involved, **B2**.1206 (Tab.),
　　　B2.1213–16
　　transmission, **B2**.1206–7
　　transplant patients, **B2**.1206
　　treatment, **B2**.1221–3
　　see also individual species
　slow-growing, **B2**.1206 (Tab.)
　see also individual species
Mycobacteria, rapidly growing (RGM),
　　B2.**1236–69**
　antibacterial susceptibility testing, **B2**.1246
　clinical significance assessment, **B2**.1246
　culture, **B2**.1237
　definition, **B2**.1236
　habitats, **B2**.1236
　identification, **B2**.1236, **B2**.1238 (Tab.),
　　B2.1240–3
　　arylsulfatase, **B2**.1240
　　carbon utilization, **B2**.1240
　　chromatography, **B2**.1242–3
　　colonial morphology, **B2**.1240
　　growth rate, **B2**.1241
　　iron uptake, **B2**.1241
　　MacConkey agar without crystal violet,
　　　B2.1241
　　molecular methods, **B2**.1243–4
　　nitrate reduction, **B2**.1241
　　phenotypic, **B2**.1240–2
　　pigment production, **B2**.1241
　　polymyxin B inhibition, **B2**.1241
　　sodium chloride tolerance, **B2**.1241–2
　　staining, **B2**.1239–40
　　strain typing, **B2**.1244–6
　　temperature studies, **B2**.1242
　isolation, **B2**.1237

　pathogenicity, **B2**.1237
　phylogenetic relationships, **B2**.1237–9,
　　B2.1239 (Fig.)
　species, **B2**.1237, **B2**.1238 (Tab.),
　　B2.1239 (Fig.)
　　accounts, **B2**.1246–62
　taxonomy, **B2**.1237–9
　see also individual species
Mycobacterium
　as airborne bacteria, **B1**.188
　　sampling, **B1**.190–1
　antibacterial susceptibility/resistance
　　menaquinones, **B2**.1145
　　mycolic acids, **B2**.1145–6
　　quinolone resistance, **B1**.493 (Tab.)
　bacteriophage, **B2**.1189
　cell walls, **B1**.441
　chemical/physical agent susceptibility/
　　resistance, **B2**.1216–17
　classification, **B2**.1137–8
　definition, **B2**.1181
　fast growing *see above*
　hygiene hypothesis, **I**.739
　immune evasion
　　IL-10 induction, **I**.652
　　lysosomal killing resistance, **I**.651
　　regulatory T cells, **I**.666
　immunogenetics, **I**.589
　infection
　　bacteremia, **B1**.524
　　IL12B gene polymorphisms, **I**.582
　　immune response
　　　CD4 T cells, **I**.390
　　　CD8 T cell responses, **I**.420
　　　IL-18, **I**.290–2
　　　macrophage activation, **I**.27
　　　NK cell actions, **I**.99
　　immunodeficiency diseases/disorders,
　　　I.772–3
　　keratitis, **B1**.601
　　nosocomial infection, **B1**.399–400
　　SLC11A1 gene polymorphisms, **I**.579
　isolation/identification
　　microscopic morphology, **B2**.1141–3
　　molecular methods, **B2**.1146–7
　　staining properties, **B2**.1139–40
　nitrification, **B1**.200
　non-tuberculous *see above*
　plasmid, **B2**.1188–9
　slow growing *see above*
　see also individual species
Mycobacterium abscessus, **B2**.1238 (Tab.),
　　B2.1247–50
　antibacterial susceptibility/resistance,
　　B2.1250
　classification, **B2**.1237–9, **B2**.1246–7
　genetics, **B2**.1188
　identification, **B2**.1193–4
　　colonial morphology, **B2**.1240
　　molecular methods, **B2**.1243, **B2**.1247
　　polymyxin B inhibition, **B2**.1241
　infection, **B2**.1247–50
　pathogenicity, **B2**.1237
　strain typing, **B2**.1244–6

Mycobacterium africanum
  genetics, **B2**.1187
  habitats, **B2**.1182
  identification, **B2**.1194, **B2**.1195
Mycobacterium aichense, **B2**.1238 (Tab.),
  B2.1250–1
  classification, **B2**.1237–9
Mycobacterium alvei, **B2**.1238 (Tab.), **B2**.1251
  classification, **B2**.1237–9
Mycobacterium asiaticum, **B2**.1213–14
Mycobacterium aurum, **B2**.1238 (Tab.),
  B2.1251
  classification, **B2**.1237–9
Mycobacterium austroafricanum,
  B2.1238 (Tab.), **B2**.1251
  classification, **B2**.1237–9
Mycobacterium avium complex, **B2**.1207
  airborne bacteria, **B1**.188
  antibacterial susceptibility/resistance,
  B2.1222
    ethambutol, **B1**.481
  cell wall, barrier to antibacterial agents,
  B2.1222
  cell wall structures, **B2**.1185
  colonies, **B2**.1207, **B2**.1207 (Fig.)
  environmental prevalence, **B2**.1207
  genetics, **B2**.1188
  growth conditions, **B2**.1192
  habitats, **B2**.1182
  identification, **B2**.1193
  infection *see Mycobacterium avium* complex,
  infection
  isolation/identification, **B2**.1193, **B2**.1195
    blood cultures, **B1**.524
    serotypes, **B2**.1207
    typing, **B2**.1195
  smooth domed, **B2**.1207
  smooth transparent, **B2**.1207
  subspecies, **B2**.1207
  susceptibility/resistance to heat, **B2**.1216
Mycobacterium avium complex, infection,
  B2.1207–9
  in AIDS *see* AIDS, concomitant infection
  animals, **B2**.1207
  cervical lymphadenitis, **B2**.1208
  chest X-rays, **B2**.1208 (Fig.)
  clinical features, **B2**.1208–9
    Lady Windermere's syndrome, **B2**.1207–8
  disseminated, **B1**.524
  epidemiology, **B2**.1208
  humans, **B2**.1207–9
  IL-10 induction, **I**.653
  in immunocompromised hosts (non-AIDS),
  B2.1208
  immunogenetics, **I**.589
  keratitis, **B1**.601
  lung diseases associated, **B2**.1207–8,
  B2.1208 (Fig.)
  NK cell actions, **I**.99
  nosocomial, **B1**.399–400
  sources/transmission, **B2**.1207
  treatment, **B2**.1209, **B2**.1222
Mycobacterium avium-intracellulare complex
  (MAC), **B1**.427, **B1**.433
  immunogenetics, **I**.590

*Mycobacterium avium-Mycobacterium
  intracellulare-Mycobacterium
  scrofulaceum* (MAIS complex),
  B2.1207
Mycobacterium bohemicum, **B2**.1214
Mycobacterium bonickei, **B2**.1237–9
Mycobacterium bovis
  attenuated vaccine vectors, **I**.830–1
  carbon source, **B2**.1182
  cell wall structure, **B2**.1185
  colonies, **B2**.1198 (Fig.)
  genetics, **B2**.1187
  habitats, **B2**.1182
  identification, **B2**.1194, **B2**.1195
  immune evasion, **I**.659
  immunogenetics, **I**.589
  infection *see Mycobacterium bovis* infection
  in milk, **B1**.230
  susceptibility/resistance to heat, **B2**.1216
Mycobacterium bovis infection, **B1**.229,
  B2.1200
  cattle, **B2**.1200
    eradication, **B2**.1200
  dendritic cell infection, **I**.656
  epidemiology, **B2**.1200
  human, **B2**.1200
  mastitis, **B1**.230
Mycobacterium branderi, **B2**.1214
  genetics, **B2**.1188
Mycobacterium brumae, **B2**.1238 (Tab.),
  B2.1251
  classification, **B2**.1237–9
Mycobacterium canettii
  genetics, **B2**.1187
  habitats, **B2**.1182
  identification, **B2**.1195
Mycobacterium celatum, **B2**.1214
  genetics, **B2**.1188–9
Mycobacterium chelonae, **B2**.1238 (Tab.),
  B2.1251–3
  antibacterial susceptibility/resistance,
  B1.427, **B1**.433, **B2**.1253
  classification, **B2**.1237–9, **B2**.1251
  genetics, **B2**.1188
  identification, **B2**.1193–4
    chromatography, **B2**.1242
    colonial morphology, **B2**.1240
    molecular methods, **B2**.1243
    polymyxin B inhibition, **B2**.1241
    sodium chloride tolerance, **B2**.1241–2
    staining, **B2**.1239–40
    strain typing, **B2**.1244–6
  infection, **B2**.1251–3
    keratitis, **B1**.601
    nosocomial, **B1**.399–400
  pathogenicity, **B2**.1237
  susceptibility/resistance to heat, **B2**.1216
Mycobacterium confluentis, **B2**.1238 (Tab.),
  B2.1253
  classification, **B2**.1237–9
Mycobacterium conspicuum, **B2**.1214
Mycobacterium elephantis, **B2**.1238 (Tab.),
  B2.1254
  classification, **B2**.1237–9
Mycobacterium fallax, **B2**.1238 (Tab.), **B2**.1254
  classification, **B2**.1237–9

Mycobacterium farcinogenes, **B2**.1238 (Tab.),
  B2.1254
  classification, **B2**.1237–9
  molecular identification, **B2**.1243
Mycobacterium flavescens, **B2**.1238 (Tab.),
  B2.1254
  classification, **B2**.1237–9
Mycobacterium fortuitum, **B2**.1254–6
  antibacterial susceptibility/resistance,
  B2.1256
  characteristics, **B2**.1238 (Tab.)
  classification, **B2**.1237–9, **B2**.1246–7
  genetics, **B2**.1188
  identification
    chromatography, **B2**.1242
    molecular methods, **B2**.1245 (Fig.)
    polymyxin B inhibition, **B2**.1241
    staining, **B2**.1239–40
    strain typing, **B2**.1244–6
  infection, **B2**.1254–6
    keratitis, **B1**.601
    nosocomial, **B1**.399–400
  pathogenicity, **B2**.1237
  susceptibility/resistance to heat, **B2**.1216
  third biovariant, **B2**.1256–7
    antibacterial susceptibility/resistance,
    B2.1257
    characteristics, **B2**.1238 (Tab.)
    polymyxin B inhibition, **B2**.1241
Mycobacterium gadium, **B2**.1238 (Tab.),
  B2.1257
  classification, **B2**.1237–9
Mycobacterium gastri, **B2**.1214
  genetics, **B2**.1188
  habitats, **B2**.1182
  identification, **B2**.1193–4
Mycobacterium genavense, **B2**.1182,
  B2.1209–10
  infection, **B2**.1209–10
    in AIDS, **B2**.1209–10
  iron acquisition, **B2**.1182–3
Mycobacterium gilvum, **B2**.1238 (Tab.),
  B2.1257
  classification, **B2**.1237–9
Mycobacterium goodii, **B2**.1238 (Tab.),
  B2.1257
  classification, **B2**.1237–9
  identification
    molecular methods, **B2**.1243
    pigment production, **B2**.1241
Mycobacterium gordonae, **B2**.1214
  genetics, **B2**.1188
  habitats, **B2**.1182
  identification, **B2**.1193
  infection
    keratitis, **B1**.601
    nosocomial, **B1**.399–400
Mycobacterium haemophilium
  antibacterial susceptibility/resistance,
  B2.1218, **B2**.1222–3
  growth conditions, **B2**.1192
  infection, **B2**.1210
  iron acquisition, **B2**.1182–3
  nutritional requirements, **B2**.1182

Mycobacterium hassiacum, **B2**.1238 (Tab.), **B2**.1257
  antibacterial susceptibility/resistance, **B2**.1257
  classification, **B2**.1237–9
  temperature studies, **B2**.1242
Mycobacterium heckeshornense, **B2**.1214
Mycobacterium heidelbergense, **B2**.1214, **B2**.1215 (Fig.)
Mycobacterium hodleri, **B2**.1238 (Tab.), **B2**.1257–8
  classification, **B2**.1237–9
Mycobacterium holsaticum, **B2**.1238 (Tab.), **B2**.1258
  classification, **B2**.1237–9
Mycobacterium houstonense, **B2**.1237–9
Mycobacterium immunogenum, **B2**.1238 (Tab.), **B2**.1258
  classification, **B2**.1237–9
  polymyxin B inhibition, **B2**.1241
Mycobacterium interjectum, **B2**.1214
Mycobacterium intermedium, **B2**.1215
Mycobacterium intracellulare
  complex inclusion, **B2**.1207
  genetics, **B2**.1188
  identification, **B2**.1193
  infection, in AIDS, **B2**.1207
  susceptibility/resistance to heat, **B2**.1216
Mycobacterium kansasii, **B2**.1210–11
  antibacterial susceptibility/resistance, **B2**.1218–19, **B2**.1222
  cell wall structures, **B2**.1185
  colonies, **B2**.1210
  genetics, **B2**.1188
  habitats, **B2**.1182
  identification, **B2**.1193–4
  infection, **B2**.1210–11
    AIDS patients, **B2**.1211
    immunocompromised patients, **B2**.1206
    treatment, **B2**.1222
  susceptibility/resistance to heat, **B2**.1216
Mycobacterium lacus, **B2**.1215
Mycobacterium lentiflavum, **B2**.1215
Mycobacterium leprae
  airborne bacteria, **B1**.188
  in animals, **B2**.1182, **B2**.1204
  antibacterial susceptibility/resistance, **B2**.1218
  cell wall structure, **B2**.1183, **B2**.1185
  classification, **B2**.1181–2
  dapsone, **M**.454
  genetics, **B2**.1186–8
  habitats, **B2**.1182
  human reservoir, **B2**.1204
  immune evasion
    immunosuppression, **I**.665
    Th1/Th2 balance, **I**.665–6
  infection *see* Leprosy
  metabolism, **B2**.1183
  nutritional requirements, **B2**.1182
  tests for, **B2**.1185
  transmission, **B2**.1204
    breast milk, **B2**.1204
    nasal secretions, **B2**.1204
Mycobacterium lepraemurium, **B2**.1204

Mycobacterium mageritense, **B2**.1238 (Tab.), **B2**.1258
  classification, **B2**.1237–9
  polymyxin B inhibition, **B2**.1241
Mycobacterium malmoense, **B2**.1211
  antibacterial susceptibility/resistance, **B2**.1218, **B2**.1222–3
  habitats, **B2**.1182
  infection, **B2**.1211
    treatment, **B2**.1222–3
Mycobacterium marinum, **B2**.1211–12, **B2**.1258
  antibacterial susceptibility/resistance, **B2**.1218–19
  cell wall structures, **B2**.1185
  classification, **B2**.1236, **B2**.1237–9
  genetics, **B2**.1188
  growth conditions, **B2**.1192
  habitats, **B2**.1182
  identification, **B2**.1193–4
  infection, **B2**.1211–12, **B2**.1212 (Fig.)
    treatment, **B2**.1222–3
  susceptibility/resistance to heat, **B2**.1216
Mycobacterium microti
  genetics, **B2**.1187
  habitats, **B2**.1182
  identification, **B2**.1194, **B2**.1195
Mycobacterium moriokaense, **B2**.1258
  characteristics, **B2**.1238 (Tab.)
  classification, **B2**.1237–9
Mycobacterium mucogenicum, **B2**.1238 (Tab.), **B2**.1258–9
  classification, **B2**.1237–9
  identification
    colonial morphology, **B2**.1240
    molecular methods, **B2**.1245 (Fig.)
    polymyxin B inhibition, **B2**.1241
    sodium chloride tolerance, **B2**.1241–2
Mycobacterium neoaurum, **B2**.1238 (Tab.), **B2**.1259
  classification, **B2**.1237–9
Mycobacterium nonchromogenicum, **B2**.1182
Mycobacterium novocastrense, **B2**.1238 (Tab.), **B2**.1260
  classification, **B2**.1237–9
Mycobacterium obuense, **B2**.1238 (Tab.), **B2**.1260
  classification, **B2**.1237–9
Mycobacterium palustre, **B2**.1215
Mycobacterium parafortuitum, **B2**.1238 (Tab.), **B2**.1260
  classification, **B2**.1237–9
Mycobacterium paratuberculosis, **B2**.1212
  genetics, **B2**.1188
  habitats, **B2**.1182
  infection, **B2**.1212
    animals, **B2**.1182
    milk-borne, **B1**.243–4
  in milk, **B1**.243–4
  nutritional requirements, **B2**.1182
Mycobacterium peregrinum, **B2**.1238 (Tab.), **B2**.1260
  classification, **B2**.1237–9, **B2**.1246–7
  identification, molecular methods, **B2**.1244
  polymyxin B inhibition, **B2**.1241
Mycobacterium phlei, **B2**.1238 (Tab.), **B2**.1260
  classification, **B2**.1237–9

  susceptibility/resistance to heat, **B2**.1216
  temperature studies, **B2**.1242
Mycobacterium rhodesiae, **B2**.1238 (Tab.), **B2**.1261
  classification, **B2**.1237–9
Mycobacterium scrofulaceum, **B2**.1215
  genetics, **B2**.1188
  habitats, **B2**.1182
  susceptibility/resistance to heat, **B2**.1216
Mycobacterium senegalense, **B2**.1238 (Tab.), **B2**.1261
  classification, **B2**.1237–9
  molecular methods of identification, **B2**.1243
Mycobacterium septicum, **B2**.1238 (Tab.), **B2**.1261
  classification, **B2**.1237–9
Mycobacterium shimoidei, **B2**.1215
  identification, **B2**.1193–4
Mycobacterium simiae, **B2**.1212
  habitats, **B2**.1182
  infection, **B2**.1212
Mycobacterium smegmatis, **B2**.1261
  antibacterial susceptibility/resistance
    biocide-antibiotic linked resistance, **B1**.443–4
    triclosan action, **B1**.436–8
  characteristics, **B2**.1238 (Tab.)
  classification, **B2**.1237–9
  genetics, **B2**.1188, **B2**.1189
  identification
    molecular methods, **B2**.1243
    pigment production, **B2**.1241
  iron acquisition, **B2**.1182–3
  mycobacteriophages, **B2**.1189
  pathogenicity, **B2**.1237
  plasmids, **B2**.1188
Mycobacterium szulgai, **B2**.1212
  genetics, **B2**.1188
  infection, **B2**.1212
    treatment, **B2**.1222–3
Mycobacterium terrae, **B2**.1215, **B2**.1215 (Fig.), **B2**.1261
  airborne bacteria, **B1**.188
  classification, **B2**.1236, **B2**.1237–9
  infection, granulomatous response, **B1**.741
Mycobacterium thermoresistible, **B2**.1238 (Tab.), **B2**.1262
  classification, **B2**.1237–9
  susceptibility/resistance to heat, **B2**.1216
  temperature studies, **B2**.1242
Mycobacterium triplex, **B2**.1215–16
Mycobacterium triviale, **B2**.1193–4
Mycobacterium tuberculosis
  airborne bacteria, **B1**.188
    dispersal, **B1**.188
  antibacterial susceptibility/resistance, **B1**.433, **B1**.436–8, **B2**.1217–19
    aminoglycosides, **B1**.482
    chromosomes, **B1**.113
    rifamycins, **B1**.494
  antigens, **B2**.1185–6
  cell wall structures, **B2**.1184
  classification, **B2**.1181–2
  colonies, **B2**.1198 (Fig.)
  culture, **B2**.1191–2
    media, **B1**.524, **B2**.1191–2

Mycobacterium tuberculosis
  culture (*Continued*)
    specimens for, **B2**.1190
  enterotoxin, **I**.565–6
  genetics, **B2**.1186–9
  habitats, **B2**.1182
  Hsp 60, **B1**.690
  identification, **B2**.1189–97
    acid-fast staining, **B2**.1190
    biochemical tests, **B2**.1192
    within complex, **B2**.1194
    direct amplification tests, **B2**.1194
    handling precautions in the laboratory,
      B2.1189
    laboratory, **B2**.1189–97
    microscopy, **B2**.1190
    molecular detection/typing *see below*
    typing methods, **B2**.1192–5
  immune evasion, **B2**.1202
    antigen processing/presentation disruption,
      I.383
    Fas-mediated apoptosis, **I**.655–6
    IL-10 induction, **I**.652–3
    lysosomal killing resistance, **I**.651
    lysosome fusion inhibition, **I**.650
    MHC class I antigen presentation, **I**.660
    MHC class II antigen presentation, **I**.659
    phagocytic uptake inhibition, **I**.649
    regulatory T cells, **I**.666–7
    superantigens, **I**.668
    TNF-α suppression, **I**.652
  infection
    bone and joint infection, **B1**.684–5,
      B1.690–1
      histology, **B1**.696
    CNS infection
      intracranial abscess complication, **B1**.586
      spinal epidural abscess, **B1**.593
      subdural empyema, **B1**.591
    conjunctivitis, **B1**.598–600
    infiltration of host tissues, **B1**.152
    keratitis, **B1**.601
    nosocomial, **B1**.188
    otitis media, **B1**.617
    risk categorization, **B1**.762–3
    suppurative parotitis, **B1**.619
    see also Tuberculosis
  iron acquisition, **B2**.1182–3
  iron-dependent repression, **B1**.165–6
  lipoarabinomannan, IL-10 induction, **I**.652–3
  metabolism, **B2**.1183
  molecular detection/typing, **B1**.723 (Tab.),
    B2.1194–5
    PCR, **B2**.1195
    RFLP, **B2**.1194
    spoligotyping, **B2**.1195
    transcription-mediated amplification,
      B1.729–30
  plasmids, **B2**.1188–9
  subspecies *caprae*, **B2**.1195
  superantigens, **I**.556 (Tab.)
  tryptophan aspartate-containing coat
    protein, **B1**.152
  typing methods, **B2**.1192–5
  UV radiation susceptibility, **B1**.188, **B2**.1217
  virulence factors, **B1**.152

  virulence, IL-10 induction, **I**.653
  see also Mycobacterium tuberculosis complex
Mycobacterium tuberculosis complex
  antibacterial susceptibility/resistance,
    B2.1217
    cycloserine, **B1**.481
    isoniazid, **B1**.481
    testing, **B2**.1195–7
  culture, **B2**.1191–2
    media, **B2**.1191–2
    specimens for, **B2**.1190
  identification, **B2**.1189–90
    biochemical tests, **B2**.1192
    direct amplification tests, **B2**.1194
    genotypic markers for species within
      complex, **B2**.1194
    genotyping, **B2**.1193–4
    molecular typing, **B2**.1194–5,
      B2.1196 (Tab.)
    see also Mycobacterium africanum;
      Mycobacterium bovis; Mycobacterium
      tuberculosis
Mycobacterium tusciae, **B2**.1216
Mycobacterium ulcerans, **I**.590, **B2**.1212–13
  environmental changes and human exposure,
    B1.362
  growth conditions, **B2**.1192
  habitats, **B2**.1182
  identification, **B2**.1193–4
  infection, **B2**.1212–13, **B2**.1213 (Fig.)
  tests for, **B2**.1185
Mycobacterium vaccae, **B2**.1238 (Tab.),
  B2.1262
  classification, **B2**.1237–9
Mycobacterium wolinskyi, **B2**.1238 (Tab.),
  B2.1262
  classification, **B2**.1237–9
Mycobacterium xenopi, **B2**.1213
  antibacterial susceptibility/resistance,
    B2.1222–3
  genetics, **B2**.1188
  growth conditions, **B2**.1192
  habitats, **B2**.1182
  infection, **B2**.1213
    treatment, **B2**.1222–3
  susceptibility/resistance to heat, **B2**.1216
Mycolic acids, **B2**.1184
Mycopathologia, **M**.31
Mycoplana dimorpha, **B2**.1729 (Tab.)
Mycoplasma(s)
  cell division, **B2**.1961–2
  characteristics, **B2**.1957, **B2**.1958 (Tab.)
  classification, **B2**.1957, **B2**.1964, **B2**.1966–70,
    B2.1966 (Fig.)
    cholesterol requirement, **B2**.1969–70
    conserved genes, **B2**.1967–8
    intraspecies genetic heterogeneity,
      B2.1968–9
    metabolism, **B2**.1969–70
    phylogeny, **B2**.1966–7
    serology, **B2**.1969
    taxonomy, **B2**.1967
    taxonomy with phylogeny, **B2**.1970
    unculturable organisms, **B2**.1964
  cultivation, **B2**.1962–4
    co-cultivation with cell culture, **B2**.1963–4

  media, **B2**.1963
  cytology, **B2**.1957–62
    cell division, **B2**.1961–2
    cellular morphology/structural elements,
      B2.1957–60
    motility, **B2**.1960–1
  ecology, **B2**.1964–6
  genetic analysis, **B2**.1973–82
    comparative genomics, **B2**.1975–7,
      B2.1977 (Tab.)
    DNA replication and repair, **B2**.1978–9
    extrachromosomal elements, **B2**.1974
    gene transfer *see below*
    genome sequencing and gene annotation,
      B2.1974–5
    genome structure, **B2**.1973–4
    proteome and transcriptome analyses and
      bioinformatics, **B2**.1977–8
    rRNA sequencing, **B2**.1967, **B2**.1969
  gene transfer, **B2**.1980–2
    chromosomal rearrangements, **B2**.1982
    insertion-like elements, **B2**.1982
    restriction/modification, **B2**.1981–2
    transposition, **B2**.1981
  habitats, **B2**.1958 (Tab.), **B2**.1964–6
    animal colonization, **B2**.1965
    cell culture contaminants, **B2**.1964–5
    host and tissue specificity, **B2**.1964
    insects, **B2**.1965–6
    plants, **B2**.1965–6
  immune evasion, **B2**.1989–91
  infection *see below*
  metabolism/biochemistry, **B2**.1970–3
    cell membrane proteins, **B2**.1970
    cholesterol requirement, **B2**.1969–70
    energy-yielding pathways, **B2**.1971–3
    membrane lipids, **B2**.1970–1
    transport, **B2**.1973
  motility, **B2**.1960
  pathogenicity, **B2**.1982–91
    animal, **B2**.1965, **B2**.1983
    human, **B2**.1965, **B2**.1983
    plants, **B2**.1985–6, **B2**.1991
  transcription and translation, **B2**.1979–80
    codon usage, **B2**.1980
    ribosomes, **B2**.1980
    transcription signals, **B2**.1979–80
    transfer RNAs, **B2**.1980
Mycoplasma, **B2**.1957, **B2**.1958 (Tab.)
  antibacterial susceptibility/resistance,
    B2.1992
  cell culture contaminants, **B2**.1964–5
  cell culture contamination, **V1**.88
  cell division, **B2**.1961–2
  cell membrane proteins, **B2**.1970
  classification, **B2**.1957, **B2**.1964, **B2**.1967,
    B2.1970
  cytoskeletal elements, **B2**.1960 (Fig.)
  genetics, **B2**.1967
    adhesins, **B2**.1986–7
    comparative genomics, **B2**.1975–7
    extrachromosomal elements, **B2**.1974
    genome sequencing and gene annotation,
      B2.1974
    genome structure, **B2**.1973–4

Mycoplasma,
  genetics (*Continued*)
    proteome and transcriptome analysis and
      bioinformatics, **B2**.1977–8
    rRNA sequencing, **B2**.1967
    transcription and translation, **B2**.1979–80
  habitats, **B2**.1964–6
  metabolism/biochemistry, **B2**.1969,
    B2.1975–6, **B2**.1994
    energy-yielding pathways, **B2**.1971
    membrane lipids, **B2**.1970–1
  morphology, **B2**.1957–62, **B2**.1958 (Fig.),
    B2.1959 (Fig.)
  motility, **B2**.1960
  as normal microbiota, **B1**.296 (Tab.),
    B1.303–4
  pathogenicity, **B2**.1982–91, **B2**.1983
    adhesins, **B2**.1986
    antigenic variation, **B2**.1987–9
    clastogenic and oncogenic effects, **B2**.1985
    disease manifestations, **B2**.1983
    immune system modulation, **B2**.1989–91
    intracellular location, **B2**.1984–5
    molecular basis of, **B2**.1983–6
    oxidative damage and membrane fusion,
      B2.1983–4
  pathogenicity, adhesion to host cells,
    B2.1986–7
  see also individual species
Mycoplasma infection
  agammaglobulinemia, **I**.780
  in AIDS *see* AIDS, concomitant infection
  clinical manifestations, **B2**.1983
  cystitis, **B1**.678
  diagnosis, **B2**.1994–7
    biochemical tests, **B2**.1994
    classification, **B2**.1994
    cultivation, **B2**.1994
    PCR, **B2**.1996
    PCR *vs.* serology, **B2**.1996–7
    restriction endonuclease analysis,
      B2.1995–6
    serological techniques, **B2**.1994–5
  endocarditis, **B1**.533
  epidemiology and control, **B2**.1991–4
  human colonization, **B2**.1965, **B2**.1965 (Tab.),
    B2.1983, **B2**.1991–2
  rhinovirus infection, **V2**.873
  transmission, **B2**.1991–2
  treatment, **B2**.1992
  vaccination, **B2**.1992–4
    DNA vaccines, **B2**.1993–4
    protein vaccines, **B2**.1993
    whole cell vaccines, **B2**.1992–3
Mycoplasma agalactiae
  antigenic variation, **B2**.1988–9,
    B2.1988 (Tab.)
  cell membrane proteins, **B2**.1970
  energy-yielding pathways, **B2**.1972
Mycoplasma alvi, **B2**.1960 (Fig.)
Mycoplasma arginini, **B2**.1964–5
Mycoplasma arthritidis
  genetic analysis
    bacteriophage, **B2**.1974, **B2**.1986
    gene transfer, **B2**.1981
    pathogenicity-associated genes, **B2**.1986

immune system modulation, **B2**.1991
pathogenicity
  adhesins, **B2**.1987
  antigenic variation, **B2**.1988 (Tab.)
  genes, **B2**.1986
  superantigen, **I**.556 (Tab.), **I**.562, **I**.565–6,
    I.668
    human *vs.* murine T cell stimulation,
      I.560 (Tab.), **I**.561
    mild toxic shock syndrome, **I**.562
    T cell stimulation, **I**.562
    T cell suppression, **I**.562
Mycoplasma bovigenitalium, **B2**.1972
Mycoplasma bovis
  adhesins, **B2**.1987
  antigenic variation, **B2**.1988 (Tab.)
  energy-yielding pathways, **B2**.1972
Mycoplasma capricolum
  cell division, **B2**.1961–2
  genetic analysis, **B2**.1977
    DNA replication and repair, **B2**.1979
Mycoplasma catarrhalis, **I**.656
Mycoplasma cavipharyngis, **B2**.1968
Mycoplasma dispar, **B2**.1989–90
Mycoplasma fastidiosum, **B2**.1968
Mycoplasma fermentans
  cell culture contamination, **B2**.1964–5
  cell membrane proteins, **B2**.1970
  energy-yielding pathways, **B2**.1971
  human colonization, **B2**.1965 (Tab.)
  infection, **B2**.1965 (Tab.)
  insertion-like elements, **B2**.1982
  pathogenicity, **B2**.1982–3
    antigenic variation, **B2**.1988 (Tab.)
    clastogenic and oncogenic effects, **B2**.1985
    immune system modulation, **B2**.1990–1
    intracellular location, **B2**.1984
    oxidative damage and membrane fusion,
      B2.1984
Mycoplasma flocculare, **B2**.1987
Mycoplasma gallisepticum
  adhesins, **B2**.1987
  antigenic variation, **B2**.1988–9,
    B2.1988 (Tab.)
  cell division, **B2**.1961–2
  cellular morphology, **B2**.1959 (Fig.)
  cytoskeletal elements, **B2**.1960 (Fig.),
    B2.1961 (Fig.)
  genetic analysis
    genome sequencing and gene annotation,
      B2.1974
    transcription and translation, **B2**.1979
  gene transfer, **B2**.1980–1
  motility, **B2**.1960
  vaccines, **B2**.1993
Mycoplasma genitalium
  cell division, **B2**.1962
  cell membrane proteins, **B2**.1970
  cellular morphology, **B2**.1959
  classification, **B2**.1967
  cocultivation with cell cultures, **B2**.1964
  cytoskeletal elements, **B2**.1958 (Fig.),
    B2.1959, **B2**.1960 (Fig.)
  energy-yielding pathways, **B2**.1971–2
  genetics, **B2**.1973–4
    chromosomes, **B1**.81

comparative genomics, **B2**.1975–6
DNA replication and repair, **B2**.1978–9
genome sequencing and gene annotation,
  B2.1974, **B2**.1975 (Tab.)
genome structure, **B2**.1973–4
proteome and transcriptome analysis and
  bioinformatics, **B2**.1978
transcription and translation, **B2**.1979,
  B2.1980
transport system, **B2**.1973
transposition, **B2**.1981
infection, **B2**.1965 (Tab.)
  human colonization, **B2**.1965 (Tab.)
  urethritis, **B1**.669
metabolism, **B2**.1975–6
motility, **B2**.1960
pathogenicity
  adhesins, **B2**.1986, **B2**.1987
  disease manifestations, **B2**.1983
  intracellular location, **B2**.1984
  oxidative damage and membrane fusion,
    B2.1983–4
transport system, **B2**.1973
Mycoplasma haemofelis, **B2**.1973–4
Mycoplasma hominis
  antibacterial susceptibility/resistance, **B2**.1992
  genetic analysis, **B2**.1976
  gene transfer, **B2**.1980–1
  host and tissue specificity, **B2**.1964
  human colonization, **B2**.1965 (Tab.)
  infection, **B2**.1965 (Tab.), **B2**.1983
    bacterial vaginosis, **B1**.665, **B1**.666
    pelvic inflammatory disease, **B1**.669
    transmission, **B2**.1992
    treatment, **B2**.1992
  pathogenicity
    adhesins, **B2**.1987
    antigenic variation, **B2**.1988–9,
      B2.1988 (Tab.)
    intracellular location, **B2**.1984
Mycoplasma hyopneumoniae
  adhesins, **B2**.1987
  genome sequencing and gene annotation,
    B2.1974
  transport system, **B2**.1973
  vaccines, **B2**.1993–4
Mycoplasma hyorhinis
  cell membrane proteins, **B2**.1970
  culture, **B2**.1963
  pathogenicity
    antigenic variation, **B2**.1988 (Tab.)
    apoptosis induction, **B2**.1985
    clastogenic and oncogenic effects, **B2**.1985
Mycoplasma mobile
  culture, **B2**.1963
  motility, **B2**.1960
Mycoplasma mycoides subspecies *mycoidses*
  classification, **B2**.1968–9
  genetics, **B2**.1968–9
    genome sequencing and gene annotation,
      B2.1974
    genome structure, **B2**.1973–4
    insertion-like elements, **B2**.1982
    plasmids, **B2**.1974
  pathogenicity
    antigenic variation, **B2**.1988 (Tab.)

Mycoplasma mycoides subspecies *mycoidses*
pathogenicity (*Continued*)
  oxidative damage and membrane fusion,
    B2.1984 (Fig.)
Mycoplasma orale
  cell culture contaminants, **B2**.1964–5
  human colonization, **B2**.1965 (Tab.)
Mycoplasma penetrans
  genetic analysis, **B2**.1976
    genome sequencing and gene annotation,
      B2.1974, **B2**.1975 (Tab.)
  human colonization, **B2**.1965 (Tab.)
  infection, **B2**.1965 (Tab.)
    in AIDS and Kaposi's sarcoma, **B2**.1985,
      B2.1990
  pathogenicity, **B2**.1982–3
    adhesins, **B2**.1987
    antigenic variation, **B2**.1988 (Tab.)
    clastogenic and oncogenic effects, **B2**.1985
    immune system modulation, **B2**.1990
    intracellular location, **B2**.1984
Mycoplasma pneumoniae, **I**.30
  antibacterial susceptibility/resistance,
    B2.1992
    macrolides, **B1**.486–7
  cell division, **B2**.1961–2
  cell membrane proteins, **B2**.1970
  classification, **B2**.1967
  culture, **B2**.1963
  cytoskeletal elements, **B2**.1959,
    B2.1960 (Fig.)
  genetics
    adhesin genes, **B2**.1986, **B2**.1989
    comparative genomics, **B2**.1975–6
    DNA replication and repair, **B2**.1978–9
    gene transfer, **B2**.1981
    genome sequencing and gene annotation,
      B2.1974, **B2**.1975 (Tab.)
    genome structure, **B2**.1974
    proteome and transcriptome analysis and
      bioinformatics, **B2**.1977–8
    transcription and translation, **B2**.1979,
      B2.1980
    transport system, **B2**.1973
    transposition, **B2**.1981
  infection *see below*
  metabolism, **B2**.1975–6
    energy-yielding pathways, **B2**.1971–2
    transport system, **B2**.1973
  morphology, **B2**.1959, **B2**.1959 (Fig.)
  motility, **B2**.1960
  pathogenicity, **B2**.1983
    adhesins, **B2**.1986, **B2**.1986 (Tab.),
      B2.1987, **B2**.1989
    antigenic variation, **B2**.1989
    intracellular location, **B2**.1985
    oxidative damage and membrane fusion,
      B2.1983–4, **B2**.1984 (Fig.)
  pneumonia *see below*
Mycoplasma pneumoniae infection,
  B2.1965 (Tab.), **B2**.1983
  acute bronchitis, **B1**.647
  diagnosis, **B2**.1995, **B2**.1997
    antibody detection, **B1**.752
    complement fixation tests, **B1**.752
    EIAs, **B1**.752

serological techniques, **B2**.1995
human colonization, **B2**.1965 (Tab.)
pharyngitis, **B1**.611–12
pneumonia, **B1**.633–4, **B2**.1983
  clinical features, **B1**.633–4, **B2**.1983
  epidemiology, **B1**.633, **B2**.1992
  extrapulmonary features, **B1**.634, **B2**.1983
  infection rates, **B2**.1992
  laboratory findings, **B1**.634
  pathogenesis, **B1**.633
  periodicity, **B1**.633 (Fig.)
  prevention, **B1**.634
  rash with, **B1**.634
  therapy, **B1**.634, **B2**.1992
  transmission, **B1**.633, **B2**.1991
transmission, **B2**.1991, **B2**.1992
treatment, **B2**.1992
vaccines, **B1**.634, **I**.933 (Tab.), **B2**.1992
  proteins, **B2**.1993
  whole cell, **B2**.1992
Mycoplasma pulmonis
  antigenic variation, **B2**.1988 (Tab.)
  cell membrane proteins, **B2**.1970
  cytoskeletal elements, **B2**.1960 (Fig.)
  genetic analysis, **B2**.1976
    comparative genomics, **B2**.1976
    DNA replication and repair, **B2**.1978–9
    gene transfer, **B2**.1981
    genome sequencing and gene annotation,
      B2.1974, **B2**.1975 (Tab.)
    insertion-like elements, **B2**.1982
    restriction and modification, **B2**.1981–2
    transcription and translation, **B2**.1980
    transposition, **B2**.1981
  immune system modulation, **B2**.1989
  motility, **B2**.1960
  transport system, **B2**.1973
  vaccines, **B2**.1993
Mycoplasma salivarium
  human colonization, **B2**.1965 (Tab.)
  infection, **B2**.1965 (Tab.)
  transmission, **B2**.1992
Mycoplasma sualvi, cytoskeletal elements,
  B2.1960 (Fig.)
Mycoplasma synoviae
  adhesins, **B2**.1987
  antigenic variation, **B2**.1988 (Tab.)
Mycorrhiza, bacteria association, **B1**.197
Mycoses (journal), **M**.31
Mycosides, **B2**.1184–5
Mycotic aneurysms, infective endocarditis,
  B1.535
Mycotoxin formation, nuts, **B1**.287
Mycotoxins, *Fusarium,* **M**.754
MYC, papillomavirus E6 protein effects,
  V1.460 (Tab.)
Myelin basic protein (MP), **V2**.1415
Myelitis, VZV infection, **V2**.1422
Myeloid cell growth factors, **I**.273–9,
  I.274 (Tab.)
Myeloid leukemia, BXH-2 virus, **V1**.339–40
Myeloperoxidase (MPO), **I**.35, **I**.41–2
  Candida, **M**.590, **M**.593
  deficiency, **I**.48 (Tab.), **I**.49, **I**.770
  diagnosis, **I**.52

innate mucosal immune response, **I**.521
  macrophages, **I**.26
  neutrophils, **I**.45
Mylotarg, licensing, **I**.355 (Tab.)
Myoblasts, DNA vaccine priming, **I**.914
Myocardial infarction
  Chlamydia pneumoniae infection, **B2**.2016
  complement pathology, **I**.155–6, **I**.155 (Tab.)
Myocarditis
  aspergillosis, **M**.141 (Fig.)
  aspergillus, **M**.700, **M**.705
  Blastoschizomyces capitatus, **M**.625
  Coxsackie virus infection, **V1**.283
  invasive aspergillosis, **M**.700, **M**.705
  pathogen induced, **I**.753 (Tab.)
  reovirus infection, **V2**.937–8
  rubella, **V2**.974
  trichinellosis, **P**.761, **P**.762
Myometrium, clostridial infection, **B2**.1111
Myoscint, licensing, **I**.355 (Tab.)
Myosin, *Taenia solium,* **P**.682–3
Myositis, trichinellosis, **P**.761
Myoviridae, **V1**.26, **V1**.378
  classification, **V1**.27 (Tab.), **V1**.42,
    V1.43 (Tab.)
  see also specific viruses
Myoviridae bacteriophage, **B2**.1535
Myringitis, **B1**.629
Myxococcus xanthus, **B1**.81
Myxoma growth factor (MGF), **V1**.257
Myxomatosis, **V1**.588
Myxoma virus (MYXV), **V1**.588
  emerging infection, **V2**.1651 (Tab.)
    host resistance changes, **V2**.1656–7
  genome sequence, **V1**.588
  herd immunity, **V2**.1657
  host susceptibility, **V1**.265
  immune evasion
    apoptosis mitochondrial pathways,
      V1.324–5
    chemokine binding proteins, **V1**.320,
      I.622–3
    IFN receptor, **V1**.315, **I**.619, **I**.687
    MHC interference, **V1**.619
    receptor homologues, **I**.620–1
    secreted cytokine receptors, **V1**.318
    serpins, **V1**.623
  phylogenetic comparison, **V1**.584 (Fig.)
Myxomycota, **M**.49, **M**.50 (Tab.)
Myxoviruses, classification, **V1**.26
Myxozoa, structure, **P**.166–8, **P**.168 (Fig.)

N_0 value, **B1**.446
N95 masks, **B1**.764
  severe acute respiratory syndrome, **B1**.373
NADH dehydrogenase, **B1**.64
NADPH oxidase
  macrophages, **I**.26
  measurement, **I**.51–2
  neutrophils, **I**.41, **I**.42 (Fig.)
  nitroblue tetrazolium reaction, **I**.51 (Fig.),
    I.52
Naegleria, **P**.187
  classification, **P**.197
  immune response, **P**.87, **P**.232

Naegleria ameba cytopathogenic material (NACM), **P**.232, **P**.233
Naegleria fowleri, **P**.226
　amoebostomes, **P**.227
　cell composition, **P**.230
　cell differentiation, **P**.229–30
　classification, **P**.226
　culture, **P**.232
　cysts, **P**.227, **P**.228 (Fig.)
　DNA, **P**.230
　encystment, **P**.229–30
　enflagellation, **P**.230
　　prevention, **P**.230
　flagellated forms, **P**.227, **P**.227 (Fig.)
　genetics, **P**.231
　immunology, **P**.87, **P**.232
　　antibodies, **P**.232
　infection
　　chemotherapy, **P**.236–7
　　clinical features, **P**.231–2
　　cytopathic effect, **P**.232
　　diagnosis, **P**.234–5
　　epidemiology/control, **P**.235–6
　　neutrophils, **I**.43
　　pathogenicity, **P**.232–3
　　pathology, **P**.233
　　vaccination, **P**.237
　life-cycle, **P**.228, **P**.229 (Fig.)
　phagocytosis by, **P**.232
　reproduction, **P**.227, **P**.231
　respiratory metabolism, **P**.230
　structure, **P**.227
　transmission, **P**.235–6
　trophozoites, **P**.227, **P**.227 (Fig.)
Naegleria gruberi, **B1**.762
Naftifine, **M**.183 (Tab.), **M**.184, **M**.233
　mechanism of action, **M**.70
Nagana, **P**.15, **P**.30, **P**.351
NA gene, Influenza virus B, **V1**.641, **V1**.642
Nagler reaction, **B1**.756–7
NAH plasmid, **B2**.1597
Nail infection *see* Onychomycosis
Nairobi sheep disease, **V2**.1046
Nairovirus, **V2**.1025
　characteristics, **V1**.129 (Tab.)
　classification, **V1**.50, **V2**.1026
　G1 glycoprotein, **V2**.1034, **V2**.1038
　genome structure
　　consensus sequences, **V2**.1031 (Tab.)
　　gene organization, **V2**.1033 (Fig.)
　see also Nairoviruses
Nairoviruses
　genome structure, **V2**.1034
　transcription, **V2**.1035
　see also Nairovirus; Nanoviridae
Nalidixic acid
　spectrum of activity, **B1**.470–1, **B1**.499 (Tab.)
　　Brucella, **B2**.1742
　　Enterobacter, **B2**.1484–5
　　Ewingella, **B2**.1493
　　Leclercia, **B2**.1495
　　Moellerella, **B2**.1496
　　Yokenella, **B2**.1498
　structure, **B1**.494 (Fig.)
Nannizzia, **M**.229

Nannizzi, A, **M**.10–1
Nannizzia otae, **M**.10–1
Nannomonas, **P**.351
Nanophyetus, **P**.586
Nanoviridae, **V1**.27 (Tab.)
　see also Nairoviruses; *specific viruses*
NAP-2 *see* Neutrophil-activating peptide-2 (NAP-2:CXCL7)
Naphthalene degradation
　plasmids, **B1**.114
　pseudomonads, **B2**.1597
Naples virus infection, **V2**.1047
Nappy rash, **M**.596, **M**.609
Nares, normal microbiota, **B1**.295–300, **B1**.304, **B1**.628
Nariva virus, **V1**.699, **V1**.819
'Nariz de anta (tapir nose)', **P**.327
Narnaviridae, **V1**.27 (Tab.), **V1**.41 (Tab.), **V1**.51 (Tab.), **V1**.54, **V1**.54 (Tab.)
Nasal airways, anatomy, **B1**.606–7
Nasal-associated lymphoid tissue (NALT), **I**.529–30, **I**.533–4
　dendritic cells, **I**.533
　IgA responses, **I**.533–4
　intranasal vaccination, **I**.831–2
　Langerhan's cells, **I**.533
　microfold (M) cells, **I**.532
　structure, **I**.533
　see also Common mucosal immune system (CMIS)
Nasal cancer, HPV associations, **V1**.463 (Tab.)
Nasal immunization *see* Vaccination
Nasal secretions, *Mycobacterium leprae*, **B2**.1204, **B2**.1205, **B2**.1205 (Fig.)
Nasal vaccination *see* Vaccination
Nasal washings, rhinovirus infection diagnosis, **V2**.878
Nascent replicase polyproteins, *Nidovirales* order, **V1**.396
Nasopharyngeal aspirates, PCP, **M**.787
Nasopharyngeal carcinoma, **V1**.572
　clinical features, **V1**.572
　EBV infection, **V1**.349–50, **V1**.566 (Tab.), **V1**.567, **V1**.572
　environmental cofactors, **V1**.572
　epidemiology, **V1**.572
　immune response, **V1**.572
　pathogenesis, **V1**.572
　therapy, **V1**.572
Nasopharynx
　anatomy, **B1**.607
　bacterial meningitis causative agents in, **B1**.556
　infection, **B1**.628
　mucosal immunity in, **B1**.556
　normal microbiota, **B1**.295–300, **B1**.556, **B1**.609, **B1**.628
　　factors changing, **B1**.628
　pathogens in, **B1**.628, **B1**.628 (Tab.)
　secretions, *Bordetella* identification, **B2**.1791
　swabs, bacterial meningitis diagnosis, **B1**.560
Natamycin
　dacryocanaliculitis, **M**.298
　endophthalmitis, **M**.320
　keratitis, **M**.308, **M**.312

National Committee for Clinical Laboratory Standards (NCCLS), **M**.156, **M**.157–8, **M**.169–70, **M**.170 (Tab.), **B1**.722
　antibacterial susceptibility testing, **B1**.498
　antifungal susceptibility testing, **M**.156, **M**.157–8
National Health Service (UK), vaccine information, **V2**.1583
National Immunization Program, **V2**.1583
National Institute of Biological Standards and Control (NIBSC), **B1**.324
　quantification standards, **B1**.722–4
National Nosocomial Infections Surveillance (NNIS), **B1**.369, **B1**.640
National scale-up, community parasite control, **P**.120–1
'Native antigen,' *Brucella*, **B2**.1726–8
'Native hapten,' *Brucella*, **B2**.1726–8
Nattrassia toruloidea, **M**.11
Natural competence, **B1**.99–100
Natural killer (NK) cells, **P**.68, **V1**.271–2, **I.79–107**
　activating receptors, **I**.83 (Tab.), **I**.90–1, **V1**.272
　　expression patterns, **I**.91
　　ITAMs, **I**.90
　　KIR receptors *see* Killer cell immunoglobulin receptor (KIR)
　　LIR receptors, **I**.90
　　LY49 receptors, **I**.88 (Fig.), **I**.90, **I**.92, **I**.94
　　NKG2D receptors, **I**.88 (Fig.), **I**.90, **I**.94, **I**.627–8
　　NKp30, **I**.91
　　NKp46, **I**.91
　　nomenclature, **I**.90
　　specificity, **I**.91
　activation thresholds, **I**.627
　CpG stimulation, **I**.911–12
　cytokines produced, **I**.28 (Tab.), **I**.81–2, **V1**.271–2
　　granzymes, **I**.81
　　IFN-γ, **I**.287–8, **I**.478
　　IFN-γ production, **I**.99
　　IL-4, **I**.280
　　IL-5, **I**.57
　　IL-10, **I**.292
　　INFs, **V1**.271
　　lymphotoxin, **I**.286
　cytotoxic granules, **I**.474–7
　　Fas ligand, **I**.477
　　granulysin, **I**.477
　　granzymes *see* Granzyme(s)
　　killing mechanisms, **I**.479 (Fig.)
　　perforin *see* Perforin
　　serglycine, **I**.475
　in diseases/infection, **I**.94–100, **I**.99 (Fig.)
　　aspergillosis, **M**.707–8
　　in autoimmune diseases, **I**.103
　　　animal models, **I**.103
　　　'bare lymphocyte syndrome,' **I**.103
　　　diabetes mellitus, **I**.103
　　　myasthenia gravis, **I**.103
　　　red cell aplasia, **I**.103
　　　rheumatoid arthritis, **I**.103
　　　severe combined immunodeficiency, **I**.80

Natural killer (NK) cells
  in diseases/infection
    in autoimmune diseases (*Continued*)
      transporter associated with processing
        deficiency, **I**.103
    bacterial infection, **I**.79, **I**.99–100
    in cancer, **I**.100–1
      adoptive transfer experiments, **I**.101
      antibody-dependent cellular cytotoxicity,
        I.100–1
      Fas-dependent killing, **I**.100–1
      transplantable tumors, **I**.100–1
    candidiasis, **M**.260
    HCMV infection, **I**.772
    histoplasmosis capsulati, **M**.525–6,
      M.527 (Fig.)
      binding to, **M**.525–6, **M**.527 (Fig.)
      depletion of, **M**.525–6
    immunodeficiency diseases/disorders, **I**.772
    immunogenetics, **I**.576
    parasitic infection, **P**.68, **I**.79, **I**.100
      leishmaniasis, **P**.77–8
      Plasmodium, **P**.83
    viral infection, **I**.79, **I**.94–9, **I**.617–18,
      I.627–8, **V1**.618–19
      clinical observations, **I**.94–6
      experimental studies, **I**.96–7
      hepatitis B, **V1**.283
      Herpes virus infection, **V1**.272
      HHV-6 infection, **V1**.532
      HIV infection *see* HIV infection
      HSV infection, **V1**.284, **V1**.510
      Human respiratory syncytial virus
        infection, **V1**.795
      immune interference *see* Immune
        evasion, viruses
      measles, **V1**.727
      Murine cytomegalovirus infection,
        V1.272, **V1**.285
      recognition, **I**.483
      Vaccinia virus, **V1**.272
      see also individual infection
  effector functions, **I**.81–5
    animal ablation models, **I**.82, **I**.85
    antibody-dependent cell-mediated
      cytotoxicity, **I**.627, **I**.796
    cytotoxicity assays, **I**.82
    defective animal models, **I**.82–5
    Fas-mediated killing, **I**.81
    granulysin production, **I**.82, **I**.99
    perforin-dependent killing, **I**.81
    T cell activation, **I**.478
    TNF-mediated killing, **I**.81
    in vivo elimination, **I**.82
  genetics
    leukocyte receptor cluster, **I**.88, **I**.89, **I**.94,
      I.95 (Fig.)
    Ly49 genes, **I**.89
    NK gene complex, **I**.95 (Fig.)
  historical perspective, **I**.79
  IFN effects, **V1**.272, **V1**.292–3
  immune evasion *see* Immune evasion
  inhibitory receptors, **I**.83 (Tab.), **I**.87–90
    immunotyrosine inhibitory motifs, **I**.87–8
    KIR receptors, **I**.87, **I**.88–9, **I**.88 (Fig.),
      I.92, **I**.94, **I**.96 (Tab.), **I**.628, **V1**.272

LY49 receptors, **I**.87, **I**.88 (Fig.), **I**.89, **I**.92,
  I.94
MHC class I importance, **I**.88, **I**.88 (Fig.)
NKR-P1 receptors, **I**.89
NMK2A receptors, **I**.89
p75/AIRM, **I**.89
innate mucosal immune response, **I**.519
killing mechanism, **I**.479 (Fig.)
  binding, **I**.472
  inhibitory receptor lack, **I**.472
  MHC lack, **I**.472
LL37 production, **I**.175
morphology and function, **I**.472–3,
  I.473 (Fig.), **I**.474 (Fig.)
mouse models, **I**.81 (Tab.)
numbers, **I**.80
ontogeny/development, **I**.85–6
  CD2 markers, **I**.85
  CD56 markers, **I**.85
  cell surface markers, **I**.85
  deficient mice models, **I**.85
  fetal liver kinase ligand, **I**.85
  Ikaros gene, **I**.85
  IL-12, **I**.96
  IL-15, **I**.85, **I**.100
  immune tolerance development, **I**.94
  KIR receptors, **I**.85
  Ly49 receptors, **I**.92
  NOTCH-1, **I**.85
  PAX5, **I**.85
  positive selection model, **I**.93
  precursor cells, **I**.85
  receptors, **I**.92–3
  SCF, **I**.85
  sequential receptor expression model, **I**.93
  thymus, **I**.85
  type I INFs, **I**.96
in pregnancy, **I**.102–3
  cytokine production, **I**.102
  uterine cells, **I**.102
receptors/cell surface markers, **I**.79–80,
  I.80 (Tab.)
  activating receptors *see above*
  CD56, **I**.79–80, **V1**.271–2
  CD56 markers, **I**.85
  chemokine receptors, **I**.224
  cytokine receptors, **V1**.272
  FcγRI (CD64), **I**.314
  FcγRIII (CD16), **I**.79–80, **I**.627
  FcγRIIIa, **I**.315
  FcγRIII (CD16), **V1**.271–2
  gene evolution, **I**.94
  inhibitory receptors *see above*
  MHC molecule regulation, **I**.93–4
  polymorphism/complexity, **I**.92–4,
    I.96 (Tab.)
  T cells, **I**.92
regulation, **I**.85–6
  chemokines, **I**.85–6
  IFN-α, **I**.245, **I**.245 (Tab.), **I**.246 (Tab.)
  IL-2, **I**.86, **I**.279–80
  IL-7, **I**.281
  IL-12, **I**.86, **I**.288
  IL-15, **I**.85–6, **I**.282, **I**.284 (Fig.)
  IL-18, **I**.86, **I**.290

IL-21, **I**.86, **I**.283–4
integrins, **I**.85
type I INFs, **I**.86
signal transduction, **I**.87 (Tab.), **I**.91–2
  adhesion molecules, **I**.92
  cytokines, **I**.92
  ITAMs, **I**.90, **I**.91
  ITIMs, **I**.91
  redundancy of signals, **I**.91
specificity, **I**.86–94
  'missing self model,' **I**.86–7, **I**.86 (Fig.),
    I.89–90
  T helper cell interaction, **P**.95
in transplantation, **I**.101–2
  bone marrow grafts, **I**.101
  graft-versus-host disease, **I**.102
  rejection mechanisms, **I**.101–2
  UL16-binding proteins, **I**.627–8
Natural killer gene complex (NKC), **I**.95 (Fig.)
Natural waters, **B1**.213–17
NB protein, Influenza virus B *see* Influenza
  virus B
NBS gene, **I**.777
Ndumu virus (NDUV), **V2**.1010,
  V2.1011 (Tab.)
Near-patient testing *see* Immunoserology
Necator, **P**.589
  infection, **I**.682–3, **P**.715 (Tab.)
    cytokine destruction, **I**.686
    immunogenetics, **I**.600
  structure/life cycle, **P**.589
  see also individual species
Necator americanus, **P**.713
  biology/feeding, **P**.714 (Tab.), **P**.718, **P**.719
  epidemiology/population biology, **P**.722
    global distribution/abundance, **P**.42, **P**.722
    prevalence, **P**.713–14
  historical aspects, **P**.8–9
  host genetic factors, **P**.55
  infection establishment, **P**.720–1
    skin penetration, **P**.721
  life cycle, **P**.718 (Tab.), **P**.720 (Fig.)
  life expectancy, **P**.60 (Tab.)
  morphology, **P**.717
    Ancylostoma duodenale vs., **P**.717
    eggs, **P**.716 (Fig.)
  as opportunistic species, **P**.721
  see also Hookworm infection
Necator argentinus, **P**.715 (Tab.)
Necator suilus, **P**.715 (Tab.)
Necrobacillosis (Lemierre's disease), **B1**.629,
  B2.1951
Necropsies, airborne bacteria, **B1**.186 (Tab.)
Necrosis, tissue, toxoplasmosis, **P**.433–4
Necrotic granulomas (type 1), tuberculosis *see*
  Tuberculosis
Necrotizing aspergillosis, chronic, **M**.696–7
  therapy, **M**.719
Necrotizing enterocolitis, **B1**.395
Necrotizing enteropathy, **B2**.1118–19
Necrotizing fasciitis, *Apophysomyces elegans,*
  M.21, **M**.21 (Fig.)
Necrotizing funisitis, **B2**.1843
Necrotizing jejunitis (pigbel), **B2**.1118–19
Necrotizing pneumonitis *see* Pneumonitis

Needle contamination, **I**.819–20

Needle-free injectors, skin immunization, **I**.822–3

Needles, contamination by viruses, **V1**.239

Needlestick injury, **B1**.767, **B1**.767 (Tab.)
  infection transmitted by, **B1**.380, **B1**.382
  phlebotomists, **B1**.760, **B1**.767

Nef protein *see* HIV

Negative elongation factor, poxviruses, **V1**.599 (Tab.)

Negative regulating element (NRE), Hepatitis B virus, **V2**.1230

Negative selection
  B cell development, **I**.323, **I**.324
  CD4 T cells development, **I**.390, **I**.392
  T cells, **I**.379

Negative-strand RNA viruses *see* RNA viruses, negative-strand

Negishi virus, **V2**.998 (Tab.), **V2**.1004

Negri bodies, rabies, **V2**.1104, **V2**.1125

'Negro lethargy', **P**.15

Neighbor-Joining (NJ), phylogenetic analysis, **M**.47–8

Neisseria, **B2**.1270–300
  adhesins, **B1**.149
  aerobic growth, **B2**.1270, **B2**.1274–5
  animal species, **B2**.1271–3
  antibacterial susceptibility/resistance, **B2**.1291–2, **B2**.1292 (Tab.)
    evolution, **B1**.30
    plasmid-mediated, **B2**.1277
  antigens, **B2**.1278–88
    iron acquisition surface proteins, **B2**.1284–5
    lipo-oligosaccharides, **B2**.1273, **B2**.1274, **B2**.1288
    opacity-associated proteins, **B2**.1282–4
    other surface and secreted protein antigens, **B2**.1285–6
    pili, **B2**.1278–80
    polysaccharides, **B2**.1286, **B2**.1287 (Tab.), **B2**.1291
    porins, **B2**.1270, **B2**.1280–2
    reduction-modifiable protein (Rmp), **B2**.1282
    regulatory responses/proteins, **B2**.1285–6
  bacteriophage and lysogenic strains, **B2**.1278
  cell division, **B2**.1273–4, **B2**.1273 (Fig.)
  classification, **B2**.1271
  conjugation, **B1**.103
  definition, **B2**.1270
  false, **B2**.1270, **B2**.1271
  genomics, **B2**.1275–8
    cell division, **B2**.1274
    chromosome organization, **B2**.1275–6
    conjugation, **B2**.1276
    open reading frames, **B2**.1275–6
    plasmids, **B2**.1277
    small repetitive elements, **B2**.1276–7
    transduction, **B2**.1278
    transformation, **B2**.1276
    transposons, **B2**.1276–7
  growth requirements, **B2**.1274
  habitats, **B2**.1271–3
  historical perspectives, **B2**.1270–1
  human species, **B2**.1271–3, **B2**.1272 (Tab.)

infection *see Neisseria* infection; *below*
  isolation/identification, **B2**.1290–1
  metabolism, **B2**.1274–5
  morphology and structure, **B2**.1273–4, **B2**.1273 (Fig.)
    cell-wall blebs, **B2**.1274
  mutagenesis, **B2**.1277
  natural competence, **B1**.99
  non-pathogenic, **B2**.1286
    antibacterial susceptibility/resistance, **B2**.1292 (Tab.)
    as normal microbiota, **B1**.296 (Tab.), **B2**.1271–3
      nares and nasopharynx, **B1**.295–300
      nasopharynx, **B1**.609
      oral cavity, **B1**.609
      vagina, **B1**.303
    plasmids, **B2**.1276, **B2**.1277
    see also individual species
Neisseria caviae, **B2**.1270
Neisseria cinerea, **B2**.1271, **B2**.1272 (Tab.)
  conjunctivitis, **B1**.599
Neisseria cuniculi, **B2**.1270
Neisseria elongata, **B2**.1270, **B2**.1271, **B2**.1272 (Tab.)
  cell division, **B2**.1273–4
  morphology, **B2**.1273–4
  subspecies *nitroreducens*, **B2**.1271
Neisseria flavescens, **B1**.566, **B2**.1270–1, **B2**.1272 (Tab.), **B2**.1278
Neisseria gonorrhoeae
  antibacterial susceptibility/resistance, **B1**.661, **B2**.1277 (Tab.), **B2**.1291–2, **B2**.1292 (Fig.), **B2**.1292 (Tab.)
    cephalosporins, **B1**.661
    chromosomally-mediated, **B1**.661
    ciprofloxacin resistance, **B1**.661
    fluoroquinolones, **B1**.363
    β-lactamase plasmids, **B2**.1277, **B2**.1291–2
    penicillin resistance, **B1**.363, **B1**.661, **B2**.1277
    plasmid-mediated, **B1**.661
    quinolone resistance, **B1**.493 (Tab.), **B1**.661
    tetracycline, **B2**.1277, **B2**.1291–2
  antibacterial susceptibility testing, **B1**.660–1
  antigens, **B2**.1278–88
    iron acquisition surface proteins, **B2**.1284–5
    lipo-oligosaccharides, **B2**.1288
    opacity-associated proteins, **B2**.1280 (Tab.), **B2**.1282–4
    outer-membrane protein, **B1**.658–9
    pili, **B2**.1278–80
    polysaccharide capsule, **B2**.1286
    porins, **B1**.658–60, **B1**.662
    porins (PIA and PIB PorB), **B2**.1280–2
    reduction-modifiable protein (Rmp), **B2**.1282
    variation and phase transitions **B2**.1279–80, **B2**.1284
  artificial competence, **B1**.100
  cell division, **B2**.1273–4
  culture, **B1**.712–13
    agar dilution susceptibility testing, **B1**.717
    transport medium, **B1**.711–12

genomics, **B2**.1275–8
  cell division, **B2**.1274
  conjugation, **B2**.1276
  Correia elements, **B2**.1276–7
  open reading frames, **B2**.1275–6
  organization of the chromosome, **B2**.1275–6
  plasmids, **B2**.1277, **B2**.1277 (Tab.)
  small repetitive elements, **B2**.1276–7
  transformation, **B2**.1276
  transposons, **B2**.1276–7
glucose catabolism, **B1**.60
growth requirements, **B2**.1272 (Tab.), **B2**.1274
historical aspects, **B2**.1270–1
human host specificity, **B1**.658
IgA1 protease, **B2**.1286
immune evasion
  complement inhibitory proteins, **I**.664
  LPS variation, **I**.661
  outer membrane protein variation, **I**.661
infection
  adhesion to cells, **B2**.1282–3, **B2**.1288
  conjunctivitis, **B1**.599, **B1**.600
  defensin resistance, **I**.169
  epithelial cell invasion, **B2**.1283, **B2**.1288
  epithelial cell transcytosis, **B2**.1281, **B2**.1281 (Fig.)
  keratitis, **B1**.601
  pharyngitis, **B1**.611–12
  vaccines, **I**.933 (Tab.)
  see also Gonorrhea
isolation/identification, **B1**.659–61, **B2**.1274, **B2**.1290–1
  auxotyping, **B1**.662, **B2**.1274, **B2**.1290–1
  biochemical testing, **B1**.659, **B1**.659 (Tab.)
  culture, **B1**.659, **B2**.1290
  distinguishing features, **B2**.1290–1, **B2**.1290 (Tab.)
  microscopy, **B1**.659
  molecular detection *see below*
  monoclonal antibodies, **B1**.660, **B1**.662
  nucleic acid amplification tests, **B1**.660
  serotyping, **B1**.662, **B2**.1290–1
  staining/microscopy, **B2**.1270–1, **B2**.1271 (Fig.), **B2**.1290
  typing, **B1**.660, **B1**.662
metabolism, **B2**.1274–5
  nitrate reduction, **B1**.66
molecular detection, **B1**.660, **B1**.723 (Tab.)
  hybrid capture assay, **B1**.731
  probe hybridization, **B1**.725
morphology and structure, **B2**.1273
  pili, **B1**.658–9
phenotypic characteristics, **B2**.1272 (Tab.), **B2**.1290 (Tab.)
subspecies *kochii*, **B2**.1270–1, **B2**.1272 (Tab.)
as type species, **B2**.1271
Neisseria infection
  conjunctivitis, **B1**.598–9
  diagnosis
    antibody detection, **B1**.751
    immunoserology, **B1**.757
    sugar fermentation tests, **B1**.757
  entry into cells, **I**.649
  epidemiology, **B2**.1289

Neisseria infection (*Continued*)
  pathogenesis, **B2**.1290
  see also Gonorrhea; Meningococcal disease
Neisseria lactamica, **B2**.1270–1, **B2**.1272 (Tab.)
  carriage rate, **B1**.564
  habitats, **B2**.1271–3
  role in meningitis immunity, **B1**.564
Neisseria meningitidis, **B2**.1270
  antibacterial susceptibility/resistance,
    B1.499 (Tab.), **B2**.1291–2, **B2**.1292 (Tab.)
    β-lactamase, **B1**.566, **B2**.1277
    penicillin resistance, **B1**.566
    penicillin/tetracycline, **B2**.1277, **B2**.1291
    plasmids, **B2**.1277
  antigens, **B2**.1278–88
    iron acquisition surface proteins,
      B2.1284–5
    lipo-oligosaccharides, **B2**.1288
    LPS, **B1**.158, **B1**.564
    opacity-associated proteins, **B2**.1280 (Tab.),
      B2.1282, **B2**.1283
    other surface and secreted protein
      antigens, **B2**.1285–6
    pili, **B2**.1278–80
    polysaccharide capsule, **B2**.1286,
      B2.1287 (Tab.), **B2**.1291
    porins (PorA and PorB), **B2**.1280, **B2**.1282
    reduction-modifiable protein (Rmp),
      B2.1282
    variation and phase transitions,
      B2.1279–80
  carriage, **B1**.563–4
    age-specific incidence, **B1**.563, **B1**.563 (Fig.)
    smoking effect, **B1**.563–4
  carriage rates, **B1**.556, **B1**.561
    factors affecting, **B1**.563–4
    nasopharyngeal, **B1**.567
  cell division, **B2**.1273–4
  genomics, **B2**.1275–8
    conjugation, **B2**.1276
    Correia elements, **B2**.1276–7
    open reading frames, **B2**.1275–6
    organization of the chromosome,
      B2.1275–6
    plasmids, **B2**.1277
    small repetitive elements, **B2**.1276–7
    transformation, **B2**.1276
    transposons, **B2**.1276–7
  growth requirements, **B2**.1272 (Tab.),
    B2.1274
  historical aspects, **B2**.1270–1
  IgA1 protease, **B1**.556
  immune evasion
    antibody degradation/modification, **I**.662
    capsule phase variation, **I**.660–1
  infection *see* Meningococcal disease
    (meningitis); *Neisseria meningitidis*
    infection
  isolation/identification, **B2**.1291
    culture, **B2**.1291
    nasopharyngeal swabs, **B1**.560
    Neisseria gonorrhoeae vs., **B2**.1291
    serogrouping, **B2**.1286, **B2**.1287 (Tab.)
    see also individual serogroups
  laboratory worker immunization, **B1**.767

  metabolism, **B2**.1274–5
    iron-dependent repression, **B1**.165–6
    iron scavenging, **B1**.151
    nitrate reduction, **B1**.66
    protein secretion, **B1**.160
  morphology and structure, **B2**.1273
    capsules, **B1**.556, **B1**.563, **B1**.564
  as normal microbiota, **B1**.296 (Tab.),
    B2.1271–3
    nasopharynx colonization, **B1**.295–300
  pathogenicity, **B2**.1286
  phenotypic characteristics, **B2**.1272 (Tab.),
    B2.1290 (Tab.)
  serogroup A and C, **B1**.564
  serogroup B, **B1**.564
  serogroup C, notifications, **B1**.322
  vaccines *see Neisseria meningitidis* infection
  virulence factors, **B1**.556, **B2**.1286
    evolution within host, **B1**.173–4
    exopolysaccharides, **B1**.154
    phase variation, **B1**.173–4
Neisseria meningitidis infection
  attachment to host cell, **B1**.556, **B1**.563
  bacteremia, **B1**.522
  diagnosis
    EIAs, **B1**.751
    PCR, **B1**.559, **B1**.751
    serology, **B1**.757–8
  epiglottitis, **B1**.613
  immune response, **B1**.564
    blocking antibodies, **B1**.564, **B2**.1282
  immunogenetics, **I**.594
  predisposition factors, **B1**.557
  properdin deficiency, **I**.770–1
  vaccines
    BCE peptide vaccines, **I**.855 (Tab.),
      I.861 (Tab.), **I**.872–3
    capsular polysaccharides, **I**.935
    conjugate vaccines, **I**.936
    development status, **I**.933 (Tab.)
    genomic techniques, **I**.939
    group Y vaccines, **I**.936
    historical aspects/re-evaluation, **I**.15
    outer membrane proteins, **I**.872–3
    outer membrane vesicles, **I**.939–40
    proteasome vaccine carriers, **I**.839
    serogroup A and C vaccines, **B1**.568,
      B1.568 (Tab.)
    serogroup A vaccines, **I**.935, **I**.936
    serogroup B vaccines, **B1**.568–9,
      I.939–40
    serogroup C vaccines, **I**.855 (Tab.),
      I.861 (Tab.), **I**.872–3, **I**.927, **I**.936, **I**.939
    serogroup MenW135 vaccines, **I**.935, **I**.936
    serogroup Y vaccines, **I**.935
    see also Meningococcal disease
Neisseria mucosa, **B2**.1271, **B2**.1272 (Tab.)
Neisseria ovis, **B2**.1270
Neisseria perflava, **B2**.1278
  capsular polysaccharide, **B2**.1286
Neisseria polysaccharea, **B2**.1271,
    B2.1272 (Tab.)
  habitats, **B2**.1271–3
Neisseria sicca, **B2**.1271, **B2**.1272 (Tab.),
    B2.1278
Neisseria subflava, **B2**.1271, **B2**.1272 (Tab.)

Neisseria weaverii, **B2**.1270–1
  cell division, **B2**.1273–4
Neisseriaceae
  genera included, **B2**.1271
  type genus, **B2**.1271
Nelfinavir, **V2**.1624
  resistance, **V2**.1624
    HIV, **V2**.1337 (Fig.)
  structure, **V2**.1622 (Fig.), **V2**.1625 (Fig.)
Nematoda, **P**.586–95
Nematode(s), **P**.573, **I**.682–3
  characteristics, **P**.586–8
  classification, **P**.586–95, **P**.588
    Adenophorea, **P**.588–9
  historical aspects, **P**.8–9
  immunogenetics, **I**.600–1
  life cycles, **P**.587–8
  soil-transmitted *see* Nematodes,
    gastrointestinal
  structure, **P**.587 (Fig.)
  with tapeworm infection, **P**.664
  see also Lymphatic filariasis; *individual*
    species
Nematodes, gastrointestinal, **I**.682–4, **P.713–36**
  acetylcholinesterase secretion, **I**.686
  animal domestication, **P**.713–14
  biology/feeding, **P**.718–20
  classification, **P**.714–15
  clinical importance, **P**.730
  clinical manifestations, **P**.725–9
    growth stunting, **P**.725
    iron-deficiency anemia, **P**.725
    morbidity, **P**.725
    mortality, **P**.725
  control programs, **P**.43
  diagnosis, **P**.730
    fecal samples, **P**.730
    Kato–Katz smears, **P**.730
  epidemiology/population biology,
    P.46 (Tab.), **P**.713–14, **P**.721–5
    age-related prevalence, **P**.42, **P**.722–3,
      P.722 (Fig.)
    global distribution/abundance, **P**.42, **P**.722
    infection predisposition, **P**.724–5
    intensity, **P**.723–4, **P**.723 (Fig.)
    number of worms per host, **P**.724,
      P.724 (Fig.)
  historical aspects, **P**.713–14
  immune response, **P**.89–91, **P**.729–30
    experimental infection, **P**.90
  infection establishment, **P**.720–1
  life cycles, **P**.718 (Tab.), **P**.720, **P**.720 (Fig.)
  morphology, **P**.715–18
  prevention/control, **P**.730
  public health importance, **P**.40, **P**.42
    infection cost, **P**.42–3
  see also individual species
Nematodirus, **P**.595
NEMO deficiency, **I**.772
Neocallimasticales, **M**.51, **M**.53
Neocallimastigales, **M**.69
Neocomys, arenaviruses associated,
    V2.1060 (Tab.), **V2**.1061
Neodiplostomum, **P**.580, **P**.582

Neomycins
  characteristics, **B1**.482
  Citrobacter, **B2**.1476
  structure, **B1**.483 (Fig.)
Neonatal biliary atresia, reovirus infection,
  V2.938
Neonatal Fc receptor *see* FcRn (neonatal
  receptor)
Neonatal infection
  antibiotic-associated diarrhea, **B2**.1120
  aspergillosis
    amphotericin B therapy, **M**.725–6
    invasive, **M**.705–6
    therapy, **M**.725–6
  Bacillus cereus infection, **B2**.940
  bacteremia, **B1**.512–13
  candidiasis, **M**.13, **M**.14 (Fig.)
  Chlamydia trachomatis infection,
    B2.2012 (Fig.), **B2**.2013, **B2**.2019–20
  CNS infection
    intracranial abscess, **B1**.582
    meningitis, **B1**.574–5
    subdural empyema, **B1**.591, **B1**.591 (Tab.)
  Coxsackie virus, **V2**.1482–3
  diagnostic procedures, **V2**.1444–6
    PCR, **V2**.1444–5
  echoviruses, **V2**.1424, **V2**.1482–3
  enteroviruses, **V2**.871, **V2**.1482–3
  fetal infection *vs.,* **V2**.1446 (Tab.)
  HCMV, **V1**.521, **V2**.1446–54
  hepatitis viruses, **V2**.1474–82
  HIV, **V2**.1471–4
  HPV, **V2**.1483–4
  HSV, **V2**.1461–7
  LCMV, **V2**.1411–12, **V2**.1483
  Malassezia pustulosis, **M**.214
  mycoplasma diseases, **B2**.1991–2
  nosocomial infection, **B1**.394–5
  parvoviruses, **V1**.425–6, **V2**.1467
  pneumonia, **B2**.2012 (Fig.), **B2**.2013,
    B2.2019–20
  Proteus infection, **B2**.1447
  rubella *see* Rubella
  susceptibility to, **V1**.263
  transmission, **V2**.1443–4, **V2**.1444 (Tab.)
    congenital (prenatal), **V2**.1443
    gestational age, **V2**.1444
    maternal antibodies, **V2**.1443–4
    maternal infection frequency, **V2**.1443
    perinatal infection, **V2**.1443
    pregnancy loss, **V2**.1444
    Th2 immune response, **V2**.1443
  viruses, **V2**.1444 (Tab.), **V2.1443–97**
    see also specific viruses
  VZV, **V2**.1454–61
  see also Congenital infection; Postnatal
    infection; *specific infection; specific
    viruses*
Neonatal pustulosis, *Malassezia sympodialis*
  infection, **M**.214
Neonatal rat model, Borna disease virus
  infection, **V2**.1147–8
Neopterin, measles, **V1**.726
Neorickettsia
  antigens, **B2**.2056
  classification, **B2**.2026, **B2**.2048–9, **B2**.2053

genome, **B2**.2053–5
habitats, hosts and diseases, **B2**.2049 (Tab.),
  B2.2050–1
identification and typing methods, **B2**.2057
infection, **B2**.2061
isolation, **B2**.2052
microenvironment and morphology, **B2**.2051
replication, **B2**.2052
Neorickettsia helminthoeca
  classification, **B2**.2027 (Fig.)
  habitats, hosts and diseases, **B2**.2049 (Tab.)
Neorickettsia risticii
  genome, **B2**.2053–5
  habitats, hosts and diseases, **B2**.2050–1
  identification and typing methods, **B2**.2057
  infection, **B2**.2061
  microenvironment and morphology, **B2**.2051
  serological tests, **B2**.2057
Neorickettsia sennetsu
  antibiotic sensitivity, **B2**.2065–6
  classification, **B2**.2026, **B2**.2027 (Fig.)
  genome, **B2**.2053–5
  habitats, hosts and diseases, **B2**.2049 (Tab.),
    B2.2050–1
  identification and typing methods, **B2**.2057
  infection, **B2**.2061, **B2**.2063
  microenvironment and morphology, **B2**.2051
Neotestudina rosatii, **M**.27, **M**.28 (Fig.), **M**.391,
  M.392 (Tab.)
  histopathology, **M**.89 (Tab.), **M**.128 (Tab.)
Neotropical cutaneous leishmaniasis (NCL),
  P.313
Neozoa, classification, **P**.195–6
Nephropathia epidemica virus, **V1**.371 (Tab.)
Nephropathica epidemica, **V2**.1045
Nephrotic syndrome, malaria, **P**.482,
  P.501 (Tab.)
Nephrotoxicity, amphotericin B, **M**.148–9
Nerve enlargement, leprosy, **B2**.1205
Nerve growth factor (NGF), **I**.288 (Tab.)
  basophils, **I**.57
  eosinophil production, **I**.67
  HSV latency, **V2**.1418
Nerve terminals, virus release, **V2**.1405
Netilmicin
  spectrum of activity, **B1**.482
  Listeria, **B2**.957–8
  structure, **B1**.483 (Fig.)
Net reproductive success, transmission
  dynamics, **P**.58
Neural dysfunction, rabies, **V2**.1122–3
Neural receptors, rabies, **V2**.1122–3
Neural spread, **V1**.243–4, **V1**.244 (Tab.),
  V1.245, **V2**.1405
Neuraminidase (NA)
  functions, **B1**.153 (Tab.)
  influenza virus *see* Influenza viruses
  virosome vaccines, **I**.838, **I**.929
Neuraminidase inhibitors, **V2**.1626–8
  influenza therapy, **V1**.680
Neurocysticercosis
  anti-antigen 5 antibodies, **P**.689
  cancer link, **P**.700
  clinical manifestations, **P**.119, **P**.686–8
    hydrocephalus, **P**.687–8, **P**.687 (Fig.)
    late-onset epilepsy, **P**.686–7

meningeal arachnoiditis, **P**.686–7
  seizures, **P**.686–7
control, **P**.701
  animal reservoir hosts, **P**.119, **P**.119–20,
    P.122
  chemotherapy/chemoprophylaxis,
    P.144 (Tab.)
  diagnosis, **P**.143 (Tab.)
diagnosis, **P**.119, **P**.692–4
  computed tomography, **P**.692–3,
    P.693 (Fig.)
  ELISA, **P**.692, **P**.693–4
  hydrocephalus, **P**.692–3
  immunoassays, **P**.693–4
  magnetic resonance imaging, **P**.692
  serology, **P**.692–3
  Western blots, **P**.692, **P**.693–4
differential diagnosis, **P**.687–8
epidemiology, **P**.699–700
immune response, **P**.689
public health importance, **P**.105 (Tab.)
as public health problem, **P**.701
as reportable disease, **P**.689–90
treatment, **P**.696
  anti-epileptic drugs, **P**.696
  endoscopic excision, **P**.696
  surgery, **P**.696, **P**.697 (Fig.), **P**.698
  ventricular shunting, **P**.696
  ventriculoperitoneal shunting, **P**.696
see also Cysticercosis
Neurological damage, cerebral malaria, **P**.498
Neurological disease
  complement, **I**.155 (Tab.), **I**.156
  infective endocarditis, **B1**.535
  treatment with botulinum toxin, **B2**.1076
  Treponema pallidum, **B2**.1841
Neuronal cell adhesion molecule (N-CAM)
  NK cells, **I**.79–80, **I**.85
  Rabies virus receptor, **V2**.1108
Neuronal vacuoles, variant Creutzfeldt–Jakob
  disease, **V2**.1369
Neurons
  impact of CNS virus infection, **V2**.1409
  latent infection, **V1**.260–1
  virus entry, **V1**.244
Neurospora crassa, growth studies, **M**.71
Neurosyphilis, **B2**.1842 (Tab.)
  asymptomatic form, **B2**.1843
  clinical signs, **B2**.1843
  diagnosis, **B2**.1848, **B2**.1855–6
    PCR, **B2**.1852, **B2**.1855–6
  forms, **B2**.1843
  HIV patients, **B2**.1843
  treatment, **B2**.1857–8
Neurotacin (fractalkine:CX3CL1), **I**.220
Neurotoxic shellfish poisoning (NSP), **B1**.280
Neurotransmitters
  in CNS infection, **V2**.1409
  tapeworms, **P**.662
Neurotrophin-3, **I**.67
Neurotropism, **V2**.1405–7
  Canine distemper virus, **V1**.811
  Cryptococcus neoformans, **M**.645
  HHV-6, **V1**.527–8
  JC virus, **V1**.477

Neurotropism (*Continued*)
  subacute sclerosing panencephalitis (SSPE), **V1**.730
Neurovirulence, **V2**.1407
  enhancers, **V2**.1407
  nontranscribed genetic elements, **V2**.1407
  poliovirus, **V2**.1407
  promoters, **V2**.1407
Neutralizing antibodies
  alphavirus E1 glycoprotein, **V2**.1015
  arterivirus GP5 glycoprotein, **V1**.840
  Borna disease virus infection, **V2**.1141–2
  Canine parvovirus, **V1**.407–8
  CNS infection, **V2**.1412
  coronavirus spike (S) protein, **V1**.840
  Equine arteritis virus infection, **V1**.846
  filovirus infection, **V2**.1096
  Foot-and-mouth disease virus, **V2**.865
  hepatitis C, **V2**.1196, **V2**.1206–7
  HIV-1, gp120, **V2**.1332–3
  HIV vaccine development, **V2**.1332
  HPV infection, **V1**.468
  influenza, **V1**.663
  Measles virus, **V1**.715
  mumps, **V1**.751
  parvovirus capsids, **V1**.413
  polioviruses, **V2**.865
  Porcine reproductive and respiratory syndrome virus infection, **V1**.847
  Rabies virus glycoprotein (G), **V2**.1123–4
  rhinoviruses, **V2**.866
  torovirus spike (S) protein, **V1**.840
  yellow fever virus, **V2**.1412
Neutropenia, **I**.35, **I**.47, **I**.48 (Tab.), **B1**.644–5
  aspergillosis, **M**.724–5
  cyclic, **I**.765
  fluconazole, **M**.152
  G-CSF therapy, **I**.277
  GM-CSF therapy, **I**.47, **I**.50
  infantile genetic agranulosis, **I**.47
  severe combined, **I**.765
Neutrophil(s), **I.35–54**
  acute phase response, **B1**.739, **B1**.740
  adherence, thromboxane, **I**.189
  antimicrobial actions, **I**.40–2, **I**.44
    azurophil granules, **I**.165–6
    bactericidal/permeability increasing protein, **I**.115
    Candida albicans, **I**.44
    cathepsin G, **I**.41
    defensins, **I**.40–1
    experimental models, **I**.44
    Haemophilus influenzae, **I**.44
    5-hydroxyeicosatetraenoic acid, **I**.186
    Legionella pneumophilia, **I**.44
    leukotriene A$_4$ hydrolase, **I**.184
    measurement, **I**.51–2
    microbial killing assays, **I**.52
    myeloperoxidase-hydrogen peroxidase-halide system, **I**.35, **I**.41–2
    NADPH oxidase, **I**.41, **I**.42 (Fig.)
    Naegeria fowleri, **I**.43
    nonoxidative systems, **I**.40–1, **I**.40 (Tab.)
    oxidative systems, **I**.41–2, **I**.42 (Fig.)
  oxygen-dependent respiratory burst, **I**.35, **I**.41
  peptides, **I**.165
  Plasmodium falciparum, **I**.43, **I**.44
  Pseudomonas aeruginosa, **I**.44
  serpocidins, **I**.41
  Staphylococcus aureus, **I**.43, **I**.44
  Streptococcus pneumoniae, **I**.44
  apoptosis, **I**.36, **I**.45
    C5a complement protein, **I**.149
    Fas expression, **I**.45
    thrombospondin, **I**.45
    vitronectin, **I**.45
  chemokines produced, **I**.47
    growth related gene product α/β, **I**.47
    IFN-γ-inducible protein, **I**.47
  chemotaxis, **I**.38–9
    assays, **I**.50 (Tab.), **I**.51
    leukotriene B$_4$, **I**.185
  cytokines produced, **I**.45, **I**.46–7, **I**.46 (Tab.)
    α-defensin, **I**.170
    IL-1, **I**.36, **I**.46, **I**.47
    IL-3, **I**.46
    IL-6, **I**.46, **I**.47
    IL-8, **I**.47
    IL-10, **I**.46
    leukotriene B$_4$ production, **I**.184, **I**.185
    platelet-activating factor production, **I**.191
    prostaglandins, **I**.187
    stimulation, **I**.46–7
    Th1/Th2 balance, **I**.46
    TNF-α, **I**.47
  development, **I**.36–7, **I**.36 (Fig.)
    G-CSF, **I**.36, **I**.274, **I**.276–7, **I**.276 (Fig.)
    GM-CSF, **I**.36
    granule production, **I**.36–7
    IL-3, **I**.36
    IL-3 effects, **I**.275
    M-CSF, **I**.36
    surface receptors, **I**.36
    TNF-α effects, **I**.286
  diseases/infection, **I**.47–52, **I**.48 (Tab.)
    acquired, **I**.49–50
    aspergillosis, **M**.707
    candidiasis, **M**.259
      cutaneous/mucocutaneous, **M**.261–2
      oropharyngeal, **M**.262–3, **M**.263–4
      vulvovaginal, **M**.264, **M**.266
    congenital defects, **I**.47–9
    diagnosis, **I**.50–2, **I**.50 (Tab.)
    drug induced, **I**.49
    granule deficiency, **I**.48 (Tab.), **I**.49
    HIV infection, **I**.796
    immunodeficiency disease *see* Immunodeficiency diseases/disorders; *specific diseases/infection*
    myeloperoxidase deficiency, **I**.48 (Tab.), **I**.49
    therapy, **I**.50
    trichomoniasis, **P**.258, **P**.260
    tuberculosis granulomas, **I**.713
    see also individual disorders
  Enterococcus faecium resistance, **B2**.897
  inflammatory mediator production, **I**.45–7, **I**.46 (Fig.), **I**.46 (Tab.)
    lymphotoxins, **I**.45
    myeloperoxidase, **I**.45
    oxygen radicals, **I**.45
  intracellular signaling, **I**.42–3
    cJun NH$_2$-terminal kinase (JNK), **I**.43
    complement receptors, **I**.43
    extracellular signal-regulated kinase, **I**.43
    Fc receptors, **I**.42
    G proteins, **I**.42
    mitogen activated protein kinases, **I**.42, **I**.43
    p38, **I**.43
    phosphatidylinositol- kinase pathway, **I**.42
    protein kinase C, **I**.43
  lipid inflammatory mediators, **I**.46
    arachidonic acid, **I**.46
    cyclooxygenases, **I**.46
    lipoxygenases, **I**.46
    LTB, **I**.46
    platelet-activating factor, **I**.46
    prostaglandins, **I**.45, **I**.46
  lung host defence mechanism, **B1**.625
  lymphocyte interactions, **I**.45 (Fig.)
  mononuclear phagocyte interactions, **I**.45 (Fig.)
  phagocytosis, **I**.40 (Fig.), **I**.50 (Tab.), **I**.51
    autoimmune diseases, **I**.40
    Candida, **I**.40
    frustrated, **I**.40
    pathogen recognition, **I**.39–40
    Plasmodium falciparum, **I**.40
    process, **I**.39–40
  priming, **I**.35–6, **I**.43–4, **I**.44
    cyclooxygenase pathway products, **I**.44
    cytokines, **I**.43
    formyl-methionine-leucine phenylalanine receptor, **I**.44
    G-CSF, **I**.43
    GM-CSF, **I**.43, **I**.44
    IFN-β, **I**.43, **I**.44
    IFN-γ, **I**.43
    IL-1, **I**.43, **I**.44
    IL-2, **I**.43
    IL-8, **I**.43
    LTB, **I**.44
    lymphotoxin, **I**.43, **I**.44
    microbial killing, **I**.43
    properties, **I**.44 (Tab.)
    TNF-α, **I**.43, **I**.44
  receptors, **I**.39, **I**.39–40, **I**.39 (Tab.)
    C5a receptor, **I**.147
    chemokine receptors, **I**.220, **I**.223–4
    complement receptors, **I**.39, **I**.43
    CXC chemokines, **I**.223–4
    FcαR, **I**.39
    FcαRI (CD89), **I**.317
    FcγR, **I**.39, **I**.43
    FcγRIIa, **I**.314
    FcγRIIIa, **I**.315
    FcγRIIIb, **I**.315
    formyl-methionine-leucine phenylalanine receptor, **I**.43, **I**.44

Neutrophil(s) (*Continued*)
  recruitment to inflammatory sites, **I.**36,
    I.37–9, **I.**37 (Fig.)
    activation, **I.**37, **I.**38
    chemokines, **I.**37
    cytoskeleton, **I.**37–8
    diapedesis, **I.**37, **I.**38
    endothelial cell interactions, **I.**38
    inhibition, **I.**37
    margination, **I.**37
    receptors, **I.**37, **I.**38, **I.**38 (Fig.)
    rolling, **I.**38
  respiratory tract, **B1.**608
  SCF effects, **I.**275
  septic shock, **I.**699–700
  specific granules, **I.**165–6
    deficiency, **I.**769
Neutrophil-activating peptide-2 (NAP-
    2:CXCL7), **I.**218 (Tab.)
  basophil histamine release, **I.**62
  structure, **I.**217–19
    ELR motif, **I.**221
Neutrophil elastase, cathelicidin synthesis,
    I.174
Nevirapine, **V2.**1621–2
  HIV infection, **V2.**1336
  resistance, **V2.**1622
    HIV, **V2.**1336, **V2.**1337 (Fig.)
  structure, **V2.**1622 (Fig.)
Newbury agent, **V2.**926
Newcastle disease virus (NDV), **V1.**744,
    V1.815–16
  attachment (HN) protein, **V1.**706–7
  cellular susceptibility, **V1.**248
  classification, **V1.**48–9, **V1.**382–3
  clinical manifestations, **V1.**815
    age, **V1.**815
    strain of virus, **V1.**815
  control, **V1.**816
    vaccination, **V1.**815, **V1.**816
  economic impact, **V1.**815
  epizootiology, **V1.**815
  human infection, **V1.**815
  laboratory diagnosis, **V1.**816
  morphology/structure, protein structures,
    V1.70 (Tab.)
  pathology, **V1.**815
  phylogeny, **V1.**388
  transmission, **V1.**815
  virulence, **V1.**815
    fusion (F) protein, **V1.**705
New infection *see* Emerging infection
New variant antigen types (VATs), variable
    surface glycoprotein, **P.**362
New variant Creutzfeld–Jakob disease
    (nvCJD) *see* Variant Creutzfeld–Jakob
    disease (vCJD)
New World arenaviruses, **V2.**1060–1,
    V2.1060 (Tab.)
New York virus, **V2.**1666 (Tab.)
New Zealand Black/White mouse model, SLE,
    I.758–9
NF-1 protein
  BK virus, **V1.**480–1
  JC virus, **V1.**476–7

NFAT transcription factors, BCR signaling,
    I.347
NFC1 gene deficiency, **I.**769
NFC2 gene deficiency, **I.**769
NFκB *see* Nuclear factor κB (NF-κB)
NHS Direct, **B1.**319, **B1.**322
Nickel allergy desensitization, oral tolerance,
    I.545–6
Niclosamide, tapeworm chemotherapy,
    P.664
    Diphyllobothrium latum, **P.**673
Nicolle, C, **B2.**2030
Nicotinamide adenine dinucleotide phosphate
    (NADPH) oxidase, **I.**769
Nicotinic acetylcholine receptor, Rabies virus,
    V2.1108
Nidovirales, **V1.**26, **V1.**378, **V1.390–404**
  classification, **V1.**42, **V1.**51 (Tab.), **V1.**53,
    V1.390–2
    changes in, **V1.**390–2
    molecular biology, **V1.**390–2
    phylogenetic tree, **V1.**394 (Fig.)
  common features, **V1.**392–5
    gene expression, **V1.**392–3
    genome organization, **V1.**392–3
    ORF domains, **V1.**394–5, **V1.**399
    replicase *see below*
    replication, **V1.**392
    RNA structure, **V1.**392–3
    RNA synthesis, **V1.**392–3
  establishment, **V1.**378–9
  evolution/origins, **V1.**392–3, **V1.**401–2
    diversity generation, **V1.**401
    mechanisms, **V1.**401–2
    protein homology, **V1.**402
    replicative domains, **V1.**402
  genome organization, **V1.**392–3
  life cycle, **V1.**393 (Fig.), **V1.**395–7
    cell attachment, **V1.**395
    endocytosis, **V1.**395
    genome translation, **V1.**395–6
    nascent replicase polyproteins, **V1.**396
    particle assembly, **V1.**396–7
    'replication complex,' **V1.**396
    ribosomal frameshifts, **V1.**395–6
    RNA-dependent RNA polymerase, **V1.**396
    RNA synthesis, **V1.**396
  medical importance, **V1.**390
  members, **V1.**390, **V1.**392
    differences, **V1.**395
  morphology, **V1.**391 (Fig.)
  replicase/transcriptase, **V1.**394–5, **V1.**397–9
    classification consequences, **V1.**398–9
    difference between members, **V1.**398
    domain conservation, **V1.**397–8
    domain identification, **V1.**397
    sequence analysis, **V1.**397
  subgenomic RNA synthesis, **V1.**399–401,
    V1.400 (Fig.)
    'discontinuous minus strand synthesis,'
    V1.399–401
    'leader-primed transcription' model,
    V1.399–401
    models, **V1.**399–401
    noncontiguous sequences, **V1.**399
    open reading frames, **V1.**399

see also specific viruses
Nifedipine, microsporidians, **P.**550
Nifuratel, **B1.**495
Nifurtimox, Chagas disease, **P.**392–3
Nigeria, dracunculiasis eradication, **P.**832,
    P.833–4, **P.**833 (Fig.)
Nightingale, F, **B1.**370
Nigmegan breakage syndrome, **I.**777
Nikkomycin Z, **M.**511, **M.**512 (Fig.)
Nikolsky's sign, **B2.**812
Nimaviridae
  classification, **V1.**27 (Tab.), **V1.**43 (Tab.)
  see also specific viruses
9B antigen, schistosomiasis vaccine design,
    I.874
19-S regulator, **I.**411–12
Nipah virus, **V1.**816
  classification, **V1.**48–9
  C protein, **V1.**816
  emerging infection, **V2.**1648 (Tab.),
    V2.1651 (Tab.)
    agricultural practices, **V2.**1661
    species-barrier crossing, **V2.**1657 (Tab.)
  fruit bats, **V1.**817
  fusion (F) protein, **V1.**817
  genome, **V1.**816
  human infection, **V1.**817, **V1.**818
    pathogenesis, **V1.**818
  large (L) protein, **V1.**816
  phosphoprotein (P), **V1.**816
    RNA editing, **V1.**816
  species jumping, **V2.**1658
  transmission, **V1.**817, **V1.**818
  V protein, **V1.**816
  W protein, **V1.**816
Nippostrongylosis
  basophils, **I.**68
  eosinophils, **I.**65, **I.**70
  IL-13, **I.**294–7
  IL-25, **I.**292
Nisin, **B1.**139
Nitazoxanide
  Blastocystis hominis, **P.**567
  cryptosporidiosis, **P.**410
  microsporidiosis therapy, **P.**549
Nitrate reductase, **B1.**66
  Brucella, **B2.**1731
Nitrates, **B1.**429
  environmental problem, **B1.**200
  reduction, **B1.**66
    Escherichia coli, **B1.**66
    Veillonella, **B2.**1313
  respiration, **B1.**65
Nitric oxide (NO), **P.**70
  actions, **P.**68–9
  African trypanosomiasis, **P.**80
  Bordetella infection, **B2.**1795
  Burkholderia thailandensis infection, **B2.**1625
  cerebral malaria, **P.**83–4
  Chagas disease, **P.**86
  cytokine modulation, **P.**70
  eosinophils, **I.**58
  formation, **B1.**200
  formation by macrophage, **P.**68–9
  IFN-γ effects, **I.**288

Nitric oxide (NO) (*Continued*)
 leishmaniasis, **P**.77–8
 measles, **I**.804–5
 Plasmodium, **P**.83
 septic shock, **I**.697
 toxoplasmosis, **P**.79
 see also Inducible nitric oxide synthase
  (iNOS)
Nitric oxide synthase
 in Borna disease virus infection, **V2**.1410
 inducible (i-NOS), **V2**.1410
 macrophage production, **V1**.272–3
Nitrifying bacteria, **B1**.200
Nitrite, **B1**.423 (Tab.), **B1**.429
 formation, **B1**.66
  Enterobacteriaceae identification,
   B2.1319 (Tab.)
 oxidation, **B1**.200
 reduction, *Neisseria,* **B2**.1274–5
Nitrobacter, **B1**.200
Nitroblue tetrazolium (NBT) reaction,
 I.51 (Fig.), **I**.52, **B1**.740
Nitrofurans, **B1**.495–6
 mode of action, **B1**.495–6
 pharmacology, **B1**.496
 resistance, **B1**.496
 spectrum of activity, **B1**.495
 structure, **B1**.495, **B1**.496 (Fig.)
 toxicity/adverse effects, **B1**.496
 see also specific types
Nitrofurantoin
 isosporiasis, **P**.414
 pharmacology, **B1**.496
 resistance, *Proteus,* **B2**.1441
 spectrum of activity, **B1**.495, **B1**.499 (Tab.)
 structure, **B1**.496 (Fig.)
Nitrofurazone, **B1**.495
Nitrogenase, **B1**.63
 covalent modification, **B1**.76
 regulation, **B1**.63
Nitrogen fixation, **B1**.9, **B1**.200–1
 aerobic autotrophs, **B1**.200
 energy source, **B1**.201
 foliar surface, **B1**.198
 free-living bacteria, **B1**.201
 heterotrophic bacteria, **B1**.200, **B1**.201
 metabolism, **B1**.63
 plant associated bacteria, **B1**.200–1
Nitroimidazoles, **B1**.495
 mode of action, **B1**.495
 pharmacology, **B1**.495
 resistance, **B1**.495
 spectrum of activity, **B1**.495
  Campylobacter, **B2**.1548
 structure, **B1**.495, **B1**.495 (Fig.)
 toxicity/adverse effects, **B1**.495
 trichomoniasis, **P**.262
 see also specific types
Nitrophenols, **B1**.422
4-Nitrophenyl-β-D-glucuronide, **B1**.223
Nitrosamines, **B1**.429
 formation, **B1**.200
Nitrosomonas
 electron donors, **B1**.67
 nitrification, **B1**.200

Nitrous acid, as mutagen, **B1**.84–5
Nitrous oxide, formation/reduction, **B1**.66,
 B1.200
NKG2D receptors
 dendritic epidermal γδ T cells, **I**.436
 NK cells, **I**.88 (Fig.), **I**.90, **I**.94, **I**.627–8
NKp30 receptors, **I**.91
NKp46 receptors, **I**.91
NKR-P1 receptors, **I**.89
NMK2A receptors, **I**.89
N nucleotides
 somatic recombination, **I**.330
 TCR rearrangements, **I**.452–4
Nocardia, **B2**.1137–9, **B2**.1153–66
 antibacterial susceptibility/resistance,
  B2.1138, **B2**.1141, **B2**.1142 (Tab.),
  B2.1145
  menaquinones, **B2**.1145
 biochemical testing, **B2**.1141–5,
  B2.1142 (Tab.)
  lysozyme, **B2**.1144
  substrate decomposition, **B2**.1144
 bioremediation, **B1**.212
 cell wall and cell membrane composition,
  B2.1145–6
 classification, **B2**.1137–8, **B2**.1153
 cultivation, **B2**.1138–41
 culture, **B2**.1153
 definition/characteristics, **B2**.1153–4
 histopathology, **M**.128 (Tab.), **M**.140 (Fig.)
  stains, **M**.122, **M**.123 (Tab.), **M**.125
 infection, **I**.48, **B2**.1154
  clinical features, **B2**.1154
  intracranial abscess, **B1**.586
  mastitis, **B1**.230
  nosocomial, **B2**.1148–9
  treatment, **B2**.1165–6
 isolation/identification, **B2**.1138–41
  molecular, **B2**.1146–8
  other systems and methods, **B2**.1144–5
  phenotypic, **B2**.1141–3
  ribotyping, **B2**.1147
  serologic testing, **B2**.1149–50
  staining properties, **B2**.1139–40
  strain typing, **B2**.1148–9
 Lipid A, **B2**.1146
 macrophage interactions, **B2**.1149
 morphology, **B2**.1141–3, **B2**.1153
  aerial hyphae, **B2**.1143, **B2**.1153
  conidia, **B2**.1143, **B2**.1153
 mycetoma, **M**.387
 mycolic acids, **B2**.1145–6, **B2**.1153
 as opportunistic pathogen, **B2**.1154
 pathogenicity, **B2**.1149, **B2**.1153–4
 serology, **M**.391–2
 soil, **B2**.1138–9
 species, **B2**.1153–4
 superoxide dismutase, **B2**.1149
Nocardia abscessus, **B2**.1154
 antibacterial susceptibility/resistance,
  B2.1142 (Tab.)
 biochemical testing, **B2**.1142 (Tab.)
Nocardia africana, **B2**.1154–5
 identification, **B2**.1141

Nocardia asteroides, **B2**.1155–9
 antibacterial susceptibility/resistance,
  B2.1142 (Tab.)
 biochemical testing, **B2**.1142 (Tab.)
 identification, **B2**.1141, **B2**.1145
  molecular methods, **B2**.1146–7
  serologic testing, **B2**.1149
  strain typing, **B2**.1148, **B2**.1149
 infection
  in AIDS, **B2**.1157
  CNS, **B2**.1157–8
  intracranial abscess, **B1**.586
  nosocomial, **B1**.401 (Tab.)
  opportunistic, **B2**.1155–8
  predisposing factors, **B2**.1157–8
  in SLE, **B2**.1157
  in solid organ transplant patients,
   B2.1155–7
  traumatic introduction of, **B2**.1158–9
  treatment, **B2**.1165–6
 mycolic acids, **B2**.1146
 pathogenicity, **B2**.1149
Nocardia brasiliensis, **M**.387, **B2**.1159–60
 antibacterial susceptibility/resistance,
  B2.1142 (Tab.)
 biochemical testing, **B2**.1142 (Tab.)
  gelatin hydrolysis, **B2**.1144
 identification, **B2**.1141
  serologic testing, **B2**.1149
 infection, **B2**.1159–60
  treatment, **B2**.1165–6
 pathogenicity, **B2**.1149
Nocardia brevicatena, **B2**.1160
 antibacterial susceptibility/resistance,
  B2.1160
 identification, **B2**.1141
Nocardia carnea, **B2**.1160
Nocardia caviae, **B2**.1149
Nocardia corynebacterioides, **B2**.1160
Nocardia cyriacigeorgica, **B2**.1160–1
 antibacterial susceptibility/resistance,
  B2.1142 (Tab.)
 biochemical testing, **B2**.1142 (Tab.)
 identification, **B2**.1141
Nocardia farcinica, **B2**.1161–2
 antibacterial susceptibility/resistance,
  B2.1142 (Tab.), **B2**.1161
 biochemical testing, **B2**.1142 (Tab.)
  Middlebrook opacification, **B2**.1144
 identification, **B2**.1141, **B2**.1145
  molecular methods, **B2**.1147
  strain typing, **B2**.1148
 infection, **B2**.1161–2
 mycolic acids, **B2**.1146
 pathogenicity, **B2**.1149
Nocardia nova, **B2**.1162–3
 antibacterial susceptibility/resistance,
  B2.1142 (Tab.)
 biochemical testing, **B2**.1142 (Tab.), **B2**.1162
  arylsulfatase, **B2**.1143
 identification, **B2**.1141, **B2**.1145
  molecular methods, **B2**.1147
 infection, **B2**.1162–3
 mycolic acids, **B2**.1146
 pathogenicity, **B2**.1149

Nocardia otitidiscaviarum, **B2**.1163
  antibacterial susceptibility/resistance,
    B2.1142 (Tab.)
  biochemical testing, **B2**.1142 (Tab.)
    Middlebrook opacification, **B2**.1144
  identification, **B2**.1141
    molecular methods, **B2**.1146–7
    strain typing, **B2**.1149
  infection, **B2**.1163
    treatment, **B2**.1165–6
  pathogenicity, **B2**.1149
Nocardia paucivorans, **B2**.1163
Nocardia pseudobrasiliensis, **B2**.1163
  antibacterial susceptibility/resistance,
    B2.1142 (Tab.)
  biochemical testing, **B2**.1142 (Tab.)
    gelatin hydrolysis, **B2**.1144
  identification, **B2**.1141
Nocardia transvalensis, **B2**.1163–4
  antibacterial susceptibility/resistance,
    B2.1142 (Tab.)
  biochemical testing, **B2**.1142 (Tab.)
  identification, **B2**.1141
    molecular methods, **B2**.1147
  infection, **B2**.1163–5
Nocardia veterana, **B2**.1165
  identification, **B2**.1141
Nocardiopsis, **B2**.1137–8, **B2**.1166
  diaminopimelic acid and sugars, **B2**.1145
  microscopic morphology, **B2**.1143
Nocardiopsis, histopathology, **M**.128 (Tab.)
Nocardiosis, disseminated, **M**.140 (Fig.)
Nodamura virus, **V1**.53
Nodaviridae
  classification, **V1**.27 (Tab.), **V1**.51 (Tab.),
    V1.53
  see also Nodaviruses; *specific viruses*
Nodaviruses
  post-translational protein modification,
    V1.225
  see also Nodaviridae
NOD mouse model, **I**.758
NODs *see* Nucleotide-binding oligomerization
    domains (NODs)
Nodulectomy, onchocerciasis, **P**.788–9
Nodules, onchocerciasis, **P**.793
Nomenclature
  bacteria
    abbreviations, **B1**.18
    genera, **B1**.18
    species, **B1**.18, **B1**.20–2, **B1**.31–3
    see also Classification, bacteria; *individual*
      species/genera
  mycology, **M**.44, **M**.51
  viruses, **V1**.26, **V1**.35, **V1**.378
    binomial nomenclature, **V1**.35–6
    typography, **V1**.26, **V1**.35, **V1**.40, **V1**.378
    vernacular, **V1**.40
    see also Classification, viruses
Nomenspecies, **B1**.29–30
Non-A, non-B hepatitis (NANBH) *see*
    Hepatitis C
Nonbacterial thrombotic endocarditis (NBTE),
    B1.526–8
Noncapsular antigens, *Cryptococcus*
    neoformans var. *neoformans,* **M**.110

Nondermatophyte mold infection
  terbinafine therapy, **M**.189
  therapy, **M**.189
Non-endemic transmission, malaria
    epidemiology, **P**.511, **P**.514–15
Non-enveloped viruses, cellular entry, **V1**.107
Non-epidermal γδ T cells *see* γδ T-cells
Nongenital skin warts *see* Human
    papillomavirus infection
Nongonococcal urethritis, *Chlamydia*
    trachomatis infection, **B2**.2011
Nongovernmental development organizations
    (NGDO), parasite control, **P**.103–6
Nonhealth sectors, parasite control initiatives,
    P.103–6
Nonheme iron, lipoxygenase structure, **I**.184
Nonhomologous end joining (NHEJ), **I**.330
    HSV, **V1**.169–70
Nonimmune hydrops fetalis
  enterovirus infection, **V2**.1483
  fetal Parvovirus B19 virus infection, **V2**.1468,
    V2.1470
Noninvasive patch testing, onchocerciasis
    diagnosis, **P**.792
Non-ionic surfactants, **B1**.425, **B1**.432
Nonlytic viruses, high titer persistent infection,
    V1.259
Non-mammalian herpesviruses, **V1**.498
Non-melanoma skin cancer, HPV infection,
    V1.464
Non-M-Non-O (N) subtype, HIV-1, **V2**.1330–1
Nonnucleoside reverse transcriptase inhibitors
    (NNRTI), **V2**.1606, **V2**.1621–3
  hepatitis C therapy, **V2**.1216
  HIV infection therapy, **V2**.1336
  mechanism of action, **V2**.1606–7
  resistance, HIV, **V2**.1336, **V2**.1337 (Fig.),
    V2.1636
  see also specific drugs
Non-paralytic poliomyelitis, **V2**.870
Nonparametric linkage, **I**.573
Nonpeptide antigens, systemic γδ T cell
    recognition, **I**.439, **I**.440 (Fig.)
Nonproductive transformations, **V1**.205–6
Nonselective media, *Bifidobacterium,* **B2**.1025
Nonsense codons, point mutations, **B1**.86
Nonsteroidal anti-inflammatory fdrugs
    (NSAIDs), mechanism of action, **I**.186–7
Nonsteroid isoprenols, *Plasmodium,* **P**.477
Nonstructural proteins *see specific viruses*
Nontemplated nucleotide addition, **V1**.180
  respirovirus transcription, **V1**.771
Non-thymidine analogues
  HIV infection, **V2**.1334
  see also specific drugs
Nontranscribed genetic elements,
    neurovirulence, **V2**.1407
Nonulcer dyspepsia, *Helicobacter pylori*
    infection, **B2**.1580
Norfloxacin
  spectrum of activity, **B1**.470–1
    Klebsiella, **B2**.1480
    Listeria, **B2**.957–8
  structure, **B1**.494 (Fig.)
Normal human immunoglobulin (NHIG),
    V2.1566
  hepatitis A prophylaxis, **V2**.1566

Normand, Louis, **P**.9
Norovirus, **V2**.912
  see also Noroviruses
Noroviruses, **V2**.912–22
  antigenic variation, **V2**.918
    cross-challenge studies, **V2**.918
    serotyping, **V2**.918
  capsid protein, **V2**.912–13, **V2**.915–16,
    V2.915 (Fig.), **V2**.916–17
    conservation, **V2**.916–17
    soluble portion, **V2**.916
  classification, **V2**.912–13
    phylogenetic analysis, **V2**.914–15,
      V2.917 (Fig.)
  genome, **V2**.913 (Tab.)
    open reading frames, **V2**.914–15
    organization, **V2**.914–16
    sapoviruses *vs.,* **V2**.923
    structure, **V2**.916 (Fig.)
  group I, **V2**.914–15
  group II, **V2**.914–15
  historical aspects, **V2**.911–12
  isolation/propagation and identification,
    V1.98
  morphology, **V2**.912–13, **V2**.914 (Fig.),
    V2.922 (Fig.)
    cryo-electron microscopy, **V2**.913
    electron microscopy, **V2**.912
    X-ray crystallography, **V2**.913
  nomenclature, **V2**.911
  proteins, **V2**.916–17
    processing, **V2**.917, **V2**.918 (Fig.)
    protruding (P) domain, **V2**.913
    RNA-dependent RNA polymerase, **V2**.914,
      V2.917
  see also Norovirus
Noroviruses (Norwalk-type), mollusks, **B1**.280
Norovirus infection
  animals, **V2**.926–7
    prevalence, **V2**.926
  clinical manifestations, **V2**.913 (Tab.),
    V2.918–19
    projectile vomiting, **V2**.919
  emerging infection, **V2**.1648 (Tab.)
  epidemiology, **V1**.368, **V2**.919–20
    aerosol transmission, **V2**.919
    fecal–oral transmission, **V2**.919
    food borne transmission, **V2**.919–20
    mechanical transmission, **V2**.919
    seafood, **V2**.920, **V2**.922
    seasonality, **V2**.919
    water, **V2**.919–20
  innate resistance, **V2**.920–1
  laboratory diagnosis, **V2**.921–2
    electron microscopy, **V2**.921
    isolation, **V2**.921
    RT-PCR, **V2**.921–2
    serology, **V2**.921
  nosocomial infection, **B1**.374, **B1**.400
  outbreaks, **V2**.919, **V2**.922
    common-source, **V2**.922
    point-source, **V2**.919
  pathogenesis, **V2**.919
  pathology, **V2**.913 (Tab.)
  prevention/control, **V2**.922

Norovirus infection (*Continued*)
  self-limiting, **V2**.919
  seroepidemiology, **V2**.920–1
  vaccines
    development status, **I**.933 (Tab.)
    edible antigens, **I**.828
    virus-like particles, **I**.840, **I**.841
  volunteer studies, **V2**.911
Northern biotype *see Echinococcus granulosus*
Norwalk-like viruses *see* Noroviruses
Norwalk virus capsid protein (NVCP), **I**.829
NOS2A gene, **I**.582
Nose
  aspergillosis, **M**.694–5
  rhinosporidiosis, **M**.439, **M**.457, **M**.458,
    M.459, **M**.460, **M**.460 (Fig.), **M**.461 (Fig.)
  specimens, **M**.83 (Tab.), **M**.86 (Tab.)
Nosema
  classification, **P**.190–1, **P**.198, **P**.535, **P**.539–
    40
  historical aspects, **P**.539–40
  merogony, **P**.535
  public health importance, **P**.45
  ultraviolet radiation effects, **P**.550
  see also Microsporidians; Microsporidiosis
Nosema bombycis, historical aspects, **P**.18
Nosocomial infection, **M**.3, **B1**.368–9
  Absidia corymbifera, **M**.698
  age-relation, **B1**.394–5
    elderly, **B1**.394
    neonates, **B1**.394–5
  antibiotic resistance, **B1**.371
  antibiotic use, **B1**.371
  aspergillosis, **M**.692, **M**.706, **M**.729
  astroviruses, **V2**.902–3
  bacteremia, **B1**.392–4
  body sites, **B1**.384–94
    burns, **B1**.385–6
    eye, **B1**.386
    peritoneum, **B1**.386–7
    respiratory tract, **B1**.389–90
    soft tissue sites, **B1**.384–5
    surgical wounds, **B1**.384–5
    urinary tract, **B1**.388–9, **B1**.674,
      B1.674 (Tab.)
    see also specific sites/wounds/devices
  candidiasis, **M**.584, **M**.585, **M**.586, **M**.752
  chromoblastomycosis, **M**.359
  Clavispora lusitaniae, **M**.586
  consequences, **B1**.369–70
  control, **B1**.406–8
  control organization, **B1**.406–8
    Europe and USA, **B1**.406–8
    Infection Control Team, **B1**.404, **B1**.406
    subjects for control, **B1**.408 (Tab.)
    UK, **B1**.406
  cost, **B1**.369–70
  epidemiology, **V1**.357
  filovirus transmission, **V2**.1093–4
  hepatitis B, **V2**.1256
  historical perspectives, **B1**.370–3
    antibiotic era, **B1**.371–2
    early twentieth century, **B1**.371
    nineteenth century, **B1**.370–1
    recent developments, **B1**.372

Human respiratory syncytial virus infection,
  V1.798
  increase, **I**.6
  indwelling medical devices *see* Indwelling
    medical devices
  investigation and surveillance, **B1**.403–6
    epidemiological typing, **B1**.404–5
    organizations to consult, **B1**.406–8
    outbreak investigations, **B1**.403–4
    results of surveillance, **B1**.405
    sensitivity of case finding methods,
      B1.406 (Tab.)
    surveillance, **B1**.405–6
  occurrence, **B1**.369–70, **B1**.369 (Fig.)
Paecilomyces, **M**.752
  sources, **B1**.368–9
  specific pathogens, **B1**.395–403
    bacteria, **B1**.395–403, **B1**.401 (Tab.)
    fungi and protozoa, **B1**.403
    viruses, **B1**.400–3
    see also individual species
  tinea corporis, **M**.228, **M**.238–9
  transmission, **B1**.373–84, **B1**.404
    airborne spread, **B1**.373–5
    contact, **B1**.377–80
    contaminated blood, **B1**.383
    contaminated infusion fluids, **B1**.384
    environment, **B1**.378–9
    equipment, **B1**.379–80
    food-borne, **B1**.377
    inoculation, **B1**.380–4
    staff, **B1**.377–8
    tissue donation, **B1**.380–1
    waterborne, **B1**.375
  Trichophyton tonsurans, **M**.228, **M**.238–9
  zygomycosis, **M**.21
Nostoc, **B1**.201
Nostocoida limicola, **B1**.212
NOTCH-1, NK cell development, **I**.85
Notification of disease
  data collection, **B1**.319, **B1**.321 (Tab.)
  meningococcal disease, **B1**.322–3,
    B1.561 (Fig.)
  pertussis, **B1**.349 (Fig.)
  poliomyelitis, **B1**.353 (Fig.)
  UK, **B1**.321 (Tab.)
Novirhabdovirus, **V2**.1105
  characteristics, **V1**.129 (Tab.)
  classification, **V1**.385
  genome structure, **V1**.387 (Tab.)
  members, **V1**.385–6
Novobiocin, **B1**.496
Noxa protein, **I**.133
  structure, **I**.133 (Fig.)
Noxythiolin, **B1**.426–7
NP protein, Influenza virus A *see* Influenza
  virus A
N^pro protein, pestiviruses, **V2**.995–6
NRAMP1 gene *see SLC11A1 (NRAMP1)*
  gene
Nramp1 gene, leishmaniasis, **I**.596
NS1/NS2 genes, *Pneumovirinae,* **V1**.699
NS1 protein
  Erythrovirus, **V1**.415–16
  flaviviruses, **V2**.996

Human respiratory syncytial virus, **V1**.787
Influenza virus A *see* Influenza virus A
Minute virus of mice, **V1**.149 (Tab.),
  V1.157–8, **V1**.418–19
orbiviruses, **V2**.940
paramyxoviruses, **V1**.708
Parvovirus, **V1**.414–15
NS2 protein
  Hepatitis C virus *see* Hepatitis C virus
    (HCV)
  Human respiratory syncytial virus, **V1**.787
  Influenza virus A, **V1**.644 (Fig.)
  Minute virus of mice, **V1**.157–8
  orbiviruses, **V2**.940, **V2**.940 (Tab.)
  paramyxoviruses, **V1**.708
  parvovirus capsid assembly/packaging,
    V1.421–2
  pestiviruses, **V2**.995–6
NS3 protein
  Hepatitis C virus *see* Hepatitis C virus
    (HCV)
  orbiviruses, **V2**.940, **V2**.940 (Tab.)
  pestiviruses, **V2**.995–6
NS4A protein, Hepatitis C virus *see* Hepatitis
  C virus (HCV)
NS4B protein, Hepatitis C virus *see* Hepatitis
  C virus (HCV)
NS5B protein (RdRp), Hepatitis C virus *see*
  Hepatitis C virus (HCV)
NS gene, Influenza virus A, **V1**.641
NS_M protein
  Bunyamwera virus, **V2**.1039
  Bunyavirus, **V2**.1038
  orthobunyaviruses, **V2**.1031
  phleboviruses, **V2**.1033–4, **V2**.1038
  Punta Toro virus, **V2**.1033–4
  Rift Valley fever virus, **V2**.1033–4, **V2**.1039
NSP1 protein
  alphaviruses, **V2**.1012–14
  rotaviruses *see* Rotaviruses
NSP2 protein
  alphaviruses, **V2**.1012–14
  rotaviruses *see* Rotaviruses
NSP3 protein, rotaviruses *see* Rotaviruses
NSP4 protein, rotaviruses *see* Rotaviruses
NSP5 protein, rotaviruses, **V2**.946,
  V2.947 (Fig.), **V2**.948 (Tab.)
NSP6 protein, rotaviruses, **V2**.946,
  V2.947 (Fig.), **V2**.948 (Tab.)
nsp10, arterivirus replicase, **V1**.834
nsp13, coronavirus replicase, **V1**.834
NS proteins, *Parvovirus,* **V1**.414
NS_S protein
  bunyaviruses *see* Bunyaviruses
  orthobunyaviruses *see* Orthobunyaviruses
  phleboviruses *see* Phleboviruses
  Rift Valley fever virus *see* Rift Valley fever
    virus
  tospoviruses, **V2**.1038
NTPases
  Hepatitis C virus NS3 protein, **V2**.1197
  poxviruses, **V1**.603–5
  sapoviruses, **V2**.923–4
Nuclear factor 1 (NF1), adenoviruses
  replication, **V1**.160, **V1**.161–2

Nuclear factor 2 (NF2), adenoviruses
　replication, **V1**.160
Nuclear factor κB (NF-κB)
　antisense inhibition, **V1**.350
　apoptosis, **I**.135
　BCR signaling, **I**.346
　BK virus, **V1**.480–1
　CpG binding/signal transduction, **I**.911
　JC virus, **V1**.476–7
　lymphocyte-mediated cytotoxicity, **I**.471–2
　in macrophage apoptosis, **I**.138
Nuclear localization signal, astrovirus genome,
　V2.896
Nucleic acid(s)
　amplification
　　contamination control, **B1**.727
　　see also Polymerase chain reaction (PCR)
　as antibacterial agents, **B1**.437 (Tab.), **B1**.438
　Chlamydia infection diagnosis, **B2**.2018–19
　classical complement pathway activation,
　　I.142
　helical viruses, **V1**.59
　historical aspects, **V1**.6
　hybridization, **V1**.844–5
　　Enterobacteriaceae nomenclature/
　　　classification, **B2**.1332, **B2**.1334 (Fig.)
　infection diagnosis, **V2**.1535–9
　sequencing, **B1**.732–4, **B1**.735 (Fig.)
　see also DNA; RNA
Nucleic acid amplification
　advantages, **V2**.1535–6, **V2**.1536 (Tab.)
　in diagnosis, **V2**.1537–9, **V2**.1538 (Tab.)
　　commercial kits, **V2**.1538–9
　　microarrays, **V2**.1538
　　real-time methods, **V2**.1538
　　signal amplification, **V2**.1537
　HCMV detection, **V2**.1537
　Hepatitis B virus detection, **V2**.1537
　Hepatitis C virus detection, **V2**.1537
　HIV detection, **V2**.1537
　limitations, **V2**.1536 (Tab.)
　　contamination, **V2**.1538
Nucleic acid amplification tests (NAAT),
　gonorrhea diagnosis, **B1**.660
Nucleic acid metabolism
　Entamoeba histolytica, **P**.204
　Plasmodium see Plasmodium
　see also under DNA; RNA
Nucleic acid probes, **B1**.725
　Blastomyces dermatitidis identification, **M**.91
　Coccidioides immitis, **M**.91
　dimorphic fungi identification, **M**.91
　Histoplasma capsulatum identification, **M**.91
Nucleic acid sequence-based amplification
　(NASBA), **B1**.729–30, **B1**.729 (Fig.),
　V2.1537–8
Nucleic acid sequence based amplification
　(NASBA), aspergillosis diagnosis, **M**.718
Nucleic acid sequencing, **M**.94
Nucleocapsid associated protein (NP), Mumps
　virus, **V1**.745, **V1**.746 (Tab.)
Nucleocapsid proteins, **V1**.6
　arteriviruses *see* Arteriviruses
　Avian pneumovirus, **V1**.788
　bunyaviruses *see* Bunyaviruses
　coronaviruses *see* Coronaviruses

Equine arteritis virus, **V1**.840
　helical viruses, **V1**.59
　HIV *see* HIV
　Human respiratory syncytial virus, **V1**.787
　influenza virus, **V1**.71
　Marburg virus, **V1**.71
　Measles virus *see* Measles virus
　Mononegavirales order, **V1**.381
　Murine hepatitis virus, **V1**.832
　negative strand RNA viruses, **V1**.69–70
　orthobunyaviruses, **V2**.1031
　paramyxoviruses, **V1**.73
　phleboviruses, **V2**.1038
　Porcine reproductive and respiratory
　　syndrome virus, **V1**.836–7
　rabies virus, **V1**.71
　retroviruses, **V1**.77–9
　Severe acute respiratory syndrome
　　coronavirus, **V1**.832
　toroviruses, **V1**.827, **V1**.836–7
　tospoviruses, **V2**.1038
Nucleolus, protozoa, **P**.173
Nucleolysis, bacteriocins, **B1**.138
Nucleoproteins
　Borna disease virus *see* Borna disease virus
　　(BDV)
　Ebola virus, **V2**.1086–8
　filoviruses, **V1**.75, **V2**.1086–9
　Marburg virus, **V2**.1086–8
　negative-strand RNA viruses replication,
　　V1.128
　orthomyxoviruses, **V1**.71–2
　paramyxoviruses, **V1**.73, **V1**.703
　Rabies virus *see* Rabies virus (RABV)
　rhabdoviruses *see* Rhabdoviruses
　toroviruses, **V1**.836 (Tab.)
Nucleorhabdovirus, **V2**.1104–5
　characteristics, **V1**.129 (Tab.)
　classification, **V1**.49, **V1**.385
　genome structure, **V1**.387 (Tab.),
　　V2.1112 (Fig.)
　members, **V1**.385–6
Nucleoside analogue prodrugs, **V2**.1606,
　V2.1612–16
　hepatitis therapy, **V2**.1629
　toxicity, **V2**.1637–8
　see also specific drugs
Nucleoside-2'-*O*-methyltransferase, poxviruses,
　V1.599 (Tab.)
Nucleoside phosphohydrolase I, poxviruses,
　V1.599 (Tab.)
Nucleoside reverse transcriptase inhibitors
　(NRTI), **V2**.1606, **V2**.1619–21
　hepatitis B therapy, **V2**.1260–1
　HIV infection, **V2**.1334
　　resistance, **V2**.1337–8, **V2**.1337 (Fig.)
　HSV infection, **V1**.512
　see also specific drugs
Nucleotide analogues, **V2**.1616, **V2**.1625
　hepatitis therapy, **V2**.1629
　see also specific drugs
Nucleotide-binding oligomerization domains
　(NODs), **I**.114 (Tab.), **I**.115
　Blau syndrome, **I**.115, **I**.125
　Crohn's disease, **I**.115, **I**.125
　microbial recognition, **I**.23, **I**.24 (Tab.)

　as PPR, **I**.115
　single nucleotide polymorphisms, **I**.115, **I**.125
Nucleotide reverse transcriptase inhibitors
　(NTRTI)
　HIV infection, **V2**.1334–6
　　resistance, **V2**.1337 (Fig.)
　see also specific drugs
Nucleotides, ketol–enol tautomerism, **V1**.57,
　V1.58 (Fig.)
Nucleus
　microsporidians, **P**.529–31
　protozoa, **P**.172 (Fig.), **P**.173
　transfer to, **V1**.216
　　herpesviruses, **V1**.490–1
　　positive-strand RNA viruses, **V1**.142
　　retroviruses, **V2**.1592–3
NucliSens®, **B1**.723 (Tab.)
Nude phenotype, **I**.775
Number of susceptibles, incidence *vs.*, **I**.949,
　I.949 (Fig.)
Numbers per host, macroparasite
　epidemiology, **P**.52, **P**.52 (Fig.)
Numerical identification, **B1**.20, **B1**.21 (Tab.)
　black box processing, **B1**.26–7
Nurse cells
　Trichinella, **P**.761 (Fig.), **P**.762 (Fig.),
　　P.766 (Fig.)
　trichinellosis, **P**.759, **P**.760 (Fig.)
Nursery workers, **M**.368, **M**.376
Nursing homes, infection, **B1**.394
Nüsslein-Volhard, Christine, **I**.116
Nutrients
　microbial growth effect, **B1**.267
　recycling in soil, **B1**.9
Nutrition
　Balantidium coli, **P**.276
　Clonorchis sinensis, **P**.644
　Enteromonas hominis, **P**.270
　larval cestodes, **P**.681–2
　liver flukes, **P**.645
　malaria epidemiology, **P**.512
　Plasmodium see Plasmodium
Nutritional impairment, cryptosporidiosis,
　P.405
Nutritional restriction, host resistance, **B1**.176
Nutritional status
　acute phase response induction, **I**.197
　immunogenetics, **I**.572
　malaria, **P**.493
Nuts, **B1**.286–7
Nyando virus infection, **V2**.1048
Nystatin, **M**.148, **M**.182, **M**.183 (Tab.)
　Aspergillus otomycosis, **M**.700–1
　blepharitis, **M**.297
　candidiasis, **M**.257, **M**.609, **M**.611
　　oropharyngeal, **M**.189
　　vulvovaginal, **M**.189
　historical aspects, **M**.147
　mechanism of action, **M**.70
　penicilliosis marneffei, **M**.26

O antigens
　agglutination tests, **B1**.748
　Enterobacteriaceae *see* Enterobacteriaceae
　Escherichia coli, **B2**.1364

O antigens (*Continued*)
Legionella, **B2**.1770–1
Salmonella see Salmonella
Salmonella Paratyphi A, **B2**.1341–2
Salmonella Typhi, **B1**.744
Salmonella Typhimurium, **B2**.1341–2
Shigella vs. Escherichia coli, **B2**.1341
Obadhiang virus, **V2**.1105
Obesity, tinea cruris, **M**.186
Obesumbacterium, **B2**.1498
Obesumbacterium proteus, **B2**.1319 (Tab.)
'Oblique division', **P**.181, **P**.183 (Fig.)
Observational epidemiology *see* Epidemiology of infection, viral infection
Obstetric infection, Gram-positive anaerobic cocci, **B2**.910
Obstructive jaundice, liver fluke infection, **P**.649
Occult infection, acute hepatitis B, **V2**.1247–8
Occupational infection, **V2**.1518
human brucellosis, **B2**.1721–2
see also individual occupations
Ochlerotatus
Barmah Forest virus transmission, **V2**.1023
Eastern equine encephalitis virus transmission, **V2**.1019
Ross River virus transmission, **V2**.1022
Venezuelan equine encephalitis virus transmission, **V2**.1010
Western equine encephalitis virus transmission, **V2**.1020
Ochrobactrum anthropi, **B2**.1729 (Tab.)
Ochrosconis gallopavum, CNS infection, **M**.743–4
Oct-1 protein, adenoviruses replication, **V1**.160, **V1**.161–2
Octane degradation, plasmids, **B1**.114
Octreotide, microsporidiosis, **P**.548
Ocular candidiasis *see* Candidiasis, oculomycoses
Ocular cysticercosis *see* Cysticercosis
Ocular defects, congenitally acquired rubella, **V2**.973, **V2**.974 (Fig.)
Ocular histoplasmosis, AIDS, **M**.288, **M**.325, **M**.329
Ocular invasive aspergillosis, **M**.700, **M**.705
Ocular larva migrans (OLM) *see* Toxocariasis
Ocular microsporidiosis *see* Microsporidiosis
Ocular sporotrichosis, AIDS, **M**.325–6
Oculomycoses, **M**.273, **M**.273–344
AIDS, **M**.328–9
causative agents, **M**.273–90, **M**.275 (Tab.), **M**.278 (Tab.), **M**.280 (Tab.), **M**.281 (Tab.), **M**.320–1
Arthrographis kalrae, **M**.275 (Tab.), **M**.283
Aureobasidium pullulans, **M**.278 (Tab.), **M**.283–4
Bipolaris hawaiiensis, **M**.294, **M**.295, **M**.329
Bipolaris spicifera, **M**.295
Blastomyces, **M**.275 (Tab.), **M**.287–8
Cephaliophora, **M**.275 (Tab.)
Chlamydoabsidia padenii, **M**.281 (Tab.)
Chrysonilia, **M**.275 (Tab.)
Chrysosporium, **M**.275 (Tab.)
Cladorrhinum bulbillosum, **M**.278 (Tab.)
coccidioidomycosis, **M**.275 (Tab.), **M**.288, **M**.295, **M**.299, **M**.317, **M**.318, **M**.324

Colletotrichum, **M**.278 (Tab.), **M**.284, **M**.285
cryptococcosis, **M**.280 (Tab.), **M**.287, **M**.324–5, **M**.648
Cunninghamella, **M**.287
Cylindrocarpon, **M**.275 (Tab.), **M**.283
Dichotomophthora, **M**.278 (Tab.), **M**.283–4
Doratomyces, **M**.278 (Tab.)
Engyododontium alba, **M**.275 (Tab.)
Exophiala, **M**.278 (Tab.), **M**.283–4
Exserohilum rostratum, **M**.278 (Tab.)
Fonsecaea pedrosoi, **M**.278 (Tab.)
Geotrichum, **M**.280 (Tab.)
histoplasmosis, **M**.275 (Tab.), **M**.288, **M**.295, **M**.318, **M**.325, **M**.537
Lecythophora hoffmannii, **M**.283–4
Lecythophora mutabilis, **M**.278 (Tab.), **M**.283–4
Metarhizium, **M**.275 (Tab.)
Microsphaeropsis, **M**.278 (Tab.)
Microsporum canis, **M**.275 (Tab.)
Ovadendron, **M**.275 (Tab.)
Penicillium, **M**.275 (Tab.)
phaeoid (dematiaceous) fungi, **M**.278 (Tab.), **M**.283–4, **M**.301–2
Phaeoisaria, **M**.278 (Tab.), **M**.283–4
Phaeotrichonis crotalariae, **M**.278 (Tab.)
Phialophora, **M**.278 (Tab.)
Phoma oculo-hominis, **M**.278 (Tab.), **M**.283–4
Pneumocystis carinii, **M**.290, **M**.327, **M**.785
pythiosis, **M**.275 (Tab.), **M**.421, **M**.422 (Fig.)
rhinosporidiosis, **M**.457, **M**.458, **M**.459, **M**.460–1, **M**.461 (Fig.), **M**.463 (Fig.)
Rhizoctonia, **M**.275 (Tab.)
Rhizomucor, **M**.287
Saksenaea, **M**.287, **M**.290
Sarcopodium oculorum, **M**.275 (Tab.)
Scopulariopsis brevicaulis, **M**.275 (Tab.)
Sphaeropsis, **M**.278 (Tab.)
Syncephalastrum, **M**.287
Tetraploa aristata, **M**.278 (Tab.), **M**.283–4
Torulopsis, **M**.280 (Tab.)
Trichosporon asahii, **M**.280 (Tab.)
Tritirachium oryzae, **M**.275 (Tab.)
Tubercularia vulgaris, **M**.275 (Tab.)
Verticillium searrae, **M**.275 (Tab.)
Volutella cinereescens, **M**.275 (Tab.)
yeast, **M**.280 (Tab.), **M**.286–7
conjunctivitis *see* Conjunctivitis
contact lenses, **M**.329–32
cornea (keratitis) *see* Keratitis
dacryoadenitis, **M**.299
dacryocanaliculitis *see* Dacryocanaliculitis
dacryocystitis *see* Dacryocystitis
eyelid (blepharitis) *see* Blepharitis
intraocular, **M**.317–27
see also Endophthalmitis
lacrimal system, **M**.298
ocular biomaterials association, **M**.329–32
orbit *see* Orbit
post surgical, **M**.327–8
scleritis *see* Scleritis
therapy *see specific antifungals*
Odds ratio, **B1**.316

Odontogenic infection, **B1**.582–3
Oerskovia, **B2**.992
chemotaxonomic characteristics, **B2**.978 (Tab.)
habitats, **B2**.978
Oerskovia turbata, **B2**.992
biochemical characteristics, **B2**.993 (Tab.)
Oesophagostomum, **P**.594–5, **P**.811–12
classification/morphology, **P**.811
control, **P**.812
life cycle, **P**.811
transmission/epidemiology, **P**.811
prevalence, **P**.811
Oesophagostomum infection
clinical manifestations/pathology, **P**.811–12
Dapaong tumor, **P**.811–12, **P**.812 (Fig.)
helminthoma, **P**.811
diagnosis, **P**.812
barium enema, **P**.812
ELISA, **P**.812
ultrasound, **P**.811–12
Offal, microbiology, **B1**.273
Office-based tests, *Helicobacter pylori* infection diagnosis, **B2**.1574
Office buildings, airborne bacteria, **B1**.186 (Tab.)
Office International des Epizooties (OIE), **V1**.807
Office of Population Censuses and Surveys (OPCS), **B1**.317
Official Package Circular, vaccine information, **V2**.1583
Ofloxacin
spectrum of activity, **B1**.492
Borrelia, **B2**.1831 (Tab.)
Listeria, **B2**.957–8
Mycobacterium, **B2**.1217
structure, **B1**.494 (Fig.)
Ogston, A, **B1**.6
Oils, antibacterial activity, **B1**.432
Okavirus, **V1**.392
Okazaki fragments, **B1**.46
OKT3, aspergillosis risk factors, **M**.701
Old World arenaviruses, **V2**.1060 (Tab.)
Oleandomycin, structure, **B1**.486
Olecranon bursitis, protot-hecosis, **M**.398, **M**.399, **M**.401
Oleic acid–albumin medium, **B2**.1871, **B2**.1872
preparation, **B2**.1872
Olfactory mucosa, spread of viruses into CNS, **V2**.1405
Oligacanthorhynchida, **P**.597
Oligacanthorhynchidae, **P**.597
Oligella, as normal microbiota, **B1**.296 (Tab.)
2'-5' Oligo adenylate synthetase
HIV infection, **V1**.301
IFN action, **V1**.271, **V1**.294–5, **V1**.313–14
TNF-α, **V1**.296
Oligoastrocytoma, JC virus association, **V1**.479–80
Oligodendroglioma, JC virus association, **V1**.479
Oligonucleotide probes
Bifidobacterium classification, **B2**.1025–6
Burkholderia pseudomallei classification, **B2**.1619–20
Oligosaccharides, *Neisseria*, **B2**.1288

Oliveros virus, **V2**.1059

OLM (ocular larva migrans) *see* Toxocariasis

Olympus PK-TP test, **B2**.1848

Omenn syndrome, **I**.774

  molecular basis, **I**.330

OmpB gene, **I**.843

Omsk hemorrhagic fever, **V2**.1004

Omsk hemorrhagic fever virus, **V2**.998 (Tab.)

  transmission, **V1**.372 (Tab.)

Onchocerca, **P**.591

  infection *see* Onchocerciasis

  life cycle, **P**.591

  structure, **P**.587 (Fig.), **P**.591

Onchocerca lienalis infection, eosinophils, **I**.70

Onchocerca volvulus, **I**.683

  classification, **P**.782

    Dracunculus vs., **P**.782

  general biology, **P**.783

    cyclical reproductive pattern, **P**.783

  historical aspects, **P**.10

  immune evasion

    cystatin, **I**.687

    fibrous nodules, **I**.685

    glutathione *S*-transferases, **I**.686

    migration inhibitory factor homologue,
      I.687

    regulatory T cells, **I**.666

  infection *see* Onchocerciasis

  latent period, **P**.61 (Tab.)

  life cycle, **P**.781, **P**.783–4, **P**.784 (Fig.)

  life expectancy, **P**.60 (Tab.), **P**.781

  microfilariae, **P**.781, **P**.782–3

    lymph nodes, **P**.783

  morphology/structure, **P**.782–3

    cuticle, **P**.782

    eggs, **P**.782

    female worms, **P**.782

    male worms, **P**.782

  strain differences, **P**.786–7

  vector, life expectancy, **P**.61 (Tab.)

Onchocerciasis, **P.781–801**

  chemotherapy, **P**.789–90

    amocarzine, **P**.790

    diethylcarbazine, **P**.789

    ivermectin *see* Community-directed
      treatment with ivermectin (CDTI);
      Ivermectin

    moxidectin, **P**.790

    suramin, **P**.790

    Wolbachia therapy, **P**.790

  clinical features, **P**.793–4

    acanthosis, **P**.794

    depigmentation, **P**.793, **P**.794 (Fig.)

    dizziness, **P**.794

    'hanging groin,' **P**.793

    hyperkeratosis, **P**.794

    itching, **P**.793

    lesions, **P**.793

    lymph node enlargement, **P**.793, **P**.795

    musculoskeletal pains, **P**.794

    nodules, **P**.793

    onchodermatitis, **P**.793 (Fig.)

    presbyderma, **P**.794 (Fig.)

    skin effects, **P**.794

    'sowda,' **P**.793, **P**.794–5

visual effects *see* below

    weight loss, **P**.794

  complications, **P**.785

  control, **P**.40, **P**.109, **P**.787–9, **P**.787 (Tab.)

    African Programme for Onchocerciasis
      Control, **P**.110, **P**.121, **P**.788

    chemotherapy/chemoprophylaxis,
      P.144 (Tab.)

      see also Community-directed treatment
        with ivermectin (CDTI)

    conflict-related effects, **P**.107 (Tab.)

    diagnosis, **P**.130, **P**.143 (Tab.)

    ivermectin *see* Community-directed
      treatment with ivermectin (CDTI)

    nodulectomy, **P**.788–9

    OCP *see* Onchocerciasis Control
      Programme (OCP)

    Onchocerciasis Elimination Programme
      for the Americas, **P**.788–9

    stratification of disease, **P**.115, **P**.137 (Tab.)

    transmission interruption, **P**.787

    vector/reservoir control, **P**.125–6,
      P.145 (Tab.)

  diagnosis, **P**.790–2

    control program monitoring, **P**.791

    DNA-based, **P**.791–2

    immunoassays, **P**.791

    natural history effects, **P**.148–9

    parasitological, **P**.790–1

    punch biopsies, **P**.153

    rapid mapping techniques, **P**.792

    serological, **P**.791

    'skin snips,' **P**.153, **P**.782, **P**.790–1,
      P.791 (Fig.)

  differential diagnosis, **P**.783

    molecular techniques, **P**.791–2

  epidemiology, **P**.40, **P**.46 (Tab.), **P**.785–7

    annual transmission potential, **P**.785–6

    geographical distribution, **P**.785, **P**.792,
      P.792 (Fig.)

    infective biting rate, **P**.785–6

    infective density of vector, **P**.785–6

    life expectancy, **P**.792–3

    microfilariae strain differences, **P**.786–7

    monthly biting rate, **P**.785–6

    proportion of infective flies, **P**.786

    rapid epidemiological mapping of
      onchocerciasis, **P**.786, **P**.792

    socioeconomic effects, **P**.792–3

    vector biology effects, **P**.786

  historical aspects, **P**.10, **P**.781–2

  immune response/immunity, **P**.795–6

    asymptomatic individuals, **P**.795

    basophils, **I**.68

    cellular immunity, **P**.795

    concomitant immunity, **P**.795

    eosinophils, **I**.60

    humoral immune response, **P**.795

    IFN-γ, **P**.795–6

    immune individuals, **P**.795–6

    mycobacteria infection, **P**.96–7

    symptomatic individuals, **P**.795

    T cell anergy in, **P**.92

    T helper cell balance, **P**.795–6

  immunogenetics, **I**.600

    HLA genes, **I**.600–1

    immunoregulation, **P**.796

    eosinophilia, **P**.796

    IFN-γ, **P**.796

    IgE, **P**.796

    IL-10, **P**.796

    T helper cell balance, **P**.796

    transforming growth factor-β, **P**.796

  mortality, **P**.28 (Tab.), **P**.29 (Tab.)

  nodules (onchocercomata), **P**.783

    body distribution, **P**.783

  pathology/pathogenesis, **P**.794–5

    cellular infiltrates, **P**.794

    IgE, **P**.794–5

    inflammatory responses, **P**.781

    T helper cell balance, **P**.795

    Wolbachia bacteria, **P**.795

  public health importance, **P**.105 (Tab.)

  socioeconomic effects, **P**.794

  vaccines, **I**.933 (Tab.)

  vectors, **P**.781, **P**.784–5

  visual damage, **P**.793–5

    molecular mimicry, **P**.795

    postneuritic optic atrophy, **P**.793–4

    punctate keratitis, **P**.793–5

    sclerosing keratitis, **P**.793–5

    'snowflake opacities,' **P**.793–5

Onchocerciasis Control Programme (OCP),
  P.109, **P**.110, **P**.121, **P**.787–8

  epidemiological changes, **P**.115 (Fig.)

  geographical areas, **P**.115 (Fig.)

  insecticide resistance, **P**.787–8

  intentions, **P**.788

  vector control, **P**.126–7, **P**.787–8

    insecticide combinations, **P**.126–7

Onchocerciasis Elimination Programme for the
  Americas (OEPA), **P**.110, **P**.788–9

Onchocercidae, **P**.782

Onchocercidae, **P**.591–2

Onchodermatitis, onchocerciasis, **P**.793 (Fig.)

Oncogenes, **V1**.330–3, **V1**.345–6

  activation

    cell–virus interactions, **V1**.220–1

    role in neoplasia, **V1**.336

  definition, **V1**.334

  DNA tumor viruses, **V1**.336–8

  HHV-8 pathogenesis, **V1**.554

  mechanism of action, **V1**.335–6

  multi-step development of cancer, **V1**.345–6

  products, **V1**.335–6

    DNA tumor viruses, **V1**.336

  retroviral, **V1**.335–6

  see also Carcinogens/carcinogenesis

Oncogenesis

  adenoviruses, **V2**.1594–5

  epidermodysplasia verruciformis, **V1**.463–4

  Hepatitis B virus HBx protein, **V2**.1243

  papillomaviruses, **V1**.467

  see also Carcinogens/carcinogenesis

Oncogenicity, *Mycoplasma* infection, **B2**.1985

Oncolysis, reovirus infection, **V2**.938–9

Oncomelania, *Paragonimus* intermediate host,
  P.646

Oncosphere, **P**.576, **P**.577

Oncotropism, parvoviruses, **V1**.423

ONPG test, Enterobacteriaceae identification, **B2**.1319 (Tab.)

Onychocola canadensis, **M**.147, **M**.247, **M**.250
  culture, **M**.245
  infection *see* Onychomycosis
  Scytalidium dimidiatum vs., **M**.247
  Scytalidium hyalinum vs., **M**.247
Onychomycosis, **M**.246, **M**.247
  causative agents
    Acremonium infection, **M**.246
    Alternaria alternaria, **M**.246
    aspergillosis, **M**.246
    candidiasis, **M**.189, **M**.597, **M**.602, **M**.609–11
    dermatophytosis, **M**.183, **M**.221, **M**.238, **M**.244–6
    fusariosis, **M**.246, **M**.754
    Malassezia, **M**.214
    nondermatophyte mold causing, **M**.189
    rare molds causing, **M**.246 (Tab.)
    tinea unguium, **M**.228, **M**.234, **M**.238
  distal/lateral subungual, **M**.244
  dystrophy, **M**.245
  histopathology, **M**.238
  plate, **M**.244
  specimens, **M**.83 (Tab.), **M**.85, **M**.235
  superficial white, **M**.244, **M**.245
  therapy, **M**.182, **M**.187, **M**.187 (Tab.), **M**.234, **M**.252–3, **M**.609–11
    amorofine therapy, **M**.252
    fluconazole, **M**.187–8, **M**.187 (Tab.), **M**.253
    griseofulvin, **M**.187–8, **M**.253
    itraconazole, **M**.187–8, **M**.187 (Tab.)
    terbinafine, **M**.187–8, **M**.187 (Tab.)
Onygenaceae, **M**.542, **M**.811–12, **M**.820
Onygenales, **M**.55 (Tab.), **M**.811–12, **M**.820
O'nyong-nyong, **V2**.1022
O'nyong-nyong virus (ONNV), **V2**.1011 (Tab.)
Oocysts
  coccidian, **P**.166
  Cryptosporidium parvum, **P**.401–2
  Plasmodium, **P**.469
  wall composition, **P**.166
Ookinetes, *Plasmodium see Plasmodium*
Oomycota, **M**.4, **M**.49, **M**.50 (Tab.), **M**.413
Oophoritis, mumps, **V1**.748, **V1**.749
OpcP1 porin, *Burkholderia*, **B2**.1613
Open reading frames (ORFs)
  ambisense-containing negative-strand RNA viruses, **V1**.132
  arteriviruses, **V1**.827
  astroviruses, **V2**.892–3, **V2**.894 (Tab.)
  Borna disease virus, **V2**.1137–8
  Borrelia, **B2**.1825
  coronaviruses, **V1**.827
  Coxiella burnetii, **B2**.2074
  flaviviruses, **V1**.135–6
  foamy viruses, **V2**.1307
  Hepatitis B virus, **V2**.1230
  Hepatitis C virus genome, **V2**.1194–5
  HHV-8, **V1**.543–4
  HTLVs, **V2**.1287–8
  noroviruses, **V2**.914–15
  papillomaviruses, **V1**.450
  paramyxoviruses, **V1**.701

parvoviruses, **V1**.417
picornaviruses, **V1**.135–6
positive-strand RNA viruses, **V1**.135–6, **V1**.139–40
Rubella virus, **V2**.960–2
Simian hemorrhagic fever virus, **V1**.827
Torque-teno-virus, **V2**.1277
Open thorax lung biopsy, PCP, **M**.787
Operating gowns, **B1**.388
Operating theaters
  airborne bacteria, **B1**.186 (Tab.)
  infection, **B1**.374–5
    prevention, **B1**.387, **B1**.388
  ventilation, **B1**.374–5, **B1**.388
Operons, **B1**.70
  L-arabinose, **B1**.71–2
  autoinduction, **B1**.72
  coordinate control, **B1**.70
  coordinate induction, **B1**.70
  ilv-leu, **B1**.72
  inducers, **B1**.71
  organization and expression, **B1**.70
  regulation, **B1**.70–6
    attenuation, P070. **B1**.72
    cell density-dependent gene expression, **B1**.72
    repressors, **B1**.70–1
  rRNA, **B1**.47
  tryptophan, **B1**.72
Ophiostoma stenocera, **M**.371–2
Ophiostomatales, **M**.359
Ophiovirus
  characteristics, **V1**.129 (Tab.)
  classification, **V1**.27 (Tab.), **V1**.48, **V1**.127–8
Ophthalmic cryptococcosis, **M**.648
Ophthalmopathy, autoimmune thyroid disease, **I**.757
Opisthorchiasis
  clinical manifestations, **P**.649–50
    abdominal pain, **P**.649
    acute disease, **P**.649
    bile duct cancer, **P**.641, **P**.648–9, **P**.649–50
    cholangiosarcoma, **P**.649–50
    hepatomegaly, **P**.649
  control, **P**.40, **P**.654
    reinfection, **P**.654
  diagnosis
    antigen detection, **P**.653
    egg morphology, **P**.652–3
    PCR, **P**.653
  epidemiology, **P**.40, **P**.46 (Tab.)
  geographical distribution, **P**.40, **P**.41 (Fig.)
  immune response, **P**.652
  pathogenesis/pathology, **P**.651
    acute inflammatory reactions, **P**.651
    carcinogenesis, **P**.651
    cholecystitis, **P**.651
    eosinophilia, **P**.651
    histopathology, **P**.651, **P**.651 (Fig.)
  public health importance, **P**.105 (Tab.)
    economic burden, **P**.42
    travellers/immigrants, **P**.29
Opisthorchiidae, **P**.584–5
Opisthorchioidea, **P**.584–5
  features, **P**.585

Heterophyidae, **P**.584
Opisthorchiidae, **P**.584–5
Opisthorchis, **P**.584, **I**.682
  classification, **P**.641–2
  in definitive host, **P**.645
  historical aspects, **P**.11
  infection *see* Opisthorchiasis
  life cycle
    primary intermediate hosts, **P**.646
    secondary intermediate hosts, **P**.646
  morphology, **P**.642–3
    eggs, **P**.643
    flame cells, **P**.642–3
    structure, **P**.581 (Fig.)
  transmission/epidemiology
    age-related patterns, **P**.648
    location in host, **P**.648
    raw/undercooked food, **P**.647
  as zoonosis, **P**.642
  see also individual species
Opisthorchis felineus, **P**.640
  animal reservoirs, **P**.646
  historical aspects, **P**.641
  infection *see* Opisthorchiasis
  prevalence, **P**.646–7
  transmission/epidemiology, **P**.647
Opisthorchis viverrini, **P**.640
  historical aspects, **P**.641
  infection *see* Opisthorchiasis
  life cycle, **P**.644 (Fig.)
    animal reservoirs, **P**.646
  morphology
    adult, **P**.642 (Fig.)
    egg, **P**.642 (Fig.)
  prevalence, **P**.646–7
Opisthotonos, cerebral malaria in children, **P**.483, **P**.483 (Fig.)
Opossum *see Didelphis* (opossum)
Opportunistic infection, **M**.3, **M**.11–21
  fungi, **M**.3, **M**.11–21
  historical aspects/re-evaluation, **I**.8
  measles-induced immunosuppression, **V1**.727–9
  see also AIDS, concomitant infection; HIV infection, concomittant infection; *individual species*
Opsonins, in lung surfactant, **B1**.623–4
Opsonization, **I**.22–3, **I**.354, **I**.357, **I**.647
  C3b complement protein, **I**.39, **I**.146–7
  C4b complement protein, **I**.146–7
  histoplasmosis capsulati, **M**.527, **M**.529
  IgM, **I**.307
  malaria immunity, **P**.489
Opthiostomatales, **M**.61–3
OptiMAL®, malaria diagnosis, **P**.504
  treatment options, **P**.505
Optochin, *Streptococcus*, **B2**.862
Oral cancer, HPV associations, **V1**.463 (Tab.)
Oral candidiasis *see* Oropharyngeal candidiasis (OPC)
Oral cavity
  anatomy, **B1**.606
  infection, **B1**.610–15
    abscesses, **B1**.618–19

Oral cavity
  infection (Continued)
    candidiasis see Oropharyngeal candidiasis
      (OPC)
    Fusobacterium, **B2**.1950
    Leptotrichia, **B2**.1952
    Ludwig's angina, **B1**.614–15
    periodiontal abscess, **B1**.614
    spirochete, **B2**.1859–60
    stomatitis, **B1**.614
    see also individual species; specific diseases/
      infection
  normal microbiota, **B1**.609, **B1**.609 (Tab.),
    B1.628, **B2**.1859–60
    Bacteroides/Prevotella/Porphyromonas,
      B2.1932–3
    factors changing, **B1**.628
    gram-positive anaerobic cocci, **B2**.910
    site-specific, **B1**.609, **B1**.609 (Tab.)
    Veillonella, **B2**.1312–13
Oral contraceptives
  genital chlamydial infection effects, **B2**.2011
  rifamycin interference, **B1**.494
Oral epithelial dysplasia, HPV association,
  V1.465 (Tab.)
Oral hairy leukoplakia, in HIV infection,
  V2.1503
Oral poliomyelitis vaccine (Sabin: OPV),
  V2.880, **V2**.1555 (Tab.)
  adverse effects, **V2**.1564 (Tab.)
  developed countries, **V2**.1572
  development, **V2**.1571–2
  in pregnancy, **V2**.1562–3
  schedule, **V2**.1572
  virulence identification, **V1**.194–5,
    V1.196 (Fig.)
  WHO recommendations, **V2**.1572
Oral rehydration, rotavirus infection, **V2**.952,
  V2.953 (Tab.)
Oral tolerance
  αβ T cells, **I**.543–4
    clonal anergy, **I**.543
    clonal deletion, **I**.543
    regulatory T cells, **I**.543, **I**.544
    Th1/Th2 balance, **I**.544
  human examples, **I**.545–6
    autoimmune disease therapy, **I**.545
    γδ T cells, **I**.527, **I**.544–5
    mechanisms, **I**.543
    nickel allergy desensitization, **I**.545–6
  IL-4, **I**.544
  IL-10, **I**.544
  Peyer's patches, **I**.545
Oral vaccination, **I**.538–9
  advantages, **V2**.1556
  DNA vaccines, **I**.913
  HIV peptide vaccines, **I**.871
  IgA, **I**.539–40
  immune response, **V2**.1557
  live vaccines, **I**.841, **I**.899, **I**.901, **I**.903–4
    attenuated, **I**.926–7
  nasal administration vs., **I**.830 (Tab.)
  Salmonella vectors, **I**.899
  Shigella vectors, **I**.901
  Th2 cells, **I**.539
  vaccines, **I**.539

virus-like particles, **I**.840
Orán virus, **V2**.1666 (Tab.)
Orbit infection, **M**.290–6
  acute/fulminant, **M**.290
  allergic rhinosinusitis, **M**.296
  aspergillosis, **M**.673, **M**.674–5, **M**.694, **M**.695,
    M.700
  chronic invasive, **M**.294
  invasive, **M**.290
  noninvasive, **M**.290, **M**.295–6
  Paecilomyces, **M**.295
  Paecilomyces lilacinus, **M**.295
  Scedosporium apiospermum infection,
    M.294, **M**.295
Orbivirus
  classification, **V1**.47–8, **V2**.932
  superinfection exclusion, **V1**.192
  see also Orbiviruses
Orbiviruses, **V2**.939–42
  core-like particles, **V2**.941, **V2**.941 (Fig.)
  genomes, **V2**.932, **V2**.939
  guanylyltransferase, **V2**.939–40
  infection
    clinical manifestations, **V2**.942
    epidemiology, **V2**.942
    humans, **V2**.932
    pathogenesis, **V2**.942
    vaccines, **V2**.942
  NS proteins, **V2**.940, **V2**.940 (Tab.)
  proteins, **V2**.940 (Tab.)
    Bluetongue virus vs., **V2**.941 (Tab.)
    nonstructural proteins, **V2**.939, **V2**.940
    reoviruses vs., **V2**.941 (Tab.)
    rotaviruses vs., **V2**.941 (Tab.)
    structural proteins, **V2**.939
    see also specific types
  replication, **V2**.940–2
    insect cells, **V2**.940
    mammalian cells, **V2**.940
    receptor-mediated endocytosis, **V2**.933
    RNA-dependent RNA-polymerase,
      V2.933
  RNA-binding proteins, **V2**.939–40
  RNA-dependent RNA-polymerase,
    V2.939–40
  virion structure, **V2**.939–40
  virus-like particles (VLPs), **V2**.941–2,
    V2.941 (Fig.)
  VP1 protein, **V2**.939–40, **V2**.940 (Tab.)
  VP2 protein, **V2**.939–40, **V2**.940 (Tab.)
    cell attachment, **V2**.933
  VP3 protein, **V2**.939–40, **V2**.940 (Tab.)
  VP4 protein, **V2**.939–40, **V2**.940 (Tab.)
  VP5 protein, **V2**.940 (Tab.)
  VP6 protein, **V2**.939–40, **V2**.940 (Tab.)
  VP7 protein, **V2**.939–40, **V2**.940 (Tab.)
    see also Orbivirus
Orchitis, mumps, **V1**.748, **V1**.749
Orders, viral classification, **V1**.26, **V1**.35,
  V1.378
Ordination diagrams, **B1**.27 (Fig.), **B1**.28
ORF45-protein, HHV-8, **V1**.545
ORF domains, Nidovirales order, **V1**.394–5,
  V1.399

Orf virus (Contagious pustular dermatitis),
  V1.588
  classification, **V1**.583–5
  transmission, **V1**.371 (Tab.)
Organ cultures
  rhinovirus infection diagnosis, **V2**.878
  viruses, **V1**.90
Organelle disruption, apoptosis induction,
  I.131
Organic chemical pollutants, bioremediation,
  B1.201–2
Organic matter, decomposition, **B1**.9
Organochlorine insecticides, Chagas disease
  control, **P**.394–5
Organomercurial compounds resistance,
  Staphylococcus, **B2**.794 (Tab.), **B2**.804–5
Organotin compounds, **B1**.428
Organ transplants see Transplants
Oriental sore, **P**.297, **P**.313
Orientia
  classification, **B2**.2026, **B2**.2030–1, **B2**.2033
  staining, **B2**.2030
Orientia tsutsugamushi
  antibacterial susceptibility/resistance,
    B2.2043 (Tab.)
  antibiotic susceptibility testing, **B2**.2042,
    B2.2043
  cell wall composition, **B2**.2034
  classification, **B2**.2027 (Fig.), **B2**.2030–1,
    B2.2031 (Tab.)
  habitats, vectors and hosts, **B2**.2037, **B2**.2041
  infection see Scrub typhus
  pathogenicity and virulence, **B2**.2034
Origin (of viruses), **V1**.11–23
  theories, **V1**.11–4
    coevolution, **V1**.12
    fossil record absence, **V1**.11
    regressive evolution, **V1**.11
    replicons, **V1**.11
  see also Evolution/origin, viruses; specific
    viruses
Origin of replication (ORF)
  adeno-associated virus, **V1**.159
  DNA virus replication, **V1**.147–50
  HCMV, **V1**.500
  herpesviruses, **V1**.500
  HSV-1 replication, **V1**.164
  HSV type 1 (HSV-1), **V1**.500
  VZV, **V1**.500
Origin recognition proteins
  DNA virus replication, **V1**.148, **V1**.149 (Tab.)
  HSV-1 replication, **V1**.149 (Tab.)
  OriL, HSV-1 replication, **V1**.164
  OriS, HSV-1 replication, **V1**.164, **V1**.166
Orla-Jensen, S, **B1**.17–18
Ornibactins, Burkholderia, **B2**.1616–17
Ornidazole, amebiasis chemotherapy, **P**.213
Ornidyl (difluormethylornithine: DFMO:
  eflornithine) see Eflornithine
    (difluormethylornithine: DFMO:
    Ornidyl)
Ornithine decarboxylase, Enterobacteriaceae
  identification, **B2**.1319 (Tab.)
Ornithine decarboxylase, Pneumocystis, **M**.782
Ornithobilharzia, **P**.582
Ornithodoros moubata, **B2**.1753

Ornithodoros, relapsing fever transmission, **B2**.1823

Ornithosis *see Chlamydia psittaci* infection

Oronasopharynx
infection, **B1**.628–9
normal microbiota, **B1**.628

Oropharyngeal candidiasis (OPC), **M**.11–12, **M**.189, **M**.255, **M**.579, **M**.584, **M**.598, **M**.603, **M**.609, **M**.610–11
in AIDS/HIV infection *see* AIDS, concomitant infection
animal models, **M**.263
causative agents, **M**.598
diagnosis, **M**.258 (Tab.), **M**.603
epidemiology, **M**.256
history, **M**.5, **M**.7 (Fig.)
immune response, **M**.262–4, **M**.267 (Tab.)
animal models, **M**.263
cell-mediated, **M**.262–3
CTLs, **M**.263
γδ T-cells, **M**.263
humoral, **M**.260, **M**.263
Igs, **M**.260
neutrophils, **M**.262–3, **M**.263–4
T helper cells, type 1 (Th1), **M**.262–3
symptoms, **M**.258 (Tab.)
therapy, **M**.189, **M**.258 (Tab.), **M**.609, **M**.610–11
clotrimazole, **M**.189
nystatin, **M**.189

Oropharynx
factors influencing bacterial colonization, **B1**.294–5
normal microbiota, **B1**.301
viral entry, **V1**.239

Oropouche virus infection
clinical manifestations, **V2**.1043
epidemiology, **V2**.1049
transmission, **V2**.1048

Oroya fever
chloramphenicol treatment, **B2**.1891
clinical manifestations, **B2**.1888–9, **B2**.1890 (Tab.)
historical perspective, **B2**.1885
mortality, **B2**.1889
see also Carrión's disease

Orsomucoid *see* α₁-acid glycoprotein (AGP)

Ortheoreovirus, **V1**.47–8

Orthobunyavirus, **V2**.1025
characteristics, **V1**.129 (Tab.)
classification, **V1**.50, **V2**.1026
see also Orthobunyaviruses

Orthobunyaviruses
genome structure, **V2**.1031
consensus sequences, **V2**.1031 (Tab.)
M (medium) segment, **V2**.1031
potential maximization, **V1**.133
S (small) segment, **V2**.1031
Golgi transport, **V2**.1039–40
NS$_M$ protein, **V2**.1031
NS$_S$ protein, **V2**.1031
IFN effects, **V2**.1041–2
nucleocapsid (N) protein, **V2**.1031
transcription, **V2**.1035
host cell functions, **V2**.1036–7
nucleotide insertion, **V2**.1035–6

see also Orthobunyavirus

Orthoclone, licensing, **I**.355 (Tab.)

Orthohepadnavirus, **V2**.1227
classification, **V1**.46–7

Orthomyxoviridae
characteristics, **V1**.129 (Tab.), **V1**.177 (Tab.)
classification, H **V1**.27 (Tab.), **V1**.49 (Tab.), **V1**.50, **V1**.634
see also Influenza viruses; Orthomyxoviruses; *specific viruses*

Orthomyxoviruses
cell receptors, **V1**.207 (Tab.)
DNA polymerase, **V2**.1606–7
genome
segmentation, **V1**.180–1
subunit reassortment, **V1**.191, **V1**.192
infection *see* Orthomyxovirus infection
isolation/propagation and identification, **V1**.96 (Tab.), **V1**.98–9
morphology/structure, **V1**.70–2, **V1**.72 (Fig.), **V1**.73 (Fig.)
matrix protein (M1), **V1**.71
nucleoproteins, **V1**.71–2
protein structures, **V1**.70 (Tab.)
replication component, **V1**.71–2
transport component, **V1**.71
protein translation mechanisms, **V1**.114–15
replication
'cap-snatching,' **V1**.110, **V1**.131–2
nucleus, **V1**.131, **V1**.182
reverse genetics, **V1**.133–4, **V1**.189
thymidylate kinase, **V2**.1606–7
see also Orthomyxoviridae

Orthomyxovirus infection
antiviral therapy, **V2**.1606–7, **V2**.1625–8
resistance, **V2**.1636–7
BCE peptide vaccines, **I**.869–70
cell entry mechanisms, **V1**.213
immune response, IFN activity, **I**.260 (Tab.)
infection process, **V1**.241 (Tab.)
transmission, **V1**.371 (Tab.)

Orthopaedic surgical infection, **B1**.375, **B1**.686–7

Orthopedic device infection, **B1**.689
causative pathogens, **B1**.690–1
clinical features, **B1**.691–2
treatment, **B1**.696–7

Ortho-phthalaldehyde (OPA), **B1**.427, **B1**.439, **B1**.441

Orthopoxvirus
classification, **V1**.579 (Tab.), **V1**.582, **V1**.594
evolution, **V1**.585–6
phylogenetics, **V1**.583, **V1**.585, **V1**.585 (Fig.)
taxonomy, **V1**.595 (Tab.)
see also Orthopoxviruses

Orthopoxviruses
genome recombinations, **V1**.586
genome replication, **V1**.604 (Fig.)
immune evasion, **V1**.619, **V1**.620
antigen presentation, **V1**.619
complement, **V1**.619
IFN-γ (IFN-γ) receptor, **V1**.620
INFs, **V1**.619, **V1**.620
see also Orthopoxvirus

Orthoreovirus, **V2**.932

Orthoretroviridae
classification, **V1**.46 (Tab.)
nomenclature, **V2**.1305 (Tab.), **V2**.1322–3
see also Alpharetrovirus; Betaretrovirus; Deltaretrovirus; Epsilonretrovirus; Gammaretrovirus; Lentivirus

Orthotopic liver transplantation (OLT), aspergillosis, **M**.701

Oryzavirus, **V1**.47–8
classification, **V2**.932

Oryzomys
arenaviruses associated, **V2**.1060 (Tab.), **V2**.1061
Leishmania braziliensis, **P**.326

Oscillating equilibria, basic reproductive number effect, **P**.52

Oseltamivir, **V2**.1626–8
influenza therapy, **V1**.680
resistance, **V1**.680, **V2**.1637
structure, **V2**.1628 (Fig.)

Osimophilic inclusion bodies, Rubella virus, **V2**.964

Osler nodes, endocarditis, **B1**.528

Osmophiles, food, **B1**.266

OspA protein, **B2**.1825–6

OspC protein, **B2**.1825–6

Osteoarthritis, IL-13, **I**.294–7

Osteoblasts, GM-CSF production, **I**.277

Osteoclasts
IL-11 effects, **I**.279
M-CSF effects, **I**.277

Osteocytic lesions, histoplasmosis, **M**.536

Osteomyelitis
antibacterial treatment
duration, **B1**.700–1
intravenous, **B1**.698–9
oral, **B1**.699
aspergillosis, **M**.700, **M**.719
blastomycosis, **M**.489–90
causative pathogens, **B1**.685 (Tab.), **B1**.690–1
Erysipelothrix rhusiopathiae, **B2**.971
Kingella kingae, **B2**.1669–70
Proteus, **B2**.1447
children, **B1**.693
clinical features/manifestations, **B1**.685 (Tab.), **B1**.691–2
diagnosis
culture, **B1**.695
MRI, **B1**.694–5
radiology, **B1**.693
triple phase bone scan, **B1**.694, **B1**.694 (Fig.)
ultrasound, **B1**.694
Emmonsia parva, **M**.818
epidemiology, **B1**.685, **B1**.686 (Tab.)
inflammatory responses, **B1**.689
invasive aspergillosis, **M**.700, **M**.719
pressure sores due to, **B1**.684–5, **B1**.685 (Tab.), **B1**.686 (Tab.), **B1**.690
clinical features, **B1**.692
diagnosis, **B1**.692–3, **B1**.693–5
initiation and development, **B1**.687
prevention, **B1**.691
prognosis, **B1**.701
prevention, **B1**.691

Osteomyelitis (*Continued*)
  prognosis, **B1**.701
  spontaneous extrusion of sequestra, **B1**.689
  surgery, **B1**.697, **B1**.702 (Tab.)
    soft tissue cover, **B1**.697
  vertebral, spinal epidural abscess, **B1**.592–4
Osteoporosis, **I**.209–10
Osteosarcomas, SV40, **V1**.483
Ostertagia, **P**.595
Otitis
  dogs, **M**.214
  Malassezia sympodialis infection, **M**.214
Otitis externa
  Absidia corymbifera infection, **M**.247–8
  aspergillosis, **M**.247–8
  candidiasis, **M**.247–8
  coccidiomycosis, **M**.247–8
  dermatomycotic molds, **M**.247–8
Otitis media, **B1**.617, **B1**.628–9
  acute suppurative, **B1**.617, **B1**.629
  causative organisms, **M**.214, **B1**.617, **B1**.629
    Moraxella (Branhamella) catarrhalis,
      B2.1307
    Mycobacterium abscessus, **B2**.1248
    Mycobacterium chelonae, **B2**.1253
    Mycobacterium fortuitum, **B2**.1255
  chronic suppurative, **B1**.617, **B1**.629
  CNS infection
    intracranial abscess, **B1**.582, **B1**.584–5
    subdural empyema, **B1**.590, **B1**.591 (Tab.)
  epidemiology, **B1**.617
  pathogenesis, **B1**.617
  secretory (serous), **B1**.629
  spontaneous resolution, **B1**.617–18
  stages, **B1**.629
  treatment, **B1**.617–18
  viral infection, **B1**.617
Otomycoses
  aspergillosis *see* Aspergillosis
  lobomycosis, **M**.432 (Fig.)
  Pneumocystis carinii infection, **M**.785
  *see also individual species; specific diseases/
    infection*
Ourmiavirus, classification, **V1**.27 (Tab.)
Outbreak(s)
  astrovirus infection, **V2**.904
  avian astrovirus infection, **V2**.904–5
  communication of information, **B1**.330
  control, **B1**.328–30, **B1**.346–7, **B1**.347 (Tab.)
    of persons at risk, **B1**.329–30
    of source, **B1**.328–9
    of spread, **B1**.329
  Cote d'Ivoire ebolavirus infection,
    V2.1087 (Tab.)
  definition, **B1**.310, **B1**.403
  definitions, **V1**.358, **V1**.361
  Ebola virus infection, **V2**.1085–6,
    V2.1087 (Tab.)
  filovirus infection, **V2**.1085–6, **V2**.1087 (Tab.)
  investigations *see below*
  management of incidents, **B1**.327
  Marburg virus infection, **V2**.1085–6,
    V2.1087 (Tab.)
  measles, **V1**.712
  monkeypox, **V1**.587

mumps, **V1**.753
norovirus infection *see* Norovirus infection
nosocomial infection, **B1**.403
poliomyelitis, **V2**.882
Q fever, **B2**.2078
sapovirus infection, **V2**.924–5
vaccine efficacy studies, **B1**.324–5
see also individual species
'outbreak control team', **B1**.330
Outbreak investigations, **B1**.326–30
  case identification/collection/analysis,
    B1.327–8
  epidemiological/microbiological, **B1**.330
  preliminary inquiry, **B1**.326–7
    case definition, **B1**.327
    confirmation, **B1**.326–7
    diagnosis confirmation, **B1**.327
    tentative hypothesis and immediate
      control, **B1**.327
Outdoor feeding (exophagy), mosquito
  (Anopheles), **P**.470
Outer membrane (OM)
  fluidity, immune evasion, **I**.684
  gram-negative bacteria, **B1**.436, **B1**.442
  see also individual species
Outer membrane proteins (OMPs)
  Aeromonas, **B2**.1528–9
  Bordetella, **B2**.1801
  Brucella, **B2**.1724, **B2**.1728
  Brucella abortus, **B2**.1724
  Brucella melitensis, **B2**.1724
  Burkholderia cepacia complex, **B2**.1613
  Burkholderia thailandensis, **B2**.1621
  Haemophilus, **B2**.1698–9
  Haemophilus influenzae, **B2**.1698–9, **B2**.1705
  Helicobacter, **B2**.1569
  Moraxella (Branhamella) catarrhalis,
    B2.1307
  Neisseria gonorrhoeae, **B1**.658–9
  pertussis vaccines, **B1**.647
  Pseudomonas aeruginosa, **B2**.1592–3,
    B2.1595, **B2**.1599–600
  Treponema pallidum, **B2**.1840
  Yersinia, **B2**.1461, **B2**.1468–9
Outer membrane vesicles (OMV), *Neisseria
  meningitidis* B vaccines, **I**.939–40
Outlier (O) subtype, HIV-1, **V2**.1330–1
Outpatient parenteral antibiotic treatment
  (OPAT), intracranial abscess, **B1**.589
Ovadendron, oculomycoses, **M**.275 (Tab.)
Ovalbumin, as carrier protein, **I**.862–3
Ovary cancer, TCE peptide vaccines,
  I.865 (Tab.)
Overlapping reading frames, **V1**.180
  coronavirus, **V1**.827–8
Ovine astrovirus (OAstV)
  cell culture, **V2**.889
  classification, **V2**.890 (Tab.)
  genome, **V2**.894 (Tab.)
    sequencing, **V2**.899
  infection, **V2**.905
  virion-associated proteins, **V2**.891
Ovine herpesvirus type 2, **V1**.542 (Tab.)
Ovine pulmonary adenomatosis, **V1**.336
Ovomucoid, food, **B1**.267

OX-40, CD4 T cells/APC interactions,
  I.392 (Fig.), **I**.396
OX-ligand, **I**.288 (Tab.)
  CD4 T cells/APC interactions, **I**.392 (Fig.)
Oxacephems, **B1**.478–80
  structure, **B1**.471 (Fig.), **B1**.479 (Fig.)
  see also specific types
Oxacillin, structure, **B1**.474 (Fig.)
Oxalic acid, *Aspergillus*, **M**.713
Oxaloacetate, **B1**.53, **B1**.56
  as biosynthetic compound, **B1**.61
  substrate use, **B1**.56
Oxamniquine, schistosomiasis chemotherapy,
  P.622
Oxazolidinones, **B1**.489–90
  macrolide resistance association, **B1**.489
  Pasteurella multocida, **B2**.1655
  spectrum of activity, **B1**.489
Oxiconazole, **M**.183 (Tab.)
Oxidative activity, *Brucella*, **B2**.1731,
  B2.1733 (Tab.)
Oxidative phosphorylation, **B1**.64–5
Oxidative stress, **B1**.65
Oxidized metals, terminal electron acceptors,
  B1.67
Oxoline–esculin agar (OOA), **B2**.890–1
Oxygen
  hyperbaric
    experimental studies, **B2**.1115–16
    in gas gangrene, **B2**.1115–16
  toxicity, **B1**.65
  uptake, *Plasmodium see Plasmodium*
Oxygen-dependent respiratory burst
  in HIV infection, **I**.796
  neutrophils, **I**.35, **I**.41
Oxygen-derived reactive species
  malaria immunity, **P**.490–1
  malaria pathology/pathophysiology, **P**.497
Oxygen-impermeable films
  meat and meat products, **B1**.273
  poultry, **B1**.277–8
Oxygen radicals, neutrophil production, **I**.45
OxyR proteins, **B1**.65
Oxytetracycline, structure, **B1**.485 (Fig.)
Oxyuridae, **P**.592–3
Oxyuroidea, **P**.592–3
  Oxyuridae, **P**.592–3
Oysters, **B1**.280
Ozone, **B1**.429

P1 bacteriophage, **B1**.142, **B1**.143
P1 kinase (PKR), **V2**.1409–10
p6^Gag protein *see* HIV
p7 protein, Hepatitis C virus, **V2**.1196
p12^I protein, HTLVs, **V2**.1287–8
p13^II protein, HTLVs, **V2**.1287–8
p15 protein (NC), HTLVs, **V2**.1285–7
p19 protein (MA), HTLVs, **V2**.1285–7
p21^WAF/CIP1 binding, papillomavirus E7
  protein effects, **V1**.461 (Tab.), **V1**.462
P22 bacteriophage, **B1**.142
p24 antigen-capture assay, **I**.790
p24 protein (CA), HTLVs, **V2**.1285–7
p27^KIP1 binding, papillomavirus E7 protein
  effects, **V1**.461 (Tab.), **V1**.462

p38, neutrophil intracellular signaling, **I**.43

P38 promoter, parvovirus capsid assembly, **V1**.420–1

P42 protein, Influenza virus C, **V1**.644 (Fig.)

p53 tumor suppressor
latent nuclear antigen effects, **V1**.546–7
mechanism of action/role, **V1**.334
papillomavirus E6 protein effects, **V1**.459, **V1**.467

p75/AIRM, NK cells, **I**.89

p90 protein, Rubella virus, **V2**.960–2, **V2**.966

P97 promoter, HPV infection, **V1**.454

P105 promoter, HPV-18 infection, **V1**.454

p107 binding, papillomavirus E7 protein effects, **V1**.461

p110 protein, Rubella virus, **V2**.964

p130 binding, papillomavirus E7 protein effects, **V1**.461

p150 protein, Rubella virus, **V2**.960–2, **V2**.966

PACE® System, **B1**.725

Packaging (infectious materials), **V2**.1529

Paclitaxel, Kaposi's sarcoma therapy, **V1**.553

Paddy workers, rhinosporidiosis, **M**.458

Paecilomyces
antifungal susceptibility, **M**.752 (Tab.)
ecology, **M**.758
histopathology, **M**.128 (Tab.)
morphology, **M**.757

Paecilomyces infection, **M**.758
diagnosis, **M**.752
keratitis, **M**.282–3, **M**.303, **M**.316
nosocomial, **M**.752
oculomycoses, **M**.275 (Tab.), **M**.282–3
dacryocystitis, **M**.298
endophthalmitis, **M**.317
keratitis, **M**.282–3, **M**.303
orbital, **M**.295
therapy, **M**.758

Paecilomyces lilacinus, **M**.251
antifungal susceptibility, **M**.752 (Tab.)
infection
endophthalmitis, **M**.326–7, **M**.330
keratitis, **M**.316
onychomycosis, **M**.246
orbit, **M**.295
therapy, **M**.758

Paecilomyces variotii, **M**.251, **M**.251 (Fig.)
antifungal susceptibility, **M**.752 (Tab.)
infection
onychomycosis, **M**.246
therapy, **M**.758

Paenibacillus
colonies, **B2**.945–6
habitats, **B2**.924
identification, **B2**.945
taxonomy, **B2**.922–3

Paenibacillus alvei, **B2**.935 (Tab.)
colonies, **B2**.926 (Fig.), **B2**.945–6
infection, **B2**.944
microscopy, **B2**.943 (Fig.), **B2**.946
morphology, **B2**.943 (Fig.), **B2**.946
taxonomy, **B2**.922–3

Paenibacillus azotofixans, **B2**.924

Paenibacillus macerans, **B2**.935 (Tab.)
food spoilage, **B2**.923–4

habitats, **B2**.924
infection, **B2**.944
taxonomy, **B2**.922–3

Paenibacillus polymyxa, **B2**.935 (Tab.)
colonies, **B2**.926 (Fig.)
habitats, **B2**.924
infection, **B2**.944
treatment, **B2**.946
microscopy, **B2**.943 (Fig.)
morphology, **B2**.943 (Fig.)
taxonomy, **B2**.922–3

Paenibacillus popilliae, **B2**.946–7

Paget's disease, measles association, **V1**.725

Palaeacanthocephala, **P**.597–8
Echinorhynchida, **P**.597–8
Polymorphida, **P**.598

Palatal petechiae, in infectious mononucleosis (IM), **V1**.568

Pale, firm and dry (PFD) meat, **B1**.272

Palm
tinea manuum, **M**.232
tinea nigra, **M**.198

Palmidronate, **I**.440 (Fig.)

p-aminosalycylic acid (PAS), **B1**.490 (Fig.)

Pancreas
candidiasis, **M**.600
Pneumocystis carinii infection, **M**.785

Pancreatic carcinoma, **I**.865 (Tab.)

Pancreatitis, mumps, **V1**.750

Pandemics
definition, **B1**.310, **V1**.667
influenza, **V1**.367, **V1**.634–5

Pandorea, **B2**.1635

Panencephalitis, rubella, **V2**.974–5

Paneth cells, defensins, **I**.168, **I**.170

Panhandle structures, **V2**.1032 (Fig.)
adenoviruses, **V1**.441–2
arenaviruses, **V2**.1064
bunyaviruses, **V2**.1032 (Fig.)

Pannus, trachoma, **B2**.2014 (Fig.)

Panorex, licensing, **I**.355 (Tab.)

Pantoea, **B2**.1330 (Tab.)

Pantoea agglomerans
airborne bacteria, **B1**.189
biochemical activities, **B2**.1484
classification/nomenclature, **B2**.1337, **B2**.1483–4
culture, **B2**.1484
as normal microbiota, **B1**.296 (Tab.)
pathogenicity, **B2**.1487
waterborne, **B1**.220

Pantoea dispersa, **B2**.1319 (Tab.)

Pan troglotydes rhadinovirus-1, **V1**.542 (Tab.)

Papain, Ig digestion, **I**.304

Papanicolaou stain, **M**.88 (Tab.), **M**.491
mycology, **M**.87

Paper milling, waterborne bacteria, **B1**.212–13

Papilloedema, **B1**.557–8

Papillomaviridae
characteristics, **V1**.177 (Tab.)
classification, **V1**.27 (Tab.), **V1**.43 (Tab.), **V1**.45
see also Papillomaviruses; *specific viruses*

Papillomaviruses, **V1.448–72**
cell interactions, DNA maintenance, **V1**.219

classification, **V1**.449–50
changes in, **V1**.448–9
clades/supergroups, **V1**.449–50
L1 gene sequence, **V1**.449–50
phylogenetic tree, **V1**.449 (Fig.)
by species of origin, **V1**.449–50
E1 protein, **V1**.149 (Tab.), **V1**.155, **V1**.156–7, **V1**.456–7, **V1**.457–8
E2 association, **V1**.457–8
as helicase, **V1**.457
host replication factor association, **V1**.458
E2 protein, **V1**.149 (Tab.), **V1**.155, **V1**.156, **V1**.454, **V1**.456–8
DNA binding, **V1**.458
E1 association, **V1**.457–8
early promoter suppression, **V1**.458
immune response, **V1**.458
E4 protein, **V1**.458
keratin intermediate filament association, **V1**.458
E5 protein, **V1**.458–9
E6 protein, **V1**.459–60
apoptosis inhibition, **V1**.459–60
BAC degradation, **V1**.460 (Tab.)
cellular targets, **V1**.460 (Tab.)
E6 protein, **V1**.460
ERC-55 binding, **V1**.460 (Tab.)
function, **V1**.459–60
hDLG binding, **V1**.460 (Tab.)
hTERT expression, **V1**.460 (Tab.)
IFN regulatory factor-3 (IRF-3) binding, **V1**.460 (Tab.)
localization, **V1**.459
MCM7 binding, **V1**.460 (Tab.)
MYC degradation, **V1**.460 (Tab.)
oncogenesis, **V1**.467
p53 interactions, **V1**.459, **V1**.467
paxillin binding, **V1**.460 (Tab.)
structure, **V1**.459
vaccine development, **V2**.1582
E7 protein, **V1**.460–2
cellular targets, **V1**.461 (Tab.)
functions, **V1**.461–2
JUN binding, **V1**.461 (Tab.)
localization, **V1**.460–1
M2 pyruvate kinase binding, **V1**.461 (Tab.)
oncogenesis, **V1**.467
p21$^{WAF/CIP1}$ binding, **V1**.461 (Tab.), **V1**.462
p27^{KIP1} binding, **V1**.461 (Tab.), **V1**.462
p107 binding, **V1**.461
p130 binding, **V1**.461
retinoblastoma interaction, **V1**.461
S-phase entry, **V1**.459–60
structure, **V1**.460–1
TATA box-binding protein, **V1**.461 (Tab.)
vaccine development, **V2**.1582
genome, **V1**.148 (Tab.), **V1**.155, **V1**.450, **V1**.451 (Fig.), **V1**.452 (Fig.)
conservation, **V1**.450
open reading frames, **V1**.450
see also individual types
upstream regulatory region (URR), **V1**.450, **V1**.457 (Fig.)

Papillomaviruses (*Continued*)
  genome replication, **V1**.148 (Tab.), **V1**.154–7, **V1**.170 (Fig.)
    E1 protein, **V1**.149 (Tab.), **V1**.155, **V1**.156–7
    E2 protein, **V1**.149 (Tab.), **V1**.155, **V1**.156
    elongation, **V1**.157
    host-cell polymerases, **V1**.147–8
    host DNA replication machinery, **V1**.461–2
    initiation, **V1**.156–7
    initiation complex formation, **V1**.156
    origin of replication, **V1**.155–6, **V1**.156 (Fig.)
    origin recognition proteins, **V1**.149 (Tab.)
    S-phase cellular gene expression, **V1**.155
    viral proteins, **V1**.149 (Tab.), **V1**.155
  historical aspects, **V1**.448–9
  immunotherapy, **V1**.350
  infection *see* Papillomavirus infection
  L1 protein, **V1**.450, **V1**.462
  L2 protein, **V1**.450, **V1**.462
  open reading frame properties/functions *see individual types*
  polyomaviruses *vs.*, **V1**.155
  raft culture system, **V1**.456–7
  structure/morphology, **V1**.450, **V1**.450 (Fig.)
    virus-like particles (VLPs), **V1**.450
  transcription map, **V1**.452 (Fig.)
  see also Human papillomaviruses (HPVs); *Papillomaviridae; specific viruses*
Papillomavirus infection, **V1**.451–3, **V1**.452 (Fig.)
  cell entry, **V1**.451
  early gene expression, **V1**.454–6
    E2 protein, **V1**.454
    promoters, **V1**.454
  epidemiology, **V1**.373–4
  gene expression regulation, **V1**.453–7
  host range restriction, **V1**.451
  keratinocytes, **V1**.451–3
  late gene expression, **V1**.456–7
  nonproductive infection, **V1**.205–6
  oncogenic mechanisms, **V1**.342 (Tab.)
  proliferating cell nuclear antigen (PCNA) expression, **V1**.462
  target cells, **V1**.453
  temporal/spatial expression patterns, **V1**.453, **V1**.456 (Fig.)
  therapy
    antiviral drugs, **V2**.1631
    IFN-α, **V1**.295
    imiquimod, **V2**.1631
  tissue specificity, **V1**.451
  vaccines, **V1**.349
    BCG vector, **I**.845
    virus-like particles, **I**.840
  viral latency, **V1**.453
  see also Human papillomavirus infection
Papillon–Lefévre syndrome, **I**.482, **I**.770, **B2**.1663
Papovaviridae
  characteristics, **V1**.177 (Tab.)
  see also Papovaviruses; *specific viruses*
Papovaviruses
  attenuation, continuous passage, **V1**.197

gene expression, temporal control, **V1**.118–19
infection, **V1**.241 (Tab.)
  BCE peptide vaccines, **I**.872
  IFN activity, **I**.260 (Tab.)
  oncogenic mechanisms, **V1**.342 (Tab.)
  tumors associated, **V1**.332 (Tab.)
isolation/propagation and identification, **V1**.96 (Tab.), **V1**.99
mRNA synthesis, **V1**.110
splicing mechanisms, **V1**.114–15
see also Papovaviridae
Pappataci fever *see* Sandfly fever
Pap pili, *Escherichia coli*, uropathogenic, **B1**.147–8
PA protein, Influenza virus A, **V1**.643 (Tab.)
Papyrus Ebers, **P**.5
Parabasal filaments, **P**.170–2, **P**.172 (Fig.)
Parabens, **B1**.422
  action, **B1**.437 (Tab.)
Paracoccidioides brasiliensis, **M**.541
  antigens, **M**.550–1, **M**.553
  blastocondidium, **M**.542
  chitin, **M**.542
  classification, **M**.541, **M**.542
  culture, **M**.542
  ecology, **M**.24, **M**.544
    reserve areas, **M**.544
  Emmonsia, **M**.810 (Tab.), **M**.811, **M**.820
  genetics, **M**.542
  glucans, **M**.542
  gp43 glycoprotein, **M**.553
  heat shock proteins, **M**.114, **M**.542
  histopathology, **M**.89 (Tab.), **M**.126 (Tab.), **M**.128 (Tab.), **M**.133 (Fig.), **M**.543 (Fig.), **M**.553, **M**.554 (Fig.), **M**.555 (Fig.)
    periodic acid-Schiff stain, **M**.542
    stains, **M**.122, **M**.124
  Histoplasma capsulatum var. *capsulatum vs.*, **M**.532
  history, **M**.24, **M**.541
  identification, **M**.552–5
    culture, **M**.552–3
    histopathology *see above*
    microscopy, **M**.543 (Fig.), **M**.552
    molecular methods *see below*
    serology, **M**.92, **M**.113–14, **M**.553
    specimens, **M**.83 (Tab.), **M**.552
  infection *see* Paracoccidioidomycosis
  molecular studies, **M**.542
    expressed sequence tags, **M**.543
    random amplified polymorphic DNA, **M**.542
  morphology, **M**.126 (Tab.), **M**.541, **M**.543 (Fig.)
  parasitic state, **M**.542
  reproduction, **M**.542
Paracoccidioides, PCR detection, **M**.94
Paracoccidioidomycosis, **M**.541, **M.541–59**
  AIDS, **M**.550, **M**.553–4
  alcoholism, **M**.545
  animals, **M**.544
  clinical presentation, **M**.546–7, **M**.546 (Fig.)
    acute/subacute form, **M**.547, **M**.548 (Fig.), **M**.550–1
    blepharitis, **M**.297

  chronic form, **M**.548, **M**.549 (Fig.), **M**.550–1, **M**.550 (Fig.)
  CNS infection, **M**.548–9
  disseminated form, **M**.546–7, **M**.550–1
  granulomas, **M**.553, **M**.554 (Fig.)
  lymph node involvement, **M**.547, **M**.548–50
  oculomycoses, **M**.275 (Tab.), **M**.288–9, **M**.325
  opportunistic form, **M**.550
  pulmonary involvement, **M**.545–6, **M**.546 (Fig.), **M**.547, **M**.549 (Fig.)
  septicemia, **M**.547
  sequale, **M**.550
  ulceration, **M**.547, **M**.550 (Fig.)
diagnosis, **M**.125–7, **M**.434, **M**.552–5
  histopathology, **M**.128 (Tab.), **M**.133 (Fig.)
  serology, **M**.113–14
  specimens, **M**.83 (Tab.), **M**.552
epidemiology, **M**.544
  agriculture/agricultural workers, **M**.544, **M**.545
  bricklayers, **M**.545
  coffee plantation workers, **M**.545
  geographical distribution, **M**.545, **M**.546 (Fig.)
history, **M**.24, **M**.541
immune response, **M**.545–52
  HLA, **M**.545
  polymorphonuclear leukocytes, **M**.551
  T cells, **M**.550–1
immunosuppression, **M**.550
risk factors, **M**.544–5
therapy, **M**.551
  amphotericin B, **M**.551
  co-trimoxazole, **M**.551
  itraconazole, **M**.552
  ketoconazole, **M**.551
  sulfadimethoxiine, **M**.551
  sulfamethoxypyridazine, **M**.551
  voriconazole, **M**.552
vaccines, **I**.933 (Tab.)
Paracoccus denitrificans, **B1**.64
Paracolobactrum anguillimortiferum see Edwardsiella tarda
Paracrine signals, **V1**.334
Paraffin baiting technique, *Nocardia*, **B2**.1140
Parafossarulus, **P**.646
Paragonimiasis
  clinical manifestations, **P**.650
    ectopic infection, **P**.650
    hemoptysis, **P**.649
    intestinal, **P**.650
    migration, **P**.650
    tuberculosis *vs.*, **P**.650
  diagnosis, **P**.653
  epidemiology, **P**.46 (Tab.)
  geographical distribution, **P**.41 (Fig.)
  immune response, **P**.652
  pathogenesis/pathology, **P**.650–1
    eosinophilia, **P**.650–1
    granuloma formation, **P**.650–1
  public health importance, **P**.105 (Tab.)
  transmission, **P**.645
Paragonimidae, **P**.585–6

Paragonimus, **P**.585, **P**.640, **I**.682
  classification, **P**.641–2
  immune evasion
    connective tissue capsules, **I**.685
    effector cell inhibition, **I**.686
  infection *see* Paragonimiasis
  life cycle, **P**.585–6, **P**.645 (Fig.)
    animal reservoirs, **P**.646
    in definitive host, **P**.645
    life span, **P**.646
    primary intermediate hosts, **P**.646
    secondary intermediate hosts, **P**.646
    systemic migration, **P**.645
  morphology/structure, **P**.642
    spines, **P**.642
  prevalence, **P**.647
  structure, **P**.586
  transmission/epidemiology
    distribution within communities, **P**.648
    geographical distribution, **P**.647
    location in host, **P**.648
    raw/undercooked food, **P**.647–8
  see also individual species
Paragonimus africanus, **P**.647
Paragonimus heterotremus
  adult morphology, **P**.641 (Fig.)
  geographical distribution, **P**.647
Paragonimus kellicotti, **P**.647
Paragonimus mexicanus, **P**.647
Paragonimus skrjabini, **P**.647
Paragonimus uterobilateralis, **P**.647
Paragonimus westermani
  geographical distribution, **P**.647
  historical aspects, **P**.11, **P**.641
  infection *see* Paragonimiasis
  life cycle, **P**.645 (Fig.)
  morphology
    adult, **P**.641 (Fig.)
    egg, **P**.641 (Fig.)
  prevalence, **P**.647
Parainfluenza viruses
  hemagglutinin-neuraminidase (HN), **V1**.768
  isolation/propagation and identification,
    V1.99
  mixed cell culture, **V1**.88
  morphology/structure, **V1**.764 (Fig.)
  see also Human parainfluenza virus infection
Parainfluenza virus infection
  cytopathology, **V2**.1534 (Tab.)
  epidemiology, **V1**.365–6
    seasonality, **V1**.366
  in HIV infection, **V2**.1499 (Tab.)
  vaccine development, **V1**.775–6, **I**.933 (Tab.)
  see also Human parainfluenza virus infection
Paralecithodendrium, **P**.585
Paralysis
  in botulism, **B2**.1061–2, **B2**.1071,
    B2.1072 (Fig.)
  coxsackievirus infection, **V2**.871, **V2**.1423–4
  Echovirus 3 infection, **V2**.871
  enterovirus infection, **V2**.870–1, **V2**.1423–4
    enterovirus 70, **V2**.1423
  rabies in animals, **V2**.1118
  in tetanus, **B2**.1053–4, **B2**.1061–2

Paralytic poliomyelitis, **V2**.870
  post vaccination, **V2**.882, **V2**.1557
Paralytic shellfish poisoning (PSP), **B1**.280
Parametric release, **B1**.455
Paramomycin
  amebiasis, **P**.213
  anergic diffuse cutaneous leishmaniasis,
    P.342
  cryptosporidiosis, **P**.410
  Dientamoeba fragilis infection, **P**.269
  Old World leishmaniasis, **P**.307
Paramphistomatoidea, **P**.583–4
  Zygocotylidae, **P**.583–4
Paramyosin, **P**.92
  Echinococcus granulosus, **P**.682–3
  schistosomiasis, **P**.618, **P**.632 (Fig.)
    vaccine/vaccination, **P**.632–3
Paramyxoviridae, **V1**.26
  characteristics, **V1**.129 (Tab.), **V1**.177 (Tab.),
    V1.382–5
  classification, **V1**.26, **V1**.27 (Tab.), **V1**.48–9,
    V1.49 (Tab.), **V1**.699, **V1**.700 (Tab.),
    V1.783–4, **V1**.784–5, **V1**.808 (Fig.)
    characteristics, **V1**.379, **V1**.380 (Tab.)
  phylogeny, **V1**.388
  see also Paramyxoviruses; *specific viruses*
Paramyxovirinae
  characteristics, **V1**.129 (Tab.), **V1**.177 (Tab.),
    V1.382–5, **V1**.702 (Tab.)
  classification, **V1**.48–9, **V1**.49 (Tab.), **V1**.699,
    V1.700 (Tab.)
  members, **V1**.383–5
  phylogeny, **V1**.388
Paramyxovirus
  nomenclature, **V1**.40
  see also Paramyxoviruses
Paramyxoviruses, **V1.699–711**
  cell entry mechanisms, **V1**.213
    membrane fusion, **V1**.213
  cell receptors, **V1**.207 (Tab.)
    CNS, **V2**.1406 (Tab.)
  characteristics, **V1**.699
  classification, **V1**.699
    new members, **V1**.699
  fusion (F) protein, **V1**.150 (Fig.), **V1**.702,
    V1.705–6
  fusion mechanisms, **V1**.768–9
  hemagglutinin-neuraminidase (HN)
    interactions, **V1**.769 (Fig.)
  receptor binding, **V1**.768
  stabilization, **V1**.214
  virulence, **V1**.705
  virulence effects, **V1**.705
  general properties, **V1**.699–700
  genome structure/organization,
    V1.387 (Tab.), **V1**.700, **V1**.700–1,
    V1.701 (Fig.)
    M2 genes, **V1**.700
    open reading frames, **V1**.701
    potential maximization, **V1**.133, **V1**.703
    promoters, **V1**.700–1
    RNA editing, **V1**.702–4
    SH2 genes, **V1**.700
    size, **V1**.700

hemagglutinin-neuraminidase (HN), **V1**.72,
  V1.150 (Fig.), **V1**.701–2, **V1**.706–7
  conformational change, **V1**.768
  fusion (F) protein interactions,
    V1.769 (Fig.)
host range, **V1**.381–2
immune evasion, **V1**.199
immune evasion mechanisms, **V1**.199
infection
  animal infection, **V1.807–22**
    see also individual infection
  antivirals, **V2**.1625–8
  BCE peptide vaccines, **I**.868–9
  CNS *see* Central nervous system (CNS)
    infection
  IFN activity, **I**.260 (Tab.)
  infection process, **V1**.241 (Tab.)
  transmission, **V1**.700
isolation/propagation and identification,
  V1.96 (Tab.), **V1**.99
morphology/structure, **V1**.72–3, **V1**.74 (Fig.),
  V1.128–30, **V1**.699–700
  lipid rafts, **V1**.72
  nucleocapsids, **V1**.73
  nucleoproteins, **V1**.73
  polymerase, **V1**.73
  protein structures, **V1**.70 (Tab.)
  replication component, **V1**.73
  transport component, **V1**.72
mRNA transcription, **V1**.381
polypeptides, **V1**.703–9
  C proteins, **V1**.704–5
  F_1 protein, **V1**.705–6
  F_2 protein, **V1**.705–6
  M2–1 protein, **V1**.708–9
  M2–2 protein, **V1**.708–9
  matrix (M) protein, **V1**.703, **V1**.705
  NS1 protein, **V1**.708
  NS2 protein, **V1**.708
  nucleoprotein, **V1**.703
  phosphoprotein, **V1**.703–4
  RNA-dependent RNA polymerase (large
    protein), **V1**.702, **V1**.707–8
  small hydrophobic proteins, **V1**.708
  V protein, **V1**.704
  see also specific types
protein synthesis
  alternative initiation sites, **V1**.116–17
  RNA editing, **V1**.116–17
receptor binding, **V1**.213
red blood cell agglutination, **V1**.700
  attachment (H: HN: G) protein, **V1**.700
replication, **V1**.128–30, **V1**.701–3
  attachment/penetration, **V1**.701–2,
    V1.706–7
  transcription, **V1**.702–3
  virus assembly, **V1**.703
reverse genetics, **V1**.133–4, **V1**.189
RNA editing, **V1**.180
  conservation, **V1**.702–3
transcription
  alternate start sites, **V1**.180
  alternate termination sites, **V1**.180
  nucleotide insertion, **V1**.180
virus particle density, **V1**.700
see also Paramyxoviridae; Paramyxovirus

Paranasal sinuses
  anatomy, **B1**.606–7
  aspergillosis, **M**.694–6, **M**.711, **M**.711 (Fig.),
    M.719
    acute, **M**.694
    allergic fungal sinusitis, **M**.694, **M**.695,
      M.696
    diagnosis, **M**.695–6, **M**.711, **M**.711 (Fig.)
    granuloma, **M**.694
    therapy, **M**.695, **M**.696, **M**.719
  infection, **B1**.615–17
Parana virus, **V2**.1060 (Tab.)
Paraparesis, in progressive multifocal
  leucoencephalopathy (PML), **V2**.1417
Parapharyngeal abscesses, **B1**.618
Parapoxvirus, **V1**.588
  classification, **V1**.579 (Tab.), **V1**.582, **V1**.594
  genome structure, **V1**.583, **V1**.588
  phylogenetics, **V1**.583–5
  taxonomy, **V1**.595 (Tab.)
Parascardovera, **B2**.1025
Parascardovera denticolens, **B2**.1025 (Tab.)
  pathogenicity, **B2**.1026
ParaSight F dipsticks, malaria diagnosis, **P**.504,
    P.504 (Fig.)
  treatment options, **P**.505
Parasite aggregation, epidemiology effects,
    P.54–5, **P**.55–6, **P**.55 (Fig.), **P**.56 (Fig.)
Parasitemia, malaria diagnosis, **P**.500–1
Parasitemia waves
  African trypanosomiasis, **P**.363, **P**.364–5,
    P.364 (Fig.)
  malaria, **P**.471
Parasitic Diseases Group, **P**.129
Parasitic infection *see* Infection(s), parasitic
Parasitophorous vacuole, **P**.167 (Fig.), **P**.177
  Leishmania, **P**.292–4
  parasite invasion process, **P**.180–1
  Sarcocystis, **P**.443
  Toxoplasma gondii, **P**.423–5
Parasitophorous vacuole membrane (PVM),
  Plasmodium, **P**.475–6
  nutrition, **P**.475–6
Parastrongylus, **P**.592
  see also Angiostrongylus
Paratenic hosts, **P**.573
  Angiostrongylus cantonensis, **P**.803
Paratrachoma, **B2**.2012, **B2**.2013–14,
    B2.2013 (Fig.)
Paraxial rods, **P**.170–2
Parechovirus, classification, **V1**.50–2
Parechoviruses
  cell entry, **V2**.867 (Tab.)
  characteristics, **V2**.861 (Tab.)
  classification, **V2**.858
  size, **V2**.859
Parinaud's oculoglandular syndrome (POGS),
    B2.1892
Parkinson's disease, seborrheic dermatitis,
    M.211–12
Paronychia, candidiasis, **M**.189, **M**.597
Parotid gland
  mumps, **V1**.748, **V1**.749
  rhinosporidiosis, **M**.460–1
Paroxysmal nocturnal hemoglobinuria (PNH)
  decay accelerating factor deficiency, **I**.154

discovery, **I**.748
syphilis link, **I**.752–3
'Parrot fever' *see Chlamydia psittaci* infection
Parrot, J, **M**.13, **M**.14 (Fig.)
Parsimony analysis, **P**.193
Partial immunity
  epidemiology, **I**.955
  infection models, **I**.956
Partial lipodystrophy, C3 nephritic factors,
    I.153
Particle agglutination, syphilis detection,
    B2.1848–9
Particle size, astroviruses, **V2**.891
Particulate antigens, intranasal vaccination,
    I.830
Particulate matter, bioaerosols, **B1**.185–7
Partition systems *see* Plasmid(s)
Partiviridae
  classification, **V1**.27 (Tab.), **V1**.47 (Tab.),
    V1.48
  see also specific viruses
Partner notification, *Chlamydia* screening,
    B2.2021
Parvobacteria, immunoserology, **B1**.752,
    B1.757
Parvoviral initiation factor (PIF), parvovirus
  replication, **V1**.420
Parvoviridae
  characteristics, **V1**.177 (Tab.)
  classification, **V1**.26, **V1**.27 (Tab.),
    V1.41 (Tab.), **V1**.42, **V1**.408–12,
    V1.409 (Tab.)
  replication, **V1**.110
  see also Parvoviruses; *specific viruses*
Parvovirinae
  classification, **V1**.42, **V1**.408–9, **V1**.409 (Tab.)
  members, **V1**.411 (Tab.)
  phylogenetic relationships, **V1**.410 (Fig.)
  see also Parvoviruses
Parvovirus
  gene transcription, **V1**.414 (Fig.)
  genome structure, **V1**.409, **V1**.414–15,
    V1.414 (Fig.)
    accessory nonstructural proteins, **V1**.414–
      15
    NS1, **V1**.414–15
    NS proteins, **V1**.414
  historical aspects, **V1**.409
  members, **V1**.411 (Tab.)
  potential human pathogens, **V1**.425
  see also Parvoviruses
Parvovirus, **V1**.409
Parvovirus infection, **V1**.425–7
  empty capsids, **V1**.412
  epidemiology, **V1**.425
  fetal infection, **V1**.425–6
  pathogenesis, **V1**.425–6
    fetal/neonatal hosts, **V1**.425–6
    host age effects, **V1**.425
    immunocompromised hosts, **V1**.426
    mature hosts, **V1**.426
    teratogenesis, **V1**.425
Parvovirus B19 virus
  blood group P antigen binding, **V1**.432
  capsids, morphology/structure, **V1**.413
  classification, **V1**.411–12

coreceptors, **V1**.432
gene transcription, **V1**.414 (Fig.)
genome
  polymorphism, **V1**.432
  sequencing, **V1**.432
  structure, **V1**.414 (Fig.)
historical aspects, **V1**.411–12
type species, **V1**.42
in vitro culture, **V1**.432–3
Parvovirus B19 virus infection
  associated conditions, **V1**.431
  clinical manifestations, **V1**.411–12, **V1**.430–2
    arthropathy, **V1**.430
    immune complex disease, **V1**.430–1
    immune response effects, **V1**.430–1
    immunodeficiency effects, **V1**.431–2
    polyarthritis, **V1**.430
    rash, **V1**.430
    transient aplastic anemia, **V1**.411–12,
      V1.431
  diagnosis, **V1**.430
  emerging infection, **V2**.1648 (Tab.)
  epidemiology, **V1**.429–30
    global distribution, **V1**.429
    transmission routes, **V1**.429–30
  fetal infection, **V2**.1444 (Tab.)
    abortion, **V2**.1468
    associated diseases, **V2**.1468–9
    complications, **V2**.1468
    diagnosis, **V2**.1469–70
    intrauterine transmission, **V2**.1470
    long-term outcome, **V2**.1469
    management, **V2**.1470–1
    nonimmune hydrops fetalis, **V2**.1468,
      V2.1470
    pathogenesis, **V2**.1467–8
  in HIV infection, **V2**.1499 (Tab.)
  immune response, **V1**.429–30
    pathogenic effects, **V1**.430–1
  neonatal infection, **V2**.1444 (Tab.), **V2**.1467
    droplet spread, **V2**.1467
    seasonality, **V2**.1467
  in pregnancy, **V1**.431, **V2**.1444 (Tab.)
    asymptomatic, **V2**.1467
    cross-placental transmission, **V2**.1468
    delivery methods, **V2**.1470
    diagnosis, **V2**.1469
    Ig prophylaxis, **V2**.1470
    management, **V2**.1470–1
    prophylaxis, **V2**.1470–1
    vaccination, **V2**.1470
  in vitro correlation with pathology, **V1**.432–3
Parvoviruses, **V1.407–38**
  capsids, **V1**.412–13
    assembly/packaging, **V1**.420–2,
      V1.421 (Fig.)
    central pore, **V1**.413
    isocahedral symmetry, **V1**.407–8, **V1**.413
    morphology/structure, **V1**.407–8, **V1**.412,
      V1.413 (Fig.)
    neutralizing antibody-binding, **V1**.413
    replication initiator protein, **V1**.413
  characteristics, **V1**.407–8
  classification, **V1**.157
  serotypes, **V1**.407–8

Parvoviruses (*Continued*)
  gene therapy vectors, **V1**.426–7
  genome replication, **V1**.123, **V1**.157–60,
    V1.408, **V1**.418–20
    DNA polymerase δ, **V1**.418
    hairpin termini, **V1**.150
    'hairpin transfer,' **V1**.419
    host-cell polymerases, **V1**.147–8
    host cell S phase, **V1**.408
    junction resolution, **V1**.419, **V1**.420
    parvoviral initiation factor (PIF), **V1**.420
    priming, **V1**.147–8
    'rolling hairpin,' **V1**.150, **V1**.418,
      V1.419–20, **V1**.419 (Fig.)
  genome structure, **V1**.407, **V1**.413–16
    gene cassettes, **V1**.408
    open reading frames, **V1**.417
  historical aspects, **V1**.408–12
  host range, **V1**.407, **V1**.422–4
    allotropic specificity, **V1**.422
    host specificity, **V1**.422–3
    oncotropism, **V1**.423
    tissue specificity, **V1**.422–3
    transferin receptor, **V1**.422
  infection *see* Parvovirus infection
  isolation/propagation and identification,
    V1.96 (Tab.), **V1**.99–100
  mutation rates, **V1**.407
  structure, **V1**.412–16
  taxonomy, **V1**.408–12
  as vaccine vector, **V1**.427
  VP proteins, **V1**.407–8, **V1**.412
  see also Parvoviridae; Parvovirus
Parvovirus infection, **V1**.408, **V1**.416–22,
    V1.425–7, **V1**.427–9, **V1**.429–33
  acute infection, **V1**.426
  BCE peptide vaccines, **I**.871–2
  cell entry, **V1**.416–17
    acid exposure, **V1**.417
    endocytosis, **V1**.417
    multiple receptors, **V1**.416–17
  cellular S phase dependency, **V1**.418
  chronic infection, **V1**.426
  cryptic infection, **V1**.423–4
  early events, **V1**.416–8, **V1**.416 (Fig.)
  IFN activity, **I**.260 (Tab.)
  latent infection, **V1**.423–4
    detection, **V1**.424
  nuclear pore targeting, **V1**.418
  pathogenesis, **V1**.408
    hepatitis, **V1**.426
  single serotypes, **V1**.407–8
  vesicle trafficking, **V1**.417–18
Parvovirus initiation factor (PIF), Minute virus
  of mice replication, **V1**.158
Passive agglutination tests, **B1**.748
Passive immunization, **B1**.329–30, **V2**.1552,
    V2.1565–8
  adverse reactions, **V2**.1568
    allergies, **V2**.1568
    disease transmission, **V2**.1568
    live vaccine interference, **V2**.1568
  applications, **V2**.1566–8
    adenovirus infection, **V1**.446
    HHV-6 infection, **V1**.531–2

Human respiratory syncytial virus
    infection, **V2**.1567, **V2**.1567 (Tab.)
  Parvovirus B19 virus infection, **V2**.1470
  post-exposure prophylaxis, **V2**.1567–8
  pre-exposure prophylaxis, **V2**.1566–7
  rubella, **V2**.985
  therapy, **V2**.1568
  historical aspects, **V2**.1565
  Ig types, **V2**.1566, **V2**.1567 (Tab.)
    intramuscular, **V2**.1566
    intravenous (IVIG), **V2**.1566
  preparation, **V2**.1565
  see also Vaccination
Passive phagocytosis, Q fever, **B2**.2077
Pasteurella, **B2**.1651 (Tab.), **B2**.1652 (Tab.),
    B2.1653
  bone and joint infection, **B1**.690–1
  classification, **B2**.1650
  conjugation, **B1**.103
  endocarditis, **B1**.536
  habitats, **B2**.1649–50
  misclassified species, **B2**.1650, **B2**.1652 (Tab.)
  taxonomy, **B2**.1650–3
Pasteurella aerogenes, **B2**.1652 (Tab.), **B2**.1656
  antibacterial susceptibility/resistance,
    B2.1656
  infection, **B2**.1656
Pasteurella anatis, **B2**.1650
Pasteurella avium, **B2**.1651 (Tab.)
  classification, **B2**.1650
  infection in animals, **B2**.1654
Pasteurella bettyae, **B2**.1652 (Tab.), **B2**.1657
  antibacterial susceptibility/resistance,
    B2.1657
  classification, **B2**.1650
  infection, **B2**.1657
  as normal microbiota, **B1**.296 (Tab.)
Pasteurella caballi, **B2**.1652 (Tab.), **B2**.1657
  classification, **B2**.1650
Pasteurella canis, **B2**.1651 (Tab.), **B2**.1656–7
  classification, **B2**.1650
  infection in humans, **B2**.1650–3, **B2**.1656
Pasteurellaceae, **B2**.1651 (Tab.)
  taxonomy, **B2**.1650–3
Pasteurella dagmatis, **B2**.1651 (Tab.), **B2**.1657
  classification, **B2**.1650
  infection in humans, **B2**.1650–3, **B2**.1657
Pasteurella gallinarum, **B2**.1651 (Tab.),
    B2.1658
  classification, **B2**.1650
  infection in animals, **B2**.1654
  infection in humans, **B2**.1658
Pasteurella gas, **B2**.1656
Pasteurella granulomatis, **B2**.1650, **B2**.1653
Pasteurella haemolytica
  infection in animals, **B2**.1653
  pore-forming toxins, **I**.654–5
  reclassification, **B2**.1650, **B2**.1653
  vaccine, **I**.822
Pasteurella langaa, **B2**.1651 (Tab.)
  classification, **B2**.1650
  infection in animals, **B2**.1654
Pasteurella leonis, **B2**.1650–3
Pasteurella lymphangitidis, **B2**.1652 (Tab.)
  classification, **B2**.1650

Pasteurella mairiii, **B2**.1652 (Tab.)
  classification, **B2**.1650
Pasteurella multocida, **B2**.1651 (Tab.),
    B2.1654–5
  antibacterial susceptibility/resistance,
    B2.1655
  Bordetella bronchiseptica relationship,
    B2.1810
  classification, **B2**.1650
  culture and identification, **B2**.1655
  infection, **B2**.1654–5
    clinical significance, **B2**.1654–5
    epiglottitis, **B1**.613
    mastitis, **B1**.230
    pneumonia, **B1**.637
    pulmonary, **B1**.637
  infection in animals, **B2**.1654, **B2**.1810
    cattle, **B2**.1653–4
    fowl cholera, **B2**.1653–4
    mastitis, **B1**.230
    pneumonia, **B1**.637
    rabbits, **B2**.1654
    swine, **B2**.1653–4
    treatment, **B2**.1655
  as normal microbiota, **B1**.296 (Tab.)
  subspecies *gallicida*, **B2**.1651 (Tab.)
  subspecies *multocida*, **B2**.1651 (Tab.)
    infection in humans, **B2**.1650–3
  subspecies *septica*, **B2**.1651 (Tab.)
    classification, **B2**.1650
    infection in humans, **B2**.1650–3
  subspecies *tigris*, **B2**.1650–3
  virulence factors, **B2**.1653–4
    capsules, **B2**.1653–4
    lipases, **B2**.1653–4
    toxin gene, *toxA*, **B2**.1653–4
Pasteurella novicida, **B1**.99
Pasteurella phocoenarum, **B2**.1650–3
Pasteurella pneumotropica, **B2**.1652 (Tab.),
    B2.1655–6
  culture, **B2**.1656
  identification, **B2**.1656
  infection in humans, **B2**.1655–6
  transmission, **B2**.1655–6
Pasteurella seminis, **B2**.1650
Pasteurella skyensis, **B2**.1650–3
Pasteurella stomatis, **B2**.1651 (Tab.), **B2**.1656–7
  classification, **B2**.1650
  infection in humans, **B2**.1650–3, **B2**.1656
Pasteurella testudinis, **B2**.1652 (Tab.)
  classification, **B2**.1650
  infection in animals, **B2**.1654
Pasteurella trehalosi, **B2**.1652 (Tab.)
  classification, **B2**.1650, **B2**.1653
Pasteurella ureae, **B2**.1650, **B2**.1658–9
Pasteurella volantium, **B2**.1650
  infection in animals, **B2**.1654
Pasteurization, **B1**.269, **B1**.271, **B1**.446
  cream, **B1**.248
  eggs, **B1**.269, **B1**.271, **B1**.279
  milk, **B1**.232–3, **B1**.232 (Fig.), **B1**.236
  yogurt, **B1**.248
Pasteur, Louis, **V1**.3–4, **P**.4, **B1**.4–5, **B1**.5 (Fig.),
    I.6, **M**.6–8, **B1**.7, **M**.8 (Fig.), **B1**.10–11,
    M.22–3, **M**.32–3

Pastorex test
  Aspergillus, **M.**107–8, **M.**713
  Candida, **M.**100, **M.**607
  Cryptococcus, **M.**109–10
Patent ductus arteriosus, rubella, **V2.**974
Patents, species, **B1.**31–2
Pathogen-associated molecular patterns
    (PAMPs), **I.**22, **I.**110, **I.**111, **I.**652
  commensal bacteria, **I.**111
  definition, **I.**112
  double stranded RNA, **I.**896
  flagellins, **I.**896
  live vaccines, **I.**896
  LPS, **I.**896
  parasitic infection, **I.**679–80
  septic shock, **I.**696
  variation, **I.**110
Pathogenesis
  bacterial infection, **B1.**294
  viral infection, **V1.236–69**
    gastrointestinal tract, **V1.**237 (Fig.),
      V1.239, **V1.**240 (Fig.)
    historical aspects, **V1.**4
    host determinants of susceptibility,
      V1.262–5
      host genes, **V1.**264–5, **V1.**265 (Tab.)
      oncogenic viruses, **V1.**344–8
      physiological factors, **V1.**263–4,
        V1.264 (Tab.)
    infection progression, **V1.**236–50
      oncogenic viruses, **V1.**343–4
    shedding, **V1.**249
    spread/dissemination, **V1.**240–4
Pathogenicity
  bacteria, **B1.**146–7
    colonization, **B1.**147–50
      host/species-specific tropisms, **B1.**147–8
      surface adherence, **B1.**147
    definition, **B1.**146
    establishment, **B1.**7
    evolution within host, **B1.**173–5
    immune defence avoidance, **B1.**153–5
    infiltration, **B1.**152–3
    mechanisms, **B1.**147–65
    motility, **B1.**151–2
    proliferation, **B1.**150–1
      iron scavenging, **B1.**151
    sensory networks, **B1.**165–73
      iron-dependent repression, **B1.**165–6
      quorum sensing, **B1.**169–75
      two-component signal transduction
        systems, **B1.**167–9
    signal transduction subversion, **B1.**164–5
    toxins, **B1.**155–60
      see also specific toxins
    see also Virulence factors; *individual
      mechanisms; individual species*
  definition, **V1.**356
  fungi, **M.**9, **M.**79–80
    anamorphy, **M.**45–6, **M.**51
    numbers, **M.**44
    see also individual species
Pathogenicity islands (PAIs), **B1.**118–19
Pathogen-related oral spirochetes (PROS),
    B2.1859–60
Pathogens, definition, **B1.**146

Patient isolation, filovirus infection, **V2.**1097
Pattern recognition, **I.109–29**
  adaptive immunity links, **I.**123
    antigen presentation, **I.**123
    INFs, **I.**123
  APCs, **I.**112 (Fig.)
  CD14, **I.**123
  clinical implications, **I.**123–5
    therapies, **I.**123–4
  history, **I.**109–10
  microbial toxins, **I.**110
  molecular mechanisms, **I.**110
  two-step model, **I.**123
  see also Pathogen-associated molecular
    patterns (PAMPs); Pattern recognition
    receptors (PRRs); *individual systems*
Pattern recognition receptors (PRRs), **I.**22–3,
    I.24 (Tab.), **I.**113–16
  cell-surface, **I.**113–14, **I.**114 (Tab.)
  dendritic cells, **I.**750–1
  genetic polymorphisms, **I.**124–5
  Human respiratory syncytial virus infection,
    V1.793–4
  innate immunity, **I.**645
  intracellular, **I.**113–14, **I.**114–15, **I.**114 (Tab.)
  ligand recognition, **I.**112
  parasitic infection, **I.**679–80
  septic shock, **I.**695–6
  soluble, **I.**114 (Tab.), **I.**115–16
  viruses, **I.**23
  see also individual types; specific types
Paul–Bunnell test, **V1.**568–9
Paxillin, papillomavirus E6 protein effects,
    V1.460 (Tab.)
PB1-F2 polypeptide, Influenza virus A *see*
    Influenza virus A
PB1 protein, Influenza virus A, **V1.**643 (Tab.)
PB2 protein, Influenza virus A, **V1.**643 (Tab.)
pBR322 cloning vector, **B1.**119–20
PCR *see* Polymerase chain reaction (PCR)
PD-1, CD4 T cell tolerance induction, **I.**397
Peanuts, **B1.**286–7
PECAM, lymphocyte migration, **I.**508 (Tab.)
Pecluvirus, **V1.**27 (Tab.)
Pectinatus, **B2.**1930
Pectobacterium, **B2.**1330 (Tab.)
Pediococcus, intrinsic anti-glycopeptide activity,
    B1.480
Pediculus humanus, **B1.**153
Pefudensovirus, **V1.**413–14
Peliosis hepatitis
  Bartonella infection, **B2.**1894
  erythromycin treatment, **B2.**1899
Pellicle, **P.**162–4, **P.**163 (Tab.), **P.**164 (Fig.)
Pelodera, **P.**593
Pelta, **P.**170–2
Pelvic inflammatory disease
  Enterococcus, **B2.**896
  Mycoplasma hominis, **B1.**669
PenA gene, **B2.**1291
Penam, **B1.**471 (Fig.)
Penciclovir, **V2.1613–14**
  hepatitis B therapy, **V2.**1614
  herpes encephalitis, **V2.**1421
  herpesvirus infection, **V2.**1614
  infection use, **V2.**1613–14

  mechanism of action, **V2.**1613–14
  structure, **V2.**1611 (Fig.), **V2.**1613 (Fig.)
Penetration/entry of viruses *see* Cell
    attachment/entry
Penicillin(s), **B1.**473–6
  antibiotic-associated diarrhea due to,
    B2.1120
  classification, **B1.**473–5, **B1.**475 (Tab.)
  drawbacks, **B1.**473
  in gas gangrene, **B2.**1115–16
  gingivitis treatment, **B1.**614
  intracranial abscess, **B1.**588–9, **B1.**589 (Tab.)
  oral derivatives, **B1.**473
  pharmacology, **B1.**475–6
    blood–brain barrier, **B1.**475–6
  resistance
    discovery, **B1.**363
    Enterococcus, **B2.**891, **B2.**892,
      B2.892 (Tab.)
    evolution, **B1.**30
    Neisseria, **B2.**1277, **B2.**1291, **B2.**1292 (Tab.)
    Neisseria gonorrhoeae, **B1.**661
    Neisseria meningitidis, **B1.**566
    Staphylococcus, **B2.**793–801
    Streptococcus, **B2.**861–2
    Streptococcus pneumoniae, **B1.**571, **B1.**632
    Veillonella, **B2.**1315
  spectrum of activity, **B1.**473–5
    Actinobacillus actinomycetemcomitans,
      B2.1664
    Bacillus anthracis, **B2.**937–8
    Cardiobacterium hominis, **B2.**1672–3
    Edwardsiella, **B2.**1491–2
    Eikenella corrodens, **B2.**1668
    Hafnia, **B2.**1493
    Leminorella, **B2.**1496
    Listeria, **B2.**957–8
    Pasteurella multocida, **B2.**1655
    Proteus, **B2.**1441–3
    Yokenella, **B2.**1498
  in syphilis, **B1.**662–3, **B2.**1857–8
  see also specific types
Penicillinase
  Neisseria gonorrhoeae producing, **B1.**363,
    B2.1277
  plasmid resistance genes, **B1.**111
  synthesis, **B1.**111
Penicillin-binding proteins (PBPs), **B2.**1291
  β-lactam antibiotics, **B1.**471
  mecA gene (methicillin resistance), **B1.**111
Penicillin G *see* Benzylpenicillin (penicillin G)
Penicilliosis, **M.**560, **M.560–75**
  AIDS *see* AIDS
  clinical presentation, **M.**566
    bone, **M.**567
    cutaneous, **M.**567, **M.**567 (Fig.), **M.**569
    joints, **M.**567
    skin infection, **M.**567, **M.**567 (Fig.), **M.**569
  diagnosis, **M.**569–71
    antibody detection, **M.**570
    antigen detection, **M.**571
    blood culture, **M.**569, **M.**570 (Fig.)
    histopathology, **M.**567–8
    serology, **M.**570
    specimens, **M.**569

Penicilliosis (*Continued*)
  epidemiology, **M**.561–4
    bamboo rats, **M**.26, **M**.560, **M**.561,
      M.561 (Fig.), **M**.561 (Tab.), **M**.562
    children, **M**.562, **M**.564
    geographical distribution, **M**.563 (Tab.)
    histopathology, **M**.128 (Tab.), **M**.133 (Fig.)
    history, **M**.26, **M**.26–7, **M**.560–1
    immune response, **M**.568
      T cells, **M**.568
    immunosuppression, **M**.562
    oculomycoses, **M**.275 (Tab.)
      dacryocanaliculitis, **M**.298
    therapy, **M**.26, **M**.571–2
      amphotericin B, **M**.571
      corticosteroids, **M**.562
      itraconazole, **M**.569
      ketoconazole, **M**.571
      terbinafine, **M**.571
      voriconazole, **M**.571
Penicillium
  calcofluor white staining, **M**.245 (Fig.)
  differentiation, **M**.566, **M**.567 (Tab.)
  foods
    cereals, **B1**.284
    cheese spoilage, **B1**.252
    fruit, **B1**.282, **B1**.283
    herbs and spices, **B1**.287
    meat, **B1**.276
    vegetables, **B1**.281
  infection *see* Penicilliosis
  soil/plant associations, **B1**.199–200
Penicillium camemberti
  cheesemaking, **B1**.252
  cheese spoilage, **B1**.252
Penicillium citrinum, **M**.567 (Tab.)
Penicillium glaucium, **B1**.252
Penicillium janthinellum, **M**.567 (Tab.)
Penicillium marneffei, **M**.560
  classification, **M**.565
  differentiation, **M**.566, **M**.567 (Tab.), **M**.569
  ecology, **M**.561
  genetics, **M**.572
  growth, **M**.71–3, **M**.565, **M**.566 (Fig.)
  history, **M**.21, **M**.26–7, **M**.560–1
  identification, **M**.125–7, **M**.565, **M**.569–71
    culture, **M**.564, **M**.564 (Fig.), **M**.569,
      M.570 (Fig.)
    exoantigen test, **M**.566
    histopathology, **M**.126 (Tab.),
      M.128 (Tab.), **M**.133 (Fig.), **M**.567–8
    microscopy, **M**.565, **M**.565 (Fig.), **M**.569,
      M.570 (Fig.)
    PCR, **M**.94, **M**.571
  infection *see* Penicilliosis
  morphology, **M**.126 (Tab.), **M**.564,
    M.564 (Fig.), **M**.565 (Fig.), **M**.566 (Fig.)
  dimorphism, **M**.565, **M**.566, **M**.569–70
Penicillium purpurogenum, **M**.567 (Tab.)
Penicillium roqueforti
  cheesemaking, **B1**.252
  cheese spoilage, **B1**.252
Penicillium rubrum, **M**.567 (Tab.)
Penicillium vermiculatum, **B1**.283

Penis
  cryptococcosis, **M**.648
  rhinosporidiosis, **M**.459, **M**.460
Pentamidine isethionate
  African trypanosomiasis, **P**.371
  aspergillosis risk factor, **M**.705
  Old World leishmaniasis, **P**.306–7
  PCP, **M**.789
Pentatrichomonas, classification, **P**.196–7
Pentavalent antimonials, **P**.306
Pentose phosphate pathway, **B1**.57–8
  reductive (Calvin cycle), **B1**.62
Pentose–phosphate pathway, trypanosomes,
    P.359–60
Pentoses, fermentation, **B1**.57–8
  HDP pathway, **B1**.57
  heterolactic acid fermentation, **B1**.58
  hexose monophosphate pathway, **B1**.57–8
  pentose phosphate pathway, **B1**.57–8
Pentostam®, **P**.341
Pentraxins, microbial recognition, **I**.23,
    I.24 (Tab.)
Pepsin, Ig digestion, **I**.304
Peptic ulcer disease
  Helicobacter infection, **B2**.1564
  Helicobacter pylori infection, **B2**.1580
  recurrence, **B2**.1574
Peptide antibiotics, *Lactobacillus*, **B2**.866
Peptide fusion inhibitors, Human respiratory
    syncytial virus infection, **V1**.792
Peptide libraries, conformational BCE
    identification, **I**.854
Peptide-loading complex, viral immune
    interference, **I**.633–4
Peptide vaccines, **I.853–93**
  bare skin immunization, **I**.826
  B-cell epitopes, **I**.853–68, **I**.855 (Tab.)
    Alzheimer's disease, **I**.855 (Tab.), **I**.875–6
    bacterial infection, **I**.855 (Tab.), **I**.872–3
      Haemophilus influenzae, **I**.855 (Tab.),
        I.861 (Tab.)
    cancer, **I**.855 (Tab.), **I**.876
      fibrosarcoma, **I**.861 (Tab.)
      lymphoma, **I**.861 (Tab.)
    candidate vaccines, **I**.868–76
      see also individual vaccines
    carrier proteins, **I**.863
      bovine serum albumin, **I**.862–3
      covalent coupling, **I**.863
      diphtheria toxoid, **I**.862–3
      keyhole limpet hemocyanin, **I**.862–3,
        I.869
      ovalbumin, **I**.862–3
      tetanus toxoid, **I**.862–3
    chemically defined, **I**.861
    conformational, **I**.853–4
      mimotopes, **I**.854, **I**.861 (Tab.)
      stability, **I**.861–2
    contraceptive vaccines, **I**.855 (Tab.), **I**.875
    Guillain–Barré syndrome, **I**.855 (Tab.)
    history, **I**.854–61
    HIV, **I**.855 (Tab.), **I**.871
      "cluster peptides," **I**.871
      cytokine adjuvants, **I**.871
      gp41, **I**.871
      gp120, **I**.871

    oral route, **I**.871
    purified protein derivative (PPD), **I**.871
  immunogenicity, **I**.862
  measles virus, **I**.855 (Tab.), **I**.861 (Tab.),
    I.868–9
    carrier proteins, **I**.868–9
    transgenic plants, **I**.869
  multi-epitopes, **I**.863
  myasthenia gravis, **I**.855 (Tab.)
  noninvasive delivery, **I**.864
  parasites, **I**.855 (Tab.), **I**.873–5
    Cryptococcus neoformans, **I**.861 (Tab.)
    cysticercosis, **I**.855 (Tab.), **I**.874–5
    malaria, **I**.873
    Plasmodium berghei, **I**.855 (Tab.), **I**.873
    Plasmodium falciparum, **I**.855 (Tab.),
      I.873, **I**.874
    Plasmodium malariae, **I**.873
    Plasmodium ovale, **I**.873
    Plasmodium vivax, **I**.855 (Tab.), **I**.873
    Plasmodium yoelii, **I**.855 (Tab.), **I**.873
    schistosomiasis, **I**.855 (Tab.), **I**.861 (Tab.),
      I.874
    Taenia solium, **I**.855 (Tab.), **I**.874–5
  sequential, **I**.853–4
    identification, **I**.854
  TCE requirement, **I**.862–3
    design, **I**.863
    helper TCEs, **I**.862–3, **I**.862 (Tab.)
  Th2 response, **I**.864, **I**.868
  viral infection
    canine parvovirus, **I**.855 (Tab.), **I**.871–2
    feline panleukemia virus, **I**.871–2
    flaviviruses, **I**.870–1
    foot-and-mouth disease virus, **I**.854,
      I.861, **I**.855 (Tab.), **I**.870
    hepadnaviruses, **I**.872
    Hepatitis A virus, **I**.855 (Tab.), **I**.870
    Hepatitis B virus, **I**.855 (Tab.),
      I.861 (Tab.), **I**.872
    hepatitis C virus, **I**.855 (Tab.),
      I.861 (Tab.), **I**.870–1
    HIV *see above*
    HPV, **I**.855 (Tab.), **I**.872
    influenza A virus, **I**.855 (Tab.), **I**.869–70
    Japanese encephalitis virus, **I**.855 (Tab.)
    measles virus *see above*
    mink enteritis virus, **I**.855 (Tab.), **I**.871–2
    Neisseria meningitidis serogroup C,
      I.855 (Tab.), **I**.861 (Tab.), **I**.872–3
    orthomyxoviruses, **I**.869–70
    papovavirus, **I**.872
    paramyxoviruses, **I**.868–9
    parvoviruses, **I**.871–2
    picornaviruses, **I**.870
    polioviruses, **I**.855 (Tab.), **I**.870
    raccoon parvovirus, **I**.871–2
    respiratory syncytial virus, **I**.855 (Tab.),
      I.861 (Tab.), **I**.869
    retroviruses, **I**.871
    simian immunodeficiency virus,
      I.855 (Tab.)
  in vivo enzymatic degradation, **I**.862
rotaviruses, **V2**.955

Peptide vaccines (*Continued*)
  T-cell epitopes, **I**.426, **I**.865 (Tab.), **I**.876–80,
    I.877–8
    cancer, **I**.865 (Tab.)
      melanoma, **I**.865 (Tab.), **I**.877
      tumor derived material, **I**.876–7
      tumor viruses, **I**.879
    delivery systems, **I**.879
    identification of, **I**.877
    immunogenicity improvement, **I**.878–9
      adjuvants, **I**.878–9
      CD4+ T cells, **I**.878
      dendritic cell presentation, **I**.879
      peptide formulation, **I**.878–9
      peptide modification, **I**.878
Peptidoglycan (PGN), **B1**.42–3
  cross-links, **B1**.42–3
  discovery, **B1**.12
  Enterococcus, **B2**.886–7
  gram-positive bacteria, **B1**.441–2
  Shigella, **B2**.1390
  spore, **B1**.439
  synthesis, **B1**.42–3
Peptinophilus, **B2**.914–15
  classification, **B2**.904, **B2**.905 (Tab.)
  identification, **B2**.906–7
Peptinophilus asaccharolyticus, **B2**.914–15
  biochemical characteristics, **B2**.908 (Tab.)
  classification, **B2**.904–5
  clinical importance, **B2**.910
  normal microbiota, **B2**.907–10
  as normal microbiota, **B2**.910
Peptinophilus harei, **B2**.915
  biochemical characteristics, **B2**.908 (Tab.)
  classification, **B2**.905
Peptinophilus indolicus, **B2**.915
  biochemical characteristics, **B2**.908 (Tab.)
Peptinophilus ivorii, **B2**.915
  biochemical characteristics, **B2**.908 (Tab.)
  classification, **B2**.905
Peptinophilus lacrimalis, **B2**.915
  biochemical characteristics, **B2**.908 (Tab.)
  classification, **B2**.904–5
Peptococcaceae, **B2**.903–4
Peptococcus, **B2**.903–4, **B2**.915–16
  classification, **B2**.903–4, **B2**.905 (Tab.)
    changes, **B2**.904
  identification, **B2**.906–7
Peptococcus anaerobius, **B2**.904
Peptococcus niger, **B2**.904, **B2**.908 (Tab.),
    B2.915–16
  as normal microbiota, **B1**.296 (Tab.)
Peptoniphilus, **B1**.296 (Tab.)
Peptostreptococcus, **B2**.833–5, **B2**.903–4,
    B2.916
  classification, **B2**.903–4, **B2**.905 (Tab.)
    changes at genus level, **B2**.904–5,
      B2.906 (Tab.)
  identification, **B2**.906–7
  infection
    bacteremia, **B1**.523
    bacterial vaginosis, **B1**.665
    conjunctivitis, **B1**.600
    gingivitis, **B1**.614
    intracranial abscess, **B1**.584–5

oral cavity abscesses, **B1**.618
    normal microbiota, **B1**.296 (Tab.)
    oral cavity, **B1**.609
Peptostreptococcus anaerobius, **B2**.916
  biochemical characteristics, **B2**.908 (Tab.)
  classification, **B2**.904–5
  clinical importance, **B2**.910
  identification, **B2**.907
  normal microbiota, **B2**.910
  pathogenicity and virulence factors, **B2**.911
Peptostreptococcus asaccharolyticus see
    Peptinophilus asaccharolyticus
Peptostreptococcus barnesae see Gallicola
    barnesae
Peptostreptococcus harei see Peptinophilus
    harei
Peptostreptococcus heliotrinreducens, **B2**.904
Peptostreptococcus ivorii see Peptinophilus
    ivorii
Peptostreptococcus lacrimalis see Peptinophilus
    lacrimalis
Peptostreptococcus lactolyticus see
    Anaerococcus lactolyticus
Peptostreptococcus magna see Finegoldia
    magna
Peptostreptococcus micros see Micromonas
    micros
Peptostreptococcus octavius see Anaerococcus
    octavius
Peptostreptococcus prevotii see Anaerococcus
    prevotii
Peptostreptococcus productus, **B2**.904
Peptostreptococcus trisimilis, **B2**.905,
    B2.908 (Tab.), **B2**.917
Peptostreptococcus vaginalis see Anaerococcus
    vaginalis
Peracetic acid, **B1**.429
  action, **B1**.437 (Tab.), **B1**.439
  low-temperature sterilization technologies,
    B1.453
Peramivir, **V2**.1628
  structure, **V2**.1627 (Fig.)
Percutaneous aspiration–injection–re-
    aspiration (PAIR), **P**.699
Percutaneous spread of infection, **B1**.310,
    B1.329
Perfloxacin
  Haemophilus, **B2**.1710
  structure, **B1**.494 (Fig.)
Perforatorium, **P**.171 (Fig.)
Perforin, **I**.475
  calcium interaction, **I**.475, **I**.477 (Fig.)
  CTLs, **I**.422–3
    induction, **I**.478
  deficiencies, **I**.778–9
  deficiency in animal models, **I**.480–1
    autoimmunity, **I**.480
    CTL downregulation, **I**.480–1
    graft-versus-host disease, **I**.480
    tumor development, **I**.480
  deficiency in humans, **I**.481–2
  half-life, cell self-protection, **I**.477–8
  homeostatic function, **I**.478–9, **I**.480 (Fig.)
  mechanism of action, **I**.81
  pore assembly, **I**.475, **I**.475 (Fig.), **I**.477 (Fig.),
    I.478, **I**.479 (Fig.)

structure, **I**.81, **I**.475
    complement component homology, **I**.475
    domains, **I**.476 (Fig.)
  tumor rejection, **I**.482 (Tab.), **I**.483
  viral clearance, **I**.482 (Tab.)
Perforin-dependent killing, NK cells, **I**.81
Performic acid, **B1**.453–4
Pergamino virus, **V2**.1666 (Tab.)
Perianal (nappy) rash, **M**.596, **M**.609
Pericardial fluid specimens, **M**.84
Pericarditis, histoplasmosis, **M**.523, **M**.530,
    M.534–5
Pericystectomy, **P**.696–7
Perihepatitis, *Chlamydia trachomatis* infection,
    B2.2010–11, **B2**.2011 (Fig.)
Perinatal transmission, **V2**.1443, **V2**.1444 (Tab.)
  HCMV infection, **V2**.1450
  hepatitis B, **V2**.1476
  Hepatitis delta virus, **V2**.1481
  HIV infection, **V2**.1471
  see also Fetal infection
Perinephric abscess, **B1**.673
Periodic acid-Schiff (PAS) stain, **M**.33, **M**.87,
    M.88 (Tab.), **M**.123 (Tab.), **M**.235,
    M.236, **M**.491, **M**.676
  applications, **M**.122, **M**.132
  Coccidioides immitis, **M**.513, **M**.516
  Histoplasma capsulatum, **M**.533–4
  Paracoccidioides brasiliensis, **M**.542
  Tropheryma whippelii, **B2**.998–1000
Periodontal diseases
  abscesses, **B1**.614
  Actinobacillus actinomycetemcomitans,
    B2.1549–50, **B2**.1662–3
  Campylobacter, **B2**.1549–50
  Capnocytophaga, **B2**.1674
  Eikenella corrodens, **B2**.1667
  Entamoeba gingivalis infection, **P**.221
  Eubacterium, **B2**.1029–30
  spirochaetes causing, **B2**.1859–60
Periodontitis
  genetic associations, **I**.595
  immunogenetics, **I**.595
  HLA association, **I**.577
Perioral spaces, infection, **B1**.629
Peripharyngeal spaces, infection, **B1**.629
Peripheral blood mononuclear cells, HHV
    infection, **V2**.1418
Peripheral eosinophilia, *Dientamoeba fragilis*
    infection, **P**.267–8
Peripheral lymph node addressins (PNAd),
    I.506
Peripheral lymphoid organs, antigen
    presentation, **I**.378–9
Peripheral nerves, PrP^C expression, **V2**.1380
Peripheral nervous system (PNS) infection,
    Chlamydia pneumoniae infection,
    B2.2017
Peripheral neuropathy, neuro-AIDS,
    V2.1427–8
Peripheral tolerance, **I**.749–51
  activation-induced cell death, **I**.750
  extrinsic mechanisms, **I**.750–1
    dendritic cells, **I**.750–1, **I**.750 (Fig.)
    regulatory T-cells, **I**.751

Peripheral tolerance (*Continued*)
 intrinsic mechanisms, **I**.749–50
  anergy, **I**.749
  apoptosis, **I**.750
  ignorance, **I**.749
  phenotypic skewing, **I**.749
 Th1/Th2 balance, **I**.749
Periplasm, **B1**.43
Periplasmic-binding protein-dependent
 transport systems, **B1**.49
Periplasmic space, **B1**.43
Peristome, *Balantidium coli,* **P**.275–6,
 P.276 (Fig.)
Peritoneal dialysis, infection, **B1**.386–7
Peritoneal fluid specimens, **M**.84
Peritoneum, nosocomial infection, **B1**.386–7
Peritonitis
 aspergillosis, **M**.701–2
 candidiasis, **M**.600
 causative organisms
  Gordonia erythropolis, **B2**.1152
  Nocardia asteroides, **B2**.1158
 fulminating amebic colitis, **P**.207
 postoperative, **B1**.386–7
 prototothecosis, **M**.398–9, **M**.402
 Rhodotorula, **M**.627
Peritonsilar abscesses, **B1**.618, **B1**.629
Periwinkles, **B1**.280
Permeabilizing agents, **B1**.428, **B1**.436
Permeation, definition, **P**.161–2
Pernicious anemia
 Diphyllobothrium latum infection, **P**.672,
  P.673
 prevalence, **I**.748 (Tab.)
Peroxidase test for milk, **B1**.233, **B1**.234
Peroxide, spore sensitization, **B1**.439
Peroxidoredoxins, parasite immune avoidance
 mechanisms, **I**.686
Peroxisomes, **P**.177–8
Peroxygens, **B1**.423 (Tab.), **B1**.428–9
Persistence thresholds, **B1**.340–1
Persistent viral infection, **V1**.258–62
 cell–virus interactions, **V1**.205
 chronic infection, **V2**.1408
 defective interfering particles, **V1**.186–7
 epidemiology, **V1**.353–4
 high titer, **V1**.258–9, **V1**.259–60, **V1**.259 (Fig.)
  lytic viruses, **V1**.258–9, **V1**.259–60
  nonlytic viruses, **V1**.259
 influenza, **V1**.663–4
 latent infection *vs.,* **V2**.1408
 mechanisms, **V1**.258–9
 oncogenesis, **V1**.346–7
 slow virus infection, **V2**.1408
 smoldering infection, **V1**.258–9, **V1**.259 (Fig.),
  V1.261–2
  antigenic variation, **V1**.262, **V1**.263 (Fig.),
   V1.263 (Tab.)
  immunologically privileged sites, **V1**.261
  infectious immune complexes, **V1**.262
  intracellular bridges, **V1**.261
  MHC I suppression, **V1**.261–2
 viruses, **V1**.264 (Tab.)
Personal hygiene, *Enterobius vermicularis*
 control, **P**.732

Personality changes, infective endocarditis,
 B1.535
Personal protective equipment (PPE),
 V2.1518, **V2**.1520–3
Person-to-person transmission, astroviruses,
 V2.900
Pertactin (PRN), *Bordetella,* **B2**.1789,
 B2.1789 (Tab.)
Pertussis, **B1**.645–7
 causative agent, **B2**.1807–10
  see also Bordetella pertussis
 clinical course, **B2**.1808 (Fig.)
 clinical features, **B1**.646, **B2**.1807
  catarrhal and paroxysmal stages, **B2**.1807
  cough, **B1**.646
  respiratory tract infection, **B1**.627
 control, **B1**.349
  vaccine *see below*
 dendritic cell infection, **I**.656
 diagnosis, **B1**.646
 epidemics, **B1**.349
  notifications, **B1**.349 (Fig.)
 epidemiology, **B1**.645–6
  attack rates, **B2**.1807
 immunity, **B1**.349
 pathogenesis, **B1**.646, **B2**.1807–10
  sequence of events, **B2**.1808 (Fig.)
 pertussis toxin role, **B2**.1798–9, **B2**.1810
 prevention, **B1**.646–7
 transmission, **B1**.645–6, **B2**.1807
  vaccine effect on, **B1**.349
 treatment, **B1**.646, **B2**.1793–4
  immunotherapy, **B2**.1794
 vaccines/vaccination, **B1**.349, **B1**.645–6,
  B1.646–7, **B2**.1798–9, **B2**.1809–10
  acellular, **B1**.647, **B2**.1798–9, **B2**.1809–10
  adverse reactions, **B1**.325–6
  BCG vector, **I**.845
  brain damage due to, **B1**.645–7
  development status, **I**.933 (Tab.)
  effect on herd immunity, **B1**.349
  filamentous haemagglutinin, **B1**.647
  live vaccines, **I**.903
  multicomponent, **B2**.1809
  outer membrane protein, **B1**.647
  public reaction to adverse effects, **B1**.647
  Salmonella vectors, **I**.847
  schedules, **B1**.646–7
  trials, **B1**.324
  uptake and usage, **B1**.349
  Vibrio cholerae vectors, **I**.844
  whole cell, **B1**.646–7, **B2**.1809–10
Pertussis toxin (PT), **B1**.627, **B2**.1789 (Tab.),
 B2.1797–9
 activities, **B2**.1797–8, **B2**.1798 (Tab.)
 adhesin activity, **B2**.1798
 antibodies, **B2**.1792
 chemotaxis inhibition, **I**.648
 invasion of eukaryotic cell, **B2**.1798
 pertussis pathogenesis, **B2**.1798–9, **B2**.1810
 protein complex, **B2**.1798
 secretion, **B2**.1789, **B2**.1798
Pertussis toxoided form (PTd), **B2**.1798–9,
 B2.1809
Pesle, G, **M**.19

Peste-des-petits-ruminants virus (PPRV),
 V1.712–13, **V1**.810–11
 classification, **V1**.382–3
 clinical manifestations, **V1**.810
 contagious caprine pleuropneumonia *vs.,*
  V1.810
 control, **V1**.811
  sanitation, **V1**.811
  vaccination, **V1**.811
 differential diagnosis, **V1**.811
 economic importance, **V1**.810
 epizootiology, **V1**.810–11
 laboratory diagnosis, **V1**.811
 pathology, **V1**.810
 species affected, **V1**.810
 strain relationship, **V1**.811 (Fig.)
 transmission, **V1**.810–11
Pesticin II, **B2**.1467
Pestivirus
 classification, **V1**.53–4, **V2**.993
 host transcript recombination, **V1**.190
 infection, **V2**.1004–5
  border disease, **V2**.1005
  bovine viral diarrhea, **V2**.1004–5
  classical swine fever (hog cholera),
   V2.1005
 mRNA translation, **V1**.113
 protein synthesis, **V1**.115–16
Pestiviruses
 C protein, **V2**.995–6
 E1 protein, **V2**.995–6
 E2 protein, **V2**.995–6
  as antigen, **V2**.996
 E^ms^ protein, **V2**.995–6
  as antigen, **V2**.996
 genome structure, **V2**.995, **V2**.995 (Fig.)
 Hepatitis C virus *vs.,* **V2**.1190–1
 morphology, **V2**.993
 N^pro^ protein, **V2**.995–6
 NS2/NS3 protein, **V2**.995–6
 proteins, **V2**.995–6
  post-translational modification, **V2**.995–7
Petri, R J, **M**.9
Petroleum products, bioremediation, **B1**.201
Peyer's patches, **I**.505, **I**.529–30
 APCs, **I**.532
 B cells, **I**.532
 dendritic cells, **I**.538
 development, **I**.530
 as inductive site, **I**.530
 lymphocyte homing, **I**.511
 macrophages, **I**.532, **I**.538
 memory B cells, **I**.538
 microfold (M) cells, **I**.530, **I**.532
  infection route, **I**.532
 mucosal vaccination, **I**.827
 oral tolerance, **I**.545
 prion diseases, **V2**.1373, **V2**.1374
 structure, **I**.530–2, **I**.531 (Fig.)
  follicles, **I**.532
 T cells, **I**.532
  CD4 T cells, **I**.389
  memory T cells, **I**.538
  Th2 cells, **I**.538
 viral entry, **V1**.240 (Fig.)

pfcrt gene, chloroquine resistance, **P.**479, **P.**509

Pfeiffer, R, **B1.**7

P-glycoprotein, **B1.**440

pH
  antibacterial activity, **B1.**432
  Brucella culture, **B2.**1735
  macrophages, **I.**25
  microbial growth effect, **B1.**266–7
  microsporidians, **P.**550
  susceptibility/resistance to
    Campylobacter, **B2.**1545
    Mycobacterium, **B2.**1216

pH 60 α-acetolactate-synthesizing enzyme, **B1.**55

Phaeoannellomyces werneckii, **M.**128 (Tab.), **M.**139 (Fig.)

Phaeohyphomycosis, **M.**22–3, **M.739–48**
  AIDS, **M.**740, **M.**743
  CNS, **M.**743, **M.**744 (Tab.), **M.**745, **M.**746–7
  conceptual basis, **M.**27
  history, **M.**27
  hyalohyphomycosis *vs.,* **M.**740
  specimen site selection, **M.**83 (Tab.)
  therapy, **M.**745
    voriconazole, **M.**153

Phaeohyphomycosis, deep-seated (DSP)
  causative agents, **M.**741–2, **M.**741 (Tab.)
    see also individual species
  clinical concepts, **M.**740–2
  clinical manifestations, **M.**742–4
    CNS, **M.**139 (Fig.), **M.**743, **M.**744 (Tab.), **M.**745, **M.**746–7
  diagnosis, **M.**744–5
  disseminated, **M.**742, **M.**745, **M.**746–7
  future directions, **M.**746–7
  histopathology, **M.**128 (Tab.), **M.**139 (Fig.), **M.**740–2, **M.**744–5
  hyalohyphomycosis *vs.,* **M.**740
  risk factors, **M.**740, **M.**740 (Tab.)
  staining, **M.**124
  therapy, **M.**745–6

Phaeoid (dematiaceous) fungi
  description, **M.**739–40
  history, **M.**11
  oculomycoses, **M.**278 (Tab.), **M.**283–4, **M.**301–2
  pathogenesis, **M.**746
  see also individual species

Phaeoisaria, oculomycoses, **M.**278 (Tab.), **M.**283–4

Phaeosclera dematioides, chromoblastomycosis, **M.**357

Phaeotrichonis crotalariae, oculomycoses, **M.**278 (Tab.)

Phage *see* Bacteriophage(s)

Phage display, **I.**363–5, **I.**364 (Fig.)
  advantages, **I.**364–5
  affinity selection, **I.**363
  library size, **I.**363
  modification, **I.**363–4
  monoclonal antibodies, **I.**333

Phagocytes
  chemokine receptors, **I.**223–4
  chemokines, **I.**223–4
  chemotaxis, stromal-derived factor 1α, **I.**223–4

complement receptors, **I.**146–7

CXC chemokine receptors, **I.**223–4

viral infection, **V1.**241

see also Eosinophil(s); Macrophage(s); Neutrophil(s)

Phagocytosis, **P.**162
  alveolar macrophage function, **B1.**624
  antigen processing, **I.**376
  bacterial infection, **I.**645–6
    Bordetella invasion/survival, **B2.**1806
    immune interference *see* Immune evasion, bacteria
    passive, Q fever, **B2.**2077
    reactive oxygen intermediates, **I.**647–8
  discovery, **B1.**7
  FcγRI (CD64), **I.**314
  fungal infection
    aspergillosis, **M.**707, **M.**724
    candidiasis, **M.**260
    Histoplasma see Histoplasma capsulatum var. *capsulatum*
  historical aspects, **B1.**7
  HIV infection, **I.**795, **I.**796
  inhibition by, *Clostridium perfringens,* **B2.**1113
  macrophages *see* Macrophage(s)
  neutrophils, **I.**50 (Tab.), **I.**51
  parasitic infection, **P.**180–1, **P.**182 (Fig.)
    Old World *Leishmania,* **P.**292–4
    visceral leishmaniasis, **P.**300
  reduced activity and respiratory infection, **B1.**626

Phagolysosomes
  Coxiella burnetii, **B2.**2073, **B2.**2077
  Histoplasma capsulatum var. *capsulatum,* **M.**525
  Old World *Leishmania,* **P.**294

Phagosomes
  ATPase, **I.**25
  cathepsin D, **I.**25
  macrophages, **I.**25

Phaneropsolus, **P.**585

Pharmaceutical industry, airborne bacteria monitoring, **B1.**189–90

Pharmacokinetics
  ADEPT, **I.**360
  monoclonal antibody therapy, **I.**358, **I.**362

Pharyngitis, **B1.**610–12
  carriers, **B1.**611
  causative organisms, **B1.**611–12
    non-group A streptococci, **B1.**611–12
  clinical manifestations, **B1.**611
  epidemiology, **B1.**610
  pathogen identification, **B1.**610, **B1.**611
    culture, **B1.**611
    DNA assays, **B1.**611
    immunoassays, **B1.**611
  seasonality, **B1.**611
  transmission, **B1.**610
  treatment, **B1.**611

Pharynx
  abscesses, **B1.**618
  anatomy, **B1.**607

Phase-contrast microscopy, **B1.**714
  soil bacteria analysis, **B1.**207

Phase variation
  Neisseria, **B2.**1279, **B2.**1284
  Salmonella Typhimurium, **B1.**90

pH dependency, FcRn (neonatal receptor), **I.**316

Phenazine pigments, *Pseudomonas,* **B2.**1596–7

Phenethicillin, structure, **B1.**474 (Fig.)

Phenol oxidase, *Cryptococcus neoformans,* **M.**16–7, **M.**640–2

Phenols, **B1.**422, **B1.**423 (Tab.)
  actions, **B1.**437 (Tab.), **B1.**438
  concentrations, **B1.**431 (Fig.)
  pH, **B1.**432

Phenotype
  adaptation, **B1.**80–1
    permanant change, **B1.**81
    reversion, **B1.**81
  definition, **B1.**80

Phenotypes, mycology classification, **M.**46–7, **M.**46 (Tab.), **M.**49

Phenotypic analysis, herpesvirus classification, **V1.**44–5

Phenotypic mixing, **V1.**186

Phenotypic skewing, peripheral tolerance, **I.**749

Phenotypic switching, **M.**76, **M.**76 (Fig.)
  Candida, **M.**76, **M.**76 (Fig.), **M.**589
  Candida parapsilosis, **M.**76
  Candida tropicalis, **M.**76
  Cryptococcus neoformans, **M.**76

Phenotyping
  Actinomyces, **B2.**1013
  Helicobacter, **B2.**1570

2-Phenoxyethanol, **B1.**427, **B1.**438
  action, **B1.**437 (Tab.)

Phenoxymethyl penicillin, **B1.**473
  pharmacology, **B1.**475
  structure, **B1.**474 (Fig.)

Phenylalanine deaminase
  Enterobacteriaceae identification, **B2.**1319 (Tab.)
  Proteus, **B2.**1435

Phenylethanol, **B1.**427

2-Phenylphenol, **B1.**422

Pheromones
  Cryptococcus neoformans, **M.**639
  Enterococcus, **B2.**886, **B2.**896–7

Phialides, *Aspergillus,* **M.**687, **M.**689–91

Phialomonium, histopathology, **M.**128 (Tab.)

Phialophora, **M.**61–3
  histopathology, **M.**89 (Tab.)
  oculomycoses, **M.**278 (Tab.)

Phialophora verrucosa, **M.**22
  chromoblastomycosis, **M.**29–30, **M.**30 (Fig.), **M.**356, **M.**357
  ecology, **M.**357–8, **M.**358 (Tab.)
  histopathology, **M.**89 (Tab.), **M.**128 (Tab.), **M.**139 (Fig.)
  morphology, **M.**30 (Fig.), **M.**360, **M.**362 (Fig.)

Philippines, schistosomiasis control programs, **P.**628–9

Philomiragia bacterium, **B2.**1459

Phlebotomists, needlestick injury, **B1.**760, **B1.**767

Phlebotomus, **P.**283–4
  Leishmania major transmission, **P.**303

Phlebotomus, (Continued)
  Leishmania tropica transmission, **P**.304
  see also individual species
Phlebotomus argentipes, **P**.305
Phlebotomus fever *see* Sandfly fever
Phlebotomus longipes, **P**.304
Phlebotomus papatasi, **P**.303
Phlebotomus pedifer, **P**.304
Phlebovirus, **V2**.1025
  characteristics, **V1**.129 (Tab.)
  classification, **V1**.50, **V2**.1026
  genome
    ambisense coding, **V1**.181, **V1**.181 (Fig.)
    consensus sequences, **V2**.1031 (Tab.)
    gene organization, **V2**.1033 (Fig.)
    panhandle structures, **V2**.1032 (Fig.)
  Golgi transport, **V2**.1039–40
  NS$_M$ protein, **V2**.1038
  transcription, **V2**.1036
Phleboviruses
  genome, **V2**.1033–4
    ambisense coding structure, **V2**.1033–5
  genome structure
    M (medium) segment, **V2**.1033–4
    S (small) segment, **V2**.1038
  glycoproteins, **V2**.1033–4
  Golgi system transport, **V2**.1040
  NS$_M$ protein, **V2**.1033–4
  NS$_S$ protein, **V2**.1033–4, **V2**.1038
    IFN effects, **V2**.1041–2
  nucleocapsid (N) protein, **V2**.1038
  posttranslational modification, **V2**.1033–4
  transcription, **V2**.1035
  termination, **V2**.1037
Phlomobacter fragariae, **B2**.1330 (Tab.)
Phnom Penh bat virus, **V2**.998 (Tab.)
Phocine distemper virus, **V1**.712–13,
  V1.812–14, **V1**.814–15
  classification, **V1**.382–3
  clinical manifestations, **V1**.813
  control, **V1**.814–15
  emerging infection, **V2**.1657 (Tab.)
  epizootiology, **V1**.813
  historical aspects, **V1**.812–13
  transmission, **V1**.813
Phocine morbilliviruses, emerging infection,
  V2.1651 (Tab.)
Phoma oculo-hominis, oculomycoses,
  M.278 (Tab.), **M**.283–4
Phomopsis, **B1**.282
Phosphatase test of milk, **B1**.233, **B1**.234
Phosphate antigens, systemic γδ T cells,
  I.440 (Fig.)
Phosphatidylcholine, *Brucella,* **B2**.1724
Phosphatidylglycerol, *Brucella,* **B2**.1724
Phosphatidylinositol 4,5-bisphosphonate
  (PIP$_2$), **I**.344–5
Phosphatidylinositol-3- kinase (PI3-K)
  pathway
  BCR signaling, **I**.345
  CD4 T cell signaling, **I**.395
  neutrophil intracellular signaling, **I**.42
Phosphatidylserine
  apoptosis debris removal, **I**.131, **I**.136
  Vesicular stomatitis virus receptor, **V2**.1108

Phosphoenolpyruvate, **B1**.50
Phosphoenolpyruvate carboxylase, **B1**.61
Phosphoenolpyruvate phosphotransferase
  (PTS) system, **B1**.50, **B1**.71
  bacteria containing, **B1**.50
  in catabolite repression, **B1**.50, **B1**.73
  P-EI and P-EII enzymes, **B1**.50
  process, **B1**.50
Phosphofructokinase (fructose-6-
  phosphokinase), **B1**.51, **B1**.58, **B1**.59
6-Phosphogluconate, **B1**.57, **B1**.59
6-Phosphogluconate dehydrogenase, **B1**.57,
  B1.59
Phosphoglycerate kinase, **B1**.51
  Clonorchis sinensis, **P**.644
Phosphoglycerate mutase, **B1**.51
Phosphoketolase, **B1**.58
Phospholipase(s)
  Candida, **M**.587, **M**.588
  Entamoeba histolytica, **P**.204
  functions, **B1**.153 (Tab.)
  leptospires, **B2**.1873
  Naegleria fowleri culture, **P**.232–3
Phospholipase A$_2$, **I**.200
  arachidonic acid production, **I**.181–4
  innate mucosal immune response, **I**.521
Phospholipase C, *Burkholderia thailandensis,*
  B2.1624
Phospholipase Cγ2, **I**.344–5
Phospholipids
  Aspergillus, **M**.709
  cell walls, **B1**.43
  Mononegavirales order, **V1**.381
  Plasmodium, **P**.477
Phosphomycin, *Listeria,* **B2**.957–8
Phosphonoformic acid *see* Foscarnet
  (phosphonoformic acid: PFA)
Phosphoprotein (P)
  Avian pneumovirus, **V1**.788
  Borna disease virus *see* Borna disease virus
    (BDV)
  Hendra virus *see* Hendra virus
  henipaviruses *see* Henipaviruses
  Human respiratory syncytial virus, **V1**.787
  Mumps virus, **V1**.745, **V1**.746 (Tab.)
  Nipah virus *see* Nipah virus
  paramyxoviruses, **V1**.703–4
  rhabdoviruses *see* Rhabdoviruses
Phosphoprotein 65 (pp65), HCMV, **V1**.524–5
Phosphoprotein 150 (pp150), HCMV,
  V1.524–5
Phosphoribulokinase, **B1**.62
Phosphorylation
  glucose, **B1**.50–1
  Measles virus phosphoprotein (P), **V1**.717
  oxidative, **B1**.64–5
  Rabies virus nucleoprotein (N), **V2**.1113
  rhabdovirus phosphoprotein (P), **V2**.1113
  viral replication, **V1**.122
Phosphorylcholine (PC)
  C-reactive protein binding, **I**.199
  helminths, **I**.687
  lymphocyte inhibition, **I**.687
Phosphorylethanolamine, **I**.199
Photobacterium, **B2**.1330 (Tab.)
  classification, **B2**.1507

Photobacterium damselae, **B2**.1512–14,
  B2.1515 (Tab.)
  classification, **B2**.1507
  culture, **B2**.1509–10
  habitats, **B2**.1508–9
  metabolism, **B2**.1510
  molecular typing, **B2**.1516
  pathogenicity, **B2**.1517
Photochromogens, **B2**.1181
Photocoagulation, ocular cysticercosis
  treatment, **P**.696
Photophobia, trichinellosis, **P**.761–2
Photoreactivation (light repair), **B1**.87–9,
  B1.451–2
Photorhabdus, **B2**.1330 (Tab.), **B2**.1498
Photorhabdus asymbiotica
  biochemical tests, **B2**.1319 (Tab.)
  classification, **B2**.1336
Photorhabdus lumiscens
  biochemical tests, **B2**.1319 (Tab.)
  DNA hybridization group 5 *see*
    Photorhabdus asymbiotica
Photosynthesis, **B1**.67–8
  cyanobacteria, **B1**.68
  green sulfur bacteria, **B1**.68
  nitrogen fixation, **B1**.201
  purple photosynthetic bacteria, **B1**.67–8
Photosystem II, **P**.174
Phthalylsulfathiazole, **B1**.491
Phycodnaviridae
  classification, **V1**.27 (Tab.), **V1**.43 (Tab.)
  see also specific viruses
Phycomycetes, **M**.4
'Phycomycosis,' **M**.412
Phylogenetic analysis
  fungi
    dermatophytes, **M**.229–31
    Maximum Likelihood, **M**.47–8
    Maximum Parsimony, **M**.48
    Neighbor-Joining, **M**.47–8
    see also individual species
  viruses, **V1**.55
    amino acid sequences, **V1**.55
    arenaviruses, **V2**.1061 (Fig.)
    Hepatitis A virus, **V2**.1064 (Fig.),
      V2.1164–5
    noroviruses, **V2**.914–15, **V2**.917 (Fig.)
    polymerase-based, **V1**.55
    RNA-dependent RNA polymerases, **V1**.55
    sapoviruses, **V2**.917 (Fig.)
Phylogenetic tree
  herpesviruses, **V1**.498 (Fig.)
  Nidovirales order, **V1**.394 (Fig.)
Phylogeny
  Aeromonas, **B2**.1530
  Archaea, **B1**.30–1
  bacteria, **B1**.24, **B1**.26
  Bacteroides, **B2**.1917 (Fig.)
  Bordetella, **B2**.1787–8
  Cyanobacteria, **B1**.30–1
  Eukarya, **B1**.30–1
  Francisella, **B2**.1752, **B2**.1753
  Leptospires, **B2**.1876, **B2**.1877 (Fig.)
  pertussis toxin, **B2**.1788
  Porphyromonas, **B2**.1917 (Fig.)

Phylogeny (*Continued*)
  Prevotella, **B2**.1917 (Fig.)
  Pseudomonas, **B2**.1592–3
Phylograms, fungal classification, **M**.48,
    M.52 (Fig.), **M**.62 (Fig.)
Physaloptera, **P**.593
Physalopteridae, **P**.593
Physalopteroidea, **P**.593
Physalospora obtusa, **B1**.282
Physical agent susceptibility/resistance,
    B1.421–65
  picornaviruses, **V2**.869
  see also individual species; specific agents
Physical particle:plaque-forming unit ratios,
    cell–virus interactions, **V1**.203–4
Phytopathogens, classification, **M**.61–3
Phytoplasmas (undefined taxonomic status)
  characteristics, **B2**.1958 (Tab.)
  classification, **B2**.1967, **B2**.1968
  definition, **B2**.1957
Phytoreovirus, **V1**.47–8, **V2**.932
'Pian-bois,' **P**.313, **P**.329
Pichea pastoris production systems, **I**.840
Pichia guilliermondii, **M**.582
Pichia kluyveri, **B1**.282
Pichinde virus, **V2**.1059
  genome, non-coding regions, **V2**.1066
  geographical distribution/carrier and disease,
    V2.1060 (Tab.)
  infection, NK cells, **I**.96
  monoclonal antibodies, **V2**.1069
  morphology and structure, **V2**.1062
Pickling
  food processing and preservation,
    B1.268 (Tab.)
  pigs feet, **B1**.275
Picobirnavirus infection, in HIV infection,
    V2.1499 (Tab.), **V2**.1504
Picornaviridae
  characteristics, **V1**.139 (Tab.), **V1**.177 (Tab.)
  classification, **V1**.27 (Tab.), **V1**.50–2,
    V1.51 (Tab.), **V2**.858, **V2**.1161
    Hepatovirus, **V2**.1161
  defined by, **V1**.50–2
  properties of, **V2**.1162 (Tab.)
  supergroup, **V1**.52
  see also specific viruses
Picornaviruses, **V2.857–87**
  antigens, **V2**.860–1, **V2**.865–6
    see also specific types
  astroviruses *vs.,* **V2**.861
  biological properties, **V2**.860–1
  caliciviruses *vs.,* **V2**.861
  capsid assembly, **V2**.868–9
  cell entry, **V1**.109, **V1**.215, **V1**.215 (Fig.),
    V2.866
    attachment proteins, **V1**.207
    ligand conformational change, **V1**.139
    mechanisms, **V1**.213
    receptors, **V1**.207 (Tab.), **V2**.866,
      V2.867 (Tab.), **V2**.1405–6, **V2**.1406 (Tab.)
    route, **V1**.245
  characteristics, **V2**.861 (Tab.)
  classification, **V2**.858–9
    genus subclusters, **V2**.858–9
    molecular classification, **V2**.858–9

subclusters, **V2**.859 (Fig.)
  cytopathic effects, **V1**.94 (Fig.)
  directed mutagenesis, **V1**.183–4
  gene expression, **V1**.119
  genetic engineering, **V1**.195–7
  genome, **V1**.135–6, **V1**.136 (Fig.), **V2**.859,
    V2.863–5, **V2**.1161–5
    internal ribosomal entry site (IRES),
      V1.188
    open reading frame, **V1**.135–6
    replication, **V1**.124–5
    sequencing, **V2**.858
    size, **V2**.863–5
  historical aspects, **V2**.857
  infection *see* Picornavirus infection
  isolation/propagation and identification,
    V1.96 (Tab.), **V1**.100
  morphology/structure, **V1**.138, **V1**.282,
    V2.861–3, **V2**.862 (Fig.)
  mRNA, **V1**.139, **V1**.140 (Tab.)
  nonstructural proteins, **V2**.868
    see also specific types
  physical/chemical agent resistance, **V2**.869
  physical properties, **V2**.859
  post-translational protein modification,
    V1.140, **V1**.225, **V2**.867–8
    proteolytic cleavage, **V1**.121–2
  properties, **V2**.1162 (Tab.)
  protein synthesis, **V1**.115–16, **V2**.866–7
    ribosomal skipping, **V1**.117
  recombination, **V1**.15
    polioviruses, **V1**.188
  replication, **V2**.866–9
    cell binding, **V1**.138–9
    cell-specific factors, **V1**.136 (Fig.),
      V1.137
    gene expression, **V1**.110
    mRNA translation, **V1**.113
    RNA replication, **V2**.867, **V2**.868
    uncoating, **V2**.866
  togaviruses *vs.,* **V2**.861
  see also Enteroviruses; Rhinoviruses
Picornavirus infection, **V2**.869–74
  antiviral therapy, **V2**.1630–1
    resistance, **V2**.1637
  BCE peptide vaccines, **I**.870
  diagnosis, **V2**.876–8
  epidemiology, **V2**.874–6
  host cell, effects on, **V2**.869
    cell membrane metabolism, **V1**.142
    protein synthesis, **V1**.120, **V1**.141
  immune response, **V1**.282–3
    CTLs, **V1**.283
    IFN, **V1**.228, **I**.260 (Tab.)
    IgA, **V1**.282
    T cells, **V1**.282
  infection process, **V1**.241 (Tab.)
  neural spread, **V1**.244 (Tab.)
  transmission, **V1**.371 (Tab.)
  vehicles, **V1**.355
Piedra
  black *see* Black piedra
  therapy, **M**.186
  white *see* White piedra
Piedraia, **M**.195, **M**.197–8

Piedraia hortai, **M**.11, **M**.198, **M**.198 (Fig.)
  history, **M**.11
  spores, **M**.77, **M**.198, **M**.198 (Fig.)
Piedraia quintanilhae, **M**.198
Pig(s)
  atrophic rhinitis, **B2**.1653–4, **B2**.1795,
    B2.1810
  barns, airborne bacteria, **B1**.189
  infection
    Actinobacillus equuli, **B2**.1665–6
    Actinobacillus pleuropneumoniae, **B2**.1662,
      B2.1665–6
    Actinobacillus suis, **B2**.1665–6
    Campylobacter, **B2**.1550
    Pasteurella aerogenes, **B2**.1656
    Pasteurella multocida, **B2**.1653–4
    Mycoplasma hyopneumoniae vaccination,
      B2.1993–4
    pleuropneumonia, **B2**.1662, **B2**.1665–6
    proliferative enteropathies, **B2**.1550
    Yersinia enterocolitica reservoir, **B1**.274
    see also Swine
Pig-bel, **B2**.1118–19
Pigeons
  aspergillosis, **M**.18–9
  candidiasis, **M**.586
  Cryptococcus neoformans, **M**.643
Pigeon stuffers, infection, **M**.18–9
Piglets
  Escherichia coli, vero-cytotoxin-producing
    infection, **B2**.1378, **B2**.1378 (Fig.)
  hemorrhagic enteritis, **B2**.1378, **B2**.1378 (Fig.)
Pigmented retinopathy, rubella, **V2**.973
Pigment formation
  Aeromonas, **B2**.1529
  Enterobacter agglomerans complex, **B2**.1345
  Enterobacteriaceae culture, **B2**.1345
  Enterobacter sakazakii, **B2**.1345
  Leclercia adecarboxylata, **B2**.1345
  Serratia, **B2**.1345
PIgR (polymeric immunoglobulin receptor),
    I.318–19
  IgA binding/transport, **I**.318–19, **I**.537–8
  IgM binding, **I**.318–19
  J chain interactions, **I**.318–19
  mucosal immune response, **I**.525
  properties, **I**.313 (Tab.)
  structure, **I**.309 (Fig.), **I**.318–19
Pilin, **B1**.44, **B1**.101–2
  Neisseria, **B2**.1276, **B2**.1278–9
Pilus (pili)
  Aeromonas, **B2**.1528
  Bartonella henselae, **B2**.1887
  Burkholderia cepacia complex, **B2**.1614
  composition, **B1**.44
  conjugative (sex pili) *see* Conjugation,
    bacterial
  Escherichia coli, **B1**.101 (Fig.)
  Moraxella (Branhamella) catarrhalis,
    B2.1307
  Neisseria, **B2**.1278–80
  structure, **B1**.116–17
Pinocytosis, **P**.162
Pinta, **B2**.1839 (Tab.)
  clinical features, **B2**.1859
Pinworm *see Enterobius vermicularis*

Piperacillin
  Enterobacter, **B2**.1484–6
  Pasteurella multocida, **B2**.1655
  structure, **B1**.474 (Fig.)
Piperazine, *Enterobius vermicularis* infection,
  P.732
Pipestem fibrosis, schistosomiasis japonicum,
  P.630–1, **P**.630 (Fig.)
PIR-B, B-cell downregulation, **I**.348
Pirital virus, **V2**.1059
PIRO concept, **B1**.510
Piroctone olamine, seborrheic dermatitis,
  M.212
Pirodavir, **V2**.1630–1
  structure, **V2**.1626 (Fig.)
Piroplasms, **P**.189, **P**.451
  Babesia, **P**.451, **P**.453
  penetration of host, **P**.180, **P**.182 (Fig.)
Piscivirus, **V2**.1112 (Fig.)
'Pitted keratolysis,' **B2**.1151
Pittman types, **B1**.757
Pityriasis, **M**.195
Pityriasis capitis (dandruff) *see* Dandruff
  (pityriasis capitis)
Pityriasis flava, **M**.211
Pityriasis nigra, **M**.11
Pityriasis versicolor, **M**.14–5
  causative agents, **M**.203, **M**.210
    Malassezia furfur, **M**.210, **M**.211
    Malassezia globosa, **M**.210, **M**.210 (Fig.),
      M.211 (Fig.)
    Malassezia slooffiae, **M**.210
    Malassezia sympodialis, **M**.210
    see also individual species
  clinical features, **M**.210
    lesion distribution, **M**.211
  diagnosis, **M**.210, **M**.210 (Fig.), **M**.211 (Fig.)
    histopathology, **M**.128 (Tab.), **M**.138 (Fig.)
  historical perspective, **M**.202
  immune response, **M**.211
  recurrence, **M**.185
  therapy, **M**.185, **M**.185 (Tab.), **M**.211
    fluconazole, **M**.185
    itraconazole, **M**.185, **M**.211
    ketoconazole, **M**.185, **M**.211
    selenium sulfide, **M**.185
    zinc pyrithione, **M**.185
  worldwide distribution, **M**.210
Pityrosporal folliculitis therapy, **M**.185–6
Pityrosporum, **M**.14–5, **M**.202
Pityrosporum canis, **M**.14–5, **M**.202
Pityrosporum malassezi, **M**.14–5
Pityrosporum orbiculare, **M**.14–5, **M**.202
  atopic dermatitis, **M**.213
  confluent and reticulate papillomatosis of
    Gougerot–Carteaud, **M**.213–14
Pityrosporum ovale, **M**.14–5, **M**.202
  atopic dermatitis, **M**.213
Pityrosporum pachydermatis, **M**.14–5, **M**.202
Pivampicillin, **B1**.475
Pixuna virus (PIXV), **V2**.1011 (Tab.)
Placenta, *Mycobacterium leprae* transmission,
  B2.1204
Placentitis, *Chlamydia psittaci* infection,
  B2.2015
Plagiorchiida, **P**.579–80

Plagiorchiidae, **P**.586
Plagiorchioidea, **P**.585–6
  Lecithodendriidae, **P**.585
  Paragonimidae, **P**.586
  Plagiorchiidae, **P**.586
  Troglotrematidae, **P**.586
Plagiorchis, **P**.586
Plague
  in animals, **B2**.1459
  bubonic, treatment and prevention, **B2**.1466
  clinical forms, **B2**.1462
  endemic areas, **B2**.1459
  epizootic hosts, **B2**.1459
  etiology *see Yersinia pestis*
  flea vectors, **B2**.1459
  historical perspective, **B2**.1318–31
  pneumonic
    bioterrorism, **B1**.364
    emerging bacterial infection, **B1**.364
  surveillance, **B1**.317
  transmission, **B2**.1459
  treatment, **B2**.1466
  vaccines, **I**.933 (Tab.)
Planning, parasite control, **P**.111–12
Plant–bacteria interactions, **B1**.197–9
  alder–*Frankia* associations, **B1**.201
  biofilms on root surface, **B1**.199, **B1**.205–7
  biogeochemical transformations, **B1**.199–201
  biomass, **B1**.198–9
  commensal relationship, **B1**.197
  communities, **B1**.198–9
  heterogeneity, physiological and spatial,
    B1.198–9
  leaves
    new, **B1**.198
    surface, **B1**.198
    wettability, **B1**.198
  legume–rhizobia associations, **B1**.201
  metabolic activity, **B1**.198–9
  methodologies for study, **B1**.195
  mutualistic relationships, **B1**.197–8, **B1**.201
  mycorrhizal association, **B1**.197
  nitrogen status, **B1**.197
  nodule formation, **B1**.201
  parasitism, **B1**.197
  phyllosphere (aerial plant parts), **B1**.197,
    B1.198–9
    allocthonous microbes (noncolonizing),
      B1.198
    carbon and mineral source, **B1**.198
    endophytic habitats (plant interior),
      B1.198
    environmental factors impacting
      populations, **B1**.198
    epiphytic microbes (aerial colonization),
      B1.198, **B1**.201
    leachates, **B1**.198
    phylloplane (plant surfaces), **B1**.198
    recovery of populations, **B1**.204–5
    sampling, **B1**.204–5, **B1**.205–7
  relationship types, **B1**.197
  rhizodeposition, **B1**.197–8
  rhizosphere *see* Rhizosphere
  studies, **B1**.198–9
    techniques, **B1**.199

symbiotic relationships, **B1**.201
  see also individual species
Plant growth-promoting rhizobacteria (PGPR),
  B1.202–3
Plantibodies, **B2**.1994
Plant pathogens, **B1**.202, **B1**.202–4
  animals, **B1**.203–4
  diseases associated, **B1**.202
  entrance into plant, **B1**.202
  medical and veterinary significance,
    B1.203–4
  mycoplasmas, **B2**.1965–6, **B2**.1985–6
  taxonomy, **B1**.202
  utility, **B1**.202
  virulence determinants, **B1**.202
Plants, biological control
  insects, **B1**.198, **B1**.203–4
  pathogens, **B1**.198
Plant viriods, Hepatitis delta virus *vs.,* **V2**.1271
Plaque-counting, virucidal activity, **B1**.435–6
Plaque formation, *Coxiella burnetii,* **B2**.2073–4
Plaque morphology, bacteriophage analysis,
  B1.142
Plaque-reduced neutralization (PRN), measles
  diagnosis, **V1**.732
Plasma cells
  development, **I**.327
    class switching, **I**.327–8
  generation, **I**.491, **I**.493
    germinal centers, **I**.491–2
  kinetics
    primary infection, **I**.492 (Fig.)
    secondary infection, **I**.492–3
  longevity, **I**.491–2, **I**.498
  memory B cells *vs.,* **I**.491 (Tab.)
Plasma membrane, **M**.69, **M**.70–1
  fusion, **V1**.108
Plasmodium, **P**.466
Plasmaviridae
  classification, **V1**.27 (Tab.), **V1**.43 (Tab.)
  see also specific viruses
Plasmid(s), **B1**.81, **B1**.106–17
  antibiotic synthesis, **B1**.113–14
  bacteriocins, **B1**.136–7
  bacteriophage inhibition, **B1**.115–16
  biocide resistance, **B1**.442, **B1**.444
  classification, **B1**.116–17
  cloning vectors *see* Gene cloning
  conjugation genes, **B1**.110
    mob genes, **B1**.110
  copy number, **B1**.108
    high, **B1**.109
    low, **B1**.108, **B1**.109
    plasmid incompatibility, **B1**.108
  discovery, **B1**.13
  DNA vaccines *see* DNA vaccines
  DNA viruses *vs.,* **V1**.12
  electrophoretic analysis, **B1**.405
  elimination, **B1**.107
  evolution, **B1**.116–17
  generalized transduction, **B1**.105
  genes, **B1**.107–8
    antibiotic resistance, **B1**.110–11
    horizontal transmission, **B1**.110
    replication, **B1**.107

Plasmid(s)
  genes (*Continued*)
    restriction endonucleases, **B1**.115
    rolling circle replication, **B1**.107
    θ−replication, **B1**.107
    vertical transmission, **B1**.110
  historical perspective, **B1**.106
  host specificities, **B1**.116
  incompatibility groups, **B1**.116–17
    host range, **B1**.117
    pili structure, **B1**.116–17
  inheritance stability, **B1**.107
  mapping, **B1**.116
  metabolic characters, **B1**.115
  molecular biology applications, **B1**.107
  partition systems, **B1**.109
    high copy number, **B1**.109
    low copy number, **B1**.109
    par functions, **B1**.109
  post-segregational killing, **B1**.109
    low copy numbers, **B1**.109
    mode of action, **B1**.109
    resistance plasmid R1, **B1**.109
  replication, **B1**.81–2
    mediation, **B1**.108
  resistance genes (R plasmids), **B1**.106,
    B1.112 (Tab.), **B2**.1530
    β-lactamases, **B1**.111–12, **B1**.112–13
    Escherichia coli, **B2**.1276
    fluoroquinolone resistance, **B1**.113
    host specificities, **B1**.116
    mutational evolution, **B1**.113
    non-antibacterials, **B1**.114
    origins, **B1**.112–13
    penicillinase synthesis, **B1**.111
    species, **B1**.113 (Tab.)
    trimethoprim resistance, **B1**.113
    as virulence factors, **B1**.115
  Salmonella vaccine vector, **I**.901
  size, **B1**.107–8, **B1**.108 (Fig.)
  by species
    Aeromonas, **B2**.1529–30
    Bacteroides, **B2**.1931
    Borrelia, **B2**.1823–5
    Brucella, **B2**.1730
    Burkholderia cepacia, **B2**.1615
    Campylobacter, **B2**.1546
    Clostridium, **B2**.1092–3
    Coxiella burnetii, **B2**.2074–5
    Enterobacteriaceae, **B2**.1344
    Enterococcus, **B2**.886, **B2**.896
    Escherichia coli, **B2**.1276, **B2**.1371
    Haemophilus, **B2**.1697
    Helicobacter, **B2**.1567–8
    Legionella, **B2**.1770
    leptospires, **B2**.1875
    Listeria, **B2**.956
    Mycobacterium, **B2**.1188–9
    mycoplasmas, **B2**.1974
    Neisseria, **B2**.1276, **B2**.1277
    Pseudomonas, **B2**.1597
    Salmonella, **B2**.1409–10
    Staphylococcus aureus, **B2**.790–2, **B2**.791–2
    Streptococcus, **B2**.839
    Vibrio, **B2**.1512

    Yersinia, **B2**.1460–1, **B2**.1463–5, **B2**.1468
    Yersinia ruckeri, **B2**.1470
  Trypanosoma cruzi vectors, **P**.382
  viral evolution, **V1**.14
  virulence factors, **B1**.114–15
    resistance genes, **B1**.115
  visualization, **B1**.108 (Fig.)
Plasmid RP1, **B1**.118 (Fig.)
Plasminogen, **I**.203
Plasminogen activator inhibitor type I (PAI-1),
    I.204
Plasminogen activator protease, *Yersinia pestis*,
    B2.1469
Plasmodiidae, **P**.464
Plasmodium, **P**.188–9, **P**.464, **P**.473–4, **P**.474–5,
    I.676
  antigens, **P**.82–3
    antigenic variation, **P**.82, **P**.492
    gametocyte stage, **P**.83
    immunodominant, **P**.486, **P**.488
    merozoite stage, **P**.82–3
    restriction fragment length polymorphisms,
      P.491–2
  apical complexes, **P**.466
  chloroquine resistance, **P**.479, **P**.509–10
    geographical distribution, **P**.34,
      P.465 (Fig.), **P**.509–10
    historical aspects, **P**.479
    linkage analysis, **P**.479
    pfcrt gene, **P**.479
  circumsporozoite protein, **P**.82
  classification, **P**.198, **P**.464–6, **I**.675–6
    morphology, **P**.464, **P**.466
  CS protein, **P**.82
  differential diagnosis, **P**.502 (Tab.)
  drug resistance, **P**.464, **P**.479–80
    geographical distribution, **P**.465 (Fig.),
      P.481 (Fig.), **P**.509–10
    monitoring, **P**.480, **P**.481 (Fig.)
    multidrug resistance, **P**.506
    see also individual drugs
  epidemiology
    genetic diversity effects, **P**.511
    geographical distribution, **P**.473–4, **P**.474–5
    net reproductive success effects, **P**.58
  gametes, **P**.468
    exflagelation, **P**.468
    macrogametes *vs.* microgametes, **P**.468
  gametocytes, **P**.466, **P**.468, **P**.473–4,
    P.651 (Fig.)
    hyperparasitaemia, **P**.468
    structure, **P**.474 (Fig.)
  genome sequencing, **P**.478
  geographical distribution *see* Geographical
    distribution
  glycophorin-binding protein, **P**.475–6
  historical aspects, **P**.17
  host cell changes
    caveolae, **P**.473, **P**.474–5
    'knobs,' **P**.473, **P**.473 (Fig.), **P**.475
  immune evasion, **P**.491–3
    anti-disease immunity, **P**.492–3
    antigenic complexity, **I**.680
    antigenic diversity, **P**.491–2
    antigenic variation, **P**.62, **P**.82, **P**.492, **I**.681
    immune response alteration, **P**.491

    immunosuppression, **P**.491, **P**.501 (Tab.)
    poor immunogenicity, **P**.491
    sequestration, **P**.472, **P**.472 (Fig.), **P**.491
    stage-specific genes, **I**.680
  life cycle, **P**.82, **P**.466, **P**.467 (Fig.), **I**.676
    cell invasion, **P**.472
    cytoadherence, **P**.473–4
    developmental stages, **P**.466
      see also individual stages
    erythrocyte invasion, **P**.472
    erythrocytic stage, **P**.467–8
    fertilization, **P**.468–71
    hepatocyte invasion, **P**.472–3
    host cell alteration, **P**.468, **P**.473
    hypnozoites, **P**.471
    intra-erythrocytic cycle timing, **P**.468 (Fig.)
    intra-erythrocytic development, **P**.467–8
    maturation times, **P**.467
    pre-erythrocytic stage, **P**.466–7
    ring forms, **P**.473–4
    schizogony, **P**.473–4
    sporogony, **P**.468–71
    synchronicity, **P**.469, **P**.471–2
    transmission, **P**.469–70
  major surface protein, **P**.82–4
    vaccine, **P**.84–5
  merozoites, **P**.466
    development, **P**.466–7
    immune response, **P**.82–3
    structure, **P**.82–3, **P**.466
  metabolic pathways, **P**.468, **P**.475–8
    carbohydrate metabolism, **P**.476
    ion metabolism, **P**.477–8
    lipid metabolism, **P**.477
    nucleic acid metabolism, **P**.476–7
    oxygen uptake, **P**.478
    polyamine synthesis, **P**.476
    protein synthesis, **P**.476
    redox status, **P**.478
  microgametes, **P**.468
  mitochondria, **P**.466
  molecular biology/genetics, **P**.478–80
    antifolate resistance, **P**.479–80
    apicoplast, **P**.479
    chloroquine resistance, **P**.479
    drug resistance epidemiology, **P**.480
    extrachromosomal DNA, **P**.479
    genetic recombination, **P**.479
    genome structure, **P**.478–9
  morphology, **P**.474 (Fig.)
  nutrition, **P**.466, **P**.475–6
    access, **P**.475–6
    glycophorin-binding protein, **P**.475–6
    hemoglobin digestion, **P**.466, **P**.468, **P**.475
    new permeation pathways, **P**.475
    parasitophorous vacuole membrane,
      P.475–6
    secretion pathways, **P**.475–6
    serine-rich protein, **P**.475–6
    transmembrane gradients, **P**.475
  oocytes, **P**.470 (Fig.)
  ookinetes, **P**.466
  parasitophorous vacuole membrane, **P**.475–6
  plasma membrane, **P**.466
  polymorphisms, **P**.474–5

Plasmodium, (Continued)
public health importance, **P**.44
schizonts, **P**.466
development, **P**.466–7
structure, **P**.468 (Fig.), **P**.474 (Fig.)
sequestration, **P**.471, **P**.472, **P**.472 (Fig.),
P.473–4, **P**.491
serine-rich protein, **P**.475–6
sporozoites, **P**.466–7
structure, **P**.82, **P**.466
subgenera, **P**.192
surface proteins, **I**.676, **I**.681
thrombospondin related adhesion protein,
P.82
trophozoites
development, **P**.466–7
sequestration, **P**.472
structure, **P**.82, **P**.474 (Fig.)
see also Malaria; *individual species*
Plasmodium berghei, **I**.855 (Tab.), **I**.873
Plasmodium falciparum, **P**.188–9, **P**.464,
P.473–4
antigenic variation, **P**.492
chloroquine resistance, **P**.509–10
circumsporozoite protein, **P**.82, **I**.862 (Tab.)
cytoadherence, **P**.473–4
differential diagnosis, **P**.502 (Tab.)
epidemiology
genetic diversity effects, **P**.511
geographical distribution, **P**.473–4
fusidic acid effects, **B1**.488
genome sequencing, **P**.478
infection *see* Malaria, falciparum (malignant
tertian)
intra-erythrocytic development, **P**.467–8
life cycle, **P**.82, **P**.467 (Fig.)
erythrocyte invasion, **P**.472
gametocytes, **P**.468, **P**.473–4, **P**.651 (Fig.)
host cell changes, **P**.473, **P**.473 (Fig.)
intra-erythrocytic cycle timing, **P**.468 (Fig.)
latent period, **P**.61 (Tab.)
ring forms, **P**.473–4
schizogony, **P**.473–4
morphology, **P**.474 (Fig.)
sequestration, **P**.471, **P**.472, **P**.473–4
vector, life expectancy, **P**.61 (Tab.)
Plasmodium malariae, **P**.464, **P**.475
differential diagnosis, **P**.502 (Tab.)
erythrocyte invasion, **P**.472
gametocytes, **P**.468
host cell changes, **P**.473, **P**.473 (Fig.), **P**.475
infection *see* Malaria, malariae (quartan)
intra-erythrocytic development, **P**.467–8
morphology, **P**.474 (Fig.)
sequestration, **P**.471
Plasmodium ovale, **P**.464, **P**.475
differential diagnosis, **P**.502 (Tab.)
erythrocyte invasion, **P**.472
gametocytes, **P**.468
host cell changes, **P**.473
hypnozoites, **P**.471
infection *see* Malaria, vivax/ovale (benign
tertian)
intra-erythrocytic development, **P**.467–8
morphology, **P**.474 (Fig.)

Plasmodium vivax, **P**.464, **P**.474–5
chloroquine resistance, **P**.509–10
differential diagnosis, **P**.502 (Tab.)
erythrocyte invasion, **P**.472
gametocytes, **P**.468, **P**.651 (Fig.)
geographical distribution, **P**.474–5
host cell changes, **P**.473, **P**.474–5
hypnozoites, **P**.471
infection *see* Malaria, vivax/ovale (benign
tertian)
intra-erythrocytic development, **P**.467–8
morphology, **P**.474 (Fig.)
polymorphisms, **P**.474–5
Plasmodium vivax hibernans, **P**.474–5
Plasmodium vivax multinucleatum, **P**.474–5
Plasmotomy
Blastocystis hominis, **P**.560–1
microsporidians, **P**.531–2
Plastics, bioremediation, **B1**.201–2
Plastic surgery, post-operative infection
Mycobacterium abscessus, **B2**.1247–8
Mycobacterium chelonae, **B2**.1252
Mycobacterium smegmatis, **B2**.1261
Plate count test
for milk, **B1**.233–4
for water, **B1**.222
Platelet-activating factor (PAF), **I**.190–1
actions/effects, **I**.190–1
basophil chemotaxis, **I**.60
basophil histamine release, **I**.62
eosinophil chemotaxis, **I**.61
eosinophil rolling, **I**.60
leukocytes aggregation, **I**.191
platelet aggregation, **I**.191
smooth muscle contraction, **I**.191
in diseases/infection
airway hypersensitivity pathology, **I**.731–2
septic shock, **I**.699
inactivation mechanisms, **I**.190–1
metabolism, **I**.191
production, **I**.190, **I**.191
eosinophils, **I**.191
macrophages, **I**.191
monocytes, **I**.191
neutrophils, **I**.46, **I**.191
P-selectin effects, **I**.190–1
receptors, **I**.191
structure, **I**.190
Platelet derived growth factor (PDGF), adeno-
associated virus binding, **V1**.416–17
Platelet endothelial cell adhesion molecule-1
(PECAM-1:CD31)
CD31 gene, **I**.600
diapedesis, **I**.38
macrophage development, **I**.21
Platelets
acute phase response, **I**.207
aggregation
platelet-activating factor production,
I.191
thromboxane, **I**.189
cytokines produced, **I**.28 (Tab.)
septic shock, **I**.699–700
thromboxane production, **I**.189

Platyhelminthes, **P**.573, **P**.574–86, **P**.677
classification, **P**.574–86
Pleckstrin homology (PH) domains, **I**.345
Pleconaril, **V2**.1630–1
enterovirus control, **V2**.878
mechanism of action, **V2**.1630 (Fig.)
resistance, **V2**.1637
Plectin, **I**.136
Pleistophora
classification, **P**.198, **P**.535, **P**.542
fish infection, **P**.541–2, **P**.544
human infection, transmission, **P**.544
structure/life cycle
meront, **P**.535
sporophorous vesicles, **P**.532–3, **P**.535
see also Microsporidians; Microsporidiosis
Plenodomus avramii, **M**.391
Pleocytosis
measles, **V1**.723
mumps, **V1**.748, **V1**.749–50, **V1**.756
Pleomorphic fungi, nomenclature, **M**.77
Pleomorphism, *Trypanosoma brucei,*
P.356–7
Plerocercoid stage, **P**.576
Plesiomonas, **B2**.1330 (Tab.)
classification, **B2**.1507
changes to, **B2**.1336
enterobacterial common antigen,
B2.1343–4
Plesiomonas shigelloides, **B2**.1512–13,
B2.1513 (Tab.)
biochemical tests, **B2**.1319 (Tab.)
intestinal infection, **B2**.1347
Pleural effusion, pneumonia complication,
B1.641
Pleurodynia (Bornholm disease), **V2**.871
Ploidy, *Trypanosoma brucei,* **P**.361–2
Pneumococcal meningitis, **B1**.569–74
bacteremia, **B1**.519, **B1**.569
clinical features, **B1**.570
epidemiology, **B1**.569
risk factors, **B1**.570
incidence, **B1**.569, **B1**.570 (Fig.)
management of contacts, **B1**.571
maternal immunization effect, **B1**.572
mortality and morbidity, **B1**.569, **B1**.570
outcome, **B1**.570
prevention, **B1**.571–2
antibiotic prophyaxis, **B1**.572
antibiotic prophylaxis, **B1**.572
vaccination, **B1**.571–2
recurrent, **B1**.571
treatment, **B1**.571
antibiotics, **B1**.571
contact management, **B1**.571
steroids, **B1**.571
Pneumococci *see Streptococcus pneumoniae*
Pneumocystis, **M**.763, **M**.764–9
adhesion, **M**.778, **M**.785–6, **M**.792–3
antigens, **M**.792
biochemistry, **M**.772, **M**.780–3
carbohydrates, **M**.772, **M**.783
cholesterol, **M**.772, **M**.780, **M**.781
coenzyme Q homologues, **M**.781
dihydrofolate reductase, **M**.790

Pneumocystis,
biochemistry (*Continued*)
fatty acids, **M.**781
glucans, **M.**765, **M.**783
lipids, **M.**772
nucleic acids, **M.**783, **M.**788
polyamines, **M.**782
proteins, **M.**782–3
replication, **M.**783
sterols, **M.**772, **M.**780, **M.**781
transport systems, **M.**782
classification, **M.**771–8, **M.**775 (Tab.),
M.777–8, **M.**778 (Tab.), **M.**779 (Fig.),
M.796
Ascomycetes, **M.**772–4, **M.**778,
M.778 (Tab.), **M.**796
ferrets, **M.**775–6
genetics, **M.**772–4
antigens, **M.**792
diversity, **M.**774, **M.**775 (Tab.),
M.776 (Fig.), **M.**777 (Tab.)
elongation factor 3, **M.**774
genome, **M.**783
Genome Project, **M.**769, **M.**771, **M.**783,
M.796–7
life cycle, **M.**768–9
major surface glycoproteins, **M.**774, **M.**775,
M.792
mitochondrial genes, **M.**772–4, **M.**777,
M.788
growth pattern, **M.**70
history, **M.**763–4
identification
fluorescein-isothiocyanate, **M.**788
Giemsa stain, **M.**787–8
life cycle, **M.**764–5, **M.**768, **M.**769 (Fig.),
M.772, **M.**783, **M.**791
excystation, **M.**765, **M.**767–8
sporogenesis, **M.**766–8, **M.**769 (Fig.)
morphology, **M.**764–5
cyst, **M.**766–7, **M.**767 (Fig.), **M.**768 (Fig.),
M.769 (Fig.), **M.**786 (Fig.), **M.**787
pre-cyst, **M.**765–6, **M.**767 (Fig.),
M.769 (Fig.)
taxonomy, **M.**771–2
trophic form, **M.**765, **M.**766 (Fig.), **M.**768,
M.769 (Fig.), **M.**787
motility, **M.**765
nomenclature, **M.**763, **M.**777,
M.778 (Tab.)
prototype and variant, **M.**775
ribosomal RNA, **M.**772, **M.**775
in vitro propagation, **M.**778–80
cell-free systems, **M.**778–9
monolayers, **M.**778
Pneumocystis carinii, **P.**189
biochemistry, **M.**780–2
carbohydrates, **M.**783
nucleic acids, **M.**783
polyamines, **M.**782–3
transport, **M.**782
classification, **M.**4, **M.**69, **M.**796
genetics, **M.**772–4
antigens, **M.**793
diversity, **M.**775–6, **M.**775 (Tab.),
M.776 (Fig.), **M.**777 (Tab.)
mitochondrial genes, **M.**772–4

history, **M.**763
identification, **M.**788
histopathology, **M.**126 (Tab.),
M.128 (Tab.), **M.**134 (Fig.), **M.**140 (Fig.)
stains, **M.**123 (Tab.)
infection *see below*
life cycle, **M.**768–9, **M.**769 (Fig.)
morphology, **M.**126 (Tab.), **M.**786 (Fig.)
cyst, **M.**786 (Fig.)
trophic form, **M.**766 (Fig.)
nomenclature, **M.**763, **M.**777, **M.**778
phylogenetic tree, **M.**772, **M.**773 (Fig.)
ribosomal RNA, **M.**4, **M.**772, **M.**774
transport, **M.**782
Pneumocystis carinii complex, **M.**69
Pneumocystis carinii infection, **M.**785
adrenal glands, **M.**785
animals, **M.**775–6
bone marrow, **M.**785
ears, **M.**785
gastrointestinal tract, **M.**785
genitourinary tract infection, **M.**785
heart, **M.**785
in HIV infection, **I.**795
HTLV infection, **I.**802–3
IL-2 pathway, **I.**772–3
immune response, **M.**794–5
regulatory T cells, **I.**666–7
immunogenetics, **I.**595–6
nosocomial infection, **B1.**403
oculomycoses, **M.**290, **M.**327, **M.**785
endophthalmitis, **M.**317
SCID, **I.**774
X-linked hyper-IgM-CD40 ligand deficiency,
I.778
see also Pneumocystis pneumonia (PCP)
Pneumocystis infection
diagnosis, EIAs, **M.**793–4
histopathology, **M.**121–2, **M.**125–7,
M.128 (Tab.), **M.**134 (Fig.), **M.**140 (Fig.)
stains, **M.**123 (Tab.)
host range, **M.**764, **M.**769–71, **M.**770 (Tab.)
immune response, **M.**784, **M.**792–5
cell-mediated, **M.**784, **M.**794
humoral, **M.**784, **M.**793
pneumonia *see Pneumocystis* pneumonia
(PCP)
Pneumocystis jirovecii, **M.**764
biochemistry, **M.**772
cytochrome *b,* **M.**764, **M.**790–1, **M.**796
classification, **M.**796
colonization, **M.**792
dihydropteroate synthase, **M.**764, **M.**790,
M.791–2, **M.**796
epidemiology, **M.**791, **M.**792
genetics, **M.**796
antigens, **M.**793
cytochrome *b* mutants, **M.**764, **M.**790–1,
M.796
DHPS mutants, **M.**764, **M.**790, **M.**791–2,
M.796
diversity, **M.**775 (Tab.), **M.**776–7,
M.776 (Fig.)
selective drug pressure and mutations,
M.790

identification, **M.**788, **M.**792
PCR, **M.**94
infection, **M.**785
immune response, **M.**793–5
see also Pneumocystis infection;
Pneumocystis pneumonia (PCP)
nomenclature, **M.**763, **M.**777, **M.**778
Pneumocystis murina
classification, **M.**796
genetics
antigens, **M.**793
diversity, **M.**775 (Tab.), **M.**776 (Fig.)
immune response, **M.**795
nomenclature, **M.**763, **M.**778
Pneumocystis pneumonia (PCP), **M.**140 (Fig.),
M.783–8, **M.763–806**
AIDS *see* AIDS
animal models, **M.**793, **M.**795–6
clinical features, **M.**784
diagnosis, **M.**786, **M.**786 (Fig.)
arterial blood gas, **M.**788
bronchoalveolar lavage, **M.**784, **M.**787,
M.792, **M.**794
culture, **M.**788
lung biopsy, **M.**787
microscopy, **M.**787
molecular methods, **M.**788
pulmonary function tests, **M.**788
sample collection, **M.**787
serology, **M.**788
epidemiology, **M.**763–4, **M.**791–2
glucose-6-phosphate dehydrogenase
deficiency, **M.**789
histopathology, **M.**785–6, **M.**786 (Fig.)
history, **M.**763–4
immune response, **M.**792–5
CD4 cells, **M.**792, **M.**793, **M.**796
cell-mediated, **M.**784, **M.**794
humoral, **M.**784, **M.**793
immunocompetence, **M.**785, **M.**792
immunosuppression, **M.**764, **M.**784, **M.**785,
M.791, **M.**792, **M.**793, **M.**795–6
animal models, **M.**793, **M.**795–6
see also AIDS
incidence, **M.**783–4
pathogenesis, **M.**785
presentation, **M.**784
adults, **M.**784
children, **M.**784, **M.**791–2
extrapulmonary, **M.**784–5
risk factors, **M.**784
therapy, **M.**764, **M.**789–91
corticosteroids, **M.**784, **M.**789–91
co-trimoxazole *see* Co-trimoxazole
(trimethoprim-sulfamethoxazole)
HAART, **M.**764, **M.**783–4
Pneumocystis wakefieldiae
animals, **M.**775–6
classification, **M.**796
genetics
antigens, **M.**793
diversity, **M.**775–6, **M.**776 (Fig.),
M.777 (Tab.)
nomenclature, **M.**763, **M.**778
Pneumolysin, chemotaxis inhibition, **I.**648

Pneumonia, **B1**.629–45, **V1**.777
 acute aspergillus bronchopneumonia, **M**.699
 animals, *Rhodococcus equi* causing, **B2**.1167
 aspiration, **B1**.641, **B1**.643 (Tab.)
  causative organisms, **B1**.643 (Tab.)
 blastomycosis, **M**.489
 caspase deficiency, **I**.776
 causative organisms
  Chlamydia pneumoniae, **B2**.2016
  Chlamydia psittaci, **B2**.2014–15
  Streptococcus pneumoniae see
   Streptococcus pneumoniae infection
 chronic, **B1**.644
 classification, **B1**.629
 clinical manifestations, **V1**.777
 community-acquired bacterial, **B1**.629–30
  causative organisms, **B1**.630–7,
   B1.631 (Tab.)
   Coxiella burnetii, **B1**.636
   Haemophilus influenzae, **B1**.636–7
   Legionella pneumophila, **B1**.634–6
   Mycoplasma pneumoniae, **B1**.633–4
   Staphylococcus aureus, **B1**.636
   Streptococcus, **B1**.637
   Streptococcus pneumoniae, **B1**.630–3
  gram-negative bacillary, **B1**.637
  incidence, **B1**.629–30
  management, **B1**.638
   antibacterial therapy, **B1**.638
  mortality, **B1**.630, **B1**.630 (Tab.)
  other causes, **B1**.637
  severe cases, **B1**.638–40
  symptoms, **B1**.630
 complications, **B1**.641–4
  empyema, **B1**.641–3
  necrotizing pneumonitis and lung abscess,
   B1.643–4
  pleural effusion, **B1**.641
 cryptococcal, **M**.646–7, **M**.649–50,
  M.650 (Fig.)
 diagnosis, **V1**.777
 etiology, **V1**.777
 HCMV infection in transplants, **V1**.521–2
 in HIV infection, **B1**.645
 immunocompromised patients, **B1**.644–5
 influenza complications, **V1**.367
 nosocomial, **B1**.389, **B1**.640–1
  causative organisms, **B1**.389, **B1**.640–1,
   B1.640 (Tab.)
  conditions predisposing, **B1**.389–90
  definition, **B1**.640
  elderly, **B1**.393
  frequency and factors increasing, **B1**.640
  mortality, **B1**.640
  pathogenesis, **B1**.640
  prevention, **B1**.390, **B1**.641
  treatment, **B1**.641, **B1**.642 (Tab.)
  viral, **B1**.640–1
 pathology, **B1**.629
 Pittsburgh, **B1**.635
 Pneumocystis see Pneumocystis pneumonia
  (PCP)
 primary atypical, **B1**.633
  Mycoplasma pneumoniae, **B2**.1983
  see also Mycoplasma pneumoniae

 varicella, **V1**.513
 viral *vs.* bacterial, **V1**.777
Pneumonia virus of mice, **V1**.385
Pneumonic pasteurellosis
 cattle, **B2**.1654
 sheep, **B2**.1654
Pneumonitis
 in AIDS/HIV infection
  HCMV infection, **V2**.1505
  Respiratory syncytial virus, **V2**.1505–6
 chemical, **B1**.641
 immunosuppressed patients, HSV infection,
  V2.1506
 necrotizing, **B1**.643–4
  causative agents, **B1**.644
  diagnosis and treatment, **B1**.644
 Q fever, **B2**.2076
Pneumoviridae
 classification, **V1**.808 (Fig.)
 intergenic regions, **V1**.701
 see also Pneumovirinae
Pneumovirinae
 characteristics, **V1**.129 (Tab.), **V1**.177 (Tab.),
  V1.385, **V1**.701 (Tab.)
 classification, **V1**.48–9, **V1**.49 (Tab.), **V1**.382,
  V1.699
  NS1/NS2 genes, **V1**.699
 members, **V1**.385
 phylogeny, **V1**.388
 see also Pneumoviridae; Pneumoviruses
Pneumovirus, **V1.783–806**
 animal models, **V1**.790
 characteristics, **V1**.129 (Tab.), **V1**.701 (Tab.)
 classification, **V1**.48–9, **V1**.382, **V1**.700 (Tab.)
 genome structure/organization,
  V1.387 (Tab.), **V1**.701 (Fig.),
  V1.785 (Fig.), **V1**.789
 members, **V1**.385
 mRNA transcription, **V1**.790
 proteins, **V1**.785–7
 type species *see* Human respiratory syncytial
  virus (HRSV)
 virus assembly, **V1**.790
 virus replication, **V1**.789–90
 in vitro culture, **V1**.790
Pneumoviruses
 attachment (G) protein, **V1**.706, **V1**.707
 genome structure, **V1**.387 (Tab.)
 immune evasion, **V1**.199
 immune evasion mechanisms, **V1**.199
 small hydrophobic proteins, **V1**.708
 see also Pneumovirinae
P (palindromic) nucleotides
 somatic recombination, **I**.330
 TCR rearrangements, **I**.452–4
Podoviridae, **V1**.26, **V1**.378
 classification, **V1**.27 (Tab.), **V1**.42,
  V1.43 (Tab.)
 see also specific viruses
Podoviridae bacteriophage, **B2**.1535
Point mutations, **B1**.84–6
 antigenic variation, **I**.660
 base analogue incorporation, **B1**.84–5
 base pair substitutions, **B1**.84
  intergenic suppression, **B1**.86–7
  pseudorevertants, **B1**.86

 frame-shift mutations, **B1**.84, **B1**.85
  acridine dyes, **B1**.85
  pseudoreversion, **B1**.85
 mis-sense mutations, **B1**.86
  reversion mutants, **B1**.87
 nonsense codons, **B1**.86
 tautomeric shifts, **B1**.84, **B1**.85 (Fig.)
 transitions, **B1**.84–5
 transversions, **B1**.84
 spontaneous, **B1**.85
Point-of-care tests, influenza diagnosis, **V1**.675
Point-source outbreaks, **V1**.358 (Fig.)
 definition, **V1**.358
 norovirus infection, **V2**.919
Poisson distribution, cell–virus interactions,
 V1.203, **V1**.204 (Tab.)
Polar events, transposable elements, **B1**.94
Polarized cells, viral receptors, **V1**.209
Polaroplast, microsporidians, **P**.529–31
Polar tubes, **P**.529–31, **P**.531 (Fig.)
 emergence, **P**.531, **P**.531 (Fig.)
pol gene
 foamy viruses, **V2**.1308
 HTLVs, **V2**.1285–7
pol II-dependent transcriptase, viral gene
 transcription, **V1**.113–14
Poliomyelitis, **V2**.870, **V2**.1422–3
 'abortive' illness, **V2**.870, **V2**.1422–3
 biphasic illness, **V2**.1422–3
 clinical features, **V2**.1422–3
 emerging infection, **V2**.1648 (Tab.)
 host age, **V2**.1655
 entry route, **V2**.1404–5
 epidemics, **B1**.353–4, **B1**.353 (Fig.)
 epidemiology
  age-relation, **V1**.356–7
  fecal–oral transmission, **V1**.368–9
  global distribution, **V2**.883 (Fig.)
  infection route and spread, **V2**.1407–8,
   V2.1422
  outbreaks, **V2**.882
 eradication, **B1**.345, **B1**.346, **B1**.353–4,
  V2.879–83, **V2**.1573
  wild strains, **V2**.880–1
 future prospects, **V2**.870
 host cell, effects on
  cell membrane metabolism, **V1**.142
  persistent infection, **V2**.869
  protein synthesis, **V1**.203, **V1**.223–4
 hygiene control, **B1**.353–4
 immune response, **V1**.283
 inapparent infection, **V2**.870
 infection/spread, **V1**.237 (Fig.), **V2**.1422
 laboratory worker immunization, **B1**.767
 'minor' illness, **V2**.870
 neurovirulence, **V2**.1406, **V2**.1407
 neutralizing antibodies, **V2**.865
 non-paralytic, **V2**.870, **V2**.1422–3
 notifications, **B1**.353 (Fig.)
 paralytic, **V2**.870, **V2**.1423
  bulbar, **V2**.1423
  incidence, **V2**.879 (Fig.)
 pathogenesis, **V2**.869, **V2**.1407–8, **V2**.1423
  virulence relationship, **V2**.1406
 pathology, **V2**.1407–8, **V2**.1423

Poliomyelitis (*Continued*)
post-polio syndrome, **V2**.870, **V2**.1423
silent infection, **V2**.1422–3
transmission, **V2**.1404–5
vaccines/vaccination, **B1**.339, **I**.424 (Tab.),
  V2.879–83, **V2**.1571–3
  attenuated vaccine vectors, **I**.830–1
  BCE peptide vaccines, **I**.855 (Tab.), **I**.870
  cessation of, **V2**.881–2
  chronic excretion, **V1**.368–9, **V2**.882–3
  efficacy, **V2**.879 (Fig.)
  history, **V1**.8 (Tab.)
  inactivated (Salk: IPV) *see* Inactivated
    poliomyelitis vaccine (Salk: IPV)
  live oral (Sabin: OPV) *see* Oral
    poliomyelitis vaccine (Sabin: OPV)
  paralysis, **V2**.882, **V2**.1557, **V2**.1563–4,
    V2.1572
  persistence, **V2**.882
  programs, **V2**.1559 (Tab.)
  quality assurance, **V2**.881
  recombination events, **V2**.881–2
  schedules, **V2**.1560–1
  SV 40 transmission, **V1**.482, **V2**.1557
  tropical countries, **V2**.880–1
  USA schedules, **V2**.1559–60, **V2**.1560 (Fig.)
  VP1 protein, **I**.870
viremia, **V1**.242 (Fig.)
  determining virulence, **V1**.245, **V1**.252
Poliovirus, **V1**.50–2
cell receptors, **V1**.207
  virus release, **V1**.211–12
cytocidal infection, **V1**.205
immune evasion, **V1**.230
Polioviruses, **V1**.254–5
antibacterial agents, **B1**.440
antigens
  infectious particles, **V2**.865
  isolate variation, **V2**.865
  monoclonal antibodies, **V2**.865
  neutralizing antibodies, **V2**.866 (Tab.)
attenuated strains, **V1**.253, **V1**.254–5,
    V1.254 (Tab.)
  5' non-translated regions, **V1**.254–5,
    V2.1406
  mutations, **V1**.255
  structural/non-structural proteins, **V1**.255
capsids
  antigens, **V2**.865
  assembly, **V2**.868–9
  structure, **V2**.862–3, **V2**.864 (Fig.)
cell entry, **V1**.109, **V2**.866
  inhibition by antibody, **V1**.277
  ligand conformational change, **V1**.139
  receptor *see below*
characteristics, **V1**.135
genome, **V2**.863–5
  replication, **V1**.143
historical aspects, **V2**.857
host range, **V2**.869
immune evasion, **V1**.295
infection *see* Poliomyelitis
isolation systems, **V2**.877 (Tab.)
morphology/structure, **V2**.862, **V2**.862 (Fig.),
  V2.863 (Fig.)
multifunctional gene products, **V1**.136–7

nonstructural proteins, **V2**.863–5
  see also specific types
particle assembly/release, **V1**.144
post-translational protein modification,
  V1.140, **V2**.867
receptors, **V1**.207 (Tab.), **V1**.246 (Fig.),
  V1.247, **V2**.866
  antibody-blocking, **V1**.209
  CNS receptors, **V2**.1406 (Tab.)
  ICAM-1, **V2**.866
  poliovirus receptor, **V1**.209
recombination, **V1**.15, **V1**.187
  picornaviruses, **V1**.188
replication
  cell-specific factors, **V1**.136 (Fig.)
  RNA replication, **V2**.868
structural proteins, **V2**.863–5
  see also specific types
vaccine *see* Poliomyelitis
as vaccine vector, **I**.846–7, **I**.899
virulence, **V1**.251 (Tab.)
  genetic determinants, **V1**.254–5
VP1 protein, **V2**.862–3, **V2**.864 (Fig.)
VP2 protein, **V2**.862–3, **V2**.864 (Fig.)
VP3 protein, **V2**.862–3, **V2**.864 (Fig.)
VP4 protein, **V2**.862–3
Pollution
atmospheric
  denitrification process contribution, **B1**.200
  respiratory tract infection, **B1**.626
bioremediation, **B1**.199, **B1**.201–2, **B1**.212
Poloxamers, **B1**.425
Pol (polymerase) protein, **V1**.78–9, **V1**.147–8
foamy viruses, **V2**.1307
paramyxoviruses, **V1**.73
retroviruses, **V1**.78, **V2**.1322–3, **V2**.1591
rhabdoviruses, **V1**.74
Poly-3-hydroalkanoates, **B2**.1594
Polyacrylamide gel electrophoresis (PAGE)
Actinomyces identification, **B2**.1013
Bacillus, **B2**.945
Bifidobacterium, **B2**.1025–6
Haemophilus, **B2**.1705
Leptonema, **B2**.1877
rotavirus infection diagnosis, **V2**.952
sodium dodecyl sulfate, **B1**.25
  Bacillus cereus flagella antigen, **B2**.929
  Enterococcus, **B2**.890, **B2**.890 (Fig.)
see also Pulse-field gel electrophoresis
  (PFGE)
Polyadenylation, gene expression, **V1**.112–13
Polyamine synthesis, *Plasmodium*, **P**.476
Polyarthritis, Parvovirus B19 virus infection,
  V1.430
Polycistronic mRNAs, respirovirus
  transcription, **V1**.771
Polyclonal antibodies
monoclonal antibody therapy *vs.*, **I**.353–4
reactivity range, **I**.353
Polydnaviridae
classification, **V1**.27 (Tab.), **V1**.43 (Tab.)
see also specific viruses
Polyenes, **M**.148–9, **M**.169 (Tab.), **M**.171,
  M.182
ergosterol, **M**.172

lipid vehicles, **M**.149
mechanism of action, **M**.70, **M**.182
resistance, **M**.170–2
  candidiasis, **M**.170–1, **M**.611
therapy
  blastomycosis, **M**.497
  candidiasis, **M**.182
  keratitis, **M**.307–8
see also individual agents
Polygenic variation, emerging viral infection,
  V2.1652
Polyhexamethylene biguanides (PHMB),
  B1.426
action, **B1**.437 (Tab.), **B1**.438
mycotic keratitis therapy, **M**.306–7
Polyhydroxybutyric acid (PHB), **B1**.42
  Pseudomonas accumulation, **B2**.1594
Polymerase-based viral classification, **V1**.55
Polymerase chain reaction (PCR), **B1**.25,
  B1.26, **B1**.721–2, **B1**.725–7
adenoviruses, **V1**.446
aerobic actinomycetes, **B2**.1146–7
Aeromonas, **B2**.1532, **B2**.1534
African trypanosomiasis, **P**.367
airborne bacteria, **B1**.191
amebiasis, **P**.211, **P**.220
American visceral leishmaniasis, **P**.335
Anaplasma phagocytophilum, **B2**.2064–5
Aspergillus, **M**.94, **M**.105, **M**.108, **M**.715–16
  A. fumigatus, **M**.108, **M**.715–16
  bronchoalveolar lavage, **M**.715
  ELISA *vs.*, **M**.715
  genetic analysis, **M**.715–16
  light cycler, **M**.716
  nested, **M**.716
  two-step, **M**.716
astroviruses, **V2**.906
avian infectious bronchitis virus, **V1**.844
babesiosis, **P**.457
Bacillus anthracis, **B2**.937
bacterial meningitis, **B1**.559–60
Bartonella, **B2**.1895–7
Bartonella henselae, **B2**.1897
Blastomyces, **M**.94, **M**.491
Bordetella pertussis, **B2**.1792
Borrelia, **B2**.1821
botulinum toxin, **B2**.1063
Brucella, **B2**.1721
bunyaviruses, **V2**.1050
Burkholderia cepacia, **B2**.1614–15
Burkholderia pseudomallei, **B2**.1619–20
Burkholderia thailandensis, **B2**.1620–1
Candida, **M**.94, **M**.101–2, **M**.584
  C. albicans, **M**.101–2
  C. fumigatus, **M**.104
  C. glabrata, **M**.102, **M**.103
  C. krusei, **M**.102, **M**.103–4
  C. parapsilosis, **M**.102–3, **M**.103–4
  C. tropicalis, **M**.102, **M**.103–4
Carrión's disease, **B2**.1890
cat-scratch disease, **B2**.1895–7
Chlamydia, **B2**.2006–7, **B2**.2018–19
clonorchiasis, **P**.653
Coccidioides, **M**.94
Corynebacterium diphtheriae, **B2**.984

Polymerase chain reaction (PCR) (*Continued*)
  Cryptococcus, **M**.94, **M**.110
    C. neoformans, **M**.110
  cyclosporiasis, **P**.415
  in diagnosis/detection, **B1**.755–6, **V2**.1537–8
    see also specific diseases/infection
  Ehrlichia chaffeensis, **B2**.2064–5
  endophthalmitis, **B1**.603
  Enterobacteriaceae, **B2**.1351
  enteroviruses, **V2**.877
  Erysipelothrix rhusiopathiae, **B2**.970
  fetal infection, **V2**.1444–5
  filoviruses, **V2**.1097 (Tab.)
  giardiasis, **P**.250–1
  gram-positive anaerobic cocci, **B2**.907
  Haemophilus, **B2**.1704, **B2**.1704 (Fig.),
    B2.1710
  Haemophilus ducreyi, **B1**.664
  HCMV infection, **V1**.526
    breastmilk, **V2**.1451
    fetal infection, **V2**.1451
    neonatal, **V2**.1451–2
  Helicobacter pylori, **B1**.174, **B2**.1574
  hepatitis B, **V2**.1252
  hepatitis C, **V2**.1190, **V2**.1213–14
  HHV-6, **V1**.532–3
  HHV-7, **V1**.532–3
  Histoplasma, **M**.94
    H. capsulatum, **M**.94, **M**.112
  HIV, **I**.790, **V2**.1472–3
  HSV, **V2**.1465, **V2**.1466
  HTLV, **V2**.1294, **V2**.1294 (Fig.), **V2**.1542
  human brucellosis, **B2**.1739, **B2**.1740
  isosporiasis, **P**.413
  juvenile laryngeal papillomatosis, **V2**.1484
  keratitis, mycotic, **M**.306
  Legionella pneumophila, **B2**.1774
  Leishmania, **P**.284–5, **P**.301–2
  leptospires, **B2**.1879, **B2**.1880
  Lyme borreliosis, **B2**.1829
  lymphatic filariasis, **P**.777
  malaria, **P**.504–5, **P**.505 (Fig.)
    blood transfusions, **P**.506
    sensitivity, **P**.505
    treatment options, **P**.505
  methicillin-resistant *Staphylococcus aureus,*
    B2.807–8
  microsporidiosis, **P**.547
  Mycobacterium, **B2**.1193
  Mycobacterium tuberculosis, **B2**.1195
  Mycoplasma, **B2**.1996–7
  Neisseria meningitidis, **B1**.751
  non-diagnostic applications, **B1**.725–7
    amplicon recovery, **B1**.121
    antiviral susceptibility testing, **V2**.1543
    contamination and contamination control,
      B1.727
    directed mutagenesis, **V1**.183–4
    emerging viral infection recognition,
      V2.1646–7
    genotyping, **V2**.1542
      astrovirus, **V2**.899
      poxvirus identification, **V1**.583
    HLA immunogenetics, **I**.576–7
    protozoa classification, **P**.193

  site-directed mutation, **B1**.89–90,
    B1.90 (Fig.)
  soil bacteria analysis, **B1**.206–7
  onchocerciasis, **P**.791–2
  opisthorchiasis, **P**.653
  Parvovirus B19 virus infection, **V1**.430,
    V2.1469–70
  parvovirus infection, **V1**.424
  PCP diagnosis, **M**.788
  Penicillium marneffei, **M**.571
  Pneumocystis jirovecii, **M**.788, **M**.792
  principle, **B1**.725–7
  process, **B1**.725–6
  Proteus, **B2**.1445–6
  Q fever, **B2**.2077
  rapidly growing mycobacteria, **B2**.1244
  restriction endonuclease analysis (REA),
    Malassezia, **M**.215
  Rickettsia and *Orientia,* **B2**.2036
  sample type
    blood, **B1**.559–60
    cerebrospinal fluid, **B1**.559
    fecal samples, **P**.151
    target DNA quantity, **B1**.725
  sarcocystosis, **P**.449
  Shigella, **B2**.1391
  Stenotrophomonas maltophilia, **B2**.1637
  Streptobacillus moniliformis, **B2**.1911
  Streptococcus pyogenes, **B2**.858
  Toxocara infection, **P**.751
  toxoplasmosis, **P**.435
  Trichomonas vaginalis infection, **P**.261
  Tropheryma whippelii, **B2**.999, **B2**.1000–2
  Tropheryma whipplei, **B2**.1147–8
  Trypanosoma cruzi genetic diversity,
    P.382–3
  tularemia, **B2**.1754
  type
    broad-range bacterial, **B1**.726 (Tab.)
    modifications, **B1**.726–7, **B1**.726 (Tab.)
    multiplex, **B1**.726 (Tab.)
    nested, **M**.491, **B1**.726 (Tab.), **B2**.1147–8
    quantitative, **B1**.191, **B1**.726 (Tab.)
    quantitative competitive, **B1**.726 (Tab.)
    real-time *see* Real-time polymerase chain
      reaction (RT-PCR)
    repetitive element sequence-based,
      B1.726 (Tab.)
    RFLP, **B1**.207
    semi nested, **B2**.1147
    semiquantitative or limiting dilution,
      B1.726 (Tab.)
    in situ, **B1**.726 (Tab.)
  yellow fever, **V2**.1000
  Yersinia, **B2**.1463–5
Polymerase (Pol) protein *see* Pol (polymerase)
  protein
Polymeric bioparticles, DNA vaccine delivery,
  I.918
Polymeric IgA, mucosal immune response,
  I.524–5
Polymeric IgM, mucosal immune response,
  I.524–5
Polymeric substrate particles (PLSP), **I**.831
Polymers, cellular, **B1**.42

Poly-methylmethacrylate (PMMA) beads,
  B1.699–700, **B1**.700 (Fig.)
Polymorphida, **P**.598
Polymorphidae, **P**.598
Polymorphism information content (PIC),
  linkage, **I**.573
Polymorphisms, genetic *see* Genetic
  polymorphisms
Polymorphonuclear leukocytes (PMNLs)
  acute phase response, **I**.206–7
  complement receptor 1, **I**.151
  histoplasmosis capsulati, **M**.525
  paracoccidioidomycosis, **M**.551
  phagocytosis of *Histoplasma capsulatum* var.
    capsulatum, **M**.525
  respiratory burst, **M**.525
  respiratory tract, **B1**.608
  see also Eosinophil(s); Neutrophil(s)
Polymyxin(s), **B1**.496–7
  mode of action, **B1**.496
  pharmacology, **B1**.496
  resistance, **B1**.496
  spectrum of activity, **B1**.496
    Listeria, **B2**.957–8
    Serratia, **B2**.1488–9
  structure, **B1**.496, **B1**.497 (Fig.)
  toxicity/adverse effects, **B1**.497
  see also specific types
Polymyxin B, spectrum of activity,
  B1.499 (Tab.)
Polymyxin E *see* Colistin (polymyxin E)
Polymyxin-lysozyme-EDTA-thallous acetate
  (PLET) agar, *Bacillus anthracis,* **B2**.934,
  B2.948
Polynuclear aromatic compounds,
  bioremediation, **B1**.201
Polyomaviridae
  classification, **V1**.27 (Tab.), **V1**.43 (Tab.),
    V1.45
  see also Polyomaviruses; *specific viruses*
Polyomaviruses, **V1**.473–87
  cell entry, **V1**.213, **V1**.473–4
  genome, **V1**.151, **V1**.473–4
    DNA regulatory sequence, **V1**.474
  genome replication, **V1**.151 (Fig.)
    host-cell polymerases, **V1**.147–8
  historical aspects, **V1**.150–1
  host cell interaction, S-phase entry, **V1**.217,
    V1.218
  human, **V1**.474–83
  large T antigen, **V1**.218
  middle T antigen, **V1**.336
  protein transcription, **V1**.473–4
  protein translation mechanisms, **V1**.114–15
  replication, **V1**.150–4
  T-antigen, **V1**.473–4
  in vitro replication systems, **V1**.151
  see also Polyomaviridae; specific viruses
Polyomavirus infection, **V1**.473–4
  bone marrow transplants, **V2**.1509
  cell surface receptors, **V1**.473–4
  early phase, **V1**.474
  immunodeficient patients (non-HIV),
    V2.1509–10
  late phase, **V1**.474
  nonproductive infection, **V1**.205–6

Polyomavirus infection (*Continued*)
  oncogenesis, **V1**.338 (Tab.)
    mechanisms, **V1**.342 (Tab.)
  species infected, **V1**.473
  T antigen, **V1**.473–4
Polyomavirus transcription, **V1**.180
Polyoma virus vaccine, **I**.840
Polyphasic taxonomy, **B1**.22 (Tab.), **B1**.26,
  B1.30, **B1**.33
Poly(A)polymerase, poxviruses, **V1**.599 (Tab.)
Polyp(s), rhinosporidiosis *see* Rhinosporidiosis
Polyribosomes, **P**.175–6
Polysaccharide B, *Brucella*, **B2**.1724, **B2**.1728
Polysaccharide intercellular adhesin (PIA)
  synthesis, biofilm formation, **B1**.149–50
Polysaccharides
  Brucella, **B2**.1726–8
  discovery/history, **B1**.12
  vaccines *see* Subunit vaccines
Polysomes, **P**.175–6
Polysorbates, **B1**.425, **B1**.432
Polythetic class, viral species, **V1**.31–2,
  V1.32 (Fig.)
n-3 Polyunsaturated fatty acids, **I**.197
n-6 Polyunsaturated fatty acids, **I**.197
Pomovirus, **V1**.27 (Tab.)
Pontiac fever, **B1**.635
  clinical findings, **B2**.1765
  history, **B2**.1761–4
  mode of spread, **B1**.188
  see also Legionella pneumophila;
    Legionellosis
Pony bites, *Pasteurella caballi* infection,
  B2.1657
Pooled human immunoglobulin, **V2**.1566
Populations
  classification, **I**.954–5
  definition, **I**.953
  individual *vs.*, **I**.948
Population, world estimates, **B1**.360 (Fig.)
Porcine astrovirus (PAstV)
  cell culture, **V2**.906
  classification, **V2**.890 (Tab.)
  genome, **V2**.894 (Tab.)
  virion-associated proteins, **V2**.891
Porcine circovirus 1, **V1**.41
Porcine endogenous retrovirus (PoEV),
  xenotransplantation risk, **V2**.1297
Porcine epidemic diarrhea virus (PEDV)
  accessory proteins, **V1**.835–6
  infection, **V1**.841 (Tab.)
Porcine hemagglutinating encephalomyelitis
  virus (HEV)
    hemagglutinin-esterase (HE), **V1**.838–9
    infection, **V1**.841 (Tab.)
Porcine parvovirus (PPV), **B1**.434
  allotropic specificity, **V1**.422
  infection, **V1**.426
  morphology/structure, **V1**.412
  pathogenic potential, **V1**.422
Porcine reproductive and respiratory syndrome
  virus (PRRSV), **V1**.825, **V1**.847–8
    classification, **V1**.53, **V1**.392
    genome
      non-translated region, **V1**.827
      subgenomic RNA, **V1**.831–2

glycoproteins, **V1**.827
  GP$_2$ glycoprotein, **V1**.839
  GP$_4$ glycoprotein, **V1**.836 (Tab.)
    antibodies, **V1**.840
  infection, **V1**.841 (Tab.), **V1**.847–8
    diagnosis, **V1**.847–8
    emerging infection, **V2**.1651 (Tab.)
    neutralizing antibodies, **V1**.847
    transmission, **V1**.847
    vaccines, **V1**.847–8
  major surface glycoprotein (MSG), **V1**.838
  nucleocapsid (N) protein, **V1**.836–7
  replicase (RNA polymerase), **V1**.833 (Fig.)
Porcine respiratory coronavirus (PRCoV),
  V1.824–5
    morphology/structure, **V1**.76 (Fig.)
Porcine rubellavirus, **V1**.382–3
Porcine rubulavirus, **V1**.744
Porcine teschovirus, **V1**.50–2
Porcine torovirus (PToV)
  infection, **V1**.841 (Tab.)
  tissue culture, **V1**.846
Pore-forming toxins
  apoptosis modulation, **I**.654–5
  Pasteurella haemolytica, **I**.654–5
Porins, **B1**.43
  Aeromonas, **B2**.1528–9
  β-lactam antibiotics resistance, **B1**.473
  Brucella, **B2**.1724, **B2**.1728
  Burkholderia, **B2**.1613
  Helicobacter, **B2**.1569
  Neisseria, **B2**.1280–2
  Pseudomonas aeruginosa, **B2**.1592–3,
    B2.1600
Porphyrin test, *Haemophilus*, **B2**.1701
Porphyromonas, **B2**.1924 (Tab.), **B2**.1926–9
  antibacterial susceptibility/resistance,
    B2.1930–1, **B2**.1935–6
    mechanisms, **B2**.1935
  antigens, **B2**.1936–7
  cell wall composition, **B2**.1915
  classification, **B2**.1913–17
    criteria, **B2**.1914–15
    phylogenetic tree, **B2**.1917 (Fig.)
    rRNA sequence analysis, **B2**.1915–17
  infection
    gingivitis, **B1**.614
    oral cavity abscess, **B1**.618
  molecular analysis, **B2**.1931–2
  normal microbiota, **B1**.296 (Tab.), **B1**.301,
    B2.1932–4
  oral cavity, **B1**.609, **B2**.1933
  pathogenicity, **B2**.1936–8
  pigment production, **B2**.1916 (Fig.), **B2**.1926
  see also individual species
Porphyromonas asaccharolytica,
  B2.1924 (Tab.), **B2**.1926–7
  normal microbiota, **B2**.1934
Porphyromonas cangingivalis, **B2**.1924 (Tab.),
  B2.1927
Porphyromonas canoris, **B2**.1924 (Tab.),
  B2.1927
Porphyromonas cansulci, **B2**.1924 (Tab.),
  B2.1927
Porphyromonas catoniae, **B2**.1924 (Tab.),
  B2.1927

Porphyromonas circumdentaria,
  B2.1924 (Tab.), **B2**.1928
Porphyromonas crevioricans, **B2**.1924 (Tab.),
  B2.1928
Porphyromonas endodontalis, **B2**.1924 (Tab.),
  B2.1928
Porphyromonas gingivalis, **B2**.1924 (Tab.),
  B2.1928
  immune evasion
    antibody degradation/modification, **I**.662
    complement cleavage, **I**.663–4
    nonlysosomal organelles, **I**.650
  infection, gingivitis, **B1**.614
  normal microbiota, **B2**.1932
  pathogenicity, **B2**.1936–8
    adhesion, **B2**.1937
    environmental factors, **B2**.1936
    exotoxins, **B2**.1937
    invasion, **B2**.1937–8
    LPS, **B2**.1936–7
    neutrophil and monocyte responses,
      B2.1938
    proteases/protease inhibitors, **B2**.1938
  TLR-2 LPS receptor, **I**.119
  vaccines
    BCE peptide vaccines, **I**.855 (Tab.)
    development status, **I**.933 (Tab.)
Porphyromonas gingivicans, **B2**.1928
Porphyromonas gulae, **B2**.1924 (Tab.)
Porphyromonas levii, **B2**.1928–9
  distinguishing feature, **B2**.1924 (Tab.)
Porphyromonas macacae, **B2**.1924 (Tab.),
  B2.1929
Porpoise morbillivirus (PMV), **V1**.712–13
Portal hypertension, liver fluke infection, **P**.649
Posaconazole, **M**.155
  Acremonium infection, **M**.758
  fusariosis, **M**.755
  histoplasmosis capsulati, **M**.531
  Paecilomyces infection, **M**.758
  phaeohyphomycosis, **M**.745
  Scedosporium, **M**.757
  systemic zygomycosis, **M**.677–8
Posadas, A, **M**.24–6
Positive elongation factor, poxviruses,
  V1.599 (Tab.)
Positive selection model
  αβ TCRs, **I**.456
  B cell development, **I**.491
  CD4 T cells development, **I**.390, **I**.392
  NK cell development, **I**.93
  T cells, **I**.379
Positive-strand RNA viruses *see* RNA viruses,
  positive-strand
Positron emission tomography (PET), **I**.360
Pospiviridae, **V1**.54 (Tab.)
Post-abortion pelvic inflammatory disease,
  Chlamydia trachomatis infection,
  B2.2012
Post-bypass syndrome, **I**.157
Post-exposure prophylaxis, rabies, **V2**.1127
Postgonococcal urethritis, *Chlamydia
  trachomatis* infection, **B2**.2011
Post-herpetic neuralgia, **V1**.514, **V1**.515
Postinfectious encephalitis (PIE) *see* Measles

Postinfectious encephalomyelitis, mumps, **V1**.748, **V1**.749–50

Post kala-azar leishmaniasis (PKDL) *see* Leishmaniasis, Old World

Postnatal infection
  HCMV infection, **V2**.1450
  Hepatitis B virus, **V2**.1476
  see also Neonatal infection

Postneuritic optic atrophy, onchocerciasis, **P**.793–4

Postoperative enterocolitis, **B2**.1119

Postoperative infection, **B1**.374–5, **B1**.384–5
  prevention, **B1**.387–8
  see also specific infection

Post-polio syndrome, **V2**.870, **V2**.1423

Post-replication recombination, DNA repair, **B1**.451–2

Post-segregational killing *see* Plasmid(s)

Post-translational modification, recombinant gene expression, **B1**.123

Posttranslational modifications
  arterivirus replicase, **V1**.832, **V1**.834
  Borna disease virus glycoprotein (G), **V2**.1142
  bunyavirus glycoproteins, **V2**.1038
  coronavirus replicase, **V1**.832, **V1**.834
  foamy virus core antigen (GAG), **V2**.1310
  foamy virus envelope antigens, **V2**.1307
  Hepatitis C virus E2 protein, **V2**.1195, **V2**.1196
  Hepatitis C virus NS2 protein, **V2**.1195
  Hepatitis C virus NS3 protein, **V2**.1195
  Hepatitis delta virus replication, **V2**.1270
  large T antigen, **V1**.152–3
  picornaviruses, **V2**.867–8
  positive-strand RNA viruses, **V1**.140
  rhabdovirus glycoprotein (G), **V2**.1115
  Rubella virus proteins, **V2**.964
  torovirus replicase (RNA polymerase), **V1**.832

Postviral fatigue syndrome (myalgic encephalomyelitis), **V2**.871

Potamon, **P**.646

Potassium cyanide growth, Enterobacteriaceae identification, **B2**.1319 (Tab.)

Potassium hydroxide, **M**.87, **M**.88 (Tab.), **M**.235

Potassium iodide
  pythiosis, **M**.425
  sporotrichosis, **M**.28, **M**.368–9, **M**.379
  zygomycosis, **M**.352

Potassium metabolism, *Plasmodium,* **P**.477

Potatoes, spoilage, **B1**.267

Potato leafroll virus, **V1**.15–6

Potato yellow dwarf virus (PYDV), **V2**.1105

Potential transmission, effective reproduction number *(R),* **I**.956

Potexvirus, **V1**.27 (Tab.)

Potyviridae, **V1**.27 (Tab.), **V1**.51 (Tab.), **V1**.52
  see also specific viruses

Poult enteritis mortality syndrome (PEMS), **V2**.904–5

Poultry, **B1**.276–8
  chicks and poults, **B1**.276–7
  infection
    Pasteurella gallinarum, **B2**.1654
    Pasteurella multocida, **B2**.1653–4

infection, waterborne bacteria, **B1**.212, **B1**.218, **B1**.223–4

normal microbiota, **B1**.277–8, **B2**.1934

predominant pathogens, **B1**.276

preservation
  ionizing radiation, **B1**.271–2, **B1**.278
  oxygen-impermeable films, **B1**.277–8

production, **B1**.276–8
  bacterial resistance emergence, **B1**.363
  carbon dioxide in atmosphere, **B1**.277–8
  chilling, **B1**.277
  dressing procedures, **B1**.277
  feed, **B1**.276–7
  killing after purchase, **B1**.277
  live, **B1**.277
  modern slaughter operations, **B1**.277
  new stock quarantine, **B1**.276
  plucking (picking), **B1**.277
  post-evisceration washing, **B1**.277
  scalding, **B1**.277
  stress, **B1**.277
  transmission of microorganisms between birds, **B1**.277
  washing, **B1**.277

safety assurance, **B1**.288–9
  government reforms, **B1**.289

Salmonella infection
  breeder stock feed, **B1**.276
  chick and poults colonization, **B1**.276–7
  eggs, internal contamination, **B1**.276
  improvement programs, **B1**.276
  irradiation, **B1**.278
  litter, **B1**.277
  live poultry and symptomless excreters, **B1**.277
  new stock quarantine, **B1**.276
  other sources, **B1**.276
  safety assurance, **B1**.289
  slaughter operations, **B1**.277

spoilage causes, **B1**.277–8

Poultry barns, airborne bacteria, **B1**.189

Povidone-iodine solutions, **B1**.425

Powassan virus, **V2**.998 (Tab.), **V2**.1004

Poxviridae
  characteristics, **V1**.177 (Tab.)
  classification, **V1**.26, **V1**.27 (Tab.), **V1**.42–4, **V1**.43 (Tab.), **V1**.579 (Tab.), **V1**.582, **V1**.594
  taxonomy, **V1**.595 (Tab.)
  see also Poxviruses; *specific viruses*

Poxviruses, **V1**.594–633, **V1**.578–93
  apoptosis inhibition, **V1**.603 (Fig.), **V1**.624–5
    MC66, **V1**.624
    MC159R, **V1**.624–5
  bioterrorism, **V1**.581, **V1**.589–90
  BIR serine/threonine protein kinase, **V1**.605
  capping enzyme, **V1**.599 (Tab.)
  cell-associated enveloped virus, **V1**.596–7
    maturation, **V1**.612–14
  characteristics, **V1**.578
  classification, **V1**.582, **V1**.594–600
    conserved genes, **V1**.594–5, **V1**.603–4, **V1**.606
    distinguishing features, **V1**.594
    historical aspects, **V1**.26

new genera, **V1**.582

conserved genes, **V1**.583

cytoplasmic replication, **V1**.600, **V1**.601–2, **V1**.607–8

directed mutagenesis, **V1**.183–4

DNA structure, **V1**.600–1
  concatemeric intermediates, **V1**.600, **V1**.602, **V1**.605 (Fig.)
  terminal inverted sequence region, **V1**.601, **V1**.602–3, **V1**.603 (Fig.), **V1**.606 (Fig.)

enzymes, **V1**.599 (Tab.)
  see also specific enzymes

epidermal growth factor (EGF), **V1**.257

extracellular enveloped virus, **V1**.596–7, **V1**.613 (Fig.)
  intracellular mature virus *vs.,* **V1**.597
  maturation, **V1**.612–14

gene expression
  regulation, **V1**.607–12
  temporal control, **V1**.118–19

genetic manipulation, **V1**.615–17
  marker rescue mapping, **V1**.615–16
  mutant construction, **V1**.616
  protein overexpression, **V1**.616–17
  reverse genetics, **V1**.615–16
  transient protein expression, **V1**.617
  vaccine vectors, **V1**.617

genome replication, **V1**.123, **V1**.168–9, **V1**.601–3
  A20 protein, **V1**.169 (Tab.)
  A48 protein (thymidylate kinase), **V1**.169 (Tab.)
  A50 protein, **V1**.169 (Tab.)
  B1 protein, **V1**.168–9, **V1**.169 (Tab.)
  concatemeric intermediates, **V1**.169
  D4 protein, **V1**.169 (Tab.)
  D5 protein, **V1**.168–9, **V1**.169 (Tab.)
  DNA biosynthesis, **V1**.217
  DNA ligase, **V1**.168, **V1**.605–6
  DNA polymerases, **V1**.147–8, **V1**.168, **V1**.169 (Tab.), **V1**.603–4
  dUTPase, **V1**.169 (Tab.)
  E9 protein, **V1**.168–9
  enzymes, **V1**.603–6
  genes, **V1**.607 (Tab.)
  H6 protein (topoisomerase), **V1**.169 (Tab.)
  initiation, **V1**.602
  J2 protein (thymidine kinase), **V1**.169 (Tab.)
  origins of replication, **V1**.168
  processivity factors, **V1**.168
  protein kinases, **V1**.168
  protein phosphatase, **V1**.168
  recombination, **V1**.606
  ribonucleotide reductase, **V1**.169 (Tab.)
  topoisomerase, **V1**.168–9
  viral proteins, **V1**.168–9, **V1**.169 (Tab.)

genome sizes, **V1**.583

genome structure, **V1**.168, **V1**.596 (Fig.)
  gene structure, **V1**.601
  promoters, **V1**.607

glutaredoxin, **V1**.598–600

growth cycle, **V1**.596 (Fig.)

historical aspects, **V1**.578–9

Poxviruses (*Continued*)
  host range control, **V1**.595, **V1**.603 (Fig.),
    V1.623–4
    CHOHR genes, **V1**.624
    E3L gene, **V1**.620, **V1**.624
    K3L gene, **V1**.620, **V1**.624
    serpin SP-1, **V1**.623–4
  hosts, **V1**.578
  host shutoff, **V1**.612
  identification, **V1**.583
    PCR, **V1**.583
  immune evasion, **V1**.199, **V1**.595,
    V1.603 (Fig.), **V1**.617–23, **V1**.619
    antigen presentation, **V1**.229–30, **V1**.619,
      V1.622–3
    apoptosis interference, **V1**.287
    caspase inhibitors, **I**.627
    chemokine receptor homologues, **I**.622
    chemokines, **V1**.288, **V1**.619, **V1**.622
    complement, **V1**.230, **V1**.287, **V1**.313,
      V1.619–20, **I**.639
    cytokine receptor analogues, **V1**.229–30,
      V1.287, **V1**.314–15, **V1**.318–19, **I**.620,
      V1.620–1, **I**.621
    cytokines, **V1**.288, **V1**.298 (Tab.), **V1**.316–
      17, **V1**.619, **I**.620, **V1**.621–3
    cytotoxicity blocking, **I**.483
    death-receptor inhibitors, **I**.626–7
    3β-Hydroxysteroid hydrogenase, **V1**.622
    IFN binding proteins, **V1**.230, **I**.619
    IL-1β, **V1**.621
    IL-18 binding proteins, **V1**.314–15,
      V1.318–19, **V1**.620–1
    INFs, **V1**.199, **V1**.230, **V1**.286–7, **V1**.619,
      V1.620
    macrophage avoidance, **I**.30
    MHC control, **V1**.619
    mitochondrial apoptosis inhibitors, **I**.627
    semaphorin, **V1**.622–3
    serpins, **V1**.623
    TNF-α, **V1**.621–2
    viral TNF-α receptor, **V1**.287
  infection *see* Poxvirus infection
  intracellular enveloped virus, **V1**.596–7,
    V1.613 (Fig.)
  intracellular mature virus, **V1**.597–600,
    V1.613 (Fig.)
    electron microscopy, **V1**.597
    envelope, **V1**.597
    enzyme content, **V1**.598–600
    extracellular enveloped virus *vs.*, **V1**.597
    maturation, **V1**.612–14
    membrane formation, **V1**.614–15
    precursors, **V1**.612–14
    wall composition, **V1**.597–8
  intracellular nucleotide pool conservation,
    V1.606
  isolation/propagation and identification,
    V1.96 (Tab.), **V1**.100
  late transcription factors, **V1**.599 (Tab.)
  medically significant, **V1**.594
  morphogenesis, **V1**.612–15
    membrane formation, **V1**.614–15
    viral DNA packaging, **V1**.615
  mRNA capping, **V1**.609
    D1R gene, **V1**.609

D12L gene, **V1**.609
    enzymes, **V1**.599 (Tab.)
    J3R gene, **V1**.609
  mRNA polyadenylation
    E1L gene, **V1**.609
    enzymes, **V1**.599 (Tab.)
  myxoma growth factor (MGF), **V1**.257
  negative elongation factor, **V1**.599 (Tab.)
  nomenclature, **V1**.595–6
  NTPase, **V1**.603–5
  nucleoside-2'-*O*-methyltransferase,
    V1.599 (Tab.)
  nucleoside phosphohydrolase I,
    V1.599 (Tab.)
  packaging, **V1**.169
  phylogenetic relationships, **V1**.583–6
    conserved genes, **V1**.583–5
    genome size, **V1**.583
  poly(A)polymerase, **V1**.599 (Tab.)
  positive elongation factor, **V1**.599 (Tab.)
  protein kinases, **V1**.598–600
  protein phosphatase, **V1**.598–600
  replication, **V1**.217
    in cytoplasm, **V1**.112
  resolvase, **V1**.606
  ribonucleotide reductase, **V1**.606
  RNA helicase, **V1**.598–600
  RNA polymerases, **V1**.599 (Tab.), **V1**.608–9
    structural forms, **V1**.608–9
  RNA turnover, **V1**.612
  serine/threonine protein kinase, **V1**.603–4
  thiol oxidoreductases, **V1**.598–600
  thymidine kinase, **V1**.606
  thymidylate kinase, **V1**.606
  TNF receptors, **V1**.257
  topoisomerase, **V1**.598–600, **V1**.606
  transcription, **V1**.607–12
    early genes, **V1**.609–10
    intermediate genes, **V1**.610–11
    late genes, **V1**.611–12
    mRNA capping *see above*
    polyadenylation, **V1**.609
    regulation, **V1**.607
    temporal measurement, **V1**.607,
      V1.608 (Fig.)
  uracil DNA glycosylase, **V1**.603–5
  as vaccine vector, **I**.897–8
  viral early transcription factor (VETF),
    V1.599 (Tab.), **V1**.610
    packaging, **V1**.611
  'viral factories,' **V1**.612–14, **V1**.612 (Fig.)
  viral intermediate transcription factors
    (VITF), **V1**.599 (Tab.), **V1**.609–10,
    V1.610–11
    D1R/D12L capping enzyme, **V1**.610–11
    transcription, **V1**.610
  viral late transcription factors (VLTF),
    V1.599 (Tab.), **V1**.610, **V1**.611
  viral termination factor (VTF),
    V1.599 (Tab.), **V1**.610
  virion structure, **V1**.586, **V1**.596–7,
    V1.598 (Fig.)
    see also specific types
  'viroplasm,' **V1**.612–14
  virulence, genes of cellular origin, **V1**.257
  see also Poxviridae; specific viruses

Poxvirus infection, **V1**.241 (Tab.)
  antiviral therapy, **V1**.590, **V2**.1631
    cidofovir, **V2**.1616
  cell interactions, **V1**.220
  diseases, **V1**.586–9
    see also specific diseases/infection
  immune response, IFN-γ, **I**.260 (Tab.),
    V1.620
  receptor-mediated endocytosis, **V1**.216–17
  transmission, **V1**.371 (Tab.)
  tumors associated, **V1**.257, **V1**.332 (Tab.)
PR-39 *see* Cathelicidins
Praomys, arenaviruses associated,
    V2.1060 (Tab.), **V2**.1061
Prawns, **B1**.279–80
Praziquantal
  clonorchiasis, **P**.654
  cystic echinococcosis, **P**.698–9
  cysticercosis, **P**.119–20, **P**.697–8
  opisthorchiasis, **P**.654
  schistosomiasis, **P**.125, **P**.607, **P**.622, **P**.635
  tapeworm infection, **P**.664
    Diphyllobothrium latum, **P**.673
    Taenia solium, **P**.669
Pre-BCR *see* B-cell receptor (BCR)
Precipitin reaction, **B1**.719
  aspergillosis, **M**.717
  Streptococcus pneumoniae detection, **B1**.756
Prednisone
  allergic aspergillosis, **M**.718
  PCP, **M**.789–90
Pre-erythrocytic stage, *Plasmodium*, **P**.466–7
Pre-exposure prophylaxis, rabies, **V2**.1127
Pregnancy
  bacterial vaginosis, **B1**.668
  bacteriuria, **B1**.679
  Carrión's disease, **B2**.1889
  Chagas disease, **P**.385
  Chlamydia trachomatis infection, **B2**.2011
  coccidioidomycosis, **M**.508–9, **M**.511
  Group B streptococci colonization, **B1**.668
  Listeria monocytogenes, **B1**.669
  malaria *see* Malaria
  NK cells *see* Natural killer (NK) cells
  Pneumocystis jirovecii colonization, **M**.792
  syphilis, **B2**.1842, **B2**.1856, **B2**.1857
  vaccinations during, **V2**.1562–3
    hepatitis B, **V2**.1562–3
    inactivated poliomyelitis vaccine,
      V2.1562–3
    influenza, **V2**.1562–3
    live oral poliomyelitis vaccine, **V2**.1562–3
    measles, **V1**.736
    measles, mumps and rubella (MMR)
      vaccine, **V2**.1562–3
    Parvovirus B19 virus infection, **V2**.1470
    rubella, **V2**.985
    tetanus, **B2**.1065
    varicella, **V2**.1562–3
  viral infection
    BK virus, **V1**.480–1
    enteroviruses, **V2**.870
    influenza, **V1**.661
    Lassa fever, **V2**.1070
    Parvovirus B19 virus, **V1**.431

Pregnancy
  viral infection (*Continued*)
    Venezuelan equine encephalitis, **V2**.1021
  vulvovaginal candidiasis, **M**.598–9
Preintegration complex (PIC), HIV
  replication, **V2**.1323
Premature infants, vaccination, **V2**.1561–2
Premunition *see* Concomitant immunity
  (premunition)
Prenatal screening, toxoplasmosis, **P**.435
Preoperative preparation
  antiseptic treatment, **B1**.387
  surgical wounds, **B1**.384–5
Pre-patency period, malaria epidemiology,
  P.511
Presbyderma, onchocerciasis, **P**.794 (Fig.)
Preservation, definition, **B1**.421
Pressure, hydrostatic, **B1**.450, **B1**.454
Pressure sores, osteoyelitis *see* Osteomyelitis
Presumed ocular histoplasmosis syndrome
  (POHS), **M**.525
  therapy, **M**.531
Preterm birth, bacterial vaginosis association,
  B1.668
Prevalence
  definition, **B1**.310
  incidence *vs.*, **I**.948, **I**.948 (Fig.)
  period, **B1**.310
  point, **B1**.310
  studies, **B1**.313–14, **B1**.314 (Fig.)
  see also Epidemiology
Prevotella, **B2**.1921–6
  antibacterial susceptibility/resistance,
    B2.1930–1, **B2**.1935–6
    mechanisms, **B2**.1935
  cell wall composition, **B2**.1915
  classification, **B2**.1913–17
    criteria, **B2**.1914–15
    phylogenetic tree, **B2**.1917 (Fig.)
    rRNA sequence analysis, **B2**.1915–16
  distinguishing features, **B2**.1924 (Tab.)
  genus definition, **B2**.1921–6
  infection
    bacterial vaginosis, **B1**.665
    gingivitis, **B1**.614
    oral cavity abscess, **B1**.618
  non-pigmented species, **B2**.1921
  normal microbiota, **B1**.296 (Tab.), **B1**.301,
    B2.1932–4
    oral, **B1**.609, **B2**.1932, **B2**.1933
    vagina, **B2**.1934
  pathogenicity, **B2**.1936–8
  pigments, **B2**.1916 (Fig.), **B2**.1921, **B2**.1932–3
  see also individual species
Prevotella albensis, **B2**.1925
Prevotella bivia, **B2**.911, **B2**.1925, **B2**.1934
Prevotella brevis, **B2**.1925
Prevotella bryantii, **B2**.1925–6
Prevotella buccae, **B2**.1925
Prevotella buccalis, **B2**.1923
Prevotella corporis, **B2**.1923, **B2**.1924 (Tab.)
Prevotella dentalis, **B2**.1925
Prevotella denticola, **B2**.1922, **B2**.1924 (Tab.)
Prevotella disiens, **B2**.1925, **B2**.1934
Prevotella enoeca, **B2**.1925
Prevotella gulae, **B2**.1928

Prevotella heparinolytica, **B2**.1925
Prevotella intermedia, **B2**.1922–3
  adhesion, **B2**.1937
  distinguishing features, **B2**.1924 (Tab.)
  invasion, **B2**.1937–8
  normal microbiota, **B2**.1932, **B2**.1934
Prevotella loescheii, **B2**.1922, **B2**.1924 (Tab.),
  B2.1932
  adhesion, **B2**.1937
Prevotella melaninogenicus, **B2**.1922,
  B2.1924 (Tab.)
  infection
    intracranial abscess, **B1**.584–5
    stomatitis, **B1**.614
  normal microbiota, **B2**.1934
Prevotella nigrescens, **B2**.1922–3, **B2**.1938
  distinguishing feature, **B2**.1924 (Tab.)
Prevotella oralis, **B2**.1923
Prevotella oris, **B2**.1925
Prevotella oulora, **B2**.1925
Prevotella pallens, **B2**.1923, **B2**.1924 (Tab.)
Prevotella ruminicola, **B2**.1925, **B2**.1934
Prevotella salivae, **B2**.1926
Prevotella shahii, **B2**.1926
Prevotella tannerae, **B2**.1924 (Tab.), **B2**.1925
Prevotella veroralis, **B2**.1923
Prevotella zoogleoformans, **B2**.1923–5
Primaquine, **M**.789
  mechanism of action, **P**.478
Primary amebic meningoencephalitis (PAM),
  P.226
  chemotherapy, **P**.236–7
  clinical features, **P**.231
  diagnosis, **P**.234–5
  epidemiology/control, **P**.235–6
  immune response, **P**.232
  pathology, **P**.233, **P**.233 (Fig.)
Primary atypical pneumonia (PAP), **B1**.633
Primary effusion lymphoma, HHV-8 infection,
  V1.550, **V1**.553–4
Primary health care, malaria control, **P**.517–18
Primary infection, cellular immune response,
  I.493–4, **I**.494 (Fig.)
Primary influenza pneumonia, influenza,
  V1.661
Primary intermediate hosts *see* Intermediate
  hosts
Primary lymphoid organs, **I**.504–5
Primates (non-human)
  Balantidium coli infection, **P**.280–1
  Borna disease virus infection, **V2**.1148
  bovine spongiform encephalopathy
    transmission, **V2**.1363
  virus propagation, **V1**.90
Prime-and-realign model, hantavirus
  transcription, **V2**.1035–6
'Prime-boost immunization,' **I**.846–7
  cell-mediated immunity, **I**.846
  DNA vaccines, **I**.846, **I**.919
  HIV vaccines, **I**.846
  influenza virus vectors, **I**.846
  live vaccines, **I**.898–9
  malaria vaccines, **I**.846
  Plasmodium yoelii vaccine, **I**.846
  tuberculosis vaccines, **I**.846
Primoinfection, **I**.9

Prion(s), **V1**.7, **V2**.**1346–400**
  definition, **V2**.1388
  diseases *see* Prion diseases
  gene targeting, **V2**.1354–5
  historical aspects, **V2**.1348–9
  infectivity bioassays, **V2**.1348–9
    incubation time, **V2**.1373 (Fig.)
  lower organisms, **V2**.1387–8
  nerve transport, **V2**.1381–2
  nomenclature introduction, **V2**.1349
  propagation, **V2**.1352–4
    transgenic mice, **V2**.1352
  properties, **V2**.1346–57
  strains, **V2**.1356–7
    disease *vs.*, **V2**.1356
    incubation period differentiation, **V2**.1356
    molecular basis, **V2**.1357
  transgenetics, **V2**.1354–5
    GSS modeling, **V2**.1355
    PrP gene ablation, **V2**.1354–5,
    V2.1356 (Fig.)
  see also Prion protein (PrP)
Prion diseases, **V2**.1361–72
  adaptive immunity, **V2**.1384–6
  Alzheimers disease *vs.*, **V2**.1367
  brain damage, **V2**.1372–3
  CNS spread, **V2**.1382–3
  diagnosis, **V2**.1386–7
    cell culture, **V2**.1387
    inoculating serial dilutions, **V2**.1387
    sodium phosphotungstic precipitation
      detection, **V2**.1386–7
  discovery/historical aspects, **V1**.7
  human disease, **V2**.1347 (Tab.), **V2**.1364–71
    diagnosis, **V2**.1364–5
    epizoonotic, **V2**.1371
    inherited, **V2**.1367–9
    see also Creutzfeldt–Jakob disease (CJD);
      Fatal familial insomnia (FFI);
      Gerstmann–Sträussler–Scheinker disease
      (GSS); Kuru
  immunization, **V2**.1386
  immunology, **V2**.1387
  incubation periods, **V2**.1356
  innate immunity, **V2**.1383–4
    complement, **V2**.1383–4
    macrophages, **V2**.1383
    Toll-like receptors, **V2**.1383
  lymphocytes, **V2**.1374, **V2**.1376–7
    B cells, **V2**.1376–7, **V2**.1379
    deficient mice, **V2**.1376 (Tab.)
    T cells, **V2**.1376
  lymphoid organs, **V2**.1377–9
    follicular dendritic cells, **V2**.1377–8,
    V2.1378 (Fig.), **V2**.1379
    innervation patterns, **V2**.1381,
    V2.1381 (Fig.), **V2**.1382 (Fig.)
    lymphotoxin effects, **V2**.1378,
    V2.1379 (Fig.), **V2**.1380
  lymphotropism, **V2**.1380
  oral administration, **V2**.1373–4
    M cells, **V2**.1374, **V2**.1375 (Fig.)
    Peyer's patches, **V2**.1373, **V2**.1374
  peripheral pathogenesis, **V2**.1373–6
  pre-exposure prophylaxis, **V2**.1384–6
  skin uptake, **V2**.1374–6

Prion diseases (*Continued*)
strain *vs.,* **V2**.1356
sympathetic nerves, **V2**.1380–3
transmission, **B1**.381
spiroplasma association, **B2**.1966
see also Bovine spongiform encephalopathy
(BSE); Chronic wasting disease (CWD)
of deer and elk; Scrapie
Prion protein (PrP), **V1**.7
amyloid, **V2**.1350
disease diagnosis, **V2**.1365
antibodies to, **V2**.1355, **V2**.1384–6,
V2.1385 (Fig.)
autoimmune disease, **V2**.1385
chemical modification, **V2**.1351–2
discovery, **V2**.1349–50
historical aspects/re-evaluation, **I**.6
mutations, **V2**.1369 (Tab.)
E200K mutation, **V2**.1368
familial prion disease, **V2**.1367–9
Gerstmann–Sträussler–Scheinker disease,
V2.1367
polymorphisms, **V2**.1371–2
codon 129, **V2**.1371–2
codon 219, **V2**.1371–2
Prnd gene, **V2**.1350 (Fig.), **V2**.1358–61
conservation, **V2**.1358–9
deficient mice, **V2**.1359
fertility, **V2**.1359–61, **V2**.1361 (Fig.)
functions, **V2**.1359
protein function, **V2**.1359–61
spermatozoa, **V2**.1360–1, **V2**.1360 (Fig.),
V2.1361 (Fig.)
PRNP gene, **I**.589, **V2**.1349–50,
V2.1350 (Fig.)
ablation, **V2**.1354–5, **V2**.1356 (Fig.)
chromosome 20, **V2**.1350
mutations *see above*
polymorphism *see above*
polymorphisms, **I**.589
PrP, **V2**.1372–3
PrP^C, **V2**.1346, **V2**.1388
conversion to PrP^Sc, **V2**.1346–7,
V2.1350–2, **V2**.1355 (Fig.)
discovery, **V2**.1349
functions, **V2**.1357–8
glycosylation, **V2**.1358 (Fig.)
molecular interactions, **V2**.1358
in pathogenesis, **V2**.1372
peripheral nerve expression, **V2**.1380
recirculation, **V2**.1351, **V2**.1351 (Fig.)
structure, **V2**.1352, **V2**.1353 (Fig.),
V2.1354 (Fig.)
PrP^Sc, **V2**.1346, **V2**.1388
discovery, **V2**.1349
formation of, **V2**.1350–2, **V2**.1351 (Fig.)
human disease diagnosis, **V2**.1364
as 'informational molecule,' **V2**.1356
intracellular accumulation, **V2**.1351
monoclonal antibodies, **V2**.1365
in pathogenesis, **V2**.1372
PrP^C conversion, **V2**.1346–7, **V2**.1350–2,
V2.1355 (Fig.)
sodium phosphotungstic precipitation
detection, **V2**.1386–7
structure, **V2**.1352, **V2**.1354 (Fig.)

Western blotting, **V2**.1365
structure, **V2**.1352, **V2**.1353 (Fig.)
electron microscopy, **V2**.1354 (Fig.)
transgenic mice, **V2**.1347–8
see also Prion(s)
Prions, **P**.159, **B1**.434–5
transmission prevention, **B1**.380
Pristinamycin, **B1**.489
Privileged site infection, **B1**.747–8
Prnd gene *see* Prion protein (PrP)
PRNP gene *see* Prion protein (PrP)
Probability, **B1**.316
Probe hybridization, **B1**.725
applications, **B1**.725–6
definition, **B1**.725
Procaine benzypenicillin, *Bacillus anthracis,*
B2.937–8
Procalcitonin, acute phase response, **I**.208
Procalcitonin levels, acute phase response,
B1.740
Procaspase(s)
mitochondria apoptosis, **I**.132
mitochondrial apoptosis, **I**.624
Procercoid larvae, **P**.577
definition, **P**.576
Processivity factors, poxvirus replication,
V1.168
Process validation, sterilization, **B1**.454–5
Procoagulant proteins, acute phase proteins,
I.203–4
Proctitis, *Chlamydia trachomatis* infection,
B2.2012–13
Proctoscopy, in diagnosis, **P**.150 (Tab.)
Procyclic forms, *Trypanosoma brucei,* **P**.357,
P.360
Procyclin, trypanosome expression in vector,
P.357
Productive infection *see* Cell–virus interactions
Productive transformation, cell–virus
interactions, **V1**.205
Proechimys, Leishmania host, **P**.320–1, **P**.326
Proflavine, as mutagen, **B1**.85–6
pro gene, HTLVs, **V2**.1285–7
Proglottids, **P**.661
Echinococcus, **P**.678
Taenia solium, **P**.678
Program assessment, control of disease, **P**.65
Programed cell death (PCD), **B1**.443
Progressive multifocal leucoencephalopathy
(PML), **V1**.477–8, **V2**.1416–18
in AIDS/HIV infection, **V1**.478, **V2**.1416,
V2.1504
causative agent, **V2**.1416
clinical features, **V2**.1417
demyelination, **V1**.477
diagnosis, **V2**.1417–18
quantitative PCR, **V2**.1418
epidemiology, **V2**.1416–17
histopathology, FIG **V1**.473
historical aspects, **V1**.477–8
immunodeficient patients (non-HIV),
V2.1510
immunosuppression, **V1**.477
mortality, **V1**.477
pathogenesis, **V1**.478, **V2**.1416

pathology, **V2**.1417–18
in absence of AIDS, **V2**.1417–18
viral reactivation, **V1**.477
Proinflammatory cytokines, **P**.72 (Tab.), **I**.193,
I.274 (Tab.), **I**.284–92, **V2**.1409
acute phase response, **I**.195–7
candidiasis, **M**.589–90
Chlamydia infection, **B2**.2009
downregulation, IL-4 effects, **I**.280
fascioliasis, **P**.652
live vaccines, **I**.903
production, IL-10 effects, **I**.292–3
septic shock, **I**.697
see also Acute phase response
Pro-inflammatory interleukin(s), **P**.70–2
Projectile vomiting, norovirus infection,
V2.919
Prokaryotes, **B1**.11, **P**.159
cellular components, **P**.160 (Tab.)
eukaryotes differences, **P**.160 (Tab.)
plant relationships *see* Plant–bacteria
interactions
see also individual species
Prokaryotic expression systems, **V1**.92
Prolactin, acute phase response, **I**.208
Proliferating cellular nuclear antigen (PCNA)
HPV replication, **V1**.457
Minute virus of mice replication, **V1**.158–9
papillomavirus infection, **V1**.462
SV40 replication, **V1**.154 (Tab.)
Proliferation, bacterial pathogenicity, **B1**.150–1
Promastigotes, **P**.285–6
Leishmania see Leishmania
metacyclic, **P**.288–9, **P**.291 (Fig.), **P**.292
Promoter genes, **V1**.113, **B1**.126
DNA vaccines, **I**.916
negative-strand RNA viruses, **V1**.132
neurovirulence, **V2**.1407
papillomaviruses, **V1**.454
paramyxoviruses, **V1**.700–1
poxviruses, **V1**.607
Promyelocyte leukemia protein (PML),
arenavirus Z protein binding, **V2**.1068
Proofreading
DNA-dependent DNA polymerases, **V1**.57
DNA virus replication, **V1**.17
RNA-dependent RNA polymerases, **V1**.57,
V1.132–3
RNA virus replication, **V1**.17
Propagated epidemics, emerging viral
infection, **V2**.1661
Propagation of viruses, **V1.86–104**
chick embryos, **V1**.4–5, **V1**.90
historical aspects, **V1**.3–4, **V1**.4–5
laboratory animals, **V1**.90
tissue/organ cultures, **V1**.90
see also specific viruses
Propamidine, **B1**.426
Propamidine isethionate
Acanthamoeba keratitis, **P**.237
microsporidiosis keratoconjunctivitis, **P**.549
Properdin, **I**.143 (Tab.)
alternate pathway activation, **I**.145,
I.145 (Fig.)
deficiency, **I**.152, **I**.770–1
deficiency, meningococcal disease in, **B1**.564

Prophenin-1, **I**.173

Prophenin-2, **I**.173

β-Propiolactone, **V1**.91, **B1**.430

  inactivated vaccines, **V2**.1553

Propionate metabolism, *Fusobacterium,*
  B2.1945, **B2**.1948

Propionibacterium, **B2**.1030–2

  antibacterial susceptibility/resistance,
    B2.1032

    metronidazole, **B1**.495

  cell walls, **B2**.1010 (Tab.), **B2**.1031

  classification, **B2**.1031 (Tab.)

    genus definition, **B2**.1030

  culture, **B2**.1031

  differential characteristics, **B2**.1032 (Tab.)

  glucose phosphorylation, **B1**.50–1

  habitats, **B2**.1031

    dairy products, **B2**.1030–1

  historical perspective, **B2**.1030–1

  isolation, **B2**.1013, **B2**.1031

  morphology, **B2**.1031

  as normal microbiota, **B1**.296 (Tab.), **B1**.303,
    B1.304

  pathogenicity, **B2**.1032

  propionic acid fermentation, **B1**.56

  virulence factors, **B2**.1032

Propionibacterium acidipropionici,
  B2.1031 (Tab.)

Propionibacterium acnes, **B1**.304,
  B2.1031 (Tab.)

  antibacterial susceptibility/resistance,
    B2.1032

  cell wall, **B2**.1031

  culture, **B2**.1031

  differential characteristics, **B2**.1032 (Tab.)

  habitats, **B2**.1031

  infection, **B2**.1030–1

    acne vulgaris, **B2**.1032

    endocarditis, **B1**.533, **B2**.1032

    endophthalmitis, **B1**.603–4

    intracranial abscess, **B1**.586

    subdural empyema, **B1**.591

  morphology, **B2**.1031

Propionibacterium australiense, **B2**.1031 (Tab.)

Propionibacterium avidum, **B1**.304,
  B2.1031 (Tab.)

  cell wall, **B2**.1031

  culture, **B2**.1031

  differential characteristics, **B2**.1032 (Tab.)

  habitats, **B2**.1031

  human disease, **B2**.1030–1

  pathogenicity, **B2**.1032

Propionibacterium cyclohexanicum,
  B2.1031 (Tab.)

Propionibacterium freudenreichii, **B2**.1030,
  B2.1031 (Tab.)

Propionibacterium granulosum, **B1**.304,
  B2.1031 (Tab.)

  culture, **B2**.1031

  differential characteristics, **B2**.1032 (Tab.)

  human disease, **B2**.1030–1

  morphology, **B2**.1031

  pathogenicity, **B2**.1032

Propionibacterium jensenii, **B2**.1031 (Tab.)

Propionibacterium microaerophilum,
  B2.1031 (Tab.)

Propionibacterium modestum, **B1**.56

Propionibacterium pentosoccium, **B1**.56

Propionibacterium propionicum,
  B2.1031 (Tab.)

  cell wall, **B2**.1031

  culture, **B2**.1031

  differential characteristics, **B2**.1032 (Tab.)

  habitats, **B2**.1031

  infection, **B2**.1030–1

  morphology, **B2**.1031

  pathogenicity, **B2**.1032

Propionibacterium propionicus, **B2**.1011–12

Propionibacterium thoenii, **B2**.1031 (Tab.)

Propionic acid, **B1**.422

  fermentations, **B1**.56

Propionic acid bacteria, **B1**.56

Propranolol, α_1-acid glycoprotein binding,
  I.205

Propylene glycol, **B1**.430

Propylene oxide, **B1**.430

3-(trimethoxysilyl)Propyloctadecyldimethyl
  ammonium chloride, **B1**.426

Prosector's wart, **B1**.382

Prospect Hill virus, **V2**.1666 (Tab.)

Prostacyclins, **I**.189

  actions, **I**.189

  biosynthesis, **I**.189

  cell types, **I**.189

  production, **I**.181, **I**.189

Prostacyclin synthetase, **I**.186–7

Prostaglandin(s) (PGs), **I**.187–9

  actions/effects, **I**.188

    acute phase response, **I**.197–8

    smooth muscle contraction, **I**.187

  production, **I**.181, **I**.187–8

    cyclooxygenase type 1, **I**.186

    neutrophils, **I**.45, **I**.46, **I**.187

  receptors, **I**.188–9

  structure, **I**.187

  see also individual types

Prostaglandin D_2, **I**.181, **I**.186–7

Prostaglandin E_2

  actions/effects, **I**.188

    arthritis, **I**.188

    asthma, **I**.188

    B cells, **I**.188

    cytokines, **I**.188

    erythropoiesis, **I**.188

    IFN-γ production, **I**.188

    IL effects, **I**.188

    inflammation, **I**.188

    inflammatory bowel disease, **I**.188

    T cells, **I**.188

    Th2 cells, **I**.188

    TNF-α, **I**.188

  production, **I**.181, **I**.183 (Fig.), **I**.187

    eosinophils, **I**.66

    IL-10 effects, **I**.292–3

    IL-17 effects, **I**.290

Prostaglandin F_2

  cell production, **I**.187

  production, **I**.181

Prostaglandin $F_2\alpha$, **I**.183 (Fig.)

Prostaglandin G_2

  half life, **I**.186–7

production, **I**.181

Prostaglandin H_2

  half life, **I**.186–7

  production, **I**.181

Prostaglandin I_2

  biosynthesis, **I**.183 (Fig.)

  production, **I**.186–7

Prostanoids, biosynthesis, **I**.183 (Fig.)

Prostascint, licensing, **I**.355 (Tab.)

Prostate carcinoma, TCE peptide vaccines,
  I.865 (Tab.)

Prostate gland

  blastomycosis, **M**.489, **M**.495

  cryptococcosis, **M**.648

  specimens, **M**.83 (Tab.)

Prostatitis

  acute, **B1**.673

  chronic, **B1**.673

Prosthesis of antibiotic loaded acylic cement
  (PROSTALAC), **B1**.700

Prosthetic joint infection

  causative pathogens, **B1**.690–1

  challenges, **B1**.684

  clinical features, **B1**.692

  diagnosis

    culture interpretation, **B1**.684, **B1**.695–6

    histology, **B1**.696

    laboratory, **B1**.693

    PCR, **B1**.696

    radiology, **B1**.693–4

    ultrasound, **B1**.694

  epidemiology, **B1**.684–5, **B1**.686 (Tab.)

  inflammatory responses, **B1**.689

  prevention, **B1**.691

  treatment, **B1**.702 (Tab.)

    debridement and excision, **B1**.697

    reconstruction, **B1**.697–8

    systemic antibacterial drugs, **B1**.698–9

Prosthetic valve endocarditis, **B2**.910

Prosthodendrium, **P**.585

Protease(s)

  Aspergillus, **M**.688, **M**.692, **M**.706, **M**.707

  A. fumigatus, **M**.692, **M**.707

  Candida, **M**.100, **M**.103, **M**.583, **M**.584,
    M.587

    C. parapsilosis, **M**.588

    C. tropicalis, **M**.588

  Coccidioides immitis, **M**.504, **M**.506 (Fig.),
    M.509, **M**.514

Protease activities, *Taenia solium,* **P**.682–3

Protease inhibitors, **V2**.1623–5

  acute phase proteins, **I**.200–2

  candidiasis, **M**.267

  CART regime, **V2**.1336

  cestodes, **I**.687

  HIV infection, **V2**.1336

    resistance, **V2**.1336, **V2**.1337 (Fig.)

  mechanism of action, **V2**.1336

  see also specific drugs

Proteases

  Burkholderia thailandensis, **B2**.1624

  Pseudomonas aeruginosa, **B2**.1600–1

  sapoviruses, **V2**.923–4

20S Proteasome, **B1**.47–8

Proteasomes, **I**.410–11
  11-S regulators, **I**.411
  20-S regulators, **I**.411
  antigen processing, **I**.412
  energy-dependence, **I**.411
  IFN-γ effects, **I**.411
  intranasal vaccine delivery, **I**.831
  MHC class I–peptide interactions, **I**.412
  structure, **I**.411
  TNF effects, **I**.411
  vaccines see Vaccine(s)
Protective immunity, **I**.489–90
  extracellular pathogens, **I**.489
  humoral vs. cellular response, **I**.489
  intracellular pathogens, **I**.489
  see also Memory
Protective transfer experiments,
    trichomoniasis, **P**.258
Protegrins see Cathelicidins
Protein(s), **B1**.42
  antibacterial agents, **B1**.438, **B1**.439
  biosynthesis, **B1**.46–8
  Borrelia metabolism, **B2**.1827–8
  cell–virus interactions
    degradation, **V1**.226
    metabolism, **V1**.221–6
    oligomerization, **V1**.224–5
    phosphorylation, **V1**.225
    protein folding, **V1**.224–5
  cleavage, **V1**.225
  degradation, regulation, **B1**.47–8
  folding, **B1**.47–8
  immune response, **I**.375–6, **I**.376 (Tab.)
  metabolism, acute phase response, **I**.207
  overexpression, poxviruses, **V1**.616–17
  SDS-PAGE analysis, **B1**.25
    see also Polyacrylamide gel electrophoresis
      (PAGE)
  secretion, **B1**.160–4, **B1**.162 (Fig.)
    gram-negative bacteria, **B1**.160–1
    inner and outer membrane translocation,
      B1.160–4
    inner membrane translocation, **B1**.160
    regulation, **B1**.48
    Sec machinery, **B1**.160
    SRP-dependent machinery, **B1**.160
    Tat machinery, **B1**.160
    type I, **B1**.160–1, **B1**.162 (Fig.),
      B1.163 (Tab.)
    type II, **B1**.161–2, **B1**.163 (Tab.)
    type III, **B1**.162, **B1**.162 (Fig.), **B1**.163–4,
      B1.163 (Tab.), **B1**.164–5
    type IV, **B1**.162–3, **B1**.162 (Fig.),
      B1.163 (Tab.), **B1**.175
    type V, **B1**.164
  synthesis, **B1**.46–8
    bacteriocins, **B1**.137, **B1**.138
  viral definition, **V1**.25–6, **V1**.25 (Fig.)
Protein A, **B1**.755
  antibody-binding, **I**.661–2
Proteinases
  Trichomonas vaginalis, **P**.257
  Trypanosoma cruzi, **P**.381
Protein-coding genes, herpesviruses, **V1**.493
Protein conservation, *Mononegavirales* order,
    V1.384 (Fig.), **V1**.388

Protein(s), crystalloid densifications, **P**.170–2
Protein C, septic shock therapy, **I**.702–3
Protein folding, isocahedral viruses, **V1**.63–5
Protein G, antibody-binding, **I**.661–2
Protein inhibition, bacteriocins, **B1**.138
Protein inhibitors, *Chlamydia trachomatis*
    infection therapy, **B2**.2020
Protein kinase C
  BCR signaling, **I**.344–5
  Hepatitis B virus, **V2**.1228–9
  neutrophil intracellular signaling, **I**.43
Protein kinase R (PKR)
  HIV infection, **V1**.301
  IFN actions, **V1**.227–8, **V1**.271, **V1**.286–7,
    V1.294–5, **V1**.313–14
  viral infection interference, **V1**.121
Protein kinases, poxviruses, **V1**.168, **V1**.598–
    600
Protein malnutrition, **I**.197
Protein metabolism
  Entamoeba histolytica, **P**.204
  Fasciola hepatica, **P**.644
Protein phosphatase
  poxviruses, **V1**.598–600
  poxvirus replication, **V1**.168
Protein S, 022.44
Protein synthesis
  adenoviruses, **V1**.118
  cell–virus interactions see Cell–virus
    interactions
  Cryptosporidium parvum, **P**.403
  flaviviruses, **V1**.115–16
  Hepacivirus, **V1**.115–16
  orthomyxoviruses, **V1**.114–15
  Pestivirus, **V1**.115–16
  Plasmodium see *Plasmodium*
  polyomaviruses, **V1**.473–4
  positive-strand RNA viruses see RNA
    viruses, positive-strand
Protein tyrosine kinases, BCR signaling,
    I.342–3
Proteinuria, babesiosis, **P**.455
Protein vaccines, mycoplasma, **B2**.1993
Proteobacteria, **B2**.1331 (Fig.), **B2**.1332 (Fig.),
    B2.1532, **B2**.2072–3
Proteolytic cleavage, **V1**.121–2
  flaviviruses, **V1**.121–2
Proteus, **B2**.1435–47
  antibacterial susceptibility/resistance, **B1**.433,
    B2.1441, **B2**.1443–4
    cefamandole resistance, **B2**.1441–3
    β-lactamases, **B2**.1441–4
    nitrofurantoin resistance, **B2**.1441
  antigens, **B2**.1444–5
  anti-swarming agents, **B2**.1438–9
  cell envelope composition, **B2**.1444–5
  characteristics, **B2**.1435
  colonies, **B2**.1439
    Phase A/B/C, **B2**.1439
  culture, **B2**.1436–9
    colonial appearances, **B2**.1439
    media, **B2**.1436
    morphology, **B2**.1345, **B2**.1345 (Tab.)
  definition, **B2**.1435–6
  extracellular products, **B2**.1440

  fimbriae, **B2**.1342–3, **B2**.1436, **B2**.1437–8,
    B2.1446
  flagella, **B2**.1436–9
  habitats, **B2**.1440
  H antigens, **B2**.1444–5
  hemolysins, **B2**.1446, **B2**.1447
  infection
    animals, **B2**.1447
    bacteremia, **B2**.1447
    endophthalmitis, **B1**.603
    intestinal, **B2**.1347
    intracranial abscess, **B1**.585
    keratitis, **B1**.601
    neonatal, **B2**.1447
    nosocomial infection, **B1**.398 (Tab.),
      B1.404–5
    septic lesions, **B2**.1447
    urinary tract, **B2**.1446–7
  isolation/identification, **B2**.1440–1,
    B2.1443 (Fig.)
    biochemical tests, **B2**.1442 (Tab.)
    deoxyribonuclease production, **B2**.1351
    gelatin liquefaction, **B2**.1351
    historical perspective, **B2**.1351
    screening tests, **B2**.1349 (Tab.)
  lactose fermentation, plasmids, **B1**.115
  LPS, **B2**.1444
    Rickettsia homology, **B2**.1444
  metabolism, **B2**.1440
  migration, **B2**.1438
  morphology, **B2**.1436
  as normal microbiota, **B1**.296 (Tab.)
  O antigens, **B2**.1444–5
  pathogenicity, **B2**.1446–7
  peptidoglycan, **B2**.1444
  peritrichate flagella, **B2**.1436
  peritrichous fimbriae, **B2**.1436
  physical and chemical agents susceptibility,
    B2.1441
  proteinase, **B2**.1447
  quorum sensing, **B2**.1436–7
  species, **B2**.1435–6
  sterilization, ionizing radiation, **B1**.271
  swarm cells, **B2**.1437–9
    chemotaxis, **B2**.1438–9
  swarming, **B1**.152, **B2**.1436–9
    cause, **B2**.1438–9
    continuous, **B2**.1438, **B2**.1438 (Fig.)
    discontinuous, **B2**.1438, **B2**.1438 (Fig.)
    factors and genes involved, **B2**.1436–7,
      B2.1437 (Fig.)
    process, **B2**.1436–8
    virulence associated, **B2**.1447
  typing methods, **B2**.1445–6
    bacteriocin typing, **B2**.1445
    bacteriophage typing, **B2**.1445
    Dienes, **B2**.1445, **B2**.1445 (Fig.), **B2**.1446
    PCR, **B2**.1445, **B2**.1446
    P/S, **B2**.1446
    ribotyping with pulsed field gel
      electrophoresis, **B2**.1445, **B2**.1446
  urease, **B2**.1446, **B2**.1447
  vegetative cells, **B2**.1436–9
  virulence factors, **B2**.1439, **B2**.1446–7

Proteus, (Continued)
water
biofilms, **B1**.220
bioremediation, **B1**.212
Proteus hauseri, **B2**.1435–6
biochemical tests, **B2**.1441, **B2**.1442 (Tab.)
EDTA-sensitive metalloproteinase, **B2**.1440
Proteus inconstans see Providencia
alcalifaciens; Providencia stuartii
Proteus mirabilis, **I**.172, **B2**.1435–6
antibacterial susceptibility/resistance,
B2.1441–4
intrinsic, **B2**.1352 (Tab.)
β-lactamases, **B2**.1441–4
biochemical tests, **B2**.1441, **B2**.1442 (Tab.)
EDTA-sensitive metalloproteinase, **B2**.1440
fimbriae, **B2**.1436, **B2**.1446
flagella, genes, **B2**.1436
hemolysins, **B2**.1446, **B2**.1447
HpmA and HlyA, **B2**.1440, **B2**.1447
infection, **B2**.1446, **B2**.1447
burns, **B2**.1447
extraintestinal, **B2**.1346–7
nosocomial infection, **B1**.398 (Tab.)
RA association, **B2**.1447
urinary tract, **B1**.674, **B1**.676–7, **B1**.680,
B2.1446–7
isolation/identification, **B2**.1440–1
biochemical tests, **B2**.1319 (Tab.)
screening tests, **B2**.1349 (Tab.)
typing, **B2**.1445, **B2**.1446
pathogenicity, **B2**.1446–7
physical and chemical agents susceptibility,
B2.1441
swarming, **B1**.152
urease, **B1**.676–7, **B2**.1446, **B2**.1447
virulence factors, **B2**.1446–7
Proteus morganii see Morganella morganii
Proteus myxofaciens, **B2**.1435–6
antibacterial susceptibility/resistance,
B2.1441
biochemical tests, **B2**.1319 (Tab.), **B2**.1441,
B2.1442 (Tab.)
habitats, **B2**.1440
Proteus penneri, **B2**.1435–6
antibacterial susceptibility/resistance,
B2.1441–4
biochemical tests, **B2**.1319 (Tab.), **B2**.1441,
B2.1442 (Tab.)
EDTA-sensitive metalloproteinase, **B2**.1440
Proteus rettgeri see Providencia rettgeri
Proteus vulgaris, **B2**.1435–6
antibacterial susceptibility/resistance,
B2.1441–4
intrinsic, **B2**.1352 (Tab.)
biochemical tests, **B2**.1319 (Tab.), **B2**.1441,
B2.1442 (Tab.)
EDTA-sensitive metalloproteinase, **B2**.1440
identification
DNA–DNA analysis, **B2**.1338
screening tests, **B2**.1349 (Tab.)
infection, **B2**.1447
nosocomial, **B1**.398 (Tab.)
Prothecal olecranon bursitis, **M**.135 (Fig.)
Proticins, **B2**.1445
Protists, **P**.159–60

Protoctista, **M**.4, **M**.44 (Fig.), **M**.49, **M**.50 (Tab.)
Proton-motive force (pmf), **B1**.64, **B1**.69,
B1.438
bacteriocins, **B1**.137–8
Proton pump inhibitors (PPIs), *Helicobacter*
pylori infection treatment, **B2**.1575
Proto-oncogenes, **V1**.330–3
retroviruses, **V1**.335 (Tab.)
role in tumor development, **V1**.336, **V1**.340
Protoplast fusion, **B1**.106
Protoscolices, *Echinococcus granulosus,*
P.681 (Fig.)
Prototheca, **M**.396
antifungal resistance, **M**.402
culture, **M**.402–3
ecology, **M**.396–7
histopathology, **M**.406–7
identification, **M**.404–5
infection *see* Prototheccosis
morphology, **M**.403
sporangia, **M**.403, **M**.404 (Fig.),
M.406 (Fig.), **M**.407 (Fig.)
sporangiospores, **M**.403, **M**.404 (Fig.),
M.406 (Fig.), **M**.407 (Fig.)
physiology, **M**.403–4
Prototheca isolation medium (PIM), **M**.402–3,
M.403 (Tab.), **M**.405
Prototheca moriformis, **M**.401, **M**.403
Prototheca stagnora, **M**.403
Prototheca ulmea, **M**.403
Prototheca wickerhamii, **M**.4, **M.396–411**
AIDS/HIV, **M**.399
culture, **M**.402–5, **M**.405 (Tab.)
ecology, **M**.396–7
histopathology, **M**.128 (Tab.), **M**.135 (Fig.),
M.405 (Fig.), **M**.406, **M**.406 (Fig.),
M.407 (Fig.)
identification, **M**.405, **M**.405 (Tab.), **M**.406
infection
antibiotic therapy, **M**.402
experimental, **M**.401
human infection, **M**.396–7, **M**.397–9
immune response, **M**.401
morphology, **M**.403, **M**.403 (Fig.)
physiology, **M**.403–4
sporangiospores, **M**.406
Prototheca zopferi
sporangia, **M**.407
sporangiospores, **M**.407
Prototheca zopfii, **M**.4, **M.396–411**
animal infection, **M**.396, **M**.399–400
bovine mastitis, **M**.399–400, **M**.407
experimental, **M**.401
culture, **M**.402–3, **M**.405, **M**.405 (Tab.)
ecology, **M**.396–7
histopathology, **M**.128 (Tab.), **M**.142 (Fig.),
M.407, **M**.407 (Fig.)
human infection, **M**.397–8, **M**.398–9, **M**.407
EIAs, **M**.400
see also Prototheccosis
identification, **M**.405, **M**.405 (Tab.)
physiology, **M**.403–4
Prototheccosis, **M.396–411**
animals, **M**.397, **M**.398, **M**.399–400
bovine mastitis, **M**.399–400, **M**.407
cats, **M**.398, **M**.400

dogs, **M**.398, **M**.400, **M**.407
causative agents, **M**.396
clinical presentation, **M**.397–9
cutaneous, **M**.397 (Fig.), **M**.398, **M**.399,
M.401, **M**.402
diarrhoea, **M**.398–9
foot, **M**.397–8
gastrointestinal tract, **M**.398–9
olecranon bursitis, **M**.398, **M**.399, **M**.401
opportunistic, **M**.399, **M**.401
systemic, **M**.399, **M**.401
wound infection, **M**.398, **M**.399, **M**.401
diagnosis, **M**.402–8
histopathology, **M**.128 (Tab.)
epidemiology, **M**.396–7
agriculture/agricultural workers, **M**.397,
M.399
AIDS, **M**.399
dairy farming, **M**.396–7, **M**.399–400
history, **M**.396
immune response, **M**.397–402
immunosuppression, **M**.398, **M**.399, **M**.401
predisposition to, **M**.401
therapy, **M**.401–2
amphotericin B, **M**.402
azoles, **M**.402
fluconazole, **M**.402
Prototypic foamy virus (PFV), **V2**.1295,
V2.1306
gene vectors, **V2**.1314
genome, **V2**.1307–8
transient immunosuppression, **V2**.1295–6
Protozoa
antibacterial susceptibility/resistance, **B1**.434,
B1.445
cellular organization, **P**.160–72
cell membrane, **P**.160–2, **P**.162 (Fig.),
P.168
cyst walls, **P**.165–8, **P**.178–9
cytoplasm, **P**.169–72
cytoplasmic inclusions, **P**.173–81
cytoskeleton, **P**.169–70
inner membranes, **P**.162
micropores, **P**.164, **P**.165 (Fig.),
P.166 (Fig.)
microtubules, **P**.162, **P**.169–72
motility of cytoplasm, **P**.169–70
organelles *see below*
pellicles, **P**.162–4, **P**.163 (Tab.), **P**.164 (Fig.)
subpellicular microtubules, **P**.162,
P.163 (Tab.), **P**.165 (Fig.), **P**.170–2
unique skeletal elements, **P**.169–70,
P.170–2
characteristics/structure, **P**.160–72,
P.161 (Fig.), **P**.186
classification, **P.186–99**
below species level, **P**.192
Corliss' (utilitarian) (1994), **P**.189–90,
P.194–5
currently used, **P**.195–6
genera/species name stability, **P**.190–2
instability in phyla and classes, **P**.190
kingdoms, **P**.189–90
molecular and biochemical, **P**.192–3,
P.195–6

Protozoa
  classification (*Continued*)
    Society of Protozoologists' (1964/1980),
      P.190
    subgenus and subspecies levels, **P**.191,
      P.192
    techniques used in, **P**.284–5
    traditional, **P**.190, **P**.194
    Whittaker's 5 kingdoms, **P**.189–90
  definition, **P**.160, **P**.186–7
  historical aspects, **P.13–8**
    recently discovered species, **P**.18–9
  infection, **P**.187–9
    amebae, **P**.187
    antigenic complexity, **P**.74–5
    chronicity, **P**.74–5
    historical aspects, **P.13–8**, **P**.4–5
    HIV co-infection, **P**.74–5, **P**.298–9, **P**.301
    immune evasion *see* Immune evasion
    infection comorbidities, **P**.97
    nosocomial infection, **B1**.403
    piroplasms, **P**.189
    T helper cell polarization, **P**.73
    *see also individual species; specific diseases/
      infection*
  intracellular, discovery, **P**.13
  invasion processes, **P**.180–1
  locomotion *see* Locomotion, protozoa
  motility *see* Locomotion, protozoa
  nature of, **P**.160, **P**.186–7
  nuclear division, **P**.173
  organelles, **P**.173–81
    endoplasmic reticulum, **P**.174–5
    Golgi-adjunct body, **P**.174, **P**.175 (Fig.)
    Golgi apparatus, **P**.176–7, **P**.177 (Fig.)
    lysosomes, **P**.177
    microbodies, **P**.177–8
    micronemes, **P**.178
    mitochondria, **P**.173–4, **P**.174 (Fig.)
    nuclear pores, **P**.173, **P**.173 (Fig.)
    nucleolus, **P**.173
    nucleus, **P**.172 (Fig.), **P**.173
    ribosomes, **P**.175–6
    vacuoles and storage elements, **P**.179
    wall-forming bodies, **P**.178–9
  origin of name, **P**.160
  parasitic, species included, **P**.187–9
  reproduction, **P.181–5**, **P**.186
    binary fission, **P**.181
    multiple divisions, **P**.181–5, **P**.184 (Fig.)
    rosette-like multiplication, **P**.181
  species number, **P**.186
  surface interactions and penetration,
    P.180–1, **P**.182 (Fig.)
  see also individual species
Protozoa Kingdom, classification, **P**.196
Protozoology
  establishment, **P**.13
  historical aspects, **P**.189–90
Protruding (P) domain, noroviruses, **V2**.913
Providencia, **B2**.1450–2
  antibacterial susceptibility/resistance,
    B2.1452
  antigens, **B2**.1451
  biochemical groups, **B2**.1442 (Tab.), **B2**.1450

  characteristics, **B2**.1435
  classification, **B2**.1450
  definition, **B2**.1450
  differentiating characteristics, **B2**.1450–1
  general properties, **B2**.1450–2
  identification
    screening tests, **B2**.1349 (Tab.)
    typing methods, **B2**.1451
  infection, **B2**.1451–2
    nosocomial, **B1**.398 (Tab.)
  motility, **B2**.1450
  normal microbiota, **B1**.296 (Tab.)
  species, **B2**.1450
Providencia alcalifaciens, **B2**.1450
  antibacterial susceptibility/resistance,
    B2.1452
  biochemical tests, **B2**.1319 (Tab.),
    B2.1442 (Tab.)
  biogroup 3 *see Providencia rustigianii*
  identification, **B2**.1451
  infection, diarrhea, **B2**.1451
*Providencia friedericiana see Providencia
  rustigianii*
Providencia heimbachae, **B2**.1450
  biochemical tests, **B2**.1319 (Tab.),
    B2.1442 (Tab.)
  identification, **B2**.1451
Providencia rettgeri, **B2**.1450
  antibacterial susceptibility/resistance,
    B2.1452
    intrinsic, **B2**.1352 (Tab.)
  biochemical tests, **B2**.1319 (Tab.),
    B2.1442 (Tab.)
  classification, **B2**.1450
  groups, **B2**.1451
  infection, **B2**.1452
Providencia rustigianii (friedericiana), **B2**.1450
  biochemical tests, **B2**.1319 (Tab.),
    B2.1442 (Tab.)
  classification, **B2**.1450
  identification, **B2**.1451
  infection, **B2**.1452
Providencia stuartii, **B2**.1450
  antibacterial susceptibility/resistance, **B1**.433,
    B2.1452
    chlorhexidine resistance, **B1**.442
  biochemical tests, **B2**.1319 (Tab.),
    B2.1442 (Tab.)
  biogroups, **B2**.1442 (Tab.)
  infection, **B2**.1451
  MR/K fimbriae, **B2**.1451
  nosocomial infection, **B1**.398 (Tab.)
  properties, **B2**.1451
  typing, **B2**.1451
Provirus, retroviral, **V1**.7, **V1**.338, **V1**.345
Prozone reaction, syphilis serological tests,
  B2.1846
PrP^C *see* Prion protein (PrP)
PrP^{CJD} *see* Prion protein (PrP), PrP^{Sc}
PrP^{Sc} *see* Prion protein (PrP)
Prunes, spoilage, **B1**.283
Pyronaridine, **P**.506
Psammomys obesus, **P**.303
  eradication of, **P**.118
P-selectin, **I**.505–6
  lymphocyte migration, **I**.506–7, **I**.508 (Tab.)

  platelet-activating factor effects on, **I**.190–1
  Th1 cells, **I**.400
P-selectin glycoprotein ligand-1 (PSGL-1),
  I.506–7, **I**.508 (Tab.)
Pseudallescheria, **M**.19, **M**.20
*Pseudallescheria boydii see Scedosporium
  apiospermum*
Pseudallescheriasis, **M**.19–20
  histopathology, **M**.128 (Tab.)
Pseudoacanthocephalus, **P**.598
Pseudoapolysis, *Diphyllobothrium latum,*
  P.671–2
Pseudobacteremia, **B1**.393
Pseudochaetosphaeronema larense, **M**.391
Pseudocowpox virus, **V1**.588
Pseudodiploid form, retrovirus genome,
  V1.188
Pseudogenes
  Borrelia, **B2**.1823–4
  lyssaviruses, **V2**.1112
Pseudoglobin, **I**.141
Pseudohyphal growth
  histopathology, **M**.88 (Fig.), **M**.89 (Tab.)
  Saccharomyces cerevisiae, **M**.75
Pseudoknots
  arteriviruses, **V1**.827–8
  coronavirus genome, **V1**.827–8
  formation, protein synthesis, **V1**.117,
    V1.117 (Fig.)
Pseudomembranous colitis, **B1**.396–7, **B2**.1119
Pseudomonaceae, cereals, **B1**.284–5
Pseudomonads
  aerobic
    cell envelopes, **B2**.1594
    growth temperatures, **B2**.1595
    habitats, **B2**.1593
    metabolism, **B2**.1598–603
    as opportunistic pathogens, **B2**.1591,
      B2.1593
    plasmids, **B2**.1597
    xenobiotic compounds degradation,
      B2.1598
    see also Pseudomonas
  infection, risk categorization, **B1**.762
  phytopathogenicity, **B1**.202
  poultry, **B1**.277–8
  vegetables, **B1**.281
Pseudomonas
  adhesins, **B1**.149
  airborne bacteria, **B1**.189
    concentrations in facilities, **B1**.186 (Tab.)
  chromopeptides, **B2**.1596
  classification, **B2**.1591–2
    phylogeny, **B2**.1592–3
  conjugation, **B1**.103
  diversity, **B2**.1598
  E. coli phylogenetic relationship, **B2**.1592–3
  fluorescent and non-fluorescent species,
    B2.1591, **B2**.1592
  in foods
    butter, **B1**.250
    fish, **B1**.279
    meat and meat products, **B1**.273
    milk, **B1**.230, **B1**.233
    pH, **B1**.266–7
    poultry, **B1**.277–8

Pseudomonas (Continued)
  glucose catabolism, **B1**.59–60
    oxidative pathway for hexoses, **B1**.59–60
    phosphorylated routes, **B1**.59
  habitats, **B1**.211, **B1**.220, **B1**.224–5, **B2**.1593
  historical perspective, **B2**.1591–3
  identification, **B2**.1592–3
    anaerobic arginine degradation, **B2**.1598
    antigenic epitope, **B2**.1595
    culture characteristics, **B2**.1595–6
    DNA-DNA hybridization studies, **B1**.25,
      B2.1592
    DNA GC content, **B2**.1591, **B2**.1602
    EDTA sensitivity, **B2**.1595
    fatty acids and ubiquinone, **B2**.1597
    incompatibility groups, **B2**.1597
    metabolic diversity, **B2**.1592
    ribosomal RNA groups, **B2**.1592, **B2**.1597
    rRNA, **B2**.1593
    rRNA-DNA hybridization, **B2**.1592–3
    of species, **B2**.1592–3
  infection
    endophthalmitis, **B1**.603
    intracranial abscess, **B1**.585
    keratitis, **B1**.601
    nosocomial, **B1**.376–7, **B1**.401 (Tab.),
      B2.1593
    otitis externa, **M**.247–8
    pneumonia, **B1**.637
  mercury resistance, **B1**.114
  metabolism, **B2**.1598–603
    arginine dihydrolase pathway, **B2**.1598
    carbohydrates, **B2**.1598
    carbon sources, **B2**.1591–2
    catabolic plasmids, **B2**.1597
    fatty acid composition, **B2**.1597
    glucose catabolism *see above*
    nitrification, **B1**.200
    substrate changes and colonization,
      B1.199–200
  monoclonal antibodies, **B2**.1595
  morphology and structure, **B2**.1593–6
    fimbriae/pili, **B2**.1594
    flagella, **B2**.1593
    mesosomes and rhapidosomes, **B2**.1594
    refractile granules, **B2**.1594
    siderophores, **B2**.1596
    ubiquinones, **B2**.1597
  natural competence, **B1**.99
  nomenclature, **B2**.1592
    changes, **B1**.32
  as normal microbiota, **B1**.301
  pigmentation, **B2**.1596–7
    fluorescent, **B2**.1596
    lemonnierin, **B2**.1597
    phenazine, **B2**.1596–7
  plasmids, **B2**.1597
    TOL and NAH, **B2**.1597
  as soil pathogens, **B1**.203
    phytopathogenicity, **B1**.202
  sterilization, ionizing radiation, **B1**.271
  virulence factors, LPSs, **B1**.158–9
  waterborne, **B1**.221
Pseudomonas acidovorans see Delftia
  (Comamonas) acidovorans

Pseudomonas aeruginosa
  active efflux, **B2**.1599–600
  adhesins, **B1**.627
  antibacterial susceptibility/resistance, **B1**.422,
    B1.425–6, **B1**.433, **B1**.438, **B1**.442,
    B1.499 (Tab.), **B2**.1599–600
    aminoglycosides, **B1**.482
    biocide-antibiotic linked, **B1**.444
    biofilms, **B1**.443
    chloramphenicol, **B1**.484
    modification reactions, **B2**.1600
    quinolone resistance, **B1**.492–3,
      B1.493 (Tab.)
    tetracycline resistance, **B2**.1600
  antigenic epitope, **B2**.1595
  aspergillus allergy, **M**.693–4
  bacteriocins, **B1**.136–8
  cellular structure, **B2**.1593–6, **B2**.1598–9,
    B2.1599 (Fig.)
    alginate, **B1**.627
    biofilms, **B1**.149, **B1**.688, **B2**.1594
    fimbriae/pili, **B2**.1594, **B2**.1601
    flagella *see below*
    outer-membrane proteins, **B2**.1592–3,
      B2.1595, **B2**.1599–600
    porins, **B2**.1592–3, **B2**.1600
  culture, **B2**.1594, **B2**.1595
    growth temperatures, **B2**.1595
  in cystic fibrosis, *Burkholderia cepacia* co-
    infection, **B2**.1617
  enterotoxin, **I**.565–6
  exotoxin A, **I**.556 (Tab.)
    as vaccine carrier, **I**.936–7
  exotoxins, **B2**.1600
  57RP strain, **B2**.1594
  flagella, **B2**.1593–4
    genetic control, **B2**.1593–4
    monotrichous cells, **B2**.1598–9,
      B2.1599 (Fig.)
    virulence, **B2**.1601
  genetics, chromosomes, **B1**.81
  habitats, **B1**.215, **B1**.216 (Tab.), **B1**.224–5
  immune evasion
    capsule phase variation, **I**.660–1
    complement cleavage, **I**.663–4
    MHC class II antigen presentation, **I**.659
    phagocytic uptake inhibition, **I**.649
  infection
    agammaglobulinemia, **I**.780
    animal models, **I**.593–4
    bacteremia due, **B1**.521
    blue pus, **B2**.1594
    bone and joint infection, **B1**.690–1
    chronic sinusitis, **B1**.615
    conjunctivitis, **B1**.599
    corneal, **B2**.1600
    in cystic fibrosis, **B1**.399, **B1**.650
    endocarditis, **B1**.526, **B1**.532
    Ig deficiencies, **I**.781–2
    induced apoptosis, **I**.138
    intracranial abscess, **B1**.585
    keratitis, **B1**.601
    leukocyte adhesion deficiency type 1,
      I.47–8
    lung, **B2**.1601
    malignant external otitis, **B1**.618

  neutrophils, **I**.44
  nosocomial infection *see below*
  opportunistic, **B2**.1593, **B2**.1598–600
  otitis media, **B1**.617
  respiratory tract, virulence factors
    promoting, **B1**.627
  spinal epidural abscess, **B1**.593
  vaccines
    BCE peptide vaccines, **I**.855 (Tab.),
      I.873
    development status, **I**.933 (Tab.)
    live vaccine, **I**.903
    see also Nosocomial infection (below)
  iron-dependent repression, **B1**.165–6
  metabolism, **B2**.1598
    alkaline protease, **B1**.650
    catabolite repression, **B1**.73
    elastase, **B1**.650, **B2**.1600–1
    iron scavenging, **B1**.151
    oxidative pathway for hexoses, **B1**.60
    proteases, **B2**.1600–1
  monoclonal antibodies, **B2**.1595
  morphology, **B2**.1593–6
  motility, **B2**.1594
    chemotaxis, **B2**.1594, **B2**.1601
    salicylate effect, **B2**.1594
    swarming, **B2**.1593–5
    swimming, **B2**.1594
    twitching, **B2**.1594, **B2**.1601
  mucoid colonies, **B2**.1595
  as normal microbiota, **B1**.296 (Tab.)
  nosocomial infection, **B1**.372, **B1**.397–9,
    B2.1593
    burns, **B1**.385, **B1**.397–9
    food-borne, **B1**.377
    neonates, **B1**.395
    pneumonia, **B1**.389, **B1**.640–1,
      B1.640 (Tab.),
    sinusitis, **B1**.615
    spread, **B1**.397–9
  Opr F, **B2**.1592–3, **B2**.1600
  phenotypes, **B2**.1594
  pigments, **B1**.650, **B2**.1596–7
  sensory networks, **B1**.165
    quorum-sensing, **B1**.170–2, **B1**.171 (Fig.),
      B2.1602
  signal transduction
    subversion of host cell, **B1**.164
    two-component systems, **B1**.167–8
  superantigens, **I**.556 (Tab.)
  toxins, **B1**.627
  tritrpticin sensitivity, **I**.172
  typing, **B1**.399, **B2**.1602
    bacteriocins, **B2**.1602
    DNA restriction analysis, **B2**.1602
    serology, **B2**.1602
  virulence factors, **B1**.627, **B2**.1600–2
    adhesins, **B1**.149
    biofilms, **B1**.149, **B1**.171–2
    exopolysaccharides, **B1**.154
    type IV pili, **B1**.149
Pseudomonas alcaligenes, **B2**.1591
  metabolism, **B2**.1598
Pseudomonas cepacia see Burkholderia cepacia
Pseudomonas denitrificans, **B1**.200

Pseudomonas diminuta see Brevundimonas diminuta

Pseudomonas fluorescens, **B2**.1591, **B2**.1592, **B2**.1602–3
biological control agent against plant pathogens, **B1**.202–3, **B1**.203–4
biovars, **B2**.1595–7, **B2**.1602–3
culture characteristics, **B2**.1595
denitrification, **B2**.1603
EDTA sensitivity, **B2**.1603
in food, chilling, **B1**.264
genetically engineered, plant frost injury protection, **B1**.198
infection, Crohn's disease, **B2**.1603
oxidative pathway for hexoses, **B1**.59
catabolite repression, **B1**.73
pigment, **B2**.1597, **B2**.1602–3
root population estimates, **B1**.204
slime formation, **B2**.1603
waterborne, **B1**.224–5

Pseudomonas mallei see Burkholderia mallei

Pseudomonas marginalis, **B1**.281

Pseudomonas marginata see Burkholderia gladioli

Pseudomonas mendocina, **B2**.1603
metabolism, **B2**.1598

Pseudomonas pseudoalcaligenes, **B2**.1591, **B2**.1594
metabolism, **B2**.1598

Pseudomonas putida, **B2**.1591, **B2**.1592
culture odor, **B2**.1595
plasmids, **B2**.1597
waterborne, **B1**.224–5

Pseudomonas stutzeri, **B2**.1591, **B2**.1603
culture characteristics, **B2**.1595–6
flagella, **B2**.1593–4
genetic control, **B2**.1593–4
metabolism, **B2**.1598
waterborne, **B1**.224–5

Pseudomonas syringae
genetically engineered, **B1**.198
phytopathogenicity, **B1**.202

Pseudomonas thermotolerans, **B2**.1593

Pseudomycetoma, **M**.138 (Fig.), **M**.385–6, **M**.392, **M**.394
dermatophytic, **M**.232, **M**.238
dermatophytoses *see* Dermatophytoses

Pseudonocardia, **B2**.1150

Pseudo-outbreaks, **B1**.403

Pseudopeptidoglycan (pseudomurein), **B1**.44

Pseudophyllidea, **P**.576–7
Diphyllobothriidae, **P**.576–7
features, **P**.576

Pseudopodia, protozoa, **P**.179

Pseudoramibacter alactolyticus
differential characteristics, **B2**.1029 (Tab.)
pathogenicity, **B2**.1029–30

Pseudoreversion
base pair substitutions, **B1**.86
frame-shift mutations, **B1**.85

Pseudoterranova, **P**.590

Pseudoterranova decipens
classification/morphology, **P**.814, **P**.814 (Fig.)
clinical manifestations, **P**.816
life cycle, **P**.814, **P**.815 (Fig.)
see also Anisakis

Pseudotypes, formation, **V1**.186

Pseudoviridae
classification, **V1**.27 (Tab.), **V1**.46 (Tab.), **V1**.47
infectivity, **V1**.45–6
reverse transcription, **V1**.181–2
see also specific viruses

Psittacosis *see Chlamydia psittaci* infection

Psophora, Venezuelan equine encephalitis virus transmission, **V2**.1010

Psoralens, **B1**.281

Psychiatric units, *Balantidium coli* infection, **P**.279, **P**.281

Psychrophiles
Aeromonas, **B2**.1529
temperature range for growth, **B1**.264

Psychrotrophs
fish and fish products, **B1**.279
meat and meat products, **B1**.273, **B1**.274–5
temperature
freezing, **B1**.269, **B1**.270
range for growth, **B1**.264
vegetables, **B1**.282

pTP, adenoviruses replication, **V1**.149 (Tab.), **V1**.161

PU.1, B cell development, **I**.324

Public health importance, **P**.105 (Tab.)
babesiosis, **P**.454
Chagas disease, **P**.389
emerging bacterial infection, **B1**.364

Public Health Laboratory Service (PHLS), Meningococcal Reference Unit, **B1**.322

Public–private partnerships, parasite control, **P**.103–6, **P**.110

PubMed, **B2**.1339

pUC cloning vectors, **B1**.120

Puerperal fever, **B2**.910

Pulex irritans, **B2**.2037

Pullunase secretion system, **B1**.48

Pulmonary arterio-venous (AV) malformations, **B1**.583

Pulmonary ascariasis, **P**.726

Pulmonary aspergillosis *see* Aspergillosis

Pulmonary blastomycosis, **M**.489, **M**.490–2, **M**.497

Pulmonary cryptococcosis *see* Cryptococcosis

Pulmonary edema
babesiosis, **P**.454
falciparum malaria, **P**.482
malaria in pregnancy, **P**.484, **P**.484 (Fig.)

Pulmonary function tests, PCP diagnosis, **M**.788

Pulmonary involvement, infective endocarditis, **B1**.535

Pulmonary sporotrichosis, **M**.367, **M**.375

Pulmonary zygomycosis, **M**.20–1, **M**.674, **M**.674 (Tab.), **M**.678

Pulse-field gel electrophoresis (PFGE), **B1**.81
Cryptosporidium parvum, **P**.403
epidemiological strain typing, **B1**.735–6
hospital acquired infection investigation, **B1**.404–5
Malassezia, **M**.215
species detected
Bordetella, **B2**.1792–3
Campylobacter, **B2**.1549

Enterobacteriaceae typing, **B2**.1352
Enterococcus, **B2**.894
Legionella, **B2**.1776
Nocardia, **B2**.1148–9
rapidly growing mycobacteria, **B2**.1244–6
Salmonella molecular typing, **B2**.1409, **B2**.1410–11
Salmonella Typhi, **B2**.1410
Salmonella Typhimurium, **B2**.1410
Salmonella Typhimurium antibacterial resistance, **B2**.1413

Pulse vaccination regimes, vaccination models, **I**.962, **I**.962 (Fig.)

Puma protein, **I**.133
structure, **I**.133 (Fig.)

Punch biopsies
Borrelia infection, **B2**.1828
onchocerciasis diagnosis, **P**.153

Punctate keratitis, onchocerciasis visual damage, **P**.793–5

Punta Toro virus
G2 glycoprotein, **V2**.1038
genome structure
ambisense coding, **V1**.181, **V1**.181 (Fig.)
panhandle structures, **V2**.1032 (Fig.)
infection, **V2**.1047
NS_M protein, **V2**.1033–4
transcription termination, **V2**.1037

Purified Protein Derivative of Tuberculin (PPD), **B2**.1185
HIV peptide vaccines, **I**.871
IL-10 induction, **I**.652–3

Purine nucleoside phosphorylase deficiency, **I**.775

Purines, synthesis, **B1**.60–1

Purine synthesis, *Trypanosoma brucei,* **P**.360

Purple bacteria
photosynthesis, **B1**.67–8
sulfur oxidation, **B1**.201

Purtilo's syndrome *see* X-linked lymphoproliferative disease (XLP)

Pus, specimens, **M**.84

Pustulosis, neonatal, **M**.214

Putidaredoxin, **P**.256

Putrefaction
definition, **B1**.4–5
historical aspects, **B1**.4–5

'Putrid poison,' **I**.109

pUT transposon vectors, **B1**.125
limitations, **B1**.125

Puumula virus (PUUV), **V2**.1666 (Tab.)
infection, **V2**.1045
immune response, **V2**.1041
transmission, **V1**.371 (Tab.)

pX region, leukaemogenic retrovirus genome, **V1**.335–6

Pycnomonas, **P**.351

Pyelonephritis, acute, **B1**.673, **B1**.675
clinical features, **B1**.673
Escherichia coli, uropathogenic adherence specificity, **B1**.147–8
pregnancy, **B1**.679
Proteus, **B2**.1446
treatment, **B1**.679

Pyocins, **B1**.138, **B2**.1602

Pyocyanin, **B1**.650, **B2**.1596–7, **B2**.1601–2

Pyomelanin, **B2**.1596

Pyorubin, **B2**.1596

Pyoverdines, **B2**.1596

Pyrantel palmoate

Enterobius vermicularis infection, **P**.732

Oesophagostomum control, **P**.812

Pyrazinamide (PZA), **B1**.481

Mycobacterium, **B2**.1197, **B2**.1218

Pyrenochaeta, **M**.391

Pyrenochaeta mackinnonii, **M**.391

Pyrenochaeta romeroi, **M**.28 (Fig.),
M.89 (Tab.), **M**.387–8, **M**.390 (Tab.),
M.391

histopathology, **M**.128 (Tab.)

Pyridine nucleotide transhydrogenase,
Entamoeba histolytica, **P**.202

Pyridione, substituted, **M**.183 (Tab.)

Pyrimethamine

babesiosis, **P**.459

mechanism of action, **P**.477

resistance

dhfr-ts gene, **P**.480

historical aspects, **P**.479

linkage, **P**.480

toxoplasmosis, **P**.437, **P**.438–9

Pyrimethamine–sulfadiazine, isosporiasis,
P.414

Pyrimidines

keratitis therapy, **M**.308

salvage, *Plasmodium*, **P**.477

synthesis, **B1**.60–1

Pyrin domain (PYD), caspases, **I**.134

Pyrithione zinc, seborrheic dermatitis, **M**.212

Pyrogenic exotoxins (PET), **I**.555, **I**.556–62,
I.556 (Tab.)

biological significance, **I**.561–2

autoimmunity, **I**.562

enterotoxic activity, **I**.562

immunosuppression, **I**.561–2

pathogenicity role, **I**.561–2

as virulence factors, **I**.561

dimerization, **I**.559

homologies, **I**.557

isolate frequency, **I**.557–8

mechanism of action, **I**.558–60

MHC class II binding, **I**.558–9

non-MHC receptors, **I**.559

TCR interactions, **I**.558–9, **I**.560

polymorphisms, **I**.557

Streptococcus see Streptococcal pyogenic
exotoxins (SPE)

structure, **I**.558, **I**.558 (Fig.)

MHCα binding sites, **I**.558–9

MHCβ binding sites, **I**.559

zinc binding site, **I**.558, **I**.559

Pyrophosphate analogues, **V2**.1616–17

resistance, **V2**.1634–5

structure, **V2**.1617 (Fig.)

Pyrophosphate, inorganic, *Entamoeba
histolytica*, **P**.204

Pyrrolidonyl-β-naphthylamide (PYR), **B2**.882

Pyruvate, **B1**.54

formation from glucose by KDPG pathway,
B1.58

glyceraldehyde-3-phosphate conversion to,
B1.51–2

lactate formation, **B1**.54

oxidation and decarboxylation, **B1**.55–6

Pyruvate carboxylase, **B1**.61

Pyruvate decarboxylase, **B1**.54

Pyruvate dehydrogenase (PDH) complex,
B1.52

Pyruvate:ferredoxin oxidoreductase, **B1**.55–6

Pyruvate kinase, **B1**.52

Pyruvate metabolism, *Dientamoeba fragilis*,
P.267

Pyruvate phosphate dikinase (PPDK),
Entamoeba histolytica, **P**.204

Pythiosis, **M**.412–29

animals, **M**.412–13, **M**.416–17, **M**.418–21

cats, **M**.420, **M**.421 (Fig.)

cattle, **M**.420, **M**.421 (Fig.)

diagnostic inoculation, **M**.425

dogs, **M**.419–20, **M**.420 (Fig.)

horses, **M**.412–13, **M**.418–19, **M**.419 (Fig.),
M.425 (Fig.)

immune response, **M**.421–2

vaccination, **M**.422

clinical features, **M**.418–21

bone, **M**.418–19, **M**.419 (Fig.)

cutaneous granulomas, **M**.418–19,
M.419 (Fig.), **M**.421

eye infection, **M**.421, **M**.422 (Fig.)

keratitis, **M**.301–2, **M**.305, **M**.316

oculomycoses, **M**.275 (Tab.), **M**.289–90

diagnosis, **M**.422–5

animal inoculation, **M**.425, **M**.425 (Fig.)

DNA-based assays, **M**.423

EIAs, **M**.424

ELISA, **M**.424

histopathology, **M**.419–23, **M**.426–7,
M.427 (Fig.)

immunodiffusion test, **M**.423–4

immunohistochemistry, **M**.424–5

serology, **M**.423–5

Western blotting, **M**.424

epidemiology, **M**.416–17

geographical distribution, **M**.417,
M.417 (Fig.), **M**.420–1

hemoglobinopathies, **M**.420–2

spread, **M**.418

history, **M**.412–13

immune response, **M**.421–2, **M**.426–7,
M.427 (Fig.)

eosinophils, **M**.421, **M**.422

kunkers, **M**.418–19, **M**.419 (Fig.), **M**.421

pathogenesis, **M**.427 (Fig.)

pathological signs, **M**.418–21

therapy, **M**.425–7

amphotericin B, **M**.425–6

drug therapy, **M**.425–6

flucytosine, **M**.425–6

immunization, **M**.422, **M**.426–7,
M.426 (Fig.)

surgery, **M**.425

Pythium, **M**.412, **M**.413

hair, **M**.416–17

infection *see* Pythiosis

phylogenetics, **M**.414, **M**.416 (Fig.)

Pythium destruens, **M**.413

Pythium gracile, **M**.413

Pythium insidiosum, **M**.21, **M**.412–29

classification, **M**.4, **M**.49, **M**.413

developmental stages, **M**.413–14,
M.414 (Fig.), **M**.417–18

ecology, **M**.416–17, **M**.417–18

identification, **M**.413, **M**.424 (Fig.)

infection *see* Pythiosis

life cycle, **M**.415 (Fig.), **M**.417–18

plant host, **M**.416–17, **M**.417–18

morphology, **M**.413–16

oogonia, **M**.414

sporangia, **M**.413, **M**.414 (Fig.), **M**.415 (Fig.),
M.417–18

spread, **M**.418

taxonomy, **M**.413–16

zoospores, **M**.413–14, **M**.414 (Fig.),
M.415 (Fig.), **M**.418

infectivity, **M**.418

Pythium insidiosum vaccines, **I**.933 (Tab.)

Qa-1, CD8+ T-cells interactions, **I**.443, **I**.445,
I.444 (Fig.)

*Qac*A genes, **B1**.442, **B1**.444

*Qac*B genes, **B1**.442, **B1**.444

*Qac*C genes, **B1**.442

*Qac*G genes, **B1**.442

*Qac*H genes, **B1**.442

Q fever, **B1**.231, **B1**.636

clinical features, **B1**.636

endocarditis, **B1**.533, **B1**.534, **B1**.536,
B1.537, **B1**.748, **B2**.2076

hepatitis, **B2**.2076

control, **B2**.2079

disinfectants, **B2**.2079

risk reduction, **B2**.2079

vaccine *see below*

diagnosis, **B1**.636, **B1**.748, **B2**.2077

associated risks, **B2**.2077

direct immunofluorescence, **B2**.2077

indirect immunofluorescence, **B2**.2077

PCR, **B2**.2077

retrospective serology, **B2**.2077

endocarditis, **B1**.748, **B2**.2076

epidemiology, **B2**.2078–9

incubation period, **B2**.2076

outbreaks, **B2**.2078

as zoonosis, **B2**.2076, **B2**.2078

history, **B2**.2072

pathogenesis, **B2**.2077

acid phosphatase, **B2**.2077

Mip protein, **B2**.2077

pneumonia, **B1**.636

pneumonitis, **B2**.2076

reinfection immunity, **B2**.2076

self-limiting, **B2**.2078

transmission, **B2**.2076

passive phagocytosis, **B2**.2077

treatment, **B1**.636, **B2**.2077–8

doxycycline, **B2**.2078

fluoroquinolones, **B2**.2078

tetracyclines, **B2**.2078

vaccine, **B2**.2073, **B2**.2075

chloroform-methanol residue vaccines,
B2.2075

Qinghaosu
  malaria therapy, **P**.128
  mechanism of action, **P**.478
QS-21 adjuvant, **I**.930
  monophosphoryl lipid combination, **I**.930
  TCE peptide vaccines, **I**.878–9
  T helper cell response, **I**.930
  vaccines used, **I**.930
Qualitative traits, immunogenetics, **I**.572
Quality assurance/control, infection diagnosis,
  V2.1547–8
Quality assurance materials, biosafety, **B1**.761
Quality control, chemotherapy/
  chemoprophylaxis, **P**.128
Quantitative buffy coat (QBC), malaria
  diagnosis, **P**.501, **P**.503 (Fig.)
  treatment options, **P**.505
Quantitative polymerase chain reaction
  (QPCR)
  airborne bacteria detection, **B1**.191
  mumps diagnosis, **V1**.754
Quantitative prediction, vaccination models,
  I.964
Quantitative traits, immunogenetics, **I**.572
Quarantine, **B1**.347
  rabies control, **V2**.1126
  rinderpest control, **V1**.810
Quartan malaria see Malaria; Malaria,
  malariae (quartan)
Quasi-species
  biological significance, **V1**.17–9
  definition, **V1**.17, **V1**.55
  emergence of new viruses/viral infection,
    V1.193
  fitness variations, **V1**.18–9
  foot-and-mouth disease virus, **V1**.19
  generation, **V1**.17
  misnomer, **V1**.33
  RNA viruses, **V1**.192–3
  variability, **V1**.192–3
Quaternary ammonium compounds (QACs),
  B1.423 (Tab.), **B1**.426
  action, **B1**.437 (Tab.), **B1**.439
  resistance to, **B1**.442, **B1**.444
  see also specific compounds
Queensland tick fever, clinical manifestations,
  B2.2039 (Tab.), **B2**.2040
Quellung reaction, **B1**.631–2
  Streptococcus pneumoniae detection, **B1**.756
Questionnaires, epidemiological, **B1**.311
  design, **B1**.311
Quinacrine
  giardiasis, **P**.251
  prion disease therapy, **V2**.1387
Quincke's edema, Gnathostoma doloresi, **P**.823
Quinine
  α₁-acid glycoprotein binding, **I**.205
  Babesia microti infection treatment, **P**.459
  malaria therapy, **P**.506
Quinoline derivatives, **B1**.428
Quinolones, **B1**.492–4
  in gas gangrene, **B2**.1116
  intracranial abscess, **B1**.588
  mode of action, **B1**.492
    DNA gyrase (topoisomerase II), **B1**.492

pharmacodynamics, dose-dependency,
  B1.469–70
pharmacology, **B1**.493
resistance, **B1**.492–3
  Campylobacter, **B1**.493 (Tab.)
  Campylobacter jejuni, **B1**.492–3
  chromosomal mutation, **B1**.492–3
  Enterococcus, **B2**.892 (Tab.)
  Enterococcus faecalis, **B1**.493 (Tab.)
  Escherichia coli, **B1**.493 (Tab.)
  mechanisms, **B1**.493 (Tab.)
  Neisseria gonorrhoeae, **B1**.661
  prevention, **B1**.470
spectrum of activity, **B1**.492
  Campylobacter, **B2**.1548
  Chlamydia, **B1**.492, **B2**.2021
  Legionella, **B2**.1777
  mycobacteria, **B1**.492
  Mycoplasma, **B2**.1992
structure, **B1**.492, **B1**.494 (Fig.)
toxicity/adverse effects, **B1**.493–4
see also specific types
Quinones, **B1**.63, **B1**.64, **B1**.67–8, **B1**.427–8
  chemotaxonomy, **B1**.24
Quinupristin, **B1**.489
  spectrum of activity, **B1**.499 (Tab.)
  structure, **B1**.489 (Fig.)
Quorum-sensing, **B1**.167 (Fig.), **B1**.169–73
  Burkholderia cepacia complex, **B2**.1617
  Proteus, **B2**.1436–7
  Pseudomonas aeruginosa, **B1**.170–2,
    B1.171 (Fig.), **B2**.1602
  staphylococcal AGR system, **B1**.172–3,
    B1.173 (Fig.)
  system, **B1**.72

RING-finger domains, inhibitors of apoptosis,
  I.135
R61837, rhinovirus infection therapy, **V2**.879
Rabbit hemorrhagic disease virus (RHDV),
  V2.912
  emerging infection, **V2**.1651 (Tab.)
Rabbit infectivity testing (RIT), syphilis
  diagnosis, **B2**.1851
  PCR vs., **B2**.1852
Rabbit kidney vacuolating virus (RKV),
  V1.473
Rabbits
  Actinobacillus capsulatus infection,
    B2.1665–6
  Francisella infection, **B2**.1753
Rabies, **V2**.1117–20
  in animals
    clinical aspects, **V2**.1118
    paralysis, **V2**.1118
    prodromal period, **V2**.1118
  clinical aspects, **V2**.1117–18
    determining factors, **V2**.1117
    species susceptibility, **V2**.1117, **V2**.1118–19
  CNS, **V2**.1120–2
    axonal transport, **V2**.1122
    gene expression changes, **V2**.1123
    histopathology, **V2**.1122, **V2**.1122 (Fig.)
    neural dysfunction, **V2**.1122–3
    neural receptor modulation, **V2**.1122–3

  spongiform lesions, **V2**.1122, **V2**.1122 (Fig.)
  spread to, **V2**.1120–1
  transsynaptic passage, **V2**.1121–2
  vacuolation, **V2**.1122, **V2**.1122 (Fig.)
control, **V2**.1126–7
  exclusion controls, **V1**.370–1
  geographic isolation, **V1**.370–1
  quarantine, **V2**.1126
  vaccine see below
diagnosis, **V2**.1125–6
  immunofluorescence, **V2**.1125
  molecular biology, **V2**.1125
  Negri bodies, FIG **V2**.1104, **V2**.1125
  virus variant identification, **V2**.1125–6
emerging infection, **V2**.1648 (Tab.),
  V2.1664–5
epidemiology, **V1**.370–1, **V2**.1118–20
  in bats, **V2**.1120
  in dogs, **V2**.1119
  epizootiology, **V2**.1104, **V2**.1118–20
  geographic distribution, **V2**.1119–20
  transmission, **V2**.1117, **V2**.1119
  wild carnivores, **V2**.1119–20
in humans
  clinical features, **V2**.1117–18
  epidemiology, **V2**.1120
  incubation period, **V2**.1117–18
immune response, **V2**.1123–5
  cell-mediated immunity, **V2**.1115–16,
    V2.1124–5
  immunopathology, **V2**.1125
  neutralizing antibodies, **V2**.1115–16,
    V2.1123–4
  nucleocapsid (N) protein, **V2**.1124
immunopathology, **V1**.279 (Tab.)
immunosuppression, **V2**.1124–5
infection route, **V1**.238 (Fig.), **V1**.239
laboratory worker immunization, **B1**.767
pathogenesis/pathology, **V2**.1120–7, **V2**.1409
  cellular apoptosis, **V2**.1123
  GABA release, **V2**.1409
  inoculation site, **V2**.1120, **V2**.1120 (Fig.)
  Negri bodies, FIG **V2**.1104
  nonnervous tissue infection, **V2**.1123
  virus spread, **V2**.1120–2
prophylaxis, **V2**.1127
  post-exposure, **V2**.1127
  pre-exposure, **V2**.1127
vaccines/vaccination, **V2**.1552 (Tab.),
  V2.1578
  adverse effects, **V2**.1578
  DNA vaccines, **V2**.1116, **V2**.1554
  domestic animal vaccination, **V1**.370,
    V2.1126
  history, **B1**.7, **V1**.8 (Tab.), **V2**.1578
  inactivated live, **V2**.1126
  oral live attenuated, **V2**.1126–7
  post-exposure prophylaxis, **V2**.1578
  programs, **V2**.1559 (Tab.)
  replication, **V2**.1111
  wild animal vaccination, **V2**.1126–7
Rabies immunoglobulin (HRIG), **V2**.1566,
  V2.1567 (Tab.)
Rabies virus (RABV)
  attenuation, **V1**.253

Rabies virus (RABV) (*Continued*)
  cell receptor, **V2**.1108
  cellular protein packaging, **V2**.1106
  classification, **V1**.385–6
  CNS receptors, **V2**.1406 (Tab.)
  genome structure, **V2**.1112 (Fig.)
  genotype 1 (classic), **V2**.1103–4
  glycoprotein (G)
    as antigen, **V2**.1115–16
    cell entry, **V2**.1108
    cell receptor binding, **V2**.1115
    CNS spread, **V2**.1121–2
    immune response to, **V2**.1125
    neutralizing antibodies, **V2**.1123–4
  matrix (M) protein, **V2**.1114
  morphology/structure, **V2**.1105,
    V2.1106 (Fig.)
  nucleocapsids, **V1**.71
  nucleoprotein (N)
    as antigen, **V2**.1115, **V2**.1116
    immune response to, **V2**.1125
    phosphorylation, **V2**.1113
  receptor, **V2**.1405–6
  reverse genetics, **V1**.133–4
  superantigens, **I**.563–4
  transcription–replication switch, **V2**.1111
  transmission, **V1**.371 (Tab.)
  vaccine *see* Rabies
RAC-2 deficiency, **I**.769
Raccoon parvovirus, BCE peptide vaccines,
  I.871–2
Racemose cysticercus, *Taenia solium,* **P**.679–
  80, **P**.685–8
Rac GTPase
  apoptosis debris removal, **I**.136
  BCR signaling, **I**.346
  Vav activation by, **I**.345–6
Racial differences, immunogenetics, **I**.572
Racoonpox virus, **V1**.614
Radermecker complexes, **V2**.1432
Radiation
  susceptibility/resistance to
    Azotobacter, **B1**.46
    chromosomal polyploidy, **B1**.46
    Legionella, **B2**.1777
    Mycobacterium, **B2**.1217
    virus inactivation, **V1**.91, **V1**.91 (Tab.)
  see also Ionizing radiation
Radiation-attenuated parasites, schistosomiasis
  vaccine, **P**.620
Radiation-induced pulmonary injury, **I**.279
Radiation-sensitive severe combined
  immunodeficiency (RS-SCID), **I**.330
Radioactivity label release assays, cell-
  mediated immune response, **V2**.1545
Radiography
  adiaspiromycosis diagnosis, **M**.814,
    M.814 (Fig.)
  chronic necrotizing pulmonary aspergillosis,
    M.697
  Histoplasma capsulatum var. *duboisii,* **M**.536
Radioimmunoassays (RIAs), **M**.35, **B1**.719–20,
  V2.1545
  amebiasis, **P**.211–12
  in diagnosis, **V2**.1535
    mumps, **V1**.754

enteroviruses, **V2**.877
histoplasmosis, **M**.532
human brucellosis diagnosis, **B2**.1739–40
malaria diagnosis, **P**.503
  antigen detection, **P**.504
vaccine response, **V2**.1558
Radioimmunoconjugates, **I**.359–60
  antibody fragments, **I**.369
  imaging, **I**.359–60
  therapy, **I**.359
Radiology
  alveolar echinococcosis, **P**.688–9
  Anisakis diagnosis, **P**.817
  ascariasis diagnosis, **P**.730
  bone and joint infection, **B1**.693–4,
    B1.693 (Fig.)
  paragonimiasis diagnosis, **P**.653
Radiotherapy, immunodeficiency, **I**.788 (Tab.)
Rae expression, **I**.437
Raffinose fermentation
  Enterobacteriaceae identification,
    B2.1319 (Tab.)
  plasmids, **B1**.115
Raft culture system, papillomaviruses, **V1**.456–
  7
Rafting cells, bioaerosols, **B1**.185–7
RAG proteins
  B cell development, **I**.324
  mutations, **I**.330
  RAG-1 deficient mice, **I**.330
    airway hypersensitivity, **I**.734
  RAG-2 proteins
    αβ TCRs, **I**.456
    deficient mice, **I**.330
  somatic hypermutation, **I**.327
  somatic recombination, **I**.328–30
  TCR rearrangements, **I**.451
  upregulation, **I**.327
Rahnella, **B2**.1496–7
  antibacterial susceptibility/resistance,
    B2.1497
  biochemical tests, **B2**.1496
  culture, **B2**.1496
  definition, **B2**.1496
  habitats, **B2**.1497
  pathogenicity, **B2**.1497
Rahnella aquatilis, **B2**.1496
  biochemical tests, **B2**.1319 (Tab.)
  DNA–DNA analysis, **B2**.1338
  habitats, **B2**.1497
  pathogenicity, **B2**.1497
Raillietina, **P**.577–8
Rain, bacteriology of, **B1**.211–12,
  B1.212 (Tab.), **B1**.213
Ralstonia, **B2**.1635
Ralstonia eutrophica, **B2**.1635
Ralstonia metallidurans, **B2**.1635
Ralstonia pickettii, **B2**.1635
  nosocomial infection, **B2**.1635
Ralstonia solanacearum, **B2**.1635
Ramichloridium obovoideum infection
  CNS, **M**.743–5
  therapy, **M**.745
Ranavirus, **V1**.44

Random amplified polymorphic DNA
  (RAPD)
  aerobic actinomycetes, **B2**.1147
  Aeromonas, **B2**.1535
  Burkholderia thailandensis, **B2**.1623
  classification, **M**.47
  Enterococcus, **B2**.894
  Escherichia, **B2**.1371
  Helicobacter, **B2**.1570
  Malassezia, **M**.215
  microsporidiosis diagnosis, **P**.547
  Mycobacterium abscessus, **B2**.1248–9
  Paracoccidioides brasiliensis, **M**.542
  principle, **B1**.726 (Tab.)
  protozoa classification, **P**.193
  Salmonella, **B2**.1409, **B2**.1411
  Sporothrix schenckii, **M**.379
  Yersinia, **B2**.1467
Random cloned sequence (RCCS) typing,
  Salmonella, **B2**.1409
Randomized controlled trials, **B1**.313
Random mutagenesis, genetic analysis, **V1**.183
Random transmission, infection models,
  I.948–9
RANTES (CCL5), **I**.218 (Tab.)
  antagonists, inflammatory disease therapy,
    I.231
  CNS expression, **V2**.1409
  dendritic epidermal γδ T cell, **I**.437
  DNA vaccine co-administration, **I**.918,
    I.918 (Tab.)
  effects
    basophil chemotaxis, **I**.58
    basophil cytokine production, **I**.66
    basophil histamine release, **I**.62
    CD8+ T cells, in HIV infection, **I**.793
    eosinophil chemotaxis, **I**.61
    T cell chemotaxis, **I**.224
  immunogenetics, **I**.582
  intradermal DNA vaccine delivery, **I**.912–13
  receptor *see* CC chemokine receptors, CCR5
  structure, **I**.217–19
Rap1 GTPase, BCR signaling, **I**.346
Rapamycin, immunodeficiency, **I**.788 (Tab.)
Rapid epidemiological mapping of
  onchocerciasis (REMO), **P**.786, **P**.792
Rapidly growing mycobacteria (RGM) *see*
  Mycobacteria, rapidly growing (RGM)
Rapid mapping techniques, onchocerciasis
  diagnosis, **P**.792
RapIDonE test, **B2**.1463
Rapid plasma reagin (RPR) test, **B1**.663,
  B2.1845–6, **B2**.1846 (Tab.), **B2**.1858
'Rapid progressors,' HIV infection, **I**.790
Rapid rabies enzyme immunodiagnosis
  (RREID), **V2**.1125
Rapid urease test, *Helicobacter pylori,* **B2**.1571
  (Tab.), **B2**.1572,
Raptiva, licensing, **I**.355 (Tab.)
Ras GTPase
  activation, **I**.346
    Grb2, **I**.346
  BCR signaling, **I**.346
Rashes/exanthem
  bacterial meningitis, **B1**.559, **B1**.565–6
  bunyavirus infection, **V2**.1042

Rashes/exanthem (*Continued*)
congenitally acquired rubella, **V2**.973, **V2**.974 (Fig.)
Coxsackie virus infection, **V2**.872
echovirus infection, **V2**.872
enterovirus infection, **V2**.872
infectious mononucleosis (IM), **V1**.568
Parvovirus B19 virus infection, **V1**.430
perianal, **M**.596, **M**.609
pneumonia with, **B1**.634
varicella (chickenpox), **V1**.512–13, **V1**.513 (Fig.)
VZV infection, **V1**.514, **V2**.1421
Rat-bite fever
causative organism *see Spirillum minus*
Spirillum minus, **B2**.1908
Streptobacillus moniliformis, **B2**.1908, **B2**.1911
Rat coronavirus (RtCoV) infection, **V1**.841 (Tab.)
Rat cytomegalovirus, genome sequences, **V1**.494 (Tab.)
Rational drug design, antiviral chemotherapy, **V2**.1606–7
Rats
bamboo, *Penicillium marneffei,* **M**.26, **M**.560, **M**.561, **M**.561 (Fig.), **M**.561 (Tab.), **M**.562
Borna disease virus model, **V2**.1145–7
Leishmania braziliensis, **P**.326
Leishmania infantum chagasi, **P**.320
listeriosis, **B2**.963
Pneumocystis, **M**.770 (Tab.), **M**.774, **M**.775, **M**.793, **M**.796
Raulin, J, **M**.8–9
Raw food *see* Undercooked/raw food
Reaction centers, Cyanobacteria, **B1**.68
Reactive arthritis
Clostridium difficile infection, **B2**.1121–2
HLA association, **I**.577
HLA-B27, **I**.752, **I**.752 (Tab.)
HLA-DR, **I**.752 (Tab.)
immunogenetics, **I**.594–5
microbial infection, **I**.594–5
pathogen induced, **I**.753 (Tab.)
Shigella flexneri infection, **B2**.1387
Reactive oxygen intermediates (ROIs)
eosinophils, **I**.66
macrophages, **I**.26
malaria immunity, **P**.490
neutrophil generation, **I**.41
phagocytosis, **I**.647–8
Plasmodium, **P**.478
Reactive oxygen species (ROS)
helminth defenses, **I**.686
nicotinamide adenine dinucleotide phosphate oxidase, **I**.769
Reaginic antibody *see* Immunoglobulin E (IgE)
Real-time polymerase chain reaction (RT-PCR), **B1**.727–9, **B1**.727 (Fig.), **B2**.937
automation technologies, **B1**.729
Chlamydia detection, **B2**.2018–19
principle, **B1**.726–7, **B1**.726 (Tab.)
probes, **B1**.728–9

Reassortment, emerging viral infection, **V2**.1654
recA gene
Burkholderia, **B2**.1609, **B2**.1612
DNA damage repair, **B1**.451–2
Helicobacter, **B2**.1567–8
Recall, errors, **B1**.311
Receptor-binding proteins, viral morphology/structure, **V1**.58, **V1**.67–9
Receptor-mediated endocytosis, **V1**.206, **V1**.206 (Fig.)
Hepatitis B virus uptake, **V2**.1231
orbiviruses, **V2**.933
reoviruses, **V2**.932
Recombinant antigens, malaria vaccination, **P**.516–17
Recombinant bispecific antibodies, **I**.369–70, **I**.370 (Fig.)
Recombination, **B1**.88 (Fig.), **B1**.98 (Fig.), **V1**.187–8
astroviruses, **V2**.900
discovery, **B1**.13
DNA viruses, **V1**.14, **V1**.187–8
emerging viral infection, **V2**.1654
HIV, **V2**.1330
HIV-1, **V1**.188–9
retroviruses, **V1**.188
ribovirus evolution, **V1**.13, **V1**.15–6
viral evolution, **V1**.14–6
Recombination signal sequences (RSS)
Ig V(D)J recombination, **I**.328
somatic recombination, **I**.328–9
TCR rearrangements, **I**.451, **I**.452 (Fig.)
Record keeping, hazard analysis critical control point system, **B1**.288
Recovery rates, infection models, **I**.949–50
Recrudescences, malaria *see* Malaria
Rectal bleeding, trichuriasis, **P**.728–9
Rectal prolapse, trichuriasis, **P**.728
Rectal thermometers, nosocomial infection from, **B1**.379–80
Rectosigmoidoscopy, amebiasis, **P**.207, **P**.211
Recurrent flagellum, *Enteromonas hominis,* **P**.270
Recurrent infection, chronic granulomatous disease, **I**.26
Recurrent respiratory papillomatosis (RRP), **V1**.464
Red cell aplasia, NK cells, **I**.103
Red cells *see* Erythrocyte(s)
Red gum trees, *Cryptococcus neoformans,* **M**.643
Redmouth disease of fish, **B2**.1459
Redox potential
meat, **B1**.273
microbial growth effect, **B1**.267
Redox status
Plasmodium see Plasmodium
Trypanosoma brucei, **P**.359–60
Reductive pentose phosphate pathway (Calvin cycle), **B1**.62
Reductive TCA cycle, carbon dioxide fixation, **B1**.62
Red water disease, cattle, **B1**.203
Reed–Frost model, **B1**.337, **B1**.343
Reed–Sternberg cells, **V1**.566
Re-emerging infection *see* Emerging infection

'Refeeding malaria,' **P**.493
Reference cultures, **B1**.28–9
Reference types, **V1**.34
Refrigeration, eggs and egg products, **B1**.278
Refugees/refugee camps, emerging bacterial infection, **B1**.360
Regional lymphadenopathy, cat-scratch disease, **B2**.1891–2
Regressive evolution, **V1**.11
Regulatory cytokines, **I**.274 (Tab.), **I**.292–7
Regulatory T-cells (Treg), **P**.72–3, **I**.446
bacterial infection, **I**.647, **I**.657 (Fig.)
immune interference, **I**.666–8
IL-2, **I**.751
IL-10, **I**.751
tolerance induction, **I**.396, **I**.397 (Tab.)
oral tolerance, **I**.543, **I**.544
peripheral tolerance, **I**.751
Reinfection
babesiosis, **P**.455–6, **P**.456
clonorchiasis, **P**.654
Enterobius vermicularis control, **P**.732
isosporiasis, **P**.412–13
malaria, **P**.471 (Fig.)
opisthorchiasis, **P**.654
Reiter protein complement fixation assay, **B1**.745–6
Relapses, malaria *see* Malaria
Relapsing fever (*Borrelia*)
causative organisms, **B2**.1822
Borrelia crocidurae, **B2**.1822, **B2**.1827
Borrelia duttonii, **B2**.1822, **B2**.1827
Borrelia recurrentis, **B2**.1822, **B2**.1823, **B2**.1827
cospeciation, **B2**.1822
epidemic, **B2**.1823
epidemiology, **B2**.1823
history, **B2**.1818
relapses, **B2**.1827
serology, **B2**.1830
transmission, **B2**.1823
Relative humidity, airborne bacteria and bacterial survival, **B1**.187
Relative risk, **B1**.316
Relenza *see* Zanamivir
Religion, rhinosporidiosis, **M**.439, **M**.458
Remak, R, **M**.6
Remicade, licensing, **I**.355 (Tab.)
Removal mechanisms, host resistance to bacterial infection, **B1**.176
Renal abscess, **B1**.673
Renal diseases/infection
babesiosis, **P**.456
Encephalitozoon cuniculi infection, **P**.542
falciparum malaria, **P**.481
infective endocarditis, **B1**.535
Mycobacterium abscessus, **B2**.1250
syphilis, **B2**.1842
Renal dysfunction
arenavirus infection, **V2**.1071–2
mumps, **V1**.748–50
Renal failure, secondary amyloidosis due to leprosy, **B2**.1204
Renal fusariosis, **M**.138 (Fig.)
Renal insufficiency, amphotericin B causing, **M**.148–9

Renal transplants
  aspergillosis, **M**.701
  EBV infection, **V2**.1507
  Nocardia asteroides infection, **B2**.1156
  polyomavirus infection, **V2**.1509
Renal tubule scarring, leptospire infection,
  B2.1881
Renon, R, **M**.18–9
ReoPro, licensing, **I**.355 (Tab.)
Reoviridae
  characteristics, **V1**.177 (Tab.)
  classification, **V1**.27 (Tab.), **V1**.47–8,
    V1.47 (Tab.), **V2**.932
    common features, **V2**.932
  see also Reoviruses; *specific viruses*
Reoviruses, **V2**.933–9
  cell receptors, **V1**.207 (Tab.)
    junctional adhesion molecule 1 (JAM1),
      V2.933
  cellular entry, **V1**.108–9, **V1**.215–16
  epidemiology, **V2**.933
  gene expression, **V1**.120
  genetic determinants of virulence, **V1**.255–6
    gene segments, **V1**.256, **V1**.256 (Tab.)
  genome
    segmentation, **V1**.180–1
    size, **V2**.932
    structure, **V2**.933
    subunit reassortment, **V1**.191–2
  immune evasion, **V2**.936
    IFN inhibition, **V1**.286–7, **V1**.315
  infection *see* Reovirus infection
  isolation/propagation and identification,
    V1.96 (Tab.), **V1**.100
  λ1 protein, **V2**.933, **V2**.934 (Tab.)
    in transcription, **V2**.936
  λ2 protein, **V2**.933, **V2**.934 (Tab.)
    as RNA polymerase, **V2**.936
  λ3 protein, **V2**.933, **V2**.934 (Tab.)
    in transcription, **V2**.936
  mRNA translation, **V1**.113
  μ1 protein, **V2**.933, **V2**.934 (Tab.)
  μ2 protein, **V2**.933, **V2**.934 (Tab.)
    in transcription, **V2**.936
  proteins, **V2**.933, **V2**.938 (Fig.)
    nonstructural proteins, **V2**.933,
      V2.934 (Tab.)
    orbivirus proteins *vs.*, **V2**.941 (Tab.)
    structural proteins, **V2**.933, **V2**.934 (Tab.)
    see also specific types
  replication, **V2**.933–6, **V2**.935 (Fig.)
    genome replication, **V2**.936
    receptor-mediated endocytosis, **V2**.932
    release from cell, **V2**.936
    translational templates, **V2**.936
  σ1 protein, **V2**.933, **V2**.935 (Fig.)
    cell attachment, **V2**.933, **V2**.936–7
    in pathogenesis, **V2**.939 (Tab.)
    virion structure, **V2**.934 (Tab.)
  σ2 protein, **V2**.933, **V2**.934 (Tab.)
  σ3 protein, **V2**.933, **V2**.934 (Tab.)
    degradation, **V2**.936
    immune evasion, **V1**.315, **V2**.936
    virion structure, **V2**.934 (Tab.),
      V2.935 (Fig.)

type, **V1**.3–4
  virion structure, **V2**.933, **V2**.935 (Fig.)
  see also Reoviridae
Reovirus infection
  apoptosis, **V2**.936–7
  epidemiology, **V2**.938–9
  in humans, **V2**.932, **V2**.938
    myocarditis, **V2**.937–8
    neonatal biliary atresia, **V2**.938
    neural spread, **V1**.244 (Tab.)
    systemic disease, **V2**.937
  immune response, IFN activity, **I**.260 (Tab.),
    I.619
  infection process, **V1**.241 (Tab.)
  oncolysis, **V2**.938–9
  pathogenesis, **V2**.937–8
    CNS invasion, **V2**.937
    encephalitis, **V2**.937
    serotype specific, **V2**.937
Reovirus type 3, **V1**.207 (Tab.)
Rep40 protein, adeno-associated viruses,
  V2.1599
Rep52 protein, adeno-associated viruses,
  V2.1599
Rep68 protein
  adeno-associated viruses, **V1**.159, **V1**.418–19,
    V2.1599
  Dependovirus, **V1**.415
Rep78 protein
  adeno-associated viruses, **V1**.159, **V1**.418–19,
    V2.1599
  Dependovirus, **V1**.415
Repeated infection, transmission dynamics,
  P.62
Repetitive element sequence (REP)-
  polymerase chain reaction,
  Enterococcus, **B2**.894
Rep gene deletion, adeno-associated virus
  gene vectors, **V2**.1599–600
Replica plating, **B1**.84
Replicase (RNA polymerase)
  arteriviruses *see* Arteriviruses
  coronaviruses *see* Coronaviruses
  Equine arteritis virus *see* Equine arteritis
    virus (EAV)
  Equine torovirus (EToV: Berne virus),
    V1.833 (Fig.)
  Human coronavirus, **V1**.833 (Fig.)
  Infectious bronchitis virus, **V1**.833 (Fig.)
  Murine hepatitis virus *see* Murine hepatitis
    virus (MHV)
  Nidovirales see Nidovirales
  Porcine reproductive and respiratory
    syndrome virus, **V1**.833 (Fig.)
  Severe acute respiratory syndrome
    coronavirus *see* Severe acute respiratory
    syndrome coronavirus (SARS-CoV)
  toroviruses *see* Toroviruses
  see also Pol (polymerase) protein;
    RNA-dependent RNA polymerase
Replicate organism detection and counting
  (RODAC), **B1**.190
Replication
  bacteria
    errors, mutations, **B1**.87, **B1**.88 (Fig.)
    plasmid genes, **B1**.107

viruses, **V1**.241–2, **V1**.105–26
  in blood cells, **V1**.243 (Tab.)
  cellular attachment, **V1**.105–6, **V1**.106–7,
    V1.107 (Fig.)
    conformational changes, **V1**.106
  cellular entry, **V1**.107–9
    cell compartment distribution, **V1**.108–9
    endocytosis, **V1**.107–8
    enveloped viruses, **V1**.107–8,
      V1.108 (Fig.)
    non-enveloped viruses, **V1**.107
    plasma membrane fusion, **V1**.108
    protein conformational changes,
      V1.107–8, **V1**.108–9
  in CNS, **V2**.1405, **V2**.1412
  in endothelial cells, **V1**.242–3
  gene expression *see* Gene expression
  genome replication, **V1**.122–5
  historical aspects, **V1**.6
  infection initiation, **V1**.106–7
  protein processing, **V1**.121–2
    glycosylation, **V1**.122
    phosphorylation, **V1**.122
    proteolytic cleavage, **V1**.121–2
    sulfation, **V1**.122
    N-terminal myristoylation, **V1**.122
  protein synthesis, **V1**.105–6, **V1**.120–2
    alternative reading frames, **V1**.116–17
    host protein synthesis, **V1**.120–1
    pseudoknot formation, **V1**.117,
      V1.117 (Fig.)
    ribosomal skipping, **V1**.117
    RNA editing, **V1**.116–17
    splicing, **V1**.114–15
  protein transport, **V1**.121
  release from cell, **V1**.105–6
  translation, **V1**.114–8
    splicing mechanisms, **V1**.114–15
  see also specific viruses
Replication and transcription activator
  (ORF50/K-RTA), **V1**.545
Replication compartments/centers, **V1**.170–1
'Replication complex,' *Nidovirales* order,
  V1.396
Replication factor C (RF-C), **V1**.153–4,
  V1.154 (Tab.)
Replication forks, **B1**.46
Replication initiator protein, parvovirus
  capsids, **V1**.413
Replication protein A (RPA)
  HPV replication, **V1**.457
  papillomavirus replication, **V1**.156–7
  SV40 genome replication, **V1**.153,
    V1.154 (Tab.)
Replication protein C (RPC), HPV
  replication, **V1**.457
Replication switch, respirovirus transcription,
  V1.771–2
Replicative elements, DNA viruses *vs.*, **V1**.12
Replicative form (RF) intermediates
  Minute virus of mice replication, **V1**.158
  positive-strand RNA virus replication,
    V1.138
Replicative transposition, **B1**.93 (Fig.), **B1**.95
Replicons
  Burkholderia cepacia complex, **B2**.1610

Replicons (*Continued*)

viral evolution, **V1**.11

The Report of the Committee on Infectious Diseases of the American Academy of Pediatrics (Red Book), **V2**.1583

Repressors, in operons, **B1**.70–1

lactose, **B1**.70–1

Reproduction *see individual species*

Reproduction numbers, vaccination models, **I**.957–8

Reproductive capacity, African trypanosomiasis, **P**.366

Reproductive success *see* Transmission dynamics

Reproductive systems *see individual species*

Reptile importation, **B1**.360

Rescriptor *see* Delavirdine

Reservoir hosts

Afipia, **B2**.1900–1

alphavirus transmission, **V2**.1017

Balantidium coli, **P**.275, **P**.280–1

Blastocystis hominis, **P**.557

Borna disease virus, **V2**.1143

Chilomastix mesnili, **P**.272

Clonorchis sinensis, **P**.646

Colorado tick fever virus, **V2**.942

control, **P**.112, **P**.118–20, **P**.125–7, **P**.145 (Tab.)

African trypanosomiasis, **P**.125, **P**.145 (Tab.), **P**.368

alveolar echinococcosis, **P**.119

Chagas disease, **P**.126, **P**.145 (Tab.)

cysticercosis, **P**.119, **P**.119–20, **P**.122

dracunculiasis, **P**.145 (Tab.)

echinococcosis, **P**.119

International Commission for Disease Eradication, **P**.118

leishmaniasis, **P**.118–19, **P**.145 (Tab.)

lymphatic filariasis, **P**.145 (Tab.)

malaria, **P**.145 (Tab.)

neurocysticercosis, **P**.119, **P**.119–20, **P**.122

onchocerciasis, **P**.125–6, **P**.145 (Tab.)

schistosomiasis, **P**.127, **P**.145 (Tab.), **P**.635–6

Eastern equine encephalitis virus, **V2**.1017

Entamoeba chattoni, **P**.219, **P**.222

Entamoeba polecki, **P**.219

glanders, **B2**.1633

Leishmania, **P**.318

Leishmania infantum, **P**.118

Leishmania major, **P**.118

melioidosis, **B2**.1628

Opisthorchis, **P**.646

Paragonimus, **P**.646

Sindbis virus, **V2**.1017

Taenia, **P**.119

Venezuelan equine encephalitis virus, **V2**.1017

Western equine encephalitis virus, **V2**.1017

'Reservosomes', **P**.175

Resiquimod, **V2**.1618

structure, **V2**.1618 (Fig.)

Resistance genes

plasmids *see* Plasmid(s)

transposons, **B1**.111–12

Resistance/nodulation/cell division family (RND), **B1**.440

Resolvase, **B1**.96

poxviruses, **V1**.606

Resourcing, parasite control, **P**.111–12

Respiration, **B1**.63–7

aerobic, **B1**.63–5

Respiratory chains, **B1**.63–4

Respiratory distress syndrome, prophenin therapy, **I**.173

Respiratory epithelium

anatomy, **B1**.606

Burkholderia intracellular infection, **B2**.1615–16

Respiratory equipment, contamination, **B1**.390

Respiratory failure, tetanus, **B2**.1065–6

Respiratory syncytial virus *see* Human respiratory syncytial virus (HRSV)

Respiratory tract, **M**.5 (Fig.)

anatomy, **B1**.606–7

ethmoid sinus, **B1**.606–7

frontal sinus, **B1**.606–7

infundibulum, **B1**.606–7

lacrimal duct, **B1**.606–7

middle ear, **B1**.606

nasal airways, **B1**.606–7

oral cavity, **B1**.606

paranasal sinuses, **B1**.606–7

respiratory epithelium, **B1**.606

sinuses, **B1**.606

sphenoid sinus, **B1**.606–7

stratified squamous epithelium, **B1**.606

turbinate, **B1**.606–7

B cell, **B1**.608

candidiasis, **M**.600

colonization, **B1**.625–6

in cystic fibrosis, **B1**.649–50

goblet cells, **B1**.623 (Fig.)

host defence defects, **B1**.608, **B1**.625–6

cellular immune defects, **B1**.626

environmental influences, **B1**.626

epithelial barriers and reflexes, **B1**.626

Ig deficiency, **B1**.626

mucociliary clearance defects, **B1**.626

phagocytic activity reduction, **B1**.626

host defence mechanisms, **B1**.607–8, **B1**.622–5, **B1**.622–5

airway architecture, **B1**.622–3

alveolar macrophage, **B1**.624–5

antibacterial secretions, **B1**.607–8

cellular mechanisms, **B1**.608

complement, **B1**.624

epithelial barrier, **B1**.623

factors in airway secretions, **B1**.623–4

Igs, **B1**.624

mucociliary clearance, **B1**.623

mucus, **B1**.607–8

primary, **B1**.607

recruited, **B1**.622, **B1**.625

resident, **B1**.622–5

secondary, **B1**.607

secretory IgA, **B1**.607–8

infection *see below*

normal microbiota, **B1**.295–302, **B1**.302, **B1**.609, **B1**.628

secretions, **B1**.623–4

specimen collection, **M**.83 (Tab.), **M**.84, **M**.86 (Tab.)

Respiratory tract infection, **B1.622–56**

acute bronchitis, **B1**.647

agammaglobulinemia, **I**.780

basophils, **I**.71

bronchiectasis, **B1**.649

children, **B2**.1669

in day-care centers, **B1**.361

chronic, in immunodeficiency, **B1**.626

emerging bacterial infection, **B1**.361

Encephalitozoon hellem, **P**.542, **P**.543

epidemiology, **V1**.365–7

by age, **V1**.366 (Fig.)

lower, **B2**.1654–5

Human coronaviruses, **V1**.841–2

influenza, **V1**.661

rhinoviruses, **V2**.873

morbidity, **P**.26 (Fig.)

mortality, **P**.26 (Fig.), **P**.28 (Tab.), **P**.29 (Tab.)

nosocomial, **B1**.389

prevalence and mortality, **B1**.389

pathogenesis, **B1**.625–8

bacterial virulence, **B1**.626–8

upper tract *see below*

viruses

adenoviruses, **V1**.160, **V1**.443–4

arenavirus, **V2**.1071–2

enteroviruses, **V2**.872

entry, **V1**.239–40, **V1**.241 (Tab.)

role in bacterial meningitis pathophysiology, **B1**.556

shedding, **V1**.249, **V1**.249 (Fig.)

see also individual species; specific diseases/ infection; specific viruses

Respiratory tract infection, upper, **B1**.628–9

airborne bacteria, **B1**.188

bacterial virulence mechanisms, **B1**.608–9

colonization, **B1**.608

Pasteurella multocida, **B2**.1654–5

pathogenesis, **B1**.608

antibacterial therapy, **B1**.608

environmental effects, **B1**.608

trauma, **B1**.608

vitamin A deficiency, **B1**.608

specimens, **B1**.609–10

collection, **B1**.609–10

culture, **B1**.610

Gram stain, **B1**.610

transport, **B1**.610

see also individual species; specific diseases/ infection

Respirovirus

characteristics, **V1**.129 (Tab.), **V1**.702 (Tab.)

classification, **V1**.48–9, **V1**.382, **V1**.700 (Tab.), **V1**.808 (Fig.)

members, **V1**.382–3

renaming, **V1**.40

see also Respiroviruses

Respiroviruses, **V1.763–82**

assembly/budding, **V1**.773

cell entry, **V1**.701–2, **V1**.764–9

fusion (F) protein, **V1**.764, **V1**.766–8, **V1**.767 (Fig.)

Respiroviruses
  cell entry (*Continued*)
    receptor molecules, **V1**.765–6
    viral interference, **V1**.766
    see also Below, hemagglutinin-
      neuraminidase (HN)
  classification, **V1**.763
  features, **V1**.763
  C proteins, **V1**.704–5, **V1**.763–4, **V1**.771
  fusion (F) protein, **V1**.763–4
    activation, **V1**.768–9
    in capsid, **V1**.773
    cell entry, **V1**.764, **V1**.766–8, **V1**.767 (Fig.)
    cleavage, **V1**.766–8
    fusion mechanisms, **V1**.768–9
    hemagglutinin-neuraminidase (HN)
      interactions, **V1**.769 (Fig.)
    host range, **V1**.766–8
    receptor binding, **V1**.768
    structure, **V1**.765 (Fig.)
    tissue tropisms, **V1**.766–8
  genome structure/organization,
    V1.387 (Tab.), **V1**.701 (Fig.), **V1**.763–4
    conservation, **V1**.784–5, **V1**.785 (Fig.)
  hemagglutinin-neuraminidase (HN),
    V1.706–7, **V1**.763–4
    active site, **V1**.765 (Fig.)
    in capsid, **V1**.773
    cell entry, **V1**.764, **V1**.766
    conformational change, **V1**.768
    conservation, **V1**.706–7
    fusion (F) protein interactions,
      V1.769 (Fig.)
    points of action, **V1**.767 (Fig.)
    structure, **V1**.765 (Fig.)
  host cell interactions, **V1**.773–4
    apoptosis prevention, **V1**.773–4
    cell cycle alterations, **V1**.773–4
    cell machinery use, **V1**.774
    host defence evasion, **V1**.773–4
    IFN biosynthesis prevention, **V1**.773–4
  large (L) protein (RNA-dependent RNA
    polymerase), **V1**.708, **V1**.763–4, **V1**.772
    in capsid, **V1**.773
    conservation, **V1**.772
    genome replication/transcription, **V1**.771–2
    P protein complex, **V1**.772–3
    transcription, **V1**.770
  morphology/structure, **V1**.763–4,
    V1.764 (Fig.)
  M protein, **V1**.763–4
    in capsid, **V1**.773
  nucleocapsid protein (NP), **V1**.763–4, **V1**.772
    genome replication/transcription, **V1**.771–2
    transcription, **V1**.770
  phosphoprotein (P), **V1**.704, **V1**.763–4,
    V1.772–3
    in capsid, **V1**.773
    genome replication/transcription, **V1**.771–2
    large (L) protein complex, **V1**.772–3
    nucleocapsid protein (NP) complex,
      V1.772
  properties, **V1**.763–74
  replication, **V1**.769–73, **V1**.770 (Fig.)
    noncoding sequences, **V1**.769
    RNA polymerase, **V1**.770

    template, **V1**.769–70
  transcription, **V1**.770 (Fig.)
    alternate reading frames, **V1**.771
    nontemplated nucleotide addition, **V1**.771
    polycistronic mRNAs, **V1**.771
    primary, **V1**.770
    replication switch, **V1**.771–2
    RNA editing, **V1**.771
    'rule of six,' **V1**.770–1
  V proteins, **V1**.763–4
    immune evasion, **V1**.773–4
    RNA editing, **V1**.771
  see also Respirovirus
Reston ebolavirus (REBOV), **V1**.382
  animal models, **V2**.1095
  cell culture, **V2**.1091–2
  classification, **V2**.1086
  epidemiology, **V2**.1093
  genome structure, **V2**.1088
  historical aspects, **V2**.1085
  mortality, **V2**.1094
  outbreaks, **V2**.1087 (Tab.)
Restriction endonuclease analysis (REA)
  Brucella, **B2**.1729–30
  Legionella pneumophilia, **B2**.1776
  leptospires, **B2**.1880
  mycobacteria (slow-growing) identification,
    B2.1193
  Mycoplasma, **B2**.1994, **B2**.1995–6
  rapidly growing mycobacteria, **B2**.1243,
    B2.1244
Restriction enzymes *see* DNA endonucleases
  (restriction enzymes)
Restriction fragment length polymorphisms
  (RFLPs), **V2**.1542
  Actinomyces, **B2**.1017
  Aeromonas typing, **B2**.1535
  Brevibacterium, **B2**.979
  Burkholderia, **B2**.1609
  classification, **M**.47
  Corynebacterium, **B2**.979
  Coxiella burnetii, **B2**.2074
  Cryptosporidium parvum classification, **P**.400
  Enterococcus, **B2**.894
  epidemiological strain typing, **B1**.735
  fungi, **M**.47 (Tab.)
  Giardia classification, **P**.242
  Helicobacter, **B2**.1570
  Legionella pneumophilia, **B2**.1776
  Leishmania analysis, **P**.284–5
  Malassezia, **M**.215
  Mycobacterium tuberculosis, **B2**.1194
  Mycoplasma, **B2**.1995
  Plasmodium antigen diversity, **P**.491–2
  protozoa classification, **P**.193
  rapidly growing mycobacteria, **B2**.1244
  Sporothrix schenckii, **M**.378
  syphilis, **B2**.1853
  Trypanosoma brucei classification, **P**.352
  Veillonella identification, **B2**.1315
  Vibrio, **B2**.1516
  wild type *vs.* attenuated strains, **V2**.1542–3
Reticular dysgenesis, **I**.774
Reticulate body (RB), *Chlamydia*, **B2**.2007–8

Reticuloendothelial system, histoplasmosis
  capsulati, **M**.535
'Reticuloendotheliosis,' **M**.525
Retinal hemorrhages
  cerebral malaria, **P**.481, **P**.481 (Fig.)
  falciparum malaria, **P**.480–1
  malaria in children, **P**.482
Retinal lesions, congenital toxoplasmosis,
  P.430
Retinitis
  aspergillosis, **M**.323
  VZV infection in HIV infection, **V2**.1501–2
Retinoblastoma
  papillomavirus E7 protein effects, **V1**.461
  phosphorylation, **V1**.548
  temporal control, **V1**.118
Retinochoroiditis
  congenital toxoplasmosis, **P**.430, **P**.431 (Fig.)
  Toxoplasmosis, **P**.431–2
Retortamonas, classification, **P**.196–7
Retortamonas intestinalis, **P**.272–3
  classification, **P**.272
  infection, **P**.266
    autochthonous infection, **P**.273
    diagnosis, **P**.273
    epidemiology, **P**.273
    pathogenicity, **P**.273
  as normal microbiota, **B1**.296 (Tab.)
  structure/life cycle, **P**.266, **P**.272–3
    cysts, **P**.271 (Fig.)
    flagella, **P**.272–3
    trophozoites, **P**.271 (Fig.)
Retroperitoneal fibrosis rhadinoviruses, **V1**.543
  characteristics, **V1**.542 (Tab.)
Retropharyngeal abscesses, **B1**.618
Retrotransposons
  DNA viruses *vs.,* **V1**.12
  in viral evolution, **V1**.13
Retroviridae
  characteristics, **V1**.177 (Tab.)
  classification, **V1**.27 (Tab.), **V1**.46,
    V1.46 (Tab.), **V2**.1286 (Tab.)
    characteristics, **V2**.1322–3
    recent, **V2**.1285
  general properties, **V2**.1284–5
  members, **V1**.46
  nomenclature, **V2**.1305 (Tab.)
  taxonomy, **V2**.1591
  see also Alpharetrovirus; Betaretrovirus;
    Deltaretrovirus; Epsilonretrovirus;
    Gammaretrovirus; Lentivirus;
    Orthoretroviridae; Retroviruses;
    Spumavirus; specific viruses
Retroviruses, **B1**.435–6, **V2.1284–303**
  animal, xenotransplantation risks, **V2**.1297
  assembly/maturation, **V1**.78–9
    Gag cleavage, **V1**.78–9
    Gag polyprotein, **V1**.78
    Pol polyprotein, **V1**.78
  cell entry, **V1**.213, **V1**.344
  cell interactions, **V1**.219
    host RNA processing/transport, **V1**.221
  classification, **V1**.27 (Tab.)
  DNA proviruses, **V1**.338, **V1**.344
  endogenous, **V1**.182
  Env (envelope) protein, **V2**.1322–3, **V2**.1591

Retroviruses (*Continued*)
  evolution, **V1**.176
    recombination, **V1**.14–5
  Gag protein, **V1**.78–9, **V2**.1322–3, **V2**.1591
  gene expression, **V1**.111–12
  gene therapy vectors, **V1**.197–8, **V2**.1591–4, **V2**.1595 (Tab.)
    design, **V2**.1594
    hematopoietic stem cells, **V2**.1592
    history, **V2**.1591
    Rev response element, **V2**.1594
    transient infection, **V2**.1594
  gene transduction, **V1**.335, **V1**.335 (Tab.)
  genome, **V2**.1284, **V2**.1591
    long terminal repeats (LTR), **V1**.337 (Fig.)
    pseudodiploid form, **V1**.188, **V2**.1591
    replication, **V1**.123–4
    sizes, **V1**.46
  historical aspects, **V1**.7
  hypermutation, **V1**.193
  immune evasion, **V1**.313
  infection *see* Retrovirus infection
  infectivity, **V1**.45–6
  integration into host genome, **V1**.280–1, **V2**.1297–8, **V2**.1593–4
    insertional mutagenesis, **V2**.1593–4
  isolation/propagation and identification, **V1**.96 (Tab.), **V1**.100
  leukaemogenic
    oncogenic mechanism, **V1**.337 (Fig.)
    transformation by, **V1**.336
  life cycle, **V1**.280–1, **V2**.1592
    nuclear import, **V2**.1592–3
  morphology/structure, **V1**.77–9, **V1**.77 (Fig.)
    glycoproteins, **V1**.77
    lipid rafts, **V1**.77
    membrane, **V2**.1592
    protein structures, **V1**.70 (Tab.)
    replication component, **V1**.77–8
    transport component, **V1**.77
  oncogenes, **V1**.335–6, **V1**.335 (Tab.)
    identification, **V1**.338–9
  origins, **V1**.13–4
  Pol (polymerase) protein, **V1**.78–9, **V2**.1322–3, **V2**.1591
  protein synthesis, **V1**.117
  receptors, **V1**.207 (Tab.), **V1**.213, **V1**.344–5, **V2**.1592
  recombination, **V1**.188
  replication, **V2**.1284, **V2**.1285 (Fig.)
    integrase, **V1**.58
    restrictions, **V1**.344
    reverse transcriptase, **V1**.58, **V1**.181–2, **V2**.1592
  transcription, long terminal repeat (LTR) generation, **V1**.188
  transformation by, **V1**.336
  translation, splicing mechanisms, **V1**.114–15
  virulence, **V1**.253
  see also Retroviridae; Reverse-transcribing viruses; Reverse transcriptase(s); *specific viruses*
Retrovirus infection, **V2**.1285
  antiviral therapy, latent infection, **V2**.1638
  BCE peptide vaccines, **I**.871
  cancer, **V2**.1297–8

CNS infection, **V2**.1426–30
  in HIV infection, **V2**.1499 (Tab.)
  host cell DNA metabolism, **V1**.217
  host range restriction, **V1**.344–5, **V2**.1591
  immune response, **V1**.280–2
    IFN activity, **I**.260 (Tab.)
  latent, **V1**.345
  medical importance, **V1**.135
  oncogenesis, **V1**.337 (Fig.), **V1**.342 (Tab.), **V2**.1591
    cell stimulation, **V1**.341
    gene disruption, **V1**.339–40
    insertional mutagenesis, **V1**.338–40
    insertional mutagenesis modes, **V1**.339 (Fig.)
    tumors associated, **V1**.330, **V1**.331 (Tab.)
  persistent, **V1**.373
  vertical transmission, **V1**.281, **V1**.343–4
  zoonoses, **V2**.1295–6
Reverse genetics, **V1**.189–90
  arteriviruses, **V1**.830–1
  Bunyamwera virus, **V1**.189–90
  bunyaviruses, **V1**.189
  coronaviruses, **V1**.830–1
  double-stranded RNA virus, **V1**.189–90
  filoviruses, **V1**.133–4, **V1**.189
  Human respiratory syncytial virus vaccines, **V1**.793
  influenza neuraminidase (NA), **V1**.654
  negative-strand RNA viruses, **V1**.133–4, **V1**.189, **V1**.189–90, **V1**.190 (Fig.), **V1**.191 (Fig.)
  orthomyxoviruses, **V1**.133–4, **V1**.189
  paramyxoviruses, **V1**.133–4, **V1**.189
  poxviruses, **V1**.615–16
  rabies virus, **V1**.133–4
  rhabdoviruses, **V1**.189
Reverse passive latex agglutination (RPLA)
  Candida, **M**.98–100
  Cryptococcus, **M**.109, **M**.110
Reverse-transcribing viruses
  cell interactions, **V1**.219
  classification, **V1**.45–7, **V1**.46 (Tab.)
  gene expression, **V1**.111–12
  genome, **V1**.176
    replication, **V1**.123–4, **V1**.124 (Fig.)
    terminal redundancy, **V1**.181–2
  see also Retroviruses
Reverse transcriptase(s), **B1**.435–6
  assays, **V2**.1294
  discovery, **V1**.7
  HTLVs, **V2**.1285–7, **V2**.1294
  inhibitors, HIV infection, **V2**.1334–6
  retrovirus replication, **V1**.58
  sequence analysis, **V1**.113–14
  viral evolution, **V1**.14–5
  see also Retroviruses
Reverse transcription, **V1**.181–2, **V1**.188–9
Reverse transcription polymerase chain reaction (RT-PCR), **B1**.726 (Tab.)
  adenoviruses, **V1**.446
  aspergillosis, **M**.718
  astroviruses, **V2**.889, **V2**.906–7
  Borna disease virus, **V2**.1150–3
  Bovine torovirus, **V1**.846

bunyaviruses, **V2**.1050
Canine distemper virus, **V1**.812, **V1**.813–14
  in disease diagnosis, **V2**.1537–8
    croup, **V1**.775
    influenza, **V1**.676–7
    measles, **V1**.733
    mumps, **V1**.755–6
    mumps diagnosis, **V1**.756
    rinderpest, **V1**.810
    rubella, **V2**.978–9
    severe acute respiratory syndrome (SARS), **V1**.842–3
  Equine arteritis virus, **V1**.846–7
  feline coronavirus, **V1**.845
  filoviruses, **V2**.1091–2, **V2**.1096–7
  henipaviruses, **V1**.818
  Hepatitis B virus, **V2**.1254–5
  Hepatitis C virus, **V2**.1213–14
  Hepatitis G virus, **V2**.1482
  Human coronaviruses, **V1**.842
  noroviruses, **V2**.921–2
  Porcine reproductive and respiratory syndrome virus, **V1**.847–8
  Porcine transmissible gastroenteritis virus, **V1**.844–5
  Ross River virus, **V2**.1022
  rotaviruses, **V2**.952
  sapoviruses, **V2**.924–5
  syphilis detection, **B2**.1853
Reversion mutants, mis-sense mutations, **B1**.87
Review of Medical and Veterinary Mycology, **M**.31
Rev protein *see* HIV
Rev response element
  HIV, **V1**.221
  retrovirus gene therapy vectors, **V2**.1594
Rex protein *see* Human T-cell leukemia virus 1 (HTLV-1); Human T-cell leukemia virus 2 (HTLV-2)
Reyataz *see* Atazanavir
RFLP *see* Restriction fragment length polymorphisms (RFLPs)
Rhabditidae, **P**.593
Rhabditiform larvae, *Strongyloides*, **P**.738–9
Rhabditis, **P**.593
Rhabditoidea, **P**.593–4
  Rhabditidae, **P**.593
  Strongyloididae, **P**.593–4
Rhabdoviridae, **V1**.26, **V1**.385–6
  characteristics, **V1**.129 (Tab.), **V1**.177 (Tab.)
  classification, **V1**.27 (Tab.), **V1**.49, **V1**.49 (Tab.), **V1**.127–8
    characteristics, **V1**.379, **V1**.380 (Tab.)
    criteria, **V2**.1102–3
    phylogenetic tree, **V2**.1103 (Fig.)
  genera, **V1**.385
  phylogeny, **V1**.388
  serogroups, **V1**.386
  see also Ephemerovirus; Lyssavirus; Rhabdoviruses; Vesiculovirus; specific viruses
Rhabdoviruses, **V2**.**1102–36**
  antigens, **V2**.1115–16
  cell entry, **V1**.213, **V2**.1107–9
    acidification, **V2**.1108
    receptors, **V2**.1108

Rhabdoviruses (*Continued*)
cell exit, **V2**.1112
chemical composition, **V2**.1105–6
defective interfering particles, **V2**.1103
Entamoeba histolytica cylindrical particle *vs.*, **P**.203
formation of, **V1**.74–5
genome
gene expression, **V2**.1109–11
modules, **V2**.1112
size, **V2**.1111
structure, **V1**.128–30, **V1**.387 (Tab.), **V2**.1111–12
glycoprotein (G), **V2**.1105–6
cell-binding, **V2**.1115
conformational change, **V2**.1108
genes, **V2**.1112
immune response to, **V2**.1125
posttranslational modification, **V2**.1115
infection *see* Rhabdovirus infection
isolation/propagation and identification, **V1**.95, **V1**.96 (Tab.)
large (L) protein, **V2**.1106, **V2**.1113–14
genes, **V2**.1112
transcription–replication switch, **V2**.1111
life cycle, **V2**.1109 (Fig.)
matrix (M) protein, **V2**.1105–6, **V2**.1114–15
budding process, **V2**.1114
genes, **V2**.1112
ribonucleoprotein interaction, **V2**.1114
members, **V2**.1102
membrane proteins, **V2**.1114–15
morphology/structure, **V1**.73–5, **V1**.74 (Fig.), **V1**.128–30, **V1**.385, **V2**.1105, **V2**.1106 (Fig.), **V2**.1107 (Fig.), **V2**.1108 (Fig.)
DRM, **V1**.73–4
polymerase, **V1**.74
protein structures, **V1**.70 (Tab.)
replication component, **V1**.74
transport component, **V1**.73–4
mRNA transcription, **V1**.381
nucleoprotein (N), **V2**.1106, **V2**.1113
conservation, **V2**.1116
immune response to, **V2**.1124–5
phosphoprotein (P), **V2**.1106, **V2**.1113
interaction network, **V2**.1113
phosphorylation, **V2**.1113
polypeptides, **V2**.1112–15
see also specific types
properties, **V2**.1102–5
receptors, **V1**.207 (Tab.)
CNS, **V2**.1406 (Tab.)
replication, **V2**.1110 (Fig.)
reverse genetics, **V1**.189
ribonucleoprotein, **V2**.1105–6, **V2**.1113–14
matrix (M) protein interaction, **V2**.1114
structure, **V2**.1113
transcription, alternate termination sites, **V1**.180
translation, **V2**.1110 (Fig.), **V2**.1111
Rhabdovirus infection
arthropod vectors, **V2**.1102
birds, **V2**.1105
fish pathogens, **V2**.1105
host range, **V1**.381–2

IFN activity, **I**.260 (Tab.)
infection cycle, **V2**.1106–9
neural spread, **V1**.244 (Tab.)
plant pathogens, **V2**.1104–5
morphology, **V2**.1106 (Fig.)
transmission, **V1**.371 (Tab.)
Rhadinovirus
classification, **V1**.541–3, **V1**.542 (Tab.)
genome sequences, **V1**.494 (Tab.)
L-Rhamnose fermentation, Enterobacteriaceae identification, **B2**.1319 (Tab.)
Rhapidosomes, **B2**.1594
Rhesus lymphocryptovirus, **V1**.494 (Tab.)
Rhesus monkey rhadinovirus (RRV), **V1**.543
characteristics, **V1**.542 (Tab.)
genome sequences, **V1**.494 (Tab.)
Rhesus theta defensins *see* θ-Defensins
Rheumatic fever
pathogen induced, **I**.753 (Tab.)
see also Streptococcus pyogenes infection
Rheumatic heart disease, endocarditis in, **B1**.525–6
Rheumatoid arthritis (RA)
cartilage destruction/bone loss, **I**.757
complement pathology, **I**.155 (Tab.)
HLA association, **I**.577
HLA-DR, **I**.751, **I**.752 (Tab.)
IL-15, **I**.282
K/BxN mouse model, **I**.759
macrophages, **I**.31
neutrophil abnormalities, **I**.49
NK cells, **I**.103
prevalence, **I**.748 (Tab.)
Proteus mirabilis association, **B2**.1447
superantigens, **I**.564
Th1/Th2 balance, **I**.755–6
therapy
anti-inflammatory drugs, **I**.209
monoclonal antibody therapy, **I**.357
Rheumatological syndromes, histoplasmosis capsulati, **M**.523
Rhexolysis, **M**.250
Rhinitis, atrophic, in swine, **B2**.1653–4, **B2**.1795, **B2**.1810
Rhinocerebral mucormycosis *see* Rhino-orbital-cerebral zygomycosis
Rhinocerebral zygomycosis, **M**.20–1, **M**.295, **M**.673–4, **M**.674 (Tab.), **M**.678
CNS, **M**.20–1, **M**.673–4, **M**.674 (Tab.), **M**.678
Rhinocladiella aquaspersa
chromoblastomycosis, **M**.29–30, **M**.357
histopathology, **M**.89 (Tab.), **M**.128 (Tab.)
Rhino-orbital-cerebral zygomycosis
causative agents, **M**.290
Apophysomyces elegans, **M**.290, **M**.291
Mucor, **M**.290–1, **M**.292 (Fig.)
Saksenaea vasiformis, **M**.290, **M**.292
clinical features, **M**.291
diagnosis, **M**.291–2
therapy, **M**.292
amphotericin B, **M**.293
fluconazole, **M**.293–4
itraconazole, **M**.293–4
Rhino-orbital infection, amphotericin B therapy, **M**.294

Rhinoscleroma, **B1**.616–17, **B1**.629
causative organisms, **B1**.616
clinical features, **B1**.616
epidemiology, **B1**.616
in HIV infection, **B1**.616–17
treatment, **B1**.617
Rhinosinusitis, *Encephalitozoon intestinalis* infection, **P**.542
Rhinosporidiosis, **M**.69, **M**.436–75, **M**.457
animals, **M**.472
birds, **M**.447, **M**.457, **M**.470, **M**.472
cats, **M**.456–7, **M**.464, **M**.466, **M**.472
cattle, **M**.439, **M**.456–7, **M**.460, **M**.472
dogs, **M**.458
experimental, **M**.456–7
horses, **M**.456–7, **M**.472
swans, **M**.447, **M**.457, **M**.470, **M**.472
clinical presentation, **M**.460–1
ulceration, **M**.462, **M**.466 (Fig.)
concurrent diseases, **M**.465
diagnosis, **M**.125–7, **M**.469–71
cytology, **M**.471
histopathology, **M**.462, **M**.463 (Fig.), **M**.464 (Fig.), **M**.470
differential diagnosis, **M**.470, **M**.471
Microcystis aeruginosa vs., **M**.439–40
disseminated, **M**.461, **M**.463, **M**.464, **M**.465 (Fig.), **M**.466 (Fig.)
epidemiology, **M**.457
farmers/farm workers, **M**.458
geographical distribution, **M**.457, **M**.458 (Tab.)
rice paddy workers, **M**.458
genitourinary tract infection, **M**.459–60
penis, **M**.459–60
urethra, **M**.460
vulva, **M**.459–60
histopathology, **M**.121–2, **M**.128 (Tab.), **M**.136 (Fig.)
immune response, **M**.456, **M**.466–9
cell-mediated immune response, **M**.466, **M**.467 (Fig.), **M**.468 (Fig.)
delayed-type hypersensitivity, **M**.468, **M**.468 (Fig.)
humoral immune response, **M**.469
oculomycoses, **M**.275 (Tab.), **M**.289, **M**.289 (Fig.), **M**.297, **M**.457, **M**.458, **M**.459, **M**.460–1, **M**.461 (Fig.), **M**.463 (Fig.)
conjunctiva, **M**.299–300
dacryocystitis, **M**.298
polyps, **M**.459, **M**.460 (Fig.), **M**.461 (Fig.)
culture, **M**.439–40, **M**.455–6
strawberry, **M**.450, **M**.460 (Fig.), **M**.461–2, **M**.469–70
religion, **M**.439, **M**.458
sand workers, **M**.439, **M**.458–9
sites, **M**.460
bone, **M**.461–2, **M**.462 (Fig.)
CNS, **M**.462
face, **M**.460, **M**.461 (Fig.)
lymph nodes, **M**.464–5, **M**.465 (Fig.)
nose, **M**.439, **M**.457, **M**.458, **M**.459, **M**.460, **M**.460 (Fig.), **M**.461 (Fig.)
parotid gland, **M**.460–1

Rhinosporidiosis
sites (*Continued*)
skin, **M**.460, **M**.461–2, **M**.461 (Fig.), **M**.469–70
Stenson's duct, **M**.460–1
spread, **M**.459–60, **M**.464–6
therapy, **M**.471–2
dapsone, **M**.454, **M**.471–2
Rhinosporidium
growth pattern, **M**.70
infection *see* Rhinosporidiosis
Rhinosporidium pulmonale, **M**.811
Rhinosporidium seeberi infection *see*
Rhinosporidiosis
Rhinosporidosis, lymphadenitis, **M**.465, **M**.470
Rhinovirus 14, **V2**.862
Rhinovirus Collaborative Program (WHO), **V2**.858
Rhinoviruses
capsid attachment sites, **V1**.209
cell entry, **V1**.245, **V2**.867 (Tab.)
characteristics, **V2**.861 (Tab.)
classification, **V2**.858, **V2**.859 (Fig.)
neutralizing antisera, **V2**.861
genome size, **V2**.863–5
historical aspects, **V2**.858
immune evasion, **V1**.312
isolation/propagation and identification, **V1**.100
morphology/structure, **V2**.862
properties, **V2**.1162 (Tab.)
protein synthesis, **V1**.115–16
receptors, **V1**.207 (Tab.), **V1**.246 (Fig.), **V2**.867 (Tab.)
ICAM-1, **V1**.208–9, **V1**.210 (Fig.)
low-density lipoprotein receptor, **V1**.209
virus release, **V1**.211–12
shedding, **V1**.249 (Fig.)
Rhinovirus infection, **V2**.873–4
acute infection duration, **V1**.258
clinical manifestations, **V2**.873
age-related, **V2**.873
bronchitis association, **V2**.873
lower-respiratory tract, **V2**.873
diagnosis, **V2**.877–8
hemagglutination tests, **V2**.878
molecular methods, **V2**.878
nasal washings, **V2**.878
organ culture, **V2**.878
specimen transport, **V2**.878
epidemiology, **V1**.366, **V2**.875–6
seasonality, **V2**.875
etiological relationships, **V1**.365
expenditure, **V2**.873
host protein synthesis, **V1**.203, **V1**.223–4
immune response, **V2**.874
basophils, **I**.71
IgA, **V2**.874
neutralizing antibodies, **V2**.866, **V2**.866 (Tab.)
infection process, **V1**.241 (Tab.)
pathogenesis, **V2**.873–4
ciliated epithelia, **V2**.873–4
inflammation, **V2**.873
mycoplasma infection, **V2**.873
prophylaxis, **V2**.878–9

serotypes, **V2**.875–6
therapy, **V2**.878–9
antiviral drugs, **V2**.1630–1, **V2**.1630 (Fig.)
dichloroflavan, **V2**.879
disoxaril, **V2**.879
IFNs, **I**.259, **V1**.295
INFs, **V2**.879
monoclonal antibodies, **V2**.879
R61837, **V2**.879
transmission
droplets, **V1**.354
hand contact, **V2**.873
vaccine, **V2**.878
Rhipicephalus sanguineus, **B2**.2037
Rhipidomys leucodactylus, Leishmania braziliensis, **P**.326
Rhizidovirus, **V1**.27 (Tab.)
Rhizobium
legume relationship, **B1**.197
natural competence, **B1**.99
Rhizobium etli, **B1**.61
Rhizobium meliloti, **B2**.1729 (Tab.)
Rhizoctonia, oculomycoses, **M**.275 (Tab.)
Rhizomucor, **M**.660, **M**.660 (Tab.), **M**.667
history, **M**.20
oculomycoses, **M**.287
Rhizomucor microsporus var. *microsporus,* **M**.660
Rhizomucor miehei, **M**.667
Rhizomucor pusillus, **M**.660, **M**.667–8, **M**.668 (Fig.)
histopathology, **M**.128 (Tab.)
history, **M**.20
infection, **M**.667–8, **M**.674–5
experimental, **M**.677
nosocomial, **M**.21
Rhizomucor tauricus, **M**.667
Rhizomucor variabilis, **M**.659–60
Rhizopus, **M**.660, **M**.660 (Tab.), **M**.668, **M**.677
in cereals, **B1**.284
fruit, **B1**.283
groups, **M**.668
history, **M**.20
infection
desferrioxamine, **M**.13
histopathology, **M**.89 (Tab.), **M**.127 (Tab.)
nosocomial, **M**.21
oculomycoses, **M**.281 (Tab.), **M**.287
rhino-orbital-cerebral zygomycosis, **M**.290
nosocomial infection, **B1**.379
vegetables, **B1**.281
Rhizopus arrhizus
histopathology, **M**.128 (Tab.), **M**.141 (Fig.), **M**.142 (Fig.)
infection, rhino-orbital-cerebral zygomycosis, **M**.290
Rhizopus azygosporus, **M**.668, **M**.669, **M**.669 (Tab.), **M**.674
Rhizopus homothallicus, **M**.668
Rhizopus microsporus, **M**.668, **M**.669 (Tab.), **M**.670 (Fig.)
var. *microsporus,* **M**.668, **M**.669, **M**.669 (Tab.), **M**.670 (Fig.)
var. *oligosporus,* **M**.668, **M**.669, **M**.669 (Tab.), **M**.670 (Fig.), **M**.677

var. *rhizopodiformis,* **M**.660, **M**.668, **M**.669–70, **M**.669 (Tab.), **M**.670 (Fig.)
infection, **M**.20, **M**.674–5
Rhizopus oryzae, **M**.660, **M**.668, **M**.670, **M**.670 (Fig.), **M**.671 (Fig.)
identification, **M**.670 (Fig.), **M**.671, **M**.671 (Fig.)
infection, **M**.670, **M**.674–5
experimental, **M**.677
nomenclature, **M**.668
Rhizopus schipperae, **M**.668, **M**.669 (Tab.), **M**.671
Rhizopus sexualis, **M**.668
Rhizopus stolonifer, **M**.668, **M**.671–2
Rhizosphere, **B1**.197–8
classification, **B1**.197
endorhizosphere, **B1**.197
operational definition in sampling and detection, **B1**.204
recovery of populations, **B1**.204–5
rhizoplane, **B1**.197
sampling, **B1**.204–5, **B1**.205–7
size estimates, **B1**.197–8
soil ratio, **B1**.197–8
spermosphere, **B1**.197
Rho, apoptosis debris removal, **I**.136
Rhodnius prolixus, **P**.382, **P**.390–1
Rhodobacter sphaeroides
chromosomes, **B1**.46
external appendages, **B1**.44
movement, **B1**.44
Rhodococcus, **B2**.1137–8, **B2**.1166–8, **B2**.1168
antibacterial susceptibility/resistance, **B2**.1145
classification, **B2**.1137–8
identification, **B2**.1144–5
microscopic morphology, **B2**.1141–3
Middlebrook opacification, **B2**.1144
molecular methods, **B2**.1146
ribotyping, **B2**.1147
staining, **B2**.1139–40
menaquinones, **B2**.1145, **B2**.1166–7
molecular identification, **B2**.1147
mycolic acids, **B2**.1146, **B2**.1151, **B2**.1166–7
substrate decomposition, **B2**.1144
Rhodococcus equi
infection, **B2**.1167–8
horse/pig exposure, **B2**.1168
intracranial abscess, **B1**.586
nosocomial, **B1**.401 (Tab.)
pneumonia, in HIV infection, **B1**.645
pulmonary in HIV infection, **B2**.1167–8
molecular identification, **B2**.1146
strain typing, **B2**.1148
Rhodococcus fascians, **B2**.1168
Rhodococcus globerulis, **B2**.1168
Rhodosporidium, classification, **M**.63
Rhodotorula
characteristics, **M**.632, **M**.632 (Tab.), **M**.633 (Tab.)
infection, **M**.625 (Tab.), **M**.627
amphotericin B therapy, **M**.627–8
flucytosine therapy, **M**.627–8
fungemia, **M**.627
keratitis, **M**.328
oculomycoses, **M**.280 (Tab.)

Rhodotorula
  infection (*Continued*)
    peritonitis, **M**.627
Rhodotorula glutinis, **M**.627, **M**.633 (Tab.)
  characteristics, **M**.632
Rhodotorula minuta, **M**.627, **M**.633 (Tab.)
  characteristics, **M**.632
Rhodotorula rubra, **M**.627, **M**.632, **M**.633 (Tab.)
Rhombomys opimus, **P**.303
  eradication of, **P**.118
Rhoptries, **P**.178
  Babesia, **P**.452
  Toxoplasma gondii, **P**.423
RIA *see* Radioimmunoassays (RIAs)
Ribavirin, **V2**.1628
  adenovirus infection, **V1**.446
  arenavirus infection, **V2**.1078
  Borna disease virus infection, **V2**.1153
  Colorado tick fever virus, **V2**.943
  hemorrhagic fever with renal syndrome
    (HFRS) treatment, **V2**.1044–5
  henipavirus infection, **V1**.818
  hepatitis B therapy, **V2**.1629
  historical aspects, **V1**.9 (Tab.)
  mutagen, **V1**.19–20
  resistance, **V2**.1628
  respiratory syncytial virus infection, **V2**.1628
  structure, **V2**.1621 (Fig.)
Riboflavin (vitamin B2) deficiency, malaria,
    P.493
Ribonucleic acid *see* RNA
Ribonucleocapsids, bunyaviruses, **V2**.1030–1,
    V2.1030 (Fig.)
Ribonucleoprotein (RNP)
  negative-strand RNA viruses replication,
    V1.128
  rhabdoviruses *see* Rhabdoviruses
Ribonucleotide reductase
  antiviral target, **V2**.1617
  herpesviruses, **V1**.499
  HSV-1, **V1**.165 (Tab.), **V1**.499
  poxviruses, **V1**.169 (Tab.), **V1**.606
RiboPrinter®, **B1**.735
Riboprinting, amebiasis diagnosis, **P**.220
Ribose metabolism, **B1**.57, **B1**.59
Ribosomal DNA (rDNA)
  Aspergillus, **M**.108, **M**.715
  Candida albicans, **M**.103
  Candida parapsilosis, **M**.103–4
  Candida tropicalis, **M**.103–4
  Entamoeba histolytica, **P**.206
  Malassezia, **M**.215
  Sporothrix schenckii, **M**.371–2
23S Ribosomal DNA, *Coxiella burnetii,*
    B2.2072–3
Ribosomal frameshifting
  arterivirus replicase, **V1**.832
  coronavirus replicase, **V1**.832
  Nidovirales order, **V1**.395–6
  RNA viruses, **V1**.180
  torovirus replicase (RNA polymerase),
    V1.832
Ribosomal RNA (rRNA), **M**.91
  16S screening *see below*
  Aspergillus, **M**.688–9
  Candida, **M**.580, **M**.608

Coccidioides immitis, **M**.514
  content, **B1**.42
  degradation, **B1**.40
  DNA ratio, **B1**.206
  eubacterial primers, **B2**.1147–8
  gene numbers in bacteria, **B1**.47
  gene restriction pattern examination,
    B2.1947–8
  Malassezia, **M**.215
  operons, **B1**.47, **B2**.2074–5
  Pneumocystis, **M**.4, **M**.772, **M**.775
  18S rRNA genes, **M**.663
  28S rRNA genes, **M**.663
  28S rRNA genes, **M**.663
  sequencing, *Giardia* classification, **P**.242
  soil bacteria metabolism quantification,
    B1.206
16S Ribosomal RNA (rRNA) probes, gram-
    positive anaerobic cocci identification,
    B2.907
16S Ribosomal RNA (rRNA) sequencing,
    B1.22 (Tab.), **B1**.25–6
  aerobic actinomycetes, **B2**.1147
  Cedecea, **B2**.1338
  Coxiella burnetii, **B2**.2072–3
  Enterobacteriaceae, **B2**.1318, **B2**.1338
  Enterococcus, **B2**.884–5, **B2**.890
  evolution and controversy, **B1**.30–1
  groups, **B1**.31
  problems, **B1**.26, **B1**.32–3
  rapidly growing mycobacteria, **B2**.1237,
    B2.1243–4
  Veillonella identification, **B2**.1315
Ribosomal skipping
  foot-and-mouth disease virus, **V1**.117
  protein synthesis, **V1**.117
Ribosome(s)
  in arenavirus replication, **V2**.1066
  composition, **B1**.46–7
  degradation in bacterial death phase, **B1**.40
  Histoplasma capsulatum var. *capsulatum,*
    M.527
  mycoplasmas, **B2**.1980
  proteins (r-proteins), **B1**.46–7
    synthesis, **B1**.47
  proteins (r-proteins), *Candida,* **M**.591
  protozoa, **P**.175
  RNA *see above*
  scanning, coronavirus translation, **V1**.831
  translocation, **B1**.47
Ribotyping
  aerobic actinomycetes, **B2**.1147
  Burkholderia cepacia, **B2**.1614–15
  Burkholderia thailandensis, **B2**.1623
  Chlamydia, **B2**.2018–19
  Escherichia, **B2**.1371
  Legionella, **B2**.1775, **B2**.1776
  Salmonella, **B2**.1409, **B2**.1410
  Stenotrophomonas maltophilia, **B2**.1637
Riboviruses
  definition, **V1**.13
  evolution
    genome rearrangement, **V1**.16
    recombination, **V1**.13, **V1**.15–6
    origins, **V1**.13
Ribulose biphosphate carboxylase, **B1**.62

Ribulose monophosphate carboxylase (RuMP)
    pathway, **B1**.62–3
Rice, **B1**.285–6
  production, **B1**.285–6
  storage, **B1**.286
  water activity, **B1**.285–6
Rice paddy workers, infection, **M**.458
'Rice water' stools, cholera, **B2**.1516–17
Ricin, immunoconjugates *see*
    Immunoconjugates
Rickettsia
  adhesion to host cells, **B2**.2034
  antibiotic susceptibility testing, **B2**.2042–3
    arthropod model, **B2**.2042
    cell culture models, **B2**.2042–3
    embryonated egg model, **B2**.2042
  antigens, **B2**.2031–2
  cell wall composition, **B2**.2031–2, **B2**.2034
  classification, **B2**.2026, **B2**.2027 (Fig.),
    B2.2028 (Fig.), **B2**.2030–1
  escape to cytoplasm, **I**.650
  genetics, **B2**.2033–4, **B2**.2033 (Tab.)
    ATP-ADP translocase genes, **B2**.2027,
      B2.2033–4
    Omp genes, **B2**.2033–5
    open reading frames, **B2**.2033
    ProP transporter, **B2**.2033–4
  habitats and epidemiology, **B2**.2037–8,
    B2.2038 (Fig.)
  identification
    immunofluorescent antibody tests,
      B1.752–3
    immunological, **B2**.2037
    PCR, **B2**.2036–7
    phenotypic classification, **B2**.2031–3
    staining procedures, **B2**.2030, **B2**.2034–5
    Weil–Felix reaction, **B1**.752–3
  infection *see* Rickettsial diseases; Typhus
  isolation, **B2**.2034–5
  LPS, *Proteus vs.,* **B2**.1444
  metabolism, **B2**.2034
  microenvironment (intracellular), **B2**.2030
  morphology, **B2**.2030
  pathogenicity, **B2**.2034
    host cell damage, **B2**.2030
    virulence factors, **B2**.2034
Rickettsia aeschlimannii
  antibacterial susceptibility/resistance,
    B2.2043, **B2**.2043 (Tab.)
  classification, **B2**.2030–1, **B2**.2031 (Tab.),
    B2.2032
  identification, **B2**.2026–7
  infection, **B2**.2039 (Tab.), **B2**.2040
    see also Rickettsial diseases
  isolation, **B2**.2034–5
Rickettsia africae
  classification, **B2**.2030–1, **B2**.2031 (Tab.)
  detection, **B2**.2037
  geographical distribution, **B2**.2038 (Fig.)
  identification, **B2**.2026–7
  infection, **B2**.2039 (Tab.), **B2**.2040,
    B2.2040 (Fig.)
    see also Rickettsial diseases
  Western blot, **B2**.2036 (Fig.)
Rickettsia akari
  habitats, vectors and hosts, **B2**.2037

Rickettsia akari (*Continued*)
  infection, **B2**.2039 (Tab.), **B2**.2041
    see also Rickettsial diseases
  pathogenicity and virulence, **B2**.2034
    characteristics, **B2**.2033 (Tab.)
    classification, **B2**.2031–2, **B2**.2031 (Tab.)
Rickettsia amblyommii, **B2**.2030–1,
  B2.2031 (Tab.)
Rickettsia australis
  characteristics, **B2**.2033 (Tab.)
  classification, **B2**.2031–2, **B2**.2031 (Tab.)
  geographical distribution, **B2**.2038 (Fig.)
  infection, **B2**.2039 (Tab.), **B2**.2040
    see also Rickettsial diseases
Rickettsia bellii
  cell wall composition, **B2**.2034
  classification, **B2**.2031 (Tab.), **B2**.2032,
    B2.2033
Rickettsia canadensis, **B2**.2033 (Tab.)
  cell wall composition, **B2**.2034
  classification, **B2**.2031–2, **B2**.2031 (Tab.),
    B2.2033
Rickettsia conorii, **B2**.2030, **B2**.2032–3,
  B2.2033 (Tab.)
  cell wall composition, **B2**.2034
  classification, **B2**.2031–2, **B2**.2031 (Tab.)
  detection, **B2**.2037
  genetics, **B2**.2027, **B2**.2033, **B2**.2033 (Tab.)
  geographical distribution, **B2**.2038 (Fig.)
  habitats, vectors and hosts, **B2**.2031 (Tab.),
    B2.2037
  identification, **B2**.2026–7
    Western blot, **B2**.2036 (Fig.)
  infection *see* Mediterranean spotted fever
  isolation, **B2**.2034–5
  metabolism, **B2**.2034
  pathogenicity and virulence, **B2**.2034
Rickettsia cooleyi, **B2**.2030–1, **B2**.2031 (Tab.)
Rickettsia diaporica see Coxiella burnetii
Rickettsia felis
  classification, **B2**.2030–1, **B2**.2031 (Tab.)
  habitats, vectors and hosts, **B2**.2037
  identification, **B2**.2026–7
  infection, **B2**.2039 (Tab.), **B2**.2041
    see also Rickettsial diseases
  isolation, **B2**.2034–5
Rickettsia heilongjanghensis
  classification, **B2**.2031 (Tab.)
  infection, **B2**.2039 (Tab.), **B2**.2040
    see also Rickettsial diseases
Rickettsia helvetica
  classification, **B2**.2030–1, **B2**.2031 (Tab.)
  geographical distribution, **B2**.2038 (Fig.)
  identification, **B2**.2026–7
  infection, **B2**.2039 (Tab.)
    see also Rickettsial diseases
  isolation, **B2**.2034–5
Rickettsia honei
  classification, **B2**.2030–1, **B2**.2031 (Tab.)
  geographical distribution, **B2**.2038 (Fig.)
  identification, **B2**.2026–7
  infection, **B2**.2039 (Tab.), **B2**.2040
    see also Rickettsial diseases
Rickettsia japonica
  classification, **B2**.2030–1, **B2**.2031 (Tab.)

geographical distribution, **B2**.2038 (Fig.)
identification, **B2**.2026–7
infection, **B2**.2039 (Tab.), **B2**.2040
  see also Rickettsial diseases
Rickettsial diseases, **B2**.2029 (Tab.)
  antibody detection, **B1**.752–3
  clinical manifestations, **B2**.2038–42,
    B2.2039 (Tab.)
  cytopathology, **B2**.2034
  diagnosis, **B2**.2034–7
    immunofluorescent antibody tests,
      B1.752–3
    immunological, **B2**.2037
    PCR, **B2**.2036–7
    serological assays, **B2**.2035–6
    Weil–Felix reaction, **B1**.752–3
  epidemiology and natural history, **B2**.2037
  geographical distribution, **B2**.2031 (Tab.),
    B2.2037, **B2**.2038 (Fig.)
  pathogenesis, **B2**.2030, **B2**.2034
  treatment, **B2**.2043
  vaccines, **I**.933 (Tab.)
  see also Typhus
Rickettsial pox, **B2**.2039 (Tab.), **B2**.2041
Rickettsia massiliae
  characteristics, **B2**.2033 (Tab.)
  classification, **B2**.2030–1, **B2**.2031 (Tab.),
    B2.2032–3
  isolation, **B2**.2034–5
Rickettsia mongolotimonae
  classification, **B2**.2030–1, **B2**.2031 (Tab.)
  geographical distribution, **B2**.2038 (Fig.)
  identification, **B2**.2026–7
  infection, **B2**.2039 (Tab.), **B2**.2040
    see also Rickettsial diseases
  isolation, **B2**.2034–5
Rickettsia montanensis, **B2**.2032–3
  characteristics, **B2**.2033 (Tab.)
  classification, **B2**.2031–2, **B2**.2031 (Tab.)
Rickettsia parkeri, **B2**.2031–2, **B2**.2031 (Tab.)
Rickettsia peacockii, **B2**.2030–1, **B2**.2031 (Tab.)
Rickettsia prowazekii
  antibiotic susceptibility testing, **B2**.2042–3
  cell wall composition, **B2**.2034
  characteristics, **B2**.2033 (Tab.)
  classification, **B2**.2027, **B2**.2027 (Fig.),
    B2.2031–2, **B2**.2031 (Tab.)
  detection, **B2**.2037
  genetics, **B2**.2027, **B2**.2033, **B2**.2033 (Tab.)
  habitats, vectors and hosts, **B2**.2037, **B2**.2041
  infection, **B2**.2039 (Tab.), **B2**.2041
    infiltration of host tissues, **B1**.153
    see also Rickettsial diseases
  metabolism, **B2**.2034
  microbiology, **B2**.2030
  pathogenicity and virulence, **B2**.2034
  S layer, **B1**.155
Rickettsia rhipicephali
  characteristics, **B2**.2033 (Tab.)
  classification, **B2**.2031–2, **B2**.2031 (Tab.)
Rickettsia rickettsii, **B2**.2032–3
  characteristics, **B2**.2033 (Tab.)
  classification, **B2**.2027 (Fig.), **B2**.2031–2,
    B2.2031 (Tab.)
  geographical distribution, **B2**.2038 (Fig.)

habitats, vectors and hosts, **B2**.2037
infection *see* Rickettsial diseases; Rocky
  Mountain spotted fever
infiltration of host tissues, **B1**.153
isolation, **B2**.2034–5
pathogenicity and virulence, **B2**.2034
Rickettsia sibirica, **B2**.2032–3
  characteristics, **B2**.2033 (Tab.)
  classification, **B2**.2030–2, **B2**.2031 (Tab.)
  geographical distribution, **B2**.2038 (Fig.)
  infection, **B2**.2039 (Tab.), **B2**.2040
    see also Rickettsial diseases
Rickettsia slovaca
  classification, **B2**.2030–1, **B2**.2031 (Tab.)
  detection, **B2**.2037
  identification, **B2**.2026–7
  infection, **B2**.2039 (Tab.), **B2**.2040,
    B2.2040 (Fig.)
    see also Rickettsial diseases
  isolation, **B2**.2034–5
Rickettsia typhi
  characteristics, **B2**.2033 (Tab.)
  classification, **B2**.2031–2, **B2**.2031 (Tab.)
  detection, **B2**.2037
  habitats, vectors and hosts, **B2**.2037
  identification, **B2**.2026–7
  infection, **B2**.2039 (Tab.)
    see also Rickettsial diseases
  isolation, **B2**.2034–5
Rickettsiella, **B2**.2026
Rickettsiella grylli, **B2**.2027 (Fig.)
Ridley-Jopling classification, leprosy, **B2**.1204
Rifabutin
  cryptosporidiosis, **P**.410
  Mycobacterium, **B2**.1217, **B2**.1222
  spectrum of activity, **B1**.494
Rifampicin
  cat-scratch disease treatment, **B2**.1898–9
  human brucellosis treatment, **B2**.1742–3
  leprosy treatment, **B2**.1203
  resistance, *Brucella*, **B2**.1742–3
  spectrum of activity
    Actinobacillus actinomycetemcomitans,
      B2.1664
    Actinomyces, **B2**.1011
    Cardiobacterium hominis, **B2**.1672–3
    Haemophilus, **B2**.1702 (Tab.), **B2**.1703,
      B2.1710
    Listeria, **B2**.957–8
    Mycobacterium, **B2**.1218, **B2**.1222
    Mycobacterium tuberculosis, **B2**.1197,
      B2.1200, **B2**.1218
    Staphylococcus, **B2**.794 (Tab.)
  verruga peruana treatment, **B2**.1891
Rifampin
  spectrum of activity, **B1**.494, **B1**.499 (Tab.)
  structure, **B1**.494 (Fig.)
Rifamycins, **B1**.494
  mode of action, **B1**.494
  pharmacology, **B1**.494
    oral contraceptives, **B1**.494
  resistance, **B1**.494
  spectrum of activity, **B1**.494
    Mycobacterium, **B2**.1222
  structure, **B1**.494, **B1**.494 (Fig.)

Rifamycins (*Continued*)
    toxicity/adverse effects, **B1**.494
        oral contraceptive combination, **B1**.494
    see also specific types
Rift Valley fever, **V2**.1046–7
    emerging infection, **I**.7, **V2**.1648 (Tab.)
    mortality, **V2**.1046–7
    pathogenesis, **V2**.1050
    transmission, **V1**.372 (Tab.)
    vaccines, **V2**.1050–1
Rift Valley fever virus
    biosafety level 3 classification, **V2**.1526
    cell attachment/entry, **V2**.1034–5
    G1 glycoprotein, **V2**.1038
    G2 glycoprotein, **V2**.1038–9
    genome structure
        consensus sequences, **V2**.1031 (Tab.)
        panhandle structures, **V2**.1032 (Fig.)
    NS$_M$ protein, **V2**.1033–4, **V2**.1039
    NS$_S$ protein, **V2**.1038
        IFN effects, **V2**.1041–2
    transcription, **V2**.1036
        termination, **V2**.1037
Right bundle branch block, Chagas disease,
    P.386, **P**.389
Rimantadine, **V2**.1625–6
    historical aspects, **V1**.9 (Tab.)
    influenza therapy, **V1**.679–80
    mechanism of action, **V1**.679
    resistance, **V1**.679–80
    structure, **V2**.1626 (Fig.)
Rinderpest, **V1**.807–10
    clinical manifestations, **V1**.807–9
        lesions, **V1**.807–9
    control, **V1**.809–10
        attenuated vaccine, **V1**.809
        Global Rinderpest Eradication Program
            (GREP), **V1**.810
        quarantine/slaughter, **V1**.810
        sanitary measures, **V1**.809
    emerging infection, **V2**.1651 (Tab.)
    epizootiology, **V1**.809
    historical aspects, **V1**.807
    laboratory diagnosis, **V1**.810
    species affected, **V1**.807
    strain relationship, **V1**.809, **V1**.809 (Fig.)
    transmission, **V1**.809
Rinderpest virus (RPV), **V1**.712–13
    cell attachment/penetration, **V1**.701–2
    classification, **V1**.382–3
'Ring finger' motif, **V2**.1068
Ring forms, *Plasmodium*, **P**.473–4
'ring immunization', **B1**.328–9
Ring-infected erythrocyte surface antigen
    (RESA), **P**.488–9, **I**.873, **I**.874
Ring vaccination, smallpox eradication, **V1**.581
Ringworm, **M**.220
    epidemiology, **M**.225
    history, **M**.5–6
    nomenclature, **M**.228–9
    *see also individual species; specific diseases/
        infection*
Rio Mamore virus, **V2**.1666 (Tab.)
Rio Mearim virus, **V2**.1666 (Tab.)
Rio Segundo virus, **V2**.1666 (Tab.)

Risk, definition, **V1**.359
Risk quantification, microbiological risk
    assessment, **V2**.1519
Risk reduction, Q fever control, **B2**.2079
Risk, relative, **B1**.316
Ritonavir *see* Lopinavir (ritonavir)
Rituxan, licensing, **I**.355 (Tab.)
Rituximab, **I**.333, **I**.876–7
    mechanism of action, **I**.358
River blindness *see* Onchocerciasis
River water, **B1**.213–14, **B1**.215 (Tab.), **B1**.218,
    B1.221
Rivolta, S, **M**.14–5
RNA
    analysis, *Brucella*, **B2**.1730
    content, **B1**.42
    editing, **V1**.116–17, **V1**.771, **V1**.816
        genomes, **V1**.180
        Old World *Leishmania*, **P**.296
        paramyxoviruses, **V1**.116–17, **V1**.180,
            V1.702–4
        transcripts of *Trypanosoma cruzi*, **P**.381
        Trypanosoma brucei, **P**.362
    'guide', *Leishmania*, **P**.296
    historical aspects, **V1**.6
    infected cell metabolism *see* Cell–virus
        interactions
    Peste-des-petits-ruminants virus diagnosis,
        V1.811
    probes, application, **B1**.725
    ribosome *see* Ribosomal RNA (rRNA)
    sequence studies
        Corynebacterium, **B2**.979
        Listeria, **B2**.955, **B2**.958
    sigma factors *see* Sigma (σ) factors
    splicing, **V1**.221
    structure
        Mononegavirales order, **V1**.381
        Nidovirales order, **V1**.392–3
    subgenomic *see* Subgenomic RNAs
    synthesis, **B1**.46–8
        arteriviruses, **V1**.396
        coronaviruses, **V1**.396
        negative-strand RNA viruses *see* RNA
            viruses, negative-strand
        Nidovirales order, **V1**.392–3, **V1**.396
        picornaviruses, **V2**.867, **V2**.868
        regulation, **B1**.46–7
RNA-binding proteins, orbiviruses, **V2**.939–40
RNA-dependent RNA polymerase (RdRp),
    V1.114
    error frequency, **V1**.57, **V1**.132–3
    proofreading, **V1**.57, **V1**.114, **V1**.132–3
    sequence analysis, **V1**.113–14
    structure, **V1**.143
        conservation, **V1**.137–8
    viruses
        arteriviruses, **V1**.833–4
        astroviruses *see* Astroviruses
        Borna disease virus *see* Borna disease
            virus (BDV)
        classification, **V1**.55
        coronavirus, **V1**.833–4
        negative-strand RNA viruses, **V1**.128,
            V1.130
        nidoviruses, **V1**.396

        noroviruses, **V2**.914, **V2**.917
        orbiviruses, **V2**.933, **V2**.939–40
        paramyxoviruses, **V1**.702, **V1**.707–8
        rotaviruses, **V2**.949–50
        rubella virus, **V2**.962
        toroviruses, **V1**.833–4
        see also Large (L) protein; Pol
            (polymerase) protein; Replicase (RNA
            polymerase)
RNA hybridization, malaria diagnosis, **P**.504
RNA phage φ6, genome replication, **V1**.125
RNA polymerase(s)
    poxviruses, **V1**.599 (Tab.), **V1**.608–9
    proofreading lack, **V1**.229–30
    reovirus λ2 protein, **V2**.936
    respiroviruses, **V1**.770
    sapoviruses, **V2**.923–4
    subunits, **B1**.46–7
RNA polymerase II, arenavirus replication,
    V2.1066
RNA replicase, recombination, **V1**.15
RNase H1, SV40 genome replication,
    V1.154 (Tab.)
RNase L, HIV infection, **V1**.301
RNA technology
    protozoa classification, **P**.193
    ribosomal, **P**.193
    snRNA (small nuclear), **P**.193
    srRNA (small subunit ribosomal), **P**.193
RNA tumor viruses, **V1**.331 (Tab.)
RNA viruses, double-stranded
    cell interactions, RNA polymerases, **V1**.220
    characteristics, **V1**.177 (Tab.)
    double-strand *see below*
    enteric
        animal infection, **V2**.926–7
        historical perspectives, **V2**.911–12
    environmental adaptability, **V1**.17–8
    gene expression, **V1**.110–11
    genome
        replication, **V1**.124–5
        size, **V1**.176
    immune evasion
        genetic variability, **V1**.312
        mutation, **V1**.286, **V1**.311
    infection
        animal infection, **V2**.926–7
        IL-6, **V1**.297
        physical particle:plaque-forming unit
            ratios, **V1**.203–4
        TNF-α induction, **V1**.296
    in *Leishmania*, **P**.335
    negative, single strand *see below*
    origins/evolution, **V1**.13–4
        biased hypermutation, **V1**.17
        DNA viruses *vs.*, **V1**.12
        genome mutation, **V1**.16–7
    positive, single strand *see below*
    protein coding, **V1**.58
    quasi-species, **V1**.192–3
    recombination, **V1**.187
    replication, **V1**.217
        mRNA transcription, **V1**.110
        proofreading, **V1**.17
    ribosomal frameshifting, **V1**.180

RNA viruses, double-standed (*Continued*)
  RNA-dependent RNA polymerases, **V1**.110
  transcription, **V1**.110
    host enzymes, **V1**.114
    tumors associated, **V1**.331 (Tab.)
RNA viruses, double-stranded
  classification, **V1**.27 (Tab.), **V1**.40–1, **V1**.47–8, **V1**.47 (Tab.)
  gene expression control, **V1**.120
  genome
    gene reassortment, **V1**.48, **V1**.189
    replication, **V1**.125
    segmentation, **V1**.181
  innate immune response effects, **V1**.110–11
  replication, **V1**.110–11
  reverse genetics, **V1**.189–90
  see also specific viruses
RNA viruses, negative-strand
  ambisense-containing, **V1**.132, **V1**.132 (Fig.)
    open-reading frames, **V1**.132
  arenaviruses, **V2**.1059
  attenuation, **V1**.195
  biased hypermutation, **V1**.193
  'cap-snatching,' **V1**.110
  characteristics, **V1**.129 (Tab.)
  classification, **V1**.27 (Tab.), **V1**.40–1, **V1**.48–50, **V1**.49 (Tab.), **V1**.127–8
    Baltimore system, **V1**.127, **V1**.128 (Fig.)
    International Committee on Taxonomy of Viruses, **V1**.127–8
    monopartite, **V1**.48–9
    segmented, **V1**.40–1, **V1**.49–50
  gene expression control, **V1**.119–20
  genetic variation, **V1**.132–3
  genome
    potential maximization, **V1**.133
    replication, **V1**.125
    segmentation, **V1**.181
  immune evasion, **V1**.199
    IFN effects, **V1**.199
  morphology/structure, **V1**.69–79
  nonsegmented, **V1**.128–31
    morphology/structure, **V1**.128–30
  protein synthesis, **V1**.117–18
  reassortment, **V1**.133
  recombination, **V1**.133
  replication, **V1**.130 (Fig.), **V1.127–34**
    in cytoplasm, **V1**.110
    nucleoprotein, **V1**.128
    nucleus *vs.* cytoplasm, **V1**.131
    reverse genetics, **V1**.133–4
    ribonucleoprotein, **V1**.128
    RNA-dependent RNA polymerase, **V1**.128, **V1**.130
    start-stop model, **V1**.130
  reverse genetics, **V1**.189, **V1**.189–90, **V1**.190 (Fig.), **V1**.191 (Fig.)
  RNA-dependent RNA polymerases, **V1**.110
  RNA synthesis
    'cap-snatching,' **V1**.131–2
    promoters, **V1**.132
  segmented, **V1**.131–2
    replication, **V1**.131 (Fig.)
    transcription, **V1**.131 (Fig.)

transcription, nonsegmented strand, **V1**.130 (Fig.)
  translation, **V1**.130–1
  see also specific viruses
RNA viruses, positive-strand
  characteristics, **V1**.135–8, **V1**.139 (Tab.)
  classification, **V1**.27 (Tab.), **V1**.40–1, **V1**.50–4, **V1**.51 (Tab.), **V1**.135
    Baltimore, **V1**.135
    nested-set viruses, **V1**.53
    supergroups, **V1**.50
  gene expression, **V1**.111 (Fig.)
    control, **V1**.119
  genome, **V1**.135–7, **V1**.136 (Fig.)
    coding capacity, **V1**.135–7
    multifunctional gene products, **V1**.136–7
    open reading frames, **V1**.135–6, **V1**.139–40
    size, **V1**.135–7
  genome replication, **V1**.138 (Fig.), **V1**.141 (Fig.), **V1**.143
    asymmetric production, **V1**.138, **V1**.143
    cell protein dependency, **V1**.143
    initiation, **V1**.143
    negative strand synthesis, **V1**.143
  host cell, effects on, **V1**.141–2, **V1**.142 (Fig.)
    cell membrane metabolism, **V1**.142
    nucleocytoplasmic trafficking, **V1**.142
    protein synthesis, **V1**.141
  host transcript recombination, **V1**.190
  infectious DNA, **V1**.182
  medical significance, **V1**.135
  morphology/structure, **V1**.138
    protein structure conservation, **V1**.137–8
  mRNA structure, **V1**.139, **V1**.140 (Tab.)
  phylogenetics, **V1**.174
  post-translational protein modification, **V1**.139–41, **V1**.225
    proteolytic cleavage, **V1**.121–2
  protein synthesis, **V1**.115–16, **V1**.117–18, **V1**.139–41, **V1**.141 (Fig.)
    eIF4G, **V1**.140
    initiation, **V1**.140
    internal ribosome entry sites (IRES), **V1**.115–16, **V1**.116 (Fig.)
  recombination, **V1**.187–8
  replication, **V1**.58, **V1.135–46**
    cell binding, **V1**.138–9
    cell-specific factors, **V1**.136 (Fig.), **V1**.137
    genome replication, **V1**.124–5
    internal ribosome site (IRES), **V1**.58
    particle assembly/release, **V1**.143–4
  RNA-dependent RNA polymerases, **V1**.110
  see also specific viruses
RNA viruses, single-stranded
  negative strand *see above*
  positive strand *see above*
  see specific viruses
RNP complex, filoviruses, **V2**.1086–8
Robin, C, **M**.6, **M**.7 (Fig.), **M**.14–5
Rochalimaea quintana, **B2**.2026
Rocholimaea, **B2**.2026
Rocio virus (ROCV), **V2**.998 (Tab.), **V2**.1003
Rocky Mountain spotted fever
  causative organisms *see Rickettsia*
  clinical manifestations, **B2**.2038–9, **B2**.2039 (Tab.)

diagnosis, **B2**.2040
discovery, **B2**.2027–30
epidemiology and natural history, **B2**.2037, **B2**.2038
fatality rates, **B2**.2039
transmission and vectors, **B2**.2037–8
treatment, **B2**.2043
Rodent hosts, hantaviruses, **V2**.1044 (Fig.), **V2**.1049
Rodentolepis, **P**.578
Rodentolepis nana, **P**.578
Rofecoxib (Vioxx), **I**.186–7
Roll Back Malaria, **P**.110, **P**.126, **P**.518–19
  cost-effective interventions, **P**.518–19
  goals, **P**.518
  partnerships, **P**.518
Rolling-circle replication, plasmid genes, **B1**.107
Rolling-circle transposition, **B1**.95
Rolling hairpin replication (RHR)
  Minute virus of mice, **V1**.158, **V1**.418–20, **V1**.419 (Fig.)
  parvoviruses, **V1**.150, **V1**.418, **V1**.419–20
Rolling, neutrophils, **I**.38
Romana's sign, **P**.384–5, **P**.384 (Fig.)
Roniviridae, **V1**.26
  classification, **V1**.27 (Tab.), **V1**.51 (Tab.), **V1**.53, **V1**.390
  members, **V1**.392
  see also specific viruses
Ronivirus, **V1**.391 (Fig.)
Roniviruses, subgenomic RNA synthesis, **V1**.401
Ropey bread, **B1**.285
Roseolovirus, **V1**.494 (Tab.)
Rosette-like multiplication, **P**.181
Ross R., **P**.17
Ross River fever, **V2**.1022–3
  clinical features, **V2**.1022–3
  distribution, **V2**.1022
  emerging infection, **V2**.1648 (Tab.)
  history, **V2**.1022
  rubella *vs.*, **V2**.970
  transmission, **V1**.372 (Tab.), **V2**.1016–17, **V2**.1022
Ross River virus (RRV), **V2**.1011 (Tab.)
  virion structure, **V2**.1012
Rostellum, tapeworms, **P**.659
Rotavirus, classification, **V1**.47–8, **V2**.932
Rotaviruses, **V2.946–58**
  cell culture, **V2**.949–50
  cell entry, **V1**.213
  classification, **V2**.949
  genetic engineering, **V1**.195–7
  genome, **V2**.946–9
    sequences, **V2**.932
    size, **V2**.932
    subunit reassortment, **V1**.191–2
  historical aspects, **V2**.946
  host protein translation effects, **V1**.121
  infection *see Rotavirus infection*
  isolation/propagation and identification, **V1**.96 (Tab.), **V1**.98
  morphology/structure, **V2**.1580

Rotaviruses (*Continued*)

NSP1 protein, **V2**.946, **V2**.947 (Fig.), **V2**.948 (Tab.)

in pathogenesis, **V2**.951 (Tab.)

NSP2 protein, **V2**.946, **V2**.947 (Fig.), **V2**.948 (Tab.)

in pathogenesis, **V2**.951 (Tab.)

NSP3 protein, **V2**.946, **V2**.947 (Fig.), **V2**.948 (Tab.)

in pathogenesis, **V2**.951 (Tab.)

NSP4 protein, **V2**.946, **V2**.947 (Fig.), **V2**.948 (Tab.)

as antigen, **V2**.951

as enterotoxin, **V2**.951, **V2**.953 (Fig.)

in pathogenesis, **V2**.951 (Tab.), **V2**.953 (Fig.)

NSP5 protein, **V2**.946, **V2**.947 (Fig.), **V2**.948 (Tab.)

NSP6 protein, **V2**.946, **V2**.947 (Fig.), **V2**.948 (Tab.)

particle structure, **V2**.946, **V2**.947 (Fig.)

proteins

nonstructural proteins, **V2**.946

orbivirus proteins *vs.*, **V2**.941 (Tab.)

structural proteins, **V2**.946

see also specific types

replication, **V2**.949–50, **V2**.950 (Fig.)

cell receptors, **V2**.949–50

co-receptors, **V2**.949–50

particle formation, **V2**.949–50

RNA-dependent RNA polymerase, **V2**.949–50

VP1 protein, **V2**.946, **V2**.947 (Fig.), **V2**.948 (Tab.)

VP2 protein, **V2**.946, **V2**.947 (Fig.), **V2**.948 (Tab.)

VP3 protein, **V2**.946, **V2**.947 (Fig.), **V2**.948 (Tab.)

in pathogenesis, **V2**.951 (Tab.)

VP4 protein, **V2**.946, **V2**.947 (Fig.), **V2**.948 (Tab.)

in pathogenesis, **V2**.951 (Tab.)

in vaccine development, **V2**.1580

VP5 protein, **V2**.946, **V2**.947 (Fig.), **V2**.948 (Tab.)

VP6 protein, **V2**.946, **V2**.947 (Fig.), **V2**.948 (Tab.)

VP7 protein, **V2**.946, **V2**.947 (Fig.), **V2**.948 (Tab.)

in pathogenesis, **V2**.951 (Tab.)

in vaccine development, **V2**.1580

Rotavirus infection, **V2**.951–2

clinical importance, **V2**.932

clinical symptoms, **V2**.951

diagnosis, **V2**.952

emerging infection, **V2**.1648 (Tab.)

childhood infection, **V2**.1659

reassortment, **V2**.1654

epidemiology, **V1**.368, **V2**.954

fecal–oral transmission, **V1**.368

gene reassortment, **V2**.954

seasonal outbreaks, **V1**.358, **V1**.359 (Fig.), **V1**.368

strains, **V2**.954

transmission, fecal–oral transmission, **V2**.949–50

immune response, **V2**.952–3

IgA, **V2**.952–3

immunodeficient patients (non-HIV), **V2**.1508–9

pathogenesis, **V2**.950–1, **V2**.951 (Fig.)

crypt cell hyperplasia, **V2**.950

proteins, **V2**.951 (Tab.)

viral factors, **V2**.950–1

superinfection exclusion, **V1**.192

treatment, oral rehydration, **V2**.952, **V2**.953 (Tab.)

vaccine development, **I**.933 (Tab.), **V2**.954–5, **V2**.1580–1

adverse effects, **V2**.1580–1

inactivated, **V2**.955

live, attenuated, **V2**.954, **V2**.1555 (Tab.), **V2**.1580, **V2**.1581

peptide vaccines, **V2**.955

virus-like particles, **I**.840

Rothia, **B2**.991

cell wall composition, **B2**.1010 (Tab.)

chemotaxonomic characteristics, **B2**.978 (Tab.)

isolation, **B2**.1013

Rothia dentocariosa, **M**.128 (Tab.), **B2**.991

biochemical characteristics, **B2**.993 (Tab.)

disease associations, **B2**.981 (Tab.)

habitats, **B2**.977–8

as normal microbiota, **B1**.296 (Tab.)

Rothia mucilaginosa, **B2**.991

as normal microbiota, **B1**.296 (Tab.)

Roth spots, endocarditis, **B1**.528

Rototheca wickerhamii, infection *see* Prototothecosis

Rots, plant disease source, **B1**.202

Rotting vegetation, *Cryptococcus neoformans,* **M**.643

Rough mutants, *Salmonella* O antigen, **B2**.1402

Roundworms *see Ascaris lumbricoides*

Rous sarcoma virus long terminal repeat, **I**.910

Roxithromycin

Chlamydia pneumoniae infection therapy, **B2**.2021

Haemophilus, **B2**.1710

Pasteurella multocida, **B2**.1655

structure, **B1**.486

toxoplasmosis, **P**.437

Royal College of General Practitioners (RCGP), reporting system, **B1**.320, **B1**.321 (Tab.)

Royal Society of Tropical Medicine and Hygiene, foundation, **P**.9–10

R protein, Measles virus, **V1**.715–16

R/S (rhizosphere/soil) ratio, **B1**.197–8

RSS *see* Recombination signal sequences (RSS)

RT antigens (POL), foamy viruses, **V2**.1311

RTX proteins, **I**.654–5, **B2**.1796–7

Rubella, **V2**.959–92

clinical features, **V2**.968–78

complications, **V2**.969–70

congenitally acquired (CAR), **B1**.349–51, **V2**.972–8, **V2**.1444 (Tab.)

bone defects, **V2**.975

case classification criteria, **V2**.980, **V2**.980 (Tab.)

clinical features, **V2**.972–3, **V2**.973 (Tab.)

CNS defects, **V2**.974–5

deafness, **V2**.973–4

diabetes mellitus, **V2**.975

gestational age relationship, **V2**.978 (Fig.)

heart disease, **V2**.974

historical aspects, **V2**.972–3

laboratory diagnosis, **V2**.980–1

late onset disease, **V2**.975

long-term follow-up, **V2**.975–6

mechanisms of fetal damage, **V2**.976, **V2**.977

ocular defects, **V2**.973, **V2**.974 (Fig.)

pathogenesis, **V2**.976

rash, **V2**.973, **V2**.974 (Fig.)

vaccination effects, **V2**.1570

virus persistence, **V2**.976–7

control/prevention, **B1**.349–51, **V2**.981–5

vaccines, **B1**.348

see also Below, vaccination

differential diagnosis, **V2**.970

epidemics, **B1**.349–51

epidemiology, **V2**.970–1

case–control studies, **V1**.362–3

cohort studies, **V1**.363

developing countries, **V2**.970–1

epidemic periodicity, **V2**.971 (Fig.)

industrialized nations, **V2**.970

seasonality, **V2**.970

eradicable disease, **V2**.1571

historical background, **V2**.968–9

vaccine development, **V2**.969

immune response, **V2**.972

defects after, **V2**.972

incubation period, **V2**.969

laboratory diagnosis, **V2**.978–81

antibody screening, **V2**.978, **V2**.979–81

lymphoproliferative assays, **V2**.981

postnatal tests, **V2**.980–1

prenatal tests, **V2**.981

RT-PCR, **V2**.978–9

serological, **V2**.972

maternal, **B1**.349

after first trimester, **V2**.977–8

first trimester, **V2**.977

preconceptual, **V2**.978

reinfection, **V2**.972, **V2**.979

risk assessment after exposure, **V2**.979–80

risk to fetus, **V2**.977–8

panencephalitis, **V2**.974–5

passive immunization, **V2**.985

postnatally acquired, **V2**.969–72

clinical/virological features, **V2**.969–70, **V2**.971 (Fig.)

laboratory diagnosis, **V2**.979–80

in pregnancy, **B1**.349

reinfection, **V2**.972

diagnosis, **V2**.979

vaccination programs, **B1**.349–51, **V2**.976, **V2**.981–3, **V2**.1571

Europe, **V2**.982–3

males, **V2**.982

strategies, **V2**.981–3

UK, **V2**.982, **V2**.983 (Fig.)

USA, **V2**.981–2, **V2**.982 (Fig.)

Rubella
  vaccination programs (*Continued*)
    worldwide, **V2**.983 (Fig.)
  vaccines/vaccination, **I**.424 (Tab.), **V2**.981,
    V2.981–5, **V2**.1570–1
    adverse effects, **V2**.984, **V2**.1564 (Tab.),
      V2.1570
    arthralgia after, **V2**.984
    contraindications, **V2**.984–5
    coverage and congenital syndrome
      incidence, **B1**.350 (Fig.)
    development, **V2**.969
    efficacy, **V2**.984
    historical aspects, **V2**.1570
    history, **V1**.8 (Tab.)
    immune response, **V2**.983–4
    laboratory workers, **B1**.767
    live attenuated, **V2**.981, **V2**.1555 (Tab.)
    policy implications, **B1**.351
    policy options, **B1**.350
    during pregnancy, **V2**.985
    programs, **V2**.1559 (Tab.)
    recommendations, **V2**.984
    re-infection, **V2**.984
    risks/benefits of policies, **B1**.350–1
    schedules, **V2**.1560–1
    selective policy, **B1**.350
    strain antigenicity, **V2**.967–8
    universal policy, **B1**.350
    USA schedules, **V2**.1559–60
    virus excretion, **V2**.984
    see also Measles, mumps and rubella
      (MMR) vaccine
Rubella virus (RV), **V2**.959–92
  antigens, **V2**.967–8, **V2**.968 (Tab.)
    BCEs, **V2**.967
    complement-fixing, **V2**.967
    hemagglutinin, **V2**.967
    TCEs, **V2**.967
    variation, **V2**.967–8
  attachment/entry, **V2**.962
  biological/nucleic acid sequence variations,
    V2.967–8
  capsid (C) protein, **V2**.960–2, **V2**.966
    as antigen, **V2**.968 (Tab.), **V2**.972, **V2**.983
    low pH conformational change, **V2**.962
    as TCEs, **V2**.967
    translation, **V2**.964
  classification, **V2**.959
  defective interfering (DI) RNAs, **V2**.964
  E1 protein, **V2**.966
    as antigen, **V2**.968 (Tab.), **V2**.972, **V2**.983
    as BCE, **V2**.967
    coding, **V2**.960–2
    post-translational modification, **V2**.964
    as TCEs, **V2**.967
    translation, **V2**.964
  E2 protein, **V2**.966
    as antigen, **V2**.968 (Tab.), **V2**.972, **V2**.983
    coding, **V2**.960–2
    post-translational modification, **V2**.964
    as TCEs, **V2**.967
    translation, **V2**.964
  genome, **V2**.960–2, **V2**.963 (Fig.)
    base composition, **V2**.962

host cell protein interactions, **V2**.965–6
  open reading frames, **V2**.960–2
  regulatory elements, **V2**.965
genotypes, **V2**.968
historical background, **V2**.959
  isolation, **V2**.959
host cell effects, **V2**.964–5
  apoptosis, **V2**.965
  morphology, **V2**.964
  osimophilic inclusion bodies, **V2**.964
isolation/propagation and identification,
  V1.96 (Tab.), **V1**.100
life cycle, **V2**.962–6
morphology/structure, **V2**.959–60,
  V2.960 (Fig.), **V2**.961 (Tab.)
  lipoprotein envelope, **V2**.959–60
nonstructural proteins, **V2**.960–2, **V2**.966
  post-translational modification, **V2**.962
  synthesis, **V2**.962
  see also specific types
p90 protein, **V2**.960–2, **V2**.966
p110 protein, **V2**.964
p150 protein, **V2**.960–2, **V2**.966
physical properties, **V2**.961 (Tab.)
polypeptides, **V2**.966
release, **V2**.964
replication, **V2**.962–4
RNA-dependent RNA polymerase, **V2**.962
serotype, **V2**.967
structural proteins, **V2**.960–2, **V2**.966
  see also specific types
transcription, **V2**.962–4, **V2**.963 (Fig.)
translation, **V2**.962–4, **V2**.963 (Fig.)
vaccine *see* Rubella
Rubini strain, Mumps virus vaccination,
  V1.754
Rubivirus, classification, **V1**.53, **V2**.1010–12
Rubiviruses
  hepatitis E virus comparison, **V2**.1175,
    V2.1175 (Tab.)
  properties, **V2**.1175 (Tab.)
Rubulavirus, **V1**.6
  cell attachment/penetration, **V1**.701–2
  characteristics, **V1**.129 (Tab.), **V1**.702 (Tab.)
  classification, **V1**.48–9, **V1**.382, **V1**.700 (Tab.),
    V1.808 (Fig.)
  genome structure/organization,
    V1.387 (Tab.), **V1**.701 (Fig.)
    conservation, **V1**.784–5, **V1**.785 (Fig.)
    size, **V1**.700
  members, **V1**.382–3
  see also Mumps virus; Rubulaviruses
Rubulaviruses, **V1**.818–19
  attachment (HN) protein, **V1**.706–7
    conservation, **V1**.706–7
  IFN signaling inhibition, **V1**.704
  immune evasion, **V1**.704
  intergenic regions, **V1**.701
  P protein, **V1**.704
  V protein, **V1**.704
  see also Rubulavirus
Rudiviridae
  classification, **V1**.27 (Tab.), **V1**.43 (Tab.)
  see also specific viruses

'Rule of six'
  Measles virus genome, **V1**.715
  respirovirus transcription, **V1**.770–1
  Sendai virus transcription, **V1**.770–1
Rumen bacteria, **B2**.1934
Ruminobacter, **B2**.1930
  normal microbiota, **B2**.1934
Ruminobacter amylophilus, **B2**.1934
Ruminococcus, **B2**.903–4, **B2**.916
  classification, **B2**.905 (Tab.)
  growth requirements, **B2**.906
  identification, **B2**.906–7
  normal microbiota, **B2**.910
Ruminococcus flavefaciens, **B2**.904
Ruminococcus productus, **B2**.904, **B2**.916
  biochemical characteristics, **B2**.908 (Tab.)
  definition/characteristics, **B2**.916
  normal microbiota, **B1**.296 (Tab.), **B2**.910
'Runs', flagella movement, **B1**.44
Russian spring-summer encephalitis, **V2**.1003–
  4, **V2**.1424, **V2**.1426
  clinical features, **V2**.1426
  epidemiology, **V1**.373
  transmission, **V1**.372 (Tab.)
Russia, tuberculosis rates, **B1**.364
Ryanodine and ITP receptor domain,
  I.476 (Fig.)

Saaremaa virus (SAAV), **V2**.1666 (Tab.)
Sabethes, yellow fever transmission, **V2**.999
Sabía virus infection
  clinical features, **V2**.1070
  emerging infection, **V2**.1648 (Tab.)
  geographical distribution/carrier and disease,
    V2.1060 (Tab.)
  laboratory-acquired infection, **V2**.1517 (Tab.)
Sabin poliomyelitis vaccine *see* Oral
  poliomyelitis vaccine (Sabin: OPV)
Sabouraudia, **M**.31, **M**.32
Sabouraud, R., **M**.9–10, **M**.14–5, **M**.18 (Fig.),
  M.32–3
Saccharomonospora, **B2**.1139
  microscopic morphology, **B2**.1143
Saccharomyces
  characteristics, **M**.631, **M**.631 (Tab.)
  infection, **M**.625 (Tab.), **M**.628
Saccharomyces boulardii, **M**.628
Saccharomyces cerevisiae, **B1**.283
  characteristics, **M**.631
  growth, **M**.71–4
    pseudohyphal, **M**.75
  infection, **M**.628
    AIDS, **M**.628
    amphotericin B therapy, **M**.628
    fungemia, **M**.628
    mating types, **M**.768
    prion diseases, **V2**.1387–8
Saccharomyces ovalis, **M**.14–5
Saccharomyces sphaericus, **M**.14–5
Saccharomycetales, **M**.54, **M**.61, **M**.55 (Tab.)
Saccharopolyspora, **B2**.1139
  microscopic morphology, **B2**.1143
Safety *see* Laboratory safety
Safranin O, **B2**.1735

Saksenaea, **M**.20, **M**.660 (Tab.), **M**.672
　oculomycoses, **M**.287, **M**.290
Saksenaea vasiformis, **M**.21, **M**.672,
　　M.672 (Fig.), **M**.675
　identification, **M**.672, **M**.672 (Fig.), **M**.676–7
　rhino-orbital-cerebral zygomycosis, **M**.290,
　　M.292
Salem virus, **V1**.699, **V1**.819
Salibacillus, **B2**.922–3
　taxonomy, **B2**.922–3
Salicin fermentation, Enterobacteriaceae
　　identification, **B2**.1319 (Tab.)
Salicylanilides, **B1**.428, **B1**.436–8
Salicylic acid
　Burkholderia, **B2**.1616–17
　Chlamydia pneumoniae infection therapy,
　　B2.2021
Saliva
　HTLV transmission, **V2**.1292–3
　immunoserology, **B1**.753
　normal microbiota, **B1**.609 (Tab.)
Salivary gland carcinoma, EBV association,
　　V1.571
Salk vaccine *see* Inactivated poliomyelitis
　　vaccine (Salk: IPV)
Salmonella, **B2**.1398–434
　antibacterial susceptibility/resistance,
　　B2.1412–16
　　developed countries, **B2**.1412–14
　　developing countries, **B2**.1414–15,
　　　B2.1415 (Tab.)
　　food-animal use, **B2**.1412–13
　　immunocompromised patients, **B2**.1414
　　plasmid-mediated, **B2**.1412
　　quinolone resistance, **B1**.493 (Tab.)
　antigens, **B2**.1401–2
　　fimbrial antigens, **B2**.1342–3, **B2**.1407
　　flagellar antigens *see below*
　　H antigen *see below*
　　Kauffmann–White nomenclature, **B1**.757,
　　　B2.1402, **B2**.1403 (Tab.)
　　nomenclature, **B2**.1402
　　O antigen *see below*
　　Vi antigen *see below*
　　virulence effects, **B2**.1340
　　see also Below, serotyping
　biochemistry, **B2**.1319 (Tab.), **B2**.1400–1,
　　B2.1401 (Tab.)
　　differentiation, **B2**.1400 (Tab.)
　　gelatin liquefaction, **B2**.1401
　　lactose fermentation, **B1**.115
　　sugar fermentation, **B1**.115
　biotyping, **B2**.1409
　chemical agent susceptibility/resistance,
　　B2.1400
　　dyes, **B2**.1400
　classification, **B2**.1398
　　evolutionary relationships, **B2**.1318
　culture, **B2**.1399–400
　　carbon source, **B2**.1399–400
　　enrichment media, **B2**.1400
　　morphology, **B2**.1345 (Tab.)
　　screening media, **B2**.1401
　epidemiology, **B2**.1411–16
　　habitats, **B2**.1411–12
　　specific host relationships, **B2**.1411–12

extracellular slime, **B2**.1343
flagellar antigens, **B2**.1405–6
　flagellins, **B2**.1404
　triphasic strains, **B2**.1405–6
in food
　butter, **B1**.250
　cheese, **B1**.253–4
　coconuts, **B1**.287
　cream, **B1**.248
　crustacea, **B1**.279–80
　eggs, **B1**.278–9
　fruit, **B1**.283
　hazard analysis, **B1**.288
　herbs and spices, **B1**.288
　ice cream, **B1**.251
　meat and meat products, **B1**.273–5, **B1**.289
　milk, **B1**.230, **B1**.231–2, **B1**.235,
　　B1.235 (Tab.), **B1**.237–8
　milk powder, **B1**.245, **B1**.246–7
　poultry *see* Poultry
　spray drying, **B1**.269
　vegetables, **B1**.282
　wheat, **B1**.284–5
H antigen, **B2**.1401, **B2**.1404–5
　Citrobacter vs., **B2**.1402
　diphasic variation, **B2**.1404
　molecular characterization, **B2**.1407
　monophasic serotypes, **B2**.1404
　serotyping, **B2**.1403 (Tab.)
historical perspective, **B2**.1398
identification
　gelatin liquefaction, **B2**.1351
　historical perspective, **B2**.1350, **B2**.1351
　out-membrane protein typing, **B2**.1411
　problem strains, **B2**.1348–50
　screening tests, **B2**.1349 (Tab.)
　serotyping *see below*
immune evasion
　complement surface masking, **I**.662–3
　LPS variation, **I**.661
　macrophage apoptosis, **I**.655
　outer membrane protein variation, **I**.661
immunogenetics, **I**.589
infection *see* Salmonellosis
infiltration of host tissues, **B1**.152
LPS, **B1**.158
　in typing, **B2**.1411
molecular typing, **B2**.1409–11
　chromosomes, **B2**.1410–11
　enterobacterial repetitive intergenic
　　consensus, **B2**.1409, **B2**.1411
　fluorescent amplified fragment length
　　polymorphism, **B2**.1411
　insertion sequence typing, **B2**.1409,
　　B2.1410
　plasmid typing, **B2**.1409–10
　pulse-field gel electrophoresis, **B2**.1409,
　　B2.1410–11
　random amplified polymorphic DNA,
　　B2.1409, **B2**.1411
　random cloned sequence typing, **B2**.1409
　ribotyping, **B2**.1409, **B2**.1410
　single-enzyme amplified fragment length
　　polymorphism, **B2**.1411
　variable number of tandem repeat,
　　B2.1411

morphology, **B2**.1399
　fimbriae, **B2**.1342–3, **B2**.1399
motility, **B2**.1342
　nonmotile strains, **B2**.1405–6
nomenclature, **B2**.1337, **B2**.1398–9
　DNA-hybridization groups, **B2**.1398–9
　serotypes, **B2**.1399
　serotype *vs.* seovar, **B2**.1337
O antigen, **B2**.1401, **B2**.1402–4
　'chemotypes,' **B2**.1401–2
　lysogenic conversion, **B2**.1402–4
　molecular characterization, **B2**.1407
　plasmid conversion, **B2**.1404
　rough mutants, **B2**.1402
　serotype classification, **B2**.1402
　serotyping, **B2**.1403 (Tab.)
　structure, **B2**.1401–2
pathogenicity, **B2**.1424–7
　experimental studies, **B2**.1425–7
　invasive infection, **B2**.1425
　Salmonella pathogenicity island, **B1**.164,
　　B2.1425
　salmonella plasmid virulence *(spv)* genes,
　　B2.1426
　serotype-specific plasmids, **B2**.1426
　toxins, **B2**.1426–7
phenotype, **B2**.1399–407
plasmids, **B1**.115
population structure, **B2**.1407
　MLEE analysis, **B2**.1407
　multilocus sequence typing, **B2**.1407
serotyping, **B2**.1408–9
　fluorescent amplified fragment length
　　polymorphism, **B2**.1408–9
　Kauffmann–White nomenclature, **B2**.1402,
　　B2.1403 (Tab.)
　serotypes involved in gastroenteritis,
　　B1.283
　see also specific serotypes
signal transduction, **B1**.164, **B1**.167–8
　subversion of host cell, **B1**.164
subspecies II, **B2**.1403 (Tab.), **B2**.1423
subspecies IIIa, **B2**.1403 (Tab.), **B2**.1423–4
subspecies IIIb, **B2**.1403 (Tab.), **B2**.1423–4
subspecies IV, **B2**.1403 (Tab.), **B2**.1424
subspecies V, **B2**.1403 (Tab.), **B2**.1424
subspecies VI, **B2**.1403 (Tab.), **B2**.1424
as vaccine vector *see* Vaccines, live
Vi antigen, **B2**.1406
　antiphagocytic effects, **B2**.1406
　detection, **B2**.1406
　strains, **B2**.1406
virulence factors
　LPSs, **B1**.158–9
　Sips, **B1**.152
waterborne, **B1**.212, **B1**.214, **B1**.215 (Tab.),
　　B1.218–19, **B1**.236
Salmonella Agona, **B2**.1416–17
　bacteriophage typing, **B2**.1416–17
　biotyping, **B2**.1409
　MLEE typing, **B2**.1416–17
　serotyping, **B2**.1403 (Tab.), **B2**.1408
Salmonella Anatum, **B2**.1403 (Tab.)
Salmonella bongori, **B2**.1424
　biochemical tests, **B2**.1319 (Tab.),
　　B2.1400 (Tab.)

Salmonella bongori, (*Continued*)
  classification, **B2**.1398, **B2**.1399
  serotypes, **B2**.1402
Salmonella Brandenburg, **B2**.1403 (Tab.)
Salmonella Bredeney, **B2**.1403 (Tab.)
Salmonella Choleraesuis, **B2**.1417
  biochemical tests, **B2**.1319 (Tab.),
    B2.1401 (Tab.), **B2**.1417 (Tab.)
  endocarditis, **B1**.532
  flagellar antigens, mutants, **B2**.1405
  infection, **B2**.1417
    see also Salmonellosis
  MLEE analysis, **B2**.1417
  pathogenicity, serotype-specific plasmids,
    B2.1426
  serotyping, **B2**.1403 (Tab.)
Salmonella Derby, **B2**.1403 (Tab.)
Salmonella Dublin, **B2**.1417–18
  infection, **B2**.1417–18
    see also Salmonellosis
  MLEE typing, **B2**.1418
  pathogenicity
    Salmonella pathogenicity island, **B2**.1425
    serotype-specific plasmids, **B2**.1418,
      B2.1426
    Vi antigen, **B2**.1406
    virulence factors, **B1**.114, **B2**.1418
  plasmids, **B1**.114
  serotyping, **B2**.1403 (Tab.)
Salmonella Ealing, **B1**.315
Salmonella enterica
  classification, **B2**.1398
    biochemical typing, **B2**.1401
    see also individual subspecies
  immune evasion, point mutations, **I**.660
  subspecies *arizonae*, **B2**.1399, **B2**.1423–4
    biochemical typing, **B2**.1400 (Tab.)
    fimbriae, **B2**.1399
    osteomyelitis, **B1**.690
    serotypes, **B2**.1402
  subspecies *diarizonae*, **B2**.1399, **B2**.1423–4
    biochemical typing, **B2**.1400 (Tab.)
    epidemiology, **B2**.1423
    fimbriae, **B2**.1399
    serotypes, **B2**.1402
  subspecies *enterica*, **B2**.1399
    biochemical typing, **B2**.1400 (Tab.)
    classification, **B2**.1398
    serotypes, **B2**.1402
    see also individual serotypes
  subspecies *houtenae*, **B2**.1399, **B2**.1424
    biochemical typing, **B2**.1400 (Tab.),
      B2.1401
    serotypes, **B2**.1402
  subspecies *indica*, **B2**.1399, **B2**.1424
    biochemical typing, **B2**.1400 (Tab.),
      B2.1401
    serotypes, **B2**.1402
  subspecies *salamae*, **B2**.1399, **B2**.1423
    biochemical typing, **B2**.1400 (Tab.)
    fimbriae, **B2**.1399
    serotypes, **B2**.1402
  as vaccine vector, **I**.899
Salmonella enterica subspecies *arizonae see*
  Salmonella enterica

Salmonella enterica subspecies *diarizonae see*
  Salmonella enterica
Salmonella enterica subspecies *enterica see*
  Salmonella enterica
Salmonella enterica subspecies *houtenae see*
  Salmonella enterica
Salmonella enterica subspecies *indica see*
  Salmonella enterica
Salmonella enterica subspecies *salamae see*
  Salmonella enterica
Salmonella Enteritidis, **B2**.1418–19
  adhesins, **B1**.148–9
  antibacterial susceptibility/resistance,
    B2.1418–19
  bacteriophage type 4b detection, **B1**.322
  curli synthesis, **B1**.148–9
  fimbriae, **B2**.1399
  in food
    eggs, **B1**.276, **B1**.278
    ice cream, **B1**.251
  infection, **B2**.1418
    in chickens, **B2**.1418
    endocarditis, **B1**.532
    MHC class II antigen presentation, **I**.659
    reactive arthritis, **I**.594–5
    see also Salmonellosis
  molecular typing, insertion sequence typing,
    B2.1410
  nonmotile strains, **B2**.1406
  pathogenicity, serotype-specific plasmids,
    B2.1426
  plasmid typing, **B2**.1409–10
  PT4, **B1**.251
  serology, **B2**.1403 (Tab.)
  serotyping, **B2**.1408
Salmonella Gallinarum, **B2**.1419
  biochemical tests, **B2**.1319 (Tab.), **B2**.1401,
    B2.1401 (Tab.)
  culture, **B2**.1401
  nonmotile strains, **B2**.1406
  pathogenicity, serotype-specific plasmids,
    B2.1426
  serotyping, **B2**.1403 (Tab.)
Salmonella Hadar, **B2**.1419
  pathogenicity, serotype-specific plasmids,
    B2.1426
  serotyping, **B2**.1403 (Tab.), **B2**.1408
Salmonella Heidelberg, **B2**.1419–20
  flagellar antigens, **B2**.1405
  infection, **B2**.1419
    see also Salmonellosis
  insertion sequence typing, **B2**.1419–20
  multiple antibacterial resistance, **B2**.1414
  serotyping, **B2**.1403 (Tab.)
Salmonella Infantis, **B2**.1420
  infection, **B2**.1420
    see also Salmonellosis
  insertion sequence typing, **B2**.1420
  serotyping, **B2**.1403 (Tab.)
Salmonella Johannesburg, **B2**.1415 (Tab.)
Salmonella Kedougou, **B2**.1403 (Tab.)
Salmonella Livingstone
  biotyping, **B2**.1409
  serotyping, **B2**.1403 (Tab.)
Salmonella Mbandaka, **B2**.1403 (Tab.)

Salmonella Montevideo, **B2**.1420
  biotyping, **B2**.1409, **B2**.1420
  serotyping, **B2**.1403 (Tab.)
Salmonella Muenchen
  flagellar antigens, **B2**.1405
  mutants, **B2**.1405
  serotyping, **B2**.1403 (Tab.)
Salmonella Newport
  multiple antibacterial resistance, **B2**.1414
  serotyping, **B2**.1403 (Tab.)
Salmonella Oranienburg, **B1**.283
  antibacterial susceptibility/resistance,
    B2.1415 (Tab.)
Salmonella Panama, **B2**.1420
  serotyping, **B2**.1403 (Tab.), **B2**.1420
Salmonella Paratyphi A, **B2**.1420–1
  antibacterial susceptibility/resistance,
    B2.1416
    ciprofloxacin, **B2**.1421
  biochemistry, **B2**.1319 (Tab.), **B2**.1401 (Tab.),
    B2.1420
  culture, **B2**.1401
  flagellar antigen mutants, **B2**.1405
  H antigen, **B2**.1404
  MLEE typing, **B2**.1420–1
  O antigen, **B2**.1341–2
  serotyping, **B2**.1403 (Tab.)
Salmonella Paratyphi B, **B2**.1421
  bacteriophage typing, **B2**.1421
  biotyping, **B2**.1409
  culture, **B2**.1400
  gastroenteritis, **B2**.1421
  insertion sequence typing, **B2**.1410
  MLEE typing, **B2**.1421
  serotyping, **B2**.1403 (Tab.), **B2**.1408
Salmonella Paratyphi C
  biochemistry, **B2**.1417 (Tab.)
  serotyping, **B2**.1403 (Tab.)
  Vi antigen, **B2**.1406
Salmonella pathogenicity island, **B2**.1425
  Salmonella Dublin, **B2**.1425
Salmonella plasmid virulence (*spv*) genes,
  B2.1426
Salmonella Pullorum, **B2**.1419
  biochemical tests, **B2**.1319 (Tab.), **B2**.1401,
    B2.1401 (Tab.)
  culture, **B2**.1401
  nonmotile strains, **B2**.1406
  pathogenicity, serotype-specific plasmids,
    B2.1426
Salmonella Rubislaw
  flagellar antigen mutants, **B2**.1405
  serotyping, **B2**.1403 (Tab.)
Salmonella Saintpaul
  multiple antibacterial resistance, **B2**.1414
  serotyping, **B2**.1403 (Tab.)
Salmonella Salinatus, **B2**.1399
Salmonella Schwarzengrund, **B2**.1403 (Tab.)
Salmonella Sendai
  culture, **B2**.1401
  mannose-resistance and eluting
    hemagglutinins, **B2**.1399
Salmonella Senftenberg
  antibacterial resistance, **B2**.1415 (Tab.)
  serotyping, **B2**.1403 (Tab.)
Salmonella Stanley, **B2**.1403 (Tab.)

Salmonella Thompson, **B2**.1403 (Tab.)

Salmonella Typhi, **B2**.1421–2

antibacterial susceptibility/resistance, **B2**.1415–16

ampicillin, **B2**.1416

ciprofloxacin, **B2**.1416

developing countries, **B2**.1415–16

multidrug resistance, **B2**.1421

trimethoprim, **B2**.1416

conjugate vaccines, **I**.936–7

culture, **B2**.1401

flagellar antigens, **B2**.1405

food, hazard analysis, **B1**.288

genome size, **B2**.1422

H antigens, **B1**.744

monophasic serotypes, **B2**.1404–5

historical perspective, **B2**.1318–31

identification

bacteriophage typing, **B2**.1408

biochemical tests, **B2**.1319 (Tab.), **B2**.1401, **B2**.1401 (Tab.)

pulse-field gel electrophoresis, **B2**.1410

screening tests, **B2**.1349 (Tab.)

serotyping, **B2**.1403 (Tab.)

infection

animal infection, **B2**.1425

laboratory acquired, **B1**.761

see also Salmonellosis; Typhoid

intracranial abscess, **B1**.586

O antigens, **B1**.744

as vaccine vector, **I**.841–3, **I**.896–7, **I**.899–900

attenuated vectors, **I**.830–1

Vi antigen, **B1**.744, **B2**.1406, **B2**.1408

strain differentiation, **B2**.1422

Salmonella Typhimurium, **B2**.1422

adhesins, **B1**.148–9

antibacterial susceptibility/resistance, **B2**.1412–14

antibacterial use in animals, **B2**.1413–14

bacteriophage-mediated, **B2**.1412

chromosomally associated, **B2**.1413

developing countries, **B2**.1415 (Tab.)

DT 104 strain, **B2**.1412–14

multiple resistance, **B2**.1412–13, **B2**.1414, **B2**.1422

plasmid-acquired, **B1**.110, **B2**.1413

pulse-field gel electrophoresis, **B2**.1413

artificial competence, **B1**.99

covalent modification, **B1**.76

curli synthesis, **B1**.148–9

developing countries, **B2**.1414–15

DT104 bacteriophage type, **B1**.237

fimbriae, **B2**.1399

flagellar antigens, **B2**.1405

mutants, **B2**.1405

in food

cheese, **B1**.254

cream, **B1**.248

meat, **B1**.275–6

milk, **B1**.231, **B1**.235 (Tab.), **B1**.237–8

milk powder, **B1**.246

poultry, **B1**.276

H antigen, diphasic variation, **B2**.1404

identification

biotyping, **B2**.1409

molecular typing *see below*

serotyping, **B2**.1403 (Tab.), **B2**.1408

immune evasion

IL-10 induction, **I**.652

immunosuppression, **I**.665

lysosomal killing resistance, **I**.651

lysosome fusion inhibition, **I**.650

membrane attack complex inhibition, **I**.664

MHC class I antigen presentation, **I**.660

MHC class II antigen presentation, **I**.658

infection

animal infection, **B2**.1425

endocarditis, **B1**.532

IL-18, **I**.290–2

induced apoptosis, **I**.138

microfold (M) cells, **I**.532

milk-borne, **B1**.235 (Tab.)

PR-39 therapy, **I**.173

Qa-1 reactive CD8+ T-cells, **I**.443

SLC11A1 gene polymorphisms, **I**.579

see also Salmonellosis

infiltration of host tissues, **B1**.152

ion gradient-linked transport, **B1**.49

iron-dependent repression, **B1**.165–6

molecular typing

insertion sequence typing, **B2**.1410

pulse-field gel electrophoresis, **B2**.1410

nomenclature, **B2**.1399

O antigen, **B2**.1341–2

pathogenicity, serotype-specific plasmids, **B2**.1426

periplasmic-binding protein dependent transport, **B1**.49

phase variation, **B1**.90

population structure, MLEE analysis, **B2**.1407

as vaccine vector, **I**.847, **I**.899–900

Salmonella Typhisuis

biochemistry, **B2**.1401, **B2**.1417 (Tab.)

culture, **B2**.1401

Salmonella Virchow, **B2**.1422–3

antibacterial susceptibility/resistance, **B2**.1423

bacteriophage-typing scheme, **B2**.1422–3

pathogenicity, serotype-specific plasmids, **B2**.1426

serotyping, **B2**.1403 (Tab.), **B2**.1408

Salmonella Wien, **B2**.1415 (Tab.)

Salmonellosis, **B2**.1424–5

AIDS patients, **B2**.1424–5

bacteremia, **B1**.521

bone and joints, **B1**.690

day-care centers, **B1**.361

defensin resistance, **I**.169

dendritic cell infection, **I**.656

developing countries, **B2**.1414–15

diarrhea, **B2**.1426

elderly, **B1**.394

endocarditis, **B1**.532

enteric fever, **B2**.1424

entry into cells, actin cytoskeleton, **I**.649–50

immune response

CD4 T cells, **I**.390

IFN-γ, **I**.593

IL-2 pathway, **I**.772–3

macrophages, **I**.30, **I**.137–8

NK cells, **I**.99, **I**.100

TLR-5, **I**.121

immunogenetics, **I**.593–4

CFTR gene, **I**.593

IL12B gene mutations, **I**.593

IL12RB1 gene mutations, **I**.593

knockout animal models, **I**.593–4

murine models, **I**.593

transgenic animal models, **I**.593–4

induced apoptosis, **I**.137–8

intestinal, **B2**.1347

intracranial abscess, **B1**.586

mastitis, **B1**.230

nosocomial, **B1**.397

food-borne, **B1**.377

person-to-person spread, **B1**.377

subdural empyema, **B1**.591

subtype specificities, **B2**.1424

systemic disease, **B2**.1424

Salmon pancreas disease virus (SPDV), **V2**.1010, **V2**.1011 (Tab.)

Salpingitis, *Chlamydia trachomatis* infection, **B2**.2010–11, **B2**.2011 (Fig.)

Salt fish, nasopharyngeal carcinoma and, **V1**.572

Salt/salting

Campylobacter resistance, **B2**.1545

food processing and preservation, **B1**.268 (Tab.)

meat and meat products, **B1**.274–5

Sampling frame, **B1**.314, **B1**.315

Sandflies

feeding behaviour, **P**.288–9, **P**.292

gut structure, **P**.289 (Fig.), **P**.290–1

Leishmania transmission, **P**.283–4, **P**.286 (Tab.), **P**.288–9, **P**.294, **P**.305, **P**.315–16, **P**.317–18

control, **P**.339–40

life cycle in, **P**.288–92

L. infantum, **P**.286 (Tab.), **P**.305–6

L. major, **P**.286 (Tab.), **P**.303

L. tropica, **P**.286 (Tab.), **P**.304

promastigote development, **P**.289

peritrophic membrane, **P**.290

Sandfly fever, **V2**.1047

New World, **V2**.1047

transmission, **V1**.372 (Tab.)

Sand workers, rhinosporidiosis, **M**.439, **M**.458, **M**.459

Sanfelice, F, **M**.16

Sanitation

alveolar echinococcosis control, **P**.702

amebiasis transmission prevention, **P**.214

hepatitis A decline, **V2**.1172, **V2**.1173

liver fluke control, **P**.653–4

lung fluke control, **P**.653–4

Peste-des-petits-ruminants virus control, **V1**.811

rinderpest control, **V1**.809

SAP gene, **M**.103, **M**.584, **M**.587, **M**.588, **M**.605–6

Sapovirus

classification, **V2**.912

see also Sapoviruses

Sapoviruses, **V2**.922–6
  capsid protein, **V2**.923
  genome, **V2**.913 (Tab.), **V2**.923, **V2**.924 (Fig.)
    noroviruses *vs.,* **V2**.923
    sequencing, **V2**.923
  historical aspects, **V2**.922–3
  isolation/propagation and identification,
      V1.98
  morphology, **V2**.922 (Fig.)
    ultrastructure, **V2**.923
  NTPase, **V2**.923–4
  phylogenetic analysis, **V2**.917 (Fig.)
  physical characteristics, **V2**.922–3
  protease, **V2**.923–4
  proteins, **V2**.923–4
  RNA polymerase, **V2**.923–4
Sapovirus infection
  animals, **V2**.927
  at-risk groups, **V2**.925
  clinical manifestations, **V2**.913 (Tab.),
      V2.924
  epidemiology, **V2**.924–5
    seroepidemiology, **V2**.925
  incubation period, **V2**.924
  laboratory diagnosis, **V2**.925–6
    electron microscopy, **V2**.925
    immunoassays, **V2**.924–5, **V2**.925–6
    isolation, **V2**.925
    serology, **V2**.926
  outbreaks, **V2**.924–5
  pathogenesis, **V2**.924
  pathology, **V2**.913 (Tab.)
  prevalence, **V2**.925
  prevention/control, **V2**.926
  transmission, **V2**.924
  volunteer studies, **V2**.924
SAP/SH2D1A gene mutations, X-linked
    proliferative syndrome, **I**.779
Saquinavir, **V2**.1623
  historical aspects, **V1**.9 (Tab.)
  resistance, **V2**.1623
    HIV, **V2**.1337 (Fig.)
  structure, **V2**.1624 (Fig.)
Sarafloxacin, **B1**.492
Sarcina, **B2**.903–4, **B2**.917
  classification, **B2**.905 (Tab.)
  definition/characteristics, **B2**.917
  growth requirements, **B2**.906
  identification, **B2**.906–7
  normal microbiota, **B2**.910
Sarcocystis, **P**.443–50
  classification, **P**.190–1, **P**.197, **P**.443
    RNA technology, **P**.193
  historical aspects, **P**.443, **P**.444 (Tab.)
  immune response, **P**.87
  life cycle, **P**.443–8, **P**.445 (Fig.), **P**.446 (Fig.)
    bradyzoites (cystozoites), **P**.443–5
    hosts, **P**.443
    intermediate hosts, **P**.447 (Tab.)
    merozoites, **P**.443–5, **P**.446 (Fig.)
    microgamonts, **P**.174 (Fig.)
    oocysts, **P**.445, **P**.449
    schizogony, **P**.445
    schizonts, **P**.443–5, **P**.446 (Fig.)
    sporocysts, **P**.167 (Fig.), **P**.449

livestock species, **P**.447 (Tab.)
  parasitophorous vacuole, **P**.443–5
  pathogenic/non-pathogenic species, **P**.445–6
  structure, **P**.165 (Fig.), **P**.167 (Fig.), **P**.443–8,
      P.444 (Fig.)
    flagellum, **P**.170 (Fig.), **P**.180 (Fig.)
    see also Sarcocystosis; *individual species*
Sarcocystis arieticanis, **P**.447 (Tab.)
Sarcocystis bertrami, **P**.447 (Tab.)
Sarcocystis cameli, **P**.447 (Tab.)
Sarcocystis canis, **P**.446, **P**.448
Sarcocystis capracanis, **P**.447 (Tab.)
Sarcocystis cruzi
  intermediate hosts, **P**.447 (Tab.)
  life cycle, **P**.443, **P**.445 (Fig.)
Sarcocystis dubeyi, **P**.448
Sarcocystis equicanis, **P**.447 (Tab.)
Sarcocystis fayeri, **P**.447 (Tab.)
Sarcocystis fusiformis, **P**.447 (Tab.)
Sarcocystis gigantea, **P**.447 (Tab.)
Sarcocystis hircicanis, **P**.447 (Tab.)
Sarcocystis hirsuta, **P**.445–6
  intermediate hosts, **P**.447 (Tab.)
  life cycle, **P**.443
Sarcocystis hominis, **P**.188, **P**.445–6, **P**.448
  historical aspects, **P**.18
  host, **P**.445–6
  infection *see* Sarcocystosis
  intermediate hosts, **P**.447 (Tab.)
  life cycle, **P**.443
Sarcocystis horvathi, **P**.447 (Tab.)
Sarcocystis levinei, **P**.447 (Tab.)
Sarcocystis medusiformis, **P**.447 (Tab.)
Sarcocystis miescheriana, **P**.447 (Tab.)
Sarcocystis moule, **P**.447 (Tab.)
Sarcocystis neurona, **P**.446
Sarcocystis porcifelis, **P**.447 (Tab.)
Sarcocystis rileyi, **P**.447 (Tab.)
Sarcocystis suihominis, **P**.188, **P**.448
  historical aspects, **P**.18
  infection, **P**.448
    see also Sarcocystosis
  intermediate hosts, **P**.447 (Tab.)
Sarcocystis tenella, **P**.447 (Tab.)
Sarcocystosis, **P**.448, **P**.448–9
  chemotherapy, **P**.449
  clinical features, **P**.448–9
  control, **P**.449
  diagnosis, **P**.449
  epidemiology, **P**.449
  intestinal, **P**.448
    prevalence, **P**.448
  muscular, **P**.443–5
  prevalence, **P**.448, **P**.449
Sarcocysts, **P**.443–5, **P**.444 (Fig.), **P**.445
Sarcoidosis
  granulomas, histoplasmosis capsulati *vs.,*
      M.534
  IL-15, **I**.282
Sarcopodium oculorum, oculomycoses,
    M.275 (Tab.)
Saumarez reef virus, **V2**.1004
Sausages
  fermented and acidulated, **B1**.275–6
  frankfurters, **B1**.275

ionizing radiation, **B1**.271–2
  perishable raw salted, **B1**.274–5
  pickled, **B1**.275
Save the Children Fund, **P**.103–6
SBAS4 *see* Monophosphoryl lipid (MPL)
    adjuvant
SBDS gene mutations, **I**.765, **I**.767
Scabies, **B1**.403
Scaffolds
  capsid assembly, **V1**.65–7
  herpesviruses, **V1**.501
Scallops, **B1**.280
Scalp
  black piedra, **M**.197–8, **M**.198 (Fig.)
  examination, **M**.238
  mycetoma, **M**.388
  white piedra, **M**.196, **M**.197
Scardovia, **B2**.1025
Scardovia inopinata, **B2**.1025 (Tab.)
  pathogenicity, **B2**.1026
Scarlet fever
  milk-borne, **B1**.230
  see also Streptococcus pyogenes infection
Scavenger receptors, **I**.114 (Tab.)
  microbial recognition, **I**.23, **I**.24 (Tab.)
Scedosporiosis, **M**.756
  clinical manifestations, **M**.756
  CNS, **M**.138 (Fig.)
  description, **M**.741–2
  diagnosis, **M**.125–7, **M**.751, **M**.752
  histopathology, **M**.138 (Fig.)
  prognosis, **M**.757
  risk factors, **M**.756
  therapy, **M**.757
    G-CSF, **M**.757
    itraconazole, **M**.757
    miconazole, **M**.757
    posaconazole, **M**.757
    voriconazole, **M**.153
Scedosporium
  amphotericin B resistance, **M**.757
  antifungal susceptibility, **M**.752 (Tab.)
  ecology, **M**.756
  genus description, **M**.755
  histopathology, **M**.128 (Tab.)
  history, **M**.19–20
  infection *see* Scedosporiosis
  morphology, **M**.755
  pigment production, **M**.742
Scedosporium apiospermum, **M**.19, **M**.20,
    M.28 (Fig.), **M**.282 (Fig.)
  amphotericin B resistance, **M**.172
  antifungal susceptibility, **M**.752 (Tab.)
  description, **M**.755
  ecology, **M**.756
  histopathology, **M**.89 (Tab.), **M**.127 (Tab.),
      M.128 (Tab.), **M**.138 (Fig.), **M**.139 (Fig.)
  identification, **M**.390 (Fig.), **M**.390 (Tab.),
      M.391, **M**.392 (Tab.)
  infection, **M**.741–2, **M**.756
    clinical manifestations, **M**.756
    description, **M**.741–2
    diagnosis, **M**.751, **M**.752
    endophthalmitis, **M**.317, **M**.323–4
    keratitis, **M**.301–2, **M**.313–14, **M**.327–8

Scedosporium apiospermum,
infection (*Continued*)
meningitis, **M**.19
oculomycoses, **M**.275 (Tab.), **M**.279,
M.281–2
orbit, **M**.294, **M**.295
otitis externa, **M**.247–8
risk factors, **M**.756
scleritis, **M**.317, **M**.328
therapy, **M**.757
see also Scedosporiosis
morphology, **M**.755, **M**.755 (Fig.)
mycetoma, **M**.394
Scedosporium inflatum, **M**.20
Scedosporium prolificans, **M**.20, **M**.20 (Fig.)
amphotericin B resistance, **M**.172
antifungal susceptibility, **M**.752 (Tab.)
ecology, **M**.756
infection, **M**.743, **M**.756
clinical manifestations, **M**.756
CNS, **M**.743–4
diagnosis, **M**.751, **M**.752
oculomycoses, **M**.275 (Tab.), **M**.279,
M.281–2
risk factors, **M**.756
scleritis, **M**.316, **M**.328
therapy, **M**.757
see also Scedosporiosis
morphology, **M**.755, **M**.756 (Fig.)
Schaudin/polyvinyl alcohol fixative,
Dientamoeba fragilis infection, **P**.268
Schick test, **B1**.348
Schimke immuno-osseous dysplasia, **I**.777
Schistosoma, **P**.600–9, **P**.610–25, **P**.626–39,
I.682
characteristics, **P**.601 (Tab.)
classification, **P**.582, **P**.600, **P**.610, **P**.627
historical aspects, **P**.11, **P**.610
immune evasion
antibody destruction, **I**.685–6
complement inhibition, **I**.685
glutathione *S*-transferases, **I**.686
host molecule incorporation, **I**.684
outer membrane fluidity, **I**.684
infection *see* Schistosomiasis
life cycle, **P**.582, **P**.602–3, **P**.602 (Fig.), **P**.612,
P.628, **I**.682
cercariae, **P**.581 (Fig.), **P**.602–3,
P.603 (Fig.)
egg production, **P**.603
location in host, **P**.612, **P**.628
migration through tissues, **P**.603
miracidia, **P**.602
sexual maturation, **P**.603
snail intermediate hosts, **P**.602,
P.603 (Tab.)
sporocysts, **P**.602–3
morphology/structure, **P**.600–2, **P**.611–12,
P.627
gynecophoric canal, **P**.600–1
tegument, **P**.601
nutrition, **P**.601–2
Embden–Meyerhoff pathway, **P**.605–6
female nutrition, **P**.606
glucose, **P**.605–6
Krebs cycle, **P**.605–6

red cell ingestion, **P**.606
structure, **P**.581 (Fig.), **P**.582
transmission/epidemiology, **P**.628–9
see also individual species
Schistosoma bovis
characteristics, **P**.601 (Tab.)
classification, **P**.600
Schistosoma haematobium
characteristics, **P**.601 (Tab.)
classification, **P**.600
geographical distribution, **P**.43, **P**.610
historical aspects, **P**.11
infection
clinical manifestations, **P**.612–13,
P.613 (Fig.)
diagnosis, **P**.148
immune response, **P**.605
urine culture, **P**.152
urine examination, **P**.152
see also Schistosomiasis
life cycle
location in host, **P**.612
snail intermediate hosts, **P**.603 (Tab.),
P.611 (Tab.), **P**.612, **P**.612 (Fig.)
life expectancy, **P**.60 (Tab.)
morphology/structure, **P**.611
eggs, **P**.612 (Fig.)
Schistosoma incognitum, **P**.626
Schistosoma intercalatum
characteristics, **P**.601 (Tab.)
classification, **P**.600
geographical distribution, **P**.43, **P**.610
Schistosoma japonicum
characteristics, **P**.601 (Tab.), **P**.627 (Tab.)
classification, **P**.600, **P**.627
epidemiology, **P**.626
geographical distribution, **P**.43
historical aspects, **P**.11, **P**.626
infection
clinical manifestations, **P**.629–31,
P.629 (Tab.)
immune response, **P**.605
see also Schistosomiasis
life cycle
location in host, **P**.603, **P**.628
snail intermediate hosts, **P**.603 (Tab.),
P.628, **P**.628 (Fig.)
morphology/structure, **P**.601 (Fig.), **P**.627
eggs, **P**.627 (Fig.)
tegument, **P**.601
Schistosoma malayensis, **P**.626
characteristics, **P**.601 (Tab.), **P**.627 (Tab.)
classification, **P**.600, **P**.627
density dependent fecundity, **P**.61 (Fig.)
historical aspects/discovery, **P**.626–7
infection *see* Schistosomiasis
intermediate hosts, **P**.603 (Tab.), **P**.628
morphology/structure, **P**.627
Schistosoma mansoni
AIDS infection, **P**.97
characteristics, **P**.601 (Tab.)
classification, **P**.600, **P**.610
geographical distribution, **P**.43, **P**.610
historical aspects, **P**.11

infection
clinical manifestations, **P**.612–13
immune response, **P**.605
latent period, **P**.61 (Tab.)
see also Schistosomiasis
life cycle
location in host, **P**.603, **P**.612
snail intermediate hosts, **P**.61 (Tab.),
P.603 (Tab.), **P**.611 (Tab.), **P**.612,
P.613 (Fig.)
life expectancy, **P**.60 (Tab.)
morphology/structure, **P**.601 (Fig.), **P**.611
eggs, **P**.612 (Fig.)
prevalence, **P**.604
Schistosoma mattheei
characteristics, **P**.601 (Tab.)
classification, **P**.600
Schistosoma mekongi, **P**.626
characteristics, **P**.601 (Tab.), **P**.627 (Tab.)
classification, **P**.600, **P**.627
geographical distribution, **P**.43
historical aspects/discovery, **P**.626–7
infection *see* Schistosomiasis
life cycle
location in host, **P**.628
snail intermediate hosts, **P**.603 (Tab.),
P.628
morphology/structure, **P**.627
Schistosoma sinensium, **P**.626
Schistosoma spindale, **P**.626
Schistosomatidae, **P**.582
Schistosomatoidea, **P**.582
Schistosomiasis
acute, **I**.718–19
chemotherapy, **P**.607, **P**.622, **P**.635–7
artemether, **P**.607, **P**.635–6
metrifonate, **P**.622
oxamniquine, **P**.622
praziquantal, **P**.607, **P**.622, **P**.635
chronic, **I**.718–19
clinical manifestations, **P**.604–5, **P**.612–13,
P.629–31, **I**.718–19
acute infection, **P**.604–5
cerebral involvement, **P**.630–1
female genital tract disease, **P**.631
granulomas, **P**.604–5, **P**.605 (Fig.),
P.629–30
hematuria, **P**.612–13
hepatic cirrhosis, **P**.631 (Fig.)
hepatic fibrosis, **P**.612–13, **P**.630 (Fig.)
hepatosplenomegaly, **P**.612–13, **P**.630–1
hydronephrosis, **P**.612–13, **P**.613 (Fig.)
Katayama fever, **P**.629–30
physical effects, **P**.605
pipestem fibrosis, **P**.630–1, **P**.630 (Fig.)
Schistosoma haematobium, **P**.612–13,
P.613 (Fig.)
Schistosoma japonicum, **P**.629–31,
P.629 (Tab.)
Schistosoma mansoni, **P**.612–13
see also Below, immunopathology
control, **P**.607, **P**.622, **P**.635–7
albendazole, **P**.125
Cambodia control programs, **P**.636–7
chemotherapy/chemoprophylaxis, **P**.127,
P.144 (Tab.)

Schistosomiasis
  control (*Continued*)
    China control programs, **P**.628, **P**.635–6
    control programs, **P**.622
    diagnosis, **P**.143 (Tab.)
    economics, **P**.44
    Japan control program, **P**.628
    Laos control programs, **P**.636–7
    molluskicides, **P**.127, **P**.635–6
    Philippines control programs, **P**.628–9
    praziquantal, **P**.125
    reservoir hosts, **P**.635–6
    school-age children, **P**.125
    stratification of disease, **P**.115, **P**.141 (Tab.)
    vaccine development *see below*
    vector/reservoir control, **P**.127,
      P.145 (Tab.)
  diagnosis, **P**.148, **P**.606–7, **P**.621–2, **P**.635
    culture, **P**.151
    egg counts, **P**.606
    immunodiagnostics, **P**.606
    Kato–Katz smears, **P**.149–50, **P**.606
    public health effects, **P**.149–50
    sigmoidoscopy, **P**.151
    urine examination, **P**.152
  disease severity, **I**.718–19
  epidemiology *see below*
  fibrotic granulomas (type 2), **I**.710, **I**.718–23
    arginase, **I**.722
    chemokines, **I**.722–3
    collagen synthesis, **I**.722
    formation, **I**.722–3
    histology, **I**.710 (Fig.), **I**.719 (Fig.),
      I.721 (Fig.)
    IFN-γ, **I**.720
    IL-10, **I**.720
    IL-13, **I**.720, **I**.722
    macrophages, **I**.722
    mediators, **I**.720, **I**.722–3, **I**.724 (Tab.)
    morphology, **I**.720
    Th2 cells, **I**.719–20
    therapy, **I**.722, **I**.723
    transforming growth factor-β, **I**.722–3
  heterogeneity/infection predisposition
    host genetic factors, **P**.55
    human behavior, **P**.54–5, **P**.56 (Fig.)
  historical aspects, **P**.11
    Orient, **P**.626–7
  immune response, **P**.92–5, **P**.605–6, **P**.617–
    18, **P**.631–2, **I**.719–20
    acquired immunity, **P**.605
    age-dependency, **P**.94, **P**.605
    animal models, **P**.605–6
    antibody-dependent cellular cytotoxicity,
      P.94, **P**.617–18, **P**.617 (Fig.), **P**.631–2,
      I.683
    antigens, **P**.94, **P**.618
    attenuated parasite vaccine model,
      P.605–6
    basophils, **I**.68
    concomitant immunity model, **P**.94,
      P.605–6
    effector cells, **P**.617–18
    eosinophils, **I**.69–70, **P**.617–18
    experimental models, **P**.94
    genetic control, **P**.618

  humoral, **P**.94
  hypersensitivity to eggs, **P**.93, **P**.95
  IFN-γ, **I**.719
  IgE, **P**.631–2
  IL-4, **I**.68
  immunopathology *see below*
  paramyosin, **P**.618, **P**.631–2, **P**.632 (Fig.)
  Th1 cell responses, **I**.719
  T helper cells, **P**.94–5, **P**.606
  see also Below, immunopathology
  immunogenetics, **I**.601
  immunopathology, **P**.94–5, **P**.613–7
    APCs, **P**.617
    eosinophils, **P**.616
    granuloma formation, **P**.613–5, **P**.616–7
    hypersensitivity reactions, **P**.615–16
    IFN-γ, **P**.616
    IL-1, **P**.616
    IL-2, **P**.614
    IL-4, **P**.613, **P**.614-15, **I**.68
    IL-6, **P**.614–15
    IL-10, **P**.615, **P**.616
    IL-12, **P**.614–15
    IL-13, **P**.614–15
    soluble egg antigens, **P**.616
    T helper cells, **P**.613
    tumor necrosis factor, **P**.616–17
  intensity *vs.* age, **P**.57 (Fig.)
    behavioral changes, **P**.57
  intestinal, discovery, **P**.11
  life cycle, **I**.718
  mortality, **P**.28 (Tab.), **P**.29 (Tab.)
  pathogenesis/pathology, **P**.604–5, **P**.612–13,
    P.629–31, **I**.719–20
    histamine release, **I**.68–9
    Th1/Th2 balance, **I**.724
    see also Immunopathology
  prevention, **P**.607, **P**.622
  public health importance, **P**.43–4, **P**.105 (Tab.)
    economic impact, **P**.43–4
    geographical distribution, **P**.43
  transmission/epidemiology, **P**.43, **P**.46 (Tab.),
    P.600, **P**.603–4, **I**.718
    age-relation, **P**.43
    community-based studies, **P**.604,
      P.604 (Fig.)
    epidemics, **P**.142 (Tab.)
    Indonesia, **P**.629
    prevalence, **P**.43
    public heath implications, **P**.603–4
    snail intermediate hosts, **P**.603
  vaccines, **P**.94, **P**.606, **P**.618–21, **P**.632–5,
    I.941
    9B antigen, **I**.874
    BCE peptide vaccines, **I**.855 (Tab.), **I**.874
    BCG vector, **I**.845
    calpain, **P**.621, **P**.633 (Tab.), **P**.634–5
    candidates, **P**.619 (Fig.), **P**.633 (Tab.),
      P.634 (Fig.)
    development status, **I**.933 (Tab.)
    glutathione S-transferases, **P**.620,
      P.633 (Tab.), **P**.634–5
    glyceraldehyde-phosphate dehydrogenase,
      P.620
    paramyosin, **P**.632–3
    peptides, **I**.861 (Tab.)

  radiation-attenuated parasites, **P**.620
  Sm14, **P**.621, **I**.874
  Sm23, **P**.632–3, **P**.633–4, **P**.633 (Tab.)
  Sm62, **P**.620
  SMIrV1, **P**.620–1
  SMIrV5, **P**.620
  triose-phosphate isomerase, **P**.618–19,
    P.633 (Tab.), **P**.634
Schizogony
  Blastocystis hominis, **P**.560–1
  Plasmodium, **P**.473–4
  Plasmodium falciparum, **P**.473–4
Schizonts, *Plasmodium see Plasmodium*
Schizophyllum commune, **M**.77
Schizosaccharomyces pombe
  mating types, **M**.768
  Pneumocystis relation to, **M**.768, **M**.772,
    M.778
Schizotrypanum, **P**.377
Schleiden, Matthias Jacob, **P**.186–7
Schoenlein, J L, **M**.6
Schools, airborne bacteria, **B1**.186 (Tab.)
Schüffner's dots, **P**.469 (Fig.)
  Plasmodium vivax, **P**.474–5
  classification, **P**.464, **P**.465
Schwann cells, *Mycobacterium leprae,* **B2**.1204
Schwann, Theodor, **P**.186–7
Schwarz strain, Measles virus vaccine,
  V1.734–5
Scl-1 gene, leishmaniasis, **I**.596
Scleritis, **M**.316–17
  causative agents
    Absidia corymbifera, **M**.316
    Acremonium, **M**.316
    aspergillosis, **M**.316, **M**.317
    candidiasis, **M**.317
    Lasiodiplopodia theobromae, **M**.316
    Scedosporium, **M**.316, **M**.317, **M**.328
    sporotrichosis, **M**.316
  post surgical, **M**.327, **M**.328
Sclerosing cholangitis, in AIDS, **P**.405
Sclerosing keratitis, onchocerciasis, **P**.793–5
Sclerotic cells (muriform bodies), **M**.89 (Tab.),
  M.356, **M**.357 (Fig.), **M**.362–3, **M**.363–4
Sclerotina, **B1**.281
Sclerotina sclerotiorum, celery 'pink rot,'
  B1.281
Scolex, *Taenia solium,* **P**.678, **P**.679 (Fig.)
Scombroid poisoning, **B1**.280
Scopulariopsis, **B1**.276
  antifungal susceptibility, **M**.752 (Tab.)
  dacryocanaliculitis, **M**.298
  ecology, **M**.758
  histopathology, **M**.128 (Tab.)
  infection, **M**.189, **M**.758
    therapy, **M**.758–9
  morphology, **M**.757–8
Scopulariopsis acremonium, **M**.245–6
Scopulariopsis asperula, **M**.245–6
Scopulariopsis brevicaulis, **M**.78 (Fig.), **M**.245,
  M.251, **M**.251 (Fig.)
  conidiophores, **M**.78 (Fig.)
  microscopy, **M**.245
  nail dystrophy, **M**.245–6
  oculomycoses, **M**.275 (Tab.)

Scopulariopsis brevicaulis, (Continued)
  otitis externa, **M**.247–8
Scopulariopsis flava, **M**.245–6
Scopulariopsis fusca, **M**.245–6
Scopulariopsis koningii, **M**.245–6
Scotochromogens, **B2**.1181
Scrapie, **V2**.1347, **V2**.1348, **V2**.1361–2
  discovery/historical aspects, **V1**.7, **V2**.1348,
    V2.1361
  experimental, **V2**.1361
  mouse model, **V2**.1373
  'natural' infection, **V2**.1361–2
  transmission
    within flocks, **V2**.1361–2
    humans, **V2**.1371
Scraping, cell propagation, **V1**.89
Screening
  diphtheria diagnosis, **B1**.612
  Enterobacteriaceae identification, **B2**.1348,
    B2.1349 (Tab.)
  Escherichia coli identification, **B2**.1349 (Tab.)
  Hafnia identification, **B2**.1349 (Tab.)
  infection control, **B1**.347
  vaccine efficacy studies, **B1**.324–5
Screening media, *Salmonella* culture, **B2**.1401
Scrub typhus, **B2**.2030–1, **B2**.2031 (Tab.),
    B2.2041–2
  causative organism *see Orientia*
    tsutsugamushi
  clinical manifestations, **B2**.2039 (Tab.),
    B2.2041–2
  epidemiology and natural history, **B2**.2041
Scrum pox, **V1**.507
SCYA3 gene, **I**.582
SCYA4 gene, **I**.582
SCYA5 gene, **I**.582
SCYA7 gene, **I**.582
SCYA8 gene, **I**.582
SCYA11 gene, **I**.582
Scytalidium dimidiatum, **M**.245, **M**.247
  microscopy, **M**.245
  Onychocola canadensis vs., **M**.247
  onychomycosis, **M**.246
  skin infection, **M**.247
  structure and characteristics, **M**.251–2,
    M.252 (Fig.)
Scytalidium hyalinum, **M**.11, **M**.247
  Onychocola canadensis vs., **M**.247
  onychomycosis, **M**.246
  skin infection, **M**.247
  structure and characteristics, **M**.252
Scytalidium infection, **M**.189, **M**.246–7
  onychomycosis, **M**.246–7
Scytonema, **B1**.201
SDF1αβ *see* Stromal-derived factor 1α (SDF-
    1α:CXCL12)
SDF1 gene, point mutations, **I**.586
SDS-PAGE *see* Polyacrylamide gel
    electrophoresis (PAGE)
Seadornavirus, **V1**.47–8, **V2**.932
Seafood
  astrovirus infection, **V2**.900–1
  norovirus infection, **V2**.920, **V2**.922
Seals
  Canine distemper virus, **V1**.813–14
  Cetacean morbillivirus infection, **V1**.814

Seasonal outbreaks
  astroviruses, **V2**.902
  epidemiology, **V1**.358
  hepatitis A, **V1**.358
  Human coronaviruses infection, **V1**.841–2
  Human respiratory syncytial virus infection,
    V1.366, **V1**.783–4, **V1**.784 (Fig.)
  influenza, **V1**.367, **V1**.668
  meningococcal meningitis, **B1**.562
  mumps, **V1**.751–2, **V1**.751 (Fig.)
  norovirus infection, **V2**.919
  parainfluenza viruses, **V1**.366
  rain water bacteria, **B1**.212 (Tab.)
  rotavirus infection, **V1**.358, **V1**.368
  rubella epidemiology, **V2**.970
Seborrheic dermatitis, **M**.14–5, **M**.18 (Fig.),
    M.211–12
  AIDS, **M**.211–12
  animals, **M**.212–13
  causative agents, **M**.212
  clinical features, **M**.211–12
  dandruff (pityriasis capitis), **M**.211–12
  immune response, **M**.212
  immunosuppressed patients, **M**.211–12
  incidence, **M**.211–12
  multiple sclerosis, **M**.211–12
  Parkinson's disease, **M**.211–12
  therapy, **M**.185, **M**.212
SecB protein, **B1**.45
  function, **B1**.47
Secernentea, **P**.588, **P**.589
  Ancylostomatoidea, **P**.589
  Ascaridoidea, **P**.589
  Dracunculoidea, **P**.591
  Filarioidea, **P**.591–2
  Gnathostomatoidea, **P**.592
  Metastrongyloidea, **P**.592
  Oxyuroidea, **P**.592–3
  Physalopteroidea, **P**.593
  Rhabditoidea, **P**.593–4
  Spiruroidea, **P**.594
  Strongyloidea, **P**.594–5
  Thelazioidea, **P**.595
  Trichostrongyloidea, **P**.595
Secondary attack rate (SAR), definition,
    V1.356
Secondary cases, infection models, **I**.955
Secondary infection, memory B cell kinetics,
    I.492–3
Secondary intermediate hosts *see* Intermediate
    hosts
Secondary lymphoid organs, **I**.505
Secondary lymphoid tissue chemokine
    (SLC:CCL21), **I**.218 (Tab.), **I**.226
  B cell homing, **I**.226
  dendritic cell activation, **I**.393–4
  Peyer's patches production, **I**.511
Secretion pathways, *Plasmodium* nutrition,
    P.475–6
Secretory cells, **I**.473 (Fig.)
Secretory immunoglobulin A (sIgA),
    I.307–8, **I**.522, **B1**.624
  in breast milk, **P**.75
  in diseases/infection
    acute bronchiolitis pathogenesis, **V1**.776
    amebiasis, **P**.75, **P**.208

cryptosporidiosis, **P**.407
  giardiasis, **P**.76
  HIV infection, **I**.799–800
  Human respiratory syncytial virus
    infection, **V1**.794–5
  influenza, **V1**.663
  mumps, **V1**.748, **V1**.751
  Naegleria fowleri infection, **P**.232
  effector functions, **I**.311 (Tab.), **I**.537–8
    basophil histamine release, **I**.62
  epithelial cell transport, **I**.524–5
  induction, bare skin immunization, **I**.825
  molecular properties, **I**.307 (Tab.)
  mucosal vaccination, **I**.827, **I**.828
  neonatal transfer, **I**.308
  respiratory tract, **B1**.607–8
  secretory component, **I**.309–10
Secretory leukocyte protease inhibitor (SLP1)
  anti-HIV activity, **I**.521–2
  innate mucosal immune response, **I**.521
Secretory proteases, antigen processing, **I**.414
Sec system, **B1**.45
  protein secretion, **B1**.48
Sector-wide approaches to financing (SWAP),
    P.103–6
Seeds, **B1**.286–7
Segmentation, genomes, **V1**.180–1
Segregation analysis
  epidemiology, **P**.50
  immunogenetics, **I**.572
Segretain, G., **M**.19, **M**.26
SEIR (susceptible, exposed, infectious,
    resistant) model, **I**.954–5
Seizures
  HHV-6 infection, **V1**.527–8
  measles vaccination, **V1**.736
  neurocysticercosis, **P**.686–7
Selectin(s)
  basophils, **I**.59 (Tab.)
  eosinophils, **I**.59 (Tab.)
    adhesion, **I**.60
  lymphocyte migration, **I**.505–6, **I**.508 (Tab.)
  lymphocyte trafficking into CNS, **V2**.1410–11
  neutrophil interactions, **I**.38
  see also L-selectin; P-selectin
Selective decontamination of the digestive
    tract (SDD), **B1**.390
Selective media
  Aeromonas, **B2**.1532
  Borrelia, **B2**.1828
  Brucella, **B2**.1734–5, **B2**.1739
  Burkholderia cepacia complex, **B2**.1609–10
  Helicobacter pylori, **B2**.1572
Selective theory, **I**.9
Selective toxicity, antiviral chemotherapy,
    V2.1605
Selectivity, vaccination models, **I**.961
Selenium, acute phase response, **I**.208
Selenium sulfide, **M**.183 (Tab.), **M**.185
  black piedra, **M**.198
  Malassezia infection, **M**.185
  piedra, **M**.186
  pityriasis versicolor, **M**.185
  pityrosporal folliculitis, **M**.185–6
  seborrheic dermatitis, **M**.185, **M**.212

Selenium sulfide (*Continued*)
tinea capitis, **M**.188–9, **M**.234
Selenomonas, **B2**.1930
normal microbiota, **B1**.296 (Tab.)
Self-assembly, capsids, **V1**.65
'Self-complementary' gene vectors, adeno-associated viruses, **V1**.428–9
Self-limiting diarrhea, isosporiasis, **P**.412
Self/nonself discrimination, **I**.449–50
historical aspects/re-evaluation, **I**.12
Semaphorins
poxvirus immune evasion, **V1**.622–3
viral homologue, **I**.620
Semen, virus shedding, **V1**.249
'Semi-autonomous organelles', **P**.174
Semi-conservative transposition, **B1**.95
Semisulcospira, Paragonimus intermediate host, **P**.646
Semliki Forest virus (SFV), **V2**.1010, **V2**.1011 (Tab.), **V2**.1023–4
fusion protein, **V1**.214
infection
humoral immune response, **V2**.1412
immunopathology, **V1**.280
noncytopathic variant, **V2**.1012–14
Sendai virus, **V1**.763
cell receptors, **V1**.207 (Tab.), **V1**.765–6
classification, **V1**.382–3
C proteins, **V1**.705, **V1**.771
immune evasion, **V1**.773
fusion protein, **V1**.214
genome structure, **V1**.785 (Fig.)
hemagglutinin-neuraminidase (HN), **V1**.766
immune evasion, **V1**.705
infection, **I**.290–2
matrix (M) protein, **V1**.703
morphology/structure, **V1**.70 (Tab.)
multinucleated syncytia formation, **V1**.213
protein synthesis, **V1**.116–17
transcription, 'rule of six,' **V1**.770–1
V proteins, **V1**.763–4
Sendai virus C, immune evasion, **V1**.773
Sensorineural hearing loss (SNHL), congenital HCMV infection, **V2**.1449
Sensory networks, **B1**.165–73
bacterial, **B1**.165–73
Seoul virus, **V2**.1666 (Tab.)
biosafety level 3 classification, **V2**.1526
infection, **V2**.1044–5
hemorrhagic fever with renal syndrome (HFRS), **V2**.1045
transmission, **V1**.371 (Tab.)
'Separate lineage' model, αβ/γδ T cell separation, **I**.457
Sepata, classification, **P**.190–1
Sepata intestinalis see Enterocytozoon intestinalis
Sepik virus (SEPV), **V2**.998 (Tab.)
'Sepsin,' **I**.109
Sepsis
definition, **B1**.510, **B1**.511 (Tab.)
signs of, **B1**.511–12, **B1**.511 (Tab.)
Septa, **M**.72–3, **M**.72 (Fig.), **M**.73 (Fig.)
deposition, **M**.74–5
dolipores, **M**.72, **M**.73 (Fig.)

Septic arthritis
acute
epidemiology, **B1**.685, **B1**.686 (Tab.)
treatment, **B1**.702 (Tab.)
causative pathogens, **B1**.690
Kingella kingae, **B2**.1669–70
see also individual species
chronic
epidemiology, **B1**.686 (Tab.)
treatment, **B1**.702 (Tab.)
clinical manifestations, **B1**.685 (Tab.)
diagnosis, radiology, **B1**.693
prevention, **B1**.691
Septicemia
definition, **B1**.511 (Tab.)
hemorrhagic, cattle, **B2**.1653–4
listeriosis, **B1**.243
meloidosis, **B2**.1626–7
meningococcal infection, **B1**.565–6
Mycobacterium abscessus case history, **B2**.1250
paracoccidioidomycosis, **M**.547
Pasteurella multocida, **B2**.1654–5
streptococcal infection, **B1**.244
urinary tract infection, **B1**.389
Septic shock, **I**.109, **I.695–704**
cellular systems, **I**.696–7
endothelial cells, **I**.700–1
inflammatory cytokines, **I**.697
mast cells, **I**.699–700
neutrophils, **I**.699–700
platelets, **I**.699–700
TLRs, **I**.696
circulatory failure, **I**.699–701
complement
alternative pathway, **I**.697–8
C3 complement protein, **I**.698
C5 complement protein, **I**.698
classical pathway, **I**.697–8
lectin pathway, **I**.697–8
definition, **B1**.510, **B1**.511 (Tab.)
humoral systems, **I**.697–9
coagulation pathways, **I**.699
IL-1, **I**.697
inducible nitric oxide synthase, **I**.700
macrophage migration inhibitory factor, **I**.697
mannan-binding lectin, **I**.697–8
MBL-associated serine proteases, **I**.697–8
nitric oxide, **I**.697
platelet-activating factor, **I**.699
platelets, **I**.699
superoxide ions, **I**.700
tissue factor, **I**.699
TNF-α, **I**.286, **I**.697
see also individual systems
hypotension, **I**.700
microcirculation, **I**.700, **I**.701
pattern recognition, **I**.695–6
bacterial DNA, **I**.696
lipoteichoic acid, **I**.696
LPS, **I**.696
LPS-binding protein, **I**.696
pathogen-associated molecular patterns, **I**.696

pattern recognition receptors, **I**.695–6
TLR-2, **I**.696
TLR-4, **I**.696
see also Pattern recognition
therapy, **B1**.393, **I**.701–3
activated protein C, **I**.702–3
antithrombin III, **I**.701–2
coagulopathy management, **I**.701–2
corticosteroids, **I**.702
GM-CSF, **I**.702
IL-1 receptor antagonist, **I**.702
IL-4, **I**.702
IL-10, **I**.702
IL-13, **I**.702
inflammation management, **I**.702–3
tissue factor inhibitor, **I**.702
transforming growth factor-β, **I**.702
virulence factors, curli, **B1**.148–9
see also Multiple organ failure (MOF); Systemic inflammatory response syndrome (SIRS)
Sequential organ failure assessment (SOFA), **B1**.510
Sequential receptor expression model, NK cell development, **I**.93
Sequestration
malaria, **P**.472, **P**.472 (Fig.), **P**.491
see also Plasmodium
Plasmodium see Plasmodium
Plasmodium falciparum see Plasmodium falciparum
Plasmodium malariae, **P**.471
Sequiviridae
classification, **V1**.27 (Tab.), **V1**.51 (Tab.), **V1**.52
see also specific viruses
Serglycine
CTLs, **I**.475
cytotoxic granules, **I**.475
NK cell cytotoxic granules, **I**.475
Serine protease, astroviruses, **V2**.896
Serine-rich protein (SERP), *Plasmodium,* **P**.475–6
Serine-threonine protein kinases
oncogene products, **V1**.335–6
poxviruses, **V1**.603–4
Seroarcheology, influenza viruses, **V1**.635
Seroconversion, Human astrovirus, **V2**.901–2
Seroepidemiology
Bovine torovirus, **V1**.845–6
norovirus infection, **V2**.920–1
sapovirus infection, **V2**.925
Serological surveys, prevalence, **V1**.360
Serology/serological diagnosis, **M**.92, **M**.93 (Tab.), **M**.97, **M**.98 (Tab.), **P**.152–3, **P**.152 (Tab.), **B1**.718–20
Actinomyces, **B2**.1017
Actinomycetes, **M**.391–2
amebiasis, **P**.211–12
Angiostrongylus cantonensis infection, **P**.806–7
arenavirus infection, **V2**.1075
aspergillosis, **M**.92, **M**.93 (Tab.), **M**.104–9, **M**.105, **M**.712
Avian infectious bronchitis virus infection, **V1**.844

Serology/serological diagnosis (*Continued*)
babesiosis, **P**.457
basic reproductive number of infection effects, **P**.53, **P**.53 (Fig.)
Blastocystis hominis infection, **P**.563–4
blastomycosis, **M**.92, **M**.93 (Tab.), **M**.112–13, **M**.496
Borna disease virus infection, **V2**.1150, **V2**.1151 (Tab.)
candidiasis *see* Candidiasis
Carrión's disease, **B2**.1890
cat-scratch disease, **B2**.1897–8
Chagas disease, **P**.389
characterization testing, **B1**.22 (Tab.), **B1**.24
Chlamydia infection, **B2**.2019–20
   C. psittaci, **B2**.2020
   C. trachomatis, **B2**.2019–20
chromoblastomycosis, **M**.363
Coccidioides immitis, **M**.113, **M**.514
concentration techniques, **P**.152
cryptococcosis, **M**.92, **M**.93 (Tab.), **M**.109–10
culture, **P**.152–3
EBV infection, **V2**.1546, **V2**.1546 (Tab.)
echinococcosis, **P**.694
   alveolar echinococcosis, **P**.694
   cystic echinococcosis, **P**.694–6
fetal infection diagnosis, **V2**.1446 (Tab.)
filovirus infection, **V2**.1093
flavivirus infection, **V2**.1547
giardiasis, **P**.247
glanders, **B2**.1634
hantavirus infection, **V2**.1547
HCMV infection diagnosis, **V2**.1547
Helicobacter pylori infection, **B2**.1571 (Tab.), **B2**.1573
hepatitis B, **V2**.1546
hepatitis C, **V2**.1547
HHV infection, **V1**.533, **V2**.1547
histoplasmosis *see* Histoplasmosis
HPV infection, **V1**.467
HSV encephalitis, **V2**.1421
HTLV transmission, **V2**.1293–4
human brucellosis, **B2**.1739–41
Human respiratory syncytial virus infection, **V1**.791–2
influenza, **V1**.675, **V2**.1546–7
interpretation, **V2**.1547 (Tab.), **V2**.1548
measles, **V1**.732–3, **V2**.1547
methods, **B1**.718–20
microsporidiosis, **P**.536
mumps, **V1**.754, **V1**.755
Mycoplasma infection, **B2**.1969, **B2**.1994–5
   PCR *vs.*, **B2**.1996–7
neurocysticercosis, **P**.692–3
norovirus infection, **V2**.921
onchocerciasis, **P**.791
paracoccidioidomycosis, **M**.92, **M**.113–14, **M**.553
parasite control, **P**.129–30
PCP, **M**.788
penicilliosis marneffei, **M**.570
precipitin tests, **B1**.719
Q fever, **B2**.2077
relapsing fever (*Borrelia*), **B2**.1830
rubella, **V2**.972

sapovirus infection, **V2**.926
sporotrichosis, **M**.93 (Tab.), **M**.376–7
Strongyloides infection, **P**.741–2
surveillance, **B1**.324
   routine, **B1**.321–2
techniques, **M**.93 (Tab.), **M**.98 (Tab.)
toxocariasis, **P**.148
toxoplasmosis, **P**.434–5
trypanosomiasis, **P**.129–30
   African trypanosomiasis, **P**.366–7
vaccine efficacy, **B1**.324
see also Fungemia; Immunoserology; *specific assays; specific infection*
Seronegativity, HIV infection, **I**.790
Seroprevalence
astroviruses, **V2**.901–2
HHV, **V1**.529
Serotonin, in CNS infection, **V2**.1409
Serotype-specific plasmids, *Salmonella* serotypes, **B2**.1418, **B2**.1426
Serotyping/serotypes, **V2**.1542
Aeromonas, **B2**.1535
Bordetella pertussis, **B2**.1804 (Fig.)
Chlamydia, **B2**.2018
definition, **V1**.34
Foot-and-mouth disease virus, **V2**.874
hemadsorption, **V2**.1542
hemagglutination inhibition (HAI), **V2**.1542
Human astrovirus, **V2**.899
noroviruses, **V2**.918
Salmonella, **B2**.1403 (Tab.), **B2**.1408
Streptococcus pneumoniae, **B1**.570
Serovars, **B2**.1290–1
Serpins
cytotoxic cell self-protection, **I**.477–8
Myxoma virus, **V1**.623
poxvirus immune evasion, **V1**.623
Vaccinia virus effects, **V1**.623
Serpin SP-1, poxvirus host range control, **V1**.623–4
Serpocidins, neutrophils, **I**.41
Serratia, **B2**.1487–90
antibacterial susceptibility/resistance, **B2**.1488–9
   intrinsic, **B2**.1352 (Tab.)
antigens, **B2**.1489
biochemistry, **B2**.1488
characteristics, **B2**.1487
classification, **B2**.1487–8
culture, **B2**.1488
   pigment production, **B2**.1345
   temperature, **B2**.1344
definition, **B2**.1487
fimbriae, **B2**.1342–3
habitats, **B2**.1490
identification
   deoxyribonuclease production, **B2**.1351
   gelatin liquefaction, **B2**.1351
   historical perspective, **B2**.1351
   screening tests, **B2**.1349 (Tab.)
as indigenous bacteria in water, **B1**.211
infection, **B2**.1490
   bacteremia, **B1**.521
   intestinal, **B2**.1347

nosocomial infection, **B1**.372, **B1**.378, **B1**.398 (Tab.)
morphology, **B2**.1488
normal microbiota, **B1**.296 (Tab.)
pathogenicity, **B2**.1490
typing methods, **B2**.1489–90
Serratia burkholderia infection, **I**.48
Serratia entomophila, **B2**.1487–8
biochemical tests, **B2**.1319 (Tab.)
Serratia ficaria, **B2**.1487–8
biochemical tests, **B2**.1319 (Tab.)
characteristics, **B2**.1489 (Tab.)
pathogenicity, **B2**.1490
Serratia fonticola, **B2**.1487–8
biochemical tests, **B2**.1319 (Tab.)
characteristics, **B2**.1488, **B2**.1489 (Tab.)
pathogenicity, **B2**.1490
Serratia grimesii, **B2**.1487–8
Serratia liquefaciens, **B2**.1487–8
antigens, **B2**.1489
biochemical tests, **B2**.1319 (Tab.)
characteristics, **B2**.1489 (Tab.)
culture, **B2**.1488
pathogenicity, **B2**.1490
in poultry, **B1**.277–8
Serratia marcescens, **B2**.1487
antibacterial susceptibility/resistance, **B1**.433, **B2**.1488–9
   intrinsic, **B2**.1352 (Tab.)
antigens, **B2**.1489
   virulence effects, **B2**.1340
as arthropod pathogen, **B1**.203–4
characteristics, **B2**.1489 (Tab.)
classification, **B2**.1487
culture, **B2**.1488
filtration sterilization, **B1**.454 (Tab.)
habitats, **B2**.1490
historical perspective, **B2**.1318–31
identification
   biochemical tests, **B2**.1319 (Tab.)
   problem strains, **B2**.1348–50
   screening tests, **B2**.1349 (Tab.)
   typing methods, **B2**.1489–90
infection, **I**.770
   conjunctivitis, **B1**.599
   endocarditis, **B1**.532
   extraintestinal, **B2**.1346–7
   keratitis, **B1**.601
   nosocomial infection, **B1**.398 (Tab.)
iron scavenging, **B1**.151
morphology, **B2**.1488
pathogenicity, **B2**.1490
Serratia odorifera, **B2**.1487–8
biochemical tests, **B2**.1319 (Tab.)
characteristics, **B2**.1489 (Tab.)
culture, **B2**.1488
pathogenicity, **B2**.1490
typing methods, **B2**.1490
Serratia plymuthica, **B2**.1487–8
biochemical tests, **B2**.1319 (Tab.)
characteristics, **B2**.1489 (Tab.)
culture, **B2**.1488
pathogenicity, **B2**.1490
Serratia rubidaea, **B2**.1487–8
biochemical tests, **B2**.1319 (Tab.)

Serratia rubidaea, (*Continued*)
  characteristics, **B2**.1488, **B2**.1489 (Tab.)
  culture, **B2**.1488
  pathogenicity, **B2**.1490
Serum amyloid A, **I**.204–5
  acute phase response, **I**.195 (Fig.)
  high-density lipoprotein association, **I**.204–5
  isoforms, **I**.204
  production, **I**.285
Serum amyloid P, **I**.24 (Tab.)
Serum media, leptospires, **B2**.1872
Serum resistance-associated (SRA) gene,
    P.353
Serum sickness, monoclonal antibody therapy,
    I.362
Service culture collections, **B1**.28–9
Sesarma, **P**.646
Set yogurt, **B1**.248
Severe acute respiratory syndrome (SARS),
    V1.842–3, **V2**.1650–2
  clinical course, **V1**.842–3
  cytokines, **V1**.840–1
  emerging infection, **V2**.1648 (Tab.)
  epidemiology
    basic reproduction number (R_0),
      B1.340 (Tab.), **B1**.341–2
    case-finding, **B1**.347
    modeling approaches, **B1**.337–8
  infection *see* Severe acute respiratory
      syndrome coronavirus (SARS-CoV)
  laboratory-acquired infection, **V2**.1517 (Tab.)
  laboratory practices, **B1**.764
  medical importance, **V1**.135
  mortality, **V1**.842–3
  nosocomial infection, **B1**.372–3
  pathogenesis, **V1**.843
  quarantine and isolation, **B1**.347
  therapy, **V1**.843
  transmission prevention, **B1**.355, **B1**.373
Severe acute respiratory syndrome coronavirus
    (SARS-CoV), **V1**.841 (Tab.)
  accessory proteins, **V1**.835–6
  classification, **V1**.392, **V1**.398–9
  envelope (E) protein, **V1**.837
  evolution, **V1**.842–3
  genome, **V1**.828 (Fig.)
  isolation/propagation and identification,
      V1.95–8
  mutations, **V1**.17–8
  nsp15, **V1**.834
  nucleocapsid (N) protein, **V1**.832
  receptor, angiotensin-converting enzyme 2
      (ACE2), **V1**.838
  replicase (RNA polymerase), **V1**.833 (Fig.)
    post-translational modification, **V1**.834
    RNA-dependent RNA polymerase
      activity, **V1**.833–4
Severe combined immunodeficiency (SCID),
    I.774
  aetiology, **I**.774 (Fig.)
  antigen presentation, **I**.376–7
  cryptosporidiosis, **P**.404–5
  gene therapy, **V2**.1590–1, **V2**.1593–4
  infection, **I**.774
  'leaky phenotype,' **I**.774
  NK cells, **I**.80

Pneumocystis carinii infection, **I**.774
  X-linked, **I**.575
Severe combined immunodeficient (SCID)
    mice
  amebiasis, **P**.214
  babesiosis, **P**.455
  Entamoeba histolytica infection, **P**.210
Severe combined neutropenia (SCN:
    Kostmann's syndrome), **I**.765
Severe sepsis, definition, **B1**.510, **B1**.511 (Tab.)
Sewage
  bacteriology, **B1**.212, **B1**.217, **B1**.219 (Tab.),
    B1.221, **B1**.224
  tapeworm control, **P**.665
Sewage workers, giardiasis, **P**.250
Sex pheromones, *Enterococcus*, **B2**.886
Sex pili, Enterobacteriaceae, **B2**.1342, **B2**.1343
Sexual abuse, *Neisseria gonorrhoeae* typing,
    B1.662
Sexual behaviour changes, emerging bacterial
    infection, **B1**.361
Sexual intercourse, urinary tract infection,
    B1.673, **B1**.679–80
Sexually acquired reactive arthritis (SARA),
    Chlamydia trachomatis infection,
    B2.2013
Sexually transmitted diseases (STD), **V1**.237
  arenavirus infection, **V2**.1071
  behavioural prevention, **B1**.354
  definition, **I**.951 (Tab.)
  direct transmission, **V1**.354
  emerging viral infection, **V2**.1659
  epidemiological modeling, **B1**.337–8
  HCMV infection, **V2**.1502
  hepatitis B, **V1**.369
  hepatitis C, **V2**.1209, **V2**.1480
  HIV infection, **V1**.370
  HSV infection, **V1**.508, **V2**.1500
  HTLV infection, **V2**.1292
  mortality, **P**.29 (Tab.)
  Mycoplasma, **B2**.1991
  prevalence studies, **B1**.313–14, **B1**.314 (Fig.)
  reporting system, **B1**.320–1, **B1**.321 (Tab.)
  toxoplasmosis, **P**.437
  trichomoniasis, **P**.255
  see also specific diseases/infection
Sexual union (syngamy), *Balantidium coli*,
    P.277–8, **P**.279 (Fig.)
SGA medium, **M**.236
SH2 genes, paramyxoviruses, **V1**.700
Shark antibodies, **I**.368–9
'Sharps'
  laboratory safety, **V2**.1520–3
  safety precautions, **B1**.767
Shaudinn, Franz, **P**.17
Sheep
  abortion, **B2**.1549
  ewes' milk, **B1**.231–2
  infection
    Actinobacillus seminis, **B2**.1665–6
    Brucella melitensis, **B2**.1722
    Campylobacter, **B2**.1549
    listeriosis, **B2**.963, **B2**.954
    Mannheimia haemolytica, **B2**.1654
    pneumonic pasteurellosis, **B2**.1654

Shellfish
  cholera due to, **B1**.216
  cultivation, **B1**.216
  hepatitis A outbreaks, **V2**.1172
  viral transmission, **V1**.355
  see also Crustacea; Mollusks
Shell vials (cytospinning), **V2**.1540–1
Shewanella, **B1**.67
Shewanella putrefaciens
  fish, **B1**.279
  poultry, **B1**.277–8
Shiga toxin, **B2**.1390
  mechanism of action, **B1**.156 (Tab.)
  nomenclature, **B2**.1339
Shigella, **B2**.1386–97
  characteristics, **B2**.1392, **B2**.1393 (Tab.)
  classification, **B2**.1386–7
    Escherichia coli vs., **B2**.1318
    serotypes, **B2**.1388, **B2**.1392, **B2**.1393 (Tab.)
    species, **B2**.1386–7
  culture, morphology, **B2**.1345 (Tab.)
  definition, **B2**.1386–7
  diagnosis, **B2**.1391–2
    invasive phenotype, **B2**.1392
    molecular, **B2**.1392
  epidemiology, **B2**.1387–8
    in food, **B2**.1388
    crustacea, **B1**.279–80
    fruit, **B1**.283
    vegetables, **B1**.282
  genetics, **B2**.1388
  habitats, **B2**.1387
  historical perspective, **B2**.1386
  identification, **B2**.1392
    historical perspective, **B2**.1351
    screening tests, **B2**.1349 (Tab.)
  immune evasion, macrophage apoptosis,
    I.655
  infection *see* Dysentery; Shigellosis
  invasion/pathogenic mechanism, **B1**.152
    actin polymerization, **B2**.1389–90
    bacteria-host cell cross talks, **B2**.1389–90
    cell binding, **B2**.1389–90
    epithelial barrier invasion and
      inflammatory destruction, **B2**.1388–9,
      B2.1391
    macrophage apoptosis, **B2**.1388–9
    M cells, **B2**.1388–9
    polymorphonuclear cell infiltration,
      B2.1388–9
  isolation, **B2**.1391–2
    optimization, **B2**.1391
  LPS, **B1**.158, **B2**.1390
  non-motility, **B2**.1342
  O antigen, *Escherichia coli vs.*, **B2**.1341
  pathogenicity, **B2**.1388–91
    determinants, **B2**.1389
    virulence factors *see below*
  reservoirs, **B2**.1387
  serogroups, **B2**.1388, **B2**.1392, **B2**.1393 (Tab.)
    serogroup A *see Shigella dysenteriae*
    serogroup B *see Shigella flexneri*
    serogroup C *see Shigella boydii*
    serogroup D *see Shigella sonnei*

Shigella, (Continued)
transmission, **B2**.1387
fecal-oral, **B2**.1387, **B2**.1388
in foods *see above*
infective dose, **B2**.1388
routes, **B2**.1388
sexual, **B2**.1388
waterborne, **B1**.212
as vaccine vector *see* Vaccines, live
virulence factors, **B2**.1388–91
chromosomally-encoded, **B2**.1390
E-cadherin, **B2**.1390
Ipa proteins, **B2**.1389–90
Ipas, **B1**.152
Ipg proteins, **B2**.1389
N-WASP, **B2**.1390
pathogenicity island, **B2**.1389
peptidoglycan, **B2**.1390
plasmid-encoded, **B2**.1389
ShET1 enterotoxin, **B2**.1390
spa and *mxi* loci, **B2**.1389
type III secretion system, **B2**.1389
virB/virG, **B2**.1389, **B2**.1390
virulence plasmid, **B2**.1389
Shigella boydii, **B2**.1386–7
characteristics, **B2**.1393 (Tab.)
identification, **B2**.1392
biochemical tests, **B2**.1319 (Tab.)
screening tests, **B2**.1349 (Tab.)
Shigella dysenteriae, **B2**.1386–7
identification, **B2**.1392
biochemical tests, **B2**.1319 (Tab.)
screening tests, **B2**.1349 (Tab.)
infection, mucosal immune response, **I**.522–3
neuraminidase, **B1**.153 (Tab.)
serotype 1, **B2**.1388
antibacterial susceptibility/resistance,
B1.363–4
characteristics, **B2**.1393 (Tab.)
hemolytic uremic syndrome, **B2**.1387
infection, **B2**.1391
acute disasters, **B1**.360
child mortality, **B2**.1388
clinical manifestations, **B2**.1387
refugees, **B1**.360
symptoms, **B2**.1387
see also Dysentery
toxins *see* Shiga toxin
virulence factors, **B1**.153 (Tab.)
Shigella flexneri, **B2**.1386–7
antibacterial susceptibility/resistance,
plasmids, **B1**.110
characteristics, **B2**.1393 (Tab.)
fimbriae, **B2**.1342–3
genetics, **B2**.1388
identification, **B2**.1392
biochemical tests, **B2**.1319 (Tab.)
screening tests, **B2**.1349 (Tab.)
infection, **B2**.1391
infiltration of host tissues, **B1**.152–3
laboratory acquired, **B1**.761
reactive arthritis, **B2**.1387
serotype distributions, **B2**.1388
Shigella sonnei proportion *vs,* **B2**.1388

virulence factors
chromosomally-encoded, **B2**.1390
LPS, **B2**.1390
peptidoglycan, **B2**.1390
plasmids, **B2**.1389
Shigella sonnei, **B2**.1386–7
antibacterial susceptibility/resistance,
plasmids, **B1**.110
characteristics, **B2**.1393 (Tab.)
identification, **B2**.1392
biochemical tests, **B2**.1319 (Tab.)
screening tests, **B2**.1349 (Tab.)
infection
distribution, **B2**.1388
vaccines, **I**.933 (Tab.)
Shigellosis, **B2**.1387
clinical features, **B2**.1387
growth retardation in infants, **B2**.1387
entry into cells
actin cytoskeleton, **I**.649–50
escape to cytoplasm, **I**.650
epidemiology, **B2**.1387–8
day-care centers, **B1**.361
developing world, **B2**.1387–8
endemics and epidemics, **B2**.1388
international travel, **B1**.360
fatality, **B2**.1387
food, vegetables, **B1**.282
histopathological analysis, **B2**.1387
host-pathogen interaction, **B2**.1388
induced apoptosis, **I**.137–8
intestinal, **B2**.1347
macrophage infection, **I**.30
morbidity, **B2**.1387
NK cell actions, **I**.99
pathogenesis, **B2**.1388–91
prevention, **B2**.1394–5
serotype-specific protection, **B2**.1394
vaccines *see below*
treatment, **B2**.1392–4
vaccines, **B2**.1394–5
BCE peptide vaccines, **I**.855 (Tab.)
conjugate vaccines, **I**.936–7
development status, **I**.933 (Tab.)
proteasomes, **I**.839–40
Vibrio cholerae vectors, **I**.844
see also Dysentery; *individual species*
Shikimate pathway, *Cryptosporidium parvum,*
P.403
Shingles *see* Varicella-zoster virus infection
Shipping fever, **B2**.1654
see also Pneumonic pasteurellosis
Shipyard eye (epidemic keratoconjunctivitis),
V1.444, **V1**.444 (Tab.)T
Shock, **I**.210
in gas gangrene, **B2**.1114
septic *see* Septic shock
Shope fibroma growth factor (SFGF), **V1**.257
Short direct repeats (SDRs), transposable
elements, **B1**.94
Shortt, Henry, **P**.17
Shoulder joint infection, inflammatory
responses, **B1**.689
Showers, Legionnaires' disease, **B1**.375–6,
B1.634–5

SH protein, Human respiratory syncytial virus,
V1.786–7
Shrimps
freeze-drying, **B1**.269
microbiology, **B1**.279–80
Shuttle vectors, plasmid cloning vectors,
B1.121
Shuttleworthia, **B2**.1028
SHV-1 enzymes, β-lactamases, **B1**.472–3
Siadenovirus, classification, **V1**.45
Siadenoviruses, **V1**.439
Sialadentitis, **B1**.619
Sialic acid
influenza hemagglutinin binding, **V1**.652
Plasmodium cell invasion, **P**.472
structure, **V2**.1627 (Fig.), **V2**.1628 (Fig.)
trans-sialidase, *Trypanosoma cruzi,* **P**.381–2
viral receptor, **V1**.209
Sialidase activity, influenza neuraminidase
(NA), **V1**.655–6
Sialodacryoadenitis virus (SDAV), **V1**.824–5
Sialoglycoconjugates, parainfluenza virus
receptors, **V1**.765–6
Sialoglycoproteins, Minute virus of mice
binding, **V1**.416–17, **V1**.422–3
Sialy-Lewis[x] structures, **I**.506
Sicilian virus infection, **V2**.1047
Sickle cell anemia, bone and joint infection,
B1.690
Sickle-cell disease, innate malaria resistance,
P.485
mechanism of action, **P**.478
SICvar genes, *Plasmodium* antigenic variation,
P.492
Siderophores, **B2**.1793
Burkholderia cepacia complex, **B2**.1616–17
Burkholderia thailandensis, **B2**.1624
iron scavenging, **B1**.151
Pseudomonas, **B2**.1596
Yersinia ruckeri, **B2**.1470
von Siebold C.T., **P**.10–1, **P**.13
Sigma (σ) factors, **B1**.74–5
alternative, **B1**.74–5
Bacillus subtilis, **B1**.75
Escherichia coli, **B1**.74–5
σ[32] (heat shock-specific), **B1**.74, **B1**.448
σ[s] (synthesis) and resistance, **B1**.61
oxygen radical tolerance, **B1**.65
primary, **B1**.74
σ proteins *see* Reoviruses
Sigma virus, **V2**.1105
genome structure, **V2**.1112 (Fig.)
Sigmodon hispidus, **P**.326
Sigmoidoscopy, **P**.150 (Tab.), **P**.151
schistosomiasis diagnosis, **P**.151
'Signal joints'
somatic recombination, **I**.328
TCR rearrangements, **I**.452–3
Signal lymphocyte activation molecule *see*
CD150 (signal lymphocyte activation
molecule: SLAM), measles
Signal transducers and activators of
transcription (STAT)
IFN signal transduction, **V1**.294, **V1**.315
Sendai virus C protein binding, **V1**.773

Signal transduction
  acute phase response, **I**.196 (Fig.)
  bacterial subversion, **B1**.164–5
  caspase-recruitment domain, **I**.115
  CpG motifs, **I**.911
  Fcα/μR, **I**.317–18
  FcεRI, **I**.316
  FcγRI (CD64), **I**.314
  FcγRIIIa, **I**.315
  IFN receptors, **I**.247
  INFs, **V1**.227, **V1**.293–4
  NK cells *see* Natural killer (NK) cells
  pre-BCR, **I**.341
  subversion of host cell, **B1**.152, **B1**.164–5
  TLRs
    TLR-2, **I**.120 (Fig.), **I**.696
    TLR-3, **I**.119
    TLR-4, **I**.118 (Fig.), **I**.696, **I**.697 (Fig.)
    TLR-5, **I**.121
    see also Toll-like receptor(s) (TLRs)
  transforming growth factor-β, **I**.296 (Fig.)
  two-component, **B1**.75, **B1**.167–9
  type I IFN receptors, **I**.256–8, **I**.258 (Fig.)
  yeast, **M**.73, **M**.79–80
Signature-tagged mutagenesis (STM), **B1**.97, **B1**.177, **B1**.178
Silage, *Listeria*, **B2**.954
Silkworms, **M**.220
Silver, **B1**.428
  action, **B1**.437 (Tab.), **B1**.438
  resistance to, **B1**.114, **B1**.442
Silver impregnated antibacterial urinary catheters, **B1**.389
Silver nitrate, **B1**.428
Silver sulfadiazine, **B1**.428
  mycotic keratitis therapy, **M**.307
Simian foamy virus (SFV)
  evolution, **V2**.1296 (Fig.)
  gene vectors, **V2**.1314
  human infection, **V2**.1295, **V2**.1315
  infection, **V2**.1295
Simian hemorrhagic fever virus (SHFV)
  classification, **V1**.53
  genome
    open reading frames, **V1**.827
    structure, **V1**.828 (Fig.)
  infection, **V1**.841 (Tab.)
  subgenomic RNA, **V1**.831–2
Simian immunodeficiency virus (SIV)
  gene therapy vector, **V2**.1592–3
  immune evasion, **V1**.322
    CD8 interference *in vivo*, **I**.636–7
    IFN signaling, **I**.619
    MHC removal, **I**.636
  infection, **V2**.1295
    emerging infection, **V2**.1651 (Tab.)
    'species-jumping,' **V2**.1657
    IL-6, **V1**.297
    persistent infection, **V1**.259–60, **V1**.260 (Fig.)
    vaccines
      BCE peptide vaccines, **I**.855 (Tab.)
      BCG vectors, **I**.901–2
  morphology/structure, **V1**.77 (Fig.)
  oncogenic mechanisms, **V1**.342 (Tab.)

  replication, **V2**.1323
  Vpr protein, **V2**.1327
  Vpx protein, **V2**.1327
Simian T cell leukemia virus (SLTV-1), transformation by, **V1**.336
Simian varicella virus, **V1**.494 (Tab.)
Simian virus 5 (SV5), **V1**.744
  classification, **V1**.382–3
  genome structure, **V1**.785 (Fig.)
  immune evasion, **V1**.315
  protein structures, **V1**.70 (Tab.)
  small hydrophobic proteins, **V1**.708
Simian virus 10 (SV10), **V1**.382–3
Simian virus 40 (SV40), **V1**.482–3
  cell interactions
    transcription factors, **V1**.220
    viral RNA metabolism, **V1**.220
  cell transformation, **V1**.171
  genome, **V1**.151–2
    origin of replication, **V1**.482
    regulatory regions, **V1**.152 (Fig.)
    structure, **V1**.148 (Tab.), **V1**.482
    TATA box, **V1**.482
    transcription units, **V1**.482
  genome replication, **V1**.122–3, **V1**.123 (Fig.), **V1**.148 (Tab.), **V1**.151–4, **V1**.151 (Fig.), **V1**.153–4, **V1**.153 (Fig.)
    cellular proteins, **V1**.154 (Tab.)
    DNA ligase I, **V1**.154 (Tab.)
    DNA polymerase α-primase, **V1**.153, **V1**.154 (Tab.)
    DNA polymerases, **V1**.154 (Tab.)
    elongation, **V1**.153–4
    flanking regions, **V1**.152
    initiation, **V1**.153
    lagging-strand replication, **V1**.153–4
    leading-strand replication, **V1**.153–4
    origin of replication, **V1**.151, **V1**.152
    origin recognition proteins, **V1**.149 (Tab.)
    replication factor C (RF-C), **V1**.153–4, **V1**.154 (Tab.)
    replication protein A (RPA), **V1**.153, **V1**.154 (Tab.)
    RNase H1, **V1**.154 (Tab.)
    spooling, **V1**.153–4
    T antigen *see below*
    topoisomerase I, **V1**.153–4, **V1**.154 (Tab.)
    viral proteins, **V1**.149 (Tab.)
  immune evasion, **V1**.325
  large T antigen, **V1**.149 (Tab.), **V1**.151–2, **V1**.152–3, **V1**.171, **V1**.482
    nuclear localization signals, **V1**.225–6
    post-translational modifications, **V1**.152–3
    structure–function relationship, **V1**.153
  MHC class I binding, **V1**.473–4
  SELP, **V1**.473–4
  type species, **V1**.45
  VP proteins, **V1**.151
Simian virus 40 infection
  adenovirus co-infection, **V2**.1596
  cancer association, **V1**.482–3
    animal models, **V1**.482–3
    humans, **V1**.483
  human disease, **V1**.482
    transmission in poliovirus vaccine, **V1**.482, **V2**.1557

  oncogenesis, **V1**.338 (Tab.), **V1**.342 (Tab.)
  species infected, **V1**.473
Simian virus 41 (SV41), **V1**.744
  classification, **V1**.382–3
Similarity matrices, **B1**.27 (Fig.), **B1**.28
Simmons test, Enterobacteriaceae identification, **B2**.1319 (Tab.)
Simonsiella, **B2**.1271
Simple diffusion, **B1**.48–9
Simplexvirus, **V1**.494 (Tab.)
Simulect, licensing, **I**.355 (Tab.)
Simulium
  life cycle, **P**.784–5
  as onchocerciasis vector, **P**.781, **P**.783–4, **P**.784–5
    blood meals, **P**.785
    transmission ability differences, **P**.785
  seasonal population sizes, **P**.785
  windborne dispersal, **P**.785
  see also individual species
Simulium damnosum sensu lato, **P**.784
Simulium exiguum, **P**.784
Simulium guianense, **P**.784
Simulium metallicum, **P**.784
Simulium ochraceum, **P**.784
Sindbis virus (SINV), **V2**.1011 (Tab.), **V2**.1023
  antibody effects, **V1**.278
  cell receptors, **V1**.207 (Tab.), **V2**.1015
  noncytopathic variant, **V2**.1012–14
  virion structure, **V2**.1012
Sindbis virus infection
  chikungunya *vs.*, **V2**.1021–2
  CNS, **V1**.304
  IL-4, **V1**.298
  transmission, **V2**.1016–17
    reservoir hosts, **V2**.1017
Single chain Fv (scFv), **I**.367–8, **I**.367 (Fig.), **I**.368 (Fig.)
  fusion proteins, **I**.369 (Fig.)
Single domain antibodies (dAb), **I**.368, **I**.368 (Fig.)
Single-enzyme amplified fragment length polymorphism (SAFLP), **B2**.1411
Single hit relationships, cell–virus interactions, **V1**.204
Single nucleotide polymorphisms (SNPs), **M**.47, **M**.47 (Tab.)
  caspase-recruitment domain, **I**.125
  CD14, **I**.124
  chromosome 5 gene cluster, **I**.580
  immunogenetics, **I**.575
  LPS binding protein, **I**.124
  nucleotide-binding oligomerization domains, **I**.115, **I**.125
  TLRs, **I**.111, **I**.125
  see also Genetic polymorphisms
Single photon emission computed tomography (SPECT), **I**.360
Single radial hemolysis (SRH), rubella, **V2**.978
Single-strand conformational polymorphisms (SSCPs), *Aspergillus* detection, **M**.715
Sin Nombre virus, **V2**.1025, **V2**.1666 (Tab.)
  biosafety level 3 classification, **V2**.1526
  budding/transport, **V2**.1040
  genome structure, **V2**.1031–3
  transmission, **V1**.371 (Tab.)

Sin Nombre virus infection
  emerging infection, **V2**.1648 (Tab.), **V2**.1664
    recognition, **V2**.1653 (Tab.)
  hantavirus pulmonary syndrome, **V2**.1045
Sino-orbital aspergillosis
  AIDS, **M**.294–5
  amphotericin B therapy, **M**.295
Sintered glass filters, **B1**.453
Sinuses, anatomy, **B1**.606
Sinusitis, **B1**.615–16, **B1**.628
  acute, **B1**.615
  allergic fungal, **M**.672–6
    Alternaria, **M**.675
    Bipolaris, **M**.675
    Curvularia, **M**.675
    Dreschlera, **M**.675
    Exserohilum, **M**.675
  causative organisms, **B1**.615, **B1**.615 (Tab.),
    B1.628
    Moraxella (Branhamella) catarrhalis,
    B2.1307
  chronic, **B1**.615, **B1**.628
  clinical features, **B1**.616
  diagnosis, **B1**.616
  epidemiology, **B1**.615
  in HIV infection, **B1**.645
  immune deficiencies, **B1**.616
  intracranial abscess, **B1**.582, **B1**.584 (Tab.),
    B1.585
  nosocomial infection, **B1**.615
    risk factors, **B1**.616
  pathogenesis, **B1**.615
  prevention, **B1**.616
  sphenoid/frontal, **B1**.615
  subdural empyema, **B1**.590, **B1**.591–2,
    B1.591 (Tab.)
  treatment, **B1**.616
SipB, **I**.137
Siphoviridae, **V1**.26, **V1**.378
  classification, **V1**.27 (Tab.), **V1**.42,
    V1.43 (Tab.)
  see also specific viruses
Siphoviridae bacteriophage, **B2**.1535
SIR (susceptible, infectious, resistant) model,
  epidemiology, **I**.954–5
SIS (susceptible, infectious, susceptible) model,
  epidemiology, **I**.954–5
Site-directed mutagenesis *see* Mutants/
  mutations
Situation analysis, parasite control, **P**.110–11
Situs inversus, **B1**.626
6Ckine *see* Secondary lymphoid tissue
  chemokine (SLC:CCL21)
6K protein, alphaviruses, **V2**.1014
Sjögren's syndrome
  HTLV type 1 (HTLV-1) infection, **V2**.1290,
    V2.1291
  prevalence, **I**.748 (Tab.)
SKIF (PKR inhibitory factor), Vaccinia virus,
  V1.295
Skin
  anatomy, **I**.820
  as barrier to infection, **B1**.175–6, **B1**.294,
    B1.304, **I**.820
  direct transmission, **V1**.354

immune surveillance, **I**.820–1
  cytokines, **I**.820
  keratinocytes, **I**.820–1
  Langerhan's cells, **I**.820–1
  skin-associated lymphoid tissue, **I**.820
infection *see* Skin infection
normal microbiota, **B1**.304
  gram-positive anaerobic cocci, **B2**.907–10
  Staphylococcus, **B2**.775–9
vaccination *see* Vaccination, bare skin
virus entry, **V1**.236, **V1**.238 (Tab.)
virus shedding, **V1**.249
Skin-associated lymphoid tissue (SALT),
  M.262, **I**.820
Skin biopsies, **P**.153, **P**.153 (Tab.)
  onchocerciasis diagnosis, **P**.153
Skin diseases/infection
  leprosy diagnosis, **B2**.1205
  Lyme borreliosis, **B2**.1828
  onchocerciasis, **P**.794
  see also Skin infection
Skin fragments, airborne bacteria,
  B1.186 (Tab.)
Skin immunization *see* Vaccination
Skin infection
  aspergillosis, **M**.701
  blastomycosis, **M**.488, **M**.489 (Fig.), **M**.492
  candidiasis *see* Candidiasis, cutaneous/
    mucocutaneous
  cryptococcosis, **M**.647–8
  dermatomycotic molds *see* Dermatomycotic
    molds
  dermatophytic infection, **M**.244–6
  HSV infection, **V1**.507, **V1**.508–9,
    V1.508 (Fig.)
  penicilliosis marneffei, **M**.567, **M**.567 (Fig.),
    M.569
  Pneumocystis carinii infection, **M**.785
  rhinosporidiosis, **M**.460, **M**.461–2,
    M.461 (Fig.), **M**.469–70
  specimens, **M**.83 (Tab.), **M**.85, **M**.235
  systemic zygomycosis, **M**.674–5,
    M.674 (Tab.), **M**.678
  tests
    aspergillosis, **M**.711–12
    blastomycosis, **M**.484
    candidiasis, **M**.592
    chromoblastomycosis, **M**.363–4
    coccidioidomycosis, **M**.509–10, **M**.514
    histoplasmin, **M**.111, **M**.532–3
    lobomycosis, **M**.433, **M**.433 (Fig.)
    sporotrichosis, **M**.376
    tinea nigra, **M**.198–9
  see also Skin diseases/infection
Skin keratinocytes, defensins, **I**.168
Skin penetration, *Necator americanus,* **P**.721
'Skin snips,' onchocerciasis diagnosis, **P**.153,
  P.782, **P**.790–1, **P**.791 (Fig.)
Slackia, **B2**.916–17
  classification, **B2**.1028–9
Slackia exigua, differential characteristics,
  B2.1029 (Tab.)
Slackia heliotrinreducens
  biochemical characteristics, **B2**.908 (Tab.)
  classification, **B2**.904
  definition/characteristics, **B2**.916–17

SLAM *see* CD150 (signal lymphocyte
  activation molecule: SLAM), measles
Slaughter measures
  rabies control, **V2**.1126
  rinderpest control, **V1**.810
S-layers, **B1**.44, **B1**.155
  Aeromonas, **B2**.1525, **B2**.1526 (Fig.)
SLC *see* Secondary lymphoid tissue chemokine
  (SLC:CCL21)
SLC11A1 (NRAMP1) gene, **I**.579
  Chagas disease, **I**.597
  leishmaniasis association, **I**.579, **I**.597
  leprosy association, **I**.591
  polymorphisms, **I**.579
  tuberculosis association, **I**.579, **I**.591–2,
    I.592–3
Sleeping sickness, **P**.188
Slender forms, *Trypanosoma brucei,* **P**.357
Slide agglutination test, *Streptococcus
  pneumoniae* detection, **B1**.756
Sliding filament model, **P**.170–2, **P**.179–80
Slow-growing mycobacteria *see* Mycobacteria
  (slow-growing)
'Slow progressors,' HIV infection, **I**.790
Slow-reacting substances *see* Leukotriene(s)
  (LTs)
Slow viruses, infection, **V2**.1408
SLP-65 *see* BLNK (SLP-65)
Sluyter, T., **M**.14–5
SM1 gene, **I**.601
sm1 gene, **P**.55
SM2 gene, **I**.601
Sm14, schistosomiasis vaccine, **P**.621, **I**.874
Sm23, schistosomiasis vaccine, **P**.632–3, **P**.633–
  4, **P**.633 (Tab.)
Sm62, schistosomiasis vaccine, **P**.620
Smac/Diablo, mitochondria apoptosis, **I**.132
Small acid-soluble spore proteins (SASPs),
  B1.443, **B1**.448–9
Small hydrophobic (SH) protein
  Mumps virus *see* Mumps virus
  paramyxoviruses, **V1**.708
  Pneumovirinae, **V1**.708
Small intestine
  biopsy
    giardiasis, **P**.248
    microsporidiosis diagnosis, **P**.545–6,
      P.545 (Fig.)
  non-epidermal γδ T cells, **I**.438
  normal microbiota, **B1**.302
  see also Gastrointestinal tract
Small multidrug resistance family (SMR),
  B1.440
Smallpox, **V1**.586–7
  bioterrorism, **V1**.589–90
  clinical manifestations, **V1**.586
  eradication, **I**.6, **B1**.345, **V1**.578, **V1**.579–81,
    V2.1551
    calf lymph vaccine, **V1**.581
    cowpox virus, **V1**.579–80
    Edward Jenner, **V1**.579–80, **V1**.580 (Fig.)
    last natural case, **V1**.581
    pathogen dissemination, **V1**.580
    ring vaccination, **V1**.581
    vaccine supply, **V1**.580
    variolation, **V1**.579

Smallpox (*Continued*)
  historical aspects, **V1**.578–9
  human health impacts, **V1**.586
  immunodeficiency, **V1**.586–7
  mode of spread, **B1**.374
  mortality, **V1**.586–7, **V2**.1579
  naive populations, **V1**.579
  quarantine and isolation, **B1**.347
  transmission routes, **V1**.586
  vaccines/vaccination, **V1**.590–1, **V2**.1578–9
    administration, **V2**.1579
    calf lymph vaccine, **V1**.581
    complications, **V1**.589–90, **V2**.1579
    discontinuation, **V1**.589
    first-line responders, **V1**.589, **V1**.590
    history, **V1**.8 (Tab.), **V2**.1578
    live, attenuated, **V2**.1555 (Tab.)
    programs, **V2**.1559 (Tab.)
    protection correlation, **V1**.590
    ring vaccination, **V1**.581
    strains used, **V1**.590, **V2**.1578–9
    vaccine development, **V1**.591
    vaccine stocks, **V1**.589
Small repetitive elements (SRE), *Neisseria*,
  B2.1276–7
Small round structured viruses (SRSV) *see*
  Noroviruses
Small-round viruses (SRVs), historical aspects,
  V2.912
Small secreted glycoprotein (ssGP) *see* Ebola
  virus (EBOV)
Small subunit ribosomal RNA (SSR RNA)
  Blastocystis hominis, **P**.562
  Dientamoeba fragilis, **P**.267
SMAP-29, **I**.173
Smarcal gene, **I**.777
SMIrV1, schistosomiasis vaccine, **P**.620–1
SMIrV5, schistosomiasis vaccine, **P**.620
Smoking
  meat and meat products, **B1**.274–5
  tobacco *see* Tobacco smoking
Smoldering adult T-cell leukemia, **V2**.1289–90
Smoldering infection *see* Persistent viral
  infection
Smooth muscle contraction
  platelet-activating factor, **I**.191
  prostaglandins, **I**.187
Smooth muscle tumors, EBV association,
  V1.571
Snake venom, β-defensins, **I**.166
Sneezing, **B1**.176
Snow, J, **B1**.335
Snow, bacteriology of, **B1**.211–12, **B1**.213
'Snowflake opacities,' onchocerciasis, **P**.793–5
Snow mountain agent, mollusks, **B1**.280
Snowshoe hare virus
  epidemiology, **V2**.1042–3
  transcription termination, **V2**.1037
Sobemovirus, **V1**.27 (Tab.)
Social factors
  effects on population immunity, **B1**.353–5
  emerging bacterial infection, **B1**.360–1
Social mobilization, parasite control, **P**.115
Sociopolitical problems, community-directed
  treatment with ivermectin, **P**.121–2

Sodium ascorbate preserves, copper-catalysed,
  V1.91
Sodium carbonate, **B1**.422–4
Sodium dodecyl sulfate polyacrylamide gel
  electrophoresis *see* Polyacrylamide gel
  electrophoresis (PAGE)
Sodium gradient, oxaloacetate substrate use,
  B1.56
Sodium hydroxide, **B1**.422–4
Sodium hypochlorite, **B1**.422–4
  methanol, **B1**.432
Sodium iodide, pythiosis therapy, **M**.425
Sodium metabolism, *Plasmodium*, **P**.477
Sodium-motive force, **B1**.65
Sodium phosphotungstic precipitation,
  V2.1386–7
Sodium polyanethol sulfonate (SPS)
  blood cultures, **B1**.514
  gram-positive anaerobic cocci, **B2**.907
Sodium stibogluconate, Old World
  leishmaniasis, **P**.306
Soil
  bacteria *see below*
  carbon cycling, arthropods, **B1**.199
  carbon:nitrogen (C:N) ratios, **B1**.200
  clay particles, **B1**.196
  cross-sectional view, **B1**.195–6
  fertility, **B1**.200
  formation, **B1**.195–6
  horizons, **B1**.195–6
  liquid phase, **B1**.196–7
  nutrient cycling, **B1**.9
    organic matter decomposition, **B1**.9
  organic matter, **B1**.195–6
  oxygen supply, **B1**.196–7
  plant roots environment modification,
    B1.197–8
  pore size distribution, **B1**.196–7
  quality, **B1**.195–6
  structure, **B1**.196–7
  taxonomy, **B1**.195–6
  texture, **B1**.195–6
Soil bacteria
  adsorption, **B1**.196–7
  as anaerobes
    facultative, **B1**.196–7
    oxic conditions survival, **B1**.196–7
    strict, **B1**.196–7
  applications
    antibiotics, **B1**.199–200
    biological control agents, **B1**.198, **B1**.202–
      3, **B1**.203–4
    bioremediation, **B1**.199, **B1**.201–2, **B1**.202
    biotransformation, **B1**.201–2
    frost injury protection, **B1**.198
    genetically engineered microorganisms,
      B1.198, **B1**.204
  biogeochemical transformations, **B1**.199–201
    carbon cycling, **B1**.199–200
    sulfur, **B1**.201
  biomass, **B1**.195–6
  denitrification, **B1**.200
  detection/analysis, **B1**.204–7
    biofilms, **B1**.205
    biomass, **B1**.205
    direct methods, **B1**.204

    enumeration, **B1**.204–5
    indirect methods, **B1**.204
    leaf and root surface microbes separation
      methods, **B1**.204–5
    marker and reporter genes, **B1**.207
    metabolic activity in soil, **B1**.205–8
    microscopy, **B1**.207
    most probable number estimates, **B1**.204
    PCR techniques, **B1**.206–7
    propagules, **B1**.205
    quantitative estimation, **B1**.204–5
    rRNA:DNA ratio, **B1**.206
    in situ observations, **B1**.204
    spatial distribution, **B1**.205, **B1**.208
    spores, **B1**.205
    total adenine nucleotide, **B1**.206
  habitats
    quality, **B1**.195–6
    suitability, **B1**.196
  methodologies for study, **B1**.195
  nutrient limitation escape mechanisms,
    B1.199–200
  rhizosphere ratio, **B1**.197–8
  sampling, **B1**.207
    heterogeneity, **B1**.205–6, **B1**.208
    natural populations, **B1**.208
    sample scale, **B1**.208
    sample units, **B1**.208
  structure contribution, **B1**.196–7
  substrate changes and colonization, **B1**.199–
    200
  vegetable contamination, **B1**.280–1
  see also Rhizosphere; *individual species*
Soil-transmitted nematodes *see* Nematodes,
  gastrointestinal
Solenocytes (flame cells)
  liver flukes, **P**.642
  lung flukes, **P**.642
  Opisthorchis, **P**.642–3
Solex, tapeworms, **P**.659
Solid media, Enterobacteriaceae culture,
  B2.1344–5
Solid surfaces, bacterial growth, **B1**.42
Solid waste (rubbish), bacteriology of, **B1**.213,
  B1.213 (Tab.)
Solitary lymph nodes (SLNs), **I**.529–30
  as inductive site, **I**.530
Soluble (s) antigen, Borna disease virus,
  V2.1140
Soluble antigens, intranasal vaccination, **I**.830
Soluble egg antigens (SEA), **P**.616
Soluble intercellular adhesion molecules
  (sICAMs), **I**.204
Soluble vascular cell adhesion molecule
  (svCAM), **I**.204
Somatic cell count test for milk, **B1**.233
Somatic cells, DNA vaccine priming, **I**.914
Somatic hypermutation
  Igs, **I**.327–8
    RAG upregulation, **I**.327
    survival signals, **I**.327
  TCR diversity, **I**.449–50, **I**.454
Somatic rearrangement, TCR, **I**.449–50
Somatic recombination
  dendritic epidermal γδ T cells, **I**.436

Somatic recombination (*Continued*)
  Igs, **I**.328–30
    chromatin organization, **I**.328–9
    deficient animal models, **I**.330
    histone acetylation, **I**.328–9
    junctional diversity generation, **I**.330
    Ku proteins, **I**.330
    lambda chain rearrangement, **I**.329–30,
      I.329 (Fig.)
      hairpin opening, **I**.330
      TdT, **I**.330
    N nucleotides, **I**.330
    nonhomologous end joining, **I**.330
    P nucleotides, **I**.330
    RAG proteins, **I**.328–30
    recombination signal sequences, **I**.328–9
    signal joints *vs.* coding joints, **I**.328
Somatostatin, Borna disease virus infection,
    V2.1147
Somnolence, acute phase response, **I**.198, **I**.209
Sonchus yellow net virus (SYNV),
    V2.1112 (Fig.)
Sonication
  virus inactivation, **V1**.91
  virus release from culture, **V1**.91
Sorbic acid, **B1**.422, **B1**.434
  action, **B1**.437 (Tab.), **B1**.438
  pH, **B1**.432
D-Sorbitol fermentation, Enterobacteriaceae
    identification, **B2**.1319 (Tab.)
Sorbitol–MacConkey agar (SMAC),
    Enterobacteriaceae culture, **B2**.1347
Sore throats, HSV infection, **V1**.507
Sorivudine, **V2**.1614–15
  toxicity, **V2**.1638
SOS system, **B1**.440
  Ras activation, **I**.346
  UV, **B1**.451–2
Sotalia guianensis, **M**.430
'Source,' infection transmission, **I**.951
Southern blotting, **V2**.1536
'Southern cone programme', **P**.395
Southern Core Initiative, Chagas disease
    control, **P**.116 (Fig.)
Southgate's mucicarmine stain, **M**.123 (Tab.),
    M.124
'Sowda,' onchocerciasis, **P**.793, **P**.794–5
SoxABCD quinol oxidase complex, **B1**.69
SoxR proteins, **B1**.65
Sp-1 transcription factor, JC virus, **V1**.476–7
Sparganum, **P**.576
'Species-jumping,' emerging viral infection,
    V2.1657–8
Species/speciation
  bacteria, **B1**.30
    concept, **B1**.17, **B1**.20–2, **B1**.29–30
    nomenclature, **B1**.18, **B1**.20–2, **B1**.31–3
      changes, **B1**.18, **B1**.31–3
    patenting, **B1**.31–2
  viruses *see* Classification, viruses
Species-specific tropism, bacterial adherence,
    B1.147–8
Specimens
  bacteria, **B1**.711–12
    collection, **B1**.711–12
      laboratory receipt, **B1**.712

    skin antisepsis, **B1**.712
    contamination site and source, **B1**.711–12,
      B1.712 (Tab.)
    preparation, **B1**.724–5
    suitability, **B1**.724
    transport and handling, **B1**.712
    for virus detection, **B1**.724
    see also Molecular assays
  mycology
    collection, **M**.82–5
      guidelines, **M**.82–4
      site selection, **M**.83 (Tab.)
    microscopic examination, **M**.87
      detection methods, **M**.87, **M**.88 (Tab.)
      morphological diversity, **M**.87,
        M.89 (Tab.), **M**.91
    processing, **M**.85
    safety principles, **M**.92
    selection, **M**.82
    site selection, **M**.83 (Tab.)
    transport/storage, **M**.85
    see also Histopathological diagnosis
Spectinomycin
  characteristics, **B1**.482
  gonorrhea treatment, **B1**.661
  Haemophilus, **B2**.1710
  structure, **B1**.483 (Fig.)
Spermatozoa
  hCAP-18, **I**.175
  lactate dehydrogenase, **I**.875
  Prnd gene, **V2**.1360–1, **V2**.1360 (Fig.),
    V2.1361 (Fig.)
Spf vaccine (malaria), **P**.85, **P**.516–17
Sphaerophorus, **B2**.1945–6
Sphaeropsis, oculomycoses, **M**.278 (Tab.)
Sphaerotilus, **B1**.60
Sphaerotilus natans
  bioremediation, **B1**.212
  paper processing waste, **B1**.212–13
Sphagnum moss, **M**.368, **M**.369, **M**.371
S-phase *see* Cell cycle, S phase
Sphenoid sinus, anatomy, **B1**.606–7
Spheroplasts, leptospires, **B2**.1868,
    B2.1868 (Fig.)
Spherule-endospores, *Coccidioides immitis,*
    M.504, **M**.505 (Fig.), **M**.509, **M**.513,
    M.514
Spherules, **M**.89 (Tab.)
Spices, **B1**.287–8
Spike (S) protein
  coronaviruses *see* Coronaviruses
  toroviruses *see* Toroviruses
Spinal column, specimens, **M**.83 (Tab.), **M**.84,
    M.86 (Tab.)
Spinal epidural abscess, **B1**.592–4, **B1**.593 (Fig.)
  clinical features, **B1**.593–4
  diagnosis, **B1**.594
  epidemiology, **B1**.592
  management, **B1**.594, **B1**.594 (Tab.)
  pathogenesis, **B1**.593
  predisposing conditions, **B1**.592–3
Spinal poliomyelitis, **V2**.870
Spines
  Fasciola, **P**.642
  Paragonimus, **P**.642

Spiramycin
  cryptosporidiosis, **P**.410
  toxoplasmosis, **P**.437, **P**.439
Spiramycin I, structure, **B1**.486 (Fig.)
Spirillum minus, **B2**.1908–9
  antibacterial susceptibility/resistance,
    B2.1909
  definition, **B2**.1908
  habitats, **B2**.1908
  historical perspective, **B2**.1908
  infection *see* Rat-bite fever
  staining reactions and culturability,
    B2.1908–9
Spirochaeta icterogenes, **B2**.1866
Spirochaeta icterohaemorrhagiae, **B2**.1866
Spirochaeta interrogans, **B2**.1866
Spirochaetales, **B2**.1838
Spirochaeta pallida see Treponema pallidum
Spirochaetes
  infection
    antibody detection, **B1**.753
    oral, **B2**.1859–60
    syphilis *see* Syphilis
  non-pathogenic of genital region, **B2**.1860
Spirometra, **P**.576–7
Spiroplasma, **B2**.1958 (Tab.)
  classification, **B2**.1967, **B2**.1970
  energy-yielding pathways, **B2**.1971–2
  genetic analysis
    DNA replication and repair, **B2**.1979
    genome structure, **B2**.1973–4
  insect associations, **B2**.1965
  metabolism, **B2**.1969–70
  motility, **B2**.1961
  phytopathogenicity, **B1**.202
  serological techniques, **B2**.1994
  vector-transmitted plant diseases, **B2**.1965–6,
    B2.1985–6
Spiroplasma citri, **B2**.1979
  cell morphology, **B2**.1959 (Fig.)
  genetic analysis
    comparative genomics, **B2**.1976
    DNA replication and repair, **B2**.1979
    gene transfer, **B2**.1981
    genome sequencing and gene annotation,
      B2.1974
    pathogenicity associated genes, **B2**.1985–6
    transposition, **B2**.1981
  motility, **B2**.1961
  pathogenicity, associated genes, **B2**.1985–6
Spiroplasma ixodetis, **B2**.1973–4
Spiroplasma kunkelii
  genetic analysis
    comparative genomics, **B2**.1975–6
    genome sequencing and gene annotation,
      B2.1974
  metabolism, **B2**.1975–6
Spiroplasma leptinotarsa, **B2**.1963–4
Spiroplasma melliferum
  cell membrane proteins, **B2**.1970
  energy-yielding pathways, **B2**.1971–2
  genetic analysis
    DNA replication and repair, **B2**.1979
    proteome and transcriptome analysis and
      bioinformatics, **B2**.1978

Spiroplasma mirum, **B2**.1966
Spiroplasma platyhelix, **B2**.1973–4
Spiroplasma poulsonii, **B2**.1963–4
Spiruroidea, **P**.594
  features, **P**.594
  Gongylonematidae, **P**.594
Spiruroid type X larva, **P**.824–5
Spitzenkörper, **M**.71
Spleen
  aspergillosis, **M**.701, **M**.705
  aspirates in leishmaniasis detection, **P**.301
  candidiasis, **M**.595, **M**.599–600
  CD4 T cells, **I**.389
  as peripheral lymphoid organ, **I**.505
  Plasmodium sequestration, **P**.472
  Pneumocystis carinii infection, **M**.785
Splendore–Hoeppli phenomenon, **M**.122,
  M.136 (Fig.), **M**.140 (Fig.), **M**.232,
  M.238, **M**.351–2, **M**.463
  Basidiobolus, **M**.351–2, **M**.351 (Fig.)
  Coccidioides immitis, **M**.516
Splenectomy
  babesiosis after, **P**.454–5
  immunodeficiency, **I**.788 (Tab.)
Splenic invasive aspergillosis, **M**.701, **M**.705
Splenic rupture, vivax/ovale (benign tertian)
  malaria, **P**.482
Splenomegaly
  African trypanosomiasis, **P**.364, **P**.365
  babesiosis, **P**.454
  human brucellosis, **B2**.1738
  infective endocarditis, **B1**.535
  malaria in children, **P**.482
  visceral leishmaniasis, **P**.298, **P**.301
Splicing, **V1**.114–15
  adenoviruses, **V1**.114–15
  Borna disease virus, **V2**.1139–40
  herpesviruses, **V1**.493
  lentiviruses, **V1**.114–15
  papovaviruses, **V1**.114–15
Splinter hemorrhages, infective endocarditis,
  B1.534–5, **B1**.534 (Fig.)
Spoligotyping, *Mycobacterium tuberculosis*
  complex, **B2**.1195, **B2**.1196 (Tab.)
Spondweni virus (SPOV), **V2**.998 (Tab.),
  V2.1003
Spongiform lesions, rabies, **V2**.1122,
  V2.1122 (Fig.)
Spontaneous generation, theory of, **P**.5
Spontaneous mutants, genetic analysis, **V1**.183
Spontaneous transversions, point mutations,
  B1.85
Spooling, SV40 replication, **V1**.153–4
Sporadic Creutzfeldt–Jakob disease (sCJD),
  V2.1347
  diagnosis, **V2**.1386
  genetic susceptibility, **V2**.1372
  variant Creutzfeldt–Jakob disease *vs.,*
  V2.1369
  see also Creutzfeldt–Jakob disease (CJD)
Sporadic infection, definition, **B1**.310
Sporadic outbreaks, definition, **V1**.358
Sporangia, **M**.89 (Tab.)
Sporangiospore(s), **M**.79 (Fig.)
  Prototheca, **M**.403, **M**.404 (Fig.), **M**.406 (Fig.),
  M.407 (Fig.)

Prototheca wickerhamii, **M**.406
Prototheca zopferi, **M**.407
  zygomycete, **M**.77, **M**.659–61
Sporegonic stage, microsporidians, **P**.535
'Spore repair,' **B1**.452
Spores, **M**.5 (Fig.), **M**.7 (Fig.), **M**.8 (Fig.)
  Actinomycetes, **M**.5 (Fig.)
  antibacterial agents, **B1**.438–9, **B1**.441 (Tab.)
  resistance, **B1**.442–3
  Clostridium, **B2**.1091–2
  food
  freezing, **B1**.264, **B1**.270
  heating, **B1**.265–6
  heat-resistance, **B1**.449
  microsporidians, **P**.529, **P**.530 (Fig.),
  P.531 (Fig.), **P**.532–3, **P**.532 (Fig.),
  P.533 (Fig.)
  Encephalitozoon hellem, **P**.530 (Fig.),
  P.532–3, **P**.532 (Fig.), **P**.533 (Fig.)
  Enterocytozoon bieneusi, **P**.533 (Fig.)
  Trachipleistophora hominis, **P**.530 (Fig.),
  P.531 (Fig.)
  morphology, **M**.76–7
  production, **M**.76–7, **M**.78 (Fig.), **M**.79 (Fig.)
  sterilization
  biological indicators, **B1**.454
  dry heat, **B1**.449
  hydrostatic pressure, **B1**.450
  ionizing radiation, **B1**.451
  moist heat, **B1**.449
  oxic/anoxic conditions, **B1**.454
  ultraviolet radiation, **B1**.451, **B1**.452
  water content, **B1**.449
Sporicides, **B1**.433
  action, **B1**.438–9
Sporistatic agents, **B1**.433
Sporoblasts, microsporidians, **P**.532–3
Sporobolomyces
  asthma, **M**.628
  characteristics, **M**.632, **M**.632 (Tab.),
  M.633 (Tab.)
  infection, **M**.625 (Tab.), **M**.628
  amphotericin B therapy, **M**.628
Sporobolomyces holsaticus, **M**.628, **M**.632,
  M.633 (Tab.)
Sporobolomyces roseus, **M**.628, **M**.632,
  M.633 (Tab.)
Sporobolomyces salmonicolor, **M**.628, **M**.632,
  M.633 (Tab.)
  AIDS, **M**.628
Sporocysts, **P**.422
  coccidian, **P**.166
  daughter, **P**.580
  mother, **P**.580
  Sarcocystis, **P**.167 (Fig.), **P**.449
  Schistosoma, **P**.602–3
  structure, **P**.166, **P**.167 (Fig.)
  Toxoplasma gondii, **P**.422, **P**.427, **P**.429 (Fig.)
Sporogenic stage, microsporidians, **P**.532 (Fig.),
  P.534
  Brachiola, **P**.535
  Enterocytozoon, **P**.532 (Fig.), **P**.534
Sporogonial plasmodium, microsporidians,
  P.533 (Fig.)
Sporogony
  microsporidians, **P**.531, **P**.535

Plasmodium, **P**.468–71
Sporomusa, **B2**.1929–30
Sporonts, microsporidians, **P**.532–3, **P**.532 (Fig.)
Sporophorous vesicles (SPOV)
  Pleistophora, **P**.532–3, **P**.535
  Trachipleistophora, **P**.532–4
  Trachipleistophora anthropopthera, **P**.542
  Trachipleistophora hominis, **P**.533 (Fig.)
Sporoplasm, microsporidians, **P**.532 (Fig.)
  Encephalitozoon hellem, **P**.532 (Fig.)
  migration, **P**.531, **P**.531 (Fig.)
Sporopollenin, **M**.404
Sporosarcina, **B2**.922–3
Sporothrix, **M**.371–2
  morphology, **M**.371–2, **M**.374
Sporothrix cyanescens, **M**.371–2
Sporothrix schenckii, **M**.28–9, **M**.367
  culture, **M**.377–8
  dimorphism, **M**.22–3, **M**.28, **M**.29 (Fig.)
  ecology, **M**.368–71
  sphagnum moss, **M**.368, **M**.371
  epidemiology, **M**.367, **M**.368–71
  food contamination, **M**.371
  genetic analysis, **M**.369–72, **M**.378–9
  mitochondrial DNA, **M**.371–2, **M**.378,
  M.378 (Fig.)
  ribosomal DNA, **M**.371–2
  growth, **M**.73
  histopathology, **M**.89 (Tab.), **M**.128 (Tab.),
  M.134 (Fig.), **M**.375–6, **M**.375 (Fig.),
  M.376 (Fig.), **M**.377
  identification
  random amplified polymorphic DNA,
  M.379
  restriction fragment length polymorphism,
  M.378
  ribosomal DNA, **M**.371–2
  infection *see* Sporotrichosis
  morphology, **M**.372, **M**.373 (Fig.)
  asteroid bodies, **M**.375, **M**.376 (Fig.),
  M.377
  dimorphism, **M**.22–3, **M**.28, **M**.29 (Fig.)
  phylogeny, **M**.371–2
  var. *luriei,* **M**.374
  chromoblastomycosis, **M**.357
  histopathology, **M**.128 (Tab.)
  var. *schenckii,* **M**.374
  histopathology, **M**.126 (Tab.), **M**.128 (Tab.)
  morphology, **M**.126 (Tab.)
Sporotrichosis, **M**.367
  AIDS *see* AIDS
  animal vectors, **M**.370–1
  cats, **M**.367–8, **M**.369 (Tab.), **M**.370
  dolphins, **M**.371
  causative agents *see* *Sporothrix schenckii*
  clinical presentation, **M**.374–5, **M**.374 (Fig.),
  M.375 (Fig.)
  CNS, **M**.371, **M**.377, **M**.380
  dacryocanaliculitis, **M**.298
  dacryocystitis, **M**.298
  endophthalmitis, **M**.317, **M**.325–6
  keratitis, **M**.305
  meningitis, **M**.377–8
  oculomycoses, **M**.275 (Tab.), **M**.289
  pulmonary, **M**.367, **M**.375
  scleritis, **M**.316

Sporotrichosis
  clinical presentation (*Continued*)
    ulceration, **M**.367
  diagnosis, **M**.125–7, **M**.374, **M**.377–8,
      M.377 (Fig.)
    histopathology, **M**.128 (Tab.), **M**.134 (Fig.),
        M.375–6, **M**.375 (Fig.), **M**.376 (Fig.),
        M.377
    serology, **M**.93 (Tab.), **M**.376–7
    skin testing, **M**.376
    specimens, **M**.83 (Tab.)
  ecology, **M**.368–71
  epidemiology, **M**.367–8, **M**.368–71
    agriculture/agricultural workers, **M**.367–8
    animal vectors *see above*
    children, **M**.368
    farmers/farm workers, **M**.368
    miners, **M**.368–9
    spread, **M**.368
    transmission, **M**.368
    transplantation recipients, **M**.375
    veterinarians, **M**.370
  history, **M**.28–9, **M**.367–8
  immune response, **M**.376–7
  immunosuppression, **M**.375
  joints, **M**.374–5, **M**.377
  lung, **M**.367, **M**.375
  therapy, **M**.28, **M**.379–80
    amphotericin B, **M**.380
    fluconazole, **M**.379
    heat therapy, **M**.379
    itraconazole, **M**.379
    potassium iodide, **M**.28, **M**.368–9, **M**.379
    terbinafine, **M**.380
Sporozoa (Apicomplexa), **P**.464
Sporozoans
  capping phenomenon, **P**.180
  classification, **P**.197
  locomotory system, **P**.180
  structure, dense bodies, **P**.178
  tick-borne intraerythrocytic, **P**.451
Sporozoites, **P**.422
  Cryptosporidium parvum, **P**.400
  Isospora belli, **P**.411
  Plasmodium see Plasmodium
Spotted fever
  causative agents, **B2**.2030–2, **B2**.2031 (Tab.),
      B2.2033, **B2**.2041
    antibacterial susceptibility/resistance,
        B2.2043 (Tab.)
    see also Rickettsia
  clinical manifestations, **B2**.2039 (Tab.)
  treatment, **B2**.2043
  see also Rocky Mountain spotted fever
Spray drying, food preservation, **B1**.269
Spreading factors, **B1**.152, **B1**.153 (Tab.)
Springer, Tim, **I**.505
Spring waters, **B1**.215
S-protein (vitronectin), **I**.150 (Tab.), **I**.151,
    I.204
  deficiency, **I**.154
  neutrophils, **I**.45
Spt3 transcription factor, **M**.259
Spumaretroviridae
  characteristics, **V2**.1284
  classification, **V1**.46 (Tab.)

genome, **V1**.181–2
nomenclature, **V2**.1305 (Tab.)
see also Foamy viruses
Spumavirus
  animal infection, **V2**.1295
  classification, **V1**.46, **V2**.1286 (Tab.), **V2**.1295
  human disease, **V2**.1285
Sputum, **M**.84, **M**.85, **M**.86 (Tab.)
  aspergillosis, **M**.710, **M**.710 (Fig.)
  in bronchiectasis, **B1**.649
  culture, in chronic bronchitis, **B1**.648
  Mycobacterium tuberculosis
    microscopy, **B2**.1190
    primary culture, **B2**.1190
  Pneumocystis, **M**.787
  Streptococcus pneumoniae pneumonia,
      B1.631, **B1**.632
Squamous cell carcinoma (SCC), HPV
    associations, **V1**.463 (Tab.), **V1**.464
Squamous intraepithelial lesions, HPV
    infection, **V1**.463 (Tab.), **V1**.464–5,
    V1.465–7, **V1**.466 (Fig.)
Squamous papilloma, HPV associations,
    V1.465 (Tab.)
SR-A, microbial recognition, **I**.24 (Tab.)
Src tyrosine kinases, BCR signaling, **I**.343
S (small) segment, bunyavirus genome,
    V2.1028–31, **V2**.1038
ST2L, Th2 cells, **I**.400
Staff training, parenteral vaccination, **I**.819
Stage-specific genes, *Plasmodium,* **I**.680
Stage-specific proteins, *Toxoplasma gondii*
    antigens, **P**.428
Stage-specific proteins, *Trichinella,* **I**.685
Staging system, Kaposi's sarcoma, **V1**.552
Stainer–Scholte (SS) medium, **B2**.1791
Stains/staining, **M**.87, **M**.88 (Tab.)
  Actinomyces, **M**.122, **M**.123 (Tab.), **M**.124–5
  Afipia, **B2**.1903
  anti-systemic inflammation, **I**.209
  Blastocystis hominis diagnosis, **P**.565,
      P.565 (Fig.)
  Blastomyces dermatitidis, **M**.122, **M**.124,
      M.125
  Brucella, **B2**.1723
  Coccidioides immitis, **M**.122, **M**.124
  Cryptococcus neoformans, **M**.123 (Tab.),
      M.124
  cytopathology, **V2**.1533
  fecal samples, **P**.151
  Helicobacter pylori identification, **B2**.1571
  histopathology, **M**.33, **M**.87, **M**.88 (Tab.)
  Histoplasma capsulatum var. *capsulatum,*
      M.122, **M**.124, **M**.125
  Legionella, **B2**.1773
  Loboa loboi, **M**.122
  methods, **B1**.712–14, **B1**.713 (Tab.)
    historical aspects, **B1**.6–7
    Legionella, **B2**.1773, **B2**.1773 (Fig.)
  Nocardia, **M**.122, **M**.123 (Tab.), **M**.125
  Paracoccidioides brasiliensis, **M**.122, **M**.124
  Pneumocystis, **M**.123 (Tab.)
  see also Histopathological diagnosis; *specific
      methods; specific stains*
Standard tube-agglutination test (SAT),
    human brucellosis diagnosis, **B2**.1739–40

Stanley, Wendell, **V1**.25
Staphylococcal enterocolitis, **B2**.1119
Staphylococcal enterotoxins (SE), **I**.556–7,
    I.556 (Tab.), **I**.557–8
  classification, **I**.557 (Tab.)
  homology, **I**.557
  human *vs.* murine T cell binding,
      I.560 (Tab.), **I**.561
  isolate frequency, **I**.557–8
  polymorphism, **I**.557
  serotypes, **I**.556
  structure, **I**.558, **I**.558 (Fig.)
Staphylococcal scalded skin syndrome (SSSS),
    B2.786 (Tab.), **B2**.789
Staphylococci
  autoinducing peptides, **B1**.172
  coagulase-negative
    bacteremia due to, **B1**.393
    identification, **B1**.20
    infection, **B1**.518, **B2**.816
    nosocomial infection, **B1**.401 (Tab.)
    on skin, **B1**.304
  detection
    antiphospholysin test, **B1**.750
    EIAs, **B1**.750
    immunoserology, **B1**.756
  infection
    antibody detection, **B1**.750
    bacteremia, **B1**.518
    endocarditis, **B1**.531, **B1**.535, **B1**.539–40
    spreading factors, **B1**.153 (Tab.)
  as normal microbiota, **B1**.296 (Tab.), **B1**.304
    nares and nasopharynx, **B1**.295–300
    oropharynx and tonsils, **B1**.301
  quorum sensing *AGR* system, **B1**.172–3,
      B1.173 (Fig.)
  virulence factors
    hyaluronidase, **B1**.153 (Tab.)
    leukocidins, **B1**.153 (Tab.)
    staphylokinase, **B1**.153 (Tab.)
    α toxin, **B1**.153 (Tab.)
Staphylococcus, **B2**.771–832
  antibacterial susceptibility/resistance,
      B2.793–805, **B2**.794 (Tab.)
    aminoglycosides, **B2**.804
    β-lactam antibiotics, **B2**.793–802
    fluoroquinolones, **B2**.804
    macrolide, lincosamide and streptogramin,
        B2.803
    tetracycline, **B2**.803–4
    trimethoprim, **B2**.804
  biofilms, **B2**.784–5
  cellular components, **B2**.781–90
    adhesins, **B2**.782–4, **B2**.783 (Tab.)
    bacteriocins, **B2**.790
    cell membrane, **B2**.781–2
    cell wall, **B2**.782
    exocellular material, **B2**.784–5
    extracellular proteins, **B2**.785–9,
        B2.786 (Tab.)
    gene regulation, **B2**.789–90
  characteristics, **B2**.806 (Tab.)
  classification, **B2**.771–5
    as airborne bacteria, **B1**.189
    species, **B2**.772–4
    subspecies, **B2**.774–5

Staphylococcus, (Continued)
  culture, **B2**.779–80
    broth, **B2**.780
    semisolid media, **B2**.780
  definition, **B2**.772
  genetics, **B2**.790–3
    bacteriophages, **B2**.792
    genetic exchange mechanisms, **B2**.790–1
    plasmids, **B2**.791–2
  habitats, **B2**.775–9
    anterior nares, **B2**.777–9
    cutaneous skin excluding the nose, **B2**.775–7
    in milk, **B1**.230–1
  identification, **B2**.805–9
    differentiating characteristics, **B2**.906–7
    light microscopy and staining reactions, **B2**.779
    typing methods, **B2**.809
  immune evasion, **I**.661–2
  infection
    clinical significance, **B2**.808–9
    defensin resistance, **I**.169
    host range, **B2**.775, **B2**.776 (Tab.), **B2**.793–805
    keratitis, **B1**.601
    leukocyte adhesion deficiency type 1, **I**.47–8
  isolation, **B2**.805–9
  metabolism, **B2**.780–1
    amino acid biosynthesis and nitrogen requirements, **B2**.781
    carbohydrates, **B2**.780–1
    coagulase, **B2**.786 (Tab.), **B2**.789
    fibrinolytic enzymes, **B2**.786 (Tab.), **B2**.789
    heavy metal resistance, **B2**.794 (Tab.), **B2**.804–5
    respiration, **B2**.781
    thermonuclease, **B2**.786 (Tab.), **B2**.789
    urease, **B2**.786 (Tab.)
  morphology
    cellular, **B2**.779–80
    colony, **B2**.779–80
  protein A, **I**.661–2
  slime production, **B2**.784–5
  species, **B2**.772–5, **B2**.773 (Tab.), **B2**.774 (Fig.)
    subspecies, **B2**.774 (Fig.), **B2**.775 (Tab.)
  toxins, **B2**.785–9, **B2**.786 (Tab.)
Staphylococcus albus, **B2**.771–2
  upper airway abscesses, **B1**.608–9
Staphylococcus arlettae, **B2**.773 (Tab.)
  culture, **B2**.780
  host range, **B2**.776 (Tab.)
Staphylococcus aureus, **B2**.771–2, **B2**.773 (Tab.), **B2**.806 (Tab.)
  adhesins, **B1**.149
    cell surface associated and secreted, **B2**.782–4, **B2**.783 (Tab.)
    role in disease pathogenesis, **B2**.810–11
  antibacterial susceptibility/resistance, **B1**.436–8, **B1**.441–2, **B1**.499 (Tab.), **B2**.794 (Tab.)
    aminoglycosides, **B2**.804
    fluoroquinolones, **B2**.804

  gentamicin-resistance, **B1**.442, **B2**.779–80, **B2**.791, **B2**.794 (Tab.), **B2**.804
  β-lactam antibiotic resistance, **B1**.363, **B2**.793–802
  macrolide, lincosamide and streptogramin resistance, **B2**.803
  methicillin resistance *see* Methicillin-resistant *Staphylococcus aureus* (MRSA)
  multiple resistance, **B1**.395
  plasmids, **B1**.111
  quinolone resistance, **B1**.492–3, **B1**.493 (Tab.)
  small colony variants, **B2**.779–80
  trimethoprim, **B2**.804
  vanA gene spread, **B1**.363
  vancomycin resistance *see* Vancomycin-resistant *Staphylococcus aureus* (VRSA)
  bacteriophages, **B2**.792
  biocide resistance, **B1**.426, **B1**.441–2
  biofilms, **B1**.688–9
    biofilm-associated protein (Bap), **B2**.783 (Tab.)
  bone sialoprotein-binding protein (Bbp), **B2**.783 (Tab.)
  carriage, **B2**.777–9
    adherence, **B2**.778
    carriage patterns, **B2**.777
    carriage rates, **B2**.777–8
    colonization resistance, **B2**.778–9
    epithelium, **B2**.778
    eradication for prevention of infection, **B2**.813–14
    HIV-positive patients, **B2**.777–8
    host phenotype, **B2**.777
  cellular components, **B2**.781–90
    cell membrane, **B2**.781–2
    extracellular proteins, **B2**.785–9, **B2**.786 (Tab.)
    gene regulation, **B2**.789–90
  classification, epidemic strains, **B1**.395
  clumping factor A (ClfA), **B2**.783 (Tab.), **B2**.810–11
    vaccine target investigation, **B2**.815
  clumping factor B (ClfB), **B2**.778, **B2**.783 (Tab.)
  coagulase activity, **B2**.789
  collagen-binding protein Cna, **B2**.783 (Tab.)
    vaccine target candidate, **B2**.815–16
  culture, **B2**.779
  elastin-binding protein EbpS, **B2**.783 (Tab.), **B2**.784
  enterotoxins *see* Staphylococcal enterotoxins (SE)
  evolution, **B1**.30
  exofoliative toxins, **I**.556 (Tab.), **I**.564–5
  fibronectin-binding proteins A and B (FnBPA and FnBPB), **B1**.687–8, **B2**.783 (Tab.), **B2**.810–11
    infection determinants, **B2**.811
    role in disease pathogenesis, **B2**.810–11
    vaccine target investigation, **B2**.815
  in foods
    butter, **B1**.250
    cheese, **B1**.253
    cream, **B1**.248
    crustacea, **B1**.279–80
    ice cream, **B1**.251

  meat and meat products, **B1**.273–4
  milk, **B1**.230–1, **B1**.231–2, **B1**.234–5
  milk powder, **B1**.245–6
  poultry, **B1**.276
  vegetables, **B1**.282
  water activity, **B1**.266
  genetics, **B2**.790–3
    agr locus, **B1**.688
    artificial competence, **B1**.99
    conjugation, **B1**.104
    exchange mechanisms, **B2**.790–1
    genome sequence, **B2**.792–3
    ica operon, **B1**.688
    lactose operon, **B1**.71
    Map/Eap, **B2**.783 (Tab.), **B2**.784
    serine-aspartate multigene family (SdrC, SdrD and SdrE), **B2**.783 (Tab.)
    vanA gene, **B1**.363
  habitats, **B2**.777–9
  heavy metal resistance, **B2**.794 (Tab.), **B2**.804–5
  immune evasion
    capsule phase variation, **I**.660–1
    complement shedding, **I**.663
    complement surface masking, **I**.662–3
    MHC class II antigen presentation, **I**.659
    pore-forming toxins, **I**.654–5
    superantigens, **I**.668
  infection *see below*
  isolation/identification, **B2**.805–9
    ELISA, **B2**.2018
    typing, **B2**.809
  L-form cells, **B2**.779–80
  metabolism
    amino acid biosynthesis and nitrogen requirements, **B2**.781
    carbohydrates, **B2**.780–1
    respiration, **B2**.781
  morphology
    cellular, **B2**.779
    colony, **B2**.779–80
  as normal microbiota, **B1**.296 (Tab.), **B1**.304
    nares and nasopharynx, **B1**.295–300
    oropharynx and tonsils, **B1**.301
    skin, **B1**.304, **B2**.777
  pathogenicity, **B2**.772
  plasmids, **B2**.790–2
  plasmin-sensitive protein Pls, **B2**.783 (Tab.)
  poly-N-succinyl beta-6 glucosamine, **B2**.815–16
  proteases, **B2**.786 (Tab.), **B2**.789
  pyrogenic exotoxins *see* Pyrogenic exotoxins (PET)
  quorum sensing, **B1**.172–3
  signal transduction, **B1**.167–8
  small colony variants, **B1**.688–9, **B2**.779–80
    infection, **B1**.518
  staphylokinase, **B2**.789
  toxic shock syndrome *see* Toxic shock syndrome toxin-1 (TSST-1)
  toxins, **B2**.786 (Tab.)
    Alpha-toxin, **B2**.785, **B2**.786 (Tab.)
    Beta-toxin, **B2**.785, **B2**.786 (Tab.)
    Delta-toxin, **B2**.785, **B2**.786 (Tab.)

Staphylococcus aureus,
toxins (*Continued*)
exfoliative toxins (exfoliatin A &
exfoliatin B) (ETA & ETB),
B2.786 (Tab.), **B2**.789
Gamma-toxin, **B2**.785, **B2**.786 (Tab.)
pyrogenic toxin superantigens,
B2.786 (Tab.), **B2**.789
toxic shock syndrome toxin-1, **B2**.789,
B2.812–13
V factor, **B2**.1695
virulence factors
K-antigens, **B1**.154
plasmid determination, **B1**.115
staphylococcal coagulase, **B1**.153 (Tab.)
Staphylococcus aureus infection, **B2**.810–11
adhesins role, **B2**.810–11
animal models, **B2**.808
bacteremia, **B1**.517–18, **B2**.811
antibacterial susceptibility/resistance,
B1.524
hospital-acquired, **B1**.517
vaccination potential application, **B2**.815
bones/joints, **B1**.690, **B2**.811–12
adhesion, **B1**.687–8
arthritis, **B2**.811–12
bone resorption process, **B1**.690
cell and molecular basis of joint
destruction, **B1**.690
epidemiology, **B1**.685
hematogenous spread, **B1**.687
mechanisms of persistence, **B1**.688–9
osteomyelitis, **B2**.810–11, **B2**.811–12
prognosis, **B1**.701
quorum sensing, **B1**.688
carriage eradication, **B2**.813–14
clinical interpretation of cultures, **B2**.808–9
clinical manifestations, **B2**.808–9, **B2**.811–13
bacteremia *see above*
bones/joints *see above*
Brodies abscess, **B1**.740, **B1**.747
chronic granulomatous disease, **I**.48, **I**.770
chronic sinusitis, **B1**.615
conjunctivitis, **B1**.599, **B1**.600
endocarditis *see below*
epiglottitis, **B1**.613
eye, **B1**.386
genital tract, **B1**.668–9
hyper-IgE syndrome, **I**.49, **I**.770
intracranial abscess, **B1**.583–4, **B1**.584–5,
B1.588–9
Job's syndrome (hyperimmunoglobulin E
syndrome), **B2**.810
mastitis, **B1**.230
otitis media, **B1**.617
peritonsillar abscess, **B1**.618
pneumonia *see below*
pulmonary infection, **B2**.812
sinusitis, **B1**.615, **B1**.615 (Tab.)
spinal epidural abscess, **B1**.593, **B1**.594
staphylococcal scalded skin syndrome,
B2.786 (Tab.), **B2**.789, **B2**.812
subdural empyema, **B1**.591
suppurative parotitis, **B1**.619
toxic shock syndrome, **B1**.668–9, **B2**.789,
B2.812–13

urinary tract infection, **B1**.673
wound sepsis, **B1**.385
in cystic fibrosis, **B1**.650
dendritic cell infection, **I**.656
determinants, **B2**.810–11
endocarditis, **B1**.525, **B1**.526, **B1**.527, **B1**.531,
B2.811
blood culture, **B1**.537
determinants, **B2**.810–11
intravenous drug users, **B1**.527, **B1**.531
native valves, **B1**.531–2
prosthetic valves, **B1**.531–2, **B2**.813
treatment, **B1**.539–40
vaccination potential application, **B2**.815
virulence factors, **B1**.527
host factors, **B2**.810
host range, **B2**.775, **B2**.776 (Tab.)
immune response
acute phase response, **B1**.740
dysfunction, **B2**.810
evasion, **B1**.154
neutrophils, **I**.43, **I**.44
influenza, **V1**.661
management, **B2**.813
neonatal, **B1**.395
nosocomial, **B1**.395–6
airborne spread, **B1**.385
antibiotic era, **B1**.371
bacteremia, **B1**.393
burns, **B1**.385
colonization of intravascular cannulae,
B1.391
control, **B1**.396
control and antibiotic prophylaxis, **B2**.815
epidemiological typing, **B1**.404
eye, **B1**.386
nosocomial spread, **B1**.374
operating theater, **B1**.375
pneumonia, **B1**.389
role, **B1**.395
sinusitis, **B1**.615
spread by contact with staff, **B1**.378
treatment, **B1**.396
pneumonia, **B1**.636, **B2**.812
diagnosis and treatment, **B1**.636
nosocomial, **B1**.640 (Tab.), **B1**.640–1
prevention, **B2**.813–16
vaccination *see below*
prosthetic material, **B2**.810, **B2**.813
surgical wounds, **B1**.385
toxin-mediated, **B2**.812–13
vaccines, **B2**.815–16
BCE peptide vaccines, **I**.855 (Tab.)
development status, **I**.933 (Tab.)
Staphylococcus auricularis, **B1**.304, **B2**.773,
B2.773 (Tab.)
culture, **B2**.780
genetics, **B2**.791–2
habitats, **B2**.777
host range, **B2**.776 (Tab.)
Staphylococcus bovicus, **B2**.772
Staphylococcus capitis, **B2**.773 (Tab.)
cell morphology, **B2**.779
cellular components, **B2**.784–5
characteristics, **B2**.806 (Tab.)

habitats, **B2**.777
host range, **B2**.776 (Tab.)
identification, **B2**.807
infection
bacteremia, **B1**.518
endocarditis, **B1**.532
metabolism, **B2**.780–1
skin colonization, **B1**.304
slime production, **B2**.784–5
Staphylococcus caprae, **B2**.773 (Tab.)
endocarditis, **B1**.532
host range, **B2**.775, **B2**.776 (Tab.)
Staphylococcus carnosus, **B2**.773 (Tab.)
genetics, **B2**.791
host range, **B2**.776 (Tab.)
Staphylococcus carouselicus, **B2**.772
Staphylococcus caseolyticus, **B2**.772
culture, **B2**.779
Staphylococcus chromogenes, **B2**.773 (Tab.)
host range, **B2**.776 (Tab.)
metabolism, **B2**.780–1
Staphylococcus citreus, **B2**.771–2
Staphylococcus cohnii, **B2**.773 (Tab.)
antibacterial susceptibility/resistance,
B2.794 (Tab.)
macrolide and streptogramin, **B2**.803
cell morphology, **B2**.779
host range, **B2**.776 (Tab.)
Staphylococcus condimenti, **B2**.773 (Tab.)
Staphylococcus delphini, **B2**.773 (Tab.)
cellular components, **B2**.786 (Tab.), **B2**.789
host range, **B2**.776 (Tab.)
Staphylococcus epidermidis, **B2**.772,
B2.773 (Tab.)
adhesins, **B2**.784
antibacterial susceptibility/resistance, **B1**.426,
B2.794 (Tab.)
β-lactam antibiotics, **B2**.793, **B2**.801
fluoroquinolones, **B2**.804
gentamicin-resistant, **B2**.791
macrolide and streptogramin, **B2**.803
macrolide, lincosamide and streptogramin,
B2.803
methicillin, **B2**.801
trimethoprim, **B2**.804
bacteriocins, **B2**.790
bacteriophages, **B2**.792
biofilms, **B1**.149–50, **B1**.688
cellular components, **B2**.782, **B2**.784–5,
B2.786 (Tab.), **B2**.789–90
characteristics, **B2**.806 (Tab.)
culture, **B2**.780
genetics, **B2**.790, **B2**.791, **B2**.792
habitats, **B2**.777
heavy metal resistance, **B2**.804–5
identification, **B2**.807
infection *see below*
lantibiotics, **B2**.790
L-form cells, **B2**.779
metabolism, **B2**.780–1
morphology
cellular, **B2**.779
colony, **B2**.779–80
polysaccharide intercellular adhesin,
B2.779–80

Staphylococcus epidermidis, (Continued)
  quorum sensing, **B1**.172–3
  skin colonization, **B1**.304
  slime production, **B2**.784–5
  tritrpticin sensitivity, **I**.172
  virulence factors, **B1**.149–50
Staphylococcus epidermidis infection, **I**.648
  bacteremia, **B1**.518
  bone and joint infection, **B1**.688, **B1**.690
  conjunctivitis, **B1**.600
  endocarditis, **B1**.532
  endophthalmitis, **B1**.603
  eye, **B1**.386
  host range, **B2**.776 (Tab.)
  nosocomial
    colonization of intravascular cannulae,
      B1.391
    endophthalmitis, **B1**.386
    multi-resistant strains, **B1**.372
    neonates, **B1**.395
    operating theater, **B1**.375
  peritoneal, **B1**.386–7
Staphylococcus equipercicus, **B2**.772
Staphylococcus equorum, **B2**.773 (Tab.)
  culture, **B2**.780
  host range, **B2**.776 (Tab.)
  metabolism, **B2**.781
Staphylococcus felis, **B2**.773 (Tab.)
  characteristics, **B2**.806 (Tab.)
  host range, **B2**.776 (Tab.)
  identification, **B2**.807
Staphylococcus fluerettii, **B2**.773 (Tab.)
Staphylococcus gallinarum, **B2**.773 (Tab.)
  bacteriocins, **B2**.790
  Gallidermin, **B2**.790
  host range, **B2**.776 (Tab.)
Staphylococcus haemolyticus, **B2**.773 (Tab.)
  antibacterial susceptibility/resistance,
    B2.794 (Tab.)
    fluoroquinolones, **B2**.804
  bacteriocins, **B2**.790
  cellular components, **B2**.784–5, **B2**.786 (Tab.)
  characteristics, **B2**.806 (Tab.)
  genetics, **B2**.791
  habitats, **B2**.777
  host range, **B2**.776 (Tab.)
  identification, **B2**.807
  infection, bacteremia, **B1**.518
  metabolism, **B2**.780–1
  morphology, **B2**.779
  slime production, **B2**.784–5
Staphylococcus hominis, **B2**.773 (Tab.)
  antibacterial susceptibility/resistance,
    B2.794 (Tab.)
    fluoroquinolones, **B2**.804
    macrolide and streptogramin, **B2**.803
    trimethoprim, **B2**.804
  cell morphology, **B2**.779
  cellular components, **B2**.784–5
  characteristics, **B2**.806 (Tab.)
  culture, **B2**.780
  genetics, **B2**.791
  habitats, **B2**.777
  identification, **B2**.807

infection
  bacteremia, **B1**.518
  endocarditis, **B1**.532
  host range, **B2**.776 (Tab.)
  metabolism, **B2**.780–1
  slime production, **B2**.784–5
Staphylococcus hyicus
  antibacterial susceptibility/resistance,
    B2.794 (Tab.)
    macrolide, lincosamide and streptogramin,
      B2.803
  cellular components, **B2**.786 (Tab.), **B2**.789
  characteristics, **B2**.806 (Tab.)
  host range, **B2**.776 (Tab.)
  identification, **B2**.807
  metabolism, **B2**.781
Staphylococcus intermedius, **B2**.773 (Tab.)
  antibacterial susceptibility/resistance,
    B2.794 (Tab.)
    macrolide, lincosamide and streptogramin,
      B2.803
  cellular components, **B2**.781–2,
    B2.786 (Tab.), **B2**.789
  characteristics, **B2**.806 (Tab.)
  colony morphology, **B2**.779
  host range, **B2**.776 (Tab.)
  identification, **B2**.807
  infection, butter, **B1**.250
  metabolism, **B2**.780–1
Staphylococcus kloosii, **B2**.773 (Tab.)
  culture, **B2**.780
  host range, **B2**.776 (Tab.)
  metabolism, **B2**.781
Staphylococcus lentus, **B2**.773, **B2**.773 (Tab.)
  colony morphology, **B2**.779
  culture, **B2**.779, **B2**.780
  host range, **B2**.776 (Tab.)
  metabolism, **B2**.780–1
Staphylococcus lugdunensis, **B2**.773 (Tab.)
  adhesins, **B2**.784
  cadmium and zinc resistance, **B2**.794 (Tab.)
  cellular components, **B2**.784, **B2**.789–90
  characteristics, **B2**.806 (Tab.)
  culture, **B2**.780
  habitats, **B2**.777
  heavy metal resistance, **B2**.804–5
  identification, **B2**.807
  infection
    bacteremia, **B1**.518
    endocarditis, **B1**.532
    host range, **B2**.776 (Tab.)
  metabolism, **B2**.781
  quorum sensing, **B1**.172–3
Staphylococcus lutrae, **B2**.773 (Tab.),
  B2.776 (Tab.)
Staphylococcus muscae, **B2**.773 (Tab.)
Staphylococcus pasteuri, **B2**.773 (Tab.),
  B2.774–5
  host range, **B2**.776 (Tab.)
Staphylococcus piscifermentans, **B2**.773 (Tab.)
Staphylococcus saccharolyticus, **B2**.772,
  B2.773 (Tab.)
  cellular components, **B2**.789
  culture, **B2**.779
  host range, **B2**.776 (Tab.)
  metabolism, **B2**.780–1

Staphylococcus saprophyticus, **B2**.772,
  B2.773 (Tab.)
  antibacterial susceptibility/resistance
    fluoroquinolones, **B2**.804
    macrolide and streptogramin, **B2**.803
  bacteremia, **B1**.518
  cellular components, **B2**.786 (Tab.)
  characteristics, **B2**.806 (Tab.)
  habitats, **B2**.777
  heavy metal resistance, **B2**.804–5
  identification, **B2**.807
  infection, **B2**.816
    cell morphology, **B2**.779
    endocarditis, **B1**.532
    host range, **B2**.776 (Tab.)
    urinary tract, **B1**.674, **B1**.676–7
  metabolism, **B2**.780–1
  virulence factor, urease, **B1**.676–7
Staphylococcus schleiferi, **B2**.773 (Tab.)
  adhesins, **B2**.784
  cellular components, **B2**.784, **B2**.786 (Tab.),
    B2.789
  characteristics, **B2**.806 (Tab.)
  culture, **B2**.780
  genetics, **B2**.791–2
  habitats, **B2**.777
  identification, **B2**.807
  infection
    bacteremia, **B1**.518
    endocarditis, **B1**.532
    host range, **B2**.776 (Tab.)
Staphylococcus sciuri, **B2**.773, **B2**.773 (Tab.)
  antibacterial susceptibility/resistance
    fluoroquinolones, **B2**.804
    methicillin, **B2**.801
  cellular components, **B2**.789
  culture, **B2**.779, **B2**.780
  genetics, **B2**.791–2
  host range, **B2**.776 (Tab.)
  identification, **B2**.807
  infection, endocarditis, **B1**.532
  metabolism, **B2**.780–1
Staphylococcus simulans, **B2**.773 (Tab.)
  cellular components, **B2**.786 (Tab.),
    B2.789–90
  characteristics, **B2**.806 (Tab.)
  genetics, **B2**.791
  identification, **B2**.807
  infection
    bacteremia, **B1**.518
    endocarditis, **B1**.532
    host range, **B2**.776 (Tab.)
Staphylococcus succinus, **B2**.772–3,
  B2.773 (Tab.)
Staphylococcus ureolyticus, **B2**.807
Staphylococcus vitulinus, **B2**.773, **B2**.773 (Tab.)
  culture, **B2**.779, **B2**.780
  host range, **B2**.776 (Tab.)
Staphylococcus warneri, **B2**.773 (Tab.),
  B2.774–5
  cellular components, **B2**.784–5, **B2**.789–90
  characteristics, **B2**.806 (Tab.)
  fluoroquinolone /resistance, **B2**.804
  identification, **B2**.807

Staphylococcus warneri, (Continued)
  infection
    bacteremia, **B1**.518
    endocarditis, **B1**.532
    host range, **B2**.776 (Tab.)
  metabolism, **B2**.780–1
Staphylococcus xylosus, **B2**.773 (Tab.)
  antibacterial susceptibility/resistance,
    B2.794 (Tab.)
    macrolide, lincosamide and streptogramin,
      B2.803
  catabolite repression, **B1**.73–4
  cellular components, **B2**.786 (Tab.)
  heavy metal resistance, **B2**.794 (Tab.)
  host range, **B2**.775, **B2**.776 (Tab.)
  metabolism, **B2**.780, **B2**.781
Staphylokinase, functions, **B1**.153 (Tab.)
Starch granules, *Chlorella,* **M**.407–8
Start-stop model, negative-strand RNA viruses
  replication, **V1**.130
Starvation
  Bacillus subtilis response, **B1**.75
  bacterial death phase, **B1**.40
  Escherichia coli, **B1**.75
  stress response, **B1**.40
Stat4 activation, IL-23, **I**.292
Statens Seruminstitut, **V1**.86
Static agents, **B1**.421–2
Statistical analysis
  contingency table, **B1**.316, **B1**.316 (Tab.)
  epidemiology, **B1**.316
  p values, **B1**.316
  type II errors, **B1**.316
  univariate, **B1**.316
Statistics, epidemiology, **P**.50–1
Stavudine, **V2**.1619
  HIV infection, **V2**.1334
    resistance, **V2**.1337 (Fig.)
  structure, **V2**.1620 (Fig.)
STCP-1 (CCL22), **I**.218 (Tab.)
Steam, sterilization, **B1**.429–30, **B1**.445 (Tab.),
  B1.447–8, **B1**.454
Steel factor *see* Stem cell factor (SCF: *c-kit*)
Stellantchasmus, **P**.584
Stem cell factor (SCF: *c-kit*), **I**.273–5
  actions/effects
    basophil degranulation, **I**.62, **I**.63
    cell adhesion, **I**.275
    cell survival, **I**.274–5
    CNS development, **I**.274
    germ cell proliferation/migration, **I**.274
    hematopoietic effects, **I**.275 (Tab.)
    intraepithelial lymphocytes, **I**.527–8
    mast cell proliferation, **I**.275
    mucosal immune response, **I**.522–3
    neutrophil action, **I**.275
    NK cell development, **I**.85
  deficiency, **I**.770–1
  genetics, **I**.273–4
  IL-3 interaction, **I**.275
  IL-4 interaction, **I**.275
  IL-11 synergy, **I**.279
  intraepithelial lymphocytes, **I**.527–8
  receptor, **I**.274, **I**.275

Stenella araguata, **M**.199
  histopathology, **M**.128 (Tab.)
*Stenotrophomonas maltophilia (Pseudomonas
  maltophilia),* **B2**.1636–7
  antibacterial susceptibility/resistance,
    B2.1637
    β-lactam resistance, **B1**.472–3
    β-latam resistance, **B2**.1637
  classification, **B2**.1636
  habitats, **B2**.1636
  infection, **B2**.1636
    cystic fibrosis, **B2**.1637
    endocarditis, **B2**.1636–7
    in HIV infection, **B2**.1636
    nosocomial, **B1**.371, **B1**.376–7,
      B1.401 (Tab.), **B2**.1636
  typing, **B2**.1637
    PCR, **B2**.1637
    ribotyping, **B2**.1637
  waterborne, **B1**.224–5
Stenson's duct, rhinosporidiosis, **M**.460–1
Sterile fly release, African trypanosomiasis
  vector control, **P**.369–70
Sterile immunity, malaria, **P**.486
Sterile vegetation, endocarditis, **B1**.526–7
Sterility assurance level (SAL), **B1**.455
Sterilization, **B1**.445–55, **B1**.445 (Tab.)
  aseptic packaging, **B1**.271
  combined synergistic treatments, **B1**.454
  container integrity, **B1**.271
  definition, **B1**.421
  dry heat, **B1**.449, **B1**.454 (Tab.)
  filtration, **B1**.453, **B1**.454 (Tab.)
  flash, **B1**.447
  gas plasmas, **B1**.453
  historical aspects, **B1**.5
  ionizing radiation *see* Ionizing radiation
  liquid sterilization systems, **B1**.453–4
  moist heat *see* Moist heat
  new low-temperature technologies, **B1**.453–4
  surgical instruments, **B1**.388
  ultraviolet radiation, **B1**.451–2
  validation and monitoring, **B1**.454–5,
    B1.454 (Tab.)
Sterilized milk, **B1**.233
Sternal wounds, infection, **B1**.385
Steroids
  cysticercosis treatment, **P**.697–8
  Haemophilus influenzae type b (Hib)
    meningitis, **B1**.574
  HCMV infection in transplants, **V1**.521–2
  meningococcal disease treatment, **B1**.567
  pneumococcal meningitis treatment, **B1**.571
Sterol(s), **M**.70
  antifungal testing, **M**.158
  Pneumocystis, **M**.772, **M**.780, **M**.781
Sterol methyl transferase (SMT),
  Trypanosoma cruzi, **P**.381–2
Stevens-Johnson syndrome, **B1**.634
Stichosome, *Trichuris trichiuria,* **P**.718
Stickland reaction, **B2**.1095
Stieda body, **P**.166, **P**.427
Stigmatella aurantiaca, **B1**.81
Stirred yogurt, **B1**.248

St Louis encephalitis (SLE), **V2**.1001–2,
  V2.1424, **V2**.1425–6
  age-related susceptibility, **V1**.264
  epidemiology, **V2**.997
  fatality rate, **V2**.1425–6
  pathogenesis/pathology, **V2**.1425–6
  transmission, **V1**.372 (Tab.)
St Louis encephalitis virus (SLEV),
  V2.998 (Tab.), **V2**.1424
  biosafety level 3 classification, **V2**.1526
Stochastic models, **B1**.344
  αβ/γδ T cell separation, **I**.457
  infectious disease, **B1**.331–2
Stockdale, P M, **M**.10–1, **M**.32
Stokes' method, antibacterial susceptibility
  testing, **B1**.498
Stomach, normal microbiota, **B1**.302
Stomatitis, **B1**.614
Stool antigen test, *Helicobacter pylori* infection
  diagnosis, **B2**.1571 (Tab.), **B2**.1573
Stools *see* Fecal analysis
Stoxil *see* Idoxuridine
Strahlenkörper, **P**.452
Strain diversity maintenance, transmission
  dynamics, **P**.62–3, **P**.63 (Fig.)
Strains
  definition, **V1**.34
  Measles virus nucleocapsid (N) protein,
    V1.721–2
Stramenopila, **M**.413
Strand-displacement amplification (SDA),
  B1.730, **V2**.1537–8
Strand displacement synthesis, adenoviruses
  replication, **V1**.162
Stratification of disease
  African trypanosomiasis, **P**.115
  filariasis, **P**.115
  leishmaniasis, **P**.115
  malaria, **P**.115, **P**.513
  onchocerciasis, **P**.115
  schistosomiasis, **P**.115
Stratified epithelium, microfold (M) cells, **I**.827
Stratified squamous epithelium, **B1**.606
Stratum basale, skin, **I**.820
Stratum corneum, **I**.820
  immunization, **I**.821–2
Strawberry polyps, rhinosporidiosis, **M**.450,
  M.460 (Fig.), **M**.461–2, **M**.469–70
Streptobacillus moniliformis, **B2**.1909–11
  antibacterial susceptibility/resistance,
    B2.1911
  antigens, **B2**.1910
  cell wall and envelope composition, **B2**.1910
  characteristics, **B2**.1909
  classification, **B2**.1909
  culture characteristics, **B2**.1909–10
  definition, **B2**.1909
  differential characteristics, **B2**.1910 (Tab.)
  growth requirements, **B2**.1909–10
  habitats, **B2**.1909
  infection
    endocarditis, **B1**.532
    experimental, **B2**.1911
    milk-borne, **B1**.235, **B1**.244, **B2**.1911
  isolation/identification, **B2**.1911
  L-phase variant, **B2**.1909–10

Streptobacillus moniliformis, (Continued)
  metabolism, **B2**.1910
  in milk, **B1**.235, **B1**.244, **B2**.1911
  morphology, **B2**.1909
    'string of beads', **B2**.1909
  pathogenicity and virulence factors, **B2**.1911
Streptococcaceae, **B2**.833
Streptococcal pyogenic exotoxins (SPE),
    I.556–62, **I**.556 (Tab.)
  classification, **I**.556–7
  exotoxin Z, **I**.557
  homology, **I**.557
  human *vs.* murine T cell binding, **I**.560 (Tab.)
  polymorphisms, **I**.557
  structure, **I**.558
Streptococcal pyrogenic exotoxin (Spe),
    B1.157 (Tab.)
Streptococci
  group A infection
    adherence, **B1**.149
    bone and joint infection, **B1**.690
    day-care centers, **B1**.361
    see also Streptococcus pyogenes
  group B infection
    endocarditis, **B1**.530
    neonatal meningitis, **B1**.574
    pneumonia, **B1**.637
    prevention, **B1**.668
    see also Streptococcus agalactiae
  group D
    antigen, **B2**.887
    endocarditis, **B1**.529–30
  infection
    antibody detection, **B1**.750–1
    conjunctivitis, **B1**.598–9
    endocarditis, **B1**.528
    immunoserology, **B1**.756
    nosocomial, **B1**.401 (Tab.)
    spreading factors, **B1**.153 (Tab.)
  as normal microbiota, **B1**.296 (Tab.)
    nares and nasopharynx, **B1**.295–300
    oropharynx and tonsils, **B1**.301
  nutritionally variant *see Abiotrophia;*
    Granulicatella
  'pyogenic', endocarditis, **B1**.530
  viridans (oral), endocarditis, **B1**.525, **B1**.527,
    B1.528–9, **B1**.539
  virulence factors, **B1**.153 (Tab.)
Streptococcus, **B2**.833–63
  antibacterial susceptibility/resistance,
    B2.861–2
  antibacterial susceptibility testing, **B2**.862
  antigens, **B2**.842–3
  bacteriocins, **B2**.850–2
  bacteriophage, **B2**.839
  cell wall, **B2**.840–3
    carbohydrates, **B2**.840–2
    peptidoglycan, **B2**.840, **B2**.841 (Fig.)
    proteins, **B2**.842
  classification, **B2**.833–6, **B2**.843–9
    anginosus group, **B2**.846
    bovis group, **B2**.847–8
    genus definition, **B2**.833
    intrageneric structure, **B2**.843–9
    mitis group, **B2**.846–7

mutans group, **B2**.848
pyogenic group, **B2**.844–6
salivarius group, **B2**.847
species, **B2**.834 (Tab.)
competence stimulating peptide, **B2**.839
conjugation, **B1**.103
culture, **B2**.836–7
genetics, **B2**.838–40
habitats, **B2**.835–6
  in milk, **B1**.230–1
  nuts, **B1**.287
hemolysis, **B2**.837
historical perspective, **B2**.833–5
immune evasion
  antibody-binding proteins, **I**.661–2
  antibody degradation/modification, **I**.662
  pore-forming toxins, **I**.654–5
infection
  keratitis, **B1**.601
  nosocomial infection, **B1**.401 (Tab.)
isolation/identification, **B1**.223–4, **B2**.849–50,
    B2.906–7
metabolism, **B2**.837–8
  carbohydrates, **B2**.837–8, **B2**.838 (Fig.)
  other nutritional requirements, **B2**.838
  pyruvate, **B2**.837, **B2**.838 (Fig.)
morphology, **B2**.836
as normal microbiota, **B2**.852
  nasopharynx, **B1**.609
  oral cavity, **B1**.609
pasteurization, **B1**.232–3
pathogenicity, **B2**.853–61
plasmid, **B2**.839
protein G, **I**.661–2
transposons, **B2**.839–40
virulence factors, **B2**.853–61
  staphylokinase, **B1**.153 (Tab.)
waterborne, **B1**.212, **B1**.223–4
Streptococcus acidominimus
  characteristics, **B2**.834 (Tab.)
  classification, **B2**.848
Streptococcus adjacens, **B2**.862
Streptococcus agalactiae, **B2**.834 (Tab.),
    B2.849 (Tab.)
  antigens, **B2**.842, **B2**.843
  bacteriocins, **B2**.850–2
  CAMP factor, **B2**.859
  capsule, **B2**.859
  cell wall, **B2**.841, **B2**.842
  classification, **B2**.844
  culture, **B1**.668, **B2**.836
  genetics, **B2**.839–40
  hemolysin, **B2**.859
  infection
    bacteremia, **B1**.519, **B1**.520
    endocarditis, **B1**.530
    mastitis, **B1**.230
    nosocomial, **B1**.401 (Tab.)
    treatment, **B1**.668
    vaginitis, **B1**.668
  isolation/identification, **B1**.668, **B2**.849
    typing, **B2**.860
  metabolism, **B2**.837, **B2**.838
  neuraminidase production, **B2**.859
  in normal microbiota, **B1**.668, **B2**.852

pathogenicity/virulence factors, **B2**.859–60
Streptococcus alactolyticus, **B2**.834 (Tab.)
  classification, **B2**.848
Streptococcus anginosus, **B2**.834 (Tab.),
    B2.851 (Tab.)
  classification, **B2**.846
  culture, **B2**.836
  genetics, **B2**.839–40
  infection
    bacteremia, **B1**.519
    endocarditis, **B1**.529
    peritonsillar abscess, **B1**.618
  isolation/identification, **B2**.850
  metabolism, **B2**.838
Streptococcus australis, **B2**.834 (Tab.),
    B2.851 (Tab.)
  classification, **B2**.846–7
  isolation/identification, **B2**.850
Streptococcus bovis, **B2**.834 (Tab.)
  antibacterial susceptibility/resistance,
    B2.861–2
  classification, **B2**.847–8
  genetics, **B2**.839–40
  infection, endocarditis, **B1**.529, **B1**.539
  waterborne, **B1**.223–4
Streptococcus canis, **B2**.834 (Tab.),
    B2.849 (Tab.)
  classification, **B2**.844, **B2**.845
Streptococcus constellatus, **B2**.834 (Tab.),
    B2.851 (Tab.)
  classification, **B2**.846
  infection
    bacteremia, **B1**.519
    endocarditis, **B1**.529
  isolation/identification, **B2**.850
Streptococcus cricetus, **B2**.834 (Tab.)
  classification, **B2**.848
Streptococcus crista, **B2**.851 (Tab.)
  classification, **B2**.846–7
  isolation/identification, **B2**.850
Streptococcus cristatus, **B2**.834 (Tab.)
  amended name, **B2**.844
Streptococcus defectivus, **B2**.862
Streptococcus didelphis, **B2**.834 (Tab.),
    B2.849 (Tab.)
  classification, **B2**.845
Streptococcus downeii, **B2**.834 (Tab.)
  classification, **B2**.848
Streptococcus (Enterococcus) durans, **B2**.882–3
Streptococcus dysgalactiae, **B2**.834 (Tab.),
    B2.849 (Tab.)
  bacteriocins, **B2**.850–2
  cell wall, **B2**.841
  classification, **B2**.844–5
  mastitis, **B1**.230
Streptococcus entericus, **B2**.834 (Tab.)
Streptococcus equi, **B2**.834 (Tab.),
    B2.849 (Tab.)
  bacteriocins, **B2**.850–2
  cell wall, **B2**.841
Streptococcus equinus, **B2**.834 (Tab.)
  classification, **B2**.847–8
  waterborne, **B1**.223–4
Streptococcus equisimilis, **B2**.839–40, **B2**.844–5
Streptococcus faecalis see Enterococcus faecalis

Streptococcus faecium see Enterococcus faecium
Streptococcus ferus, **B2**.834 (Tab.)
  classification, **B2**.848
Streptococcus gallinaceus, **B2**.834 (Tab.)
Streptococcus gallolyticus, **B1**.529–30, **B2**.834 (Tab.)
  classification, **B2**.848
Streptococcus gordonii, **B1**.529, **B2**.834 (Tab.), **B2**.851 (Tab.)
  cell wall, **B2**.841
  classification, **B2**.846–7
  culture, **B2**.836
  genetics, **B2**.839
  infection
    bacteremia, **B1**.519
    dendritic cells, **I**.656
    endocarditis, **B1**.528–9
  isolation/identification, **B2**.850
  as vaccine vector, **I**.845–6
Streptococcus group A, vaccines
  BCE peptide vaccines, **I**.855 (Tab.), **I**.873
  development status, **I**.933 (Tab.)
Streptococcus group B, vaccines
  development status, **I**.933 (Tab.)
  subunit vaccine development, **I**.940
Streptococcus hansenii, **B2**.904
Streptococcus hyointestinalis, **B2**.834 (Tab.), **B2**.849 (Tab.)
  classification, **B2**.845
Streptococcus hyovaginalis
  characteristic, **B2**.834 (Tab.), **B2**.849 (Tab.)
  classification, **B2**.848–9
Streptococcus infantarius, **B1**.529–30, **B2**.834 (Tab.)
  classification, **B2**.847–8
Streptococcus infantis, **B2**.846, **B2**.847
  cell wall, **B2**.840–1, **B2**.841–2
  characteristics, **B2**.834 (Tab.), **B2**.851 (Tab.)
  genetics, **B2**.839
  isolation/identification, **B2**.850
Streptococcus iniae, **B2**.834 (Tab.), **B2**.849 (Tab.)
  classification, **B2**.845
Streptococcus intermedius, **B2**.834 (Tab.), **B2**.851 (Tab.)
  classification, **B2**.846
  infection
    bacteremia, **B1**.519
    endocarditis, **B1**.529
    intracranial abscess, **B1**.583–4
  isolation/identification, **B2**.850
Streptococcus intestinalis, **B2**.834 (Tab.)
  classification, **B2**.845
Streptococcus lutetiensis, **B2**.834 (Tab.)
  classification, **B2**.847–8
Streptococcus macacae, **B2**.834 (Tab.)
  classification, **B2**.848
Streptococcus macedonicus, **B2**.848
Streptococcus milleri infection
  endocarditis, **B1**.529
  intracranial abscess, **B1**.585, **B1**.588–9
  spinal epidural abscess, **B1**.593
  subdural empyema, **B1**.591

Streptococcus mitis, **B2**.834 (Tab.), **B2**.851 (Tab.)
  antibacterial susceptibility/resistance, **B2**.862
  cell wall
    carbohydrates, **B2**.840–1, **B2**.841–2
    peptidoglycan, **B2**.840
  classification, **B2**.846, **B2**.847
  genetics, **B2**.839–40
  infection
    bacteremia, **B1**.519
    endocarditis, **B1**.528–9
  isolation/identification, **B2**.850
  in normal microbiota, **B2**.852
  oral cavity, **B1**.609
Streptococcus mutans, **B2**.834 (Tab.), **B2**.851 (Tab.)
  bacteriocins, **B2**.850–2
  cell wall, **B2**.842
  classification, **B2**.848
  culture, **B2**.837 (Fig.)
  genetics, **B2**.839
  infection
    dental caries, **B1**.608–9
    endocarditis, **B1**.528–9
  metabolism, **B2**.837, **B2**.838
  in normal microbiota, **B2**.852
  oral cavity, **B1**.609
  virulence factors, exopolysaccharides, **B1**.154
Streptococcus mutans, vaccine, **I**.847
Streptococcus oligofermentans, **B2**.851 (Tab.)
  classification, **B2**.847
Streptococcus oralis, **B1**.529, **B2**.834 (Tab.), **B2**.851 (Tab.)
  antibacterial susceptibility/resistance, **B2**.862
  cell wall
    carbohydrates, **B2**.840–1, **B2**.841–2
    peptidoglycan, **B2**.840
  classification, **B2**.847
  culture, **B2**.836
  endocarditis, infection, **B1**.527, **B1**.528–9
  genetics, **B2**.839–40
  infection, bacteremia, **B1**.519
  isolation/identification, **B2**.850
  in normal microbiota, **B1**.614, **B2**.852
Streptococcus orisratti, **B2**.834 (Tab.)
  classification, **B2**.848
Streptococcus ovis, **B2**.834 (Tab.)
  classification, **B2**.849
Streptococcus parasanguis, **B2**.834 (Tab.), **B2**.851 (Tab.)
  classification, **B2**.846, **B2**.847
    amended name, **B2**.844
  infection, endocarditis, **B1**.527
  isolation/identification, **B2**.850
Streptococcus parauberis, **B2**.834 (Tab.), **B2**.849 (Tab.)
  classification, **B2**.845
Streptococcus parvulus, **B2**.904
Streptococcus pasteurianus, **B2**.834 (Tab.)
  classification, **B2**.847–8
Streptococcus peroris, **B2**.834 (Tab.), **B2**.851 (Tab.)
  classification, **B2**.846, **B2**.847
  isolation/identification, **B2**.850

Streptococcus phocae, **B2**.834 (Tab.), **B2**.849 (Tab.)
  isolation/identification, **B2**.849–50
Streptococcus pluranimalium, **B2**.834 (Tab.)
  classification, **B2**.848–9
Streptococcus pneumoniae
  adhesin, **B1**.627
  antibacterial susceptibility/resistance, **B1**.363, **B1**.499 (Tab.), **B1**.569, **B2**.861–2
    emerging bacterial infection, **B1**.360, **B1**.363, **B1**.363 (Fig.)
    international travel, **B1**.360
    penicillin, **B1**.519, **B1**.571, **B1**.632
    quinolone resistance, **B1**.493 (Tab.)
  antigens, **B2**.842, **B2**.843
    see also individual antigens
  autolysin (LytA), **B2**.861
  capsule, **B2**.860
    antibodies, **B1**.631
    swelling, **B1**.631–2
  cell wall, **B1**.557
    carbohydrates, **B2**.840–1, **B2**.841–2
    proteins, **B2**.842
  characteristics, **B2**.834 (Tab.), **B2**.851 (Tab.)
  choline binding protein A, **B1**.627
  culture, **B2**.836
  genetics, **B2**.839–40
    artificial competence, **B1**.99–100
    natural competence, **B1**.99
  habitats, **B1**.608–9
  IgA1 protease, **B2**.860–1
  immune evasion
    antibody degradation/modification, **I**.662
    chemotaxis inhibition, **I**.648
    complement, **I**.662–3, **I**.663–4
    pore-forming toxins, **I**.654–5
  infection *see Streptococcus pneumoniae* infection
  isolation/identification
    development, **B1**.751
    precipitin reaction, **B1**.756
    Quellung reaction, **B1**.756
    serology, **B1**.757–8
    slide agglutination test, **B1**.756
    typing, **B2**.861
  metabolism, **B2**.837, **B2**.838
  neuraminidases (NanA and NanB), **B2**.861
  pathogenicity, **B2**.860–1
  phosphocholine, **B2**.860
  pneumococcal surface protein (PspA), **B2**.861
  pneumolysin, **B1**.627, **B2**.861
  polysaccharides, **B1**.632
  quorum sensing, **B1**.72, **B1**.172
  serotypes, **B1**.570
  teichoic acids, **B2**.860
  virulence factors, **B1**.627, **B2**.860–1
    K-antigens, **B1**.154
  zinc-metallo-proteinases, **B2**.860–1
Streptococcus pneumoniae infection
  agammaglobulinemia, **I**.780
  asplenia, **I**.771
  bacteremia, **B1**.519, **B1**.569, **B1**.570 (Fig.), **B1**.632
  bone and joint infection, **B1**.690–1

Streptococcus pneumoniae infection (*Continued*)
 C3 deficiency, **I**.770–1
 carriage rates, **B1**.556
 chronic bronchitis, **B1**.648
 conjunctivitis, **B1**.599, **B1**.600
 emerging bacterial infection
  day-care centers, **B1**.361
  drug-resistance, **B1**.361
  international travel, **B1**.360
  Russia, **B1**.364
  USA, **B1**.364
 endocarditis, **B1**.525, **B1**.527, **B1**.530
 epiglottitis, **B1**.613
 Ig deficiencies, **I**.781–2
 immune response, **B1**.572 (Tab.)
  evasion, **B1**.154
  neutrophils, **I**.44
 influenza, **V1**.661
 intracranial abscess, **B1**.585
 nosocomial, **B1**.373–4, **B1**.401 (Tab.)
  pneumonia, **B1**.389
 otitis media, **B1**.617–18
 pneumonia, **B1**.630–3
  in AIDS, **B1**.630–1
  antibody absence, **B1**.631
  clinical features, **B1**.631, **B1**.631 (Fig.)
  complications, **B1**.632, **B1**.641–3
  epidemiology, **B1**.630–1
  laboratory findings, **B1**.631–2
  nosocomial, **B1**.640–1, **B1**.640 (Tab.)
  pathogenesis, **B1**.631
  prevention, **B1**.632–3
  therapy, **B1**.632
 predisposition factors, **B1**.557
 respiratory tract, **B1**.627
 sinusitis, **B1**.615, **B1**.615 (Tab.)
 spinal epidural abscess, **B1**.593
 vaccines, **B1**.569, **B1**.632–3
  23-valent, **B1**.571, **B1**.572, **B1**.632
  BCG vector, **I**.845
  capsular polysaccharides, **B1**.571–2, **I**.935
  conjugate vaccines, **I**.936
  CRM197 as carrier protein, **I**.936
  development status, **I**.933 (Tab.)
  multivalent, **B1**.571
  revaccination, **B1**.572
  subunit vaccine development, **I**.940
Streptococcus porcinus, **B2**.834 (Tab.), **B2**.849 (Tab.)
 classification, **B2**.845
Streptococcus pyogenes, **B2**.833–5, **B2**.834 (Tab.), **B2**.849 (Tab.)
 adherence, **B1**.149
 antibacterial susceptibility/resistance, **B1**.499 (Tab.), **B2**.861–2
  generation, **B1**.467–8
 antigens, **B2**.843
 bacteriocins, **B2**.850–2
 C5a peptidase (SCP), **B2**.857–8
 capsule, **B2**.855
 cell wall, **B2**.840
  carbohydrates, **B2**.841–2
  proteins, **B2**.842
 classification, **B2**.844

erythrotoxin B, **I**.556 (Tab.), **I**.565
 genetics, **B2**.839–40
 hyaluronidase, **B2**.858
 immune evasion
  antibody-binding proteins, **I**.661–2
  complement cleavage, **I**.663–4
  membrane attack complex inhibition, **I**.664
  superantigens, **I**.668
 infection *see Streptococcus pyogenes* infection
 isolation/identification, **B2**.849–50
  antiDNase B assays, **B1**.750–1
  antistrepsolysin O titer, **B1**.750–1
  by molecular techniques, **B1**.723 (Tab.)
  typing, **B2**.858
 metabolism, **B2**.838
 mitogenic factor, **I**.556 (Tab.), **I**.565–6
  as nuclease, **I**.565
  polymorphisms, **I**.565
 morphology, **B2**.836 (Fig.)
 M protein family, **I**.556 (Tab.), **I**.565, **B2**.853–5, **B2**.853 (Fig.), **B2**.854 (Fig.)
  cross-reactions with host tissues, **B2**.855
  discovery, **B1**.12
  function, **B2**.854–5
  pathogenesis, **B1**.610–11
 neuraminidase, **B2**.858
 in normal microbiota, **B2**.852
 nucleases, **B2**.858
 pathogenicity, **B2**.853–8
 protein F, **B2**.855–6
 pyogenic exotoxins *see* Streptococcal pyogenic exotoxins (SPE)
 pyrogenic exotoxins (Spe), **B1**.157 (Tab.), **B2**.856–7
  pyrogenic exotoxin A (SPE-A), **B2**.856
  pyrogenic exotoxin B (SPE-B), **B2**.856–7
  pyrogenic exotoxin C (SPE-C), **B2**.856
 serum-opacity factor, **B2**.858
 skin colonization, **B1**.304
 streptokinase, **B2**.857
 streptolysins, **B2**.857
 superantigens, **B2**.856
 virulence factors, **B2**.853–8
Streptococcus pyogenes infection
 bacteremia, **B1**.519, **B1**.520
 C3 deficiency, **I**.770–1
 endocarditis, **B1**.525
 keratitis, **B1**.601
 milk-borne scarlet fever, **B1**.230–1
 nosocomial
  antibiotic era, **B1**.371
  burns, **B1**.385, **B1**.401 (Tab.)
  early twentieth century, **B1**.371
  hospital spread, **B1**.374, **B1**.401 (Tab.)
  operating theater, **B1**.375
 otitis media, **B1**.617
 pathogenesis, **B2**.853–8
 peritonsillar abscess, **B1**.618
 pharyngitis *see* Pharyngitis
 sinusitis, **B1**.615, **B1**.615 (Tab.)
 vaccines
  attenuated bacterial vectors, **I**.845–6
  BCE peptide vaccines, **I**.855 (Tab.)

Streptococcus ratti, **B2**.834 (Tab.)
 name amendment, **B2**.844
Streptococcus salivarius, **B2**.834 (Tab.), **B2**.851 (Tab.)
 bacteriocins, **B2**.850–2
 cheesemaking, **B1**.252
 classification, **B2**.847
 infection, endocarditis, **B1**.528–9
 isolation/identification, **B2**.850
 in normal microbiota, **B2**.852
 oral cavity, **B1**.609
Streptococcus sanguinis, **B1**.529
 infection, endocarditis, **B1**.528–9
 in normal microbiota, **B1**.614
 oral cavity, **B1**.609
 see also Streptococcus sanguis
Streptococcus sanguis, **B2**.834 (Tab.), **B2**.851 (Tab.)
 amended name, **B2**.844
 cell wall, **B2**.841, **B2**.842
 classification, **B2**.846–7
 culture, **B2**.836
 genetics, **B2**.839–40
 infection, bacteremia, **B1**.519
 isolation/identification, **B2**.850
 metabolism, **B2**.838
 morphology, **B2**.836
 in normal microbiota, **B2**.852
 see also Streptococcus sanguinis
Streptococcus sinensis, **B2**.834 (Tab.), **B2**.851 (Tab.)
 classification, **B2**.846, **B2**.847
Streptococcus sobrinus, **B2**.834 (Tab.), **B2**.851 (Tab.)
 classification, **B2**.848
 metabolism, **B2**.838
 in normal microbiota, **B2**.852
Streptococcus suis, **B2**.834 (Tab.), **B2**.849 (Tab.)
 antigens, **B2**.843
 classification, **B2**.848
 isolation/identification, **B2**.849–50
Streptococcus thermophilus, **B2**.834 (Tab.), **B2**.851 (Tab.)
 classification, **B2**.847
 isolation/identification, **B2**.849
 as yogurt starter, **B1**.249
Streptococcus thoraltensis, **B2**.834 (Tab.), **B2**.849 (Tab.)
 classification, **B2**.848
Streptococcus uberis, **B2**.834 (Tab.), **B2**.849 (Tab.)
 classification, **B2**.845
 infection, mastitis, **B1**.230
Streptococcus urinalis, **B2**.834 (Tab.), **B2**.849 (Tab.)
 classification, **B2**.845–6
Streptococcus vestibularis, **B2**.834 (Tab.), **B2**.851 (Tab.)
 classification, **B2**.847
 isolation/identification, **B2**.850
Streptococcus zooepidemicus, **B2**.845
 in cheese, **B1**.253
 in cream, **B1**.248
 mastitis, **B1**.230
 in milk, **B1**.230, **B1**.235, **B1**.235 (Tab.), **B1**.244–5

Streptogramins, **B1**.489
  Staphylococcus resistance, **B2**.794 (Tab.), **B2**.803
Streptokinase, functions, **B1**.153 (Tab.)
Streptolysin O, **I**.654–5
Streptomyces, **B2**.1137–8, **B2**.1168–9
  antibacterial susceptibility/resistance, **B2**.1145
  classification, **B2**.1137–8
  conjugation, **B1**.103
  diaminopimelic acid and sugars, **B2**.1145
  genetics, chromosomes, **B1**.81
  identification
    microscopic morphology, **B2**.1143
    molecular methods, **B2**.1146–7
  infection, **B2**.1169
    treatment, **B2**.1169
  nitrification, **B1**.200
  phytopathogenicity, **B1**.202
Streptomyces coelicolor, **B1**.113–14
Streptomyces griseoviridis, **B1**.202–3
Streptomyces muris ratti, **B2**.1909
Streptomyces somaliensis, **M**.387–8, **M**.391–2, **B2**.1169
  histopathology, **M**.128 (Tab.)
  serology, **M**.391–2
Streptomycin
  plague, **B2**.1466
  resistance, *Coxiella burnetii* resistance, **B2**.2077–8
  spectrum of activity
    Brucella, **B2**.1742
    Citrobacter, **B2**.1476
    Enterobacter, **B2**.1484–5
    Ewingella, **B2**.1493
    Klebsiella, **B2**.1480
    Leclercia, **B2**.1495
    Listeria, **B2**.956, **B2**.957–8
    Mycobacterium, **B2**.1218–19, **B2**.1222–3
    Mycobacterium tuberculosis, **B2**.1200, **B2**.1218–19
    Streptococcus, **B2**.861–2
    Tropheryma whippelii, **B2**.1002
  structure, **B1**.483 (Fig.)
  tularemia treatment, **B2**.1755
Streptothrix madurae, **M**.386
'Stress antigen'
  intraepithelial αβ T cell recognition, **I**.441
  non-epidermal γδ T cells, **I**.438
Stress genes, **B1**.74
Strigeida, **P**.579–80
Stringent response, **B1**.40
String test, **P**.150 (Tab.), **P**.151
  cryptosporidiosis, **P**.151
  giardiasis, **P**.148, **P**.151
  Helicobacter pylori infection diagnosis, **B2**.1574
  strongyloidiasis, **P**.151
Strobila
  Echinococcus, **P**.678
  Taenia solium, **P**.678, **P**.679 (Fig.)
Stroke, complement pathology, **I**.155–6, **I**.155 (Tab.)
Stromal cells, GM-CSF production, **I**.277

Stromal-derived factor 1α (SDF-1α:CXCL12), **I**.218 (Tab.)
  actions/effects
    basophil chemotaxis, **I**.58
    phagocyte chemotaxis, **I**.223–4
  intracellular signaling, **I**.222
  receptor *see* CXC chemokine receptors
  structure, **I**.217, **I**.219 (Fig.)
  structure–function relationship, **I**.221
  T cell homing, **I**.226–7
Stromelysin, production, **I**.290
Strongyloidea, **P**.594–5
  Syngamidae, **P**.595
Strongyloides, **P**.594, **I**.682–3, **P**.737–43
  classification, **P**.737
  control, **P**.742–3
  general biology, **P**.738–9
    rhabditiform larvae, **P**.738–9
  historical aspects, **P**.737
  infection *see* Strongyloidiasis
  life cycle, **P**.594, **P**.739
    autoinfection, **P**.739
    free-living (heterogonic), **P**.738
    parasitic (homogonic), **P**.738, **P**.739
  morphology/structure, **P**.587 (Fig.), **P**.594, **P**.737–8, **P**.737 (Fig.)
  transmission/epidemiology, **P**.46 (Tab.), **P**.739–40
    geographical distribution, **P**.42, **P**.739
    HIV coinfection, **P**.739–40
    HTLV coinfection, **P**.739–40
    hyperinfection, **P**.739–40
    travellers/immigrants, **P**.29
  see also individual species
Strongyloides fuelleborni
  classification, **P**.737
  infection *see* Strongyloidiasis
  morphology/structure, **P**.737–8
  transmission/epidemiology, **P**.740
Strongyloides stercoralis
  classification, **P**.737
  historical aspects, **P**.9
  infection *see* Strongyloidiasis
  morphology/structure, **P**.737–8, **P**.737 (Fig.)
    adult female, **P**.738, **P**.738 (Fig.)
    adult male, **P**.738
    rhabditiform larvae, **P**.738, **P**.738 (Fig.)
  transmission/epidemiology, **P**.739
Strongyloidiasis
  clinical manifestations, **P**.740–1
    HTLV coinfection, **P**.740
    hyperinfection, **P**.740–1
    larva currens, **P**.740
    malabsorption syndrome, **P**.740
    'swollen-belly syndrome,' **P**.740, **P**.741
  diagnosis, **P**.741–2
    body fluids, **P**.742, **P**.742 (Fig.)
    culture, **P**.151
    duodenal aspirates, **P**.741
    fecal specimens, **P**.741, **P**.742
    in hyperinfection, **P**.742
    serology, **P**.741–2
    string test, **P**.151
  HTLV-1 coinfection, **P**.741, **I**.803

  immune response, **P**.90, **P**.741
    basophils, **I**.68
    eosinophils, **I**.70
    IgE, **P**.741
    ivermectin, **P**.789
    pathogenesis/pathology, **P**.741
Strongyloididae, **P**.593–4
Structural proteins *see specific viruses*
Structure–activity relationships, antiviral chemotherapy, **V2**.1609
Structure of viruses *see* Morphology, viruses
Study of the Efficacy of Nosocomial Infection Control (SENIC), **B1**.405
Stump-tailed macaque virus (STMV), **V1**.473
Stumpy forms, *Trypanosoma brucei*, **P**.356–7
Subacute bacterial endocarditis (SBE)
  immune response, **B1**.747–8
  pathology, **B1**.747–8
Subacute sclerosing panencephalitis (SSPE), **V1**.724, **V1**.725, **V2**.1404–5, **V2**.1408, **V2**.1431, **V2**.1432
  biased hypermutation, **V1**.193
  chorioretinitis, **V1**.725
  course, **V2**.1432
  defective interfering particles, **V1**.186–7
  disease progression, **V1**.731
  features and EEG, **V2**.1432
  incidence, **V1**.725
  intracellular spread, **V1**.261, **V1**.262 (Fig.)
  measles inclusion body encephalitis *vs.*, **V1**.724–5
  neuropathology, **V1**.725
  neurotropism, **V1**.730
  pathogenesis, **V1**.730–1
    hyperimmune humoral response, **V1**.731
    immunology, **V1**.725, **V1**.731
    virological aspects, **V1**.730–1
  persistence establishment, **V1**.730–1
  treatment, **V1**.734
Subarachnoid space, bacteria in, **B1**.557
Subcutaneous zygomycosis, immune response, **M**.350–2
Subdural empyema, **B1**.589–92, **B1**.590 (Fig.)
  bacteriology, **B1**.591, **B1**.591 (Tab.)
  clinical features, **B1**.591, **B1**.592 (Tab.)
  diagnostic methods, **B1**.591–2, **B1**.592 (Fig.)
  epidemiology, **B1**.590
  pathogenesis, **B1**.590
  treatment, **B1**.591 (Tab.), **B1**.592
Subfamilies, viral classification, **V1**.35, **V1**.39
Subgenomic RNAs
  astrovirus replication, **V2**.895, **V2**.895 (Fig.)
  Borna disease virus, **V2**.1139
  coronaviruses, **V1**.828–30
  equine arteritis virus, **V1**.830
  filovirus replication, **V2**.1092
  lactate dehydrogenase-elevating virus, **V1**.831–2
  Nidovirales order *see* Nidovirales
  Porcine reproductive and respiratory syndrome virus, **V1**.831–2
  toroviruses, **V1**.828–31
Subpellicular microtubules, **P**.162, **P**.163 (Tab.), **P**.165 (Fig.), **P**.170–2
Substance P, actions, **I**.62

Subunit reassortment, **V1**.191–2
  bunyavirus genome, **V1**.191
  influenza virus genome, **V1**.192
  orthomyxoviruses, **V1**.191, **V1**.192
  reoviruses, **V1**.191–2
  Rotavirus genome, **V1**.191–2
Subunit vaccines, **I**.424–6, **I**.488 (Tab.),
    I.932–41, **I**.933 (Tab.)
  adjuvants, **I**.425, **I**.426
  carbohydrates, **I**.424–5
  conjugate vaccines, **I**.935–7
    carrier proteins, **I**.935
    epitope suppression, **I**.935
    Hib, **I**.935–6
    limitations, **I**.935
    meningococci, **I**.936
    pneumococci, **I**.936
  definition, **I**.932
  genomics, **I**.939–41
    bacterial vaccines, **I**.939–40
    dangerous/unculturable organisms, **I**.939
    disadvantages, **I**.939
    high-throughput, **I**.939
    parasite vaccines, **I**.940–1
    protective antigen identification, **I**.940
    techniques, **I**.940
    viral vaccines, **I**.941
  immunization strategies, **I**.424–5
  polysaccharides, **I**.935
    disadvantages, **I**.935
    encapsulated bacteria, **I**.935
    vaccine produced, **I**.935
  protective antigen identification, **I**.932,
    I.934–5
  recombinant DNA techniques, **I**.937–9
    acellular pertussis vaccine, **I**.937–8
    candidate identification, **I**.937
    failures, **I**.938–9
    hepatitis B virus vaccine, **I**.937
    historical aspects/re-evaluation, **I**.15
    Lyme disease, **I**.938
  toxoids, **I**.488 (Tab.), **I**.935
    diphtheria toxoid, **I**.935
    tetanus toxoid, **I**.935
  *see also individual diseases/disorders;
    individual organisms; individual vaccines*
Succinate, **B1**.53
  production, **B1**.53
Succinate dehydrogenase (SDH), **B1**.52–3
Succinate-ubiquinone oxidoreductase, **B1**.64
Succinic acid formation, **B1**.52
Succinivibrio dextrinosolvens, **B1**.296 (Tab.)
Succinyl-CoA, **B1**.61
Suckers, oral/ventral
  liver flukes, **P**.642
  lung flukes, **P**.642
Suckling mice, virus propagation, **V1**.90, **V1**.94–5
Sucrose-acetone-BPL extraction, viral
    antigens, **V1**.92
Sucrose fermentation
  Enterobacteriaceae identification,
    B2.1319 (Tab.)
  Escherichia coli, plasmids, **B1**.115
  Neisseria detection, **B1**.757
  plasmids, **B1**.115

Porphyromonas identification, **B2**.1924 (Tab.)
Prevotella identification, **B2**.1924 (Tab.)
Sudan ebolavirus (SEBOV), **V1**.382
  animal models, **V2**.1095
  cell culture, **V2**.1091–2
  classification, **V2**.1086
  epidemiology, **V2**.1093
  historical aspects, **V2**.1085
  outbreaks, **V2**.1087 (Tab.)
Sudden infant death syndrome (SIDS)
  infant botulism *vs.*, **B2**.1070
  Pneumocystis jirovecii, **M**.791, **M**.796
Sugar cane production, waterborne bacteria,
    B1.212
Sugaring, food processing and preservation,
    B1.268 (Tab.)
Sugar metabolism, acid production, **B1**.23,
    B1.23 (Fig.)
Suicide vectors, plasmid cloning vectors,
    B1.123–4
Suipoxvirus
  classification, **V1**.579 (Tab.), **V1**.582, **V1**.594
  phylogenetics, **V1**.583
  taxonomy, **V1**.595 (Tab.)
'Suit laboratory,' biosafety level 4, **V2**.1527,
    V2.1529 (Fig.)
Sulbactam
  intracranial abscess, **B1**.588
  structure, **B1**.479 (Fig.)
Sulconazole, **M**.183 (Tab.)
Sulesomab, licensing, **I**.355 (Tab.)
Sulfadiazine, **M**.551
  babesiosis, **P**.459
  Ewingella, **B2**.1493
  Leclercia, **B2**.1495
  structure, **B1**.490 (Fig.)
  toxoplasmosis, **P**.437
  Yokenella, **B2**.1498
Sulfadimethoxiine, paracoccidioidomycosis
    therapy, **M**.551
Sulfadimidine
  pharmacology, **B1**.491
  structure, **B1**.490 (Fig.)
Sulfadoxine, **B1**.491
Sulfadoxine–pyrimethamine
  malaria therapy, **P**.506
  Plasmodium resistance, **P**.465 (Fig.)
Sulfa drugs, mechanism of action, **P**.477, **P**.480
Sulfafurazole, **B1**.490 (Fig.)
Sulfalinamide, **B1**.490 (Fig.)
Sulfamethizole, **B1**.491
Sulfamethoxazole
  pharmacology, **B1**.491
  spectrum of activity, **B1**.499 (Tab.)
    Enterobacter, **B2**.1484–5
  structure, **B1**.490 (Fig.)
  toxoplasmosis, **P**.438
Sulfamethoxypyridazine,
    paracoccidioidomycosis therapy, **M**.551
Sulfate reduction, **B1**.66, **B1**.201
Sulfation, viral replication, **V1**.122
Sulfites, **B1**.423 (Tab.), **B1**.429
  waste water, **B1**.212–13
Sulfolobus
  metabolism, **B1**.69–70
  sulfur oxidation, **B1**.201

Sulfolobus solfataricus, **B1**.70
Sulfonamides, **B1**.490–1
  antimalarial action, **P**.480
  discovery, **B1**.561
  in meningococcal diseases, **B1**.561
  mode of action, **B1**.491
  PCP, **M**.764, **M**.789, **M**.796
  pharmacology, **B1**.491
  resistance, **B1**.491
  spectrum of activity, **B1**.490–1
    Citrobacter, **B2**.1476
    Edwardsiella, **B2**.1491–2
    Escherichia, **B2**.1370
    Nocardia, **B2**.1165–6
  structure, **B1**.490–1, **B1**.490 (Fig.)
  toxicity/adverse effects, **B1**.491
  toxoplasmosis, **P**.439
  see also individual drugs; specific types
Sulfones, **B1**.471 (Fig.)
  antimalarial action, mechanism of action,
    P.480
Sulfur, biogeochemical transformations, **B1**.201
Sulfur dioxide, **B1**.429, **B1**.430
Sulfuric acid, **B1**.422
'Summer sores,' **M**.412
Summit-lesions, **B2**.1120
Sun drying, **B1**.268–9
  fruit, **B1**.283
  nuts and seeds, **B1**.287
  rice, **B1**.285–6
Sunlight, **B1**.452
Superantigens, **I**.556 (Tab.), **I.555–69**
  actions/effects, cytokine stimulation, **I**.561
  activation
    autoimmune disease, **I**.754–5
    experimental allergic encephalitis, **I**.755,
      I.759
  biological significance, **I**.561–2
    autoimmunity, **I**.562
    enterotoxic activity, **I**.562
    immunosuppression, **I**.561–2
    pathogenicity role, **I**.561–2
    as virulence factors, **I**.561
  CD4 T cells, **I**.394–5
  definition, **I**.555
  in diseases/infection
    AIDS, **I**.564
    atopic dermatitis, **I**.562
    bacterial immune interference, **I**.668
    experimental allergic encephalomyelitis,
      I.562
    Kawasaki's syndrome, **I**.562
    rheumatoid arthritis, **I**.564
  evolution, **I**.555–6, **I**.561, **I**.565–6
  HERV-K18.1, **I**.564
  human *vs.* murine T cell binding, **I**.560 (Tab.)
  IDDMK1.2, **I**.564
  mechanism of action, **I**.558–60
    MHC class II binding, **I**.558–9
    non-MHC receptors, **I**.559
    TCR interactions, **I**.558–9
  pyrogenic exotoxins *see* Pyrogenic exotoxins
    (PET)
  sources, **I**.556 (Tab.)
    EBV, **I**.563–4

Superantigens
  sources (*Continued*)
    HCMV, **I**.563–4
    human endogenous retroviruses,
      I.556 (Tab.), **I**.563–6
    *Mycoplasma arthriditis see Mycoplasma
      arthriditis,* superantigen
    rabies virus, **I**.563–4
    Yersinia enterocolitica, **I**.556 (Tab.), **I**.563
    TCR interactions, **I**.463
    see also individual bacteria; individual types
Superantigens (type 1 toxins), **B1**.157,
  B1.157 (Tab.)
  see also specific types
Supergenomic RNA, Hepatitis B virus,
  V2.1235
Supergroups
  papillomaviruses, **V1**.449–50
  picornaviruses, **V1**.52
Superinfection exclusion, **V1**.192
  Orbivirus, **V1**.192
  rotaviruses, **V1**.192
Superoxide anion, **B1**.65
Superoxide dismutase (SOD), **B1**.65, **I**.686,
  B2.1932
  Brucella, **B2**.1731, **B2**.1736
  Helicobacter pathogenicity, **B2**.1576
  Nocardia, **B2**.1149
  oxic conditions in soil, **B1**.196–7
  Plasmodium, **P**.478
Superoxide ions
  macrophages, **I**.26
  septic shock, **I**.700
Superoxidized water, **B1**.425
'Super-spreaders,' vaccination models, **I**.961–2
Supplemental essential genes, **V2**.1407–8
Supportive therapy
  filovirus infection, **V2**.1097
  Human respiratory syncytial virus infection,
    V1.792
Suppressers of cytokine synthesis (SOCS), **I**.27
Suppurative parotitis, **B1**.619
Supramolecular activation cluster (SMAC),
  I.465
Suramin
  adverse effects, **P**.370
  African trypanosomiasis, **P**.370, **P**.371
  onchocerciasis, **P**.790
Surecell®, **B2**.2019
Surface-active agents, **B1**.425–6, **B1**.432
  iodophors, **B1**.425
Surface adherence, colonization, **B1**.147
Surface projections, astroviruses, **V2**.891
Surface waters, **B1**.213–14, **B1**.215 (Tab.),
  B1.221
Surfactant protein-A (SP-A), **V1**.273
  microbial recognition, **I**.22–3, **I**.24 (Tab.)
Surfactant protein-D (SP-D), **V1**.273
  Human respiratory syncytial virus infection,
    V1.793–4
  microbial recognition, **I**.24 (Tab.)
Surfactant proteins
  aspergillosis, **M**.707
  lung, **B1**.623–4
Surfactants
  amphoteric, **B1**.423 (Tab.), **B1**.425

skin immunization, **I**.822
Surgeons
  hepatitis B, **B1**.382
  Hepatitis B virus status, **V2**.1256
  hepatitis C and HIV infection of, **B1**.382–3
  infection prevention, **B1**.387
Surgery
  cystic echinococcosis, **P**.696–7
  elective, infection after, **B1**.387
  eumycetoma therapy, **M**.393
  gas gangrene
    after, **B2**.1111, **B2**.1112–13
    treatment, **B2**.1115
  infection after, **B1**.374–5
  infection prevention guidelines, **B1**.383
  neurocysticercosis, **P**.696, **P**.697 (Fig.), **P**.698
  prophylactic antibiotics, **B1**.387–8
'surgical fever', **B1**.5–6
Surgical instruments
  nosocomial infection from, **B1**.379–80
  sterilization, **B1**.388
Surgical wounds
  'clean' and 'clean contaminated', **B1**.384
  infection
    cardiac, **B1**.385
    Mycobacterium abscessus case histories,
      B2.1247–50
    Mycobacterium chelonae, **B2**.1252
    Mycobacterium fortuitum, **B2**.1255
    Mycobacterium smegmatis, **B2**.1261
    Mycobacterium wolinskyi, **B2**.1262
    nosocomial, **B1**.384–5
    peritoneal, **B1**.386–7
    prevalence, **B1**.384
Surrogate light chains, pre-BCR, **I**.340–1
Surveillance, epidemiological, **B1**.317–26
  action consequent on, **B1**.322–3
    information dissemination, **B1**.322
  definition, **B1**.317, **B1**.405
  evaluation guidelines, **B1**.318
  historical background, **B1**.317
  importance, **B1**.317
  methods, **B1**.318
  nosocomial infection, **B1**.403–6
    process and results, **B1**.405–6
  objectives, **B1**.317–18
  principles, **B1**.318
  reporting methods, **B1**.318
  routine serological, **B1**.321–2
  targeted and selective, **B1**.405–6
  uses, **B1**.322–3
    assessment for intervention, **B1**.322–3
    early detection for rapid control, **B1**.322
    evaluation of preventive programs, **B1**.323
    new/rare disease detection, **B1**.323
    planning/costing health services, **B1**.323
    prevalent infection for clinical care, **B1**.323
'Susceptibility,' infection models, **I**.948–9
Susceptibility testing, antifungal agents, **M**.35,
  M.155–7, **M**.169–71
  agar dilution screening, **M**.158
  amphotericin B, **M**.170, **M**.172
  Candida, **M**.169–70, **M**.170 (Tab.), **M**.608,
    M.610 (Fig.)
  Candida albicans, **M**.608–9, **M**.610 (Fig.)

Cryptococcus neoformans, **M**.169–70
  early studies, **M**.156
  factors affecting, **M**.156–7
    endpoint determination, **M**.156
    incubation, **M**.156
    inoculum size, **M**.156
    media, **M**.157
  filamentous fungi, **M**.157
  fluconazole, **M**.170, **M**.170 (Tab.)
  flucytosine, **M**.170, **M**.170 (Tab.)
  itraconazole, **M**.170, **M**.170 (Tab.)
  methods, **M**.157–8
    agar dilution screening, **M**.158
    colorimetric, **M**.157
    disk diffusion, **M**.158
    E-test, **M**.158
    flow cytometry, **M**.158
    macrobroth dilution methods, **M**.156,
      M.157
    NCCLS method, **M**.156, **M**.157–8
    sterol quantification, **M**.158
  National Committee for Clinical Laboratory
    Standards, **M**.156, **M**.157–8, **M**.169–70,
    M.170 (Tab.)
  trailing endpoints, **M**.156
  in vivo–in vitro correlations, **M**.158
Susceptible, exposed, infectious, resistant
  (SEIR) model, **I**.954–5
Susceptible groups, vaccination models, **I**.963
Susceptible, infectious, resistant (SIR) model,
  I.954–5
Susceptible, infectious, susceptible (SIS)
  model, **I**.954–5
Sustiva *see* Efavirenz
Suttonella indologenes, **B2**.1668 (Tab.)
  clinical significance, **B2**.1670
  taxonomy, **B2**.1668–9
SV40 *see* Simian virus 40 (SV40)
SV40 early promoter, DNA vaccines, **I**.910
Swab cultures, candidiasis diagnosis, **M**.257
Swachman's syndrome, **I**.765, **I**.767
Swallowing reflex, failure, **B1**.626
'Swamp cancer,' **M**.412
Swans, rhinosporidiosis, **M**.447, **M**.457, **M**.470,
  M.472
Swimming
  Naegleria fowleri transmission, **P**.235–6
    control, **P**.237–8
  schistosomiasis infection, **P**.92–3
Swimming pools, **B1**.215
Swine
  erysipelas, **B2**.970–3
    see also Erysipelothrix rhusiopathiae,
      infection
  viruses, **B1**.434
  see also Pig(s)
Swine influenza, **V1**.673–4
Swine influenza virus, **V1**.371 (Tab.)
Swinepox virus, **V1**.584 (Fig.)
Swine vesicular disease (SVD), **V2**.872
'Switch' recombination regions (S regions),
  I.331, **I**.332
Swollen baby syndrome, **V2**.1070
'Swollen-belly syndrome,' strongyloidiasis,
  P.740, **P**.741

SYBR-Green I, **B1**.727 (Fig.), **B1**.728
  applications, **B1**.728–9
Syk tyrosine kinase
  BCR signaling, **I**.342–3
  structure, **I**.343 (Fig.)
Sympathetic nerves, prion diseases, **V2**.1380–3
Sympatric fungi, **M**.44–5
Symport, **B1**.49
Synagis, licensing, **I**.355 (Tab.)
Synanamorphs, **M**.45
Synapomorphy, **M**.44–5
Synaptic terminals, virus receptors, **V2**.1405–6
Syncephalastrum, **M**.660 (Tab.), **M**.672
  oculomycoses, **M**.287
Syncephalastrum racemosum, **M**.672
Synchronicity, *Plasmodium*, **P**.469, **P**.471–2
Synechocystis, **B2**.1976
Synergistic bacterial infection, gram-positive
  anaerobic cocci, **B2**.910–11
Syngamidae, **P**.595
Syngamy (sexual union), *Balantidium coli*,
  P.277–8, **P**.279 (Fig.)
Synovial fluid specimens, **M**.84
2–5A Synthases, interferon actions, **V1**.228
Synthetic antigens, malaria vaccination,
  P.516–17
Synthetic components, bioremediation,
  B1.201–2
Syphilis, **B1**.662–3, **B2**.1839 (Tab.), **B2**.1843–53
  animal studies, **B1**.662
  causative organism *see Treponema pallidum*
  chancres, **B2**.1841, **B2**.1842
  clinical features, **B1**.662, **B2**.1842–3
  congenital
    clinical signs, **B2**.1843
    diagnosis, **B2**.1848, **B2**.1855 (Tab.),
      B2.1856
  early, **B2**.1842
    diagnosis, **B2**.1854, **B2**.1854 (Tab.)
    Jarisch–Herxheimer reaction, **B2**.1857
    latent stage, **B2**.1842
    treatment, **B2**.1857
  endemic (bejel), **B2**.1839 (Tab.)
    clinical features, **B2**.1858–9
  epidemiology, **B1**.662–3, **B2**.1841
  experimental, **B1**.662
  gumma, **B2**.1842–3
  HIV-infection with, **B1**.662–3, **B2**.1843
    diagnosis, **B2**.1856–7
    treatment, **B2**.1857
  immune response, **B2**.1842
    humoral, **B1**.745–6
  late (tertiary), **B1**.662, **B2**.1842–3,
    B2.1842 (Tab.)
    diagnosis, **B2**.1855
    treatment, **B2**.1857–8
  meningitis in, **B1**.575, **B2**.1843
  paroxysmal nocturnal hemoglobinuria link,
    I.752–3
  pathology and manifestations, **B2**.1842–3
  pregnancy, **B2**.1842, **B2**.1856–7
  serology *see* Syphilis, serological tests
  sexual transmission, **B2**.1842
    men who have sex with men, **B2**.1841
  site of infection, **B2**.1842
    cardiovascular, **B2**.1855, **B2**.1855 (Tab.)

CNS *see* Neurosyphilis
  stages, **B1**.662, **B2**.1842 (Tab.)
    secondary stage, **B1**.662, **B2**.1842
  subunit vaccine development, **I**.940
  treatment, **B1**.662–3, **B2**.1857–8
    antibacterial susceptibility testing, **B2**.1858
    evaluation, **B2**.1858
Syphilis diagnosis, **B1**.663, **B1**.745–6
  congenital, **B2**.1848, **B2**.1855 (Tab.), **B2**.1856
  culture, **B1**.745–6
  direct antigen detection, **B2**.1851–3
    animal inoculation, **B2**.1851
  direct microscopy, **B1**.663, **B2**.1843–5
    darkfield microscopy, **B2**.1844
    direct fluorescent antibody techniques,
      B2.1844–5
    immunohistochemical techniques,
      B2.1844–5
  early syphilis, **B2**.1854 (Tab.)
  EIAs, **B1**.746
  fluorescent treponemal antibody test, **B1**.746
  in HIV infection, **B2**.1856–7
  late syphilis, **B2**.1855 (Tab.)
  non-treponemal tests, **B1**.663, **B2**.1845 (Tab.),
    B2.1846 (Tab.)
    false positive results, **B2**.1847 (Tab.)
    in HIV infection, **B2**.1857
    sensitivity and specificity, **B2**.1846 (Tab.)
    see also specific tests
  PCR-based tests, **B2**.1851–3
  Reiter protein complement fixation assay,
    B1.745–6
  restriction fragment length polymorphism,
    B2.1853
  serological tests, **B1**.663, **B2**.1845–51,
    B2.1845 (Tab.)
    interpretation, **B2**.1853–7
      early syphilis, **B2**.1854
      late (tertiary), **B2**.1855
      neurosyphilis, **B2**.1848
    non-treponemal tests, **B2**.1845–7
      capture-s solid phase red blood cell
        adherence assay, **B2**.1846
      flocculation tests, **B2**.1845–6
      problems, **B2**.1846–7
      sensitivity and specificity, **B2**.1845–6
      VDRL-cerebrospinal fluid, **B2**.1846
    treponemal tests, **B2**.1847–51
      EIA tests, **B2**.1849
      false positives, **B2**.1847, **B2**.1850–1
      fluorescent antibody tests, **B2**.1847–8
      hemagglutination methods, **B2**.1848
      immunoblotting, **B2**.1849–50
      immunochromatographic strip tests,
        B2.1850
      latex agglutination methods, **B2**.1849
      particle agglutination methods,
        B2.1848–9
      problems, **B2**.1850–1
  sexually acquired, **B2**.1854–5
  treponemal tests, **B1**.663, **B2**.1845 (Tab.),
    B2.1850 (Tab.)
    false positives, **B2**.1851 (Tab.)
    in HIV infection, **B2**.1857
    sensitivity and specificity, **B2**.1851 (Tab.)
    see also specific tests

Treponema pallidum immobilization test,
  B1.746
  USA case number, **B2**.1841, **B2**.1841 (Fig.)
  use and interpretation, **B2**.1853–7
Systemic γδ T cells *see* γδ T-cells
Systemic inflammation, control, **I**.209
Systemic inflammatory response syndrome
  (SIRS), **I**.193, **B1**.510, **B1**.511 (Tab.),
  I.696 (Fig.)
  definition, **I**.695
  pathogenesis, **I**.701 (Fig.)
  see also Septic shock
Systemic lupus erythematosus (SLE)
  autoantibodies, **I**.155, **I**.758
  complement, **I**.155
    C1q, **I**.149, **I**.155
    complement receptor 1, **I**.147
  etiology, **I**.756, **I**.758
  HLA-DR, **I**.758
  immune complexes, **I**.147, **I**.757
  neutrophil abnormalities, **I**.49
  New Zealand Black/White mouse model,
    I.758–9
  Nocardia asteroides infection, **B2**.1157
  prevalence, **I**.748 (Tab.)
  signs/symptoms, **I**.155
Systemic shock, disseminated intravascular
  coagulation, **I**.701

T4 bacteriophage *(Myoviridae)*, **B1**.141
Tacaribe virus, **V2**.1059–60
  genome, **V2**.1066
  geographical distribution/carrier and disease,
    V2.1060 (Tab.)
  LCMV relationship, **V2**.1069
Tacrolimus, **I**.788 (Tab.)
Taenia
  classification, **P**.579
  discovery, **P**.658
  eggs, **P**.575 (Fig.)
  epidemiology, **P**.46 (Tab.)
  geographical distribution, **P**.658
  immune evasion, **I**.685
  infection
    clinical features, **P**.579
    ELISA, **P**.664
    location in host, **P**.662
  life cycle, **P**.579
    reservoir hosts, **P**.119
  morphology/structure, **P**.575 (Fig.), **P**.579,
    P.659
  scolex, **P**.575 (Fig.)
  see also individual species
Taenia ovis, vaccine, **P**.96
Taenia rhynchus, **P**.579
Taenia saginata, **I**.682
  historical aspects, **P**.12
  infection
    immune response, **P**.663
    spontaneous cure, **P**.663
  public health importance, **P**.44
  transmission/epidemiology, prevalence,
    P.658
Taenia saginata asiatica, **P**.667–8
  control, **P**.668 (Tab.)

Taenia saginata asiatica, (Continued)
  infection, diagnosis, **P**.668
  life cycle, **P**.666 (Fig.), **P**.667–8
  morphology/structure, **P**.667
  transmission/epidemiology, **P**.668
Taenia saginata saginata, **P**.665–7
  control, **P**.667, **P**.668 (Tab.)
  general biology, **P**.665
  infection
    anal swabs, **P**.667
    clinical manifestations, **P**.666
    diagnosis, **P**.667
    economic losses, **P**.665
    immunity, **P**.667
    location in host, **P**.666
    pathogenesis/pathology, **P**.666–7
    Taenia solium vs., **P**.667, **P**.667 (Fig.)
  life cycle, **P**.665, **P**.666 (Fig.)
    intermediate hosts, **P**.665
  morphology/structure, **P**.665
  transmission/epidemiology, **P**.666
    prevalence, **P**.665
    raw/uncooked meat, **P**.665
Taenia solium, **P**.668–9, **P**.677, **I**.682
  antigen B (paramyosin), **P**.682–3
  calcareous corpuscles, **P**.681–2
  cysticercus, **P**.679, **P**.680 (Fig.)
    cellulose, **P**.679–80, **P**.685–6
    immunosuppression effects, **P**.685–6
    location in host, **P**.685–6, **P**.686 (Fig.)
    racemose, **P**.679–80, **P**.685–8
  heat stress proteins, **P**.682–3
  historical aspects, **P**.12
  immune evasion, **I**.685
  infection *see Taenia solium* infection
  life cycle, **P**.666 (Fig.), **P**.668, **P**.678–80,
    P.684 (Fig.)
    definitive host, **P**.684
    development in host, **P**.679
    intermediate hosts, **P**.668, **P**.684
  molecular taxonomy, **P**.683
  morphology/structure, **P**.668, **P**.679 (Fig.)
    eggs, **P**.678–9
    proglottids, **P**.678
    scolex, **P**.678, **P**.679 (Fig.)
    strobila, **P**.678, **P**.679 (Fig.)
  protease activities, **P**.682–3
  tegumental surface, **P**.682–3
    myosin, **P**.682–3
  transmission/epidemiology, **P**.668–9
    prevalence, **P**.658, **P**.668–9
Taenia solium infection
  clinical manifestations, **P**.669
  control, **P**.669
    BCE peptide vaccines, **I**.855 (Tab.),
      I.874–5
    chemotherapy, **P**.669
    prophylaxis, **P**.669
    transmission, **P**.669
  diagnosis, **P**.669
    brain biopsies, **P**.153
    EIAs, **P**.154
    Taenia saginata saginata vs., **P**.667,
      P.667 (Fig.)
  endocrinological effects, **P**.683

  location in host, **P**.669
  public health importance, **P**.44
Taeniidae, **P**.579, **P**.677
Tafenoquine, malaria therapy, **P**.506
Tahyna virus
  epidemiology, **V2**.1042–3
  infection, **V2**.1043
Talampicillin, **B1**.475
Tamdy virus infection, **V2**.1048
Tamiami virus
  chronic infection, **V2**.1071
  geographical distribution/carrier and disease,
    V2.1060 (Tab.)
Tamiflu *see* Oseltamivir
Tamm–Horsfall glycoprotein, **B1**.673
Tampons, toxic shock syndrome, **B1**.362
Tanapox virus, **V1**.589
  immune evasion, **V1**.318
Tandem mass spectrometry, **I**.877
Tannins, food, **B1**.267
T-antigen, polyomaviruses, **V1**.473–4
TAP2 gene, leprosy association, **I**.591
Tapeworm(s), **P**.**658–76**
  classification, **P**.659, **P**.659 (Tab.)
  general biology, **P**.661–2
    biochemistry, **P**.662
    feeding, **P**.661–2
    lifespan, **P**.661
    movement, **P**.661
    numbers per individual, **P**.661
    physiology, **P**.662
  geographical distribution, **P**.658
  historical aspects, **P**.658–63
  intestinal *see* Cestodes (intestinal
    tapeworms)
  life cycle, **P**.662
    intermediate hosts, **P**.662
  morphology/structure, **P**.659–61, **P**.660 (Fig.)
    acetabula, **P**.659
    body wall/tegument, **P**.659, **P**.660 (Fig.),
      P.661
    bothria, **P**.659
    eggs, **P**.661, **P**.661 (Fig.)
    excretory system, **P**.659–62
    muscle layers, **P**.659
    nervous system, **P**.659
    reproductive system, **P**.661
    rostellum, **P**.659
    solex, **P**.659
  transmission/epidemiology, **P**.662
    prevalence, **P**.658, **P**.662
  see also individual species
Tapeworm infection
  clinical manifestations, **P**.663
  control, **P**.664–5
    chemotherapy, **P**.664
    prophylaxis, **P**.664–5
    transmission, **P**.665
  diagnosis, **P**.664
    fecal egg counts, **P**.664
    serology, **P**.664
  immune response, **P**.663–4
    concomitant immunity, **P**.663
    other infection, **P**.664
  location in host, **P**.659, **P**.662–3

  pathogenesis/pathology, **P**.663
    eosinophilia, **P**.663
    zoonoses, **P**.667–8
  see also individual species
'Tapir nose (Nariz de anta)', **P**.327
TaqMan™, **B1**.728–9
TARC (CCL17) *see* CCL17
Tar, phenol production, **B1**.422
Tas protein *see* Foamy viruses
TATA box
  JC virus, **V1**.475–6
  SV40, **V1**.482
TATA box-binding protein, papillomaviruses,
  V1.461 (Tab.)
Tataguine virus infection, **V2**.1048
Tat protein *see* HIV
Tatum, E, **B1**.13
Tatumella, **B2**.1497
  antibacterial susceptibility/resistance,
    B2.1497
  biochemical tests, **B2**.1497
  classification, **B2**.1497
  culture, **B2**.1497
  definition, **B2**.1497
  motility, **B2**.1342
Tatumella ptyseos, **B2**.1497
  biochemical tests, **B2**.1319 (Tab.)
Tautomeric shifts, point mutations, **B1**.84,
  B1.85 (Fig.)
'Taxi-rank malaria,' **P**.511, **P**.514–15
Taxon description, **B1**.18–9
Taxospecies, **B1**.29–30
Tax protein, **V1**.336, **V1**.337 (Fig.)
  HTLV *see* Human T-cell leukemia virus 1
    (HTLV-1), Tax protein; Human T-cell
    leukemia virus 2 (HTLV-2)
Tazobactam
  Enterobacter, **B2**.1486
  structure, **B1**.479 (Fig.)
T cell(s), **V1**.274–6
  activation/proliferation
    IL-4 effects, **I**.280, **I**.281 (Fig.)
    mucosal vaccination, **I**.827, **I**.828
    Mycoplasma arthritidis superantigen, **I**.562
    Nef protein, **V2**.1329
    NK cells, **I**.478
    prostaglandin E_2 effects, **I**.188
  anergy, **P**.92, **P**.209
  antigen presentation to, **I**.378, **I**.877
    dendritic cell interactions, **I**.378
    recognition, **I**.555
  apoptosis, heat labile enterotoxin, **I**.655
  B cells *vs.,* **I**.490 (Tab.)
  β-only cells, **I**.445
    mouse knockout models, **I**.445
  chemokine receptors, **I**.224, **I**.230 (Fig.)
    CCR1, **I**.224
    CCR2, **I**.224
    CCR5, **I**.224
    CXCR3, **I**.224
  chemotaxis/homing, **I**.224
    defensins, **I**.169
    lymphoid tissue, **I**.226
    MCP-1 (CCL2), **I**.224
    nonlymphoid tissue, **I**.227

T cell(s)
  chemotaxis/homing (*Continued*)
    RANTES, **I**.224
    stromal-derived factor 1α, **I**.226–7
  cytokine effects
    IL-2, **I**.224
    IL-4, **I**.224
    IL-10, **I**.224, **I**.293–4
    IL-12, **I**.224
    IL-16, **I**.289
    IL-21, **I**.283–4
  cytokines produced, **I**.28 (Tab.), **P**.68, **P**.72–3
    GM-CSF, **I**.277
    IFN-γ, **I**.287–8
    IL-2, **I**.279
    IL-3, **I**.275
    IL-4, **I**.28 (Tab.), **I**.280
    IL-5, **I**.277
    IL-10, **I**.292
    IL-21, **I**.283–4
    IL-22, **I**.294
    IL-24, **I**.294
    IL-26, **I**.294
    lymphotoxin, **I**.286
    see also individual cytokines
  cytotoxic *see* CD8+ T-cell(s); Cytotoxic T
    cell(s)
  deficiency
    infection risk, **V1**.274
    persistent infection, **V1**.259
    pneumonia in, **B1**.644–5
  development, **I**.455–8, **I**.455 (Fig.)
    αβ/γδ separation, **I**.456 (Fig.), **I**.457
    antigen presentation, **I**.378
    CD25 expression, **I**.455
    CD44 expression, **I**.455
    clonal deletion, **I**.749
    'double-negative' cells, **I**.455
    'double-positive' cells, **I**.455
    IL-7, **I**.281
    IL-9, **I**.282, **I**.282 (Fig.)
    IL-12, **I**.288
    marker acquisition, **I**.455–6
    negative selection, **I**.379
    positive selection, **I**.379
    thymus, **I**.404
  in diseases/infection
    amebiasis, **P**.209
    aspergillosis, **M**.709
    babesiosis, **P**.456
    bacterial infection, **I**.646, **I**.664
      immune interference, **I**.664–5
    Brugia malayi infection, **I**.683
    candidiasis, **M**.590, **M**.592–3, **M**.597
    Chagas disease, **P**.385
    Chlamydia infection, **B2**.2009
    CNS infection (viral), **V2**.1412, **V2**.1413–15
    coccidioidomycosis, **M**.510
    diGeorge syndrome, **I**.774–5
    Echinococcus infection, **P**.96
    filarial nematode infection, **P**.92
    hepatitis A, **V2**.1170–1
    histoplasmosis capsulati, **M**.527–8

  HTLV-1-associated myelopathy/tropical
    spastic paraparesis (HAM/TSP),
    V2.1429–30
  immunodeficiency diseases/disorders *see*
    Immunodeficiency diseases/disorders
  influenza, **V1**.664–5
  intestinal nematode infection, **P**.90–1
  malaria, **P**.490
  measles, **V2**.1433
    immunosuppression, **V1**.727–9,
      V1.728 (Tab.), **V1**.729 (Fig.)
  Murine cytomegalovirus infection, **V1**.285
  mycetoma, **M**.387
  paracoccidioidomycosis, **M**.550–1
  PCP, **M**.794
  penicilliosis marneffei, **M**.568
  picornavirus infection, **V1**.282
  prion diseases, **V2**.1376
  helper *see* CD4+ T-cells; T-helper cell(s)
  heroin, **M**.12–3
  immune effects, **V1**.275–6
    acute viral infection clearance, **V1**.258
    persistent viral infection clearance,
      V1.260 (Fig.)
  LL37 production, **I**.175
  lung host defence mechanism, **B1**.625
  mediation, mucosal tolerance induction,
    I.542–3
  mucosal immune response *see* Mucosal
    immune response
  Peyer's patches, **I**.532
  regulatory *see* Regulatory T-cells (Treg)
  respiratory tract, **B1**.608
  skin, **I**.820
  suppression in amebiasis, **P**.209
  surface markers, **I**.495 (Tab.)
    complement receptors, **I**.147
    NK cell receptors, **I**.92
    NKG2D receptor, **I**.90
    see also specific markers/receptors
  unconventional, **I.435–48**
    conventional *vs.*, **I**.435
    definition of, **I**.435
    see also specific types
  vaccines, **V2**.1555–6
  viruses replicating in, **V1**.243 (Tab.)
  see also αβ T-cells; γδ T-cells
T-cell epitopes, **I**.853
  peptide vaccines *see* Peptide vaccines
  Rubella virus antigens, **V2**.967
T cell lymphoma, in EBV infection, **V1**.571
T-cell receptor (TCR), **I.449–69**
  αβ chains, **I**.458
    biosynthesis, **I**.459 (Fig.)
    CD3 subunit interactions, **I**.460–1
    CD4 T cells, **I**.389
    constant (C) domains, **I**.458, **I**.460–1
    crystallographic analysis, **I**.460–1
    γδ separation, **I**.456 (Fig.), **I**.457
    hypervariable regions, **I**.460–1
    intrathymic selection, **I**.456
    MHC–peptide interactions, **I**.464
    positive selection, **I**.456
    RAG2 protein degradation, **I**.456
    selection, **I**.456
    superantigen binding, **I**.559

    three-dimensional structure, **I**.461 (Fig.)
    transmembrane domains, **I**.458
    variable (V) domains, **I**.458, **I**.460–1
  abnormal ξ chain expression, **I**.756
  antigen presentation, **I**.461–3, **I**.555
    complementarity determining regions,
      I.381
    conformational change, **I**.383
    ICAM, **I**.383, **I**.384
    see also below MHC–peptide interactions
  CD4 T cells/APC interactions, **I**.392 (Fig.)
  co-receptors, NKG2D, **I**.90
  CTLs, **I**.474
  dendritic epidermal γδ T cells, **I**.436
  diversity, **I**.454–5, **I**.748–9
    combinatorial, **I**.454
    junctional, **I**.454
    non-epidermal γδ T cells, **I**.438
    restriction, **I**.454–5
    somatic hypermutation, **I**.449–50, **I**.454
    viral immune interference, **I**.636
    see also below
  γδ chains, **I**.436
    αβ separation, **I**.456 (Fig.), **I**.457
    constant (C) domains, **I**.458
    crystallographic analysis, **I**.461
    MHC–peptide interactions, **I**.464–5
    superantigen binding, **I**.559
    three-dimensional structure, **I**.461
    transmembrane domains, **I**.458
    variable (V) domains, **I**.458
    see also γδ T-cells
  gene assembly, **I**.455–8
    allelic exclusion, **I**.456–7
    chromatin remodeling, **I**.458
    cis-acting elements, **I**.458
    pre-TCR, **I**.455–6
    recombinase accessibility, **I**.457–8
    transcriptional regulation, **I**.458
    see also T cell(s), development
  genomic organization, **I**.450–5
    α/δ locus, **I**.450 (Fig.), **I**.451
    β locus, **I**.450–1, **I**.450 (Fig.)
    C elements, **I**.451
    D elements, **I**.450–1
    γ locus, **I**.450 (Fig.), **I**.451
    J elements, **I**.450, **I**.451
    V elements, **I**.450–1
  historical aspects/re-evaluation, **I**.12–3,
    I.449–50
    'altered self-model,' **I**.449–50
    gene cloning, **I**.449–50
    self-MHC restriction, **I**.449–50
    somatic rearrangement, **I**.449–50
  immunogenetics, **I**.582–3
  immunological synapse, **I**.465, **I**.466 (Fig.)
    APCs, **I**.465
    chemokine effects, **I**.465
    formation/maturation, **I**.465
    supramolecular activation cluster, **I**.465
    T-cell polarization, **I**.465
  MHC–peptide interactions, **I**.461–3,
    I.462 (Fig.), **I**.463–5
    agonism *vs.* antagonism, **I**.463–4
    alloreactivity, **I**.463

T-cell receptor (TCR)
MHC–peptide interactions (*Continued*)
complementarity-determining regions,
I.461, **I**.462–3
crystallographic analysis, **I**.461–3
topology, **I**.462
see also above antigen presentation
pyrogenic exotoxin interaction, **I**.558–9,
I.559–60
rearrangements, **I**.378, **I**.451–3
homology-guided recombination, **I**.452–3
loopingout/excision model, **I**.453–4
N nucleotides, **I**.452–4
P (palindromic) nucleotides, **I**.452–4
RAG proteins, **I**.451
recombination signal sequences, **I**.451,
I.452 (Fig.)
'signal joint' formation, **I**.452–3
TdT, **I**.452–3
V(D)J recombination, **I**.451, **I**.452 (Fig.),
I.453–4, **I**.453 (Fig.), **I**.457–8, **I**.459 (Fig.)
signaling, **I**.395
HIV infection, **I**.793
lck, **I**.395
structure, **I**.458–61
CD3 transduction complex, **I**.459 (Fig.),
I.460
CD4/CD8 co-receptors, **I**.460
complementarity determining regions,
I.381
crystallographic analysis, **I**.460–1
superantigen binding, **I**.463, **I**.558–9, **I**.559–60
adhesion molecules, **I**.560
MHC II molecules, **I**.559–60
systemic γδ T cells, **I**.439
T-dependent antigens, B cell activation, **I**.326
Technetium-labeled white cell scans,
osteomyelitis, **B1**.694
TECK *see* Thymus expressed chemokine
(TECK: CCL25)
Tectiviridae
classification, **V1**.27 (Tab.), **V1**.43 (Tab.)
see also specific viruses
Teeth
bacteria colonizing, **B1**.301
factors influencing, **B1**.294–5
normal microbiota, **B1**.609
Tego series, **B1**.425
Tegument, herpesviruses, **V1**.502
Teguments
Schistosoma, **P**.601
Schistosoma japonicum, **P**.601
Taenia solium, **P**.682–3
tapeworms, **P**.659, **P**.660 (Fig.), **P**.661
Teichoic acid, **B1**.42–3
chemotaxonomy, **B1**.24
Teichuronic acid, **B1**.43
chemotaxonomy, **B1**.24
Teicoplanin
osteomyelitis, **B1**.698–9
Staphylococcus resistance, **B2**.802–3
structure, **B1**.480 (Fig.)
Telangiectasia, hereditary hemorrhagic,
intracranial abscess complication, **B1**.583

Teleomorphs, **M**.10, **M**.45, **M**.77, **M**.221,
M.221 (Tab.), **M**.223
Aspergillus, **M**.687
Candida krusei, **M**.582
Candida lusitaniae, **M**.583
classification, **M**.45
Cryptococcus neoformans, **M**.18, **M**.639,
M.640 (Fig.)
dermatophytes, **M**.10, **M**.45–6, **M**.77, **M**.78–9,
M.221, **M**.221 (Tab.)
Telithromycin
spectrum of activity, **B1**.499 (Tab.)
structure, **B1**.486 (Fig.)
Tellurium, resistance to, **B1**.114
Telomere orientation, *Trypanosoma brucei,*
P.362
TEM-1 enzymes, **B1**.472–3
TEM-2 enzymes, **B1**.472–3
Temephos, water treatment, **P**.833–4
Temocillin
pharmacology, **B1**.475
spectrum of activity, **B1**.475
Temperate countries, *Trichuris trichiuria,*
P.718
Temperatures
antibacterial activity, **B1**.431–2, **B1**.431 (Tab.)
Brucella culture, **B2**.1735
Enterobacteriaceae culture, **B2**.1344,
B2.1345–6
food, **B1**.264–6
heat shock response, **B1**.74
hydrostatic pressure, **B1**.450
Neisseria culture, **B2**.1275
respiratory tract and viral infection, **V1**.240
susceptibility/resistance to
airborne bacteria, **B1**.187
Campylobacter, **B2**.1545
Clostridium, **B2**.1095
Haemophilus, **B2**.1695–6
Lactobacillus, **B2**.866
Legionella, **B2**.1777
Mycobacterium, **B2**.1216, **B2**.1217, **B2**.1242
Proteus, **B2**.1441
Streptococcus, **B2**.862
Temperature-sensitive mutants, **B1**.38
'Temporary immunity,' epidemiology, **I**.955
Tenofovir, **V2**.1625
HIV infection, **V2**.1334
resistance, **V2**.1337 (Fig.)
structure, **V2**.1617 (Fig.)
Tenuivirus
characteristics, **V1**.129 (Tab.)
classification, **V1**.27 (Tab.), **V1**.48, **V1**.127–8
Teratogenesis, *Parvovirus* infection, **V1**.425
Terbinafine, **M**.183 (Tab.), **M**.184, **M**.233
absorption, **M**.184
adverse effects, **M**.184
mechanism of action, **M**.70
therapy
blepharitis, **M**.297
chromoblastomycosis, **M**.364
dermatomycosis, **M**.252, **M**.253
nondermatophyte mold infection,
M.189
onychomycosis, **M**.187–8, **M**.187 (Tab.),
M.252, **M**.253

Paecilomyces infection, **M**.758
penicilliosis marneffei, **M**.571
Scopulariopsis infection, **M**.758–9
seborrheic dermatitis, **M**.212
sporotrichosis, **M**.380
superficial candidiasis, **M**.189
tinea, **M**.234, **M**.235
tinea barbae, **M**.186, **M**.187 (Tab.)
tinea capitis, **M**.188, **M**.188 (Tab.)
tinea cruris, **M**.186
tinea nigra, **M**.186
tinea pedis, **M**.186–7, **M**.187 (Tab.)
zygomycosis, **M**.352
Trichophyton rubrum resistance, **M**.175
Terconazole, vulvovaginal candidiasis, **M**.189
Tergitols, **B1**.432
Terminal inverted sequence region, poxviruses,
V1.601, **V1**.602–3, **V1**.603 (Fig.),
V1.606 (Fig.)
N-Terminal myristoylation, viral replication,
V1.122
Terminal proteins, adenoviruses replication,
V1.160
Terminal redundancy, reverse-transcribing
virus genome, **V1**.181–2
'Terminal resolution,' adeno-associated virus
genome replication, **V1**.419
Termocillin, structure, **B1**.474 (Fig.)
Ternidens, **P**.594–5
Ternidens deminutus, **P**.810–11
classification/morphology, **P**.810
control, **P**.811
infection
clinical manifestations/pathology,
P.810–11
diagnosis, **P**.811
life cycle, **P**.810
transmission/epidemiology, **P**.810
Teschovirus, **V1**.50–2
Testicular atrophy, mumps, **V1**.748, **V1**.749
Tetanospasmin *see Clostridium tetani*
Tetanus, **B1**.203, **B2**.1040–2, **B2**.1065–6
classification, **B2**.1065
cephalic, **B2**.1066
generalized, **B2**.1065–6
clinical features, **B2**.1036, **B2**.1065–6
diagnosis, **B2**.1066
epidemiology, **B2**.1041 (Tab.), **B2**.1065
etiology, **B2**.1042
historical perspective, **B2**.1037, **B2**.1040–2
immunization, **B2**.1065, **B2**.1066
laboratory workers, **B1**.767
local, **B2**.1066
milestones in understanding, **B2**.1038–42
neonatal, **B2**.1065, **B2**.1066
nosocomial, **B1**.401 (Tab.)
safety precautions, **B2**.1076
therapy, **B2**.1066
human tetanus Ig, **B2**.1066
transmission to CNS, **B2**.1065
vaccine
Salmonella vectors, **I**.842–3
USA schedules, **V2**.1560 (Fig.)
Vibrio cholerae vectors, **I**.844
Tetanus toxin, as adjuvant, **I**.925

Tetanus toxoid (TT), **B2**.1053, **B2**.1065
  as adjuvant, T-helper cell epitope,
    I.862 (Tab.)
  as carrier protein, **I**.862–3
    conjugate vaccines, **I**.935
    subunit vaccines, **I**.935
  vaccine, virosomes adjuvant, **I**.929
Tet gene, **B2**.1600
TetM gene, **B2**.1277
Tetracyclines, **B1**.485–6
  Balantidium coli infection, **P**.281
  cat-scratch disease treatment, **B2**.1898–9
  gonorrhea treatment, **B1**.662
  Helicobacter pylori infection treatment,
    B2.1575
  human brucellosis treatment, **B2**.1743
  mechanism of action, **P**.479
  mode of action, **B1**.485
  neutrophil abnormalities, **I**.49
  periodontal abscess, **B1**.614
  pharmacology, **B1**.485
  prototheccosis, **M**.401
  Q fever treatment, **B2**.2078
  resistance, **B1**.485
    Bacteroides/Prevotella/Porphyromonas,
      B2.1931
    Brucella, **B2**.1730
    Burkholderia thailandensis, **B2**.1621
    Chlamydia, **B2**.2020
    Fusobacterium, **B2**.1949
    Neisseria gonorrhoeae, **B1**.662, **B2**.1277,
      B2.1291–2
    Neisseria meningitidis, **B2**.1291–2
    Staphylococcus, **B2**.794 (Tab.), **B2**.803–4
    transposons, **B1**.485
  spectrum of activity, **B1**.485
    Actinobacillus actinomycetemcomitans,
      B2.1664
    Actinomyces, **B2**.1011
    Borrelia, **B2**.1830
    Brucella, **B2**.1742
    Campylobacter, **B2**.1548
    Cardiobacterium hominis, **B2**.1672–3
    Citrobacter, **B2**.1476
    Eikenella corrodens, **B2**.1668
    Enterobacter, **B2**.1484–5
    Escherichia, **B2**.1370
    Ewingella, **B2**.1493
    gram-positive anaerobic cocci, **B2**.912
    Haemophilus, **B2**.1702 (Tab.), **B2**.1703,
      B2.1710
    Klebsiella, **B2**.1480
    Lactobacillus, **B2**.866
    Leclercia, **B2**.1495
    Listeria, **B2**.956, **B2**.957–8
    Mycoplasma, **B2**.1992
    Pasteurella multocida, **B2**.1655
    Proteus, **B2**.1441, **B2**.1443–4
    Pseudomonas, **B2**.1600
    Streptococcus, **B2**.861–2
    Vibrio, **B2**.1514
  structure, **B1**.485, **B1**.485 (Fig.)
  syphilis, **B2**.1857–8
  toxicity/adverse effects, **B1**.485–6
  tularemia treatment, **B2**.1755

Tetradecanoylphorbol acetate (TPA), HHV-8
  cell culture, **V1**.544–5
Tetrahydromethanopterin, methanogenesis,
  B1.68, **B1**.69
Tetraploa aristata, oculomycoses, **M**.278 (Tab.),
  M.283–4
Tetrathionate reductase, bacterial
  identification, **B2**.1351
Tetrathyridium, **P**.578
Tetraviridae, **V1**.27 (Tab.), **V1**.51 (Tab.)
  see also specific viruses
Tetrazolium salts, antifungal testing, **M**.157
Tetroxoprim, **B1**.491
  structure, **B1**.491 (Fig.)
TGFB1 gene, **I**.582–3
  periodontitis association, **I**.595
Thailand virus (THAIV), **V2**.1666 (Tab.)
Thalassemias
  malaria resistance, **P**.485
    mechanism of action, **P**.478
  pythiosis, **M**.422
Thalidomide, microsporidiosis chemotherapy,
  P.549
Thallic conidiogenesis, **M**.77, **M**.79 (Fig.)
Thawing, **B1**.450
  microbial growth effect, **B1**.264–5
Theileria
  Babesia relationship, **P**.451–2
  structure, **P**.174 (Fig.)
Theileria annulata, **P**.165 (Fig.)
Theiler's murine encephalomyelitis virus
  (TMEV)
  cell-mediated immunity, **V2**.1414
  classification, **V2**.858
  immunopathology, **V1**.280
  infection, immunopathology, **V1**.279 (Tab.)
Theiler's virus, **V2**.1409–10
  infection, NK cells, **I**.96
Thelazia, **P**.595
Thelaziidae, **P**.595
Thelazioidea, **P**.595
T-helper cell(s), **P**.68
  B cell maturation/activation, **I**.348–9
  cryptosporidiosis, **P**.406
  cytokines released, **P**.68
  DNA vaccine response, **V2**.1553–4
  hepatitis C, **V2**.1206
  IL-2 effects, **I**.279–80
  intestinal nematode infection, **P**.90
  isosporiasis, **P**.412–13
  knockout mice, babesiosis, **P**.455
  schistosomiasis, **P**.94, **P**.606
  Th1/Th2 balance, **I**.29, **P**.72–3, **V1**.276,
    V1.298
    adjuvant effects, **I**.926
    antigen presentation, **I**.399
    autoimmune disease development, **I**.755–6,
      I.755 (Fig.)
    bacterial infection, **I**.665–6
    Borna disease virus infection, **V2**.1149–50
    CD1d-reactive αβ T cells, **I**.442
    common mucosal immune system, **I**.534–5,
      I.539 (Fig.)
    Crohn's disease, **I**.755–6
    delayed-type hypersensitivity, **I**.706,
      I.708–9

  dendritic cells, **I**.399, **I**.656
  diabetes mellitus type I, **I**.755–6
  granuloma formation, **I**.706
  HIV infection, **V1**.298, **V1**.300–1
  Human respiratory syncytial virus
    infection, **V1**.795–6
  IFN-γ effects, **I**.288
  IL-2 effects, **I**.279–80
  immunogenetics, **I**.580
  immunopathology, **V1**.292–3
  influenza virus infection, **V1**.298
  larval cestode diseases, **P**.690
  leishmaniasis, **I**.679
  malaria immunity, **P**.490
  multiple sclerosis, **I**.755–6
  neutrophils, **I**.46
  onchocerciasis, **P**.795–6
  oral tolerance, **I**.544
  peripheral tolerance, **I**.749
  rheumatoid arthritis, **I**.755–6
  schistosomiasis, **I**.724
  type 1 *see below*
  type 2 *see below*
  viral infection, **V1**.618–19
  see also CD4+ T-cell(s)
T-helper cells type 1 (Th1), **P**.69 (Fig.), **P**.72–3
  chemokine receptors, **I**.511–12
    CCR5, **I**.225
    CXCR3, **I**.225
  CpG effects, **I**.911, **I**.931
  cytokines produced, **P**.72–3, **P**.72 (Tab.),
    I.224, **V1**.292–3, **V1**.298
    IFN-γ, **I**.287–8
    IFN-γ secretion, **I**.397
    IL-17, **I**.290
    lymphatic filariasis, **P**.775–6
  defects, immunogenetics, **I**.576
  development/differentiation, **I**.29, **I**.397–9,
    I.398 (Fig.), **I**.399–400
    co-stimulation, **I**.399
    cytokines, **I**.398, **I**.399
    dendritic cell antigen presentation, **I**.903
    genetic background, **I**.400
    IFN-γ, **I**.398–9
    IL-12, **I**.29, **I**.398–9
    IL-12 effects, **I**.288
    IL-18, **I**.398–9
    IL-18 effects, **I**.290
    IL-23, **I**.398–9
    IL-27, **I**.398–9
  in diseases/infection
    allergic asthma, **I**.738–9
    bacterial infection, **I**.647, **I**.651,
      I.657 (Fig.)
    Brucella infection, **B2**.1736
    Burkholderia thailandensis infection,
      B2.1625–6
    candidiasis, **M**.261
      cutaneous/mucocutaneous, **M**.261–2
      gastrointestinal, **M**.262
      oropharyngeal, **M**.262–3
      vulvovaginal, **M**.264
    cerebral malaria, **P**.498
    cryptosporidiosis, **P**.406
    cystic echinococcosis, **P**.691

T-helper cells type 1 (Th1)
  in diseases/infection (*Continued*)
    filarial nematode infection, **P**.92
    granuloma formation, **I**.708–9
    HPV infection, **V1**.467–8
    intestinal nematode infection, **P**.90
    isosporiasis, **P**.412–13
    leishmaniasis, **P**.77–8
    malaria
      immunity, **P**.490–1
      pathogenicity, **P**.496
    measles, **I**.805
    Old World leishmaniasis, **P**.300
    protozoal infection, **P**.73, **P**.75
    pythiosis, **M**.426–7
    schistosomiasis, **P**.94–5, **P**.613
  functions, **I**.397–9
  historical aspects/re-evaluation, **I**.8
  IFN-γ receptor, **I**.251–2
  IgA, **I**.540 (Fig.)
  intramuscular DNA vaccine delivery, **I**.912
  mucosal vaccination, **I**.828
  NK cell interaction, **P**.94–5
  phenotypic markers, **I**.400
    CCR5, **I**.400
    E-selectin, **I**.400
    P-selectin, **I**.400
  Th2 antagonism, **I**.232
  see also T-helper cell(s), Th1/Th2 balance
T-helper cells type 2 (Th2), **P**.69 (Fig.), **P**.72–3
  chemokine receptors, **I**.511–12
    CCR3, **I**.224–5
    CCR4, **I**.225
    CCR8, **I**.225
  cytokines produced, **P**.72–3, **P**.72 (Tab.),
      V1.292–3, **V1**.298
    IL-4, **I**.224, **I**.280, **I**.397
    IL-5, **I**.224, **I**.280
    IL-6, **I**.280
    IL-10, **I**.280
    IL-13, **I**.280, **I**.294
    IL-17, **I**.290
    see also individual cytokines
  defects, immunogenetics, **I**.576
  dendritic epidermal γδ T cells, **I**.437
  development/differentiation, **I**.29, **I**.397–9,
      I.398 (Fig.), **I**.399–400
    co-stimulation, **I**.399
    cytokines, **I**.398, **I**.399
    genetic background, **I**.400
    histamine effects, **I**.66–7
    IL-4, **I**.66, **I**.280, **I**.281 (Fig.), **I**.399
    IL-10, **I**.399
    prostaglandin E₂, **I**.188
    transcutaneous immunization, **I**.837
  in diseases/infection
    airway hypersensitivity *see* Airway
        hypersensitivity/hyperreactivity
    ascariasis, **P**.729
    asthma, **I**.733–5
    bacterial infection, **I**.647, **I**.657 (Fig.)
    cryptococcosis, **M**.645
    cryptosporidiosis, **P**.406
    cystic echinococcosis, **P**.691

filarial nematode infection, **P**.91–2,
    P.93 (Fig.)
Giardia infection, **P**.76
granuloma formation, **I**.708–9
helminth infection, **I**.683, **I**.684
hookworms, **P**.729–30
intestinal nematode infection, **P**.90–1
leishmaniasis, **P**.77–8
lymphatic filariasis, **P**.776
malaria, **P**.491
measles, **V1**.726, **V2**.1433
Old World leishmaniasis, **P**.300
protozoal infection, **P**.73
pythiosis, **M**.427
schistosomiasis, **P**.94–5, **P**.613, **I**.719–20
toxocariasis, **P**.754
trichinellosis, **P**.764–5
trichuriasis, **P**.729
fetal infection transmission, **V2**.1443
functions, **I**.397–9
historical aspects/re-evaluation, **I**.8
IFN-γ receptor, **I**.251–2
phenotypic markers, **I**.400
  CCR3 (eotaxin receptor), **I**.400
  ST2L, **I**.400
responses
  aluminum salt adjuvant, **I**.926
  CpG adjuvant, **I**.926
  MF59 adjuvant, **I**.927
  monophosphoryl lipid adjuvant, **I**.929
  QS-21 adjuvant, **I**.930
  secondary lymphoid tissue, **I**.511–12
    Peyer's patches, **I**.538
  Th1 antagonism, **I**.232
  see also T-helper cell(s), Th1/Th2 balance
vaccine effects
  BCE peptide vaccines, **I**.864–8
  intradermal DNA vaccine delivery,
      I.912–13
  mucosal vaccination, **I**.828
  oral immunization, **I**.539
Therapeutic baths, **B1**.215
Therapeutic index, antiviral chemotherapy,
    V2.1610
Therapy-resistant Lyme arthritis (TRLA),
    I.753–4, **I**.754 (Fig.)
Thermal death point (TDP), **B1**.445–6
Thermal death time (TDT), **B1**.266, **B1**.270–1,
    B1.445–6
Thermized milk, **B1**.233
Thermoacidophilic Archaebacteria, **B1**.70
Thermoactiomyces, **B2**.1139
  microscopic morphology, **B2**.1143
Thermochemical treatment, **B1**.454
Thermoliability, Measles virus, **V1**.713–15
Thermophiles
  canning process, **B1**.283
  temperature range for growth, **B1**.264
Thermoplasma acidophilum
  metabolism, **B1**.70
  protein folding, **B1**.47
Thermoradiation, **B1**.454
Thermotolerance, *Mucor,* **M**.665
θ−replication, plasmid genes, **B1**.107

Thiabendazole
  adiaspiromycosis, **M**.821
  Angiostrongylus costaricensis infection,
      P.807–8, **P**.810
  chromoblastomycosis, **M**.364
  Strongyloides infection, **P**.742
  Ternidens deminutus infection, **P**.811
  trichinellosis, **P**.765–6
Thiacytidine *see* Lamivudine
Thiamphenicol
  development, **B1**.482–4
  Klebsiella, **B2**.1480
  structure, **B1**.484 (Fig.)
Thiara, Paragonimus intermediate host, **P**.646
Thienamycin, **B1**.478–80
Thièry reaction, **P**.176 (Fig.)
Thin layer chromatography (TLC), rapidly
    growing mycobacteria, **B2**.1242
Thiobacillus
  electron donors, **B1**.67
  sulfur oxidation, **B1**.201
Thiobacillus denitrificans
  denitrification, **B1**.200
  sulfur oxidation, **B1**.201
Thiobacillus novellus, **B1**.57
Thiobenzimidazolones
  HIV infection, **V2**.1336
  see also specific drugs
Thiocarbonates, **M**.233
  see also individual drugs
Thiogalactoside transacetylase, **B1**.71
Thiol oxidoreductases, poxviruses, **V1**.598–600
Thionin, *Brucella* species differentiation,
    B2.1735
Thionine blue, *Brucella* species differentiation,
    B2.1735
Thogoto virus, **V1**.50
  characteristics, **V1**.129 (Tab.)
  classification, **V1**.50
Thoracic actinomycosis, **M**.140 (Fig.)
Thorny-headed worms, **P**.595
Thosphaera, nitrification, **B1**.200
Thottapalayam virus, **V2**.1666 (Tab.)
Threadworms, **P**.593
Threonine metabolism, *Fusobacterium,*
    B2.1945, **B2**.1948
Thrombocyte growth factors, **I**.273–9,
    I.274 (Tab.)
Thrombocytopenia
  Anaplasma phagocytophilum infection,
      B2.2060
  babesiosis, **P**.455
  Bolivian and Argentine hemorrhagic fevers,
      V2.1070
  Ehrlichia chaffeensis infection, **B2**.2057–9
  malaria, **P**.501 (Tab.)
    vivax/ovale (benign tertian) malaria, **P**.482
Thrombocytopenia, IL-11, **I**.279
Thrombophlebitis, human brucellosis, **B2**.1738
Thrombospondin
  neutrophils, **I**.45
  type I repeats, **I**.476 (Fig.)
  upregulation in malaria, **P**.496–7
Thrombospondin-related anonymous protein
    (TRAP), **I**.676, **I**.873
  Cryptosporidium parvum classification, **P**.400

Thrombospondin-related anonymous protein (TRAP) (*Continued*)
Plasmodium, **P**.82
see also Malaria
Thrombotic thrombocytopenic purpura, **B1**.273–4
Thromboxane(s), **I**.189
actions, **I**.189
biosynthesis, **I**.189
cell production, **I**.189
production, **I**.189
structure, **I**.189
synthase, **I**.189
Thromboxane A$_2$ (TxA$_2$)
biosynthesis, **I**.183 (Fig.)
production, **I**.181, **I**.186–7
Thrush (oral candidiasis) *see* Oropharyngeal candidiasis (OPC)
Thymic epithelial tumors, EBV association, **V1**.571
Thymidine analogues
HIV infection, **V2**.1334
see also specific drugs
Thymidine kinase (TK)
herpesviruses, **V1**.499
HSV-1, **V1**.165 (Tab.), **V1**.499, **V1**.511–12
poxviruses, **V1**.169 (Tab.), **V1**.606
viral evolution, **V1**.14
Thymidylate kinase (TK), poxviruses, **V1**.606
Thymidylate synthase
herpesviruses, **V1**.500
HHV- 8, **V1**.500
VZV, **V1**.500
5-Thyminyl-5,6-dihydrothymine (TDHT), **B1**.452 (Fig.)
UV photoproduct, **B1**.451, **B1**.452
Thymosin, **M**.597
Thymus
antigen presentation, **I**.378–9
dendritic cells, **I**.377–8
HAART effects, **I**.798
HIV infection *see* HIV infection
NK cell development, **I**.85
T-cell development, **I**.404
Thymus-dependent areas, CD4 T cells development, **I**.393
Thymus expressed chemokine (TECK: CCL25), **I**.218 (Tab.)
CCR9 binding, **I**.227
Thyroid gland
carcinoma, TCE peptide vaccines, **I**.865 (Tab.)
PCP, **M**.785
Thyroiditis, mumps, **V1**.750
Thyroxine, acute phase response, **I**.208
'Tiacc-araña,' **P**.328
TIBO, **V2**.1621–2
structure, **V2**.1622 (Fig.)
Ticarcillin
history, **B1**.473
Pasteurella multocida, **B2**.1655
structure, **B1**.474 (Fig.)
Tick-borne encephalitis (TBE), **V2**.998 (Tab.), **V2**.1003–4, **V2**.1424, **V2**.1426
epidemiology, **V1**.373
E protein, **V2**.996 (Fig.)

incubation and clinical features, **V2**.1426
mortality, **V2**.1426
pathology, **V2**.1426
transmission, **V1**.372 (Tab.)
vaccine, **V2**.1552 (Tab.)
Tick-borne encephalitis virus (TBEV), **V2**.1424
attachment proteins, **V1**.208, **V1**.209 (Fig.)
CNS receptors, **V2**.1406 (Tab.)
glycoprotein E, **V1**.208, **V1**.209 (Fig.)
infection risk, **B1**.762
subtypes, **V2**.1424
Ticks
Anaplasma transmission, **B2**.2066–7
babesiosis transmission, **P**.458–9
prevention, **P**.460
Ehrlichia transmission, **B2**.2066–7
removal, **P**.460
repellents, **P**.460
Rickettsia isolation, **B2**.2037
Rickettsia transmission, **B2**.2037–8, **B2**.2040
van Tieghem, P E L, **M**.8–9
Tigecycline
development, **B1**.485
spectrum of activity, **B1**.499 (Tab.)
Tight junctions, disruption by bacteria, **B1**.557
T-independent antigens, B cell activation, **I**.326
Tinea
history, **M**.5–6
therapy
fluconazole, **M**.233
griseofulvin, **M**.233, **M**.234–5
itraconazole, **M**.233, **M**.234, **M**.235
ketoconazole, **M**.233–4
terbinafine, **M**.234, **M**.235
Tinea barbae
clinical presentation, **M**.231
epidemiology, **M**.228
facial hair, **M**.228, **M**.231
therapy, **M**.186, **M**.187 (Tab.)
ketoconazole, **M**.186
Tinea capitis
clinical presentation, **M**.231–2
epidemiology, **M**.227–8
folliculitis, **M**.231–2
histopathology, **M**.238
history, **M**.9–10, **M**.10–1
prevention, **M**.238
therapy, **M**.182, **M**.188, **M**.188 (Tab.), **M**.233
ciclopirox, **M**.188–9
econazole, **M**.234
ketoconazole, **M**.188–9
selenium sulfide, **M**.188–9, **M**.234
Tinea corporis
clinical presentation, **M**.231
nosocomial infection, **M**.228, **M**.238–9
prevention, **M**.239
recurrence, **M**.186
therapy, **M**.182, **M**.186, **M**.186 (Tab.), **M**.234
Tinea cruris
clinical presentation, **M**.231
epidemiology, **M**.228
groin, **M**.228, **M**.231, **M**.234, **M**.239
obesity, **M**.186
prevention, **M**.239

recurrence, **M**.186
therapy, **M**.182, **M**.186, **M**.186 (Tab.), **M**.234
fluconazole, **M**.186
griseofulvin, **M**.186
itraconazole, **M**.186
terbinafine, **M**.186
Tinea favosa
clinical presentation, **M**.232
favus, **M**.232, **M**.238
histopathology, **M**.238
Tinea imbricata, **M**.5–6
clinical presentation, **M**.232
Tinea manuum, **M**.232
hands, **M**.232
palms, **M**.232
therapy, **M**.186–7
fluconazole, **M**.186–7, **M**.187 (Tab.)
itraconazole, **M**.186–7, **M**.187 (Tab.)
terbinafine, **M**.186–7, **M**.187 (Tab.)
Tinea nigra, **M**.198–9
causative agents, **M**.195, **M**.198 (Fig.), **M**.199
clinical presentation, **M**.198
foot, **M**.198
hands, **M**.198
histopathology, **M**.139 (Fig.)
therapy, **M**.186, **M**.199
Tinea pedis, **M**.228, **M**.239
clinical presentation, **M**.231
epidemiology, **M**.228
foot, **M**.228, **M**.239
miners, **M**.228
prevention, **M**.239
therapy, **M**.186–7, **M**.187 (Tab.)
Tinea unguium
clinical presentation, **M**.232
epidemiology, **M**.228
histopathology, **M**.238
nails, **M**.228, **M**.234, **M**.238
therapy, **M**.234
see also Onychomycosis
Tinea versicolor *see* Pityriasis versicolor
Tinidazole
amebiasis, **P**.213
giardiasis, **P**.251
pharmacology, **B1**.495
structure, **B1**.495 (Fig.)
Tioconazole, **M**.234
onychomycosis/dermatomycosis therapy, **M**.252
Tioman virus, **V1**.818–19
Ti (tumor-inducing) plasmid, **B1**.202
Tipranavir, HIV resistance, **V2**.1337 (Fig.)
TIR-domain-containing adaptor protein (TIRAP), **I**.122
Tissierella, **B2**.1929
Tissierella praeacuta, **B1**.296 (Tab.), **B2**.1929
Tissue anoxia, gas gangrene pathogenesis, **B2**.1112, **B2**.1113
Tissue culture, **V1**.90
antiviral chemotherapy, **V2**.1608–9
HHV-6, **V1**.530
historical aspects, **V1**.3–4
influenza diagnosis, **V1**.674–5
virucidal activity, **B1**.435–6

Tissue donations, infection transmitted by, **B1**.381

Tissue edema, trichinellosis, **P**.761–2

Tissue factor inhibitor, septic shock therapy, **I**.702

Tissue factor, septic shock, **I**.699

Tissue migration, *Ascaris lumbricoides*, **P**.718–19

Tissue-specific tropism, bacterial adherence, **B1**.147–8

Tissues, specimens, **M**.83 (Tab.), **M**.84, **M**.86 (Tab.)

Tissue type plasminogen activator (tPA), **I**.203

T lymphocytes *see* T cell(s)

TMP-SMX therapy, PCP, **M**.764, **M**.783–4, **M**.789, **M**.790

Tn*1* transposon, **B1**.94 (Fig.)

Tn*3* transposon, **B1**.96

Tn*7* transposon, **B1**.93–4

Tn*19* transposon, **B1**.93–4

Tn*916* transposon, *Neisseria* mutagenesis, **B2**.1277

Tn*4001* transposon, **B2**.1985–6

TNF-α promoter gene, polymorphisms, malaria susceptibility, **P**.485–6

TNF gene *see* Tumor necrosis factor-α (TNF-α)

TNFRSFIA gene, mutations, **I**.571–2

Tobacco mosaic virus (TMV)
cellular entry, **V1**.215
electron microscopy, **V1**.59 (Fig.)
morphology, **V1**.6
phylogenetics, **V1**.174

Tobacco smoking
chronic bronchitis due to, **B1**.648
meningococci carriage, **B1**.563–4
Mycobacterium avium complex infection, **B2**.1207
respiratory tract infection, **B1**.626

Tobamovirus, **V1**.27 (Tab.)

Tobramycin
spectrum of activity, **B1**.482
Brucella, **B2**.1742
Enterobacter, **B2**.1485–6
Ewingella, **B2**.1493
Nocardia, **B2**.1145
structure, **B1**.483 (Fig.)

Tobravirus, **V1**.27 (Tab.)

Togaviridae
characteristics, **V1**.139 (Tab.), **V1**.177 (Tab.)
classification, **V1**.27 (Tab.), **V1**.51 (Tab.), **V1**.53
see also Togaviruses; *specific viruses*

Togaviruses, **V2.1010–24**
cell entry, **V1**.138–9
ligand conformational change, **V1**.139
classification, **V2**.1010–12
gene expression, **V1**.119
genome, **V1**.135–6, **V1**.136 (Fig.)
genome organization, **V1**.135–6
infection, **V1**.241 (Tab.)
IFN activity, **I**.260 (Tab.)
isolation/propagation and identification, **V1**.95, **V1**.96 (Tab.)
morphology/structure, **V1**.138, **V1**.395
mRNA structure, **V1**.139, **V1**.140 (Tab.)

mRNA translation, **V1**.113
particle assembly/release, **V1**.144
picornaviruses *vs.*, **V2**.861
post-translational protein modification, **V1**.140–1, **V1**.225
see also Alphaviruses; Rubivirus; *Rubivirus*, classification; Rubiviruses

Tokelau disease, **M**.5–6

Tolerance
B cell maturation/activation, **I**.348
central, **I**.749
historical aspects/re-evaluation, **I**.12
induction
dendritic cells, **I**.737
DNA vaccines, **I**.920
monoclonal antibody therapy, **I**.366
mucosal immune response *see* Mucosal immune response
mucosal vaccination, **I**.827
regulatory T-cell, **I**.396, **I**.397 (Tab.)
see also Oral tolerance
intranasal vaccination, **I**.830
mechanisms, **I**.748–51
NK cell development, **I**.94
oral *see* Oral tolerance
peripheral *see* Peripheral tolerance

Toll-like receptor(s) (TLRs), **I**.114 (Tab.), **I**.116–23, **B1**.176–7
actions/effects
acute phase response, **I**.194
antigen uptake, **I**.382
bacterial DNA recognition, **I**.696
chemokine expression, **I**.697
cytokine expression, **I**.697
dendritic cells, **I**.393–4
endothelial leukocyte adhesion molecule 1, **I**.697
inducible nitric oxide synthase, **I**.697
intercellular adhesion molecule 1, **I**.697
mucosal immune response, **I**.523–4
parasitic infection, **I**.679–80
proteasome binding, **I**.839
adjuvant effects, **I**.926
bacterial infection, **I**.652
cell expression
dendritic cells, **I**.750–1
eosinophils, **I**.64
intraepithelial αβ T cell, **I**.441
characteristics, **I**.116–18
deficiencies, **I**.771–2
discovery, **I**.116
historical aspects/re-evaluation, **I**.8
Human respiratory syncytial virus infection, **V1**.793–4
IL-1β (IL-1β) effects, **V1**.621
IL-1 receptor *vs.*, **I**.116
influenza, **V1**.662–3
ligands, **I**.119 (Tab.)
mammalian, **I**.117
microbial recognition, **I**.23–4, **I**.24 (Tab.)
lipoteichoic acid recognition, **I**.696
LPS recognition, **I**.696
prion diseases, **V2**.1383
septic shock, **I**.696
signaling, **V1**.270–1

signal transduction, **I**.116 (Fig.), **I**.117, **I**.122–3
evolutionarily conserved signaling intermediate in Toll pathways, **I**.122
IFN-regulatory factor-3, **I**.122–3
Myd88-dependent pathways, **I**.122
Myd88-independent pathways, **I**.122–3
single nucleotide polymorphisms, **I**.111, **I**.125
structure, **I**.117
tissue distribution, **I**.117–18
see also specific types

Toll-like receptor 1 (TLR-1), **I**.117 (Tab.), **I**.118–19
heterodimer formation, **I**.118–19
microbial recognition, **I**.926

Toll-like receptor 2 (TLR-2), **I**.117 (Tab.), **I**.118–19, **V1**.718–20, **V1**.719 (Tab.)
bacterial infection, **I**.652
dimerization, **I**.926
as LPS receptor, **I**.119
microbial recognition, **I**.926
septic shock, **I**.696
signal transduction, **I**.120 (Fig.), **I**.696

Toll-like receptor 3 (TLR-3), **I**.117 (Tab.), **I**.119–20, **V1**.270–1
double-stranded RNA binding, **I**.119
signal transduction, **I**.119

Toll-like receptor 4 (TLR4), **I**.117 (Tab.), **I**.120–1
bacterial infection, **I**.652
heat shock protein binding, **I**.926
LPS binding, **I**.121, **I**.926
MD-2, **I**.120–1, **I**.696
non-LPS ligands, **I**.121
respiratory syncytial virus fusion protein binding, **I**.121
septic shock, **I**.696
signal transduction, **I**.118 (Fig.), **I**.696, **I**.697 (Fig.)
TNF release, **I**.696

Toll-like receptor 5 (TLR-5), **I**.117 (Tab.), **I**.121
flagellin binding, **I**.121
in gastrointestinal disease, **I**.121
infection, **I**.121
signal transduction, **I**.121

Toll-like receptor 6 (TLR-6), **I**.117 (Tab.), **I**.118–19
heterodimer formation, **I**.118–19
microbial recognition, **I**.926

Toll-like receptor 7 (TLR-7), **I**.117 (Tab.), **I**.121–2, **V1**.270–1
bacterial infection, **I**.652
imidazoquinoline binding, **I**.121

Toll-like receptor 8 (TLR-8), **I**.117 (Tab.), **I**.121–2
imidazoquinoline binding, **I**.121

Toll-like receptor 9 (TLR-9), **I**.117 (Tab.), **I**.121–2
bacterial infection, **I**.652
DNA binding, **I**.122
CpG binding, **I**.911, **I**.926

Toll-like receptor-9 (TLR-9), **I**.896

Toll-like receptor 10 (TLR-10), **I**.118–19

Toll-like receptor 11 (TLR-11), **I**.117 (Tab.)

Tolnaftate, **M**.183 (Tab.), **M**.185, **M**.233
  mechanism of action, **M**.185
  therapy
    dermatophytoses, **M**.185
    Malassezia, **M**.185
    tinea corporis, **M**.186
    tinea cruris, **M**.186
TOL plasmids, **B2**.1597
Toludine blue O, *Pneumocystis,* **M**.787
Toludine red unheated serum test (TRUST),
    syphilis, **B2**.1845–6, **B2**.1846 (Tab.)
Toluene
  bioremediation, **B1**.201
  degradation, plasmids, **B1**.114
Tomatoes, pathogens, **B1**.282, **B1**.283
Tomato spotted wilt virus genome
  consensus sequences, **V2**.1031 (Tab.)
  panhandle structures, **V2**.1032 (Fig.)
Tombusviridae, **V1**.27 (Tab.), **V1**.51 (Tab.)
  see also specific viruses
Tonate virus (TONV), **V2**.1011 (Tab.)
TonB protein, **B1**.138–9
Tongue, normal microbiota, **B1**.609,
    B1.609 (Tab.)
Tonic signaling, BCR, **I**.342
Tonsils, **I**.533
  αβ T cells, **I**.533
  B cells, **I**.533
  biopsy, variant Creutzfeldt–Jakob disease
    diagnosis, **V2**.1386
  carcinomas, HPV infection, **V1**.464
  normal microbiota, **B1**.301
Topley, W W C, **B1**.337
Topografov virus, **V2**.1666 (Tab.)
Topoisomerase(s)
  HPV replication, **V1**.457
  Mycoplasma, **B2**.1979
  poxviruses, **V1**.168–9, **V1**.598–600, **V1**.606
  quinolones, **B1**.492
Topoisomerase I, SV40 genome replication,
    V1.153–4, **V1**.154 (Tab.)
Torovirus
  classification, **V1**.53, **V1**.390
  members, **V1**.392
  type species, **V1**.824–5
  see also Toroviruses
Toroviruses
  classification, **V1**.824–5, **V1**.824 (Tab.)
    characteristics, **V1**.823
  cyclic phosphodiesterase, **V1**.832–3
  genome, **V1**.825
    expression strategies, **V1**.829 (Fig.)
    non-translated region, **V1**.825–6
    overlaps, **V1**.827–8
    pseudoknot, **V1**.827–8
    regulatory elements, **V1**.825–6
    structure, **V1**.828 (Fig.)
    transcription-regulating sequence,
      V1.826–7
  hemagglutinin-esterase (HE), **V1**.827,
    V1.836 (Tab.), **V1**.838–9
  infection, **V1**.823, **V1**.841 (Tab.), **V1**.845–6
  membrane (M) protein, **V1**.827,
    V1.836 (Tab.)
  morphology/structure, **V1**.391 (Fig.), **V1**.825,
    V1.826 (Fig.)

nonstructural proteins, **V1**.832–6
  see also specific types
nucleocapsid (N) protein, **V1**.827, **V1**.836–7,
    V1.836 (Tab.)
replicase (RNA polymerase), **V1**.827–8,
    V1.832–5
  post-translational modification, **V1**.832
  proteinase domain, **V1**.832
  ribosomal frameshifting, **V1**.832
  RNA-dependent RNA polymerase
    activity, **V1**.833–4
  sequence analysis, **V1**.832
replication, **V1**.828–9
size, **V1**.825
spike (S) protein, **V1**.827, **V1**.836 (Tab.),
    V1.837–8
  neutralizing antibodies, **V1**.840
structural proteins, **V1**.836 (Tab.)
  see also specific types
subgenomic RNAs, **V1**.401, **V1**.828–31
transcription, **V1**.829–30
translation, **V1**.831–2
  see also Arteriviruses; Coronaviruses
TOR pathway, yeast growth/signal
    transduction, **M**.73
Torque-teno-minivirus (TTMV)
  classification, **V2**.1278 (Tab.)
  genetic heterogeneity, **V2**.1277
  genome, **V2**.1277
  infection, **V2**.1278
  laboratory diagnosis, **V2**.1280 (Tab.)
  nomenclature, **V2**.1277
  replication, **V2**.1278
Torque-teno-virus (TTV), **V2.1276–83**
  cell interactions, **V2**.1277–8
  classification, **V2**.1278 (Tab.)
  control, **V2**.1281
  discovery, **V2**.1276
  disease associations, **V2**.1280–1
  as emerging infection, **V2**.1653 (Tab.)
  epidemiology, **V2**.1280
  genetic heterogeneity, **V2**.1277
  genome, **V2**.1276–7
    open reading frames, **V2**.1277
    sequences, **V2**.1277
  infection, **V2**.1278–9
    dynamics, **V2**.1279 (Tab.)
    immune response, **V2**.1279
    self-limiting, **V2**.1278–9
    viremia, **V2**.1279
  laboratory diagnosis, **V2**.1279–80,
    V2.1280 (Tab.)
  nomenclature, **V2**.1277
  replication, **V2**.1278
  taxonomy, **V2**.1277
  virion structure, **V2**.1276–7
Torula histolytica, **M**.16, **M**.637–8
Torulopsis, oculomycoses, **M**.280 (Tab.)
Torulosis, **M**.637–8
Toscana virus infection, **V2**.1047
Tositumab, licensing, **I**.355 (Tab.)
Tospovirus, **V2**.1025
  characteristics, **V1**.129 (Tab.)
  classification, **V1**.50, **V2**.1026
  members, **V2**.1030 (Tab.)

Tospoviruses
  ambisense coding structure, **V2**.1035
  assembly/release mechanisms, **V2**.1041
  genome structure, **V2**.1034
    consensus sequences, **V2**.1031 (Tab.)
    gene organization, **V2**.1033 (Fig.)
    panhandle structures, **V2**.1032 (Fig.)
    S (small) segment, **V2**.1038
  infection, immune response, **V2**.1042
  NS$_S$ protein, **V2**.1038
  nucleocapsid (N) protein, **V2**.1038
  transport/budding, **V2**.1040
Total adenine nucleotide (TAN), **B1**.206
Total-body antiseptic treatment, **B1**.387
Total coliform bacteria test, **B1**.218
Total parenteral nutrition (TPN), nosocomial
    infection, **B1**.384
Totaviridae, *Leishmania,* **P**.335
Totiviridae, **V1**.27 (Tab.), **V1**.47 (Tab.), **V1**.48
  see also specific viruses
Toxascaris, **P**.590
Tox$^+$ bacteriophage, **B2**.984
Toxic concentration, antiviral chemotherapy,
    V2.1608–9
Toxic shock syndrome (TSS), **B1**.362, **I**.561,
    B1.668–9
  Mycoplasma arthritidis superantigen, **I**.562
  tampon association, **B1**.362
Toxic shock syndrome toxin-1 (TSST-1),
    B1.157 (Tab.), **I**.556, **I**.556 (Tab.),
    B1.668–9
  classification, **I**.557 (Tab.)
  frequency, **I**.557–8
  human *vs.* murine T cell binding,
    I.560 (Tab.), **I**.561
  nomenclature, **I**.556
  pathogenicity role, **I**.561
Toxigenicity tests, diphtheria diagnosis,
    B1.612–13
Toxin neutralization tests, **B1**.750
Toxins
  neutralization by antibody, **I**.312
  pattern recognition, **I**.110
  see also individual species; specific toxins
Toxocara, **P**.590, **P.750–6**
  general biology, **P**.750–1
    digestive physiology, **P**.750–1
    as facultative anaerobe, **P**.750–1
  infection *see* Toxocariasis
  life cycle, **P**.751–2, **P**.753 (Fig.)
    in definitive hosts, **P**.751–2
    in humans, **P**.752
  molecular biology, **P**.751
    in diagnosis, **P**.751
    internal transcribed spacer regions, **P**.751
  morphology/structure, **P**.750
    adults, **P**.750 (Fig.), **P**.751 (Fig.)
    eggs, **P**.751 (Fig.)
    larvae, **P**.751 (Fig.)
  structure/life cycle, **P**.590
  transmission/epidemiology, **P**.752
    children, **P**.752
    seasonal egg detection, **P**.752
    wild carnivores, **P**.752
  see also individual species

Toxocara canis
  immune evasion, **I**.685
  morphology/structure, **P**.750
Toxocara cati, morphology/structure, **P**.750
Toxocara malaysiensis, **P**.751
Toxocariasis
  clinical symptoms/manifestations, **P**.752–4
  control, **P**.755
    education, **P**.755
    pharmaceuticals, **P**.755
  covert, **P**.754
  diagnosis, **P**.754–5
    biopsies, **P**.754–5
    ELISA, **P**.754–5
    immunological methods, **P**.154
    life cycle effects, **P**.148
    serology, **P**.148
  historical aspects, **P**.750
  immune response, **P**.754
    basophils, **I**.68
    eosinophils, **I**.70
    granuloma formation, **P**.754
    hypersensitivity reactions, **P**.754
    IgE, **P**.754
    T helper cells type 2, **P**.754
  ocular larva migrans
    diagnosis, **P**.755
    prevalence, **P**.752
    treatments, **P**.755
    unilateral vision disorder, **P**.752
    visceral larva migrans *vs.,* **P**.752
  pathogenesis/pathology, **P**.754
    allergic manifestations, **P**.754
    asthmatic manifestations, **P**.754
    hypereosinophilic syndrome, **P**.754
    tissue dependency, **P**.754
  visceral larva migrans, **P**.750, **P**.752
    ocular larva migrans *vs.,* **P**.752
Toxoids, subunit vaccines *see* Subunit vaccines
'Toxoid', term, **B1**.155
Toxonemes *see* Micronemes (toxonemes)
Toxoplasma
  classification, **P**.197
    Isospora belli vs., **P**.411
    RNA technology, **P**.193
  immune evasion, **I**.681
  sporocysts, **P**.167 (Fig.)
  structure/life cycle, **P**.422–7
  see also Toxoplasmosis
Toxoplasma gondii, **P**.188, **I**.676–7
  AIDS, **P**.97
  antigens, **P**.428–9
  classification, **P**.192, **P**.422, **I**.675–6
  cultivation, **P**.428–9
  encystment, **I**.677
  enterotoxin, **I**.565–6
  genetic variability, **P**.429
  historical aspects, **P**.13, **P**.17–8
  immune evasion, **P**.77
  infection *see* Toxoplasmosis
  life cycle, **I**.676–7
  in milk, **B1**.231–2
  molecular biology/genetics, **P**.428–9

structure/life cycle, **P**.422–7
  bradyzoites, **P**.425, **P**.425 (Fig.),
    P.426 (Fig.)
  coccidian stage, **P**.428 (Fig.)
  enteroepithelial stages, **P**.428 (Fig.)
  gamonts, **P**.426–7, **P**.428 (Fig.)
  host cell penetration, **P**.423–5
  host cell receptors, **P**.423–5
  membranes, **P**.163 (Tab.)
  membranous tubular network, **P**.423–5
  micronemes (toxonemes), **P**.423
  oocysts, **P**.422, **P**.427, **P**.427 (Fig.),
    P.429 (Fig.), **P**.433 (Fig.)
  parasitophorous vacuole, **P**.423–5
  pellicle, **P**.423
  polar ring and conoid, **P**.423
  rhoptries, **P**.423
  schematic representation, **P**.427 (Fig.)
  sporocysts, **P**.422, **P**.427, **P**.429 (Fig.)
  surface coat, **P**.169 (Fig.)
  tachyzoites, **P**.422, **P**.424 (Fig.), **P**.427,
    P.428
  tissue cysts, **P**.425–6, **P**.425 (Fig.),
    P.426 (Fig.), **P**.427
  superantigens, **I**.556 (Tab.)
  transmission, **P**.433, **P**.436–7
  virulent strains, **P**.428, **P**.429
Toxoplasmosis, **P.422–42**
  in AIDS/HIV infection, **P**.78–9, **P**.85–6,
    P.432, **I**.676, **I**.677
    prophylactic treatment, **P**.438, **P**.438 (Tab.)
  animal infection, **P**.436, **P**.439–40
    canine, **P**.439–40
  classification, **P**.422
  clinical features, **P**.429–32, **P**.431 (Tab.)
  congenital, **P**.430–1, **P**.430 (Tab.), **P**.436
    prevalence, **P**.436–7
    socioeconomic impact, **P**.430–1
    treatment, **P**.438 (Tab.)
  diagnosis, **P**.431, **P**.432, **P**.434–5
    antibody titters, **P**.435
    ELISA, **P**.434–5
    immunological detection, **P**.154
    immunosorbent agglutination assay,
      P.434–5
    microscopy/staining, **P**.435
    PCR, **P**.435
    prenatal diagnosis, **P**.436 (Tab.)
    prenatal screening, **P**.435
    serological, **P**.434–5
  epidemiology, **P**.435–7
    incidence, **P**.429–30
    prevalence, **P**.435–6
  historical aspects, **P**.17–8, **P**.422, **P**.423 (Tab.)
  HLA association, **I**.597
  immune response, **P**.74, **P**.78–9, **P**.79, **P**.79–
    80, **P**.85–6, **P**.432–3
    acute infection, **P**.85–6
    CD8 T cell responses, **I**.420
    IL-2 pathway, **I**.772–3
    immune-mediated destruction, **P**.432
    NK cell actions, **I**.100
    tissue cyst persistence, **P**.432–3
  in immunocompromised
    immunosuppressed patients, **P**.432, **P**.433
    treatment, **P**.438 (Tab.)

nosocomial infection, **B1**.403
pathogenicity, **P**.433
pathology, **P**.433–4, **P**.434 (Fig.)
postnatally-acquired, **P**.431–2
  leukocyte transplants, **P**.432
  organ transplants, **P**.432
  reactivation, **P**.432
  risk, **P**.431
  treatment, **P**.438 (Tab.)
prevention/control, **P**.439–40
public health importance, **P**.44, **P**.45
T helper cell polarization, **P**.72–3
transmission, **P**.433
  blood transfusions, **P**.437
  routes, **P**.436–7
treatment (chemotherapy), **P**.437–9
  immunosuppressed patients, **P**.437–9
  in pregnancy, **P**.439
  prophylaxis, **P**.437–9
  schedules, **P**.438 (Tab.)
vaccination, **P**.439
  S48, RH and ts-4 strains, **P**.439
  T-263 bradyzoites, **P**.439
  vaccine development, **P**.79–80, **I**.933 (Tab.)
X-linked hyper-IgM-CD40 ligand deficiency,
  I.778
TP10, **I**.157–8, **I**.158 (Tab.)
Trabulsiella guamensis, **B2**.1498
  biochemical tests, **B2**.1319 (Tab.)
Trachea
  intubation, pneumonia after, **B1**.389–90
  normal microbiota, **B1**.302
Tracheal colonization factor (TCF), *Bordetella,*
  B2.1789 (Tab.), **B2**.1801
Tracheal cytotoxin (TCT), *Bordetella,*
  B2.1789 (Tab.), **B2**.1795
Tracheitis, **B1**.629
Tracheobronchitis
  aspergillosis, **M**.704
  dogs, **B2**.1810
  Moraxella (Branhamella) catarrhalis,
    B2.1307
Tracheobronchopneumonia, *Mycoplasma
  pneumoniae,* **B1**.633
Tracheostomy, pneumonia after, **B1**.389–90
Trachipleistophora
  classification, **P**.190–1, **P**.198, **P**.534
  infection *see* Microsporidiosis
  public health importance, **P**.45
  structure/life cycle
    binary fission, **P**.534
    meront, **P**.534
    sporophorous vesicles, **P**.532–4
  see also Microsporidians; *individual species*
Trachipleistophora anthropopthera
  human infection, **P**.542
    see also Microsporidiosis
  structure/life cycle, sporophorous vesicles,
    P.542
Trachipleistophora hominis
  classification, **P**.542
  human infection, **P**.542, **P**.543
    albendazole treatment, **P**.549–50
    insect vectors, **P**.544
    ocular infection, **P**.541

Trachipleistophora hominis
  human infection (*Continued*)
    see also Microsporidiosis
    morphology, **P**.542 (Fig.)
    structure/life cycle
      spores, **P**.530 (Fig.), **P**.531 (Fig.)
      sporophorous vesicles, **P**.533 (Fig.)
    in vitro culture, **P**.548
Trachoma, **B2**.2006, **B2**.2013–14
  blindness, **B2**.2013–14
  immune response pathology, **B2**.2009
  pannus formation, **B2**.2014 (Fig.)
  prevalence, **B2**.2010
  serotype differences, **B2**.2018
  therapy, **B2**.2021
Traditional Chinese medication, *Blastocystis hominis* infection, **P**.567
TRANCE, CD4 T cells, **I**.396
Transaldolase (TA), reactions, **B1**.57
Transbronchial biopsy, PCP, **M**.787
Trans-cobalamins, host resistance, **B1**.176
Transcription, **B1**.70
  Leishmania, **P**.296
  regulation, **B1**.122
  Trypanosoma cruzi, **P**.381
Transcriptional control sequences, HTLVs, **V2**.1285–7
Transcriptional regulation, TCR, **I**.458
Transcriptional regulators, herpesviruses, **V1**.499
Transcriptional silencing, DNA vaccines, **I**.916
Transcriptional termination sequence, DNA vaccines, **I**.910
Transcription enhancers, **V1**.113
Transcription factors
  AP-1, **V1**.335–6
  DNA virus replication, **V1**.148
  JC virus genome, **V1**.475 (Fig.), **V1**.476–7
Transcription-mediated amplification (TMA), **B1**.729–30, **B1**.729 (Fig.), **V2**.1537–8
  Chlamydia detection, **B2**.2019
Transcription-regulating sequence, arteriviruses, **V1**.826–7
Transcription signals, mycoplasmas, **B2**.1979–80
Transcription units, SV40, **V1**.482
Transcript-mediated amplification (TMA), Hepatitis C virus, **V2**.1213
Transcutaneous injection, viral infection by, **V1**.237–9, **V1**.238 (Tab.)
Transdermal powder delivery (TPD), **I**.822
Transduction, **B1**.98, **B1**.104–6
  bacteriophage analysis, **B1**.142
  discovery, **B1**.13
  generalized, **B1**.104–5
    plasmids, **B1**.105
    specialized *vs.*, **B1**.105
  oncogenes, **V1**.335
  specialized, **B1**.105–6
    generalized *vs.*, **B1**.105
Transfer factor, **M**.597, **M**.611
Transferin receptor, parvovirus binding, **V1**.422
'Transferosomes,' skin immunization, **I**.822
Transfer ribonucleic acid (tRNA), **B1**.42
  binding sites, **B1**.47

charged, **B1**.46, **B1**.47, **B1**.72
initiator, **B1**.47
Transferrin, **B1**.430
  bacterial iron sequestration of bound iron, **B1**.151
  histoplasmosis capsulati, **M**.527
  meningococcal requirement, **B1**.563
  receptors, *Neisseria gonorrhoeae*, **B2**.1284
Transferrin-binding proteins (Tbps), *Neisseria gonorrhoeae*, **B2**.1285
Transferrin receptors
  macrophages, **I**.25
  Trypanosoma brucei, **P**.355–6
  variants, **P**.363
Transfer RNA intergenic length polymorphism analysis (tDNA-PCR), **B2**.1609
Transfer RNAs, mycoplasmas, **B2**.1980
Transformation, **B1**.98, **B1**.99
  artificial competence *see* Artificial competence
  cultured cells, **V1**.330, **V1**.333 (Fig.)
  discovery, **B1**.13
  DNA fate, **B1**.100
  by DNA tumor viruses, **V1**.338
  DNA viruses, **V1**.171
  naturally competent species, **B1**.99–100
  Neisseria, **B2**.1276
  nonproductive, **V1**.205–6
  productive, **V1**.205
Transforming growth factor(s) (TGFs), **P**.70
Transforming growth factor-β (TGF-β), **I**.297
  actions/effects, **I**.28 (Tab.), **I**.296 (Fig.), **I**.297
    acute phase protein expression, **I**.197
    basophils, **I**.57
    class switching, **I**.331
    macrophage deactivation, **I**.27
    mucosal immune response, **I**.535–6
  activated fibroblasts, **M**.361
  in diseases/infection, **I**.297
    African trypanosomiasis, **P**.80
    bacterial immune interference, **I**.652–4
    Borna disease virus infection, **V2**.1150
    cryptosporidiosis, **P**.407
    experimental allergic encephalomyelitis, **I**.297
    HIV infection, **V1**.298–9, **V1**.301
    leishmaniasis, **P**.77–8, **I**.679
    lymphatic filariasis, **P**.775–6
    in neuro-AIDS, **V2**.1428
    onchocerciasis, **P**.796
    parasitic infection, **I**.297
    Plasmodium, **P**.83
    schistosomiasis granulomas, **I**.722–3
    toxoplasmosis, **P**.79
    tuberculosis, **I**.711, **I**.717
  homologue secretion, *Brugia malayi*, **I**.687
  immunogenetics, **I**.582–3
  lymphocyte migration into CNS, **V2**.1411
  production, **I**.28 (Tab.), **P**.72–3, **I**.297
    eosinophils, **I**.67
  septic shock therapy, **I**.702
  signal transduction, **I**.296 (Fig.)
  structure, **I**.297
Transfusion-acquired Chagas disease, **P**.379, **P**.392, **P**.395–6

Transfusions *see* Blood transfusions
Transgenic animals
  antibodies, **I**.365
  construction, **V1**.197
  linkage, **I**.572–3
  poliovirus receptor (PVR), **V1**.247
  prion diseases, **V2**.1352
  salmonellosis, **I**.593–4
Transgenic plants
  Escherichia coli fimbrial colonization factor CFa/I, **I**.829
  Escherichia coli heat-labile enterotoxin B, **I**.829
  hepatitis B surface antigen, **I**.828
  measles peptide vaccine, **I**.869
  murine rotavirus enterotoxin NSP4, **I**.829
  Norwalk virus capsid protein, **I**.829
Transient aplastic anemia, Parvovirus B19 virus infection, **V1**.411–12, **V1**.431
Transient infection, gene therapy, **V2**.1594
Transient protein expression, poxviruses, **V1**.617
Transitions, point mutations, **B1**.84–5
Transketolase-transaldolase (TK/TA) reactions, **B1**.57–8, **B1**.57 (Fig.), **B1**.62–3
Transmembrane activation signals, macrophages, **I**.24
Transmembrane domains
  αβ TCRs, **I**.458, **I**.460
  γδ TCRs, **I**.458, **I**.460
Transmissible gastroenteritis virus (TGEV), **V1**.392
  envelope (E) protein, **V1**.837
  genome
    packaging, **V1**.827
    structure, **V1**.831–2
  infection, **V1**.841 (Tab.)
    immune response, **V1**.840–1
  membrane (M) protein, **V1**.837
    antibody responses, **V1**.840
  replicase (RNA polymerase), **V1**.834
Transmissible gastroenteritis virus (TGEV) infection, **V1**.844—83
  diagnosis, **V1**.844–5
  epidemiology, **V1**.844
  immune response, **V1**.844
  pathogenesis, **V1**.844
  transmission, **V1**.844
Transmissible mink encephalopathy, **V2**.1363
Transmissible spongiform encephalopathies (TSEs) *see* Prion diseases
Transmission-blocking vaccination, malaria, **P**.515–16
'Transmission coefficient,' epidemiology, **I**.952–3
Transmission disequilibrium test (TDT), **I**.574
Transmission dynamics, **P**.56–63
  antigen diversity/strain structure, **P**.62–3
    antigenic change, **P**.62
    immune evasion, **P**.62
    repeated infection, **P**.62
    strain diversity maintenance, **P**.62–3, **P**.63 (Fig.)
  control of infection, **P**.64, **P**.64 (Fig.)
  cross-sectional surveys, **P**.56–7
    behavioral factors, **P**.56–7

Transmission dynamics
  cross-sectional surveys (*Continued*)
    infection resistance, **P.**56–7
    intensity *vs.* age, **P.**56–7, **P.**57 (Fig.),
      P.58 (Fig.)
    prevalence *vs.* age, **P.**54 (Fig.), **P.**56–7,
      P.58 (Fig.)
  immunity effects, **P.**61–2
    age-dependency, **P.**61, **P.**62 (Fig.)
    parasite numbers, **P.**50–1, **P.**61
    T helper cell ratios, **P.**61
  life cycles, **P.**57–9
    intermediate host effects, **P.**57–8
  parasite population growth constraints,
    P.59–61
    host immune system effects, **P.**59–61,
      P.61 (Fig.)
    life span effects, **P.**59–61
  prevalence *vs.* infection intensity, **P.**56–7
  reproductive success, **P.**57–9
    definition, **P.**58
    epidemiology, **P.**51
    life span effects, **P.**58–9, **P.**60 (Tab.),
      P.61 (Fig.)
    net reproductive success, **P.**58
    parasite population growth rate, **P.**58
    reinfection determination, **P.**58, **P.**59–61
    vector density effects, **P.**58
Transmission interruption, alphavirus control,
  V2.1018
Transmission of infection(s)s
  bacterial infection, **B1.**329
    airborne, **B1.**329
    direct contact, **B1.**329
    indirect contact, **B1.**377–80
    by inoculation, **B1.**380–4
    percutaneous, **B1.**310, **B1.**329
    spreading factors, **B1.**152, **B1.**153 (Tab.)
    waterborne, **B1.**375
      in hospitals, **B1.**375, **B1.**376
    see also Epidemiology of infection,
      bacterial infection
  classification, **I.**951, **I.**951 (Tab.)
  dynamics *see* Infection(s), mathematical
    models; Transmission dynamics
  infection mode, **I.**951
  modes, **B1.**310
  parenteral vaccination, **I.**819–20
  plasmid genes, **B1.**110
  source, **I.**951 (Tab.)
  viruses, **V1.**249–50, **V1.**354–5, **V1.**358 (Fig.)
    aerosols, **V2.**1403–4
    CNS infection, **V2.**1403–5
    direct contact, **V2.**1403–4
      influenza, **V1.**667
    direct transmission, **V1.**354, **V1.**358 (Fig.)
      aerosols, **V1.**354
      droplets, **V1.**354
      sexual contact, **V1.**354
      skin contact, **V1.**354
      vertical transmission, **V1.**354
    droplets, **V1.**239–40, **V2.**1403–4
    horizontal, **V1.**343–4
    indirect transmission, **V1.**354–5,
      V1.358 (Fig.)
      aerosol, **V1.**355

biological transmission, **V1.**355
droplet spread, **V1.**355
fomites, **V1.**354–5
infected dusts, **V1.**355
mechanical transmission, **V1.**355
vector transmission, **V1.**355
vehicles, **V1.**354–5
water-borne, **V1.**355
oncogenic viruses, **V1.**343–4
  congenital, **V1.**343–4
passive immunization, **V2.**1568
vectors, **V2.**1403–4
  see also Arthropod vectors
vertical, oncogenic viruses, **V1.**343–4
*see also specific diseases/infection; specific
  viruses*
Transmission rate, microparasite
  epidemiology, **P.**52
Transneuronal transport, viruses, **V2.**1405
Transovarian transmission, **V2.**1444 (Tab.)
  definition, **P.**452
  HCMV infection, **V2.**1448
  see also Fetal infection; Neonatal infection
Transplants, **M.**12
  adenovirus infection, **V1.**446
  aspergillosis, **M.**107–8, **M.**701–5
    invasive, **M.**701–5
    pulmonary symptoms, **M.**701–2
    risk factors, **M.**701
  chromoblastomycosis, **M.**359
  CMV intravenous Ig prophylaxis, **V2.**1566–7
  coccidioidomycosis, **M.**507–8, **M.**508–10,
    M.516
  diagnostic accuracy, **M.**82
  EBV-associated lymphomas, **V1.**570–1
  emerging bacterial infection, **B1.**362
  HCMV infection *see* Human
    cytomegalovirus (HCMV) infection
  hepatitis C transmission, **V2.**1204, **V2.**1209
  HHV-6 infection, **V1.**528–9, **V1.**529–30
  HHV-7 infection, **V1.**529–31
  intracranial abscess, **B1.**582
  microsporidiosis, **P.**537, **P.**539
  Nocardia asteroides infection, **B2.**1155–7
  rejection *see* Graft rejection
  sporotrichosis, **M.**375
  toxoplasmosis, **P.**437
  urinary tract infection, **B1.**673
  zygomycosis, **M.**21
  see also Bone marrow transplantation
    (BMT); Immunosuppressed patients;
    specific types
Transport, **B1.**48–50
  active, **B1.**49–50
    ATP-binding cassette, **B1.**49
    chemiosmotic driven transport systems,
      B1.49
    ion gradient-linked, **B1.**49
    periplasmic-binding protein-dependent,
      B1.49
    PTS system, **B1.**50
  facilitated diffusion, **B1.**48–9
    inducible, **B1.**50
  simple (passive) diffusion, **B1.**48–9
Transport (infectious materials), **V2.**1528–9
  emerging viral infection, **V2.**1658–9

Transporter associated with antigen processing
  (TAP), **I.**877
  antigen processing/presentation, **I.**413
  deficiencies, **I.**776
    chronic bronchopneumonitis, **I.**776
    NK cells, **I.**103
  DNA vaccine priming, **I.**914
  MHC class I assembly, **I.**408
  peptide selectivity, **I.**413
  polymorphisms, **I.**413
  viral immune interference, **I.**633
Transposable elements, **B1.**94
  bacteriophage Mu, **B1.**91
  F plasmid, **B1.**102
  short direct repeats, **B1.**94
Transposase, **B1.**96
Transposition
  conservative (cut-and-paste), **B1.**93 (Fig.),
    B1.95
  replicative, **B1.**93 (Fig.), **B1.**95
  rolling-circle, **B1.**95
  semi-conservative, **B1.**95
Transposition-delivery vectors, genetic
  manipulation, **B1.**124–5
Transposons, **B1.**91–4
  complex, **B1.**80, **B1.**91–2, **B1.**92–3
  composite, **B1.**80, **B1.**91–2
    classification, **B1.**93–4
  conjugative, **B1.**99
  DNA viruses *vs.*, **V1.**12
  historical perspective, **B1.**91
  insertion specificities, **B1.**94–5
  integrons, **B1.**97–8
  mutation methods, **B1.**97
    virulence genes, **B1.**97
  resistance genes, **B1.**111, **B2.**886
    β-lactamase production, **B1.**111–12
    tetracycline resistance, **B1.**485
  size, **B1.**91
  species
    Bacteroides, **B1.**93–4
    Enterococcus, **B2.**886
    Listeria, **B2.**956
    methicillin-resistant *Staphylococcus aureus*,
      B1.111
    Neisseria, **B2.**1276–7
  transposition functions, **B1.**96
  in viral evolution, **V1.**13–4
Trans-splicing
  Trypanosoma brucei, **P.**362
  Trypanosoma cruzi, **P.**381
Transsynaptic passage
  rabies, **V2.**1121–2
  viruses, **V2.**1405
Transthoracic echocardiography (TTE),
  B1.536–7
Transthyretin, **I.**205
Transversions, point mutations, **B1.**84
Traps, African trypanosomiasis vector control,
  P.369, **P.**370 (Fig.)
Trastuzumab, **I.**876–7
  licensing, **I.**355 (Tab.)
  mechanism of action, **I.**358

Trauma
  CNS infection complication
    intracranial abscess, **B1**.583, **B1**.584 (Tab.)
    subdural empyema, **B1**.591, **B1**.591 (Tab.)
  upper respiratory tract infection, **B1**.608
Travel, emerging bacterial infection, **B1**.360
Travelers
  coccidioidomycosis, **M**.506, **M**.508–9
  dermatophytosis, **M**.228–9
  laboratory safety, **M**.92
  penicilliosis marneffei, **M**.12, **M**.27, **M**.560,
    M.561, **M**.562
  tinea imbricata, **M**.5–6
Travelers' diarrhea
  Blastocystis hominis infection, **P**.563
  cyclosporiasis, **P**.415
  giardiasis, **P**.246, **P**.250
  microsporidiosis, **P**.539
  vegetables, **B1**.282
Travel history, African trypanosomiasis
  diagnosis, **P**.366
Tree nuts, **B1**.286–7
Tree shrews *(Tupaia)*, Borna disease virus
  infection, **V2**.1148
Trees, rooted/unrooted, **B1**.27 (Fig.), **B1**.28
T-regulatory (Tr) cells *see* Regulatory T-cells
  (Treg)
Trehalose
  fermentation, Enterobacteriaceae
    identification, **B2**.1319 (Tab.)
  mycobacterial cell wall structures, **B2**.1184
Trematoda, **P**.580–6
  classification, **P**.579–80, **P**.580–6
Trematodes, **P**.573, **I**.682
  classification, **P**.579–80, **P**.580–6
    Dicrocoelioidea, **P**.585
    Digenea, **P**.580–6
    Diplostomoidea, **P**.580, **P**.582
    Gymnophalloidea, **P**.582
    Opisthorchioidea, **P**.584–5
    Paramphistomatoidea, **P**.583–4
    Plagiorchioidea, **P**.585–6
    Schistosomatoidae, **P**.582
    Strigeida, **P**.579–80
    superfamilies, **P**.579–80
  life cycles, **P**.580–6, **I**.682
  structures, **P**.580–6, **P**.581 (Fig.)
  see also individual species
Tremellales, **M**.63, **M**.65 (Tab.)
Trench fever
  clinical manifestations, **B2**.1893–4
  epidemiology, **B2**.1893–4
  erythrocyte infection, **B2**.1893–4
  historical perspective, **B2**.1885, **B2**.1893–4
Trench mouth, **B1**.613–14
TrepChek, **B2**.1849
Treponema, **B2**.1858–60
  infection, **B2**.1858–9
  as normal microbiota, **B1**.296 (Tab.), **B1**.303
Treponema carateum, **B2**.1839 (Tab.)
Treponema denticola, **B2**.1859–60
  gingivitis, **B1**.614
Treponema minutum, **B2**.1860
Treponema pallidum, **B1**.662–3
  adhesins, **B1**.149, **B2**.1840–1

catabolism pathway, **B2**.1839–40
catalase absence, **B2**.1839
cellular constituents, **B1**.662
differentiating subspecies, **B2**.1853
energy metabolism, **B2**.1839
fibronectin, **B2**.1840–1
genome, **B1**.662
  sequencing, **B2**.1838–9
hemolysins, **B2**.1841
infection
  antigen masking, **B2**.1840
  cell adherence, **B1**.149, **B2**.1840–1
  conjunctivitis, **B1**.598–9
  dendritic cells, **I**.656
  macrophage phagocytosis, **B2**.1840–1
  neurotropism/neuroinvasivness, **B2**.1841
  slow recognition by host antibody, **B2**.1840
  see also Syphilis
iron sequestration, **B2**.1839
lipoproteins, **B2**.1840
molecular detection, **B2**.1851–3
  DNA probes, **B2**.1852
  early stage, **B2**.1842
  gene targets, **B2**.1852–3
  immunodominant 47kDa gene target,
    B2.1852–3
  late stage, **B2**.1843, **B2**.1855
  molecular typing, **B2**.1853
  nested primers, **B2**.1852
  polA genes, **B2**.1853
  problems, **B2**.1852
  rabbit infectivity testing *vs.,* **B2**.1852
  sensitivity, **B2**.1852
  tpr genes, **B2**.1852, **B2**.1853
morphology, **B1**.662
outer membrane proteins, **B2**.1840
purine and pyrimidine source, **B2**.1839–40
subspecies *endemicum*
  disease characteristics, **B2**.1839 (Tab.)
  molecular typing, **B2**.1853
subspecies *pallidum*
  antigens, **B2**.1859–60
  disease characteristics, **B2**.1839 (Tab.)
  molecular typing, **B2**.1853
subspecies *pertenue*
  disease characteristics, **B2**.1839 (Tab.)
  molecular typing, **B2**.1853
surface layer, **B2**.1840
tissue damage in vitro, **B2**.1841
tpr genes, **B2**.1840, **B2**.1852, **B2**.1853
virulence, fibronectin employment, **B1**.149
Treponema pallidum hemagglutination
  (TPHA) test, **B1**.663, **B2**.1848
Treponema pallidum immobilization (TPI)
  test, **B1**.746
Treponema pallidum particle agglutination
  (TP-PA) test, **B2**.1848–9
Treponema pallidum particle assay (TPPA)
  test, **B1**.663
Treponema paraluiscuniculi, **B2**.1853
Treponema pectinovorum, **B2**.1859–60
Treponema phagedenis, **B2**.1860
Treponema refringens, **B2**.1860
Treponema socranskii, **B2**.1859–60
Triatoma infestans, **P**.388–90

Triatoma sordida, **P**.390
Triatomine bugs, **P**.377 (Fig.)
  biology, **P**.390–1
  Chagas disease prevention, **P**.389, **P**.390
  control methods, **P**.394–5
    'Southern cone programme', **P**.395
    systematic approach, **P**.394–5
  insecticide resistance, **P**.394–5
  species, **P**.390
  Trypanosoma cruzi, development, **P**.379–80
Triazole antifungal agents, **M**.153
Tribromosalicylanilides, **B1**.428
Tricarboxylic acid (TCA) cycle, **B1**.52–3,
  B1.52 (Fig.)
  biosynthesis of intermediates, **B1**.61
  Neisseria gonorrhoeae, **B2**.1274–5
Tricarboxylic acid cycle, *Plasmodium*, **P**.476
Trichinella, **I**.682–3, **P.757–68**
  classification, **P**.757
  control, **P**.765–7
    chemotherapy, **P**.765–6
    prevention of infection, **P**.766
  general biology, **P**.757–8
    infectious stage, **P**.758
  historical aspects, **P**.757
  immune evasion
    outer membrane fluidity, **I**.684
    stage-specific antigens, **I**.685
  infection *see* Trichinellosis
  life cycle, **P**.588–9, **P**.758–9, **P**.763 (Fig.)
    enteric stages, **P**.760 (Fig.)
    ingestion, **P**.758–9
    migration route, **P**.758, **P**.759, **P**.759 (Fig.)
    Nurse cell formation, **P**.759, **P**.760 (Fig.)
  morphology/structure, **P**.588–9, **P**.757
    adult female, **P**.758 (Fig.), **P**.761 (Fig.)
    adult male, **P**.758 (Fig.)
    larvae, **P**.759 (Fig.)
    newborn larvae, **P**.758 (Fig.)
    Nurse cell complex, **P**.761 (Fig.),
      P.762 (Fig.), **P**.766 (Fig.)
  transmission/epidemiology, **P**.760
    prevalence, **P**.760
Trichinella spiralis, historical aspects, **P**.6–8
Trichinellidae, **P**.588–9
Trichinelloidea, **P**.588–9
  Trichinellidae, **P**.588–9
  Trichuridae, **P**.589
Trichinellosis
  clinical manifestations, **P**.761–2
    CNS, **P**.761
    'conjunctivitis,' **P**.766 (Fig.)
    dyspnea, **P**.762
    enteric stages, **P**.761, **P**.762 (Fig.), **P**.763–4
    myocarditis, **P**.761, **P**.762
    myositis, **P**.761
    parenteric stages, **P**.761–2
    photophobia, **P**.761–2
    tissue edema, **P**.761–2
  diagnosis, **P**.765
    eosinophilia, **P**.765
    immunoassays, **P**.154, **P**.765, **P**.766 (Fig.)
    muscle biopsy, **P**.153, **P**.765
  historical aspects, **P**.6–8

Trichinellosis (*Continued*)
  immune response, **P**.764–5
    anti-tyvelose reactions, **P**.764
    basophils, **I**.67–8
    eosinophils, **I**.70
    IL-s, **P**.764–5
    T helper cells type 2, **P**.764–5
  pathogenesis/pathology, **P**.762–4
    granulomas, **P**.762–3
    inflammation, **P**.762–3
Trichlorocarbanilide, **B1**.428
Trichloroisocyanuric acid, **B1**.424
Trichobilharzia, **P**.582
Trichomonad cell type, *Dientamoeba fragilis,*
  P.267
Trichomonadida, **I**.675–6
Trichomonas, **P**.187–8
  classification, **P**.196–7
  infection *see* Trichomoniasis
  see also individual species
Trichomonas foetus, immune response, **P**.76–7
Trichomonas hominis, immune response, **P**.76
Trichomonas vaginalis, **P**.187–8, **P.255–65**
  adhesion mechanism, **P**.260
  antigens, **P**.259
    adhesion to host cells, **P**.260
    antigenic drift, **P**.262
  biochemistry, **P.256–7**
    hydrolytic enzymes (proteinases), **P**.257
  'cell detachment factors', **P**.260
  classification, **P**.255, **I**.675–6
  control, **P**.262
  culture procedures, **P**.260–1
  infection *see* Trichomoniasis
  life-cycle, **P**.255–6
  molecular biology/genetics, **P.256–7**
  monoclonal antibodies, **P**.261
  nucleic acids, **P**.257
    nucleoside transport, **P**.257
    synthesis, **P**.257
  serotypes, **P**.259
  structure, **P**.255–6, **P**.256 (Fig.)
    apical pole, **P**.172 (Fig.)
    Golgi apparatus, **P**.177 (Fig.)
  transmission, **P**.259, **P**.261
  vaccines, **I**.933 (Tab.)
Trichomoniasis, **P**.255
  chemotherapy, **P**.262
  clinical features, **P**.257–8
    female, **P**.257–8
    men, **P**.257
  diagnosis, **P**.260–1
    immunological, **P**.262–1
    microscopy, **P**.260–1
    PCR method, **P**.261
    urine examination, **P**.152
  epidemiology/control, **P**.261
    prevalence, **P**.261
  epidemiology, HIV infection, **P**.261
  immune response, **P**.76–7, **P**.258–9
    antibody responses, **P**.258–9
    antigens, **P**.259
    cellular immune response, **P**.258
    immunoassays, **P**.258–9
    innate immunity, **P**.258

immunosuppression, **P**.258
integrated control, **P**.262
natural history, **P**.262
pathogenicity mechanisms, **P**.260
pathology, **P**.259–60
  histology, **P**.259–60
transmission, **P**.259, **P**.261
vaccination, **P**.262
Trichomycetes, classification, **M**.53
Trichophyton, **M**.220, **M**.221 (Tab.), **M**.222,
  M.222 (Tab.), **M**.223 (Tab.),
  M.226 (Tab.)
  classification, **M**.45–6, **M**.61, **M**.229
  growth requirements, **M**.237–8
  identification, **M**.222, **M**.237
    histopathology, **M**.128 (Tab.), **M**.238
    morphology, **M**.222, **M**.222 (Tab.),
      M.226 (Tab.)
Trichophyton ajelloi, **M**.10
  classification, **M**.229
Trichophyton concentricum, **M**.5–6,
  M.226 (Tab.), **M**.227 (Tab.)
  classification, **M**.230–1
  geographical distribution, **M**.229 (Tab.)
  infection, **M**.232
    inherited trait, **M**.232
  transmission, **M**.228
Trichophyton equinum, **M**.9–10, **M**.226 (Tab.),
  M.227, **M**.227 (Tab.)
  classification, **M**.230–1
  geographical distribution, **M**.229 (Tab.)
Trichophyton erinacei, **M**.226 (Tab.),
  M.227 (Tab.)
  epidemiology, **M**.227
  geographical distribution, **M**.229 (Tab.)
  infection, **M**.231
Trichophyton gouvilii, **M**.230
Trichophyton interdigitale, **M**.227 (Tab.)
  classification, **M**.230–1
  epidemiology, **M**.228
  geographical distribution, **M**.229 (Tab.)
  infection, **M**.231, **M**.232
Trichophyton megninii, **M**.226 (Tab.),
  M.227 (Tab.)
  classification, **M**.230–1
  geographical distribution, **M**.229 (Tab.)
  identification, **M**.237
  infection, **M**.231–2
Trichophyton mentagrophytes, **M**.6,
  M.226 (Tab.), **M**.227 (Tab.)
  classification, **M**.230–1
  epidemiology, **M**.225, **M**.227
  geographical distribution, **M**.229 (Tab.)
  germination, **M**.78–9
  griseofulvin resistance, **M**.177
  identification, **M**.237
  infection, **M**.231
    experimental, **M**.233
    inflammatory response, **M**.232
  transmission, **M**.239
  var. *erinacei see* Trichophyton erinacei
  var. *mentagrophytes,* **M**.225, **M**.227
  var. *quinckeanum*
    classification, **M**.230–1
    epidemiology, **M**.225, **M**.227
Trichophyton raubitschekii, **M**.237

Trichophyton rubrum, **M**.9–10, **M**.223,
  M.226 (Tab.), **M**.227 (Tab.)
  classification, **M**.230–1
  epidemiology, **M**.228
  geographical distribution, **M**.228–9,
    M.229 (Tab.)
  identification, **M**.237
  infection, **M**.231, **M**.232
    inflammatory response, **M**.232
    susceptibility, **M**.232
    therapy, **M**.234
  resistance
    griseofulvin, **M**.177, **M**.234
    terbinafine, **M**.175
Trichophyton schoenleinii, **M**.226 (Tab.),
  M.227 (Tab.)
  classification, **M**.230–1
  epidemiology, **M**.228
  geographical distribution, **M**.229 (Tab.)
  infection, **M**.232
Trichophyton simii, **M**.226 (Tab.), **M**.227 (Tab.)
  geographical distribution, **M**.229 (Tab.)
Trichophyton soudanense, **M**.226 (Tab.),
  M.227 (Tab.)
  classification, **M**.230
  epidemiology, **M**.225
  geographical distribution, **M**.228–9
  infection, **M**.231–2
Trichophyton tertestre, **M**.229
Trichophyton tonsurans, **M**.226 (Tab.),
  M.227 (Tab.)
  classification, **M**.230–1
  epidemiology, **M**.227–8
  geographical distribution, **M**.228–9,
    M.229 (Tab.)
  history, **M**.4
  infection, **M**.231–2
    nosocomial, **M**.228, **M**.238–9
    therapy, **M**.233
Trichophyton verrucosum, **M**.226 (Tab.),
  M.227 (Tab.)
  classification, **M**.230–1
  culture, **M**.236–7
  epidemiology, **M**.225, **M**.227
  geographical distribution, **M**.229 (Tab.)
  history, **M**.9–10
  infection, **M**.231–2
    experimental, **M**.233
    inflammatory response, **M**.232
  vaccines, **M**.233
  transmission, **M**.239
Trichophyton violaceum, **M**.226 (Tab.),
  M.227 (Tab.)
  classification, **M**.230
  epidemiology, **M**.228
  geographical distribution, **M**.229 (Tab.)
  history, **M**.9–10
  infection, **M**.231–2
Trichophyton yaoundei, classification, **M**.230
Trichosporon, **M**.195, **M**.197
  amphotericin B resistance, **M**.172
  characteristics, **M**.632, **M**.632 (Tab.)
  classification, **M**.63, **M**.65 (Tab.), **M**.632
  Filobasidiella, **M**.197
  histopathology, **M**.89 (Tab.)
  identification, **M**.197, **M**.198 (Tab.), **M**.633

Trichosporon, (*Continued*)
  infection *see* Trichosporonosis
  morphology, **M**.633
Trichosporon asahii, **M**.196, **M**.196 (Fig.),
    M.198 (Tab.), **M**.630, **M**.630 (Tab.),
    M.633
  oculomycoses, **M**.280 (Tab.)
  see also Trichosporonosis
Trichosporon asteroides, **M**.633
Trichosporon beigelii see Trichosporon
    cutaneum (T. beigelii)
Trichosporon capitatum, **M**.128 (Tab.)
Trichosporon cutaneum (T. beigelii), **M**.196,
    M.198 (Tab.), **B1**.403, **M**.632, **M**.633
  AIDS, **M**.629
  echinocandin resistance, **M**.154
  histology, **M**.629
  history, **M**.11
  identification, histopathology, **M**.128 (Tab.),
    M.135 (Fig.)
  infection, **M**.629, **M**.629 (Fig.)
    fungemia, **M**.629
    immunosuppression, **M**.109, **M**.629
    see also Trichosporonosis
  morphology, **M**.633
Trichosporon inkin, **M**.196, **M**.196 (Fig.),
    M.197 (Fig.), **M**.198 (Tab.), **M**.630,
    M.630 (Tab.), **M**.633
Trichosporon louberi, **M**.630, **M**.630 (Tab.)
Trichosporon mucoides, **M**.197, **M**.197 (Fig.),
    M.198 (Tab.), **M**.630, **M**.630 (Tab.),
    M.633
Trichosporonosis, **M**.625 (Tab.), **M**.629,
    M.629 (Fig.), **M**.630 (Tab.)
  amphotericin B therapy, **M**.629–30
  blepharitis, **M**.297
  catheter infection, **M**.629
  clinical presentation, **M**.629
  diagnosis, **M**.125–7
  fungemia, **M**.629, **M**.630
  histology, **M**.629
  histopathology, **M**.128 (Tab.), **M**.135 (Fig.)
  immunosuppression, **M**.109
Trichosporon ovoides, **M**.197, **M**.198 (Tab.),
    M.633
Trichosporon pullulans, **M**.630, **M**.630 (Tab.)
Trichostrongylidae, **P**.595
Trichostrongyloidea, **P**.595
Trichostrongylus, **P**.595, **P**.812–13
  classification/morphology, **P**.812
  clinical manifestations/pathology, **P**.813
  control, **P**.813
  diagnosis, **P**.813
  infection, **I**.60, **I**.70
  life cycle, **P**.812
    eggs, **P**.813 (Fig.)
  transmission/epidemiology, **P**.812–13
Trichovirus, **V1**.27 (Tab.)
Trichuriasis
  clinical manifestations, **P**.728–9
    growth stunting, **P**.729
    iron-deficient anemia, **P**.719–20, **P**.728–9
    morbidity, **P**.725
    rectal bleeding, **P**.728–9
    rectal prolapse, **P**.728
    secondary bacterial infection, **P**.728

  control, **P**.130
    school-age children, **P**.125
    heterogeneity/infection predisposition, host
      genetic factors, **P**.55
    immune response, **P**.90–1, **P**.729
      IL-9, **I**.282
    infection establishment, **P**.721
    morbidity, **P**.42
    mortality, **P**.28 (Tab.), **P**.29 (Tab.)
    public health importance, **P**.105 (Tab.)
Trichuridae, **P**.589
Trichuris, **P**.589, **I**.682–3
  zoonotic infection, **P**.715 (Tab.)
  see also Trichuriasis; *individual species*
Trichuris muris, **P**.88–9
Trichuris suis, **P**.715 (Tab.)
Trichuris trichiuria, **P**.713
  biology/feeding, **P**.714 (Tab.), **P**.718,
    P.719–20
  classification, **P**.715
  epidemiology/population biology, **P**.42,
    P.46 (Tab.), **P**.722
    age-related prevalence, **P**.42, **P**.722–3,
      P.722 (Fig.)
    global distribution/abundance, **P**.42, **P**.722
    infection predisposition, **P**.724
    intensity, **P**.723–4, **P**.723 (Fig.)
    number of worms per host, **P**.724,
      P.724 (Fig.)
    prevalence, **P**.713–14
    temperate countries, **P**.718
  immunity effects, age-dependency, **P**.62 (Fig.)
  immunogenetics, **I**.600
  infection *see* Trichuriasis
  life cycle, **P**.718, **P**.718 (Tab.), **P**.720 (Fig.)
  life expectancy, **P**.60 (Tab.)
  morphology, **P**.717–18
    eggs, **P**.716 (Fig.), **P**.717–18
    stichosome, **P**.718
Trichuris vulpis, **P**.715 (Tab.)
Triclabendazole, fascioliasis, **P**.654
Triclosan, **B1**.422
  handwashing, **B1**.766
  resistance, **B1**.436–8, **B1**.441
    biocide-antibiotic linked, **B1**.443
Trifluorothymidine *see* Trifluridine
Trifluridine, **V2**.1615
  structure, **V2**.1611 (Fig.)
Triiodothyronine, acute phase response, **I**.208
Trimethoprim
  mode of action, **B1**.492
  pharmacology, **B1**.492
  resistance
    Brucella, **B2**.1730
    plasmid resistance genes, **B1**.113
    Salmonella Typhi, **B2**.1416
    Staphylococcus, **B2**.794 (Tab.), **B2**.804
  spectrum of activity, **B1**.491, **B1**.499 (Tab.)
    Campylobacter, **B2**.1548
    Escherichia, **B2**.1370
    Haemophilus, **B2**.1702 (Tab.), **B2**.1703,
      B2.1704
    Listeria, **B2**.956, **B2**.957–8
  structure, **B1**.491 (Fig.)
  toxicity/adverse effects, **B1**.492

    toxoplasmosis, **P**.438
Trimethoprim–sulfamethoxazole *see* Co-
    trimoxazole (trimethoprim-
    sulfamethoxazole)
Trimetrexate, PCP, **M**.789
Trimming enzymes, antigen processing,
    I.412–13
Triose-phosphate isomerase, schistosomiasis
    vaccine, **P**.94, **P**.618–19, **P**.633 (Tab.),
    P.634
Triphenylmethane dyes, **B1**.427–8
Trismus (lockjaw), **B2**.1065
  see also Tetanus
Trisodium phosphate, **B1**.422–4
Tritirachium oryzae, oculomycoses,
    M.275 (Tab.)
Tritons, **B1**.432
Triton shell, **B2**.1959–60, **B2**.1986
Tritrpticin
  antimicrobial activity, **I**.172
  mechanism of action, **I**.172
  structure, **I**.172
Trocara virus (TROCV), **V2**.1010,
    V2.1011 (Tab.)
Trochostrongylus colubriformis infection,
    I.68
Troglotrematidae, **P**.586
'Trogocytosis', **P**.232
Tropheryma, **B2**.998, **B2**.1137–8, **B2**.1170–1
Tropheryma whippelii, **B2**.998
  antibacterial susceptibility/resistance,
    B2.1002
  classification, **B2**.998, **B2**.999–1000
    phylogeny, **B2**.999–1000
  culture, **B2**.1000–1
  definition, **B2**.998
  epidemiology and pathogenicity, **B2**.999
  genetics, **B2**.1002–3
  historical perspective, **B2**.998–9
  identification, **B2**.1001–2
    molecular, **B2**.1147–8, **B2**.1170–1
    strain differentiation, **B2**.1002
  infection
    bone and joint infection, **B1**.690–1
    endocarditis, **B1**.533
    see also Whipple's disease
  morphology, **B2**.1000 (Fig.), **B2**.1001 (Fig.)
Trophozoites
  Balantidium coli, **P**.275–6, **P**.276 (Fig.),
    P.277 (Fig.), **P**.278 (Fig.)
  Chilomastix mesnili, **P**.271 (Fig.)
  Cryptosporidium parvum, **P**.400
  Dientamoeba fragilis, **P**.267, **P**.269
  Endolimax nana, **P**.223
  Entamoeba coli, **P**.220–1
  Entamoeba gingivalis, **P**.221, **P**.221 (Fig.)
  Entamoeba moshkovskii, **P**.222, **P**.222 (Fig.)
  Entamoeba polecki, **P**.222
  Enteromonas hominis, **P**.270, **P**.271 (Fig.)
  Iodamoeba bütschlii, **P**.223–4
  Plasmodium see Plasmodium
  Plasmodium falciparum sequestration, **P**.472
  Retortamonas intestinalis, **P**.271 (Fig.)
  sequestration, **P**.472
Tropical diseases, historical aspects, **P**.4–5

Tropical pulmonary eosinophilia (TPE), lymphatic filariasis, **P**.774–5

Tropical spastic paraparesis (TSP) *see* HTLV-associated myelopathy(HAM)/tropical spastic paraparesis (TSP)

Tropical splenomegaly syndrome *see* Hyperactive malarial splenomegaly (tropical splenomegaly syndrome)

Tropism, viral, **V1**.244–9, **V2**.1405–6
  cell receptors affecting, **V1**.245–7
  mechanism, **V1**.247–8
  viral dissemination affecting, **V1**.244–5

Trousseau, A., **M**.13

TRUGENE®, **B1**.733

Trypanosoma, **P**.188
  classification, **P**.197, **I**.675–6
    anomalies/changes, **P**.191, **P**.192
    New World/Old World, **P**.191
  immune evasion
    intracellular refuge, **I**.681
    MHC inhibition, **I**.681–2
  immune evasion, antigenic change, **P**.62
  South American (New World), **P**.80, **P**.188
    infection *see* Chagas disease
  structure, **P**.162, **P**.163 (Fig.)
    flagella, **P**.179–80
    trypomastigote, **P**.163 (Fig.), **P**.165 (Fig.)
  see also individual species

Trypanosoma brucei, **P**.352–3, **I**.677–8
  biochemistry, **P**.358–61
    aerobic conditions, **P**.359
    amino acid synthesis, **P**.360
    anaerobic conditions, **P**.359
    energy metabolism, **P**.359
    glucose metabolism, **P**.359, **P**.359 (Fig.)
    glycolysis, **P**.357
    glycolytic enzymes, **P**.359
    lipids, **P**.360–1
    purine synthesis, **P**.360
    redox-regulation, **P**.359–60
    in vector, **P**.359
  classification, **P**.192, **P**.352–3
    restriction fragment length polymorphisms, **P**.352
    zymodeme analysis, **P**.352
  exo/endocytosis, **P**.355, **P**.357 (Fig.)
  immune evasion, **P**.353–5
    see also below, variable surface glycoprotein
  infection *see* Trypanosomiasis, African
  latent period, **P**.61 (Tab.)
  life cycle, **P**.80, **P**.357–8, **P**.358 (Fig.), **I**.677–8
    epimastigote, **P**.357–8
    immune response in vector, **P**.357
    metacyclic forms, **P**.357–8
    procyclic forms, **P**.357, **P**.360
    uptake by vector, **P**.357
  molecular biology/genetics, **P**.361–3
    cell division, **P**.362
    genetic information exchange, **P**.361
    ploidy, **P**.361–2
    RNA editing, **P**.362
    telomere orientation, **P**.362
    transferrin receptor variants, **P**.363
    transplicing, **P**.362

morphology, **P**.350 (Fig.)
  monomorphic forms, **P**.356–7
  pleomorphism, **P**.356–7
  slender forms, **P**.357
  stumpy forms, **P**.356–7
structure, **P**.80, **P**.353–8, **P**.353 (Fig.)
  cytoskeleton, **P**.356 (Fig.)
  flagellar pocket, **P**.355–6
  flagellum, **P**.353, **P**.355–6
  glycosome, **P**.353, **P**.359
  kinetoplast, **P**.353
  surface structure, **P**.353–5
  transferrin receptor, **P**.355–6
  Trypanosoma cruzi vs., **P**.192
  variable surface glycoprotein, **P**.353–5, **P**.354 (Fig.)
    antigenic variation, **P**.353–5, **P**.362
    gene switching, **P**.362
    metacyclic forms, **P**.362
    mutation, **P**.362
    new variant antigen types, **P**.362
    outer membrane attachment, **P**.353–5
    release from membrane, **P**.355
  vector, life expectancy, **P**.61 (Tab.)
  in vitro cultivation, **P**.358–9

Trypanosoma brucei brucei, **P**.191
  classification, **P**.351–2
    zymodeme analysis, **P**.352
  human serum effects, **P**.352–3
  infection, **P**.15, **P**.351
    see also Trypanosomiasis, African

Trypanosoma brucei gambiense, **P**.188, **P**.350
  classification, **P**.191, **P**.192, **P**.351–2
    zymodeme analysis, **P**.352
  epidemiology, **P**.368
  general biology, **P**.363 (Tab.)
  geographic distribution, **P**.352
  historical aspects, **P**.15
  immunity, **P**.80
  infection *see* Trypanosomiasis, African

Trypanosoma brucei rhodesiense, **P**.188, **P**.350
  classification, **P**.191, **P**.192, **P**.351–2
    zymodeme analysis, **P**.352
  epidemiology, **P**.368
  general biology, **P**.363 (Tab.)
  geographic distribution, **P**.352
  historical aspects, **P**.15
  immunity, **P**.80
  infection *see* Trypanosomiasis, African
  serum resistance-associated gene, **P**.353

Trypanosoma congolense, **P**.352
  human serum effects, **P**.352
  infection, **P**.15, **P**.351

Trypanosoma cruzi, **P**.188, **I**.678, **P.376–98**
  AIDS, **P**.97
  amastigotes, **P**.378–9
    fusiform transformation, **P**.379
    orbicular cycle transformation, **P**.379
  antigens, cross-reactive, **P**.387–8
  attenuated strains, **P**.393–4
  biochemistry, **P**.380–4
    proteinases, **P**.381
  classification, **P**.191, **P**.192, **P**.377
  culture, **P**.379

epidemiology
  'clonal hypothesis,' **P**.383
  geographical distribution, **P**.391
epimastigotes, **P**.378
experimental models, **P**.379
genetic diversity, **P**.382–4, **P**.382 (Fig.)
  PCR analyses, **P**.382–3
genetic exchange between strains, **P**.383
historical aspects, **P**.13, **P**.15–6, **P**.376–7
immune response, **P**.77, **P**.80, **P**.86–7
  immune evasion, **P**.77, **P**.86, **P**.87, **P**.385–6
  resistance to, **P**.385
infection *see* Chagas disease
life cycle, **P**.86, **P**.377–80, **P**.378 (Fig.), **I**.680
  development in triatomine bugs, **P**.379–80
  hosts, **P**.391
  insect vectors, **P**.382
  mammalian species infected, **P**.391
  pseudo-cyst, **P**.378, **P**.378 (Fig.)
  survival in host, **P**.385
molecular biology, **P**.381–2
  discontinuous transcription, **P**.381
  gene cloning, **P**.381–2
  mini-exon genes, **P**.381
  plasmic/cosmid shuttle vectors, **P**.382
  RNA editing of transcripts, **P**.381
reference strains, **P**.382–3
structure, **P**.377–80
  extranuclear DNA, **P**.377–8
  flagellum, **P**.377–8
  glycosome, **P**.377–8
  kinetoplast, **P**.377–8
  'reservosomes', **P**.177–8
transmission, **P**.86, **P**.376, **P**.379
  blood transfusions, **P**.27–9, **P**.379, **P**.392, **P**.395–6
  congenital, **P**.379, **P**.392
  non-vectorial, **P**.392
  oral, **P**.379, **P**.392
  sexual, **P**.379
  silvatic cycles, **P**.391–2
  vectors, **P**.390–1
Trypanosoma brucei vs., **P**.192
Trypanosoma rangeli vs, **P**.388–9
trypomastigotes, **P**.378, **P**.378 (Fig.)
types, **P**.379
zymodemes, **P**.382–3, **P**.383–4
  Z1, **P**.383–4
  Z1, Z2 and Z3 strains, **P**.383
Trypanosoma equiperdum, classification, **P**.352
Trypanosoma evansi, classification, **P**.352
Trypanosomal macrophage activating factor (TMAF), **P**.80
Trypanosoma rangeli, **P**.188, **P**.376–7
  life-cycle, **P**.379–80
  Trypanosoma cruzi vs, **P**.388–9
Trypanosomatida, **P**.350
Trypanosomatidae, **P**.283
Trypanosoma vivax, **P**.352
  flagellum, **P**.180 (Fig.)
  human serum effects, **P**.352
  infection, **P**.15, **P**.351
  kinetoplast, **P**.174 (Fig.)
  structure, surface coat, **P**.169 (Fig.)

Trypanosome-derived lymphocyte triggering factor (TLTF), **P.**80

Trypanosomes, African, **P.**80, **P.**188
  antigenic variation, **P.**80, **P.**169
    discovery, **P.**15
  classification, **P.**351–3
  historical aspects, **P.**15
  immune evasion
    antigen variation, **I.**680
    variant surface glycoproteins, **I.**680
  immunity, **P.**80–1
    killing/lysis mechanisms, **P.**80–1
  infection *see* Trypanosomiasis, African
  structure, **P.**162, **P.**163 (Fig.)
    pellicles, **P.**162, **P.**163 (Tab.)
    surface coat, **P.**168 (Fig.), **P.**169, **P.**169 (Fig.)
    variant surface glycoprotein, **P.**80, **P.**169
  variant antigen types, **P.**80, **P.**169
  see also Trypanosoma brucei; Trypanosoma brucei gambiense; Trypanosoma brucei rhodesiense

Trypanosomiasis
  control
    diagnosis, **P.**143 (Tab.)
    serology, **P.**129–30
    stratification of disease, **P.**133 (Tab.)
    vector elimination, **P.**109
  HLA association, **I.**597
  immune response, NK cell actions, **I.**100
  South American *see* Chagas disease
  vaccines, **I.**933 (Tab.), **I.**941

Trypanosomiasis, African, **P.350–75**
  causative organism *see Trypanosoma brucei*
  chemotherapy, **P.**370–1, **P.**372 (Tab.)
    azathioprine, **P.**371
    difluormethylornithine, **P.**371
    drug-resistant strains, **P.**371
    melarsoprol, **P.**371
    pentamidine isethionate, **P.**371
    suramin, **P.**370, **P.**371
    surveillance/detection, **P.**370
  clinical aspects, **P.**363–4, **P.**364 (Tab.)
    chancre, **P.**363–4
    CNS, **P.**365
    edema, **P.**365
    encephalopathy, **P.**365
    fibrosis, **P.**365
    inflammatory lesions, **P.**365
    lymphadenopathy, **P.**365
    'Morula cells of Mott,' **P.**365
    parasitemia waves, **P.**363, **P.**364–5, **P.**364 (Fig.)
    phase 1 disease, **P.**363–4
    phase 2 disease, **P.**364
    phase 3 disease, **P.**364
    reproductive capacity, **P.**366
    splenomegaly, **P.**364, **P.**365
    variant specific antibody, **P.**364–5
  control, **P.**368–70
    chemotherapy/chemoprophylaxis, **P.**30, **P.**144 (Tab.)
    conflict-related effects, **P.**107 (Tab.)
    economics, **P.**30, **P.**370
    environmental conditions, **P.**368–9

Global Alliance for African Human Trypanosomiasis, **P.**110
    individual surveillance/treatment, **P.**368–9
    reservoir host removal, **P.**125, **P.**368
    stratification of disease, **P.**115
    vector control *see below*
  diagnosis, **P.**366–7
    immunoassays, **P.**367
    lymph node biopsy, **P.**367
    serology, **P.**366–7
    symptoms, **P.**366
    travel history, **P.**366
    in vitro cultivation, **P.**367
  epidemiology, **P.**46 (Tab.), **P.**363, **P.**368, **P.**368 (Tab.)
    epidemics, **P.**142 (Tab.)
    geographical distribution, **P.**29–30, **P.**350, **P.**351, **P.**367
    incidence, **P.**367
    prevalence, **P.**29–30, **P.**367
    travellers, **P.**29–30
  historical aspects, **P.**15, **P.**351
  immune mechanisms, **I.**681
  immunology/pathology, **P.**80–1, **P.**364–6
    Arthus reaction, **P.**365
    B cell depletion, **P.**80–1
    CTLs, **P.**81
    cytokine network, **P.**81 (Fig.)
    encephalopathy, **P.**365
    humoral response, **P.**80–1
    IgG, **P.**365
    IgM, **P.**365
    immunodepression, **P.**80–1
    immunosuppression, **P.**365–6
    macroglobulinemia, **P.**365
    resistant hosts, **P.**366
    susceptible hosts, **P.**364–6
    variant-specific antibody, **P.**81
  incidence, **P.**351
  mortality, **P.**28 (Tab.), **P.**29 (Tab.)
  public health importance, **P.**29–30, **P.**105 (Tab.), **P.**351
    economic effects, **P.**30
  signs/symptoms, **I.**677–8
  vaccination, **P.**371
  vector *see* Tsetse flies (*Glossina*)
  vector control, **P.**125, **P.**145 (Tab.), **P.**368–70
    disposable screens, **P.**369, **P.**370 (Fig.)
    insecticide application, **P.**369
    secondary host insecticide dipping, **P.**369
    sterile fly release, **P.**369–70
    traps, **P.**369, **P.**370 (Fig.)

Trypanothione, *Trypanosoma cruzi* metabolism, **P.**380

Trypanozoon, **P.**351

Trypsin, **B2.**1924 (Tab.)

Tryptophan deaminase, *Proteus,* **B2.**1435

Tryptophan operon, regulation, **B1.**72

Tsetse flies (*Glossina*), **P.**350–1
  elimination, **P.**125
  trypanosomiasis discovery, **P.**15

TSST-A, CD4 T cell interactions, **I.**394–5

Tst-1 transcription factor, JC virus, **V1.**476–7

Tsukamurella, **B2.**1137–8, **B2.**1171–4
  antibacterial susceptibility/resistance, **B2.**1145
  classification, **B2.**1137–8
  lysozyme, **B2.**1144
  microscopic morphology, **B2.**1141–3
  staining properties, **B2.**1139–40
  substrate decomposition, **B2.**1144
  temperature studies, **B2.**1144

Tsukamurella inchonensis, **B2.**1173

Tsukamurella paurometabola, **B2.**1171–3
  infection, **B2.**1172–3
  strain typing, **B2.**1148, **B2.**1171–2

Tsukamurella pulmonis, **B2.**1173

Tsukamurella strandjordae, **B2.**1174

Tsukamurella tyrosinosolvens, **B2.**1173–4

TTM viruses *see* Torque-teno-minivirus (TTMV)

TT viruses *see* Torque-teno-virus (TTV)

Tubal factor infertility, *Chlamydia trachomatis* infection, **B2.**2010–11

Tubercularia vulgaris, oculomycoses, **M.**275 (Tab.)

Tuberculins, **B2.**1185

Tuberculin skin tests, **B1.**746–7, **B2.**1185

Tuberculomas, **B2.**1201
  subpial, **B1.**575

Tuberculosis, **B2.**1197–203
  in AIDS *see* AIDS, concomitant infection
  bcg allele, **B2.**1203
  bovine *see Mycobacterium bovis* infection
  causative agents, **B2.**1198
    see also Mycobacterium bovis; Mycobacterium tuberculosis
  cell infection
    complement, **I.**649
    dendritic cells, **I.**656
    macrophages, **I.**30
    microfold (M) cells, **I.**532
  in children, **B2.**1200–1
  chronic necrotizing pulmonary aspergillosis, **M.**697
  clinical features, **I.**710–11, **B2.**1200–2
    melioidosis *vs.,* **B2.**1627–8
    postprimary, **B2.**1201–2
    primary, **B2.**1200–1
  diagnosis, **B2.**1189–97
    cross-reactivity, **B1.**746–7
    evoked gamma IFN assays, **B1.**747
    Heaf test, **B1.**746
    laboratory, **B2.**1189–97
    latent infection, **B1.**746
    Mantoux test, **B1.**746
    microscopic, **B2.**1190
    specimens for, **B2.**1190
    tuberculin skin tests, **B1.**746–7
  drug-resistant, **B2.**1199–200
    refugees, **B1.**360
  emerging bacterial infection
    breakdown in public-health infrastructure, **B1.**364
    refugees, **B1.**360
  epidemiology, **B2.**1198–9
    drug resistance, **B2.**1199–200
    impact of HIV pandemic, **B2.**1199
    Mycobacterium bovis disease, **B2.**1200

Tuberculosis
  epidemiology (*Continued*)
    transmission, **I**.711
  gastrointestinal nematode infection, **P**.730
  genetic resistance, **I**.711
  granulomas
    calcification, **B2**.1201 (Fig.)
    formation, **B2**.1202
  hematogenous spread, **B2**.1200–1
  historical aspects, **B2**.1197–8
  in HIV infection *see* AIDS
  HLA association, **I**.591
    HLA-A9, **I**.592
    HLA-B14, **I**.592
    HLA-DPB1, **I**.592
    HLA-DQA1, **I**.592
    HLA-DQB1, **I**.592
    HLA-DR2, **I**.592
    HLA-DR3, **I**.592
  immune response
    αβ T cells, **I**.445
    cellular immunity, **B2**.1202
    genetic factors, **B2**.1203
    HLA-E reactive CD8+ T-cells, **I**.443
    immunity, **I**.711–3
    macrophage activation, **B2**.1202
    NK cell actions, **I**.99
    protective immunity, **B2**.1202–3
    tissue-necrotizing hypersensitivity, **B2**.1202–3
  immunodeficiency, **I**.713
  immunogenetics, **I**.591–3
    HLA association *see above*
    IL1 gene cluster, **I**.591–2
    MBL gene, **I**.591–2, **I**.592–3
    SLC11A1 (NRAMP1) gene, **I**.591–2, **I**.592–3
    twin studies, **I**.591
    UBE3A gene, **I**.591–2
    VDR gene, **I**.591–3
  miliary, **I**.711
  morbidity, **P**.26 (Fig.)
  mortality, **P**.26 (Fig.), **P**.28 (Tab.), **P**.29 (Tab.)
  necrotic granulomas (type 1), **I**.709–10, **I**.710–17
    animal models, **I**.714–15, **I**.715 (Fig.), **I**.716 (Fig.)
    caseation, **I**.713, **I**.715 (Fig.)
    chemokines, **I**.724–5
    collagen degradation, **I**.717
    cytokines, **I**.713
    formation, **I**.712 (Fig.), **I**.713–7
    granulocytes, **I**.717
    histology, **I**.710 (Fig.), **I**.713 (Fig.), **I**.714 (Fig.), **I**.716 (Fig.)
    macrophage necrosis, **I**.712–13
    mediators, **I**.718 (Tab.), **I**.724 (Tab.)
    metalloproteinases, **I**.717
    morphology, **I**.713
    neutrophils, **I**.713
    therapy, **I**.717
    transforming growth factor-β, **I**.717
  nosocomial, **B1**.373, **B1**.399
    airborne spread, **B1**.373
    risk of infection, **B1**.399

paragonimiasis *vs.,* **P**.650
pathogenesis, **I**.711–3, **I**.724–5
  local mediator release, **I**.711
  T cell proliferation, **I**.711
  tubercules, **I**.711
post-primary disease, **I**.711
prevention, **B2**.1219
  contact tracing, **B2**.1219
  see also BCG vaccine
protective immunity, **I**.711–12
  IFN-γ, **I**.711
  transforming growth factor-β, **I**.711
reactivation, measles, **I**.804
as systemic disease, **I**.711
therapy
  standard chemotherapy regimen, **B2**.1219
  WHO regimens, **B2**.1219
types
  cerebral, **B2**.1201 (Fig.)
  endogenous reactivation, **B2**.1199
  exogenous reinfection, **B2**.1199
  miliary, **B2**.1200–1
  milk-associated, **B1**.229
  multidrug-resistant, **B1**.399
  post-primary, **B2**.1201–2
  'primary complex', **B2**.1201
  pulmonary, **B2**.1200, **B2**.1201 (Fig.)
  skin, **B1**.382
  spinal, **B2**.1201 (Fig.)
  urinary tract, **B1**.678
vaccines, **I**.903, **I**.933 (Tab.)
  DNA vaccines, **I**.717
  MPL/QS-21 adjuvant, **I**.930
  'prime-boost immunization,' **I**.846
  subunit vaccine development, **I**.938, **I**.940
  see also BCG vaccine
Tuberculostearic acid (TBSA), **B2**.1184
Tularemia
  bioterrorism, **B1**.768
  causative agents, **B2**.1752
    see also Francisella
  clinical features, **B2**.1754–5
    conjunctivitis, **B1**.598–9
    endocarditis, **B1**.532
    pharyngitis, **B1**.611–12
    ulceroglandular, **B2**.1754–5
  diagnosis, **B2**.1754
    EIAs, **B1**.752
  geographical distribution, **B2**.1752, **B2**.1753
  historical aspects, **B2**.1752
  immune response, **B2**.1756–8
    animal models, **B2**.1756
    immunity to, **B2**.1756–7
  laboratory exposure, **B2**.1753, **B2**.1754, **B2**.1757
  immunization, **B1**.767
  in macrophage, **B2**.1755
  mortality, pre-antibiotics, **B2**.1755
  pathogenesis, **B2**.1754–5
  risk categorization, **B1**.762–3
  routes of infection, **B2**.1754–5
  treatment, **B2**.1755
  vaccine development, **B2**.1757–8
Tula virus, **V2**.1666 (Tab.)
'Tumbling', flagella movement, **B1**.44

Tumor necrosis factor(s) (TNFs), **P**.70–2, **V1**.296
  babesiosis, **P**.456
  Lassa virus, **V2**.1072
  poxvirus receptors, **V1**.257
  viral receptor homologues, **V1**.318
Tumor necrosis factor-α (TNF-α), **P**.70, **I**.285–6, **I**.288 (Tab.), **M**.794–5
  actions/effects, **I**.28 (Tab.), **P**.68–9, **I**.286, **I**.287 (Fig.)
    acute phase response, **I**.194–5, **I**.195 (Fig.)
    AIDS, **I**.286
    antigen presentation, **I**.384
    basophils, **I**.57, **I**.58
    cachexia, **I**.286
    death-inducing signaling complex assembly, **I**.134
    defensin induction, **I**.520–1
    dendritic cells, **I**.378, **I**.393–4
    dependent-kiling, NK cells, **I**.81
    eosinophils, **I**.58, **I**.60
    eotaxin release, **I**.61
    E-selectin expression, **I**.506–7
    ICAM-1 upregulation, **I**.60
    IL-13 suppression, **I**.294–7
    IL-17 synergy, **I**.290
    lung host defence mechanism, **B1**.625
    monocytes, **I**.286
    neutrophils, **I**.37, **I**.43, **I**.44, **I**.286
    nitric oxide synthase regulation, **P**.73
    2'-5' oligo adenylate synthetase, **V1**.296
    prostaglandin, **I**.187
    tumors, **I**.286
    vascular endothelial growth factor upregulation, **I**.286
  bacterial immune interference, **I**.652
  cells producing, **V1**.296
  CNS expression, **V2**.1409–10
  in diseases/infection
    AIDS-dementia complex (ADC), **V1**.304
    candidiasis resistance, **M**.259–60
    cerebral malaria, **P**.83–4, **P**.498
    Chagas disease, **P**.86
    Dengue fever, **V1**.296
    DNA virus infection, **V1**.296
    EBV, **V1**.296, **V1**.301–2, **V1**.302–3
    granuloma formation, **I**.708
    hepatitis B, **V1**.284, **V1**.303
    HHV-6, **V1**.296
    histoplasmosis capsulati, **M**.528
    HIV, **V1**.299, **V1**.300
    HSV-1, **V1**.301–2
    HTLV-1-associated myelopathy/tropical spastic paraparesis (HAM/TSP), **V2**.1429–30
    Human respiratory syncytial virus, **V1**.296
    influenza, **V1**.296
    intestinal nematode infection, **P**.90
    leishmaniasis, **P**.77–8, **I**.596
    malaria, **P**.495–6
      immunity, **P**.490–1
      pathology/pathophysiology, **P**.495–6, **P**.496 (Fig.), **P**.497–8
    measles, **V1**.727
    microsporidiosis in AIDS, **P**.539
    neurocysticercosis, **P**.690

Tumor necrosis factor-α (TNF-α)
in diseases/infection (*Continued*)
Plasmodium, **P**.83
poxviruses, **V1**.621–2
RNA virus infection, **V1**.296
schistosomiasis, **P**.94–5, **P**.616–17
septic shock, **I**.286, **I**.697
toxoplasmosis, **P**.78–9
tuberculosis, **I**.715, **I**.717
Vaccinia virus, **V1**.621–2
Variola virus, **V1**.621–2
viral CNS infection, **V1**.303–4, **V2**.1410
in viral infection, **I**.286
Yersinia infection, **I**.138
IL-6, **V1**.296
mucosal immune response, **I**.522–3, **I**.525
polymorphisms, malaria epidemiology, **P**.512
production, **I**.28 (Tab.), **I**.285–6
CD8 T cells, **I**.421–2
CpG effects, **I**.911, **I**.931
eosinophils, **I**.67
intradermal DNA vaccine delivery,
I.912–13
keratinocytes, **I**.820–1
macrophages, **P**.68–9, **V1**.272–3
neutrophils, **I**.47
NK cells, **I**.81
prostaglandin E$_2$ effects, **I**.188
superantigen stimulation, **I**.561
TLR-4 stimulus, **I**.696
proteasomes, **I**.411
receptor analogue secretion, **V1**.621–2
receptors, **I**.286
IL-10 effects, **I**.292–3
viral homologues, **I**.620–1
structure, **I**.285
suppression, heat labile enterotoxin, **I**.652
therapeutic uses
DNA vaccine co-administration, **I**.918,
I.918 (Tab.)
monoclonal antibody blocking, **I**.357
septic shock treatment, **B1**.393
TNF gene
leishmaniasis association, **I**.596, **I**.597
malaria association, **I**.598–9
polymorphisms, **I**.577–8
hepatitis C, **I**.587–8
HTLV infection, **I**.586
nematode infection, **I**.600–1
Tumor necrosis factor-β (TNF-β:
lymphotoxin), **P**.70–2, **I**.286–7,
I.288 (Tab.)
actions/effects, **I**.286–7
eosinophil apoptosis, **I**.58
eotaxin release, **I**.60–1
neutrophil priming, **I**.43, **I**.44
cerebral malaria, **P**.495
gene *see LTA* gene
granuloma formation, **I**.708
HHV-6 infection, **V1**.301–2
LTα, **I**.286–7
apoptosis induction, **I**.286–7
receptor, **I**.286–7
LTβ, **I**.286–7
malaria immunity, **P**.491

prion diseases, **V2**.1378, **V2**.1379 (Fig.),
V2.1380
production, **I**.286, **V1**.296
eosinophils, **I**.67
neutrophils, **I**.45
Th1 cells, **I**.224
structure, **I**.286
Tumors *see* Cancer(s)
Tumor suppressor genes, **V1**.334
DNA vaccine effects, P048.
Tumor virology, **V1.330–52**
historical background, **V1**.330–4
implication in cancer etiology
genetic susceptibility, **V1**.344–5
host response, **V1**.346–7
multi-step oncogenesis, **V1**.345–6
new viruses, **V1**.347
non-cytolytic virus-host interactions,
V1.345
virus infection/transmission, **V1**.343–4
incidence, **V1**.330–3, **V1**.331 (Fig.)
management principles, **V1**.347–50
infection prevention, **V1**.347–9
neoplasia development prevention, **V1**.349
therapy, **V1**.349–50
multi-step development of cancer, **V1**.345–6
retrovirus-associated tumors, **V1**.330,
V1.331 (Tab.)
risk factors, **V1**.341–3, **V1**.343 (Fig.)
RNA viruses associated, **V1**.331 (Tab.)
see also Tumor viruses; *specific viruses*
Tumor viruses
antiviral therapy, **V1**.349
carriers, **V1**.347–8
direct pathogenic mechanisms, **V1**.334
gene disruption, **V1**.339–40
'hit and run', **V1**.340
insertional mutagenesis, **V1**.336–40,
V1.339 (Fig.)
oncogenes, **V1**.334–6, **V1**.345–6
proto-oncogenes role, **V1**.340
DNA viruses, **V1**.332 (Tab.)
genome integration, **V1**.345
immunity, **V1**.348–9
immunotherapy, **V1**.349–50
indirect pathogenic mechanisms, **V1**.340–1
cell death, **V1**.341
growth factor synthesis, **V1**.341
immune impairment, **V1**.341, **V1**.342 (Tab.)
superantigens, **V1**.341
infection prevention, **V1**.347–9
new, **V1**.347
pathogenic mechanisms, **V1**.334–41,
V1.342 (Tab.)
direct *see above*
indirect *see above*
risk factors, **V1**.341–3, **V1**.343 (Fig.)
RNA viruses, **V1**.331 (Tab.)
susceptibility, **V1**.344–5
transmission/infection, **V1**.343–4
vaccines, **V1**.348–9
virulence, **V1**.253–4
Tupaia virus, **V1**.699, **V1**.819
Tupaiid herpesvirus, **V1**.494 (Tab.)
Turbinate, anatomy, **B1**.606–7

Turicella, **B2**.990–1
chemotaxonomic characteristics,
B2.978 (Tab.)
identification, **B2**.979
Turicella otitidis, **B1**.296 (Tab.), **B2**.990–1
biochemical characteristics, **B2**.993 (Tab.)
habitats, **B2**.977–8
Turkey astrovirus (TAstV), **V2**.888–9
classification, **V2**.890 (Tab.)
genome, **V2**.894 (Tab.)
sequencing, **V2**.899
infection, **V2**.904–5
Turkey coronavirus (TCOV)
hemagglutinin-esterase (HE), **V1**.838–9
infection, **V1**.841 (Tab.)
Turkey herpesvirus, **V1**.494 (Tab.)
Turkey meningo-encephalitis virus, **V2**.997
Turkey rhinotracheitis virus *see* Avian
pneumovirus (APV)
Turkeys
coryza, **B2**.1810–11
rhinotracheitis, **B2**.1810–11
Turneria, **B2**.1865–6
definitions, **B2**.1865–6
morphology, **B2**.1867–8
Turneria parva, **B2**.1871
serovars/serogroups, **B2**.1878 (Tab.)
Tursiops truncatus, **M**.430
Tweens, **B1**.425
12*D* process, canning, **B1**.265–6
12/23 rule, Ig V(D)J recombination, **I**.328
20-S, proteasomes, **I**.411
Twin arginine translocator (TAT), **B1**.160
Twin studies
autoimmune disease, **I**.752
immunogenetics, **I**.572
leprosy, **I**.590
tuberculosis immunogenetics, **I**.591
Two-component signal transduction systems
(TCSTS), **B1**.167–9, **B1**.168 (Tab.)
Two-dimensional immunoelectrophoresis,
M.34
Two-dose schedule, Measles virus vaccine,
V1.734, **V1**.735–6
Twort, F, **B1**.9
'Two-signal' hypothesis, APC-T cell
interaction, **I**.383
Two-well chambers, chemokine activity
measurement, **I**.223
Tymoviridae, **V1**.27 (Tab.), **V1**.51 (Tab.)
see also specific viruses
'tyndallization', **B1**.5
Type III secretion system (TTSS)
apoptosis modulation, **I**.655
phagocytic uptake inhibition, **I**.649
Type concept, **B1**.28–9
Type III secretion system, *Bordetella*,
B2.1789 (Tab.), **B2**.1801
Type I-IV secretion systems, bacterial protein
secretion, **B1**.48
Typhoid, **B1**.521, **B2**.1421
antibiotic resistance, **B2**.1415–16
ampicillin, **B2**.1416
chloramphenicol, **B2**.1415–16
ciprofloxacin, **B2**.1416
multiple resistance, **B2**.1415–16

Typhoid
  antibiotic resistance (*Continued*)
    plasmids, **B2**.1416
  historical perspective, **B2**.1318–31
  ice cream, **B1**.251
  immune response, **B1**.744
  infection process, **B1**.744
  laboratory worker immunization, **B1**.767
  treatment
    azithromycin, **B2**.1416
    cefotaxime, **B2**.1416
    ceftriaxone, **B2**.1416
  vaccines/vaccination, **B1**.744
    capsular polysaccharides, **I**.935
    development status, **I**.933 (Tab.)
  Widal reaction, **B1**.744
  see also Salmonella Typhi
Typhus
  causative agents, **B2**.2030–2, **B2**.2031 (Tab.), **B2**.2033
    antibacterial susceptibility/resistance, **B2**.2043 (Tab.)
    see also Rickettsia
  epidemiology and natural history, **B2**.2037
  historical aspects, **B2**.2027–30
  louse-borne, **B2**.2041
    clinical manifestations, **B2**.2039 (Tab.), **B2**.2041
    epidemiology and natural history, **B2**.2041
  murine, **B2**.2040–1
    clinical manifestations, **B2**.2039 (Tab.), **B2**.2040–1
    epidemiology and natural history, **B2**.2037, **B2**.2040
    see also Rickettsia typhi
  treatment, **B2**.2043
Typography, viral nomenclature, **V1**.26, **V1**.35, **V1**.40
Tyrocidine, **B1**.497
Tyrosine hydromlysis, Enterobacteriaceae identification, **B2**.1319 (Tab.)
Tyuleniy virus, **V2**.1004
Tyzzer, Edward Ernest, **P**.18

UBE3A gene, tuberculosis association, **I**.591–2
Ubiquinol-cytochrome *c* oxidoreductase, **B1**.64
Ubiquinones
  Brucella, **B2**.1724
  candidiasis therapy, **M**.580
  cycling, *Plasmodium*, **P**.478
  Pneumocystis infection, **M**.781
  Pseudomonas, **B2**.1597
Ubiquitin, **I**.411–12
  apoptosis, **I**.135
  DNA vaccine modulation, **I**.917
Ubiquitin hydrolases, **I**.411–12
Ubiquitin–proteasome pathway, **I**.410–2
  antigenic peptide generation, **I**.412
Ubiquitin proteasome system (UPS) *see* HIV
UFD1L gene, diGeorge syndrome, **I**.774–5
UL5/UL8/UL52, HSV-1 replication, **V1**.165, **V1**.165 (Tab.)
UL9, HSV-1 replication, **V1**.149 (Tab.), **V1**.165, **V1**.166
UL16-binding proteins, NK cells, **I**.627–8

UL30/UL40, HSV-1 replication, **V1**.165, **V1**.165 (Tab.)
UL42, HSV-1 replication, **V1**.165 (Tab.)
'Úlcera de Bauru,' **P**.327
Ulcerative blepharitis, candidiasis, **M**.257, **M**.296, **M**.297
Ulcerative colitis, IL-15, **I**.282
Ulcers/ulceration
  amebiasis, **P**.206 (Fig.), **P**.207, **P**.210, **P**.210 (Fig.)
  aspergillosis, **M**.701
  Chiclero's, **P**.313, **P**.323, **P**.323 (Fig.)
  dracunculiasis, **P**.831–2
  gastrointestinal zygomycosis, **M**.674
  lobomycosis, **M**.431
  lymphogranuloma venereum, **B2**.2012
  paracoccidioidomycosis, **M**.547, **M**.550 (Fig.)
  protothecosis, **M**.398
  rhinosporidiosis, **M**.462, **M**.466 (Fig.)
  sporotrichosis, **M**.367
  tularemia, **B2**.1754–5
U_L, HSV-1 genome, **V1**.163–4
Ultra-heat-treated (UHT) milk, **B1**.233
Ultrasonography
  alveolar echinococcosis, **P**.694
  Anisakis, **P**.817
  ascariasis, **P**.730
  bone and joint infection diagnosis, **B1**.694
  echinococcosis, **P**.694
  fascioliasis, **P**.650
  fetal infection diagnosis, **V2**.1445 (Tab.)
    HCMV infection, **V2**.1451
    Parvovirus B19 virus infection, **V2**.1470
  with glutaraldehyde, **B1**.454
  lymphatic filariasis, **P**.773, **P**.777
  paragonimiasis, **P**.653
  VZV infection, **V2**.1457
Ultraviolet (UV) radiation, **B1**.452
  microsporidians, **P**.550
  mutation, **B1**.82, **B1**.87–9
  sterilization, **B1**.451–2
    applications, **B1**.445 (Tab.), **B1**.452
    DNA repair, **B1**.451–2
    mechanisms of action, **B1**.451, **B1**.452 (Fig.)
    microbial sensitivity, **B1**.451
  susceptibility/resistance to
    Campylobacter, **B2**.1545
    Mycobacterium, **B2**.1217
    plasmids, **B1**.114
Umbavirus, classification, **V1**.27 (Tab.)
Una virus (UNAV), **V2**.1011 (Tab.)
Uncinocarpus reesii, **M**.820
Undercooked/raw food
  clonorchiasis, **P**.647
  dracunculiasis, **P**.834
  fascioliasis, **P**.647–8
  lung flukes, **P**.647
  Opisthorchis, **P**.647
  Opisthorchis felineus, **P**.647
  Paragonimus, **P**.647–8
Undulant fever, milk-associated, **B1**.229
Unheated serum reagin (USR) test antigen, **B2**.1845
Unilateral vision disorders, ocular larva migrans, **P**.752

Uniport, **B1**.49
United Kingdom (UK)
  Communicable Disease Control Services, **B1**.404
  epidemiological surveillance, **B1**.317
  food-borne botulism, **B2**.1069
  nosocomial infection
    incidence, **B1**.369, **B1**.369 (Fig.)
    surveillance, **B1**.405
  notification of disease, **B1**.319, **B1**.321 (Tab.)
  rabies quarantine, **V2**.1126
  sexually transmitted diseases reports, **B1**.320–1
  vaccination programs, **V2**.1560
    measles, **B1**.351–3
    rubella, **B1**.351, **V2**.982, **V2**.983 (Fig.)
United Nations Childrens' Fund, **V2**.1583
United States of America (USA)
  bacteremia statistics, **B1**.509
  epidemiological surveillance, **B1**.317
  food-borne botulism, **B2**.1066–7
  measles elimination, **V1**.735–6
  nosocomial infection
    control, **B1**.406
    incidence, **B1**.369, **B1**.369 (Fig.)
    surveillance, **B1**.405
  notification of disease, **B1**.319
  syphilis case number, **B2**.1841 (Fig.)
  tetanus incidence, **B2**.1065
  tuberculosis cases, **B1**.364
  vaccination programs, **V2**.1559–60, **V2**.1562 (Fig.)
    rubella, **B1**.351, **V2**.981–2, **V2**.982 (Fig.)
Universal Postal Union (UPU), infectious material transport, **V2**.1528–9
Universal System of Virus Taxonomy, **V1**.38–54, **V1**.378–9
  genome strategy, **V1**.40–1
  see also Classification, viruses
Unlinked Anonymous HIV Prevalence Monitoring Program, **B1**.321–2
Unna band, lobomycosis, **M**.433–4
Unpasterized milk, restrictions on sale of, **B1**.234
Unsaturated fatty acids, skin immunization, **I**.822
Unstained preparations, *Blastocystis hominis*, **P**.565
Unweighted Pair-Group Method with Arithmetic Mean (UPGMA), **M**.48
Upper respiratory tract infection *see* Respiratory tract infection, upper
Upper respiratory tract infection, influenza, **V1**.661
Upstream regulatory region (URR), papillomaviruses, **V1**.450, **V1**.457 (Fig.)
UQ_A, **B1**.67–8
UQ_B, **B1**.67–8
Urabe Am 9 strain, Mumps virus vaccination, **V1**.753–4
Uracil-DNA glycosylase
  herpesviruses, **V1**.500
  HSV type 1 (HSV-1), **V1**.500
  poxviruses, **V1**.603–5
Uracil N glycosylase, HSV-1 replication, **V1**.165 (Tab.)

Urbanization
　　emerging bacterial infection, **B1**.359–60
　　epidemics, **P**.117
　　　leishmaniasis, **P**.117
Urea breath test, *Helicobacter pylori* infection
　　diagnosis, **B2**.1571 (Tab.), **B2**.1572–3
Urea hydrolysis
　　bacterial identification, **B2**.1351
　　Enterobacteriaceae identification,
　　　B2.1319 (Tab.)
Ureaplasma
　　characteristics, **B2**.1958 (Tab.)
　　classification, **B2**.1967
　　genetics, **B2**.1968–9
　　　genome structure, **B2**.1973–4
　　infection, **B2**.1983
　　metabolism/biochemistry, **B2**.1969, **B2**.1994
　　　energy-yielding pathways, **B2**.1972
　　pathogenicity, **B2**.1983
Ureaplasma parvum, **B2**.1968–9
Ureaplasma urealyticum
　　antibacterial susceptibility/resistance,
　　　B2.1992
　　cell division, **B2**.1962
　　cell membrane proteins, **B2**.1970
　　classification, **B2**.1968–9
　　culture, **B2**.1963
　　genetic analysis
　　　comparative genomics, **B2**.1976
　　　genome sequencing and gene annotation,
　　　　B2.1974, **B2**.1975 (Tab.)
　　host and tissue specificity, **B2**.1964
　　infection, **B2**.1965 (Tab.), **B2**.1983
　　　human colonization, **B2**.1965 (Tab.)
　　　transmission, **B2**.1991, **B2**.1992
　　　treatment, **B2**.1992
　　as normal microbiota, **B1**.296 (Tab.), **B1**.303
　　pathogenicity, **B2**.1983
　　　apoptosis induction, **B2**.1985
　　　clastogenic and oncogenic effects, **B2**.1985
　　transport system, **B2**.1973
Urease
　　Brucella, **B2**.1731
　　Cryptococcus, **M**.640–1
　　Helicobacter pathogenicity, **B2**.1576
Uredinales, **M**.63
Urediniomycetes, **M**.63, **M**.65 (Tab.)
Ureibacillus, **B2**.922–3
Urethra
　　flora, **B1**.673, **B1**.677
　　normal microbiota, **B1**.303
　　rhinosporidiosis, **M**.460
Urethral syndrome, **B1**.673
Urethritis
　　microsporidiosis, **P**.550
　　non-gonococcal
　　　Mycoplasma genitalium, **B1**.669, **B2**.1983
　　　Ureaplasma urealyticum causing, **B2**.1983
Uridylic acid (UMP), **B1**.60–1
Urinals, nosocomial infection from, **B1**.379–80
Urinary tract, **B1**.672–3
　　anatomical considerations, **B1**.672
　　bladder calculi, **B2**.1446
　　host defence mechanisms, **B1**.672–3
　　physiological flora, **B1**.677

Urinary tract infection (UTIs), **B1**.672–80
　　acute cystitis, **B1**.673
　　acute pyelonephritis, **B1**.673
　　asymptomatic, **B1**.672, **B1**.673
　　bacteremia due to, **B1**.520
　　blastomycosis, **M**.489, **M**.495
　　causative organisms
　　　Enterobacteriaceae, **B2**.1346–7
　　　Enterococcus, **B2**.896
　　　Escherichia coli, **B1**.520
　　　Escherichia coli, uropathogenic,
　　　　B2.1379–80
　　　Proteus mirabilis, **B2**.1446–7
　　clinical syndromes, **B1**.673
　　complicated *vs.* uncomplicated, **B1**.672
　　cryptococcosis, **M**.648
　　diagnosis, **B1**.677–9
　　　culture, **B1**.677–9
　　　sample collection, **B1**.677
　　　specimens unacceptable for, **B1**.678–9
　　　specimen transport, **B1**.677
　　　see also Urine, culture
　　Enterobius vermicularis, **P**.731
　　epidemiology, **B1**.672
　　hospital-acquired, **B1**.388, **B2**.896
　　management, **B1**.679–80
　　　prophylaxis, **B1**.679–80
　　microbiology, **B1**.674, **B1**.674 (Tab.)
　　pathogenesis, **B1**.674–7
　　　adhesion, **B1**.674–6
　　　cytotoxic necrotizing factor 1, **B1**.676
　　　hemolysin, **B1**.676
　　　iron siderophores, **B1**.676
　　　organization of virulence factors, **B1**.677
　　perinephric abscess, **B1**.673
　　Pneumocystis carinii infection, **M**.785
　　renal abscess, **B1**.673
　　rhinosporidiosis, **M**.459, **M**.460
　　special hosts, **B1**.673
　　tuberculosis, **B1**.678
　　urethral syndrome, **B1**.673
　　urine specimens, **M**.83 (Tab.), **M**.84,
　　　M.86 (Tab.)
　　vaccine development, **B1**.680
　　see also Genital tract infection;
　　　Genitourinary tract infection
Urine
　　babesiosis, **P**.454
　　'coca-cola'-like, **V2**.1171
　　collection, **B1**.677
　　culture, **B1**.677–8
　　　antibacterial substances, **B1**.678
　　　colony-forming units, **B1**.677–9
　　　filter paper method, **B1**.678
　　　interpretation, **B1**.679
　　　rarely encountered species, **B1**.678
　　midstream clean-voided specimen, **B1**.677,
　　　B1.678, **B1**.679
　　samples, **B1**.677
　　　unacceptable specimens for laboratory,
　　　　B1.678–9
　　schistosomiasis diagnosis
　　　culture, **P**.152
　　　examination, **P**.152
　　suprapubic aspiration, **B1**.677, **B1**.679

　　virus shedding, **V1**.249
Uroid, **P**.201–2
Urokinase plasminogen activator (uPA), **I**.203
Uropathogenic *Escherichia coli see Escherichia coli*, uropathogenic (UPEC)
URR structure, HPV-16, **V1**.457 (Fig.)
US Department of Transport, infectious
　　material transport, **V2**.1528
Usevir *see* Sorivudine
U_S, HSV-1 genome, **V1**.163–4
Ustilaginales, **M**.63, **M**.65 (Tab.)
Ustilaginomycetes, **M**.63
Ustilago, **M**.633
　　characteristics, **M**.632 (Tab.)
　　infection, **M**.625 (Tab.), **M**.630
　　　catheters, **M**.630
Ustilago esculenta, **M**.630
Ustilago maydis, **M**.630
Usutu virus (USUV), **V2**.998 (Tab.), **V2**.1003
'Uta,' **P**.313, **P**.328
Uukuniemi virus
　　assembly/release mechanisms, **V2**.1040
　　G1 glycoprotein, **V2**.1034
　　G2 glycoprotein, **V2**.1034
　　genome structure, **V2**.1033–4
　　transcription termination, **V2**.1037
Uveitis, **M**.317
　　Chlamydia trachomatis infection, **B2**.2013
　　Yersinia pseudotuberculosis infection, **I**.563
Uvitex 2B staining, microsporidiosis diagnosis,
　　P.546
Uvitex 2B whitening agent, **M**.123 (Tab.),
　　M.125

vacA gene
　　Helicobacter pylori pathogenicity, **B2**.1577
　　Helicobacter typing, **B2**.1570
VacA protein, **B1**.174–5
Vaccination, **I.819–35**, **V2.1551–89**
　　autoimmune disease, **I**.759–60
　　bare skin immunization *see* Vaccination,
　　　bare skin
　　controlled trials, **V1**.365
　　edible vaccines (transgenic plants), **I**.828–30
　　　bacterial antigens, **I**.829
　　　cost, **I**.828
　　　degradation protection, **I**.828
　　　hepatitis C virus, **I**.870–1
　　　safety, **I**.828
　　　viral antigens, **I**.828–9, **I**.870–1, **V2**.1553
　　historical aspects/re-evaluation, **I**.13, **I**.14,
　　　I.490–5, **V1**.579–81, **V2**.1551
　　　'variolation,' **I**.487
　　humoral *vs.* cellular protection, **I**.489,
　　　I.490 (Fig.)
　　international travelers, **V2**.1563
　　mathematical models *see* Vaccination,
　　　mathematical models
　　molecular biology, **I**.14–6
　　mucosal routes, **I**.537–41, **I**.827–32
　　　antigen uptake, **I**.827
　　　B cell induction, **I**.827
　　　cellular immune response, **I**.828
　　　edible *see above*
　　　epithelia, **I**.827, **I**.827 (Tab.)

Vaccination
  mucosal routes (*Continued*)
    gut-associated lymphoid tissue, **I**.827
    humoral immune response, **I**.828
    mucosa-associated lymphoid tissue, **I**.827–8
    nasal administration *see below*
    oral immunization *see* Oral vaccination
    Peyer's patches, **I**.827
    secretory IgA, **I**.827, **I**.828
    T cell activation, **I**.827, **I**.828
    T helper cells, **I**.828
    tolerance induction, **I**.827
    see also individual routes
  nasal administration, **I**.540–1, **I**.830–2
    adjuvants, **I**.830, **I**.831–2, **I**.864
    advantages, **I**.831, **V2**.1556–7
    attenuated vaccines, **I**.830–1
    CpG motifs, **I**.864
    DNA vaccines, **I**.913
    immune response, **V2**.1557
    immunostimulating complexes, **I**.864
    live vaccines *see* Vaccines, live
    nasal-associated lymphoid tissue, **I**.831–2
    oral administration *vs.*, **I**.830 (Tab.)
    particulate antigen, **I**.830
    proteasomes, **I**.839
    soluble antigen, **I**.830
    tolerance *vs.* immunity, **I**.830
    vectors, **I**.541, **I**.830–1
  needle-free delivery, **I**.819–20
    advantages, **I**.819–20
    compliance, **I**.819
    see also individual methods
  oral administration *see* Oral vaccination
  parenteral routes
    cost, **I**.819
    disadvantages, **I**.819–20
    disease transmission, **I**.819–20
    staff training, **I**.819
  in pregnancy *see* Pregnancy
  premature infants, **V2**.1561–2
  programs *see below*
  routine
    age at infection, **B1**.345
    control of infectious disease by, **B1**.345–6
    honeymoon periods, **B1**.346, **B1**.346 (Fig.)
  skin immunization *see* Vaccination, bare skin
  transcutaneous immunization *see*
    Vaccination, bare skin
  see also Passive immunization; *specific*
    diseases/infection
Vaccination Act (1898), **V1**.580–1
Vaccination, bare skin, **I**.820–7, **I**.823–7,
  I.824 (Fig.), **I**.837–8
  adjuvants, **I**.824–5, **I**.837–8
    CpG oligodeoxynucleotides, **I**.824, **I**.825
    CT, **I**.823, **I**.824, **I**.826, **I**.826 (Fig.)
    cytokines, **I**.824
    LT, **I**.823, **I**.824, **I**.826, **I**.826 (Fig.)
  antigen absorption, **I**.821–3, **I**.821 (Fig.),
    I.826
  APCs, **I**.837
  in children, **I**.838
  dimethyl sulfoxide, **I**.822
  DNA vaccines, **I**.825

eczematous reactions, **I**.826–7
electroporation, **I**.822
hair follicles, **I**.822, **I**.825
immune response variation, **I**.825–6,
  I.826 (Fig.)
liposomes, **I**.822
mucosal immunity induction, **I**.825
needle-free injectors, **I**.822–3
skin hydration, **I**.823–4
  glycerol, **I**.823–4
  water, **I**.823–4
stratum corneum penetration, **I**.821–2, **I**.837
surfactants, **I**.822
transdermal powder delivery, **I**.822
'transferosomes,' **I**.822
unsaturated fatty acids, **I**.822
vaccines, **I**.823
  peptides, **I**.826
  see also individual organisms
Vaccination, mathematical models, **I.947–65**
  age effects, **I**.960–1
    age at infection rise, **I**.949, **I**.960
    disease nature effects, **I**.960–1
    susceptible individual age, **I**.961
  applications, **I**.963–4
    evolution, **I**.964
    health economics, **I**.964
    hepatitis B vaccination programs, **I**.963–4
    MMR vaccination programs, **I**.963
    quantitative prediction, **I**.964
  delivery, **I**.961–2
    age effects, **I**.961
    cost–benefit implications, **I**.962
    failure rate, **I**.961
    randomness, **I**.961–2
    selectivity, **I**.961
    'super-spreaders,' **I**.961–2
  herd immunity/community immunity, **I**.957–
    8, **I**.959 (Fig.)
  introduction into endemic situations, **I**.958,
    I.959 (Fig.)
  repeated campaigns, **I**.962–3
    age gateways, **I**.962
    frequency, **I**.962–3
    pulse vaccination regimes, **I**.962,
      I.962 (Fig.)
    susceptible groups, **I**.963
  reproduction numbers, **I**.957–8
  time (dynamic effects), **I**.960
  vaccine characteristics, **I**.961
    degree, **I**.961
    duration, **I**.961
    take, **I**.961
  see also Infection(s), mathematical models
Vaccination programs, **B1**.347–53, **V2**.1558–65
  adolescents, **V2**.1559
  campaigns, **B1**.346
  cost-effectiveness, **V2**.1558–9
  diphtheria, **B1**.348–9
  disease eradication, **V2**.1558
  epidemiological aspects, **V2**.1558
  historical aspects, **V2**.1551
  infants, **V2**.1559
  influenza, **V1**.367
  measles, **B1**.351–3

monitoring, **V2**.1564–5
percentage of cases vaccinated, **B1**.324–5,
  B1.325 (Fig.)
pertussis, **B1**.349
rubella *see* Rubella
schedules, **V2**.1559–61
  adults, **V2**.1561, **V2**.1562 (Fig.)
  infants, **V2**.1559–61
  UK, **V2**.1560
  USA, **V2**.1559–60, **V2**.1562 (Fig.)
simultaneous vaccine administration,
  V2.1561
surveillance, **B1**.323–6
  vaccine efficacy, **B1**.324–5
  vaccine safety, **B1**.325–6
  vaccine uptake, **B1**.326
see also individual organisms
Vaccine(s), **I**.488 (Tab.), **V2.1551–89**
  adverse effects, **B1**.325–6, **V2**.1564 (Tab.)
    monitoring, **V2**.1565
  anti-idiotypic antibodies, **V2**.1553
  conjugate, immunosuppressed, **V2**.1563
  development, **I**.423–6
    gene cloning, **B1**.127
    genetic analysis, **V1**.197
  DNA *see* DNA vaccines
  effectiveness, **V1**.363–4
  efficacy monitoring, **B1**.324–5
    antigens, **B1**.324
    calculation, **B1**.324–5
    causative organisms, **B1**.324
    cold-chain monitors, **B1**.324
    epidemiological studies, **B1**.324–5
    handling/storage, **B1**.324
    potency testing, **B1**.324
    serological studies, **B1**.324
  examples, **I**.424 (Tab.)
  handling/storage, **V2**.1565
  historical aspects, **B1**.7, **V1**.8, **V1**.8 (Tab.)
    introduction dates, **V1**.8 (Tab.)
  immune response, **V2**.1555–8
    adjuvants, **V2**.1555–7
    antibody response, **V2**.1556
    antigen processing/presentation, **V2**.1556
    host factors, **V2**.1557–8
    measurement of, **V2**.1558
    T-cell response, **V2**.1555–6
  inactivated (killed), **I**.423–4, **I**.488 (Tab.),
    V1.678–9, **V1**.752, **V1**.925, **V2**.955,
    V2.1552–3, **V2**.1576–8
    adjuvants, **V2**.1552–3
    advantages, **V2**.1552–3, **V2**.1556
    adventitious agents, **V2**.1556
    cell-mediated immune response, **V2**.1556
    disadvantages, **V2**.1556
    handling/storage, **V2**.1565
    immune response, **V2**.1556
    immunosuppressed, **V2**.1563
    methods, **V2**.1553
  information sources, **V2**.1583
  injury compensation, **V2**.1563–4
  live *see below*
  mechanism of action, **V2**.1552
  oral *see* Oral vaccination
  peptide *see* Peptide vaccines

Vaccine(s) (*Continued*)
  prelicensure evaluation, **V2**.1558
  proteasomes, **I**.839–40
    nasal route, **I**.839
    outer membrane proteins, **I**.839
    safety/immunogenicity, **I**.839
    TLRs, **I**.839
  recombinant, **V1**.349, **V1**.573, **V2**.1076–7,
      V2.1174–5
    immunosuppressed, **V2**.1563
    vaccinia virus use in, **V1**.573, **V2**.1174–5
  retrovirus risks, **V2**.1297
  safety, **V2**.1563–4
    monitoring, **B1**.325–6
  subunit *see* Subunit vaccines
  toxoids, **B1**.155
  types, **V2**.1552–8, **V2**.1552 (Tab.)
    see also specific types
  uptake, **B1**.326
  vectors
    parvoviruses, **V1**.427
    poxviruses, **V1**.617
  virosomes, **I**.838–9, **I**.838 (Fig.)
    CTL responses, **I**.838
    DNA vaccines, **I**.839
    hemagglutinin, **I**.838
    MHC class I pathway, **I**.838
    MHC class II pathways, **I**.838
    targeting, **I**.838
  virus-like particles, **I**.840–1
    baculovirus production systems, **I**.840
    clinical trials, **I**.840–1
    definition, **I**.840
    immune response, **I**.840
    manufacture, **I**.840
    Pichea pastoris production systems, **I**.840
    plant production systems, **I**.840
    structure, **I**.840
    *see also individual organisms; individual
        species; specific vaccines; specific viruses*
Vaccine-related poliomyelitis, **V2**.882,
    V2.1557, **V2**.1563–4, **V2**.1572, **V2**.1574
  epidemiology, **V1**.198
Vaccines, live, **I.895–908**
  advantages, **I**.895
  attenuated, **I**.424, **I**.488 (Tab.), **V2**.1554–5,
      V2.1555 (Tab.)
    advantages, **V2**.1556–7
    development, **V2**.1554–5
    disadvantages, **V2**.1556–7
    handling/storage, **V2**.1565
    immune response, **V2**.1556–7
  attenuated bacterial vectors, **I**.488,
      I.488 (Tab.), **I**.845–6, **I**.897 (Tab.), **I**.899
    DNA vaccines, **I**.913
    Listeria monocytogenes vectors, **I**.902
    mechanism of action, **I**.896–7
    nasal administration, **I**.830–1
  attenuated vectors, **I**.488, **I**.488 (Tab.), **I**.841–
      6, **I**.842 (Fig.), **I**.895–6, **I**.897 (Tab.)
    bacterial *see above*
    mechanism of action, **I**.896–7
    multipathogen vaccines, **I**.895–6
    viral *see below*

attenuated viral vectors, **I**.488, **I**.488 (Tab.),
    I.489 (Tab.), **I**.897–9, **I**.897 (Tab.),
    V2.1554–5
  adenoviruses, **I**.830–1, **I**.897–8, **I**.897 (Tab.),
      I.899
    advantages, **I**.897–8
  canarypox virus, **I**.846, **I**.898, **I**.902,
      V2.1555
  clinical trials, **I**.898–9
  cytokine administration, **I**.898
  disadvantages, **I**.898
  fowlpoxviruses, **I**.846, **I**.898
  mechanism of action, **I**.896–7
  modified vaccinia virus Ankara *see*
      Modified vaccinia virus Ankara (MVA),
      as vaccine vector
  nasal routes, **I**.830–1
  polio virus, **I**.830–1, **I**.846–7, **I**.899
  poxviruses, **I**.897–8
  'prime-boost strategy' *see* 'Prime-boost
      immunization'
  type I herpesvirus glycoprotein D, **I**.898
  vaccinia virus, **I**.830–1, **I**.896–7, **I**.897–8,
      I.897 (Tab.), **I**.902
  yellow fever virus, **I**.899
  see also individual types
BCG vectors, **I**.844–5, **I**.897 (Tab.), **I**.901–2
  intranasal, **I**.901–2, **I**.904
  MHC class II presentation, **I**.844
delivery route, **I**.895, **I**.903–4
  intranasal, **I**.901–4
  mucosal, **I**.841
  Salmonella vectors, **I**.899
  Shigella vector, **I**.901
directed mutagenesis, **V2**.1554–5
immune system targeting, **I**.902–3
  adenovirus vectors, **I**.902, **I**.903
  BCG vectors, **I**.902
  canarypox virus vectors, **I**.902
  CTL responses, **I**.902
  dendritic cells, **I**.903
  Listeria monocytogenes vectors, **I**.902
  MHC class I antigen presentation, **I**.902
  proinflammatory cytokines, **I**.903
  Salmonella vectors, **I**.902
  vaccinia virus vectors, **I**.902
immunogenicity, **I**.896
  pathogen-associated molecular patterns,
      I.896
immunosuppressed, **V2**.1563
Listeria vector, **I**.845
oral *see* Oral vaccination
rational attenuation, **I**.895
related strains, **V2**.1554–5
Salmonella vectors, **I**.540, **I**.841–3,
    I.897 (Tab.), **I**.899–901, **I**.900 (Fig.), **I**.902
  DNA vaccines, **I**.913
  intranasal, **I**.830–1, **I**.904
  MHC class I, **I**.899–901
  plasmids, **I**.901
  S. enterica, **I**.899
  sifA gene, **I**.899–900, **I**.900 (Fig.)
  S. typhi, **I**.830–1, **I**.841, **I**.841–3, **I**.896–7,
      I.899–900
  S. typhimurium, **I**.847, **I**.868, **I**.899–900
sequential vaccination, **V2**.1555

Shigella vectors, **I**.843, **I**.897 (Tab.), **I**.901
  advantages, **I**.843
  disadvantages, **I**.843
  DNA vaccines, **I**.901, **I**.913
  guaBA operon, **I**.843
  intranasal route, **I**.830–1
  iuc gene, **I**.843
  mutants, **I**.901
  ompB gene, **I**.843
  types, **I**.488 (Tab.), **I**.896–902
Vibrio cholerae vectors, **I**.843–4
  intranasal route, **I**.830–1
  virulence gene knockouts, **I**.895
  *see also individual organisms; individual
      species*
Vaccinia
  IL-18, **I**.290–2
  NK cells, **I**.96
Vaccinia immunoglobulin (VIG), **V2**.1566,
    V2.1567 (Tab.)
  in therapy, **V2**.1568
Vaccinia virus
  biomedical contributions, **V1**.582
  capping enzyme, **V1**.112
  cell interactions
    DNA degradation, **V1**.219
    host protein synthesis, **V1**.223
    host protein synthesis inhibition, **V1**.203
    host RNA degradation, **V1**.221
  classification, **V1**.583
  extracellular enveloped virus, **V1**.586
  gene delivery system, **V1**.304–5
  genome replication, **V1**.148 (Tab.)
    origins of replication, **V1**.168
    viral proteins, **V1**.149 (Tab.)
  genome structure, **V1**.148 (Tab.), **V1**.583,
      V1.602 (Fig.)
  host range, **V1**.603 (Fig.)
  identification, **V1**.581–2
  immune evasion, **V1**.198–9
    apoptosis regulation, **V1**.603 (Fig.)
    caspase inhibition, **V1**.324
    chemokine binding proteins, **V1**.320,
        V1.622, **I**.622–3
    complement, **V1**.257, **V1**.313, **V1**.619–20,
        I.639
    cytokines, **V1**.288, **V1**.316–17, **V1**.317–18,
        I.620, **I**.623
    dendritic cells, **I**.632
    genes, **V1**.603 (Fig.)
    3β-Hydroxysteroid hydrogenase, **V1**.286,
        V1.622
    identification, **V1**.198–9
    IFN interference, **V1**.230, **V1**.286–7,
        V1.295, **V1**.315, **I**.619
    IFN receptor, **I**.619
    IL-1β binding protein, **V1**.318, **V1**.585–6,
        V1.621
    inflammation inhibition, **V1**.286
    receptor homologues, **I**.620–1
    secreted cytokine receptors, **V1**.318
    serpins, **V1**.623
    TNF-receptor analogue secretion,
        V1.621–2
  intracellular mature virus, **V1**.586

Vaccinia virus (*Continued*)
  isolation/propagation and identification,
    V1.100
  LC16m8 strain, **V1**.591
  MVA strain, **V1**.591
  NK cells, **V1**.272
  origins, **V1**.581–2
    confusions over, **V1**.581
  phylogenetic comparison, **V1**.584 (Fig.)
  receptor-mediated endocytosis, **V1**.216–17
  replication in cytoplasm, **V1**.112
  SKIF (PKR inhibitory factor), **V1**.295
  as vaccine vector, **I**.830–1, **I**.896–7, **I**.897–8,
    I.897 (Tab.), **I**.902
    for EBV, **V1**.573
    hepatitis A, **V2**.1174–5
  viral complement control protein, **V1**.313
  virion structure, **V1**.586
  virulence, genes of cellular origin,
    V1.257 (Fig.)
Vacuolar form, *Blastocystis hominis*, **P**.557,
    P.557 (Fig.), **P**.558 (Fig.)
Vacuolating cytotoxin gene, *Helicobacter*,
    B2.1567–8
Vacuoles, **P**.179
Vacuum packing (VP), food processing and
    preservation, **B1**.268 (Tab.)
VACV *see* Valaciclovir (VACV)
Vagina
  Candida colonization *see* Vulvovaginal
    candidiasis (VVC)
  'frothy' discharge, trichomoniasis, **P**.257–8
  Fusobacterium in, **B2**.1946
  normal microbiota, **B1**.303
    Bacteroides/Prevotella/Porphyromonas,
      B2.1933–4
    gram-positive anaerobic cocci, **B2**.910
Vaginitis, *Trichomonas vaginalis*, **P**.257–8
  histology, **P**.259–60
Vaginosis, causative organisms, **B1**.303
Vagococcus, **B2**.833–5
Vagococcus fluvialis, **B2**.888 (Tab.), **B2**.889
Valaciclovir (VACV), **V2**.1615–16
  biochemical properties, **V2**.1614 (Tab.)
  herpes encephalitis, **V2**.1421
  HSV infection, **V2**.1501
  structure, **V2**.1613 (Fig.)
  VZV infection, **V1**.517, **V2**.1507
    in HIV infection, **V2**.1502
    in pregnancy, **V2**.1460
Valganciclovir
  congenital HCMV infection, **V2**.1453
  HCMV infection, **V1**.526–7, **V2**.1619
  structure, **V2**.1613 (Fig.)
Validation Lists of Bacterial Names, **B1**.18
Valinomycin, **B1**.497
Valtres *see* Valaciclovir (VACV)
Vanbreuseughem, R, **M**.10
Vancomycin
  in pneumococcal meningitis, **B1**.571
  resistance
    Bacillus, **B2**.946–7
    Enterococcus see Vancomycin-resistant
      enterococci (VRE)
    Staphylococcus aureus see Vancomycin-
      resistant *Staphylococcus aureus* (VRSA)

vanR gene, **B1**.111
vanS gene, **B1**.111
spectrum of activity, **B1**.499 (Tab.)
  Actinomyces, **B2**.1011
  Clostridium, **B2**.1064–5
  Clostridium difficile, **B2**.1123
  gram-positive anaerobic cocci, **B2**.907
  Lactobacillus, **B2**.866
  Listeria, **B2**.957–8
  Pasteurella multocida, **B2**.1655
  Streptococcus, **B2**.861–2
  structure, **B1**.480 (Fig.)
Vancomycin-resistant enterococci (VRE),
    B1.396, **B2**.891, **B2**.892–3, **B2**.892 (Tab.)
  antibacterial agents, **B1**.433
  detection by molecular technology,
    B1.723 (Tab.)
    cycling probe technology, **B1**.731–2
  emergence, **B1**.363
  identification, **B2**.891
Vancomycin-resistant *Staphylococcus aureus*
    (VRSA), **B2**.794 (Tab.), **B2**.802–3
  infection
    emerging bacterial infection, **B1**.363
    nosocomial, **B1**.363
van Durme, Paul, **P**.9
van Leeuwenhoek, A, **M**.6, **M**.20
van Leeuwenhoek, Antony, **B1**.3, **P**.13, **P**.241
  protozoa, **P**.186–7
vanR gene, vancomycin resistance, **B1**.111
vanS gene, vancomycin resistance, **B1**.111
'Van Tieghem cell,' **M**.9 (Fig.)
van Tieghem, P E L, **M**.8–9
Vantocil, **B1**.426
VAP-1, lymphocyte migration, **I**.508 (Tab.)
vapA gene, *Aeromonas* genetics, **B2**.1525
Vapor-phase disinfectants, **B1**.423 (Tab.),
    B1.429–30
var genes, *Plasmodium* antigenic variation,
    P.492
Variable (V) domains
  αβ TCRs, **I**.458, **I**.460–1
  γδ TCRs, **I**.458
  Ig heavy chains, **I**.305
  Ig light chains, **I**.304
  interactions, **I**.305
Variable number of tandem repeat (VNTR)
    loci
  ILA1 gene cluster, **I**.578
  Salmonella molecular typing, **B2**.1411
  Tropheryma whippelii, **B2**.1002
Variables, in epidemiology, fixed and
    continuous, **B1**.311–12, **B1**.312 (Fig.)
Variable surface glycoprotein (VSG),
    *Trypanosoma brucei see Trypanosoma
    brucei*
Variance component methods, linkage, **I**.573
Variant Creutzfeld–Jakob disease (vCJD),
    V2.1347, **V2**.1369–71
  bovine spongiform encephalopathy *vs.*,
    V2.1369–70
  carrier status, **V2**.1371
  clinical signs, **V2**.1369
  diagnosis, tonsil biopsy, **V2**.1386
  emerging infection, **V2**.1648 (Tab.)
  historical aspects/discovery, **V1**.7

immunogenetics, **I**.589
incidence, **V2**.1370 (Tab.), **V2**.1371 (Fig.)
  sporadic Creutzfeldt–Jakob disease *vs.*,
    V2.1369
  see also Creutzfeldt–Jakob disease (CJD)
Variant Creutzfeldt–Jakob disease (vCJD),
    transmission, **B1**.381
Variant specific antibody, African
    trypanosomiasis, **P**.364–5
Variant surface glycoproteins (VSGs)
  Leishmania, **I**.680
  Trypanosoma brucei complex, **I**.680
Variant surface proteins (VSPs), *Giardia
    lamblia*, **I**.681
Varibaculum, **B2**.1016 (Tab.)
  classification, **B2**.1005
Varibaculum cambriensis
  classification, **B2**.1005
  pathogenicity, **B2**.1007 (Tab.)
Varicella, **V1**.512, **V2**.1421
  clinical features, **V1**.512–13, **V1**.515
    adults, **V1**.513, **V1**.513 (Fig.)
    CNS involvement, **V1**.513
    pneumonia, **V1**.513
  epidemiology, **V1**.514
    epidemics, **V1**.514
  fetal infection, **V2**.1444 (Tab.), **V2**.1454–6
    see also Congenital varicella syndrome
      (CVS)
  health impact, **V2**.1582–3
  immunocompromised patients, **V1**.513
  incubation period, **V1**.512–13
  neonatal infection, **V1**.513, **V2**.1444 (Tab.),
    V2.1456
  in pregnancy, **V1**.513
  vaccines/vaccination, **V1**.516, **I**.933 (Tab.),
    V2.1574–5
    adverse effects, **V2**.1575
    complication prevention, **V2**.1582–3
    contraindications, **V2**.1562–3
    healthcare workers, **V2**.1575
    history, **V1**.8 (Tab.)
    in HIV infection, **V2**.1505
    in immunosuppressed patients, **V2**.1506,
      V2.1575
    live, attenuated, **V2**.1555 (Tab.)
    Oka strain, **V1**.516
    in pregnancy, **V2**.1458–60, **V2**.1562–3
    programs, **V2**.1559 (Tab.), **V2**.1575
    USA schedules, **V2**.1559–60,
      V2.1560 (Fig.), **V2**.1575
  see also Varicella-zoster virus infection
Varicella-zoster immunoglobulin (VZIG),
    V1.516, **V2**.1566, **V2**.1567 (Tab.)
  in HIV infection, **V2**.1502
  immunodeficient patients (non-HIV),
    V2.1506
  post exposure prophylaxis, **V2**.1567–8
  in pregnancy, **V2**.1444 (Tab.), **V2**.1458
Varicella-zoster virus (VZV)
  characteristics, **V1**.489 (Tab.)
  culture, **V1**.516
  detection
    cytospinning, **V2**.1540–1
    ELISA *see* Enzyme-linked immunosorbent
      assay (ELISA)

Varicella-zoster virus (VZV) (*Continued*)
  DNA replication, **V1**.500
  genome, **V1**.492–3, **V1**.493 (Fig.),
    V1.494 (Tab.)
  host relationship, **V2**.1421–2
  initial immune response, **V1**.261
  isolation/propagation and isolation, **V1**.98
  medical importance, **V1**.162
  nucleotide metabolism, **V1**.500
  reactivation, **V2**.1421–2
  shell vial culture, **V1**.87
  vaccine *see* Varicella
Varicella-zoster virus infection, **V1**.506,
    V1.512–7
  bone marrow transplants, **V2**.1506
  chemotherapy (aciclovir), **V1**.516–17
    in pregnancy, **V2**.1460
  clinical features, **V1**.512–4
  CNS complications, **V2**.1421–2
    clinical features, **V2**.1421–2
    pathogenesis, **V2**.1422
  control/therapy, **V1**.516–17
    chemotherapy (aciclovir) *see above*
    epidemiological, **V1**.516
    passive immunization, **V1**.516, **V2**.1458–61
  diagnosis, **V1**.516
    cytopathology, **V2**.1534 (Tab.)
    ELISA *see* Enzyme-linked immunosorbent
      assay (ELISA)
    serological assays, **V1**.516
    skin test, **V1**.516
  epidemiology, **V1**.514
  fetal infection, **V1**.513, **V2**.1454–6,
    V2.1454–61
    diagnosis, **V2**.1457
    see also Congenital varicella syndrome
      (CVS)
  in HIV infection, **V2**.1499 (Tab.), **V2**.1501–2
    in children, **V2**.1505
    clinical features, **V2**.1501–2
    prophylaxis/treatment, **V2**.1502
  Ig (VZIG), **V1**.516
    in pregnancy, **V2**.1458, **V2**.1461
  immune response, **V1**.515–16, **V2**.1421
    antibodies, **V1**.516
    NK cells, **I**.94–6
    T cells, **V1**.515–16
  immunodeficient patients (non-HIV),
    V2.1506–7
  infection route, **V1**.514
  latency, **V1**.513, **V1**.515, **V2**.1421–2, **V2**.1501
  latent infection, **V1**.260
  in leukemia, **V1**.516
  neonatal infection
    breastfeeding, **V2**.1461
    diagnosis, **V2**.1457
    fatality, **V2**.1456
    intrauterine infection, **V2**.1456
    management, **V2**.1461
    maternal antibodies, **V2**.1456
    nosocomial exposure, **V2**.1461,
      V2.1462 (Tab.)
  nosocomial, **B1**.400
  pathogenesis and pathology, **V1**.515
  persistent, **V1**.373
  phlebotomists, transmission, **B1**.760

  in pregnancy, **V2**.1454
    abortion, **V2**.1454
    adverse effects, **V2**.1454
    diagnosis, **V2**.1456–7
    exposure, **V2**.1459 (Tab.), **V2**.1460 (Tab.)
    incidence, **V2**.1454
    management, **V2**.1458–60, **V2**.1459 (Tab.)
    pneumonia, **V2**.1454
    reactivation, **V1**.261, **V1**.513, **V1**.515,
      V2.1421–2
    recurrence, **V1**.515
    shingles, **V1**.512
      clinical features, **V1**.513 (Fig.), **V1**.514,
        V1.515
      complications, **V1**.514, **V2**.1421–2
      cranial, **V1**.513, **V1**.514
      epidemiology, **V1**.514
      mandibular, **V1**.514 (Fig.)
      thoracic, **V1**.513, **V1**.513 (Fig.)
      VZV reactivation, **V2**.1421–2
    vaccine *see* Varicella
    see also Varicella
Varicellovirus, **V1**.494 (Tab.)
Varicosavirus, **V1**.27 (Tab.), **V1**.48
Variolation, **I**.487, **V2**.1551
  smallpox eradication, **V1**.579
Variola virus, **V1**.594
  accidental escape, **V1**.581
  classification, **V1**.583
  immune evasion, **I**.639
    chemokine receptor analogues, **V1**.622
    complement, **V1**.313, **V1**.619–20
    INFs, **V1**.620
    TNF-receptor analogue secretion,
      V1.621–2
  infection *see* Smallpox
  phylogenetics, **V1**.585
  viral complement control protein, **V1**.313
Vascular cell adhesion molecule 1 (VCAM-1)
  airway hypersensitivity, **I**.733–4
  basophil binding, **I**.58
  cell adhesion, **I**.275
  eosinophil adhesion, **I**.60
  lymphocyte migration, **I**.508 (Tab.)
  macrophage development, **I**.21
  malaria upregulation, **P**.496–7
  upregulation, **I**.60
    IL-4, **I**.60, **I**.280
Vascular endothelial growth factor (VEGF),
  TNF-α effects, **I**.286
Vascular endothelium, prostacyclin
  production, **I**.189
Vasculating cytotoxin, *Helicobacter*
  pathogenicity, **B2**.1577
Vasculitis, hepatitis C, **V2**.1207
Vaseitis, *Chlamydia trachomatis* infection,
  B2.2012–13
Vasoconstriction
  dermonecrotic toxin of *Bordetella*, **B2**.1795
  thromboxane, **I**.189
Vasodilation, prostacyclins, **I**.189
Vav
  activation, **I**.345–6
  BCR signaling, **I**.345–6
  JNK pathway activation, **I**.345–6
Vav1, **I**.345

Vav2, **I**.345
Vav3, **I**.345
VCAM-1 *see* Vascular cell adhesion molecule
  1 (VCAM-1)
VDR gene, **I**.582–3
  dengue virus infection, **I**.588
  leprosy association, **I**.591
  periodontitis association, **I**.595
  tuberculosis association, **I**.591–3
VDRL test, syphilis diagnosis, **B1**.745
VE-cadherin, diapedesis, **I**.512–13
Vectavir *see* Penciclovir
Vector(s)
  CNS infection route, **V2**.1403–4
  control *see below*
  definition, **I**.951 (Tab.)
  life expectancy, **P**.61 (Tab.)
  microsporidiosis, **P**.544
  onchocerciasis, **P**.781, **P**.784–5
  viruses, **V1**.355
  Wuchereria bancrofti, **P**.772
  see also Arthropod vectors; *individual
    vectors; specific diseases/infection*
Vector control, **P**.112, **P**.118–20, **P**.125–7,
  P.145 (Tab.)
  African trypanosomiasis *see*
    Trypanosomiasis, African
  alphavirus control, **V2**.1018–19
  bacterial disease, **B1**.354–5
  Chagas disease, **P**.126, **P**.145 (Tab.)
  community parasite control, **P**.121
  dracunculiasis, **P**.145 (Tab.)
  echinococcosis, **P**.109
  leishmaniasis, **P**.145 (Tab.)
  lymphatic filariasis, **P**.109, **P**.122–3,
    P.145 (Tab.), **P**.778
  malaria, **P**.109, **P**.125–6, **P**.145 (Tab.)
  onchocerciasis, **P**.125–6, **P**.145 (Tab.)
    Onchocerciasis Control Programme,
      P.126–7
  schistosomiasis, **P**.127, **P**.145 (Tab.)
  trypanosomiasis, **P**.109
  Wuchereria bancrofti, **P**.109
Vector Control Research Centre (VCRC),
  P.124
Vectorial competence, mosquito (*Anopheles*),
  P.470
Vegetables, **B1**.280–3
  bacterial spoilage, **B1**.281–2
  biofilms, **B1**.282
  blanching, **B1**.281–2
  canned, **B1**.283
  carbon dioxide in atmosphere, **B1**.282
  chilling, **B1**.281
  containers, **B1**.281
  contamination sources, **B1**.281
  control of quality, **B1**.280–1
  crushing, bruising and puncturing, **B1**.281
  cut produce, **B1**.281
  dried, **B1**.282
  emerging bacterial infection, **B1**.360
  equipment sanitation, **B1**.281
  food-borne disease outbreaks, **B1**.282
  freezing, **B1**.281–2
  fungal spoilage, **B1**.281, **B1**.282
  handling, **B1**.281

Vegetables (*Continued*)
humidity control, **B1**.281
irradiation, **B1**.271
large scale agricultural operations, **B1**.280–1
leafy, **B1**.281
microbiology, **B1**.280–3
modified atmosphere packaging, **B1**.281, **B1**.282
nutrients, **B1**.281
pH, **B1**.281
predominant pathogens, **B1**.282
rots, **B1**.281
salads, **B1**.281, **B1**.282
selection and grading, **B1**.280–1
storage, **B1**.281–2
stress metabolites, **B1**.281
transport, **B1**.281
vacuum packaging, **B1**.281
washing, **B1**.281
water activity, **B1**.281
Vegetation
Cryptococcus neoformans, **M**.643
epidemics, **P**.117
Vehicle of infection, **B1**.310
indirect transmission, **V1**.354–5
Veillonella, **B2**.1312–16
antibacterial susceptibility/resistance, **B2**.1315
penicillin resistance, **B2**.1315
biochemical detection, **B2**.1312
nitrate reduction, **B2**.1313
propionic acid fermentation, **B1**.56
cell walls, **B2**.1314
classification, **B2**.1312
differential characteristics, **B2**.1313 (Tab.)
genetic makeup, **B2**.1312
culture, **B2**.1314
fluorescence, **B2**.1314
Gram staining, **B2**.1314
habitats, **B2**.1312–13
historical perspective, **B2**.1312
isolation/identification, **B2**.1314–15
biochemistry, **B2**.1314–15
Gram staining, **B2**.1314–15
molecular methods, **B2**.1315
laboratory maintenance, **B2**.1314
LPS, **B2**.1314
as normal microbiota, **B1**.296 (Tab.), **B1**.303, **B2**.1313
mouth, **B1**.609
oropharynx, **B1**.301
as opportunist pathogen, **B2**.1313–14
dental caries, **B2**.1314
infection, **B2**.1313–14
virulence factors, **B2**.1314
Veillonella,, antibody degradation/modification, **I**.662
Veillonella atypica, **B2**.1312–13
biochemical identification, **B2**.1314–15
Veillonella caviae, **B2**.1312–13
Veillonellaceae, **B2**.1312
Veillonella criceti, **B2**.1312–13
biochemical identification, **B2**.1314–15
Veillonella dispar, **B2**.1312–13
biochemical identification, **B2**.1314–15

possible infection, **B2**.1313–14
Veillonella parvula, **B2**.1312–13
biochemical identification, **B2**.1314–15
possible infection, **B2**.1313–14
Veillonella ratti, **B2**.1312–13
Veillonella rodentium, **B2**.1312–13
V elements, TCR, **I**.450–1
Veneering, monoclonal antibody therapy, **I**.365–6
Venereal Disease Research Laboratory (VDRL) antigen, **B2**.1845–6, **B2**.1846 (Tab.)
Capture-S solid phase red blood cell adherence, **B2**.1846
cerebrospinal fluid variation, **B2**.1846
Venereal Disease Research Laboratory (VDRL) test, **B1**.663
Venezuelan encephalitis virus, **V2**.1648 (Tab.)
Venezuelan equine encephalitis, **V2**.1020–1
adults, **V2**.1021
children, **V2**.1021
clinical features, **V2**.1020–1
distribution, **V2**.1020
history, **V2**.1020
in pregnancy, **V2**.1021
transmission, **V1**.372 (Tab.), **V2**.1016–17, **V2**.1020, **V2**.1021 (Fig.)
aerosols, **V2**.1018
reservoir hosts, **V2**.1017
Venezuelan equine encephalitis virus (VEEV), **V2**.1010, **V2**.1011 (Tab.)
biological warfare agent, **V2**.1018
cell receptors, **V2**.1015
enzootic strains, **V2**.1021
virion structure, **V2**.1012
Venezuelan hemorrhagic fever, **V2**.1070
Ventilator-associated pneumonia (VAP), hospitals, **B1**.640
Ventral disc, **P**.170–2
Ventricular septal defects (VSDs), rubella, **V2**.974
Ventricular shunting, neurocysticercosis treatment, **P**.696
Ventriuloperitoneal (VP) shunts
cryptococcosis therapy, **M**.652
CSF withdrawal, **M**.652
intracranial pressure reduction, **M**.652
neurocysticercosis treatment, **P**.696
Verapamil, α_1-acid glycoprotein binding, **I**.205
Verluma, licensing, **I**.355 (Tab.)
Vernacular nomenclature, **V1**.40
Vero cell line
filovirus cell culture, **V2**.1091
Rubella virus culture, **V2**.964
Vero-cytotoxin-producing *Escherichia coli* (VTEC) *see Escherichia coli,* verotoxigenic (VTEC)
Verona imipenemase, carbapenem resistance, **B1**.478–80
Verruca vulgaris, HPV associations, **V1**.465 (Tab.)
Verruga peruana
clinical manifestations, **B2**.1889
historical perspective, **B2**.1885
prevalence, **B2**.1889
rifampicin treatment, **B2**.1891
see also Carrión's disease

VERSANT®, **B1**.722, **B1**.723 (Tab.), **B1**.733–4
Vertical transmission, **V1**.354
hepatitis B, **V1**.369
HPV-16, **V1**.467
HTLV transmission, **V2**.1292
malaria in pregnancy, **P**.484
plasmid genes, **B1**.110
retroviruses, **V1**.281
Verticillium searrae, oculomycoses, **M**.275 (Tab.)
Vesicles
HSV infection, **V1**.508–9, **V1**.508 (Fig.)
trafficking, Canine parvovirus, **V1**.417
varicella (chickenpox), **V1**.512–13, **V1**.513 (Fig.), **V1**.515
VZV, **V1**.514
Vesicle trafficking, parvovirus infection, **V1**.417–18
Vesicular exanthema of swine virus, **V2**.912
Vesicular stomatitis Indiana virus, type species, **V1**.385–6
Vesicular stomatitis virus (VSV)
attenuation, **V1**.195, **V1**.197 (Fig.)
gene vector development, **V1**.197–8
cell interactions
host protein synthesis inhibition, **V1**.203
host RNA synthesis, **V1**.220–1
cellular protein packaging, **V2**.1106
defective interfering particles, **V1**.186
gene expression, **V1**.119–20
genome structure, **V1**.128–30, **V2**.1112 (Fig.)
glycoprotein (G), **V2**.1115
vaccines, **V2**.1117
hypermutation, **V1**.193
infection
cytocidal infection, **V1**.205
defensin actions, **I**.168
INFs, **V1**.271
matrix (M) protein
auto-association, **V2**.1114
budding process, **V2**.1114
cell morphology, **V2**.1115
membrane-binding, **V2**.1114
posttranslation processing, **V2**.1114
viral genome transcription inhibition, **V2**.1114
morphology/structure, **V1**.74 (Fig.), **V1**.75
M proteins, **V1**.69–70
protein structures, **V1**.70 (Tab.)
receptors, **V1**.207 (Tab.), **V2**.1108
RNA-dependent RNA polymerase, **V1**.130
transcription–replication switch, **V2**.1111
type species, **V2**.1103
Vesiculovirus
characteristics, **V1**.129 (Tab.)
classification, **V1**.385, **V2**.1103
members, **V1**.385–6
type species *see* Vesicular stomatitis virus (VSV)
see also Vesiculoviruses
Vesiculoviruses
genome
size, **V2**.1111
structure, **V1**.387 (Tab.), **V2**.1112 (Fig.)

Vesiculoviruses (*Continued*)
  infection, **V2**.1116–17
    in animals, **V2**.1116
    in humans, **V2**.1116–17
    transmission, **V2**.1117
    vaccines, **V2**.1117
  matrix (M) protein, in replication, **V2**.1109
  morphology, **V2**.1106 (Fig.)
Vesivirus, **V2**.912
  phylogenetic analysis, **V2**.917 (Fig.)
Veterinarians
  blastomycosis, **M**.484, **M**.488
  sporotrichosis, **M**.370
Veterinary pathogens, bunyaviruses, **V2**.1042
Veterinary practice, cleaning surfaces, **B1**.424,
    B1.425
V factor, *Haemophilus,* **B2**.1695
vFLIPs *see* Viral FLICE inhibitory proteins
    (vFLIPs)
V genes, Igs, **I**.328
Viable but nonculturable (VBNC) state,
    Aeromonas hydrophila, **B2**.1529
Vi antigen *see Salmonella*
Vibrio, **B2**.1507–20
  adhesins, **B1**.149
  antibacterial susceptibility/resistance,
    B2.1514
  bacteriophages, **B2**.1511, **B2**.1512, **B2**.1518
    typing, **B2**.1516
  biofilms, **B2**.1508–9
  cellular organization, **B2**.1510–11
    capsules, **B2**.1509, **B2**.1511
    cell wall, **B2**.1511
    chromosomes, **B2**.1511–12
    flagella, **B2**.1510
    pili, **B2**.1511
    plasmids, **B2**.1512
  characteristics, **B2**.1330 (Tab.)
  classification, **B2**.1507
    genus, **B2**.1508
  culture, **B2**.1509–10
    growth requirements, **B2**.1509–10
  definition, **B2**.1508
  environmental change adaption, **B2**.1509
  genetics, **B2**.1511–12
  habitats, **B2**.1508–9
  infection
    in fish, **B1**.279, **B2**.1508–9
    mollusks, **B1**.280
    shellfish, **B2**.1508–9
    undercooked/raw seafood consumption,
      B2.1508
    see also Cholera
  integrons, **B2**.1512
  isolation/identification, **B2**.1512–14
    biotypes, **B2**.1514
    genus, **B2**.1512–13
    molecular typing methods, **B2**.1516
    species, **B2**.1513–14
  metabolism, **B2**.1510
  morphology, **B2**.1509
    colonies, **B2**.1509
    microscopic, **B2**.1509
  in normal microbiota, **B2**.1516
  pathogenicity, **B2**.1516–17

  species, **B2**.1508, **B2**.1513–14
  typing, **B2**.1514–16
    bacteriophage typing, **B2**.1516
    molecular typing, **B2**.1516
    serotyping, **B2**.1514–16
  viable but nonculturable state, **B2**.1509
  virulence factors, **B2**.1517–20
    LPS, **B1**.158–9
Vibrio aerogenes
  growth requirements, **B2**.1510
  metabolism, **B2**.1510
Vibrio alginolyticus
  bacteriophages, **B2**.1512
  characteristics, **B2**.1513–14, **B2**.1515 (Tab.)
  culture, **B2**.1509–10
    growth requirements, **B2**.1510
  flagella, **B2**.1510
  mollusks, **B1**.280
  morphology, **B2**.1509
  pathogenicity, **B2**.1517
Vibrio anguillarum
  classification, **B2**.1507
  growth requirements, **B2**.1510
  habitats, **B2**.1508–9
  pathogenicity, **B2**.1517
  serotyping, **B2**.1514–16
Vibrio cholerae, **B2**.1507–8
  antibacterial susceptibility/resistance,
    B2.1514
  bacteriophages, **B2**.1512
    typing, **B2**.1516
  BCE peptide vaccines, **I**.855 (Tab.)
  cellular organization, **B2**.1510–11
    cell wall, **B2**.1511
    flagella, **B2**.1510
    pili, **B1**.149, **B2**.1511
  characteristics, **B2**.1512–14, **B2**.1513 (Tab.),
    B2.1515 (Tab.)
  colonization factors, **B2**.1511
  culture, **B2**.1509, **B2**.1509–10
    growth requirements, **B2**.1510
  foods
    hazard analysis, **B1**.288
    vegetables, **B1**.282
  genetics, **B2**.1511–12
    cep genes, **B2**.1511
    chromosomes, **B2**.1511–12
  habitats, **B1**.212, **B2**.1508–9
  infection *see* Cholera
  iron-dependent repression, **B1**.165–6
  isolation/identification
    biotypes/biotyping, **B2**.1514
    molecular typing, **B2**.1516
    serotyping, **B2**.1514
    typing, **B2**.1514–16
  mannose-sensitive hemagglutinin, **B2**.1511
  morphology, **B2**.1509
    wrinkled, or rugose colonies, **B2**.1509
  non-epidemic (non-O1, non-O139), **B1**.280,
    B1.363
  in normal microbiota, **B2**.1516
  pathogenicity, **B2**.1516–17
  phenotype switching, **B2**.1509
  sensory networks, **B1**.165
  signal transduction, **B1**.167–9

  toxins, **B2**.1517–20
    accessory cholera enterotoxin, **B2**.1516–17,
      B2.1518
    NAG-ST, **B2**.1518–19
    similarity to *Escherichia coli* enterotoxin,
      B2.1517–18
    toxin coregulated pilus, **B2**.1511, **B2**.1512,
      B2.1518
    zonnula occludens toxin, **B2**.1516–17,
      B2.1518
    see also Cholera toxin (CT)
  as vaccine vectors *see* Vaccines, live
  virulence factors, **B2**.1517–19
    cholera toxin, **B1**.156 (Tab.)
    neuraminidase, **B1**.153 (Tab.)
    toxin-coregulated pilus, **B1**.149
Vibrio cholerae O1
  bacteriophages, **B2**.1512
  biotypes/biotyping, **B2**.1514
  cell wall, **B2**.1511
  El Tor biotype
    culture, **B2**.1510
    pilii, **B2**.1511
  isolation/identification, **B2**.1513
Vibrio cholerae O139, **B2**.1507–8
  antibacterial susceptibility/resistance,
    B2.1512, **B2**.1514
  bacteriophages, **B2**.1512
  cell wall, **B2**.1511
  emerging bacterial infection, **B1**.363
  epidemic cholera, **B2**.1507–8
  integrons, **B2**.1512
  pili, **B2**.1511
  plasmids, **B2**.1512
  SXT elements, **B2**.1512
Vibrio cincinnatiensis, **B2**.1512–14,
    B2.1515 (Tab.)
  culture, **B2**.1509–10
Vibrio diabolicus, flagella, **B2**.1510
Vibrio fischeri
  autoinduction, **B1**.72
  flagella, **B2**.1510
  habitats, **B2**.1508–9
Vibrio fluvialis, **B2**.1513–14, **B2**.1515 (Tab.)
  culture, **B2**.1509–10
  mollusks, **B1**.280
  pathogenicity, **B2**.1517
  serotyping, **B2**.1514–16
Vibrio furnissii, **B2**.1513–14, **B2**.1515 (Tab.)
  bacteriophage typing, **B2**.1516
  metabolism, **B2**.1510
  pathogenicity, **B2**.1517
  serotyping, **B2**.1514–16
Vibrio harveyi
  bacteriophages, **B2**.1512
  characteristic, **B2**.1515 (Tab.)
  flagella, **B2**.1510
  morphology, **B2**.1509
  signal transduction, **B1**.167–8
Vibrio hollisae, **B2**.1513–14, **B2**.1515 (Tab.)
  culture, **B2**.1509–10
  mollusks, **B1**.280
  pathogenicity, **B2**.1517
Vibrio logei, **B2**.1510

Vibrio metschnikovii, **B2**.1513–14,
    B2.1515 (Tab.)
  culture, **B2**.1509–10
  growth requirements, **B2**.1510
Vibrio mimicus, **B2**.1513–14, **B2**.1513 (Tab.),
    B2.1515 (Tab.)
  culture, **B2**.1509–10
    growth requirements, **B2**.1510
  habitats, **B2**.1508–9
  pathogenicity, **B2**.1516–17
Vibrionaceae, fish spoilage, **B1**.279
'Vibrion septique', **B1**.9–10
Vibrio parahaemolyticus, **B2**.1513–14,
    B2.1515 (Tab.)
  bacteriophages, **B2**.1512
  cell wall, **B2**.1511
  chromosomes, **B2**.1511–12
  culture, **B2**.1509–10
  flagella, **B2**.1510
  habitats, **B2**.1508–9
  infection, **B2**.1508
    climate changes, **B1**.362
  morphology, **B2**.1509
  pathogenicity, **B2**.1517
  pili, **B2**.1511
  serotyping, **B2**.1514–16
  in shellfish, **B2**.1508
    crustacea, **B1**.279–80
    mollusks, **B1**.280
  virulence factors, **B2**.1519–20
Vibrio pectenicida, **B2**.1510
Vibrio salmonicida, **B2**.1510
Vibrio tapetis, **B2**.1517
Vibrio vulnificus
  bacteriophages, **B2**.1512
  biotypes/biotyping, **B2**.1514
  cell wall, **B2**.1511
  characteristics, **B2**.1513–14, **B2**.1515 (Tab.)
  culture, **B2**.1509–10
  flagella, **B2**.1510
  habitats, **B2**.1508–9
  infection, **B2**.1508, **B2**.1517
  morphology, **B2**.1509
  pathogenicity, **B2**.1517
  pili, **B2**.1511
  in shellfish, **B2**.1508, **B2**.1517
    crustacea, **B1**.279–80
    mollusks, **B1**.280
  virulence factors, **B2**.1519
Vidarabine, **V2**.1615
  structure, **V2**.1611 (Fig.)
Villous atrophy
  ascariasis, **P**.727
  cryptosporidiosis, **P**.407, **P**.408
  isosporiasis, **P**.413
Vinca alkaloids, Kaposi's sarcoma therapy,
    V1.553
Vincent's disease, **B1**.613–14
Vioxx (rofecoxib), **I**.186–7
Viracept *see* Nelfinavir
Viral clearance
  granzymes, **I**.482 (Tab.)
  IFN-γ, **I**.478
  perforin, **I**.482 (Tab.)

Viral early transcription factor (VETF) *see*
    Poxviruses
'Viral factories,' poxviruses, **V1**.612–14,
    V1.612 (Fig.)
Viral FLICE inhibitory proteins (vFLIPs)
  definition, **V1**.624–5
  Herpesvirus saimiri (HVS), **V1**.287
  HHV-8, **V1**.546, **V1**.548, **V1**.549 (Tab.)
  Kaposi's sarcoma-associated herpesvirus,
    V1.287, **V1**.323
  Molluscum contagiosum virus, **V1**.323
Viral genes that interfere with antigen
    presentation (VIPR), **I**.633
Viral hemorrhagic fevers, nosocomial
    infection, **B1**.400
Viral hemorrhagic septicemia virus (VHSV)
  cell receptor, **V2**.1108
  classification, **V1**.385–6
Viral intermediate transcription factors (VITF)
    see Poxviruses
Viral late transcription factors (VLTF) *see*
    Poxviruses
Viral termination factor (VTF), poxviruses,
    V1.599 (Tab.), **V1**.610
Viramune *see* Nevirapine
Virchow, R, **M**.18–9, **M**.19 (Fig.)
Viread *see* Tenofovir
Viremia, **V1**.240–3
  active, **V1**.240–1
  acute hepatitis B, **V2**.1247
  acute hepatitis C, **V2**.1203
  cell-associated, **V1**.242
  hepatitis D, **V2**.1272
  passive, **V1**.240
  persistent, **V1**.242 (Fig.)
  plasma, **V1**.240, **V1**.241
  primary/secondary, **V1**.240
  Torque-teno-virus infection, **V2**.1279
  virulence reduction, **V1**.246 (Fig.), **V1**.252
  virus localization affected by, **V1**.245
vir genes, *Plasmodium* antigenic variation,
    P.492
Virgibacillus, **B2**.922–3
Virgibacillus pantothenticus, **B2**.935 (Tab.)
  taxonomy, **B2**.922–3
Virginiamycin, **B1**.489
Viricides, **B1**.434
  regulations, **B1**.434
  tests, **B1**.435–6, **B1**.435 (Tab.)
Virions
  concept, **V1**.6
  viruses *vs.,* **V1**.26
Virion structural protein (VP), filoviruses,
    V2.1086–8
Viroceptors, **V1**.256–7
Viroids, **P**.159
  Hepatitis D virus *vs.,* **V1**.12–3
  origins, **V1**.12–3
  structure, **V1**.12
Virokines, **V1**.256–7
Viropexis, **V2**.1065
'Viroplasm,' poxviruses, **V1**.612–14
Viroptic *see* Trifluridine
Virosomes *see* Vaccine(s)
Virudox *see* Idoxuridine

Virulence, **V1**.250–8
  carcinogenesis, **V1**.253–4
  definition, **B1**.146, **V1**.250, **V1**.356
  emerging viral infection, **V2**.1655
  experimental manipulation, **V1**.251–2
  genes of cellular origin, **V1**.256–8,
    V1.257 (Fig.)
  genetic analysis, **V1**.194–5
  genetic determinants, **V1**.254–6
  measures, **V1**.250–1
    quantitative comparison, **V1**.252 (Fig.)
  mechanisms, **B1**.626–8
    respiratory tract infection, **B1**.626–8
  neural spread affecting, **V1**.253
  Newcastle disease virus, **V1**.815
  pathogenic mechanisms, **V1**.252–4
  persistent infection *see* Persistent viral
    infection
  precise estimates, **V1**.251
  protein secretion *see* Protein(s), secretion
  relative nature, **V1**.250
  for target organs, **V1**.253, **V1**.254 (Tab.)
  tropism and host range, **V1**.253
  viremia determining, **V1**.246 (Fig.), **V1**.252
  see also individual species
Virulence factors
  Agrobacterium tumefaciens, **B1**.115
  Aspergillus fumigatus, **M**.79
  Aspergillus nidulans, **M**.79–80
  Bifidobacterium, **B2**.1026
  Borrelia, **B2**.1825
  Brucella, **B2**.1726
  Burkholderia, **B2**.1614
  Burkholderia cepacia complex, **B2**.1615
  Candida, **M**.79–80, **M**.258–9, **M**.586–7,
    M.598–9
  cloning, **I**.14
  Cryptococcus neoformans, **M**.79, **M**.641–2,
    M.646
  Escherichia coli, **B1**.114
  genomic studies, **B1**.177–8
  K-antigens, **B1**.154
  Leishmania, **I**.678
  MAP kinases, **M**.79–80
  plasmid resistance genes, **B1**.115
  Propionibacterium, **B2**.1032
  pyrogenic exotoxins, **I**.561
  quorum sensing, **B1**.72
  Salmonella Dublin, **B1**.114, **B2**.1418
  Staphylococcus aureus, **B1**.115
  superantigens, **I**.561
  Veillonella, **B2**.1314
Virulence genes, transposon, **B1**.97
Viruria, **V1**.249
Virus associated (VAI) RNAs, host protein
    synthesis effects, **V1**.121
Viruses, **P**.159
  antibacterial agents, **B1**.434, **B1**.439–40
    biocide interactions, **B1**.440
    resistance, **B1**.445
  immune evasion *see* Immune evasion, viruses
  infection *see* Infection(s)
  mollusks, **B1**.280
  neutralization by antibody, **I**.312
  pattern recognition receptors, **I**.23

Viruses (*Continued*)
  sterilization, ultraviolet radiation, **B1**.451
  sunlight, **B1**.452
  as vaccine vectors *see* Vaccines, live
Virus-like particles (VLPs)
  Bluetongue virus, **V2**.941 (Fig.)
  Leishmania, **P**.335
  orbiviruses, **V2**.941–2, **V2**.941 (Fig.)
  papillomaviruses, **V1**.450
  in vaccines *see* Vaccine(s)
Virus neutralization assays, antibody analysis,
    V2.1545
Virus particles, viruses *vs.,* **V1**.26
*Virus Taxonomy: VIIIth Report of the
    International Committee on the
    Taxonomy of Viruses,* **V1**.38–9
Visceral larva migrans (VLM) *see* Toxocariasis
Visceral leishmaniasis *see* Leishmaniasis, Old
    World, visceral (kala-azar)
Visna-maedi virus
  antigenic variation, **V1**.262
  viremia, **V1**.243 (Fig.)
Vistide *see* Cidofovir
Visual damage, onchocerciasis *see*
    Onchocerciasis
Vitamin(s)
  requirements, Enterobacteriaceae culture,
    B2.1345
  synthesis by intestinal bacteria, **B1**.293–4
Vitamin A
  acute phase response, **I**.207–8
  deficiency
    malaria, **P**.493
    upper respiratory tract infection, **B1**.608
Vitamin B2 (riboflavin) deficiency, malaria,
    P.493
Vitamin B$_{12}$ absorption, *Diphyllobothrium
    latum,* **P**.663, **P**.672
Vitamin D-binding protein, **I**.203
Vitamin D receptor
  gene *see* VDR gene
  immunogenetics, **I**.582–3
Vitek enteric pathogens card, **B2**.1463
VITF-1, poxviruses, **V1**.599 (Tab.)
VITF-3, poxviruses, **V1**.599 (Tab.)
Vitiligo, prevalence, **I**.748 (Tab.)
Vitivirus, **V1**.27 (Tab.)
Vitrectomy, toxocariasis therapy, **P**.755
Vitreous body
  fungal infection, **M**.317–27
  specimens, **M**.84
Vitronectin *see* S-protein (vitronectin)
Vittaforma
  animal models, **P**.540
  classification, **P**.198, **P**.535, **P**.540
  structure, **P**.535
  see also Microsporidians; Microsporidiosis
Vittaforma corneae
  corneal infection, **P**.543
  meronts, **P**.540 (Fig.)
  in vitro culture, **P**.548
V(D)J recombination
  class switching, **I**.330
  Ig diversity generation, **I**.328
  recombination signal sequences, **I**.328

TCR rearrangements, **I**.451, **I**.452 (Fig.),
    I.453–4, **I**.453 (Fig.), **I**.457–8, **I**.459 (Fig.)
  12/23 rule, **I**.328
VLA-4 *see* Integrin α$_4$β$_1$ (VLA-4)
VLTF-1, poxviruses, **V1**.599 (Tab.)
VLTF-2, poxviruses, **V1**.599 (Tab.)
VLTF-3, poxviruses, **V1**.599 (Tab.)
VLTF-4, poxviruses, **V1**.599 (Tab.)
Voges–Proskauer test
  Aeromonas, **B2**.1532
  Brucella, **B2**.1731
  Enterobacteriaceae, **B2**.1319 (Tab.)
Volunteer studies
  astrovirus infection, **V2**.904
  community parasite control, **P**.121
  norovirus infection, **V2**.911
Volutella cinereescens, oculomycoses,
    M.275 (Tab.)
von Siebold C.T., **P**.10–1, **P**.13
Voriconazole, **M**.153, **M**.182–3
  activity, **M**.153
  coccidioidomycosis therapy, **M**.511
  drug interactions, **M**.153
  mechanism of action, **M**.70
  safety, **M**.153
  therapy
    Acremonium infection, **M**.758
    Alternaria infection, **M**.153
    aspergillosis, **M**.153, **M**.723, **M**.726
    Bipolaris infection, **M**.153
    candidiasis, **M**.613
    fusariosis, **M**.153, **M**.755
    histoplasmosis capsulati, **M**.531
    Paecilomyces infection, **M**.758
    paracoccidioidomycosis, **M**.552
    penicilliosis marneffei, **M**.571
VP1 protein
  Erythrovirus, **V1**.415–16
  Minute virus of mice (MVM), **V1**.157–8
  orbiviruses, **V2**.939–40, **V2**.940 (Tab.)
  polioviruses, **V1**.109, **V2**.862–3
  rotaviruses, **V2**.946, **V2**.947 (Fig.),
    V2.948 (Tab.)
VP2 protein
  Erythrovirus, **V1**.415–16
  Minute virus of mice (MVM), **V1**.157–8
  polioviruses, **V2**.862–3
  rotaviruses, **V2**.946, **V2**.947 (Fig.),
    V2.948 (Tab.)
VP3 protein
  Minute virus of mice (MVM), **V1**.157–8
  orbiviruses, **V2**.939–40, **V2**.940 (Tab.)
  polioviruses, **V2**.862–3
  rotaviruses *see* Rotaviruses
VP4 protein
  orbiviruses, **V2**.939–40, **V2**.940 (Tab.)
  polioviruses, **V2**.862–3
  rotaviruses *see* Rotaviruses
  N-terminal myristolaytion, **V1**.122
VP5 protein
  orbiviruses, **V2**.940 (Tab.)
  rotaviruses, **V2**.946, **V2**.947 (Fig.),
    V2.948 (Tab.)
VP6 protein
  orbiviruses, **V2**.939–40, **V2**.940 (Tab.)

rotaviruses, **V2**.946, **V2**.947 (Fig.),
    V2.948 (Tab.)
VP7 protein
  orbiviruses, **V2**.939–40, **V2**.940 (Tab.)
  rotaviruses *see* Rotaviruses
VP16 protein, herpesviruses, **V1**.498
VP24 protein, **V1**.75–6, **V2**.1091
VP30 (minor nucleoprotein), **V2**.1090–1
VP35 (polymerase cofactor), **V2**.1089
VP40 matrix protein, **V1**.75–6, **V2**.1089
VP protein(s)
  foot-and-mouth disease virus *see* Foot-and-
    mouth disease virus
  parvoviruses, **V1**.407–8, **V1**.412
VP proteins, poliovirus, **I**.870
Vpre-B, pre-BCR, **I**.340–1
V proteins
  Bovine parainfluenza virus 3, **V1**.763–4
  Hendra virus, **V1**.816
  henipaviruses, **V1**.816
  Measles virus, **V1**.715–16, **V1**.717
  Nipah virus, **V1**.816
  paramyxoviruses, **V1**.704
  respiroviruses *see* Respiroviruses
  Sendai virus, **V1**.763–4
Vpr protein, **V2**.1327
Vpu protein *see* HIV-1
Vpx protein, **V2**.1327
Vsp proteins, *Borrelia* antigenic variation,
    B2.1827
Vuillemin, P, **M**.16
Vulva, rhinosporidiosis, **M**.459, **M**.460
Vulvovaginal candidiasis (VVC), **M**.189,
    M.579–80, **M**.584, **M**.593, **M**.598–9,
    M.603, **M**.603 (Fig.), **M**.609, **M**.610,
    M.611
  animal models, **M**.264, **M**.265–6
  causative agents, **M**.599
  diagnosis, **M**.258 (Tab.), **M**.603
  epidemiology, **M**.257
  immune response, **M**.264–7, **M**.593,
    M.267 (Tab.)
    animal models, **M**.264, **M**.265–6
    cell-mediated immunity, **M**.264, **M**.265–6
    humoral immune response, **M**.260, **M**.266
    IgA, **M**.260, **M**.266
    IgG, **M**.266
    independent compartmentalization
      concept, **M**.264
    innate immunity, **M**.266
    neutrophils, **M**.264, **M**.266
    T-cells, **M**.265
    T helper cells, type 1 (Th1), **M**.264
  incidence, **M**.255
  pregnancy, **M**.598–9
  recurrence, **M**.257, **M**.599, **M**.610
  symptoms, **M**.258 (Tab.)
  therapy, **M**.189, **M**.258 (Tab.), **M**.609, **M**.610

Wall-forming bodies, **P**.178–9
Wangiella dermatitidis
  chromoblastomycosis, **M**.357
  histopathology, **M**.89 (Tab.)
  infection
    CNS, **M**.743–4

Wangiella dermatitidis
infection (*Continued*)
therapy, **M**.745
melanin, **M**.746
pathogenicity, **M**.746
virulence, **M**.746
Wanowrie virus infection, **V2**.1048
War *see* Civil unrest
Warthin–Starry stain
Bartonella, **B2**.1898
Bartonella bacilliformis, **B2**.1890–1
WASP gene
glycogenosis Ib, **I**.767
Wiskott–Aldrich syndrome, **I**.777–8
Wassermann reaction, **B1**.745
Waste, laboratory safety, **V2**.1528
Waste, solid, **B1**.213, **B1**.213 (Tab.)
Wastewater treatment, airborne bacteria,
B1.186 (Tab.)
Wastewater workers, protothecosis, **M**.397
Water, **B1.211–28**
airborne bacteria, **B1**.185–7, **B1**.189
bacteriological analysis of, **B1**.220–5
bare skin immunization, **I**.823–4
biofilms in, **B1**.220
bottled, **B1**.215–16, **B1**.217 (Tab.), **B1**.224–5
cistern, **B1**.215, **B1**.216 (Tab.)
coastal, **B1**.217, **B1**.220, **B1**.224
contamination
hepatitis A, **V2**.1172, **V2**.1173
hepatitis E, **V2**.1180
Naegleria fowleri transmission, **P**.236
Schistosoma transmission, **P**.92–3
contributed bacteria, **B1**.211–3
endotoxin-free, for cell culture, **V1**.87
estuarine areas, **B1**.216
ground waters, **B1**.214–15, **B1**.224
hardness, antibacterial activity, **B1**.432
indigenous bacteria, **B1**.211
natural self-purification, **B1**.213, **B1**.219–20
norovirus infection, **V2**.919–20
pasteurization, **B1**.236
pathogenic bacteria, **B1**.217–19, **B1**.225
purification
hepatitis A prevention, **V2**.1173
hepatitis E prevention, **V2**.1180
quality criteria for, **B1**.220
surface waters, **B1**.213–14, **B1**.215 (Tab.), **B1**.221
swimming pools, **B1**.215
testing for, **B1**.220–5
treatment
dracunculiasis eradication, **P**.833–4
giardiasis prevention, **P**.251–2
Naegleria fowleri prevention, **P**.237–8
Water activity, microbial growth effect,
B1.266
Waterborne infection
bacteria, **B1**.212 (Tab.), **B1**.310, **B1.211–28**
bacteriological analysis, **B1**.220–5
Clostridium perfringens, **B1**.224
Escherichia coli, **B1**.223
fecal coliforms, **B1**.223
fecal streptococci, **B1**.223–4
heterotrophic bacteria, **B1**.221

Pseudomonas, **B1**.224–5
stressed organisms, **B1**.221
total coliform bacteria, **B1**.222–3
biofilms, **B1**.220
bottled water, **B1**.215–16, **B1**.217 (Tab.), **B1**.224–5
characterization, **B1**.211–13
cisterns, **B1**.215, **B1**.216 (Tab.)
coastal waters, **B1**.217, **B1**.220, **B1**.224
contributed, **B1**.211–13, **B1**.212 (Tab.)
ecological changes encouraging resurgence
of infection, **B1**.362
estuarine areas, **B1**.216
ground waters, **B1**.214–15, **B1**.224
indigenous, **B1**.211
nosocomial, **B1**.375, **B1**.376
pathogens, **B1**.217–19, **B1**.225
pathways, **B1**.218–19
persistence, **B1**.219
seasonal variation, **B1**.212 (Tab.)
surface waters, **B1**.213–14, **B1**.215 (Tab.), **B1**.221
swimming pools, **B1**.215
transmission, **B1**.310
Helicobacter pylori infection, **B2**.1579
Legionnaires' disease, **B1**.634–6
Legionnaires' disease due to, **B1**.375
Leptospira, **B2**.1879
tularemia, **B2**.1753
viruses, **V1**.355
*see also individual species; specific diseases/
infection*
Waterhouse–Friderikson syndrome, **B2**.1674–5
Watermelons, **B1**.283
Watsonius, **P**.583
Watson, J D, **B1**.13
Wayson's dye mixture, **B2**.1460
Weapons of mass destruction (WMD),
airborne bacteria, **B1**.189
Weeksella virosa, **B1**.296 (Tab.), **B1**.303
as normal microbiota, **B1**.296 (Tab.), **B1**.303
Wegener's granulomatosis, histoplasmosis
capsulati *vs.*, **M**.534
Weight loss, onchocerciasis, **P**.794
Weil–Felix reaction, **B2**.2030, **B2**.2035
Rickettsia detection, **B1**.752–3
Weil's disease, **B2**.1866
Well water, **B1**.214–15, **B1**.224
Werner–Hiss disease *see* Trench fever
Wesselsbron virus (WESSV), **V2**.997, **V2**.998 (Tab.), **V2**.1003
West-Caucasian bat virus (WCBV), **V2**.1104
Western blotting, **B1**.720, **V2**.1545
Bartonella detection, **B2**.1897, **B2**.1898
Borrelia detection, **B2**.1829, **B2**.1830 (Tab.)
cysticercosis diagnosis, **P**.690
filovirus infection diagnosis, **V2**.1096–7, **V2**.1097 (Tab.)
foamy virus detection, **V2**.1315–16
HTLV, **V2**.1293–4
human brucellosis diagnosis, **B2**.1740
microsporidiosis, **P**.536
neurocysticercosis diagnosis, **P**.692, **P**.693–4
PrP^{Sc}, **V2**.1365
Pythium insidiosum, **M**.424, **M**.424 (Fig.)
Rickettsia detection, **B2**.2035

syphilis test, **B2**.1849–50
see also Immunoblotting
Western equine encephalitis, **V2**.1020
clinical features, **V2**.1020
distribution, **V2**.1020
history, **V2**.1020
transmission, **V1**.372 (Tab.), **V2**.1017 (Fig.), **V2**.1020
reservoir hosts, **V2**.1017
Western equine encephalitis virus (WEEV), **V2**.998 (Tab.), **V2**.1010, **V2**.1011 (Tab.)
biological warfare agent, **V2**.1018
genetic subtypes, **V2**.1020
West Nile virus (WNV), **V2**.998 (Tab.), **V2**.1002, **V2**.1425
animal models, **I**.588–9
ELISA, **V2**.1425
geographical distribution, **V2**.1424, **V2**.1425
immune evasion, **V1**.296
infection
chikungunya *vs.*, **V2**.1021–2
clinical symptoms, **V2**.1425
emerging infection, **V2**.1648 (Tab.), **V2**.1651 (Tab.)
ecological changes, **V2**.1662–3
recombination, **V2**.1654
laboratory-acquired infection, **V2**.1517 (Tab.)
medical importance, **V1**.135
mortality, **V2**.1425
rubella *vs.*, **V2**.970
vaccine development, **I**.933 (Tab.), **V2**.1555
replication, cell-specific factors, **V1**.136 (Fig.)
transmission, **V1**.372 (Tab.)
transmission control, **B1**.355
West Nile virus, immune evasion, **V1**.296
Whataroa virus (WHAV), **V2**.1011 (Tab.)
Wheat, **B1**.284–5
harvesting, **B1**.284
normal microbiota, **B1**.284
production, **B1**.284
storage, **B1**.284–5
water activity, **B1**.284
Whelks, microbiology, **B1**.280
Whipple's disease
causative agent *see Tropheryma whippelii*
clinical features, **B2**.999, **B2**.1170
diagnosis, **B2**.1001–2, **B2**.1147–8
problems, **B2**.1170
epidemiology and pathogenicity, **B2**.999
etiology, **B1**.365
investigations, **B2**.998–9
intestinal involvement, **B2**.999, **B2**.1001–2, **B2**.1001 (Fig.)
treatment, **B2**.1171
antibacterial agents, **B2**.1002
Whipworms *see Trichuris trichiuria*
White fluids, **B1**.422
Whitening agents, **M**.123 (Tab.), **M**.125
White piedra, **M**.196–7, **M**.196 (Fig.)
animal infection, **M**.196
axilla, **M**.196
causative agents, **M**.195, **M**.196–7, **M**.198 (Tab.)
see also individual species

White piedra (*Continued*)
  clinical presentation, **M**.196, **M**.196 (Fig.)
  facial hair, **M**.196
  genitourinary tract infection, **M**.196, **M**.197
  history, **M**.10–11
  therapy, **M**.186, **M**.197
Whitewater Arroyo virus, **V2**.1059
Whitfield's ointment, tinea nigra, **M**.186
Whittaker's 5 kingdom classification, **P**.189–90
WHN gene, nude phenotype, **I**.775
Whole-cell vaccines
  mycoplasmas, **B2**.1992–3
  Q fever, **B2**.2075
Widal test, **B1**.748, **B1**.751
  enteric fever diagnosis, **B1**.744
  Salmonella Vi antigen, **B2**.1406
  typhoid diagnosis, **B1**.744
Wig cleaners, aspergillosis, **M**.18–9
Wigglesworthia glossinidia, **B2**.1330 (Tab.)
Wild carnivores, rabies, **V2**.1119–20
Wildlife refuges, waterborne bacteria,
  B1.218–19
Wilson, G S, **B1**.337
Wilts, plant disease source, **B1**.202
WIN 54954, structure, **V2**.1626 (Fig.)
Wiskott–Aldrich syndrome, **I**.777–8
  encapsulated bacteria infection, **I**.777–8
  WASP gene, **I**.777–8
Wistar-King-Aptekman (WKA) rats, **V2**.1430
Wistar rats, Borna disease virus infection,
  V2.1145
Witebsky, Ernest, **I**.748
Wolbachia
  classification, **B2**.2026, **B2**.2048–9, **B2**.2053
  habitats, hosts and diseases, **B2**.2049 (Tab.)
  human disease association, **B2**.2061
  identification and typing methods, **B2**.2057
  isolation, **B2**.2052
  onchocerciasis, **P**.790, **P**.795
  replication, **B2**.2052
  surface antigen genes, **B2**.2053–5
Wolbachia melophagi, **B2**.2026
Wolbachia persica, **B2**.1753
  classification, **B2**.2026, **B2**.2027 (Fig.)
Wolbachia pipientis, **B2**.2027 (Fig.)
Wolbachia pipientis-like symbionts
  antibiotic sensitivity, **B2**.2065–6
  genome, **B2**.2053
  habitats, hosts and diseases, **B2**.2049 (Tab.)
Wolf, Arne, **P**.17–8
Wolhynia fever *see* Trench fever
Wolinella succinogenes, terminal electron
  acceptors, **B1**.67
Women, emerging bacterial infection, **B1**.361
Woodchuck Hepatitis B virus (WHV)
  discovery, **V2**.1227
  HBx protein, **V2**.1242
  Hepatitis delta virus interactions, **V2**.1271
  infection
    hepatocellular carcinoma, **V2**.1244
    insertional mutagenesis, **V1**.338–9
Wood sugars (cyclitols), waterborne bacteria,
  B1.212–13
'Working cultures,' Enterobacteriaceae,
  B2.1346

World Health Organization (WHO), **I**.6
  emerging bacterial infection, **B1**.365
  essential drugs, antibacterial therapy, **B1**.467,
    B1.467 (Tab.)
  International Standards, **B1**.722–4
  leprosy, prevalence, **B2**.1203
  measles virus strain assignation, **V1**.721–2
  parasite control initiatives, **P**.103–6
  reference cell lines, **V1**.86
  SPf66 malaria vaccine approval, **P**.85
  vaccination schedule recommendations,
    V2.1560–1, **V2**.1561 (Tab.)
    hepatitis B, **V2**.1574
    influenza, **V1**.677–8
    poliomyelitis, **V2**.1572
  vaccine information, **V2**.1583
  vaccine potency testing, **B1**.324
World-wide web, nomenclature changes, **B1**.32
Wounds
  debridement, **B2**.1115
  infection
    clostridial, **B2**.1112
    Clostridium botulinum, **B2**.1072 (Fig.),
      B2.1073, **B2**.1112, **B2**.1113
    Clostridium perfringens, **B2**.1111–16
      see also Gas gangrene
    Enterococcus, **B2**.896
    tissue anoxia, **B2**.1112, **B2**.1113
  management, tetanus prevention, **B2**.1066
W protein, **V1**.816
  henipaviruses, **V1**.816
Wright stain, **M**.88 (Tab.)
  mycology, **M**.87
Wuchereria bancrofti, **P**.591, **I**.683, **P**.769
  characteristics, **P**.771 (Tab.)
  control, vector elimination, **P**.109
  epidemiology, **P**.39, **P**.769
  historical aspects, **P**.9, **P**.769–71
  immune evasion
    host molecule incorporation, **I**.684
    migration inhibitory factor homologue,
      I.687
  infection *see* Lymphatic filariasis
  ivermectin, **P**.789
  latent period, **P**.61 (Tab.)
  life expectancy, **P**.60 (Tab.)
  morphology, **P**.769, **P**.771 (Fig.)
  structure/life cycle, **P**.591, **P**.758 (Fig.),
    P.771–2
    intermediate hosts, **P**.771
    vectors, **P**.772
  vector, life expectancy, **P**.61 (Tab.)

Xanthomonads, vegetables, **B1**.281
Xanthomonas
  nuts, **B1**.287
  phytopathogenicity, **B1**.202
Xanthomonas phaseoli, **B1**.99
XC chemokines, **I**.217
  receptor, **I**.510 (Tab.)
XCL1 *see* Lymphotactin (XCL1:XCL2)
XCL2 *see* Lymphotactin (XCL1:XCL2)
Xenobiotic compounds
  aerobic pseudomonads degradation, **B2**.1598
  bioremediation, **B1**.201–2

Xenodiagnosis, Chagas disease, **P**.388–9
Xenopsylla cheopis, **B2**.2037
Xenorhabdus, **B2**.1330 (Tab.), **B2**.1498
Xenorhabdus luminescens see Photorhabdus
Xenorhabdus nematophilus, biochemical tests,
  B2.1319 (Tab.)
Xenotransplantation, risks, **V2**.1297
Xerophiles, **B1**.266
X factor, *Haemophilus*, **B2**.1694–5
XIAP, caspases inhibition, **I**.135
X-linked agammaglobulinemia (Bruton's
  disease), **I**.779, **I**.780–1
  btk gene mutations, **I**.780
  common variable immunodeficiency *vs.*,
    I.781
  pre-BcR signaling, **I**.323–4
X-linked autoimmunity-allergic dysregulation
  syndrome (XLAAD), **I**.752
X-linked hyper-IgM syndrome, **I**.326–7, **I**.778
X-linked lymphoproliferative disease (XLP),
  V1.568, **I**.779, **V2**.1508
  EBV infection, **I**.779
  hypogammaglobulinemia, **I**.779
  NK cells, **I**.95
  SAP/SH2DIA gene mutations, **I**.779
X-linked severe combined immunodeficiency,
  IL-2 receptor, **I**.575
Xolair, licensing, **I**.355 (Tab.)
X-protein *see* Borna disease virus (BDV)
X-ray crystallography
  isocahedral viruses, **V1**.62
  noroviruses, **V2**.913
X-rays
  irradiated sporozoites, malaria vaccination,
    P.516–17
  mutation, **B1**.82
  see also Radiology
XTT (tetrazolium salt), antifungal testing,
  M.157
Xylene, bioremediation, **B1**.201
Xylenols, **B1**.422
Xylose
  Enterobacteriaceae identification,
    B2.1319 (Tab.)
  metabolism, **B1**.57, **B1**.59

Y_0 value, **B1**.446
Yaba-like disease virus (YLDV), **V1**.589
  phylogenetic comparison, **V1**.584 (Fig.)
Yaba monkey tumor virus, **V1**.589
YAC clones, type I interferon receptors, **I**.253
Yatapoxvirus, **V1**.589
  classification, **V1**.579 (Tab.), **V1**.582, **V1**.594
  phylogenetics, **V1**.583
  taxonomy, **V1**.595 (Tab.)
Yaws, **B2**.1839 (Tab.)
  clinical features, **B2**.1859
Yeast(s)
  antibacterial agents, **B1**.433–4
  food
    fruit spoilage, **B1**.282, **B1**.283
    water activity, **B1**.266
  growth pattern, **M**.70, **M**.70 (Fig.), **M**.73
    budding, **M**.70 (Fig.), **M**.73
    fission, **M**.73

Yeast(s) (*Continued*)
 histopathology, **M**.87, **M**.87 (Fig.),
  M.89 (Tab.)
 infection
  oculomycoses, **M**.280 (Tab.), **M**.286–7
  uncommon species, **M**.624
  see also specific types
 morphological media, **M**.91, **M**.91 (Tab.)
 plants, **B1**.198
 serology, **M**.93 (Tab.)
 see also under Saccharomyces
Yellow cards, adverse reaction reporting,
  B1.325
Yellow fever, **V2**.999–1000
 emerging infection, **I**.6, **V2**.1648 (Tab.),
  V2.1663
  ecosystem alteration, **V2**.1662
 epidemiology, **V1**.372, **V2**.997
 neutralizing antibodies, **V2**.1412
 transmission, **V1**.372 (Tab.)
 vaccines/vaccination, **V1**.372, **V2**.997,
  V2.1579–80
  adverse effects, **V2**.1579–80
  history, **V1**.8 (Tab.)
  live, attenuated, **V2**.1555 (Tab.)
  programs, **V2**.1559 (Tab.)
  recommendations, **V2**.1580
  schedules, **V2**.1560–1
  SV 40 transmission, **V2**.1557
Yellow fever virus (YFV), **V2**.998 (Tab.),
  V2.999–1000, **B2**.1866
 17D strain, **V1**.251
 classification, biosafety level 3, **V2**.1526
 Hepatitis C virus *vs.*, **V2**.1190
 public health importance, **V2**.997
 vaccine *see* Yellow fever
 as vaccine vector, **I**.899
Yellow head virus (YHV), **V1**.825
 classification, **V1**.398
Yellow pigment production,
  Enterobacteriaceae identification,
  B2.1319 (Tab.)
'Yellows' disease, **B2**.1966
Yersinia, **B2**.1458–70
 antibacterial susceptibility/resistance,
  B2.1465–6
 antigens, **B2**.1461
  F1, V and W antigens, **B2**.1461
  LPS, **B2**.1461
  outer-membrane proteins, **B2**.1461,
   B2.1468–9
 bacteriocins, **B2**.1467–8
 bacteriophage, **B2**.1467–8
 biochemistry/metabolism, **B2**.1460, **B2**.1463,
  B2.1464 (Tab.)
  association with virulence, **B2**.1465 (Tab.)
  as facultative anaerobe, **B2**.1458
 biogroup 3A *see Yersinia mollaretii*
 biogroup 3B *see Yersinia bercovieri*
 biogroup X2 *see Yersinia aldovae*
 cell wall and envelope composition, **B2**.1461
 classification, **B2**.1461–2
  DNA–DNA analysis, **B2**.1338
  evolutionary relationships, **B2**.1318
  genus/species definition, **B2**.1458
  species, **B2**.1458

culture, **B2**.1460, **B2**.1463
 growth requirements, **B2**.1460
genetics, **B2**.1460
 conjugation, **B1**.103
habitats, **B2**.1459
historical perspective, **B2**.1458–9
immune evasion
 IL-10 induction, **I**.653
 macrophage avoidance, **I**.30
 MHC class II antigen presentation, **I**.659
 outer membrane protein variation, **I**.661
 phagocytic uptake inhibition, **I**.649
 type III secretion system, **I**.655
infection
 clinical disease, **B2**.1462
 host cell signal transduction subversion,
  B1.164
 IFN-γ, **I**.138
 immune response, **B2**.1462
 induced apoptosis, **I**.138
 infiltration of host tissues, **B1**.152
 intestinal, **B2**.1347
 macrophage apoptosis, **I**.138
 NK cell actions, **I**.100
 prevention, **B2**.1466
 TNF-α, **I**.138
 treatment, **B2**.1466
isolation/identification, **B2**.1462–5
 PCR, **B2**.1463–5
 screening tests, **B2**.1349 (Tab.)
 serology, **B1**.757
 typing methods, **B2**.1466–7
morphology, **B2**.1460
as normal microbiota, **B2**.1468
pathogenicity, **B2**.1458, **B2**.1468–70
plasmids, **B2**.1460–1, **B2**.1463–5, **B2**.1468
stress proteins, **B2**.1469
as vaccine vector, **I**.897 (Tab.)
virulence factors, **B2**.1460–1, **B2**.1468–70
 invasin, **B1**.152
waterborne, **B1**.212, **B1**.218–19
Yop protein secretion system, **B1**.48
Yersinia aldovae
 biochemical tests, **B2**.1319 (Tab.),
  B2.1464 (Tab.)
 historical perspective, **B2**.1459
Yersiniabactin (yersinio-phore), **B2**.1469
Yersinia bercovieri
 biochemical tests, **B2**.1319 (Tab.),
  B2.1464 (Tab.)
 habitats, **B2**.1459
Yersinia enterocolitica, **B2**.1458
 antibacterial susceptibility/resistance,
  B2.1465–6
 β-lactamases, **B2**.1465–6
 autoagglutination, **B2**.1465
 bacteriocins, **B2**.1467, **B2**.1467–8
 bacteriophage, **B2**.1467–8
 biogroup 3, **B2**.1459
 biotypes, **B2**.1461–2
  antibacterial susceptibility/resistance,
   B2.1465–6
 classification, **B2**.1461–2
 culture, **B2**.1460
  morphology, **B2**.1345 (Tab.)

temperature, **B2**.1344
in foods
 butter, **B1**.250
 meat and meat products, **B1**.273–5
 milk, **B1**.230–1, **B1**.235, **B1**.245
 poultry, **B1**.278
 storage temperature, **B1**.264
 vegetables, **B1**.282
 yogurt, **B1**.249
habitats, **B2**.1459
historical perspective, **B2**.1458–9
immune evasion
 IL-10 induction, **I**.652
 membrane attack complex inhibition, **I**.664
 superantigens, **I**.668
 TNF-α suppression, **I**.652
infection
 from blood products, **B1**.362
 clinical disease, **B2**.1462
 entry into cells, bacterial proteins, **I**.649
 IL-18, **I**.290–2
 immune response, **B2**.1462
 milk, **B1**.245
 mucosal immune response, **I**.522–3
 prevention, **B2**.1466
 reactive arthritis, **I**.594–5
 treatment, **B2**.1466
invasin, **B2**.1468
iron-regulated proteins (HMWP1 and 2),
  B2.1469
iron storage, **B2**.1469
isolation/identification, **B2**.1462–5
 biochemical tests, **B2**.1319 (Tab.),
  B2.1464 (Tab.)
 PCR, **B2**.1463–5
 screening tests, **B2**.1349 (Tab.)
 typing methods, **B2**.1466–7
morphology, **B2**.1460
 L-form, **B2**.1460
Myf, **B2**.1469
in normal gut flora, **B2**.1468
O and H antigens, **B2**.1461
pathogenicity, **B2**.1468, **B2**.1468–70
plasmids, **B2**.1460–1, **B2**.1463–5
 lactose fermentation, **B1**.115
serogroups, **B2**.1461–2
serotypes, **B2**.1461
superantigens, **I**.556 (Tab.), **I**.563
toxin, **B2**.1468
transmission, **B2**.1459
virulence factors, **B2**.1468–70
virulent *vs.* avirulent strains, **B2**.1465
Yersinia enterocolitica-like group, **B2**.1459
Yersinia frederiksenii
 biochemical tests, **B2**.1319 (Tab.),
  B2.1464 (Tab.)
 habitats, **B2**.1459
 historical perspective, **B2**.1459
 isolation/identification, **B2**.1463
Yersinia intermedia
 bacteriocins, **B2**.1467
 biochemical tests, **B2**.1319 (Tab.),
  B2.1464 (Tab.)
 historical perspective, **B2**.1459

Yersinia kristensenii
- bacteriocins, **B2**.1467
- biochemical reactivity, **B2**.1464 (Tab.)
- historical perspective, **B2**.1459
- isolation/identification, **B2**.1463

Yersinia mollaretii
- biochemical tests, **B2**.1319 (Tab.), **B2**.1464 (Tab.)
- habitats, **B2**.1459

Yersinia pestis
- antibacterial susceptibility/resistance, **B2**.1466
- antigens, **B2**.1461
  - LcrV antigen, **B2**.1469
  - pH6 antigen, **B2**.1469
- bacteriocins, **B2**.1467
- bacteriophage, **B2**.1467
- biochemical tests, **B2**.1319 (Tab.), **B2**.1464 (Tab.)
- biogroups, **B2**.1462
- bioterrorism, **B1**.189, **B1**.364–5
- culture, **B2**.1460
- habitats, **B2**.1459
- historical perspective, **B2**.1331, **B2**.1458–9
- infection, **B2**.1462
  - immune response, **B2**.1462
  - pneumonia, **B1**.637
  - *see also* Plague
- iron-dependent repression, **B1**.165–6
- isolation/identification, **B2**.1462–3
- morphology, **B2**.1460
- non-motility, **B2**.1342
- pharyngitis, **B1**.611–12
- plasmids, **B2**.1460–1, **B2**.1468, **B2**.1469
- plasminogen activator protease, **B2**.1469
- transmission, **B2**.1459
- typing methods, **B2**.1466–7
- viability, **B2**.1459
- virulence factors, **B2**.1468–70

Yersinia pseudotuberculosis
- antibacterial susceptibility/resistance, **B2**.1466
- bacteriocins, **B2**.1467
- bacteriophage, **B2**.1467
- classification, **B2**.1461–2
- culture, **B2**.1460
- habitats, **B2**.1459
- historical perspective, **B2**.1318–31, **B2**.1460
- immunosuppression, **I**.665
- infection, **B2**.1462
  - erythema nodosum, **I**.563
  - immune response, **B2**.1462
  - Kawasaki's disease, **I**.563
  - reactive arthritis, **I**.563
  - symptoms, **I**.563
  - treatment and prevention, **B2**.1466
  - uveitis, **I**.563
- isolation/identification, **B2**.1463–5
  - biochemical tests, **B2**.1319 (Tab.), **B2**.1464 (Tab.)
  - typing methods, **B2**.1466–7
- mitogen, **I**.556 (Tab.), **I**.563
- mitogen (YPM), **B2**.1468
- O and H antigens, **B2**.1461
- pathogenicity, **B2**.1468–70

pH6 antigen, **B2**.1469
- serotypes, **B2**.1461
- subspecies *pestis see Yersinia pestis*
- superantigens, **I**.556 (Tab.), **I**.563
- toxin, **B2**.1468
- transmission, **B2**.1459
- virulence factors, **B2**.1468–70

Yersinia rohdei
- biochemical tests, **B2**.1319 (Tab.), **B2**.1464 (Tab.)
- habitats, **B2**.1459
- historical perspective, **B2**.1459

Yersinia ruckeri
- antibacterial susceptibility/resistance, **B2**.1466
- biochemical tests, **B2**.1319 (Tab.), **B2**.1464 (Tab.)
- historical perspective, **B2**.1459
- plasmids, **B2**.1470
- virulence factors, **B2**.1469–70

Y intercept, **B1**.446
Yogurt, **B1**.248–50
- microbiological quality of, **B1**.249–50
Yokenella, **B2**.1497–8
- antibacterial susceptibility/resistance, **B2**.1498
- biochemical tests, **B2**.1498
- culture, **B2**.1498
- definition, **B2**.1497
- habitats, **B2**.1498
- pathogenicity, **B2**.1498

Yokenella regensburgei, **B2**.1497
- antibacterial susceptibility/resistance, **B2**.1498
- biochemistry, **B2**.1319 (Tab.), **B2**.1498
- culture, **B2**.1498
- habitats, **B2**.1498
- pathogenicity, **B2**.1498

YopJ/P, macrophage apoptosis, **I**.138
Yop protein, *Yersinia* secretion system, **B1**.48
YO-PRO-1 nucleic acids staining, **B2**.1000, **B2**.1001 (Fig.)

Zaire ebolavirus (ZEBOV), **V1**.382
- animal models, **V2**.1095
- cell culture, **V2**.1091–2
- classification, **V2**.1086
- epidemiology, **V2**.1093
- genome structure, **V1**.381, **V2**.1088
  - gene overlap, **V2**.1088
- glycoprotein (GP), **V2**.1089
- historical aspects, **V2**.1085
- large (L) protein, **V2**.1091
- mortality, **V2**.1094
- non structural glycoproteins, **V2**.1091
- nucleoprotein (NP), **V2**.1086–8
- outbreaks, **V2**.1085–6, **V2**.1087 (Tab.)
- VP24, **V2**.1091
- VP30 (minor nucleoprotein), **V2**.1090–1
- VP35 (polymerase cofactor), **V2**.1089
- VP40 (matrix protein), **V2**.1089
Zalcitabine, **V2**.1620
- HIV infection, **V2**.1334
  - point mutation resistance, **V2**.1337 (Fig.)
- structure, **V2**.1620 (Fig.)

Zanamivir, **V2**.1626–8
- influenza therapy, **V1**.680
- resistance, **V1**.680, **V2**.1637
- structure, **V2**.1627 (Fig.)
ZAP-70
- deficiency, **I**.775
- immunoreceptor tyrosine-based activation motif binding, **I**.775
Zelitrex *see* Valaciclovir (VACV)
Zenapax, licensing, **I**.355 (Tab.)
Zevalin, licensing, **I**.355 (Tab.)
Ziagen *see* Abacavir
ZIC3 gene mutations, **I**.771
Zidovudine *see* Azidothymidine (AZT)
Ziehl–Neelsen stain, **B1**.714
- modified, **M**.123 (Tab.)
- *Mycobacterium leprae* detection, **B2**.1205
Zika virus (ZIKV), **V2**.998 (Tab.)
Zinc, acute phase response, **I**.208
Zinc-binding protein, arenaviruses, **V2**.1068
Zinc deficiency, malaria, **P**.493
'Zinc-finger' motif, influenza M1 protein, **V1**.657
Zinc-metalloproteases, **B2**.1040, **B2**.1061
Zinc pyrithione
- piedra, **M**.186
- pityriasis versicolor, **M**.185
- seborrheic dermatitis, **M**.185
Zinc resistance, *Staphylococcus*, **B2**.794 (Tab.), **B2**.804–5
Zona pellucida glycoproteins, contraceptive vaccines, **I**.875
Zoogloea ramigera, **B1**.212
Zoonoses
- bunyavirus infection, **V2**.1048
- epidemiology *see* Epidemiology of infection
- filovirus infection, **V2**.1093
- *Helicobacter pylori* infection, **B2**.1578
- historical aspects, **P**.4–5
- New World leishmaniasis, **P**.314
- retroviruses, **V2**.1295–6
- transmission prevention, **B1**.355
- trypanosomiasis, African, **P**.15, **P**.351
- *see also specific diseases/infection; specific viruses*
Zoophilic dermatophytes, **M**.45–6, **M**.223–5, **M**.225–7, **M**.227 (Tab.), **M**.239
Zoophthora, **M**.347
Zoster immunoglobulin (ZIG) *see* Varicella-zoster immunoglobulin (VZIG)
Zoster sine herpete, **V1**.514
Zostrex *see* Brivudin
Zovirax *see* Aciclovir (ACV)
Z value, **B1**.266, **B1**.446, **B1**.446 (Tab.), **B1**.449
Zygocotylidae, **P**.583–4
Zygomycetes, **M**.659–61
- Chlamydoconidia, **M**.659–60
- classification, **M**.53, **M**.54 (Tab.), **M**.659, **M**.660 (Tab.)
- culture, **M**.91 (Tab.), **M**.661, **M**.676–7
- ecology, **M**.659
- history, **M**.20–1
- hyphae, **M**.659, **M**.676, **M**.676 (Fig.)

Zygomycetes (*Continued*)
  identification, **M**.659, **M**.661, **M**.675–7
    histopathology, **M**.89 (Tab.), **M**.127 (Tab.),
      M.136 (Fig.), **M**.141 (Fig.), **M**.142 (Fig.),
      M.676, **M**.676 (Fig.)
    immune response, **M**.677
    microscopy, **M**.676, **M**.676 (Fig.)
    specimens, **M**.83 (Tab.), **M**.85, **M**.676
  pathogenicity, **M**.677
  reproduction, **M**.659
  sporangiospores, **M**.77, **M**.659–61
  see also individual species
Zygomycosis (Zygomycetes infection),
    M.672–5, **M**.674 (Tab.)
  causative agents, **M**.661–72
    see also individual species
  clinical presentation, **M**.672–5, **M**.674 (Tab.)
  CNS, **M**.673–5
  concomitant diseases
    AIDS, **M**.661, **M**.674–5
    diabetes mellitus, **M**.20–1, **M**.674–5, **M**.677,
      M.678
    enteral candidiasis, **M**.142 (Fig.)
  cutaneous, **M**.674–5, **M**.674 (Tab.), **M**.678
  desferrioxamine, **M**.13, **M**.20–1
  diagnosis, **M**.675–7
  disseminated, **M**.136 (Fig.), **M**.674 (Tab.),
    M.675, **M**.678
  epidemiology, **M**.20–1
  experimental infection, **M**.677

gastrointestinal tract, **M**.20–1, **M**.674,
    M.674 (Tab.), **M**.678
  esophagus, **M**.20–1
histopathology, **M**.128 (Tab.), **M**.136 (Fig.),
    M.142 (Fig.), **M**.676, **M**.676 (Fig.)
history, **M**.20–1
immunosuppression, **M**.21, **M**.672–3
nosocomial infection, **M**.21
oculomycoses, **M**.280 (Tab.), **M**.281 (Tab.),
    M.287, **M**.287 (Fig.)
  endophthalmitis, **M**.326
pulmonary, **M**.20–1, **M**.136 (Fig.), **M**.674,
    M.674 (Tab.), **M**.678
rhinocerebral, **M**.20–1, **M**.295, **M**.673–4,
    M.674 (Tab.), **M**.678
  chronic, **M**.295
rhino-orbital-cerebral *see* Rhino-orbital-
    cerebral zygomycosis
serology, **M**.677
skin infection, **M**.674–5
subcutaneous *see below*
terminology, **M**.659–60
therapy, **M**.677–8
  amphotericin B, **M**.677–8
  IFN-γ, **M**.678
  posaconazole, **M**.677–8
Zygomycosis, subcutaneous, **M**.347
  causative agents, **M**.347–50
    see also individual species
  diagnosis, **M**.351–2
    culture, **M**.352
    histopathology, **M**.351–2

immune response, **M**.352
microscopy, **M**.351–2
serology, **M**.352
immune response, **M**.350–1
therapy, **M**.352
  amphotericin B, **M**.352
  azoles, **M**.352
  co-trimoxazole, **M**.352
  fluconazole, **M**.352
  itraconazole, **M**.352
  ketoconazole, **M**.352
  potassium iodide, **M**.352
  terbinafine, **M**.352
  see also Entomophthoromycosis
    (entomophthoramycosis)
Zygomycota, **M**.44 (Fig.), **M**.49, **M**.51,
    M.52 (Fig.), **M**.53
  see also individual species
Zygosaccharomyces bisporus, **B1**.283
Zygosaccharomyces rouxii, **B1**.283
Zygospores, **M**.659
Zymodemes, **P**.200–1, **P**.284
  definition, **P**.284
  Entamoeba histolytica, **P**.200–1, **P**.211
  Giardia, **P**.247
  Leishmania, **P**.284, **P**.286 (Fig.)
  Trypanosoma cruzi, **P**.382–3, **P**.383–4
  see also Isoenzyme characterization
Zymomonas, **B1**.60
Zymomonas mobilis, **B1**.60